162.00

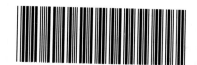

369 0289818

KU-627-841

Harris & Harris'
The Radiology of Emergency Medicine

FIFTH EDITION

Harris & Harris'
The Radiology of Emergency Medicine

FIFTH EDITION

EDITED BY

Thomas L. Pope, Jr., MD, FACR

Formerly: Professor of Radiology and Orthopaedics, University of Virginia (Charlottesville, VA), Professor of Radiology and Orthopaedics, Wake Forest University School of Medicine (Winston-Salem, NC) and Professor of Radiology and Orthopaedics and former Chair of Radiology, Medical University of South Carolina (Charleston, SC)
Presently: Consulting Radiologist
Clinical Specialty Board
Radisphere National Radiology Group
Beachwood, OH and Westport, CT

COEDITOR

John H. Harris, Jr., MD, DSc, FACR, FRACR (Hon)

Distinguished Emeritus Professor of Radiology
The University of Texas Medical School at Houston
Houston, Texas
Professor of Radiology
St. Joseph's Hospital and Medical School
Phoenix, Arizona

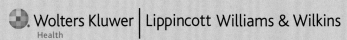

Wolters Kluwer | Lippincott Williams & Wilkins
Health
Philadelphia • Baltimore • New York • London
Buenos Aires • Hong Kong • Sydney • Tokyo

Senior Executive Editor: Jonathan W. Pine, Jr.
Product Manager: Amy G. Dinkel
Vendor Manager: Alicia Jackson
Senior Manufacturing Manager: Benjamin Rivera
Senior Marketing Manager: Kimberly Schonberger
Designer: Teresa Mallon
Production Service: Absolute Service, Inc.

© 2013 by LIPPINCOTT WILLIAMS & WILKINS, a WOLTERS KLUWER business
Two Commerce Square
2001 Market Street
Philadelphia, PA 19103 USA
LWW.com

Printed in China

Library of Congress Cataloging-in-Publication Data

Harris & Harris' radiology of emergency medicine / edited by Thomas L. Pope Jr. ; co-editor John H. Harris Jr. — 5th ed.
   p. ; cm.
  Radiology of emergency medicine
  Rev. ed. of: Radiology of emergency medicine / John H. Harris Jr., William H. Harris. 4th ed. c2000.
  Includes bibliographical references and index.
  ISBN 978-1-4511-0720-3 (hardback : alk. paper)
  I. Pope, Thomas Lee. II. Harris, John H., 1925- III. Harris, John H., 1925- Radiology of emergency medicine. IV. Title: Radiology of emergency medicine.
  [DNLM: 1. Emergencies. 2. Emergency Medicine—methods. 3. Radiography—methods. WB 105]

  616.07'572—dc23
        2012030187

To purchase additional copies of this book, call our customer service department at (800) 638-3030 or fax orders to (301) 223-2320. International customers should call (301) 223-2300.

Visit Lippincott Williams & Wilkins on the Internet: at LWW.com. Lippincott Williams & Wilkins customer service representatives are available from 8:30 am to 6 pm, EST.

10 9 8 7 6 5 4 3 2 1

CCS0912

I dedicate this book to the uncountable number of fellows, residents, and medical students with whom I have interacted in my career. All of them have taught me aspects of lifelong learning in some way which all humans, especially physicians, should embrace and practice with enthusiasm and commitment; to my two sons, David and Jason, whom I know live their lives by this basic principle; and lastly, to my significant other, Dr. Jennifer Newcomb Cranny, who is a constant and solid pillar of support for me personally and professionally.

—TLP, Jr.

To the members of the Church of the Red Rocks (Sedona, Arizona), whose steadfast love and support sustained my wife, Cathy, and I during her terminal illness, and which will sustain me the rest of my life.

—JHH, Jr.

CONTENTS

CONTRIBUTORS

Diane Armao, MD
Research Instructor
Department of Radiology
University of North Carolina School of Medicine
Chapel Hill, North Carolina

Dominic A. Barron, MB, BS
Department of Clinical Radiology
Leeds Teaching Hospitals NHS Trust
Leeds, United Kingdom

Alexander B. Baxter, MD
Assistant Professor
Department of Radiology
NYU Langone Medical Center
New York, New York

Mark P. Bernstein, MD
Assistant Professor, Trauma and Emergency Radiology
Department of Radiology
NYU Langone Medical Center/Bellevue Hospital
Assistant Professor
Department of Radiology
New York University
New York, New York

Robert S.D. Campbell, FRCR
Department of Radiology
Royal Liverpool University Hospital
Honorary Clinical Lecturer
Liverpool University
Liverpool, United Kingdom

Mauricio Castillo, MD, FACR
Attending Neuroradiologist
Professor of Radiology
University of North Carolina
Chapel Hill, North Carolina

Ne-Siang Chew, MRCP, FRCR
Consultant Interventional Musculoskeletal Radiologist
Department of Radiology
Bradford Royal Infirmary
Bradford, United Kingdom
Honorary Senior Lecturer
Leeds Institute of Molecular Medicine
Faculty of Medicine and Health
University of Leeds
Leeds, United Kingdom

Richard H. Daffner, MD, FACR
Director
Division of Emergency, Musculoskeletal, and Trauma
    Radiology
Allegheny General Hospital
Pittsburgh, Pennsylvania
Adjunct Clinical Professor
Diagnostic Radiology
Temple University School of Medicine
Philadelphia, Pennsylvania

Roberta diFlorio, MD
Staff Radiologist
Dartmouth-Hitchcock Medical Center
Lebanon, New Hampshire
Assistant Professor
Radiology and Obstetrics and Gynecology
Dartmouth Medical School
Hanover, New Hampshire

Robert D. Harris, MD
Co-Director of Ultrasound Education and Research
Department of Radiology
Dartmouth-Hitchcock Medical Center
Lebanon, New Hampshire
Professor of Radiology and Obstetrics/Gynecology
Geisel School of Medicine
Hanover, New Hampshire

Benjamin Y. Huang, MD
Assistant Professor
Department of Radiology
University of North Carolina
Chapel Hill, North Carolina

Amanda M. Jarolimek, MD
Diagnostic Radiologist
The University of Texas Health Sciences Center at
    Houston
Houston, Texas

Bruce E. Lehnert, MD
Radiologist
Department of Radiology
University of Washington
Seattle, Washington

Ken F. Linnau, MD, MS
Staff Emergency Radiologist
Department of Radiology
Harborview Medical Center
Assistant Professor
Department of Radiology
University of Washington
Seattle, Washington

Eugene McNally, FRCPI, FRCR
Consultant Radiologist
Department of Radiology
Nuffield Orthopaedic Centre
Honorary Senior Lecturer
Oxford University
Oxford, England

Stuart E. Mirvis, MD, FACR
Director of Emergency Radiology
Department of Diagnostic Radiology and Nuclear
    Medicine
Professor of Radiology and Nuclear Medicine
University of Maryland Medical Center
Baltimore, Maryland

Johnny U. V. Monu, MB, BS
Director, Musculoskeletal Radiology
Imaging Sciences
Strong Memorial Medical Center
Professor of Imaging and Orthopedics
University of Rochester
Rochester, New York

Curtis R. Partington, MD, PhD
Radiologist
Imaging Center of Louisiana
Baton Rouge, Louisiana

Philip Robinson, MB, ChB(Hons), MRCP, FRCR
Department of Musculoskeletal Radiology
Leeds Teaching Hospitals
Leeds, United Kingdom

Emma L. Rowbotham, MB, BS
Department of Clinical Radiology
Leeds Teaching Hospitals NHS Trust
Leeds, United Kingdom

J. Keith Smith, MD, PhD
Attending Radiologist
Department of Radiology
University of North Carolina Memorial Hospital
Associate Professor of Radiology
University of North Carolina School of Medicine
Chapel Hill, North Carolina

Jorge A. Soto, MD
Associate Professor of Radiology
Vice-Chairman of Radiology
Boston University School of Medicine
Boston, Massachusetts

Eric J. Stern, MD
Professor of Radiology
Adjunct Professor of Medicine
Department of Radiology
University of Washington
Seattle, Washington

Leonard E. Swischuk, MD
Pediatric Radiology
The University of Texas Medical Branch
Galveston, Texas

O. Clark West, MD, FACR
Diagnostic Radiologist
Memorial Hermann Hospital
Texas Medical Center
Houston, Texas

Anthony J. Wilson, MB, ChB, FRANZCR
Retired Professor of Radiology
Spanaway, Washington

Sarah Yanny, MRCP, FRCR
Consultant Radiologist
Department of Radiology
Stoke Mandeville Hospital
Buckinghamshire, United Kingdom

FOREWORD

It is indeed a pleasure and an honor to be asked to write the introduction for the fifth edition of *The Radiology of Emergency Medicine*, edited by Thomas L. Pope, Jr., and John H. Harris, Jr. This "classic" textbook was well known to me as a resident in general surgery during my rotation in the emergency department (ED). Also, when Dr. Harris "retired" from his position at the University of Texas-Houston and came to Arizona, he was introduced to me as the "guy who wrote the book on emergency radiology." I soon realized that this statement was true, both literally and figuratively. For the past 40 years, Dr. John Harris' dedication to his colleagues in radiology and his intellectual connection to emergency medicine physicians and trauma surgeons make this textbook "the standard reference" for diagnostic imaging for emergency medicine and trauma. He is one of those rare radiologists who comes out of the "bat cave" into the light of the trauma bay and the ED to give real-time interpretations and discussions of patient images. On countless occasions, I have found Dr. Harris in our trauma receiving area, reviewing radiographs and teaching our residents and attendings the nuances of interpreting conventional radiographs.

The fifth edition has again strived to keep up with the changing technology in diagnostic imaging in addition to emphasizing current practice in EDs and trauma centers. New chapters on imaging of skull fractures, maxillofacial trauma, chest trauma, and the acetabulum have been added to this volume to emphasize the importance of these areas with respect to imaging techniques and changes in clinical diagnosis and practice. In addition to redefining the importance of standard radiographs, the fifth edition has incorporated high-quality multidetector computed tomographic (CT) images, 3-D reformations, and magnetic resonance imaging to provide new information with evolving clinical practice. For example, the chapter dedicated to chest trauma not only highlights the importance of technical factors in interpreting emergency chest radiographs but also emphasizes the increasing reliance on CT diagnosis. Moreover, the chapter has added numerous sources of practical information not only for the radiologist but also for clinicians involved in the direct care of the patient.

Finally, the editors' devotion to fields as dynamic as radiology and emergency care is evident in the effort that has been taken to contemporize the fifth edition. It will continue to be requisite reading for radiology residents, experienced radiologists, and clinicians alike. Also, the images that are available on the online version of this edition will provide ongoing, valuable educational resources for residents, radiology and emergency medicine faculty, and frontline physicians for years to come.

Scott R. Petersen, MD, FACS
Professor of Surgery, Creighton University
Clinical Professor of Surgery
University of Arizona
Medical Director, ACS Level I Trauma Center
St. Joseph's Hospital and Medical Center
Phoenix, Arizona

I am very proud to welcome Tommy Pope, MD—an internationally recognized musculoskeletal radiologist—as coeditor of the fifth edition of *The Radiology of Emergency Medicine.* Tommy's reputation throughout the world radiologic community precludes the need for a more formal introduction here.

It was Dr. Pope's recommendation that we obtain new coauthors for nearly every chapter, which has been accomplished. It was Dr. Pope's suggestion that we should recruit non-American musculoskeletal chapter authors. That, also, has been accomplished, and their contributions are beautifully visible in the chapters dealing with the appendicular skeleton. So, Dr. Pope is the logical choice to perpetuate *The Radiology of Emergency Medicine* in future editions.

It is interesting to reflect that in the first edition of this book, published by Williams and Wilkins in 1975, it contained 14 chapters and nearly 500 pages. The first chapter on the "Skull" consisted of 24 pages and 39 figures devoted to conventional radiography of the skull, including such topics as the distinction between skull fractures and sutures, the various radiographic appearance of skull fractures, and methods of determining pineal gland displacement as a manifestation of increased intracranial pressure or midline shift.

In 1975, conventional radiography was the primary diagnostic tool of the emergency department physician and what few subspecialists there were at that time. Also, very few clinical radiologists and radiologic physicists had more than an inkling of what the future of imaging would become in the 21st century. Today, imaging is the cornerstone of emergent diagnosis. It is now common, because of multiplanar computed tomography (MPCT) in, or adjacent to, the trauma bay and the availability of MPCT in the evaluation of nontrauma emergency department patients, that the patient's definitive diagnosis is established or confirmed before leaving the trauma bay or the emergency department.

The fifth edition of *The Radiology of Emergency Medicine* consists of 23 chapters, including six new chapters and approximately 1,000 pages replete with state-of-the-art MPCT and ultrasound (US) images germane to conditions which prompt patient emergency department or trauma visits. Each chapter has been extensively revised to include contemporary imaging indications and protocols. This edition contains more than 2,000 images or schematic anatomic drawings of the manuscript.

While I believe each chapter to be a vast improvement of those in the fourth edition, some, in my opinion, deserve special recognition. Anthony Wilson, MD, has, as his final academic effort, prepared for the readers the clearest, most succinct, and the most understandable descriptions of both the Letournel classification of acetabular fractures and of the Lauge-Hansen classification of ankle injuries I have ever read.

Chapter 4, "Face, Including Intraorbital Soft Tissues and Mandible," is one of my favorite topics and one which I think I have explained well in prior editions. Dr. Mark Bernstein's revision of this chapter has elevated the bar of intellectual sophistication while, at the same time, continuing to present the imaging aspects of the complex concepts of facial trauma in a lucent, understandable, and practical fashion.

Dr. Richard Daffner's revision of the "Cervical Spine," Chapter 5, is an exemplary example of blending his concepts of cervical spine injuries with mine, which have been somewhat at variance over the years, into a traditionally organized and beautifully written chapter. Dr. Daffner's revision should provide the reader with a clear understanding of the complexities of cervical spine.

A very significant positive addition to the fifth edition is the contribution of our non-American authors; although the images of musculoskeletal trauma are universally similar, their description and understanding from the unique European perspective provides interesting and occasionally challenging reading. The addition of the European authors to our work has enhanced the stature of our text.

The purpose of the fifth edition of *The Radiology of Emergency Medicine* is to present to the reader, regardless of their experience in interpreting images of acutely ill and injured patients, the contemporary concepts and philosophies of the imaging of any patient presenting to the imaging department. It is intended for imagers but could also be appreciated by any and every physician who sees patients in the emergency setting. It is our sincere hope that, by virtue of its contemporary and authoritative contents, emergent patient care will be in some way enhanced and that the patients seen in this setting will receive better and more complete care because of all of our efforts.

John H. Harris, Jr., MD, DSc

Radiology, and the radiologist, can be of invaluable assistance in the assessment of the acutely ill or injured patient. The radiology of emergency medicine occupies a minor position in the curriculum of most medical schools and radiology training programs. Consequently, physicians involved in the care of emergency patients have varied experience and training in the radiology related to this aspect of medicine.

The purpose of this work is to describe the role of radiology in the appraisal of the acutely ill or injured patient, to emphasize and illustrate its value as well as its limitations, and to guide the physician in the roentgen diagnosis of the emergency patient. It is hoped that this will provide a better understanding of appropriate roentgen examination to be requested and the information that the study can be reasonably expected to provide.

It is not our intent to present radiographic examples of every disease entity that might prompt an emergency department patient visit, nor is it our intent to present any entity described herein exhaustively.

Many textbooks and articles exist which do provide such comprehensive roentgen descriptions.

Rather, it is our purpose to focus upon those radiologic aspects of emergency medical care which, in our experience, have acted as "pitfalls" to the examination, diagnosis, and understanding of emergency medical problems. Every illustration has been chosen from our personal practices to illustrate a point which, at some time or other, has presented some degree of difficulty. Emphasis has always been placed upon objective, although frequently subtle, changes which should lead to the correct radiographic diagnosis.

While the prime motivation for this effort has been a desire to be of assistance to emergency department physicians, it is hoped that the book will be of value to physicians of all disciplines involved in the diagnosis and management of the acutely ill or injured patient.

John H. Harris, Jr., MD, DSc
William H. Harris, MD

ACKNOWLEDGMENTS

As the historical author of Harris and Harris' *The Radiology of Emergency Medicine*, I have usurped the privilege of preparing the Acknowledgments.

First and foremost, this 5th Edition would not have seen the light of day were not for the interest, wisdom, and guidance of Charlie Mitchell, previously of LWW, or without the enthusiastic, energetic participation of Tommy Pope, my co-editor, who is personally responsible for recruiting many new authors including those wonderful UK authors whose European concepts illuminate several chapters of this edition.

Tommy and I deeply appreciated the work done by all the first-time authors, many of whom are members of The Society of Emergency Radiology, and we look forward to their continued involvement in the perpetuation of this text.

Anthony Wilson's contributions to this edition have been previously described. However, Dr. Wilson's work is notable for two reasons: his concepts of the Letournel classification of acetabular fractures and of the Lauge-Hansen classification of ankle fractures, and his ability to convey these complex concepts in understandable language is truly unique. For the first time, in my experience, these classifications are comprehendible. Further, his contributions to this edition complete his life-long advancement of Radiologic knowledge, thus making this text the sole published source of Dr. Wilson's remarkable understanding of these difficult concepts.

On the technical side, Tommy and I thank Jonathan Pine, Senior Executive Editor, Ryan Shaw, former Product Manager, and Amy Dinkel, Product Manager, all of Lippincott Williams & Wilkins, and Teresa Exley of Absolute Service, Inc. Personally, I thank Wendy Hansen and Peggy Keys-Farley, Sedona (Arizona) Photo for their accurate and a gracious production of images required for my work when that service was not otherwise available.

Tommy Pope, MD, Co-Editor
John H. Harris, Jr., MD, DSc, Co-Editor

CHAPTER 1

Skull Fractures

Ken F. Linnau ■ John H. Harris Jr.

CONTEXT AND EPIDEMIOLOGY

Since ancient times, humans are believed to have treated trauma to the head and skull. Anthropologic evidence suggests that the Incas in Peru have used trepanation techniques for treatment of skull fractures as early as 200 BC, and current treatment techniques have evolved from the observations and practices of Greek and Roman physicians.[1,2]

This chapter illustrates and describes the imaging characteristics of acute injury of the cranial bones at the initial patient encounter in the emergency center. The true incidence of skull fractures in children and adults presenting to emergency departments (ED) is unknown and much of the data is derived from traumatic brain injury (TBI) evaluation, which affects about 1.7 million patients every year and accounts for up to 1.4 million annual ED visits in the United States (2006 data).[3] About 300,000 TBI patients are hospitalized annually and about 4% of patients treated for head trauma have a skull fracture.[4] The most common causes of TBI include falls (35%), motor vehicle crashes (MVC) (17%), assaults (10%), and being struck by or against an object. Falls show the highest rates in children less than 4 years and adults older than 75 years of age. MVC injury is the leading cause of TBI-related death, particularly in young adults who are less than 24 years old.

In children, intentional injury (i.e., non-accidental trauma, abusive head trauma) represents an important cause of skull fractures and associated morbidity such as intracranial hemorrhage and retinal bleeding.[5]

INDICATIONS FOR IMAGING AND SUPPORTING EVIDENCE

Indiscriminate use of skull radiographs triggered one of the earliest assessments for rational imaging use. In 1987, a prospective study of ED patients was performed to validate an expert guideline, which recommended that low-risk patients should not undergo routine skull radiography after head trauma in order to reduce radiation exposure and imaging cost.[6,7] Today, computed tomography (CT) is the imaging modality of choice in the initial evaluation of patients with emergent cranial and intracranial signs and symptoms. The need for imaging is usually based on the severity of head injury as indicated by initial Glasgow Coma Scale (GCS) (Table 1.1). With this scale, the three main aspects of neurologic function evaluated are (1) opening of the eyes to external stimuli, (2) verbal response, and (3) motor response to stimuli. Strong evidence supports the use of urgent head CT imaging for severe TBI (based on a GCS of 3 to 8) to identify lesions requiring surgical intervention. Clinical prediction rules, such as the Canadian Head CT rule and the New Orleans criteria, derived and validated using sophisticated scientific methodology inform evidence-based imaging recommendations with CT for mild TBI. The reader is directed to the

TABLE 1.1	Glasgow Coma Scale
Eye opening	
Spontaneous	4
To voice	3
To pain	2
None	1
Verbal response	
Oriented	5
Confused	4
Inappropriate words	3
Incomprehensible words	2
None	1
Motor response	
Obeys commands	6
Localized pain	5
Withdraw (pain)	4
Flexion (pain)	3
Extension (pain)	2
None	1

fractures and are superfluous if a CT of the head has been obtained. For depiction of linear skull fractures, which may be overlooked on axial CT images, scout view images (topograms), which are included in every CT scan, can be used as a substitute for radiographs (Figs. 1.1, 1.3, and 1.4) or 3D renderings from CT (Figs. 1.2 to 1.5) can be helpful. Limited indications for skull radiographs include penetrating injuries, particularly for the course, location, and number of gunshot fragments; the location of other foreign bodies; and the presence of depressed skull fragments. In cases of suspected child abuse, skull radiographs are sometimes obtained as part of the skeletal survey for documentation or screening of injury. The absence of skull fractures on these radiographs does not reliably exclude intracranial hemorrhage.

Because of their low cost and low radiation, skull radiographs in two planes may have use in the pre-magnetic resonance imaging (MRI) screening evaluation of obtunded or unreliable trauma patients, if MRI-incompatible foreign material is suspected (e.g., ferromagnetic shrapnel).

original citations for details.[8,9] Tong et al. have recently summarized the available evidence guiding imaging for TBI.[10]

In the initial assessment of any trauma patient, rapid identification and stabilization of life-threatening traumatic injuries is the primary goal. Airway protection and control of bleeding are mandated during this primary survey. To control bleeding from scalp lacerations, it is sometimes necessary to staple them closed in the prehospital setting to obtain adequate hemostasis.

Identification of skull fractures increases the chance of detecting associated cervical spine injuries to 15% or more, mandating prehospital spine precautions and careful evaluation of the craniocervical junction.

Radiography

Radiographs previously played a major role in the evaluation of skull and brain lesions but now have a very limited role for the evaluation of skull

Computed Tomography and Magnetic Resonance Imaging

CT has become the imaging modality of choice for the initial evaluation of TBI.[11] Using thin-slice multidetector CT (MDCT) acquisition with isovolumetric voxels allows for multiplanar image reconstruction (usually in the coronal and sagittal plane) in bone and brain reconstruction algorithms allowing for identification of all clinically important skull fractures.[12] Three-dimensional surface-rendered (SR) image reconstructions can be helpful and are more intuitive for clinical communication. Some data suggest increased sensitivity for fracture detection of the cranial vault and skull base with the use of curved maximum intensity projections (MIPs).[13,14] At our institution, SR image reconstruction of all head CTs of young children (<5 years) is performed to aid in the depiction of fractures and avoid the confusion of sutures with nondisplaced skull fractures (Fig. 1.2). Thin-section CT imaging is the initial

(text continues on page 7)

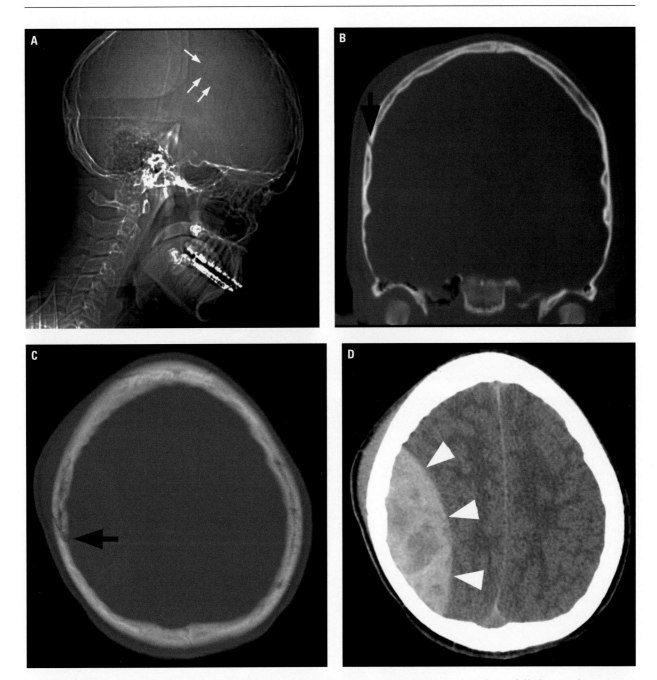

Figure 1.1. Lateral scout from CT of the head (**A**) of a 15-year-old skateboarder after a fall shows a lucent jagged line *(small white arrows)* suggestive of fracture. Coronal (**B**) and axial (**C**) CT images confirm a linear right parietal skull fracture *(black arrow)*. Brain window of the same CT (**D**) shows a large heterogeneous epidural hematoma *(arrow heads)*, which required surgical evacuation.

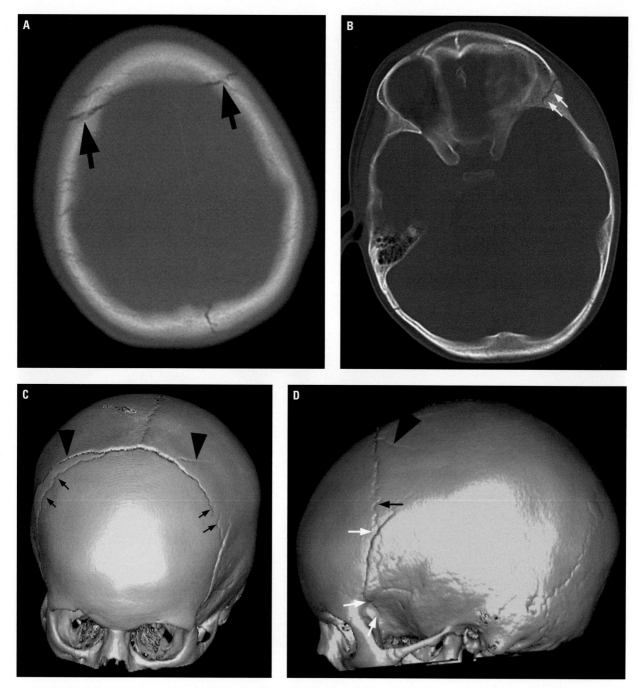

Figure 1.2. On axial CT (**A**) of a 3-year-old boy who fell 12 feet out of a window, bilateral parietal fractures *(black arrows)* could easily be mistaken for the coronal suture. Fracture extension into the sphenoid bone *(small white arrows)* is subtle on axial CT images (**B**). 3D surface renderings of the calvarium (**C**) easily allow differentiation of bilateral parietal fractures *(black arrowheads)* from the coronal suture *(small black arrows)*. Lateral 3D surface rendering (**D**) shows fracture extension across the coronal *(small black arrow)* and frontosphenoid suture into the greater wing of the left sphenoid bone *(small white arrows)*. Left high-parietal linear skull fracture is again shown *(black arrowhead)*.

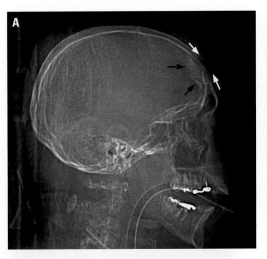

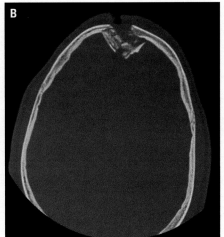

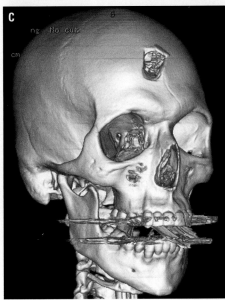

Figure 1.3. Lateral scout image from cranial CT (**A**) of a man involved in a motorcycle crash shows a frontal soft tissue defect *(small white arrows)* and multiple linear double densities in the frontal bone *(small black arrows)*, which extend deep to the inner table, indicative of a compound depressed skull fracture. Findings are easily confirmed and visualized on axial (**B**) and 3D surface-rendered (**C**) CT images. The injury was treated surgically.

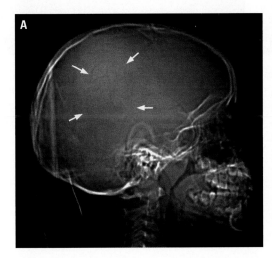

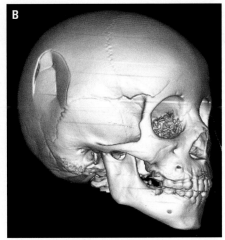

Figure 1.4. Lateral CT scout image (**A**) of a 5-year-old girl who fell shows the "wagon–wheel" appearance *(small white arrows)* of a mildly depressed skull fracture. 3D surface renderings (**B**) from the same CT confirm a simple depressed skull fracture, which was treated nonoperatively.

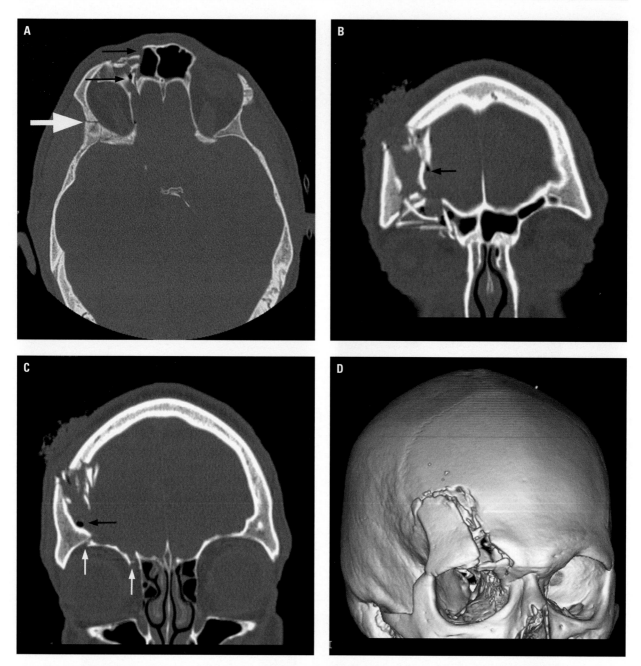

Figure 1.5. Axial CT image (**A**) of a man who was hit with a rake shows an orbital roof fracture with disruption of the inner and outer table of the right frontal sinus and associated small pneumocephalus *(small black arrows)*. Fracture extension into the greater wing of the sphenoid bone *(white arrow)* is present. Coronal CT reformations (**B and C**) confirm pneumocephalus *(small black arrows)* and violation of the anterior skull base at the right orbital roof *(white arrows* in **C**) of this complex open skull fracture. The extent of the injury is easily appreciated on 3D surface renderings (**D**).

imaging modality of choice for the identification and characterization of skull base fractures.[4] Thin-bone algorithm reconstructions can be obtained from the initial head CT data set as long as the relevant anatomy is included.

Depiction of brain parenchyma and extra-axial spaces on CT allows for ready identification of subarachnoid, subdural, and epidural hemorrhage. MRI should be considered as a secondary imaging modality reserved for cases requiring clarification, particularly when vascular, ligamentous, or parenchymal damage (e.g., diffuse axonal injury [DAI]) is suspected in the setting of blunt or penetrating trauma. Fractures themselves can be occult on MRI.

CT angiography (CTA) is commonly used for evaluation of intracranial vasculature in the setting of trauma. Only limited scientific evidence exists to guide in the use of CTA in the presence of skull fractures, but diagnostic accuracy is now believed to be similar to catheter angiography.[15] At our institution, CTA will be obtained for any fracture of the skull base, which extends into the carotid canal.

CLASSIFICATION OF SKULL FRACTURES

Skull fractures most commonly occur in the parietal, temporal, occipital, and frontal bones. Skull fractures can be classified as linear, depressed, or skull base fractures. In closed skull fractures, the intact scalp provides an effective barrier protecting the brain parenchyma. In open skull fractures, this barrier between the environment and the intracranial tissue is disrupted, thus increasing the risk of infection.

Linear Skull Fractures

Linear skull fractures usually extend through both tables of the flat bones of the calvarium (Figs. 1.1 and 1.2). Most linear skull fractures have minimal clinical significance. The clinical suspicion alone of a linear, nondepressed skull fracture is *not* an indication for plain skull radiography because it is an established fact that a linear skull fracture by itself does not alter patient management. Similarly, a linear, nondepressed skull fracture on a conven-

tional radiographic examination of the face, for example, also is not an absolute indication for head CT. However, such a fracture involving the inferior portion of the greater wing of the sphenoid bone (Fig. 1. 2) should prompt a high index of suspicion for tearing of the middle meningeal artery and an epidural hematoma.

The radiographic diagnosis of a nondepressed fracture may be confirmed on the basis of the following: (1) fracture line is more lucent than a vascular groove, (2) fracture lines are usually straight or jagged, (3) fracture lines may cross sutures, and (4) a fluid level in the sphenoid sinus or opacification of the mastoid is usually an indication of fracture involving the skull base.

Depressed Skull Fractures

Depressed skull fractures occur when bone fragments are driven below the level of the adjacent skull bones. These fractures are more likely to involve injury to the brain parenchyma and carry a higher risk of infection, seizure, intracranial hemorrhage, and death if not diagnosed early and managed appropriately.

Most depressed skull fractures are open fractures and then are referred to as compound skull fractures (Fig. 1.3). When the overlying scalp tissue is not disrupted, a simple depressed skull fracture is present (Fig. 1.4).

The force necessary to create a depressed skull fracture is substantial and usually results from a blunt or penetrating object directed at a small area of skull surface. The sharp edges of bone fragments driven into the brain parenchyma can easily disrupt the dura mater, resulting in potential cerebrospinal fluid (CSF) leakage and increased risk of central nervous system (CNS) infection. Indications for surgical treatment of depressed skull fractures include dural penetration, substantial intracranial hematoma, bone depression greater than 1 cm, frontal sinus involvement, gross cosmetic deformity, wound infection, pneumocephalus, or gross wound contamination. For patients without any of these findings, nonoperative treatment is appropriate.[16] Depressed fractures may show multiple irregular lines radiating from a central point to a round peripheral fracture line, that is, "wagon–wheel" fracture (Fig. 1.4).

Skull Base Fractures

Basilar skull fractures involve at least one part of the skull base, which is comprised of (1) the occipital bone, (2) the sphenoid bone, (3) the squamous and petrous portion of the temporal bone, (4) the orbital roof, and (5) the cribriform plate.

Pneumocephalus is the presence of air or gas in the cranial cavity, which is usually caused by trauma to the head and/or face. Posttraumatic air in the cranial cavity indicates a communication between intracranial and extracranial spaces like paranasal sinuses, mastoid air cells, or ambient air (Fig. 1.5). Pneumocephalus commonly heralds an occult basilar skull fracture and portends significant complications such as meningitis or CSF leak. CT is highly sensitive in the detection of pneumocephalus, being able to detect as little as 0.5 mL (a few bubbles). It is postulated that air gains entry into the cranial cavity either through a dural defect during increase in paranasal sinus pressure such that occurs with sneezing, blowing the nose, or the Valsalva maneuver, or when a CSF leak causes a decrease in intracranial pressure allowing for influx of air into the cranial cavity. Each head CT should be scrutinized in lung windows for the presence of pneumocephalus, especially if a skull base fracture is suspected clinically (rhinorrhea, otorrhea, hemotympanum, raccoon eyes, or Battle sign).

The most important complications related to skull base fractures include cranial nerve injury, hearing loss, CSF leak, posttraumatic infection, and injury to the vascular structures of the skull base. Vascular injury carries a high risk of trauma-related stroke. The temporal bone, which is intimately related to cranial nerves VII and VIII, inner ear, middle ear, sigmoid, transverse, petrous sinus, and petrous portion of the carotid artery is most commonly injured accounting for 14% to 22% of skull fractures.

Temporal bone fractures have been classified as transverse or longitudinal according to the long axis of the fracture line with respect to the long axis of the petrous bone (petrous ridge). Transverse fractures extend perpendicular to the long axis of the pars petrosa of the temporal bone. Longitudinal fractures are parallel to the petrous ridge. However, this classification does not correlate well with clinical complications of temporal bone fractures such as hearing loss and cranial nerve palsies. Most temporal bone fractures are more complex and oblique to be described in such a planar fashion. The Brodie classification of temporal bone fractures distinguishes fractures as involving or sparing the otic capsule. Otic capsule violating injuries extend through the labyrinth (i.e., semicircular canals, vestibule, and cochlea), whereas otic capsule sparing injuries do not. Associated intracranial injury (epidural and subarachnoid hemorrhage) and clinical complications of temporal bone fracture (hearing loss, CSF leaks, perilymphatic fistula, facial nerve palsy, and vascular complications) are more likely when the otic capsule is disrupted. Because commonly used temporal bone fracture classifications are limited in predicting clinical outcomes and aiding in clinical decision making, radiologists should understand these classifications for the purpose of communication with other providers while addressing specific issues of the individual case in their reporting. Describing involvement of a relevant individual anatomic structure is more important than assigning the fracture into a general category in order to help determine the extent and nature of the injury (Fig. 1.6).

Isolated fractures of the orbital roof are uncommon. These fractures usually occur in combination with other fractures involving the facial bones or the skull. Orbital roof fractures may extend into the frontal or ethmoidal sinuses. An isolated fracture involving the anterior wall of the frontal sinus probably has no great clinical significance. However, a fracture involving both tables of the frontal sinus is considered "open" with the potential of meningeal contamination. Fractures of the orbital roof should be evaluated by CT (Fig. 1.5).

Skull Fractures in Penetrating Trauma

In penetrating trauma, CT or radiography of the head can be helpful to determine the missile path for therapeutic or forensic considerations (Fig. 1.7). Radiographs obtained in the trauma bay can be helpful to identify retained bullet fragments. The outcome of penetrating trauma and gunshot wounds to the head will be determined by the specific brain structures wounded, which is discussed in a subsequent chapter of this book.

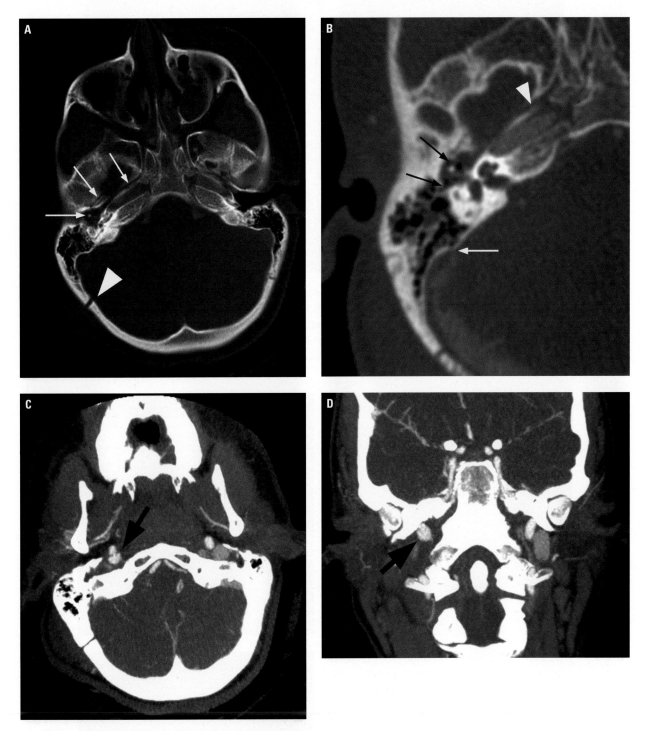

Figure 1.6. Axial image from noncontrast head CT (**A**) of an 11-year-old girl hit by a car shows diastasis of the lambdoid suture *(white arrow head)* and a temporal bone fracture through the middle ear, extending toward the carotid canal *(white arrows)*. Subsequently obtained thin-section CTA images of the neck (**B**) confirm a temporal bone fracture extending through the opacified mastoid air cells *(white arrow)*—the middle ear—which is fluid filled *(black arrows)* and extension into the transverse portion of the carotid canal *(white arrow head)*. Axial (**C**) and coronal (**D**) maximum intensity projections (MIPs) from CTA of the neck show a traumatic pseudoaneurysm of the right internal carotid artery at the skull base *(black arrow)*, complicating the temporal bone fracture.

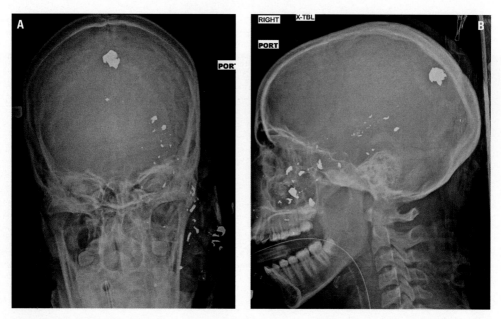

Figure 1.7. Frontal (**A**) and lateral (**B**) skull radiographs of a 16-year-old gunshot victim obtained in the trauma bay shows a left-to-right (**A**) and anteroposterior upward (**B**) bullet trajectory through the face and into the skull outlined by multiple small metallic projectile fragments, also referred to as a "snowstorm of lead." The biggest fragment of the mushroomed bullet is lodged intracranially at the midline (**A**).

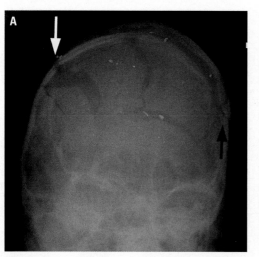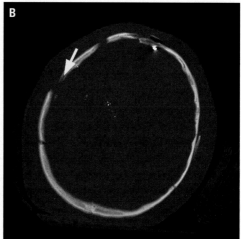

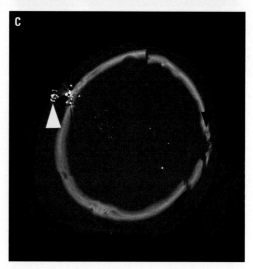

Figure 1.8. The frontal skull radiograph (**A**) of a 24-year-old man who suffered a devastating self-inflicted gunshot injury shows multiple displaced skull fractures. Bone fragmentation with inward beveling on the right side of the skull (*white arrow*) and outward beveling on the left side of the skull (*black arrow*) suggest a right-to-left trajectory and right-handedness of the victim. Axial CT images (**B and C**) confirm inward beveling on the right side of the skull (*white arrow*), indicating the entry wound. The exit wound on the left calvarium (**C**) shows outward beveling (*black arrows*) with a wider defect at the outer table of the skull than on the inner table. Note the skin staples on the right side of the skull (*white arrow head*) placed for hemostasis.

Inward beveling (wider on the inside) on the calvarial defect at the bullet entry site and outward beveling of the skull at the exit wound are typical.[17] Characteristic fracture patterns of the skull may aid in the identification of entry and exit wounds (Fig. 1.8). A nearly spent bullet is often arrested in the subcutaneous tissue of the scalp without a visible exit wound owing to the elastic properties of the skin.

REFERENCES

1. Andrushko VA, Verano JW. Prehistoric trepanation in the Cuzco region of Peru: a view into an ancient Andean practice. *Am J Phys Anthropol.* 2008;137(1):4–13.
2. Kshettry VR, Mindea SA, Batjer HH. The management of cranial injuries in antiquity and beyond. *Neurosurg Focus.* 2007;23(1):E8.
3. Centers for Disease Control and Prevention. Injury prevention & control: traumatic brain injury. CDC Web site. http://www.cdc.gov/TraumaticBrainInjury/index.html. Updated June 27, 2011. Accessed June 30, 2011.
4. Saraiya PV, Aygun N. Temporal bone fractures. *Emerg Radiol.* 2009;16(4):255–265.
5. Hedlund GL, Frasier LD. Neuroimaging of abusive head trauma. *Forensic Sci Med Pathol.* 2009;5(4):280–290.
6. Thornbury JR, Campbell JA, Masters SJ, et al. Skull fracture and the low risk of intracranial sequelae in minor head trauma. *AJR Am J Roentgenol.* 1984;143(3):661–664.
7. Masters SJ, McClean PM, Arcarese JS, et al. Skull x-ray examinations after head trauma. Recommendations by a multidisciplinary panel and validation study. *N Engl J Med.* 1987;316(2):84–91.
8. Haydel MJ, Preston CA, Mills TJ, et al. Indications for computed tomography in patients with minor head injury. *N Engl J Med.* 2000;343(2):100–105.
9. Stiell IG, Wells GA, Vandemheen K, et al. The Canadian CT head rule for patients with minor head injury. *Lancet.* 2001;357(9266):1391–1396.
10. Tong KA, Oyoyo U, Holshouser BA, et al. Neuroimaging for traumatic brain injury. In: Medina LS, Blackmore CC, eds. *Evidence-Based Imaging: Optimizing Imaging in Patient Care.* 1st ed. New York, NY: Springer Publishing; 2006:233–259.
11. Provenzale J. CT and MR imaging of acute cranial trauma. *Emerg Radiol.* 2007;14(1):1–12.
12. Sodickson A, Okanobo H, Ledbetter S. Spiral head CT in the evaluation of acute intracranial pathology: a pictorial essay. *Emerg Radiol.* 2011;18(1):81–91.
13. Ringl H, Schernthaner R, Philipp MO, et al. Three-dimensional fracture visualisation of multidetector CT of the skull base in trauma patients: comparison of three reconstruction algorithms. *Eur Radiol.* 2009;19(10):2416–2424.
14. Ringl H, Schernthaner RE, Schueller G, et al. The skull unfolded: a cranial CT visualization algorithm for fast and easy detection of skull fractures. *Radiology.* 2010;255(2):553–562.
15. Utter GH, Hollingworth W, Hallam DK, et al. Sixteen-slice CT angiography in patients with suspected blunt carotid and vertebral artery injuries. *J Am Coll Surg.* 2006;203(6):838–848.
16. Letarte P. The brain. In: Feliciano D, Mattox K, Moore E, eds. *Trauma.* 6th ed. Philadelphia, PA: McGraw-Hill Companies, Inc; 2008:397–418.
17. Hollerman JJ, Fackler ML, Coldwell DM, et al. Gunshot wounds: 2. Radiology. *AJR Am J Roentgenol.* 1990;155(4):691–702.

CHAPTER **2** | Imaging of Brain Trauma

J. Keith Smith ■ Diane Armao ■ Mauricio Castillo

NORMAL ANATOMY

Brief Overview, Computed Tomography

Computed tomography (CT) is the most commonly used imaging method in the patient with acute neurological deficits, acute onset of severe headache, or cranial trauma. The examinations are generally obtained using 3 to 5 mm thick sections in the axial plane. We now use spiral (helical) technique for all trauma brain CT studies. These are acquired by 0.6 mm slice thickness (pitch = 1) and reconstructed by 4 or 5 mm slice thickness. Examinations performed for trauma or acute mental status changes generally do not require contrast administration. The images are obtained beginning at the base of the skull and extending to the vertex. Generally, the images are presented with soft tissue window settings (width: 110 to 120 for the posterior fossa and 80 for the cerebral hemispheres, level: 40) and bone window settings (width: 3,500, level: 700). The so-called "blood" or intermediate windows (width: 250, level: 80) are helpful for identification of small extra-axial (between the brain and skull) collections of acute blood. The normal gray matter measures approximately 25 to 40 Hounsfield units and the normal white matter approximately 25 to 30 units. In newborns and young children, the white matter is relatively hypodense compared to that of adults.

The normal fourth ventricle appears in the midline as an inverted U-shaped structure (Fig. 2.1A) which may contain calcified choroid plexus. In older individuals, the perimedullary, prepontine, and cerebellopontine angle cisterns are clearly seen and are low (fluid) density (Fig. 2.1B). All cerebrospinal fluid (CSF) containing spaces have a CT density of 0 to 20 units. The tentorium cerebelli separates the infratentorial and supratentorial compartments.

The tentorium is slightly denser than the brain and has an inverted V shape. This structure may be difficult to visualize in the absence of calcification, contrast administration, or acute blood layering on it. Structures lateral to the tentorium are supratentorial, while all structures medial to it are infratentorial in location. The interpeduncular cistern is located at the level of the midbrain (Fig. 2.1B). This is an important landmark because subarachnoid hemorrhage (SAH) tends to accumulate in this location. Anterior to this cistern is the suprasellar cistern. This CSF-filled structure has either a five-point or six-point appearance. Its borders are formed anteriorly by the gyri recti, laterally by the temporal lobe unci, and posteriorly by the cerebral peduncles. The most important structures contained in the suprasellar cistern are the optic chiasm and the apex of the basilar artery. The Sylvian fissures are generally symmetrical and of CSF density. Medial to these fissures are the insulae—subinsular regions (which contain the extreme capsules, claustra, and external capsules). The structures within the subinsular regions are not usually individually identifiable on CT. Each lentiform nucleus comprising the putamen (laterally) and the globus pallidus (medially) has, as its name implies, a lens shape with its apex directed medially (Fig. 2.1C). These structures are of slightly higher density than the surrounding white

13

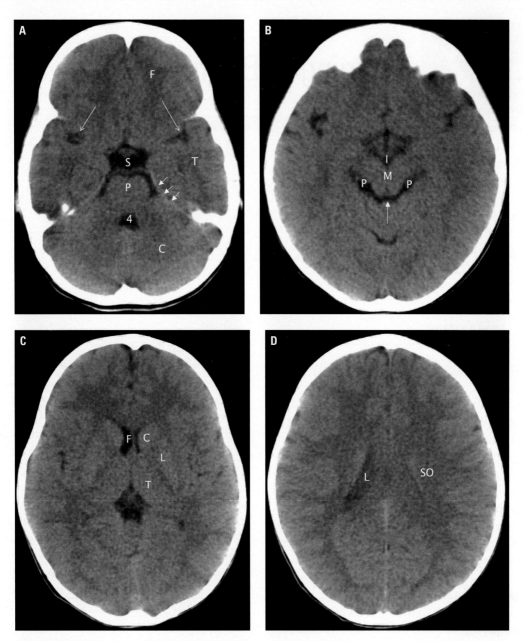

Figure 2.1. Normal noncontrast CT in a 3-year-old, soft tissue window settings. **A:** Axial slice shows the fourth ventricle *(4)*, hyperdense tentorium *(small closed arrows)*, frontal lobes *(F)*, temporal lobes *(T)*, pons *(P)*, and cerebellum *(C)* Sylvian fissures *(long open arrows)* have CSF attenuation. **B:** Axial slice at the level of the midbrain *(M)* *(superior to A)* shows quadrigeminal plate cistern *(arrow)*, which continues laterally to the ambient and perimesencephalic *(P)* cisterns. The interpeduncular cistern *(I)* lies between the cerebral peduncles. **C:** Axial slice through the level of the basal ganglia shows the head of the caudate nucleus *(C)*, the thalamus *(T)*, and lentiform nucleus *(L)*. The frontal horn *(F)* of the lateral ventricle is indented by the head of the caudate. Some degree of size asymmetry between the left and right lateral ventricles such as is seen in this patient is a common normal variant. **D:** Axial slice at the level of the centrum semi-ovale *(SO)* demonstrates the normal gray–white density difference. The body of the right lateral ventricle is partially visible *(L)*.

matter. The third ventricle is a linear-shaped structure in the midline. The pineal gland and habenular calcifications are present in most adults at the posterior aspect of the third ventricle. Posterior and inferior to these calcifications is the quadrigeminal plate and its accompanying cistern (Fig. 2.1B). The quadrigeminal cistern has a W shape and continues laterally with the ambient cisterns and the perimesencephalic cisterns. The lateral ventricles are visualized in a piecemeal fashion. The frontal horns are indented laterally by the head of the caudate nuclei (Fig. 2.1C). The frontal horns have a narrow angle between them and are separated from each other by the septum pellucidum. Inferiorly, the temporal horns are visible in images that demonstrate the temporal lobes. The occipital horns are seen slightly superior and contiguous with the trigones (atria). The trigones are the largest part of the lateral ventricles and contain the commonly calcified glomi of the choroid plexi. The cephalad-most portion of the lateral ventricles are the bodies (Fig. 2.1D). The white matter tracts adjacent to the lateral ventricles consist of commissural fibers from the corpus callosum and projection fibers from the corona radiata. When the brain is sectioned horizontally, above the level of the lateral ventricles, deep white matter is seen as a semi-oval shaped area comprising intersecting bundles of commissural, projection, and association fibers known as the centrum semiovale. The interhemispheric fissure contains the falx cerebri, which may become calcified in adults.

TRAUMATIC BRAIN EMERGENCIES

Acute Hemorrhage

Computed Tomograpy

On CT, the normal gray matter has an attenuation value of 25 to 40 H units, whereas fresh blood in a patient with a normal hematocrit measures 40 to 70 units. This difference in density allows for recognition of fresh blood.

Magnetic Resonance Imaging

On magnetic resonance imaging (MRI), the signal characteristics of blood depend on the biochemical and oxidation characteristics of hemoglobin. The appearance of blood on MRI is extremely complex and also dependent on imaging parameters used. The following description applies only to intracerebral blood as imaged on 1.5T MR units. Freshly extravasated blood contains fully oxygenated hemoglobin (oxyhemoglobin) within intact red blood cells. This results in a weak diamagnetic effect, and the imaging appearance of a hyperacute hematoma is similar to that of CSF (isointense to gray matter in T1-weighted images [T1WIs] and hyperintense on T2-weighted images [T2WIs]). During the first few hours following a hemorrhage, oxyhemoglobin loses oxygen and becomes deoxyhemoglobin, which is still contained within intact erythrocytes. Deoxyhemoglobin has a diamagnetic effect and is of slightly low signal intensity on T1WI and low signal intensity on T2WI. This hypointensity is more pronounced on T2-weighted gradient recalled echo (T2*) sequences or susceptibility weighted images. The deoxyhemoglobin is oxidized into methemoglobin. Intracellular methemoglobin (3 to 7 days) is paramagnetic and is hyperintense on T1WI and hypointense on T2WI and T2*-weighted images. During the following days (>5 days) and beginning at the periphery of the hematoma, erythrocytes lyse, liberating their contents. Extracellular methemoglobin is paramagnetic and is bright on T1- and T2-weighted sequences. Phagocytes ingest the methemoglobin and store it as ferritin. Once their capacity to store ferritin is reached, iron is stored as hemosiderin. Both of these compounds are paramagnetic and result in very low signal intensity on T1WI, T2WI, and T2*-weighted images. To further complicate this sequence of events, the signal characteristics of blood also depend on the state of hydration and retraction of the clot. The sequence of events described previously occurs in that order in the presence of uncomplicated hematomas. Deviations from this sequence may suggest the presence of an underlying lesion such as a tumor or a vascular malformation or rebleeding into a hematoma.

EXTRACEREBRAL TRAUMA

Epidural Hematoma

The potential epidural space is located between the outer layer of dura (periosteum) and the inner table of the skull. The dura is attached to the bone by Sharpe's fibers and a forceful dissection is needed to strip it away and create a space. The dura is also firmly attached at the level of the cranial sutures. Epidural hematomas result from laceration of the

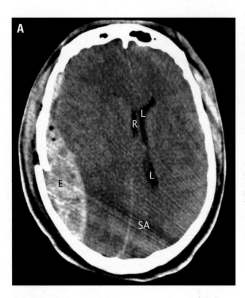 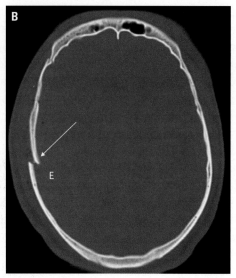

Figure 2.2. Epidural hematoma. **A:** Axial noncontrast CT shows biconvex high-density blood collection *(E)* in the right temporoparietal region. Right lateral ventricle *(R)* is compressed and shifted to the left side. The left lateral ventricle *(L)* is slightly enlarged, probably because of obstruction of CSF drainage at the foramen of Monro. Streak artifact *(SA)* is caused by a radiodense object outside the scanners' field of view, such as a metal fastener in the trauma board. **B:** In the same patient, axial CT (bone window settings) shows fracture *(arrow)* in the right temporal squama, which resulted in laceration of the middle meningeal artery and an epidural hematoma *(E)*.

meningeal arteries and/or dural venous sinuses. The most common location (75%) for epidural hematomas is at the level of the middle meningeal artery and is caused by fractures involving the squamosal portion of the temporal bone. Approximately 95% of epidural hematomas have underlying fractures. The fractures per se, are of little clinical significance unless they are depressed. Most epidural hematomas are unilateral and supratentorial. Epidural hematomas have a better prognosis than subdural hematomas because the brain parenchyma is often less severely injured compared to patients with subdural hemorrhage.

The imaging method of choice in head trauma patients is CT. Acute epidural hematomas have a density ranging from 50 to 70 units. Their shape is typically biconvex and their margins stop at the cranial sutures (Fig. 2.2A). Bone window settings allow for identification of underlying fractures (Fig. 2.2B). Because epidural hematomas are located outside of the dura, they may cross the midline and the venous sinuses. Epidural hematomas in the posterior fossa are more common in children than in adults. When an epidural hematoma is located nearby or above and below the tentorium, tear of the transverse sinus

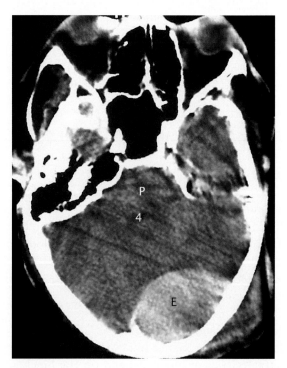

Figure 2.3. Venous epidural hematoma. Axial CT at the level of the pons *(P)* shows extra-axial high-density blood collection *(E)* in the left posterior fossa arising from a transverse sinus laceration. The fourth ventricle *(4)* is compressed and displaced toward the right by the mass effect.

should be strongly suspected (Fig. 2.3). Approximately 20% of patients with epidural hematomas also show blood in the subdural space. Eight percent of epidural hematomas are found in follow-up imaging studies and do not present acutely (delayed epidural hematomas).

Subdural Hematoma

These collections are located between the inner layer of the dura and the arachnoid membrane. Because this space is easily dissected, subdural hematomas tend to be extensive. They arise from injury to the bridging veins (crossing between the arachnoid membrane and the dura) and most are located primarily in the frontoparietal regions. Approximately 10% to 15% of subdural hematomas are bilateral. Brain contusions, hemorrhages, and shearing injuries are present in 50% of patients with subdural hematomas. The mortality because of subdural hematomas with concomitant brain injuries is high (60% to 90%). The mortality for isolated subdural hematomas is lower (20%). Bilateral convexity or interhemispheric subdural hematomas in a child should raise the suspicion of non-accidental trauma (see NAHI: Child Abuse, subsequently).

Acute subdural hematomas (<7 days) are usually hyperdense and measure 50 to 70 units (Fig. 2.4A). Subdural hematomas have a crescentic shape. They

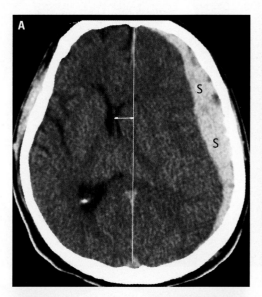

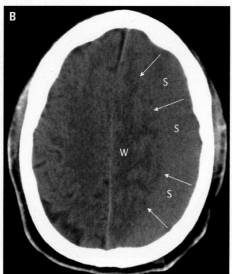

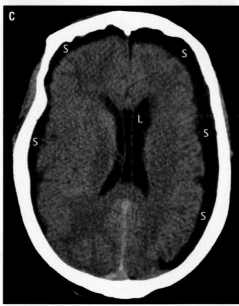

Figure 2.4. Subdural hematoma. **A:** Axial CT shows **acute hyperdense** left hemispheric subdural hematoma *(S)*. Note effacement of the left lateral ventricle. The midline brain structures are shifted to the right of the cranial vault midline *(thin line)*, compatible with a subfalcine herniation. **B:** In a different patient, axial CT shows a left hemispheric **subacute, isodense** subdural hematoma *(S)*. The subdural blood is similar in density to the gray matter, but can be detected by noticing the shift of the gray–white junction *(arrows)* away from the inner table of the skull. The white matter of the centrum semiovale *(W)* is compressed. **C:** In a different patient, axial CT shows a bilateral hemispheric **chronic, low density** subdural hematomas *(S)*. Attenuation of the subdural collections are similar to the CSF in the lateral ventricle *(L)*.

are generally accompanied by significant mass effect. Between 1 and 3 weeks, subdural hematomas become isodense with respect to brain and may be difficult to visualize. In these patients, recognizing the displacement of the gray–white junction away from the inner table of the skull may facilitate the diagnosis (Fig. 2.4B). Chronic subdural hematomas (>3 weeks) are hypodense with respect to brain (Fig. 2.4C). Identification of small subdural hematomas can be aided by the use of intermediate (blood) window settings (width: 250 and level: 40)

(Fig. 2.5A). Subdural hematomas may follow the dural reflections and be seen along the falx anteriorly or posteriorly (Fig. 2.5A), the tentorium (Fig. 2.5B), or in the interhemispheric fissure superiorly (Fig. 2.5C). Repeated episodes of bleeding into a subdural hematoma may result in a layered or swirled appearance. Delayed subdural hematomas are less common than delayed epidural hematomas. Although MRI does not play a role in the initial diagnosis of these lesions, it is extremely helpful in the identification of subacute and chronic subdural

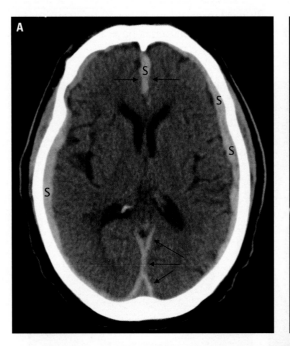

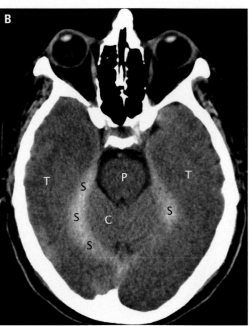

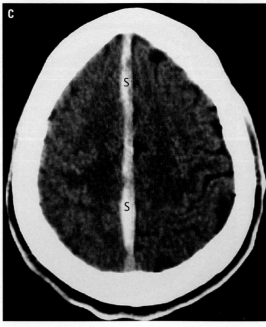

Figure 2.5. Subdural hematoma following dural reflections. **A:** Axial CT shows **acute hyperdense** bilateral hemispheric subdural hematomas *(S)*. The subdural hematoma over the hemispheres is continuous with hematoma following the dural reflection into the falx anteriorly and posteriorly *(arrows)* into the interhemispheric fissure. **B:** In a different patient, axial CT at the level of the pons *(P)* shows acute subdural hematoma *(S)* along the tentorium, between the temporal lobes *(T)* laterally and the cerebellum *(C)* medially. **C:** In a different patient, axial CT at the vertex shows an interhemispheric **acute hyperdense** subdural hematoma *(S)*, which is following the dural reflection along the falx.

hematomas. MRI is particularly helpful when attempting to establish the presence of subdural hematomas of varying ages. In cases of inflicted head trauma in child abuse, MRI is essential for assessing subacute and chronic injury.

Subdural Hygroma

A collection of CSF in the subdural space is termed a hygroma. They are thought to result from laceration of the arachnoid membrane and extravasation of nonbloody CSF into the subdural space. The incidence of subdural hygroma is not known, but they are less common than subdural hematomas. Subdural hygromas have a shape similar to subdural hematomas, but their CT density is equal to that of CSF (Fig. 2.6). By CT, subdural hygromas may be indistinguishable from chronic subdural hematomas or widened subarachnoid spaces in the elderly or other patients with significant brain atrophy. Small subdural hygromas do not require evacuation and resolve spontaneously within several months.

Subarachnoid Hemorrhage

Trauma is the most common cause of SAH. SAH is seen with most moderate and severe head injuries. The blood arises from superficial brain contusions or laceration of small veins crossing the subarachnoid space. Hydrocephalus may complicate SAH.

CT detects more than 90% of all subarachnoid bleeds within the initial 24 hours (Fig. 2.7). Most CT studies return to normal about 3 days after the hemorrhage, depending on the quantity of blood. The location of the SAH may be remote to the site of trauma as blood becomes diluted by CSF rapidly and extends throughout the subarachnoid spaces. In some patients, CT may show greater concentrations of blood in the interpeduncular cistern, Sylvian fissures, and along the tentorium and posterior extension of the falx cerebri. Subarachnoid blood, which has settled posteriorly, may outline the posterior part of the sagittal sinus, creating the "pseudo-delta" sign

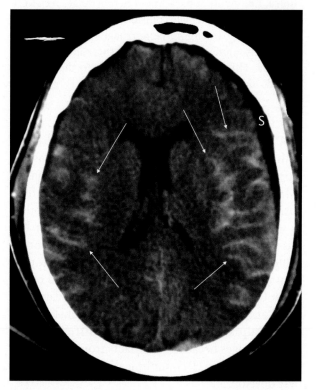

Figure 2.7. Acute subarachnoid hemorrhage. Axial CT in an adult motor vehicle collision victim shows diffuse subarachnoid hemorrhage *(arrows)*. Subarachnoid location of hemorrhage is confirmed by the location within the cortical sulci, fissures, and cisterns. This patient also had an acute subdural hygroma *(S)*, which nicely demonstrates the separation of the subdural and subarachnoid spaces.

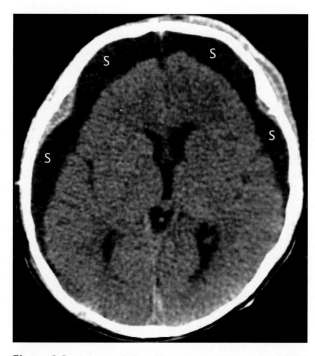

Figure 2.6. **Acute subdural hygroma** CT scan in a child motor vehicle collision victim shows **acute low density** subdural collections *(S)*. Imaging appearance may be indistinguishable from a chronic hematoma, but in this case, collections developed immediately after the episode of trauma.

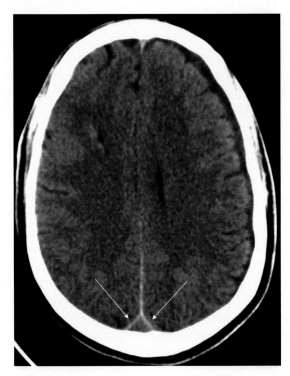

Figure 2.8. Acute subarachnoid hemorrhage. Axial CT in an adult motor vehicle collision victim shows a small amount of subarachnoid hemorrhage *(arrows)* layered posteriorly along the margins of the superior sagittal sinus. This appearance has been given the name of "pseudo-delta" sign.

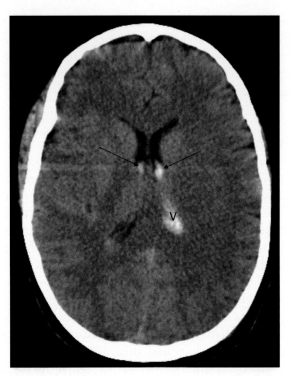

Figure 2.9. Intraventricular hemorrhage. Axial noncontrast CT in an adult who fell from a horse shows hyperdense acute hemorrhage in both lateral ventricles *(arrows*, and *V)*.

(Fig. 2.8) (the true "delta" sign is seen in a patient with sagittal sinus thrombus outlined by contrast on a post contrast CT). Although magnetic resonance (MR) is not the imaging method of choice in these patients, new sequences have improved its ability to visualize acute SAH. Fluid attenuation inversion recovery (FLAIR) images allow for identification of acute blood in the subarachnoid space. FLAIR may even allow for identification of subarachnoid blood when CT has returned to normal. Identification of small amounts of blood around the brainstem and in the suprasellar cistern may be difficult using FLAIR images because of artifacts from CSF pulsations. After an SAH, communicating hydrocephalus may develop.

Intraventricular Hemorrhage

Intraventricular blood may be found in up to 35% of patients with moderate-to-severe head trauma (Fig. 2.9). It is believed to arise from tearing of the subependymal veins and is more commonly found within the lateral ventricles. It may also be the result of extension from an adjacent parenchymal hemorrhage or retrograde extension of SAH. Intraventricular hemorrhage is relatively common in patients with injuries of the corpus callosum. Intraventricular hemorrhage may result in acute noncommunicating hydrocephalus secondary to clot obstructing the normal circulation pathway of CSF (Fig. 2.10). CT clearly demonstrates high-density clot inside the ventricles and is the imaging method of choice. MRI may show this type of hemorrhage, and the use of FLAIR images greatly facilitates its identification.

Pneumocephalus

In this condition, there is a communication between the intracranial and extracranial compartments allowing the passage of air into the intracranial space. Skull fractures, particularly those involving the base of the skull, are responsible for most pneumocephalus cases. Pneumocephalus may also be postsurgical because of gas-producing microorganisms or

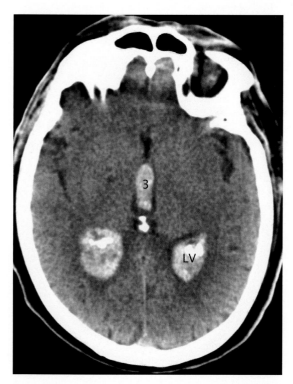

Figure 2.10. Intraventricular hemorrhage. Axial noncontrast CT in an adult shows hyperdense acute hemorrhage in both lateral ventricles *(LV)* and third ventricle *(3)*. The ventricles are dilated.

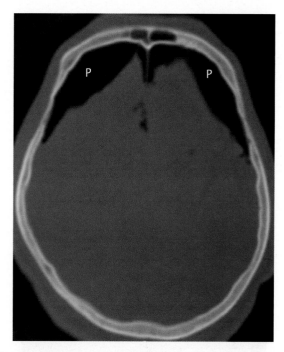

Figure 2.11. Tension pneumocephalus. Axial CT bone window in a patient with a severe skull base fracture shows large bifrontal collections of air *(P)* with compression of the underlying brain.

idiopathic. Air accumulates in the subarachnoid spaces and/or in the ventricles. In most cases, pneumocephalus resolves spontaneously in a matter of days. Tension pneumocephalus comprises less than 10% of all cases of pneumocephalus. In this condition, a large amount of intracranial air results in compression of the brain parenchyma and the ventricles (Fig. 2.11). Surgical evacuation is required to treat tension pneumocephalus. CSF rhinorrhea or otorrhea commonly accompanies pneumocephalus.

INTRACEREBRAL TRAUMA

Contusions

This type of injury may be either hemorrhagic or nonhemorrhagic. Contusions involve the crowns of gyri and spare the deep white matter. They are found in 5% to 10% of all patients with moderate-to-severe head trauma. Contusions tend to involve the regions of the brain that are in close proximity with crests of bone. As such, contusions are more commonly found in the anterior and basal frontal, temporal, and occipital lobes, and occasionally in the posterior cerebellar hemispheres (Figs. 2.12 and 2.13). Contusions may also be the direct result of a depressed fracture (Fig. 2.14). Contusions occurring at the site of impact are termed "coup," whereas those located opposite to the site of impact are termed "contrecoup." Contusions are multiple in 30% of patients. Hemorrhagic contusions are well demonstrated by CT and appear as areas of increased density (50 to 70 units) generally following the configuration of gyri. Hemorrhagic contusions are surrounded by a thin halo of edema. CT obtained 24 to 48 hours post-trauma often show contusions to be larger and more numerous than on the initial CT scans.

Shearing Injuries

Shearing brain injuries result from sudden acceleration and rotation of the brain within the cranial vault leading to shear forces at the gray–white matter interfaces and resulting in hemorrhagic and nonhemorrhagic injuries (Fig. 2.15). Common sites

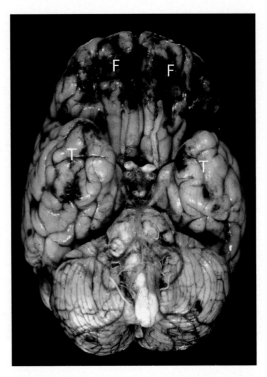

Figure 2.12. Cerebral contusions. Gross anatomic specimen of brain viewed from undersurface from a patient who died following severe head injury shows the typical distribution pattern of brain contusions from closed head injury *(darker areas of hemorrhage)* on the anterior and undersurface of the frontal *(F)* and temporal *(T)* lobes.

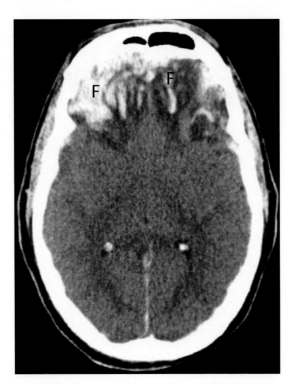

Figure 2.13. Cerebral contusions. Axial noncontrast CT study from an adult victim of motor vehicle collision shows multiple acute hemorrhagic contusions with hypodense surrounding edema in the inferior frontal lobes *(F)*.

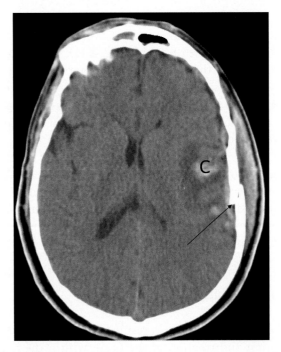

Figure 2.14. Cerebral contusions. In a patient with a depressed left temporal skull fracture *(arrow)* there is an acute brain contusion *(C)* in the underlying brain parenchyma.

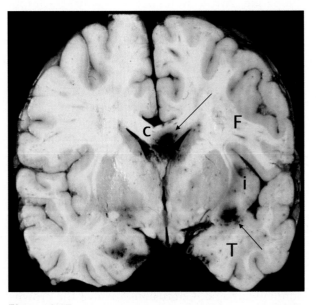

Figure 2.15. Shearing injuries. Gross brain specimen from a patient who died following high-speed motor vehicle collision shows shear hemorrhages *(arrows)* at the gray–white junction in the insula *(i)*, and temporal lobe *(T)* and in the corpus callosum *(C)*. Frontal lobe *(F)*.

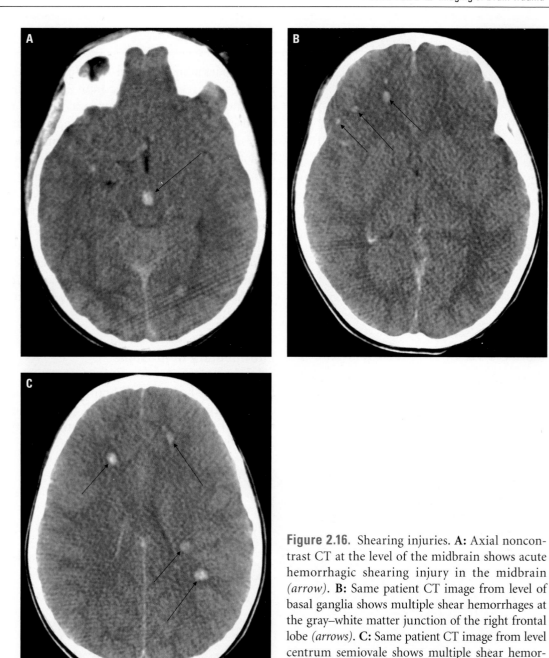

Figure 2.16. Shearing injuries. **A:** Axial noncontrast CT at the level of the midbrain shows acute hemorrhagic shearing injury in the midbrain *(arrow)*. **B:** Same patient CT image from level of basal ganglia shows multiple shear hemorrhages at the gray–white matter junction of the right frontal lobe *(arrows)*. **C:** Same patient CT image from level centrum semiovale shows multiple shear hemorrhages at the gray-white matter junction of both frontal lobes and the left parietal lobe *(arrows)*.

of shearing injuries are the subcortical gray–white junction, internal capsules, centrum semiovale, brainstem, subependymal regions, septum pellucidum, and corpus callosum (Figs. 2.16 and 2.17). Shearing injuries in patients less than 2 years of age should raise the suspicion of non-accidental trauma.

Shearing injuries are accompanied by diffuse axonal injury, which may be difficult to detect on acute imaging studies. They are associated with a signifi-

cant morbidity (persistent coma) and high mortality. The possibility of diffuse axonal injury should be considered in patients who are severely neurologically depressed with small hemorrhages or diffuse edema. MRI is sensitive in the detection of nonhemorrhagic and hemorrhagic shearing injuries. The use of susceptibility weighted images facilitates the identification of hemorrhagic shearing injures by virtue of their increased sensitivity to magnetic susceptibility effects from blood.

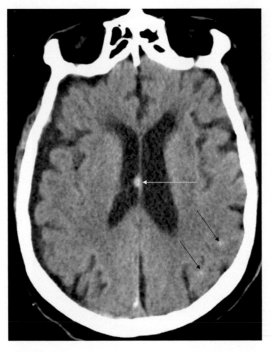

Figure 2.17. Shearing injuries. Axial noncontrast CT at the level of the lateral ventricles shows acute hemorrhagic shearing injury in the septum pellucidum *(white arrow)* and at the gray–white matter junction on the left *(black arrows)*.

Diffuse Edema

Diffuse edema may be seen with diffuse axonal injury or with severe hypoxic injury. This can be a difficult diagnosis for the inexperienced CT reader because the images are symmetric and there may be no visible hemorrhage. The diagnosis may be made by noticing the lack of distinction between the gray and white matter and effacement or absence of the cortical sulci and cisterns (Fig. 2.18). Occasionally, especially in young children, the cerebellum, brainstem, and deep gray nuclei may be relatively spared. In this case, these relatively normal density structures may appear abnormally dense compared to the surrounding edematous (low density) tissue. This has been termed the "white cerebellum" sign (Fig. 2.19).

Intermediary Contusions

Intermediary hemorrhagic brain lesions are an uncommon type of shearing injury and are found in the basal ganglia and thalami. Patients with this

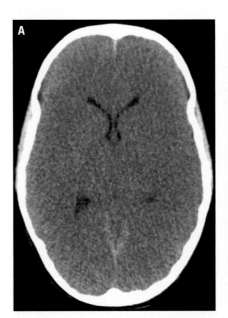

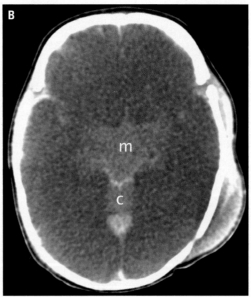

Figure 2.18. Diffuse edema. **A:** Axial noncontrast CT at the level of the basal ganglia from an adult victim of high-speed motor vehicle collision shows effacement of all cortical sulci and loss of the normal density difference between gray and white matter at the cortex and deep gray matter nuclei. The patient had severe diffuse axonal injury. **B:** A child victim of motor vehicle collision with diffuse edema. Axial noncontrast CT at the level of the basal ganglia shows loss of the normal density difference between gray and white matter at the cortex and effacement of all cortical sulci. In this case, the cerebellum *(C)* and parts of the midbrain *(m)* and deep gray matter nuclei were relatively spared. This can make the relatively brighter cerebellum seem abnormally bright to the inexperienced viewer—the so-called "white cerebellum" sign.

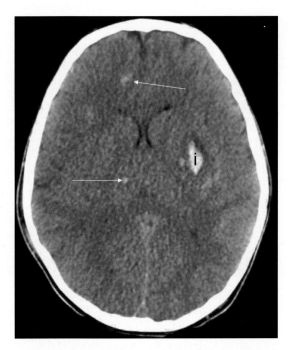

Figure 2.19. Intermediary hemorrhage. Axial CT shows acute intermediary hemorrhage *(i)* in the left lentiform nucleus. Other shear hemorrhages *(arrows)* are present in the right thalamus and right frontal lobe gray–white junction.

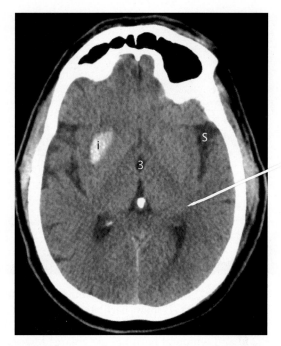

Figure 2.20. Intermediary hemorrhage. Axial CT of a different patient shows acute intermediary hemorrhage *(i)* in the right lentiform nucleus. Normal third ventricle *(3)* and Sylvian fissure *(S)*.

type of injury have a very poor prognosis. By CT, intermediary contusions have a fairly typical appearance tending to be hyperdense, often bilateral and confined to the lentiform nuclei and/or thalami (Figs. 2.19 and 2.20).

Cerebral Herniations

The skull is a rigid vault enclosing noncompressible tissues, (brain, blood, and CSF). Regulation of cerebral blood flow and production of CSF act as compensatory mechanisms in the presence of increased intracranial pressure. When these mechanisms are overwhelmed, brain herniation occurs. Brain herniation represents displacement of tissue from one compartment into another. The classification of brain herniation is arbitrary but based on a description of the tissue displaced or the brain compartments or adjacent structures involved.

The most common type of herniation is subfalcine (Figs. 2.21A,B). The cingulate gyrus is displaced inferiorly—under the falx—and shifted toward the opposite side. The CT signs of subfalcine herniation include displacement of the corpus callosum and corresponding lateral ventricle toward the opposite

side. This type of herniation may result in compression of the callosomarginal branch of the anterior cerebral artery (ACA) and subsequent infarction. Subfalcine herniation may lead to dilatation of the opposite lateral ventricle secondary to occlusion of its foramen of Monro.

The second most common type of herniation is uncal (downward transtentorial). In uncal herniation, the mesial aspect of one temporal lobe is forced across the tentorial incisura and the herniated brain compresses the ipsilateral perimesencephalic cistern and midbrain (Fig. 2.22). The corresponding side of the suprasellar cistern may also be obliterated in early uncal herniation. In severe or late instances, the entire suprasellar cistern may become effaced. With more posteriorly located lesions (typically in the occipital or posterior temporal regions), effacement of the quadrigeminal plate and ambient cisterns without effacement of the suprasellar cistern (caused by herniation of the hippocampus rather than the uncus) may be the earliest signs. As herniation worsens, progressive obliteration of the basal cisterns will develop. Compression of the corresponding posterior cerebral artery (PCA) by the herniated uncus may lead to cerebral infarction. Early compression of a third

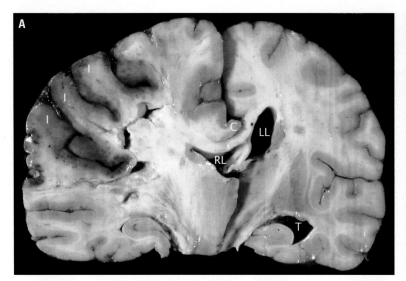
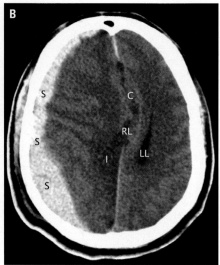

Figure 2.21. Subfalcine herniation. **A:** Gross anatomic brain specimen from a patient who died from a cerebral infarct *(I)* shows herniation of the right cingulate gyrus *(C)* across the midline under the falx. The right lateral ventricle *(RL)* is compressed and displaced across the midline. The left lateral ventricle body *(LL)* and temporal horn *(T)* are enlarged because of obstruction of CSF flow. **B:** Axial noncontrast CT image at the level of the lateral ventricles from a patient with acute traumatic subdural hematoma *(S)* shows displacement of the right lateral ventricle *(RL)* and cingulate gyrus *(C)* across the midline. The left lateral ventricle is enlarged *(LL)*. There is an area of low density from an infarct *(I)* in the medial frontoparietal junction likely caused by obstruction of distal branches of the anterior cerebral artery as they were pinched by the subfalcine herniation.

cranial nerve results in decreased function of the pupilloconstricting fibers and dilatation of the ipsilateral pupil.

Transalar herniation occurs when brain tissue is displaced over the ridge of the greater sphenoid ala (wing), which separates the anterior and middle cranial fossae. Two types of transalar herniation are commonly described. A descending transphenoidal herniation occurs when a frontal lobe is pushed posteriorly and below the greater wing of the sphenoid bone into the middle cranial fossa. In descending transphenoid herniations, the ipsilateral gyrus rectus is displaced inferiorly, and the middle cerebral artery and Sylvian fissure are displaced posteriorly. An ascending transphenoidal herniation occurs when a temporal lobe is displaced superiorly and anteriorly over the greater wing of the sphenoid into the anterior cranial fossa. In ascending transphenoid herniation, the Sylvian fissure is displaced superiorly over the greater wing of the sphenoid bone. The least common type of supratentorial brain herniations is the external type, which occurs when the brain is forced outside of the cranium (fungus cerebri). It is most commonly seen when edematous brain is displaced outwardly via a surgical bone defect.

In the posterior fossa, herniations may be descending, ascending, or both. Descending cerebellar herniation is characterized by downward displacement of the cerebellar tonsils through the foramen magnum (Fig. 2.23). It may be secondary to space-occupying supratentorial lesions or infratentorial lesions. Compression of the brainstem may occur and has a grave prognosis. Ascending (upward) transtentorial herniation occurs when the medial cerebellar hemispheres and superior vermis are displaced upward through the tentorial incisura. Findings on cross sectional imaging include effacement of the superior cerebellar cistern, displacement of the superior vermis through the incisura, compression of the midbrain, and forward displacement of the pons against the clivus (Fig. 2.23). Hydrocephalus can occur in both ascending and descending transtentorial herniation as a result of compression of the cerebral aqueduct in the midbrain.

Penetrating Trauma

Most bullets used by civilians are of the semijacketed lead type. These bullets deform easily on

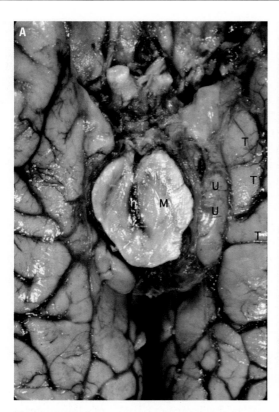

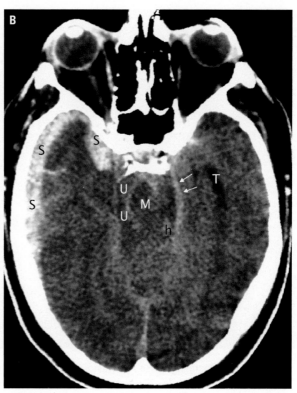

Figure 2.22. Downward transtentorial herniation. **A:** Gross anatomic brain specimen from a patient who died from cerebral trauma, viewed from the undersurface at the level of the cut midbrain shows herniation of the left uncus *(U)* compressing the midbrain *(M)*. There is a notch between the rest of the temporal lobe *(T)* and the uncus caused by the edge of the tentorium (removed to allow brain fixation). There is a hemorrhage *(h)* in the center of the compressed midbrain. **B:** Axial noncontrast CT image at the level of the midbrain from a patient with a right-sided subdural hematoma *(S)* shows herniation of the right uncus *(U)* through the tentorial opening, compressing the midbrain *(M)*. There is a small hemorrhage in the left midbrain *(h)*. Subarachnoid blood is present in the perimesencephalic cistern *(arrows)*, which outlines the midbrain. The tip of the temporal horn of the left lateral ventricle *(T)* is enlarged because of obstruction of CSF flow through the cerebral aqueduct.

impact resulting in an increase in their diameter. A deformed and enlarged bullet creates a cavity 3 to 4 times its diameter. As a bullet slows down, its energy is transmitted to the neighboring tissues increasing the damage. This damage is further aggravated by cavitation and displacement of bone fragments along the bullet's pathway. Injuries produced by bullets include fractures and fragmentation of the skull, intra-axial hematomas, SAH, intraventricular hemorrhage, pneumocephalus, pulped brain (Fig. 2.24), vessel dissection, and pseudoaneurysm formation. Gunshot wounds to the posterior fossa are uniformly fatal. Injuries confined to one cerebral lobe or to one hemisphere have, approximately, a 50% mortality. Injuries involving both hemispheres or multiple lobes are fatal in nearly all patients. CT

is commonly degraded by artifacts produced by the bullets.

NON-ACCIDENTAL HEAD INJURY (CHILD ABUSE)

It is estimated that more than 79,000 children are victims of physical abuse and some 2,000 children die annually in the United States from abuse.[1,2] These statistics are almost certainly underestimated because cases go unreported and physicians miss the diagnosis. Non-accidental head injury (NAHI) may involve impact and/or acceleration–deceleration forces (shaken baby syndrome) and is characterized by the triad of subdural hemorrhage, retinal hemorrhage, and encephalopathy.

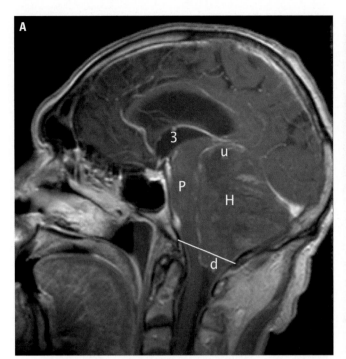

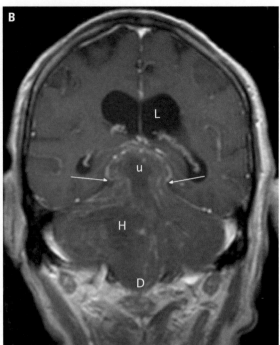

Figure 2.23. Posterior fossa herniations. **A:** Sagittal enhanced T1WI in a patient with a large cerebellar hemorrhage *(H)* with both upward transtentorial herniation and downward tonsillar herniation. Note complete effacement of the superior cerebellar cistern caused by displacement of the cerebellum upward *(u)* as well as compression of the pons *(P)* and fourth ventricle. The cerebellar tonsil is displaced downward *(d)* below the foramen magnum *(demarcated by the white line)*. **B:** Coronal gadolinium enhanced T1WI demonstrates the upward herniation of the cerebellum *(u)* through the tentorial incisura *(arrows)* and downward *(D)* displacement of the tonsil by mass effect from a large hematoma *(H)*. The lateral ventricles *(L)* are enlarged because of obstruction of CSF flow through the cerebral aqueduct and fourth ventricle.

The diagnosis of abusive head trauma is easily missed in infants and toddlers because of nonspecific symptoms. Importantly, head injuries, particularly in young children and infants, may present without any localizing neurologic signs and symptoms. Likewise, skull radiographs are an unreliable source of screening because serious intracranial pathology may occur in the absence of skull fractures. Children with significant inflicted brain injury may even have no external signs of trauma on presentation and may lack visible retinal hemorrhages and fractures on skeletal survey. In light of this, the most recent American College of Radiology guidelines[3] recommends that all clinicians should maintain a low threshold for performing CT or MRI of the head in all cases of suspected abuse. Neuroimaging is also important in elucidating findings that may point to other diagnoses, including accidental trauma, infection, coagulopathy, and rare metabolic diseases. Imaging is vital when cases of NAHI require emergent neurosurgical intervention and provides critical data

for hospital child protective services and, in cases of child fatality, forensic and medicolegal investigation.

Patterns of Injury: Clinical Implications and Diagnostic Neuroimaging

The major components of inflicted head trauma are variable and may include skull fracture, subdural hemorrhage, SAH, contusion, intraparenchymal hemorrhage, hypoxic-ischemic damage, and diffuse axonal injury. However, certain patterns of neuroimaging abnormalities are strongly associated with abuse.

Subdural Hemorrhage

In cases of child abuse, the most commonly detected intracranial abnormality on imaging is subdural hemorrhage (SDH) (Figs. 2.25 to 2.27). SDH is

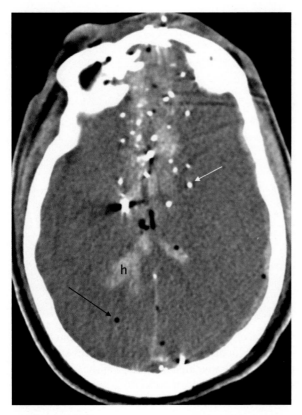

Figure 2.24. Gunshot wound. Axial CT in a victim of a shooting shows multiple bullet fragments *(white arrow)* along the bullet track, some producing considerable streak artifacts. Gas *(pneumocephalus)* is also present *(black arrow)*, along with extensive hemorrhage *(h)*.

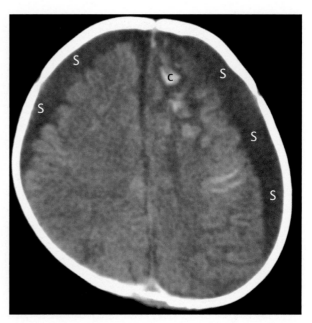

Figure 2.25. Child abuse. Axial noncontrast CT image at the level of the centrum semiovale from a victim of child abuse shows bilateral low density subdural collections *(S)* and acute parenchymal hemorrhagic contusions *(C)* in the left frontal lobe.

present in up to 95% of fatal abusive head trauma. In most cases, the SDH is diffusely distributed over one or both cerebral convexities. The interhemispheric fissure is another common site. A key finding on imaging is the presence of SDH at multiple sites or of different ages or SDH with concomitant diffuse cerebral edema. The incidence of non-abusive SDHs in neonates following vaginal delivery is well recognized, occurring in up to 26% of vaginal births at full term. However, these non-abusive SDHs are small, peritentorial in location (in contrast to the cerebral convexity and interhemispheric pattern of child abuse), resolve shortly after birth (~1 month), and do not rebleed on longitudinal follow-up.

It is important to note the high correlation of retinal hemorrhages (RH) with SDH, warranting a retinal examination in every case of suspected inflicted head injury. Although the incidence of RH with abusive head trauma is extremely high, the incidence of RH with proven severe accidental trauma (high-force motor vehicle accidents), seizures, chest

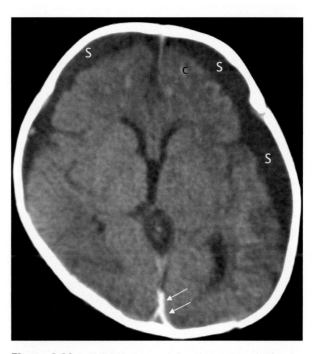

Figure 2.26. Child abuse. Axial noncontrast CT image at the level of the basal ganglia from a victim of child abuse shows bilateral low density subdural collections *(S)* and acute subdural blood along the posterior falx *(arrows)*; there is a small parenchymal contusion *(c)* in the left frontal lobe.

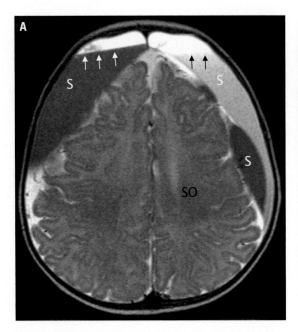
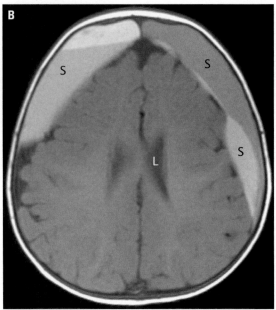

Figure 2.27. Child abuse. **A:** T2-weighted MR image at the level of the centrum semiovale *(SO)* from a victim of child abuse shows bilateral subdural hematomas *(S)* with loculations containing different stages of blood breakdown and debris/fluid levels *(arrows)*. **B:** Same patient T1-weighted MR image at the level of the body of the lateral ventricles *(L)*. Subdural location, large collections, bilateral collections, and collections with differing stages of blood breakdown products should each raise suspicion for child abuse.

compressions, forceful vomiting, and severe persistent vomiting is very low.

Skull Fractures

One of the most common histories proffered by caregivers in cases of NAHI is of an alleged accidental fall at home to various surfaces from items of household furniture. Helfer et al. studied two groups of children in the home and hospital setting.[4] Out of 176 falls at home, there were 2 skull fractures, whereas 85 falls in the hospital resulted in 1 skull fracture. No fracture was diastatic and no fracture was greater than 1 mm in width. None of the children suffered serious head injury with neurologic complications. No children had evidence of epidural hemorrhage or SDH. Even in more serious falls, Barlow et al. investigated falls of 61 children from heights of at least one story.[5] Skull fractures occurred in 17 but there was only 1 SDH. Thus, the evidence suggests that skull fractures can occur after accidental trauma, including minor domestic accidents, but are not usual and seldom cause serious intracranial pathology. Further, certain fracture characteristics occur significantly more often in NAHI. These in-

clude multiple or comminuted fractures, depressed or widely diastatic (>1 mm) fractures, or involvement of more than one bone or fractures involving bones other than the parietal bone. If a comminuted or diastatic fracture is seen on a radiologic study of an infant's skull where the supposed mechanism of injury is a simple household accident, it is reasonable for the radiologist to consider the possibility of abuse and clearly communicate such findings to the clinical team, thereby enlisting the support of child protective services.

Neuroimaging Protocol Guidelines

The Royal College of Radiologists has developed a neuroimaging schedule to be followed in cases of NAHI: According to the UK-based guidelines, every child with suspected NAHI should receive a CT scan within 24 hours of admission, MRI of the brain and spine within 5 days of presentation, and a second follow-up MRI brain exam at 3 to 4 months. Skull radiography is recommended as part of the skeletal survey. In addition to children presenting with neurologic symptoms, neuroimaging should be undertaken in all children younger than the age of

1 year with evidence of physical abuse. According to the American College of Radiology guidelines, every child 2 years of age or younger with suspected physical abuse without neurologic signs or symptoms deserves an x-ray skeletal survey and CT or MRI of the head. All cases of potential inflicted head trauma should be reviewed and reported by a radiologist with expertise in neuroimaging and experience with patterns of abuse.

Increasing attention to cervical spinal injury, especially in cases of shaking and whiplash mechanisms of inflicted trauma, has motivated some centers to include the cervical spine MRI along with their cranial MRI protocols. Both brain and spine MRI is recommended in all cases with positive cranial CT findings and in selected cases with normal CT results but strong clinical suspicion.

Although changing CT attenuation or MRI signal characteristics may be helpful in providing a general timeline in differentiating between acute and chronic hematoma, findings should be interpreted with caution. Anatomic factors such as size and location of hemorrhage, combined with physiologically dynamic influences, such as varying rates of hemoglobin degradation and mixing of hematoma with CSF, have variable impacts on signal characteristics and preclude precise dating of hematoma.

Delayed MRI at 3 to 4 months provides important information regarding the extent of end stage brain damage following NAHI. During this period, MRI reliably detects late complications such as hydrocephalus and enlarging chronic subdural effusions that may require surgical intervention.

SUMMARY

In cases of suspected NAHI, significant ethical and professional responsibility rests with the radiologist. Radiologists may be the first to raise the possibility of abuse, especially if the clinical history is discrepant with the nature or pattern of neuroimaging findings. The duty of a radiologist is to generate a detailed description of the imaging findings, provide differential diagnoses when appropriate, and clearly communicate concern for NAHI to the primary care team in an efficacious manner.

REFERENCES

1. U.S. Department of Health and Human Services, Administration on Children, Youth and Families. *Child maltreatment 2007.* Available at: http://www.acf.hhs.gov/programs/cb/pubs/cm07/cm07.pdf
2. McClain PW, Sacks JJ, Froehike RG, et al. Estimates of fatal child abuse and neglect, United States, 1979 through 1988. *Pediatrics.* 1993;91:338–343.
3. Meyer JS, Gunderman R, Coley BD, et al. ACR Appropriateness Criteria(®) on suspected physical abuse-Child. *J Am Coll Radiol.* 2011;8(2):87–94.
4. Helfer RE, Slovis TL, Black M. Injuries resulting when small children fall out of bed. *Pediatrics.* 1977;60:533–535.
5. Barlow B, Niemirska M, Gandhi RP, et al. Ten years of experience with falls from a height in children. *J Pediatr Surg.* 1983;18:509–511.

SUGGESTED READINGS

1. Bradley WG Jr. MR appearance of hemorrhage in the brain. *Radiology.* 1993;189(1):15–26.
2. Gentry LR. Imaging of closed head injury. *Radiology.* 1994;191(1):1–17.
3. Klufas RA, Hsu L, Patel MR, et al. Unusual manifestations of head trauma. *AJR Am J Roentgenol.* 1996;166(3):675–681.
4. Johnson PL, Eckard DA, Chason DP, et al. Imaging of acquired cerebral herniations. *Neuroimag Clin N Am.* 2002;12(2):217–228.
5. Kleinman PK. Diagnostic imaging in infant abuse. *AJR Am J Roentgenol.* 1990;155(4):703–712.
6. Meyer JS, Gunderman R, Coley BD, et al. ACR Appropriateness Criteria(®) on suspected physical abuse-child. *J Am Coll Radiol.* 2011;8(2):87–94.
7. Rajaram S, Batty R, Rittey CD, et al. Neuroimaging in non-accidental head injury in children: an important element of assessment. *Postgrad Med J.* 2011;87(1027):355–361.
8. Section on Radiology, American Academy of Pediatrics. Diagnostic imaging of child abuse. *Pediatrics.* 2009;123(5):1430–1435.
9. Jaspan T. Current controversies in the interpretation of non-accidental head injury. *Pediatr Radiol.* 2008;38(suppl 3):S378–S387.
10. Stoodley N. Neuroimaging in non-accidental head injury: if, when, why and how. *Clin Radiol.* 2005;60(1):22–30.

CHAPTER 3

Nontraumatic Intracranial Emergencies

Benjamin Y. Huang ■ Mauricio Castillo

GENERAL CONSIDERATIONS

The list of nontraumatic intracranial processes that commonly present on an emergent basis encompasses a wide range of pathologies, which, although disparate etiologically, often present with very similar symptoms and signs that include headaches, seizures, dizziness, alterations in mental status, or focal neurologic deficits. For these reasons, accurate diagnosis of specific intracranial abnormalities on purely clinical grounds is frequently impossible. Imaging therefore plays a crucial role in the workup and triage of patients with suspected central nervous system (CNS) pathology. In most cases, unenhanced head computed tomography (CT) is the initial imaging test of choice because of its widespread availability and its ability to reliably rule out most gross pathology such as hemorrhage or large mass lesions. Additional studies such as contrast-enhanced CT, CT angiography (CTA), or magnetic resonance imaging (MRI) largely play an ancillary role in the emergency room setting and are generally reserved for cases in which (1) an abnormality is identified on unenhanced CT that requires further characterization, or (2) intracranial pathology is still suspected despite a negative head CT.

In this chapter, we review the radiologic evaluation of nontraumatic intracranial processes that commonly present as neurologic emergencies. From an organizational standpoint, these entities are grouped in this chapter into general categories, including (1) vascular emergencies, (2) hydrocephalus and associated conditions, (3) CNS infections, and (4) miscellaneous processes including toxic exposures and pituitary apoplexy.

VASCULAR EMERGENCIES

Vascular emergencies affecting the brain can be divided into those caused by aberrations in brain perfusion, which primarily result in edema (e.g., ischemic infarctions, spontaneous arterial dissections, venous thrombosis, posterior reversible encephalopathy) and those manifesting primarily with intracranial hemorrhage (ICH) (e.g., hypertensive bleeds, ruptured aneurysms, or vascular malformations). In some cases, such as in hemorrhagic venous infarcts or hemorrhagic transformation of ischemic infarctions, both processes occur, but in these instances the primary pathologic mechanism is vessel occlusion; therefore, these entities are discussed in the category of primarily nonhemorrhagic vascular diseases.

Predominantly Nonhemorrhagic Vascular Disorders

Ischemic Infarctions

After ischemic heart disease and cancer, stroke is the third leading cause of death in the United States. Roughly 80% to 87% of clinically evident acute strokes are caused by cerebral ischemia, with the remainder being caused by ICHs. Acute strokes typically manifest with sudden onset of a focal neurologic deficit, although some patients may experience a more gradual or stepwise progression of symptoms. Specific neurologic deficits caused by stroke depend on the vascular territory affected. Anterior circulation strokes commonly present with symptoms such as unilateral weakness or sensory loss, aphasia, dysarthria, and neglect. Patients with anterior circulation infarcts usually demonstrate normal or only slightly impaired consciousness. Posterior circulation infarcts, which account for approximately 20% of ischemic events, may cause dizziness, vertigo, headache, vomiting, ataxia, bilateral weakness, or hemianopia.

With the widespread availability of intravenous (IV) thrombolytics, rapid diagnosis is now critical to optimize outcomes in patients with acute ischemic stroke. The landmark 1995 National Institute of Neurological Disorders and Stroke tissue plasminogen activator (NINDS-tPA) trial demonstrated that patients receiving IV tPA within 3 hours of stroke onset were 30% more likely to have little or no disability at 3 months than patients receiving placebo. The subsequent European Cooperative Acute Stroke Study III (ECASS III) trial showed that clinical outcomes are also improved in patients receiving IV tPA up to 4.5 hours after stroke onset, but, generally speaking, there is a gradually diminishing benefit with increasing time from ictus. Intra-arterial recanalization techniques, including direct intra-arterial thrombolysis and use of mechanical clot retrieval devices, are also becoming more widely available and are generally considered for patients presenting outside of the effective window for IV thrombolysis up to 6 hours from the onset of stroke symptoms and in some cases beyond.

All patients with suspected acute ischemic cerebral infarctions in whom recanalization therapy is being considered should undergo emergent cross-sectional brain imaging. The primary goals of imaging in the acute setting are (1) to identify the presence of hemorrhage, (2) to identify a large vessel occlusion, and (3) to assess the volume of irreversibly injured brain tissue. Secondarily, imaging may also be performed to estimate the presence of a clinically relevant ischemic penumbra.

Computed Tomography in Acute Stroke

In clinical practice, unenhanced CT is usually the first imaging study performed in patients presenting with acute stroke symptoms given its speed and widespread availability. Within the first 6 hours of an ischemic stroke (the hyperacute stage), CT will demonstrate an abnormality in approximately 50% to 80% of patients. Early CT findings of ischemic infarctions include a hyperdense artery, parenchymal hypodensity, local brain swelling, or loss of gray–white differentiation. Because these findings can be extremely subtle when viewed with traditional brain CT windows, viewing the CT images with narrow "stroke windows" (W = 30, L = 30) often increases the conspicuity of these findings (Fig. 3.1). Although the sensitivity of CT is relatively low, its primary utility in the acute setting is to identify findings that would preclude initiation of thrombolytic therapy—specifically, acute hemorrhage (for which CT is quite sensitive) or significant parenchymal hypodensity indicating irreversible tissue injury (usually defined as hypodensity involving >1/3 of the middle cerebral territory).

Magnetic Resonance Imaging in Acute Stroke

Magnetic resonance (MR) diffusion weighted imaging (DWI) is the most sensitive imaging technique for diagnosing ischemic infarcts, identifying 88% to 100% of infarcts in the hyperacute setting. DWI signal alterations usually become apparent in infarcting tissue within 30 minutes of arterial occlusion. This is in contradistinction to conventional MR sequences (T1-weighted, T2-weighted, and fluid attenuation inversion recovery [FLAIR]), which, like CT, may miss a substantial proportion of hyperacute infarcts. Ischemic infarcts demonstrate high-signal intensity on DWI, reflecting restriction of the random motion or diffusion of extracellular water molecules caused by cell swelling and subsequent reduction in the volume of the extracellular space. When one is interpreting DWI, it is important to keep in mind that the signal characteristics displayed on the trace image reflect a combination of both T2 and diffusion effects. Therefore, DWI image sets should always be viewed in conjunction with their corresponding apparent diffusion coefficient (ADC) maps to exclude the phenomenon of "T2 shine through," which refers to the phenomenon in which tissues with a long T2 but normal or increased diffusion appear hyperintense on DWI. Infarcted tissues with truly decreased diffusion will demonstrate decreased signal intensity on the ADC map in addition to high-signal intensity on

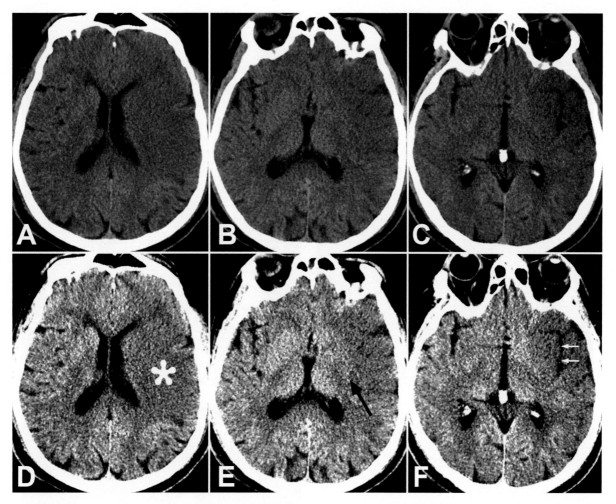

Figure 3.1. Comparison of different CT windows in acute stroke. **A to C:** Multiple CT images through the head displayed in standard brain windows (W = 80, L = 40) in a patient with an acute left MCA territory infarct. **D to F:** The same levels displayed using narrow "stroke" windows (W = 30, L = 30). The infarcted region (*asterisk* in **D**) is more easily seen with stroke windows and demonstrates hypodensity, sulcal effacement, and loss of normal gray–white differentiation. Effacement of the basal ganglia *(black arrow* in **E**) and loss of the normally dense insular ribbon *(small white arrows* in **F**) are also more conspicuous using the narrower window settings.

the DWI sequence (Fig. 3.2), whereas tissues demonstrating T2 shine through will appear isointense or hyperintense on the ADC map.

Conventional MR images usually become abnormal around 3 to 6 hours after stroke onset. On FLAIR and T2-weighted images (T2WIs), infarcts demonstrate increased tissue swelling and high-signal intensity edema (Fig. 3.2). Replacement of normal arterial flow voids with high-signal intensity in the occluded vessels is another early sign. Unenhanced T1-weighted images (T1WIs) are usually normal in early ischemic strokes but may demonstrate subtle blurring of gray–white interfaces. Contrast-enhanced T1WI may demonstrate arterial enhancement within 2 to 4 hours (Fig. 3.3) secondary to slow flow, collateral flow, or hyperperfusion following early recanalization.

Computed Tomography Angiography and Magnetic Resonance Angiography

Noninvasive angiographic imaging with CTA or MR angiography (MRA) is frequently undertaken in patients with acute ischemic strokes to identify and characterize large vessel occlusions and to assess the degree of collateral flow to at risk territories. This information is helpful for prognosis and may be useful in acute treatment planning, as recent studies have suggested that patients presenting with

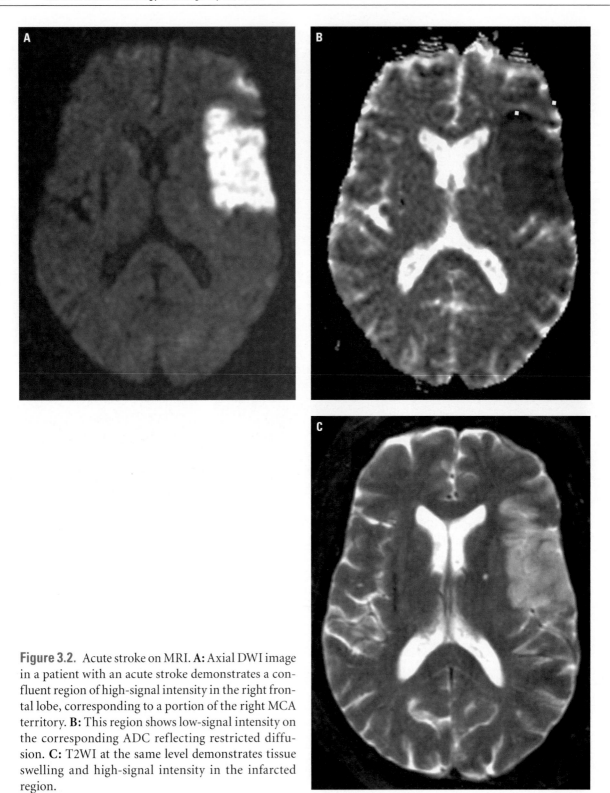

Figure 3.2. Acute stroke on MRI. **A:** Axial DWI image in a patient with an acute stroke demonstrates a confluent region of high-signal intensity in the right frontal lobe, corresponding to a portion of the right MCA territory. **B:** This region shows low-signal intensity on the corresponding ADC reflecting restricted diffusion. **C:** T2WI at the same level demonstrates tissue swelling and high-signal intensity in the infarcted region.

large vessel occlusions on CTA have poorer overall outcomes and may benefit more from intra-arterial thrombolysis than IV thrombolysis. The choice of technique (CT vs MR) primarily depends on institutional preference. With both modalities, images are frequently displayed as three-dimensional surface shaded or maximum intensity projection (MIP) reconstructions, which are similar to traditional digital subtraction angiographic (DSA) images (Fig. 3.4).

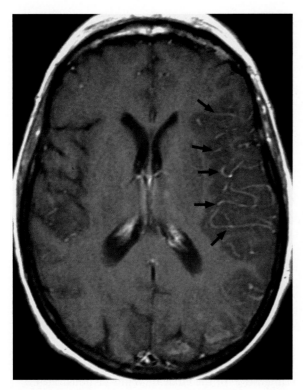

Figure 3.3. Acute stroke on MRI. Axial post-contrast T1WI shows abnormal intravascular enhancement in the left Sylvian region *(arrows)* in a patient with an acute left MCA infarction.

Extracranial imaging is also commonly performed to identify potentially thrombotic or embolic causes of stroke, including atherosclerotic plaques and arterial dissections. Overall, the diagnostic performance for CTA and MRA

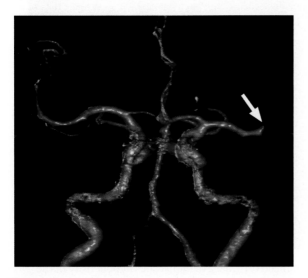

Figure 3.4. Acute MCA occlusion on CTA. Three-dimensional surface shaded reconstruction of a CTA of the head demonstrates abrupt cutoff of the left MCA *(arrow)* in a patient with an acute infarct.

for detecting cervical arterial stenoses and dissections is probably comparable. MRA and MRI are particularly useful for identifying acute carotid dissections, which can present with strokes or ipsilateral Horner's syndrome. Fat-suppressed, unenhanced axial T1WI or T2WI through the neck should be obtained in cases of suspected dissection and classically demonstrate an eccentric crescent of high-signal intensity thrombus along the wall of the dissected vessel (the so-called crescent sign) (Fig. 3.5). MRA is useful for depicting length of vessel involvement. Although the sensitivity of the MR crescent sign for carotid dissections is quite high (>90%), its sensitivity is considerably lower for vertebral artery dissections (<60%). In the latter setting, CTA may be the better noninvasive option. CTA findings of arterial dissection include vessel wall irregularity, presence of an intimal flap or pseudoaneurysms, and vessel wall thickening.

Computed Tomography and Magnetic Resonance Perfusion Imaging

There has been increasing interest recently in the use of CT and/or MR perfusion imaging to better select stroke patients for potential revascularization therapy, particularly in instances in which the time from ictus to presentation is unknown or falls outside of the currently accepted windows for attempted reperfusion. Ischemic strokes are the result of severe reductions in blood flow to the brain, with areas severely deprived of blood flow (lower than 12 mL/100 g tissue) undergoing cell death within minutes. This infarct core is what is represented as the area of reduced diffusion on DWI and to a lesser degree as the area of visible hypoattenuation on CT. In the acute stage of ischemic infarctions, there may be a peripheral zone of impaired but viable tissue that is supported by collateral circulation referred to as the "ischemic penumbra," which contains cells that theoretically may be salvaged with prompt reperfusion. The penumbra can be estimated using physiologic perfusion maps that can be obtained either with CT or MR perfusion imaging. The penumbra is represented by the area of mismatch observed between the volume of hypoperfused tissue on perfusion maps (typically the cerebral blood flow or time-to-peak maps) and the volume of the infarct core (as assessed on DWI or unenhanced CT) (Fig. 3.6).

Existing data on outcomes for stroke patients triaged to delayed thrombolysis on the basis of CT or

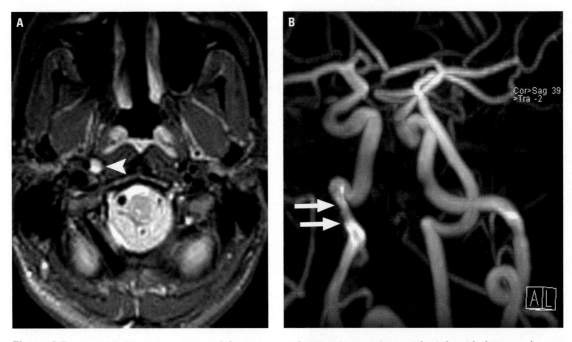

Figure 3.5. Carotid dissection. **A:** Axial fat-suppressed T2WI in a patient with right-sided Horner's syndrome demonstrates an eccentric crescent of high signal along the medial wall of the right ICA *(arrowhead)*, consistent with intramural thrombus. **B:** The corresponding MRA of the circle of Willis demonstrates narrowing and irregularity of the distal petrous segment of the ICA *(arrows)*.

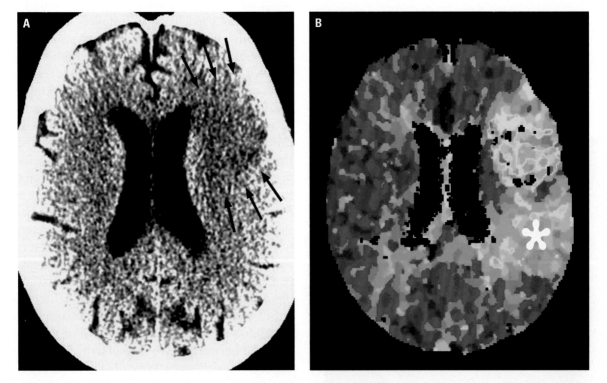

Figure 3.6. Perfusion mismatch in acute stroke. **A:** Unenhanced CT image demonstrates hypodensity in the left MCA territory *(arrows)* compatible with an acute infarct. The hypodense region represents the infarct core. **B:** Time-to-peak map from a CT perfusion study demonstrates a perfusion mismatch with viable but hypoperfused tissue, primarily displayed in green *(asterisk)*, posterior to the infarct core.

MR perfusion mismatches are conflicting because some studies suggest a potential benefit, whereas others report no benefit. Delayed thrombolysis appears to be associated with increased rates of recanalization, but has not been shown definitively to be associated with improved patient outcomes. Therefore, perfusion weighted imaging currently remains an investigational tool in acute stroke patients.

Specific Ischemic Stroke Patterns
Middle Cerebral Artery Infarctions

More than half of ischemic cerebral infarctions involve the middle cerebral artery (MCA) territory. Early CT findings of an MCA infarction include hyperdensity of the MCA trunk or its branches (Fig. 3.7) and parenchymal hypodensity, local brain swelling, or loss of gray–white differentiation in the territory supplied by the MCA. Effacement of the normally slightly hyperdense basal ganglia (the "disappearing basal ganglia" sign) or insular cortex (the "insular ribbon" sign) are subtle findings suggestive of an acute MCA infarction (Fig. 3.1).

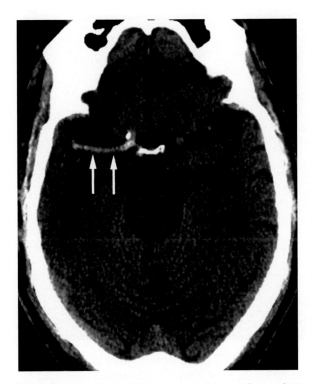

Figure 3.7. The dense MCA sign. Axial unenhanced CT demonstrates an asymmetric hyperdense right MCA, reflecting the presence of acute intravascular clot.

Anterior Cerebral Artery Infarctions

Infarctions of the anterior cerebral artery (ACA) territory account for up to 5% of ischemic strokes. They are often seen in combination with MCA infarctions, and isolated ACA infarctions are uncommon. Unlike MCA infarctions, most ACA strokes result from primary vessel disease (e.g., atherosclerosis, vasculitis, or vasospasm related to aneurysmal subarachnoid hemorrhage [SAH]) rather than an emboli. ACA infarcts may also occur as a result of subfalcine herniation as the ACA becomes compressed under the falx cerebri. On unenhanced CT, ACA infarctions appear as hypodensities involving the medial aspect of the superior frontal and parietal lobes adjacent to the falx, whereas MRI will demonstrate restricted diffusion and T2 shortening in these regions (Fig. 3.8). A hyperdense ACA may also be observed in some cases, indicating acute thrombus within the vessel (Fig. 3.9).

Posterior Circulation Infarctions

Posterior circulation strokes are caused by obstruction of the vertebral, basilar, or posterior cerebral arteries (PCAs) and their branches and may involve the brainstem, the cerebellum, or the posterior portions of the cerebrum. They account for roughly 20% of ischemic infarctions. Of these, PCA infarctions account for roughly 30%. On imaging, isolated PCA infarctions classically involve the ipsilateral occipital lobe, medial and posterior temporal lobe, or the thalamus (Fig. 3.10).

Thrombosis of the basilar artery is a potentially catastrophic occurrence that carries a mortality rate of 80% to 90% if left untreated. Even with thrombolytic therapy, the survival rate of patients with basilar thrombosis only increases to approximately 50%. The clinical and imaging manifestations of basilar artery thrombosis can be quite variable and depend on the location and extent of thrombus and on the degree of collateral flow. In addition to feeding the PCAs and the anterior–inferior and superior cerebellar arteries, the basilar artery also gives off multiple perforators directly supplying the pons and midbrain. Complete thrombosis of the basilar artery therefore results in infarcts to all of the structures supplied by these vessels including the pons and midbrain, mid and upper cerebellum, thalami, and the posterior limbs of the internal capsules. Infarcts of the portions of the cerebrum supplied by the PCAs may also be present. Complete basilar occlusion is generally rapidly fatal and rarely goes on to imaging.

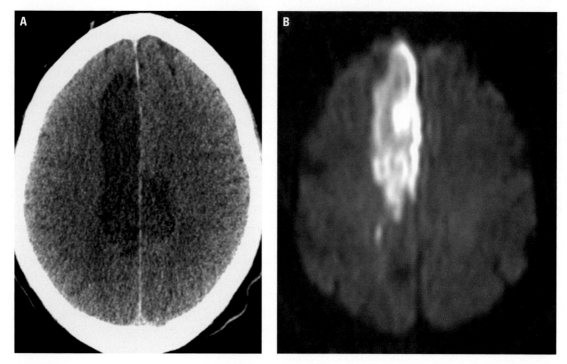

Figure 3.8. Anterior cerebral artery infarctions. **A:** Axial unenhanced CT demonstrates a large right ACA infarct and a smaller left ACA infarct, which appear as hypodensities in medial aspects of the frontal and parietal lobes. **B:** An axial DWI image in a different patient demonstrates high-signal intensity in the right ACA territory.

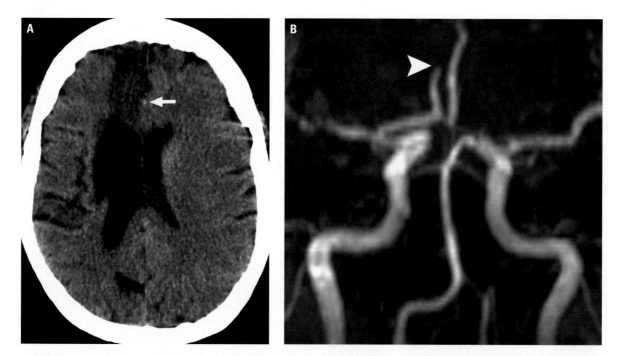

Figure 3.9. Anterior cerebral artery infarction. **A:** Axial unenhanced CT image demonstrates hypodensity in the right ACA territory compatible with an acute infarct. The right ACA is hyperdense *(arrow)* indicating the presence of thrombus. **B:** TOF-MRA demonstrates abrupt cutoff of the A2 segment of the right ACA *(arrowhead)*.

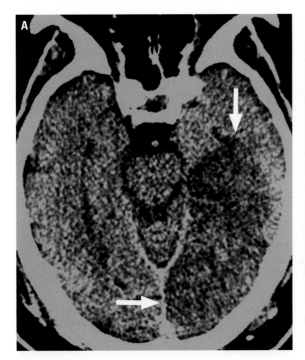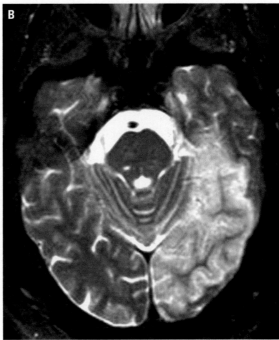

Figure 3.10. Posterior cerebral artery infarction. **A:** Unenhanced axial CT image demonstrates hypodensity within the left occipital lobe and medial left temporal lobe *(arrows)* in the territory of the left PCA. **B:** Axial T2WI in the same patient demonstrates gyral swelling and hyperintensity in the infarcted region.

Patients with less extensive thromboses may present acutely or with a gradual or stuttering course. Imaging in these patients shows a more limited distribution of infarctions. Occlusion of the proximal and midportions of the basilar artery may result in a "locked in" state caused by infarction of the upper ventral pons. This syndrome is characterized by complete loss of voluntary movement, with the exception of vertical eye movement, and preserved consciousness (caused by sparing of the pontine tegmentum). Thrombosis involving only the distal basilar artery produces the "top-of-the-basilar" syndrome, with infarcts of the midbrain, thalami, and temporal and occipital lobes classically causing visual, oculomotor, and behavioral abnormalities, usually without significant motor dysfunction. Unlike more proximal basilar thromboses, which are usually the result of atherosclerotic disease, distal basilar thrombosis is usually caused by embolism.

On unenhanced CT, thrombus within the basilar artery may appear hyperdense (Fig. 3.11), and the appearance of a dense artery may precede the development of parenchymal hypodensity. As with infarcts of the anterior circulation, DWI is more sen-

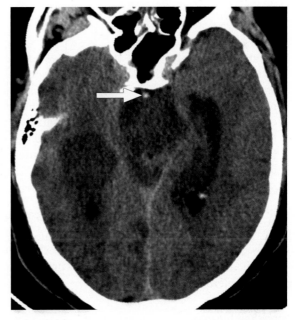

Figure 3.11. Basilar artery thrombosis. Unenhanced axial CT image demonstrates multiple hypodensities in the pons, cerebellum, medial temporal lobes, and right occipital lobe compatible with posterior circulation infarcts. The basilar artery is hyperdense, indicating intraluminal thrombus *(arrow)*.

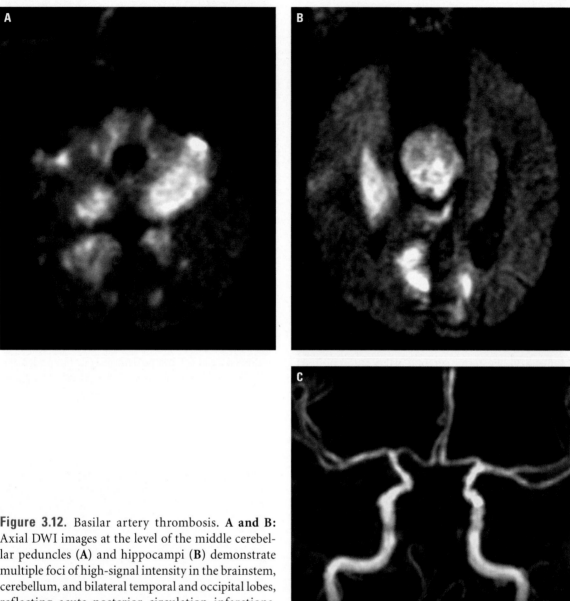

Figure 3.12. Basilar artery thrombosis. **A and B:** Axial DWI images at the level of the middle cerebellar peduncles (**A**) and hippocampi (**B**) demonstrate multiple foci of high-signal intensity in the brainstem, cerebellum, and bilateral temporal and occipital lobes, reflecting acute posterior circulation infarctions. **C:** TOF-MRA demonstrates absent flow within the basilar artery and its branches.

sitive and better delineates the extent of infarction in the acute setting (Fig. 3.12). CTA and MRA both effectively demonstrate the location and extent of occlusion and may document potentially predisposing atherosclerotic changes.

Watershed Infarcts

"Watershed" infarctions occur in the boundary zones between major arterial territories and account for approximately 10% of ischemic strokes. The pathogenesis of these infarcts is debated, but it is likely that they involve multiple factors including systemic hypotension, arterial stenosis or occlusion, and microembolization. Hypoperfusion in combination with severe occlusive disease of the internal carotid arteries (ICA) can cause both embolization and decreased brain perfusion, which is most pronounced at the arterial border zones. Decreased perfusion may, in turn, alter blood flow currents, encouraging microemboli to lodge in these watershed areas.

Like other ischemic infarcts, acute watershed infarcts are hypodense on CT and demonstrate high-signal intensity on DWI, T2-weighted, and FLAIR sequences. Anterior watershed infarctions between the ACA and MCA territories manifest as multiple ischemic lesions involving a linear strip of frontal

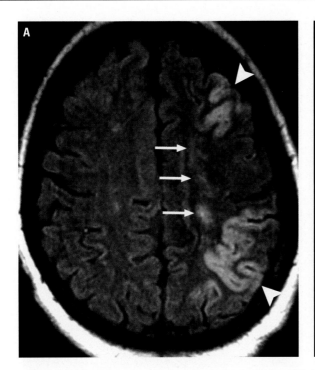 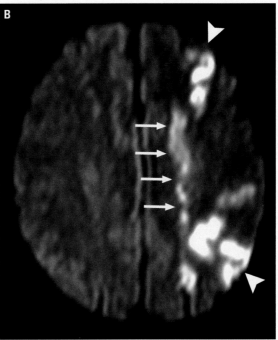

Figure 3.13. Watershed infarctions. **A:** Axial FLAIR image demonstrates wedge-shaped areas of cortical hyperintensity in the left frontal and parietal lobes *(arrowheads)* and foci of deep white hyperintensity in a parasagittal distribution *(arrows)*, corresponding to the external and internal watershed regions. **B:** These areas show restricted diffusion on the DWI image indicating they represent acute infarcts.

cortex on the superior convexity close to the interhemispheric fissure (referred to as the external or cortical watershed region) as well as the white matter along and slightly above the lateral ventricle, including portions of the corona radiata between the territories of the deep and superficial perforators of the MCA and the centrum semiovale between the superficial perforators of the ACA and MCA (known as the internal watershed region) (Fig. 3.13). Posterior watershed infarcts develop between the ACA, MCA, and PCA territories and affect a parieto-temporo-occipital wedge of tissue extending from the occipital horn of the lateral ventricle to the parieto-occipital cortex (Fig. 3.13). The infarcts may be unilateral or bilateral.

Identification of a watershed pattern of infarctions by imaging should prompt one to perform vascular imaging of the intracranial and extracranial vascular imaging with Doppler ultrasound, CTA, or MRA to rule out the presence of contributory arterial occlusions or flow limiting stenoses.

Lacunar Infarcts

Lacunar infarcts account for 20% to 25% of all strokes and most often occur in patients with a longstanding history of diabetes mellitus or hypertension.

They are usually caused by occlusion of small penetrating arteries and, as a result, are typically small (≤1.5 cm) and associated with little or no mass effect or edema. They most frequently occur in the basal ganglia, thalami, internal capsule, pons, and centrum semiovale. Symptoms related to lacunar infarcts can be quite variable depending on their location, and most are clinically silent. Despite the prevailing belief that most lacunar infarcts are caused by small vessel thrombosis, the NINDS-tPA trial showed that patients with lacunar infarcts are just as likely to benefit within the 3-hour IV thrombolysis window as patients with other ischemic stroke subtypes. Therefore, identification of a lacunar infarct on imaging does not preclude the initiation of IV tPA.

Acute lacunar infarcts are often difficult to appreciate on unenhanced CT. They frequently occur in the background of more extensive white matter disease or may be difficult to distinguish from enlarged perivascular spaces. When visible on CT, they appear as small, round or ovoid hypodensities within one of the characteristic locations listed earlier (Fig. 3.14). As with other ischemic infarcts, acute lacunar infarcts are most easily detected on DWI, which has a reported accuracy of approximately

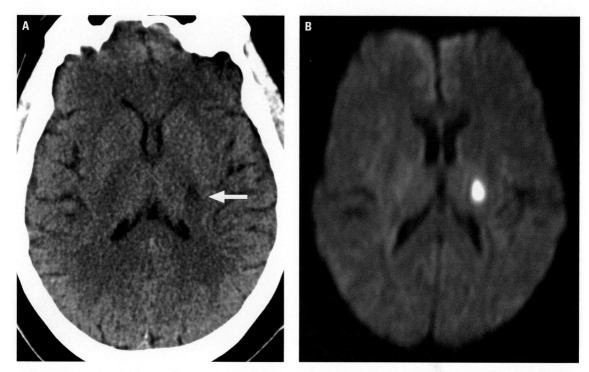

Figure 3.14. Acute lacunar infarct. **A:** Axial unenhanced CT image demonstrates an ovoid area of hypodensity centered in the posterior limb of the left internal capsule. **B:** A corresponding DWI image demonstrates high-signal intensity, reflecting restricted diffusion in an acute lacunar infarct.

95% and will demonstrate a small, isolated focus of restricted diffusion in a characteristic location (Fig. 3.14). Acute lacunar infarcts may be difficult to distinguish from chronic lacunes on conventional MR sequences, particularly in patients with underlying chronic small vessel disease.

Hypoxic-Ischemic Brain Injury

Hypoxic-ischemic encephalopathy (HIE) is characterized by diffuse ischemic brain injury caused by global hypoperfusion or a severe disturbance in blood oxygenation. In children, HIE is commonly the result of drowning, choking, accidental asphyxiation, or non-accidental trauma, whereas in adults, HIE is usually a consequence of cardiac arrest or cerebrovascular disease in combination with severe or prolonged hypotension. Two basic and often overlapping patterns of brain injury are seen in patients with HIE: (1) hemodynamic (watershed) infarcts at the confluences of the MCA, PCA, and ACA territories, which are usually the result of mild to moderate hypoxic-ischemic events; and (2) generalized cortical and deep gray matter injury, which is generally caused by severe anoxic insults. Because imaging of watershed infarcts was discussed earlier, here we shall focus primarily on the latter pattern of injury.

Gray matter structures preferentially involved in severe cases of HIE include the basal ganglia, thalami, cerebral cortex (with a predilection for the sensorimotor and visual cortices), cerebellum, and hippocampi. Although MRI is better for evaluating the extent of injury in patients with HIE, CT is usually the first study ordered in the emergency department setting. Findings of severe HIE on CT include diffuse cerebral edema causing effacement of the cerebrospinal fluid (CSF)-containing spaces, decreased cortical gray matter density with loss of normal gray–white differentiation, and decreased density in the bilateral basal ganglia (Fig. 3.15). A minority of patients may demonstrate the so-called reversal sign in which there is reversal in the normal CT densities of gray and white matter with white matter being of higher density than the cortical gray matter. Another well-described but relatively insensitive CT sign of severe HIE is the "white cerebellum" sign, in which the cerebellum and brainstem demonstrate apparent high attenuation because of the development of diffuse cerebral edema (Fig. 3.16).

DWI is extremely sensitive for HIE and demonstrates restricted diffusion in injured structures, usually evident within minutes of the anoxic event and lasting for approximately 1 week (Fig. 3.17).

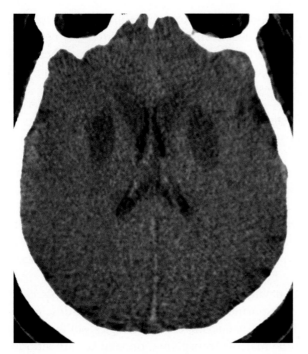

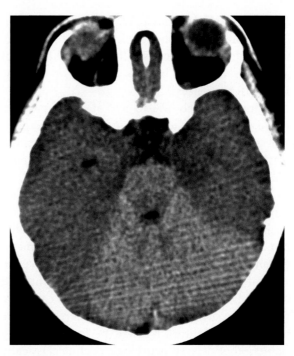

Figure 3.15. Hypoxic ischemic encephalopathy. Unenhanced axial CT image demonstrates symmetric basal ganglia hypodensity and diffuse cerebral edema with complete loss of gray–white differentiation.

Figure 3.16. The "white cerebellum" sign. Unenhanced axial head CT in a child who suffered a severe hypoxic-ischemic insult demonstrates higher attenuation in the brainstem and cerebellum relative the cerebral hemispheres.

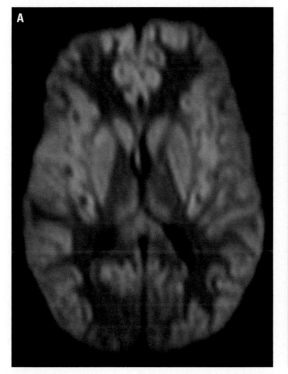

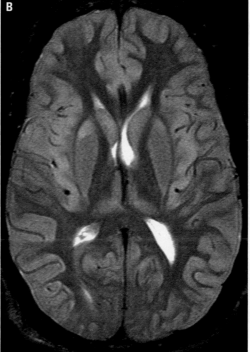

Figure 3.17. Hypoxic-ischemic encephalopathy. **A:** Axial DWI image demonstrates diffusely increased signal intensity in the basal ganglia, thalami, and cerebral cortex, reflecting diffusely reduced gray matter diffusion. **B:** The corresponding T2WI demonstrates diffusely increased gray matter signal intensity and swelling.

Conventional T1WI and T2WI are usually normal or show only subtle changes in the first 24 hours. After 24 hours, cortical swelling and blurring of gray–white interfaces become apparent on conventional MR sequences.

In approximately 2% to 3% of cases, patients with a global hypoxic-ischemic insult may experience a syndrome of delayed white matter injury. This syndrome, termed *postanoxic leukoencephalopathy*, is characterized by a period of relative clinical stability or even improvement followed by an acute neurologic decline, usually 2 to 3 weeks after the initial insult. Patients may demonstrate delirium, personality changes, intellectual impairment, movement disorders, or, rarely, seizures. In typical cases of postanoxic encephalopathy, conventional MR and DWI immediately following the causative insult fail to demonstrate significant cerebral white matter abnormalities, but MR performed during the period of delayed neurologic decline classically demonstrates symmetric, confluent cerebral white matter hyperintensity on T2-weighted and FLAIR sequences with corresponding restricted diffusion on DWI (Fig. 3.18). Approximately 75% of patients

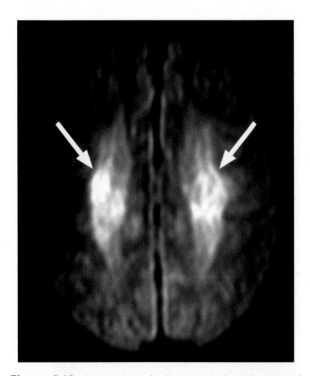

Figure 3.18. Postanoxic leukoencephalopathy. Axial DWI image in a patient who presented with an acute neurologic decline weeks after a hypoxic event demonstrates symmetric confluent cerebral white matter hyperintensity, indicating reduced white matter diffusion.

with postanoxic leukoencephalopathy go on to complete or near complete recovery over the next 6 to 12 months. In the remainder of patients, there may be residual dementia. Rarely, the condition may progress to paresis, a vegetative state, or death.

Posterior Reversible Encephalopathy Syndrome

Posterior reversible encephalopathy syndrome (PRES) is a clinicoradiologic entity characterized by a distinct pattern of typically reversible brain edema that primarily affects the parietal and occipital lobes. It frequently occurs in the setting of moderate-to-severe hypertension (seen 70% to 80% of patients with PRES) and was therefore previously referred to as hypertensive encephalopathy. Additional risk factors for PRES include eclampsia, renal disease, treatment with immunosuppressant therapies (especially cyclosporine A and tacrolimus) or high-dose multi-drug antineoplastic chemotherapies, solid organ or bone marrow transplantation, and certain autoimmune diseases including lupus. PRES can also occur in the setting of infection, sepsis, or shock. Women are affected more commonly than men.

Although the pathophysiology of PRES is not well understood, the prevailing theory is that severe hypertension overwhelms compensatory mechanisms regulating cerebral blood flow, ultimately resulting in vasodilatation and edema. More recently, it has been suggested that PRES may be caused by circulating toxic substances that induce endothelial injury, blood–brain barrier breakdown, and edema. Why PRES predominantly involves the posterior portions of the brain is also uncertain, but it has been hypothesized that the relatively limited sympathetic innervation of the posterior circulation reduces its ability to protect against marked increases in blood pressure compared to the anterior circulation.

Symptoms of PRES may develop acutely or over several days. Patients commonly present with headaches, visual disturbances, seizures, and/or alterations in mental status. Focal neurologic deficits such as paresis can also occasionally occur. With appropriate therapy, the prognosis for PRES is usually excellent, with most patients experiencing complete resolution of clinical and radiographic findings. Rarely, however, PRES may progress to irreversible ischemia and infarction.

The characteristic CT findings of PRES are bilateral—often symmetric—cortical and sub-cortical areas of low attenuation on CT, predominantly affecting the parietal and occipital lobes.

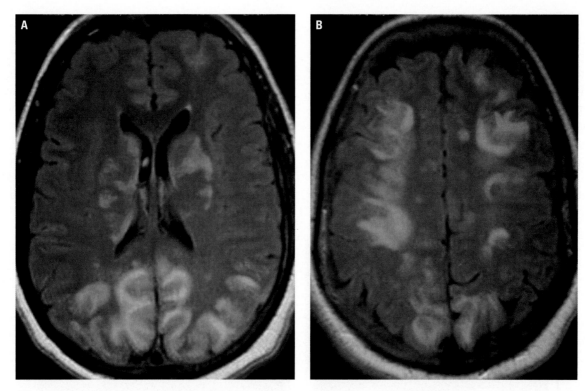

Figure 3.19. Posterior reversible encephalopathy syndrome. **A:** Axial FLAIR image through the lateral ventricles demonstrates symmetric cortical and subcortical high-signal intensity predominantly affecting the occipital lobes. Patchy signal abnormalities are also present in the basal ganglia. **B:** Axial FLAIR image superior to (**A**) demonstrates additional areas of involvement in the parietal and frontal lobes.

MR is much more sensitive for detecting PRES and shows high-signal intensity in these regions on T2-weighted and FLAIR images (Fig. 3.19). The affected areas usually do not demonstrate significant reductions in ADC on DWI. Diffusion abnormalities, when present, usually appear as small, patchy, or punctate areas within much larger areas of vasogenic edema. Although PRES classically affects the parietal and occipital lobes, involvement of other locations is not uncommon. Frontal lobe involvement is seen in roughly two-thirds of patients with PRES, and the basal ganglia, brainstem, cerebellum, and deep white matter may also be affected (Fig. 3.19).

MRA in cases of PRES frequently shows evidence of vasculopathy, demonstrated as vessel irregularity with alternating areas of vasoconstriction and vasodilatation. Like the areas of edema in PRES, these angiographic findings are usually reversible.

Venous Thrombosis and Venous Infarction

Cerebral venous thrombosis (CVT) accounts for up to 2% of adult strokes and an even higher proportion of strokes in younger patients. The diagnosis of CVT is often overlooked or delayed because the disorder can present with a wide range of complaints that often mimic other processes. Common signs and symptoms include headache, seizures, focal neurologic deficits, altered consciousness, and papilledema, which can present in isolation or in association with other symptoms. Predisposing conditions to the development of CVT include dehydration, genetic or acquired prothrombotic disorders, cancer, inflammatory bowel diseases, collagen vascular diseases, pregnancy and puerperium, and oral contraceptive use.

CVT is generally classified as involving the deep or superficial venous systems, and often both are simultaneously involved. The deep cerebral veins include the thalamic veins, thalamostriate veins, internal cerebral veins, basal veins of Rosenthal, vein of Galen, and the straight sinus. These veins are responsible for drainage of the thalami, basal ganglia, and deep white matter. Venous return from the small thalamic and thalamostriate veins is collected by the internal cerebral veins and basal veins of Rosenthal, which in turn drain into the vein of Galen. The vein of Galen then joins with the inferior sagittal sinus to form the straight sinus, which communicates with the dural venous sinuses at the torcular Herophili. Occlusion of the deep venous system is seen in roughly 16% of patients with CVT.

The superficial venous system is made up of the cortical veins of the cerebrum and the more superficially located dural venous sinuses, which include the superior sagittal sinus, transverse sinuses, and sigmoid sinuses. The superficial veins drain blood from the superficial surfaces of the cerebral hemispheres into the dural sinuses.

Diagnosis of CVT relies on neuroimaging. CVT causes venous congestion and vasogenic edema, which varies in extent and distribution depending on the veins involved. Most patients demonstrate parenchymal abnormalities on imaging, manifesting as focal areas of edema with or without hemorrhage (often referred to as "venous infarctions"). Roughly, a third of patients with CVT will demonstrate hemorrhagic lesions. In cases of deep CVT, the characteristic finding is symmetric bilateral thalamic involvement (Fig. 3.20), which

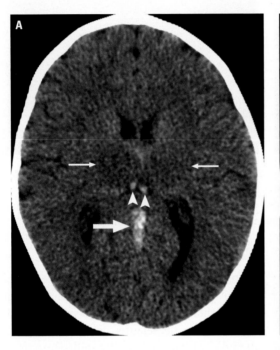

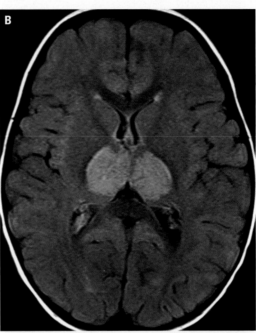

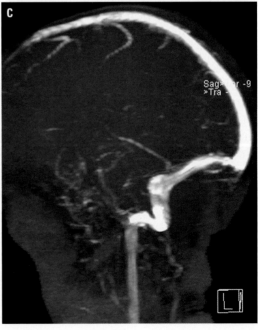

Figure 3.20. Deep cerebral venous thrombosis. **A:** Unenhanced axial CT image demonstrates symmetric thalamic hypodensity *(small arrows)*. The straight sinus *(large arrow)* and internal cerebral veins *(arrowheads)* are hyperdense due to intraluminal thrombus. **B:** Axial FLAIR image in the same patient demonstrates swollen, hyperintense thalami. **C:** Lateral projection MIP image from a 2D TOF-MRV demonstrates absent flow-related enhancement in the deep venous system as well as in the right transverse and sigmoid sinuses, reflecting both deep and superficial venous thrombosis.

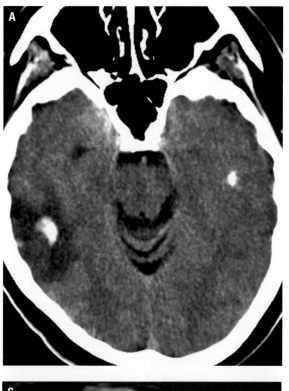

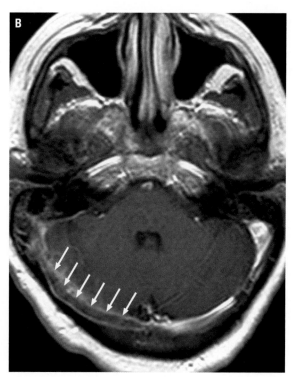

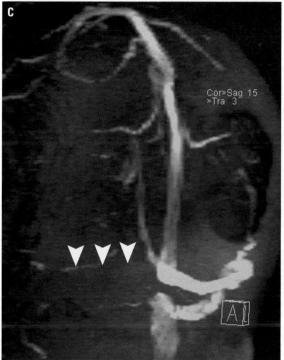

Figure 3.21. Hemorrhagic venous infarction caused by superficial sinus thrombosis. **A:** Unenhanced axial CT image demonstrates a hyperdense hemorrhage with substantial surrounding edema in the right temporal lobe. **B:** An axial post-contrast T1WI demonstrates a filling defect in the right transverse sinus *(small arrows)*. **C:** Right posterior oblique projection MIP image from a 2D TOF-MRA demonstrates lack of flow in the right transverse *(arrowheads)* and sigmoid sinuses.

may extend into the basal ganglia, midbrain, and adjacent deep white matter. Parenchymal lesions related to superficial CVT are usually cortical and subcortical, and their location depends on the specific veins that are occluded. Thrombosis of the superior sagittal sinus or veins normally draining into it typically causes lesions in the parasagittal frontal and parietal lobes. Transverse sinus thrombosis typically gives temporal or occipital lobe lesions (Fig. 3.21). Contrast-enhanced CT and MRI may also demonstrate parenchymal or leptomeningeal enhancement.

Restricted diffusion can be seen in the edematous regions on DWI, presumably representing areas of cytotoxic edema; however, the diffusion weighted signal abnormality in venous infarctions is often much less impressive than changes seen in cases of arterial infarction, usually involves a relatively small portion of the edematous tissue, and is frequently reversible.

Thrombus within a cortical vein or venous sinus is evident on unenhanced CT in roughly 25% of cases of CVT, appearing as high-density material within the occluded vein (the so-called cord sign) (Figs. 3.20 and 3.22). On contrast-enhanced CT or MR, an intraluminal filling defect can often be seen within an occluded sinus (Fig. 3.21). One well-described finding on contrast-enhanced studies is the "empty delta" sign that appears as a central filling defect in the triangular superior sagittal sinus surrounded by enhancing collateral venous channels in the dural envelope (Fig. 3.22).

On MRI, thrombus is suggested by the absence of a normal flow void in the occluded venous structure. Acute thrombus (0 to 5 days) is predominantly isointense on T1WI and hypointense on T2WI, whereas subacute thrombus (6 to 15 days) becomes increasingly hyperintense on both T1WI and T2WI. Sequences susceptible to blood may also be useful for detecting thrombosed veins, which will appear markedly hypointense on susceptibility weighted imaging (SWI) and T2* images.

Phase contrast or time-of-flight MR venography (MRV) in patients with CVT demonstrate absence of normal venous flow-related signal (Figs. 3.20 and 3.21). In some cases, however, time-of-flight MRV may appear falsely negative because of high signal from thrombus being mistaken as normal flow. In these cases, contrast-enhanced CT or MRV usually clearly depicts the filling defect.

Outcomes in patients with CVT are usually favorable with mortality rates falling far lower than 10%. CVT of the deep venous system is associated with a poorer prognosis than purely superficial thromboses, largely because of the fact that the deep system lacks a substantial collateral anastomotic drainage pathway, unlike the superficial system. Anticoagulation is the mainstay of treatment even in cases of hemorrhagic venous infarction. In patients with severe neurologic deterioration, catheter-directed

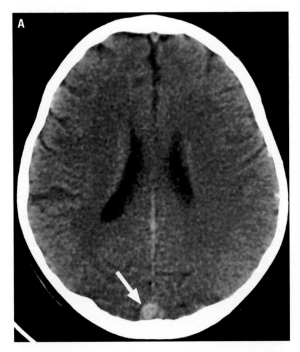
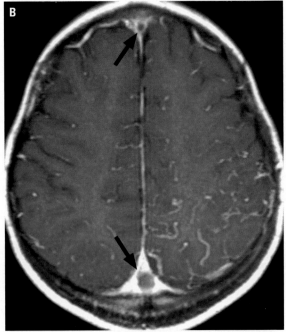

Figure 3.22. Superior sagittal sinus thrombosis. **A:** Unenhanced axial CT demonstrates high-density thrombus (the so-called cord sign) in the superior sagittal sinus *(white arrow)*. **B:** Axial post-contrast T1WI in the same patient demonstrates central filling defects in the sagittal sinus *(black arrows)* surrounded by enhancing collateral venous channels in the dural envelope. There is also prominent leptomeningeal enhancement, likely reflecting venous congestion.

thrombolytic therapy or open surgical thrombectomy may be warranted.

Cavernous Sinus Thrombosis

Cavernous sinus thrombosis (CST) warrants its own mention. CST is a septic thrombophlebitis, which is most commonly a complication of sinusitis and other infections of the middle third of the face. The cavernous sinuses are paired collections of thin-walled veins on either side of the sella turcica that receive venous return from the superior and inferior orbital veins and drain into the superior and inferior petrosal sinuses. They contain the ICAs and are intimately related with several cranial nerves (CN), including the oculomotor nerve (CN III), the trochlear nerve (CN IV), the abducens nerve (CN VI), and divisions of the trigeminal nerve (CN V). The freely anastomosing valveless venous system of the paranasal sinuses allows spread of infection to the cavernous sinus in a retrograde fashion via the superior and inferior ophthalmic veins.

Most patients with CST develop fever, ptosis, proptosis, chemosis, and external ophthalmoplegia (because of dysfunction of CNs III, IV, and VI).

Obstruction of venous drainage from the retina can also result in papilledema, retinal hemorrhages, and visual loss. In addition, thrombophlebitis can propagate into other dural venous sinuses resulting in CVT or may incite thrombosis of the cavernous ICA—resulting in ischemia.

CST can be diagnosed with contrast-enhanced CT or MR, which will typically demonstrate a dilated, thrombosed superior ophthalmic vein and filling defects in an enlarged cavernous sinus (Fig. 3.23). The contralateral cavernous sinus may also be involved because of propagation of thrombus across intercavernous sinuses located anterior and posterior to the sella, and images should also be scrutinized for evidence of extension into other dural sinuses or involvement of the ICA. A primary source of infection, usually the adjacent paranasal sinuses, will often be evident.

Staphylococcus aureus is the most common organism identified in CST, accounting for 60% to 70% of cases. Less common pathogens include streptococcal species, gram-negative bacilli, anaerobes, and fungi such as *Aspergillus* (discussed subsequently) or *Mucor*. Prior to the widespread availability of

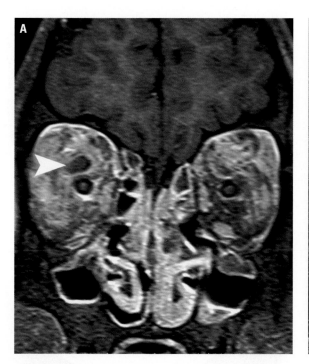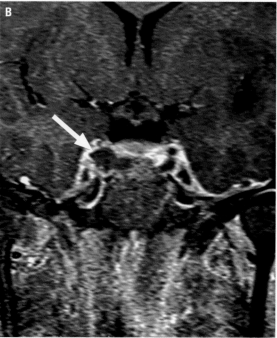

Figure 3.23. Cavernous sinus thrombosis. **A:** Fat-suppressed coronal post-contrast T1WI through the orbits demonstrates a thrombosed right superior ophthalmic vein *(arrowhead)*, which is enlarged and nonenhancing. There is diffuse sinonasal inflammatory disease and diffusely abnormal enhancement of the orbital soft tissues bilaterally, reflecting postseptal orbital cellulitis. **B:** Post-contrast coronal T1WI through the cavernous sinuses demonstrates a right cavernous sinus filling defect *(arrow)*.

antibiotics, CST was almost universally fatal, but mortality rates in the modern antibiotic era have dropped significantly to less than 20%.

Nontraumatic Hemorrhagic Disorders

Like traumatic hemorrhages, nontraumatic ICH can be classified as intra-axial (or intraparenchymal) or extra-axial. Primary intra-axial hemorrhages usually originate from the spontaneous rupture of small vessels damaged by long-standing hypertension or amyloid angiopathy and account for 78% to 88% of nontraumatic parenchymal hemorrhages. Secondary hemorrhages, which make up the minority of cases, may be caused by vascular anomalies (malformations or aneurysms), tumors, coagulopathies, or vasculitis.

Nontraumatic extra-axial hemorrhages are usually localized to the subarachnoid space or subdural space. Atraumatic SAH is usually caused by a ruptured aneurysm. Subdural hematomas (SDH) can occur spontaneously or as a result of trivial trauma. Causes of spontaneous SDH include intracranial hypotension, hemorrhagic dural metastases, anticoagulation, and bleeding diatheses. These SDHs can present in the subacute or chronic stages and may therefore demonstrate mixed densities (suggesting multiple repeated hemorrhages) on unenhanced CT or density lower than expected for acute hemorrhage, at times isodense to adjacent brain parenchyma. Nevertheless, they are otherwise identical in location and configuration to SDH occurring in the setting of acute trauma and are, therefore, not discussed in detail here.

Hypertensive Hemorrhage

Chronic hypertension is the leading cause of spontaneous intraparenchymal hemorrhage in adults. Hypertensive hemorrhages occur most frequently in the sixth and seventh decades of life and more commonly in men than women. Long-standing hypertension induces proliferation and eventual death of the smooth muscle cells in the walls of small penetrating arteries with eventual collagenous replacement. Depending on the rate of collagen deposition, vascular occlusion or ectasia may result. In the latter case, focal arteriolar dilatations are referred to as Charcot-Bouchard aneurysms, and it has long been theorized that hypertensive hemorrhages are caused by rupture of these aneurysms. However, more recent evidence suggests that hemorrhage may be the result of ischemic damage to the arterial wall,

which usually occurs in areas of previous ischemic damage. Mortality associated with spontaneous intracerebral hemorrhage is between 23% and 58%, and large hematoma size and intraventricular extension are associated with a higher likelihood of mortality.

Acute hypertensive hemorrhages are characteristically ovoid or mildly lobulated and homogeneously hyperdense on unenhanced CT. Common sites of hypertensive hemorrhage include the basal ganglia, the thalami, the brainstem, and the dentate nuclei of the cerebellum (Figs. 3.24 and 3.25). Large cerebellar hematomas (>3 cm in diameter) may compress the brainstem or cause rapidly progressive hydrocephalus (because of compression of the fourth ventricle), which often requires emergent surgical evacuation. Hypertensive lobar white matter hemorrhages also occur, although less frequently than those arising from the more typical sites. It is quite common for intraparenchymal hematomas to expand within the first few hours of symptom onset, a finding that is associated with poor outcomes. Therefore, any deterioration in clinical status in a patient with a parenchymal hemorrhage requires emergent reimaging to determine whether the hematoma has grown.

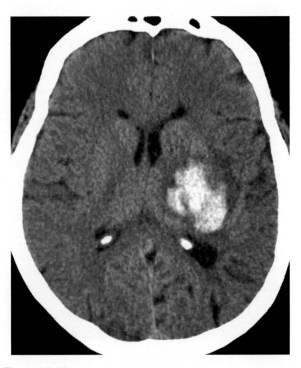

Figure 3.24. Hypertensive hemorrhage. Unenhanced axial CT image demonstrates a hyperdense parenchymal hematoma centered in the left basal ganglia, which is a typical location for hypertensive hemorrhages.

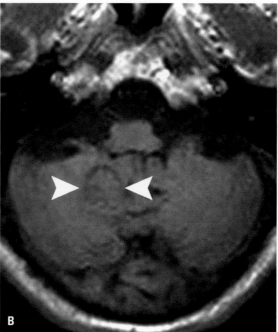

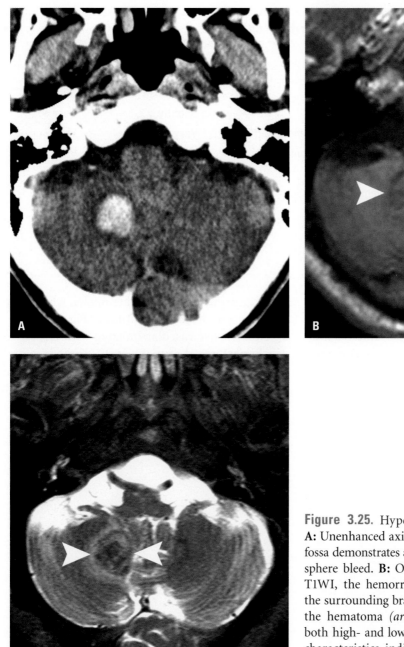

Figure 3.25. Hypertensive cerebellar hemorrhage. **A:** Unenhanced axial CT image through the posterior fossa demonstrates a hyperdense right cerebellar hemisphere bleed. **B:** On the corresponding unenhanced T1WI, the hemorrhage *(arrowheads)* is isodense to the surrounding brain parenchyma. **C:** On the T2WI, the hematoma *(arrowheads)* demonstrates areas of both high- and low-signal intensity. These MR signal characteristics indicate the hematoma consists primarily of acute blood products (oxyhemoglobin or deoxyhemoglobin).

Subsequent deterioration at 24 to 48 hours after hemorrhage onset is often caused by worsening cerebral edema.

On MRI, the signal characteristics of intraparenchymal hemorrhage depend on the age of the hemoglobin breakdown products contained within the hematoma (Table 3.1). Although it is useful to describe the evolution of hematomas in well-defined stages, multiple hemoglobin breakdown products often coexist within a given hemorrhage. Acute hematomas mostly contain oxyhemoglobin and deoxyhemoglobin and are therefore hypointense to isointense to brain on T1WI and either hyperintense (oxyhemoglobin) or hypointense (deoxyhemoglobin) on T2WI (Fig. 3.25). Enhancement is not seen in acute hypertensive hemorrhages, and the presence of contrast enhancement within or adjacent to a

TABLE 3.1	Appearance of Parenchymal Hemorrhage on MR		
Stage of Hemorrhage	**Blood Product**	**SI on T1WI**	**SI on T2WI**
Hyperacute (<24 h)	Oxyhemoglobin	Isointense	Slightly ↑
Acute (1–3 d)	Deoxyhemoglobin	Slightly ↓	Very ↓
Early subacute (3–7 d)	Intracellular methemoglobin	Very ↑	Very ↓
Late subacute (>7 d)	Extracellular methemoglobin	Very ↑	Very ↑
Chronic (>14 d)			
Center	Hemichromes	Isointense	Slightly ↑
Rim	Hemosiderin	Slightly ↓	Very ↓

SI: signal intensity

hematoma on MRI should prompt a workup to exclude alternative diagnoses such as a tumor or vascular malformation (Fig. 3.26). Gradient echo, T2*-weighted, or susceptibility-weighted images are useful sequences to include in MRI protocols because they may demonstrate the presence of remote microhemorrhages in the brainstem, deep gray nuclei, and dentate nuclei, which would support a hypertensive etiology (Fig. 3.27).

Noninvasive vascular imaging with CTA is routinely performed at many institutions in patients with intracerebral hemorrhages to exclude underlying vascular abnormalities (see the following texts), particularly when the clinical or imaging features

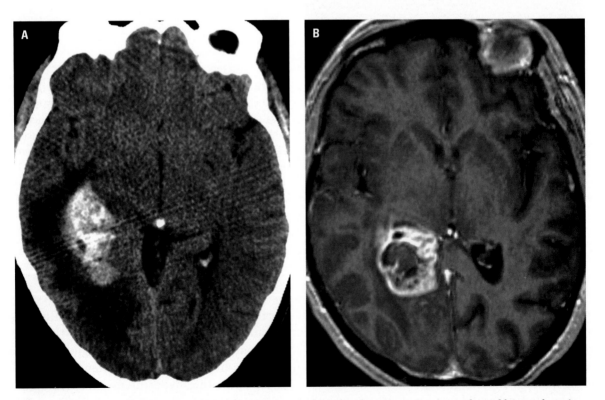

Figure 3.26. Hemorrhagic tumor. **A:** Axial unenhanced CT image demonstrates a parenchymal hemorrhage in the right temporal lobe with surrounding edema. The location of the hematoma is atypical for hypertensive hemorrhage. **B:** Axial post-contrast T1WI demonstrates an enhancing mass adjacent to the hematoma subsequently proven to be a glioblastoma.

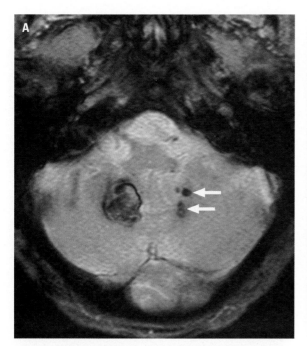

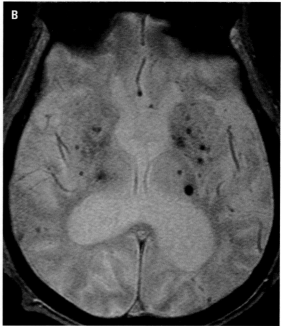

Figure 3.27. Hypertensive microhemorrhages on gradient echo imaging. **A:** Axial gradient echo T2WI through the cerebellum in the same patient from Figure 3.25 again demonstrates the right cerebellar hemorrhage. In addition, there are small areas of signal void in the left cerebellar hemisphere *(arrows)* indicating remote microhemorrhages. **B:** Gradient echo image through the level of the lateral ventricles demonstrate numerous additional remote microhemorrhages in the basal ganglia and thalami. This distribution of hemorrhages is typical of chronic hypertension.

are atypical for hypertensive hemorrhage. Additionally, evidence of contrast extravasation on CTA images, the so-called spot sign, predicts early hematoma growth in patients with spontaneous ICH.

ICHs similar to hypertensive ICH can occur in association with drug abuse (most commonly cocaine, methamphetamine, or ecstasy). These hemorrhages tend to occur in a younger population than classic hypertensive bleeds and have a greater tendency to have intraventricular extension. The exact mechanisms underlying drug-induced ICH are unclear and likely are multifactorial, including processes such as vasospasm, cerebral vasculitis, and hypertensive surges associated with altered cerebral autoregulation. Several studies have also reported a relatively high incidence of underlying vascular lesions in patients with drug-associated ICH and therefore recommend that these patients undergo vascular imaging to exclude an aneurysm or arteriovenous malformation (AVM).

Cerebral Amyloid Angiopathy

Cerebral amyloid angiopathy (CAA) is a disorder characterized by the accumulation of amyloid in the walls of small and medium-sized arteries in the brain and leptomeninges. CAA is observed in approximately 50% of individuals older than 80 years, many of whom are asymptomatic, suggesting that amyloid deposition may be a feature of "normal" aging. When severe, however, CAA can cause weakening of vessel walls leading to rupture and intracerebral hemorrhage or can occlude vessel lumens leading to ischemia. Hemorrhages caused by CAA primarily occur in patients older than the age of 60 years, and CAA is estimated to account for between 5% and 20% of spontaneous cerebral hemorrhages in elderly patients.

CAA-related hemorrhages are classically described as lobar, cortical, or cortico-subcortical hemorrhages—often multiple and recurrent—occurring in normotensive patients older than the age of 55 years. They are frequently large, demonstrate irregular or lobulated borders and occasional hematocrit levels, and may extend into the subarachnoid space or ventricles (Fig. 3.28). CAA hemorrhages show a slight frontal and occipital lobe predominance and typically spare regions commonly affected by hypertensive hemorrhages (deep gray matter, brainstem, and cerebellum). An important clue to the diagnosis is the presence of multiple

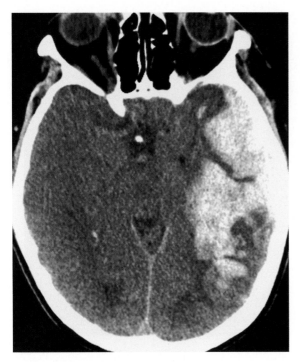

Figure 3.28. Amyloid angiopathy related hemorrhage. Unenhanced axial CT image in an elderly patient demonstrates a large left temporal lobe hemorrhage with irregular, lobulated margins.

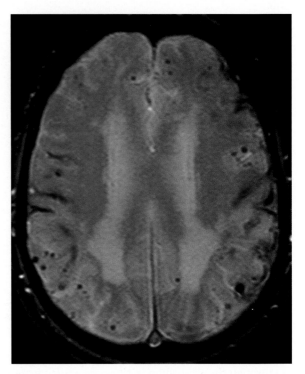

Figure 3.29. Microhemorrhages caused by amyloid angiopathy. Axial gradient echo T2WI demonstrates multiple punctate microhemorrhages, predominantly distributed in the cortex and subcortical white matter. This distribution is characteristic of amyloid angiopathy and helps to distinguish it from chronic hypertension. (Image courtesy of Dr. John Grimme.)

cortical and subcortical microhemorrhages, which are best seen on gradient echo T2-weighted, T2*-weighted, or susceptibility-weighted MR sequences (Fig. 3.29). These microhemorrhages are often not evident on CT or conventional spin-echo or fast spin-echo MR sequences.

CAA is also a recognized cause of spontaneous convexity SAHs in the elderly, and another occasional imaging finding in patients with CAA is the presence of subarachnoid and superficial cortical siderosis, which appears as a thin stripe of low-signal intensity in the leptomeninges and cortical surface on T2WI or other blood-sensitive sequences (Fig. 3.30). This finding presumably represents hemosiderin deposition caused by prior episodes of SAH and/or primary bleeding in the superficial cortical layers.

According to proposed guidelines for the diagnosis of CAA-related hemorrhages (the Boston criteria), definitive diagnosis of CAA hemorrhage can only be made on postmortem examination. Using entirely noninvasive criteria, CAA is considered "probable" when there are imaging findings of multiple cortico-subcortical hemorrhages in a patient 55 years of age or older, there is appropriate clinical history, and there is no other clinical or radiologic

cause of hemorrhage identified. The term "possible" CAA is used when there is a single cortico-subcortical hemorrhage in a patient 55 years of age or older, there is clinical data suggesting CAA, and there is no other identifiable cause of hemorrhage. The clinical diagnosis "probable" CAA has a reported positive predictive value (PPV) of 100%, whereas "possible" CAA has a PPV of 62%.

Vascular Malformations

Vascular malformations account for approximately 20% of all spontaneous ICHs and are the most common cause of nontraumatic ICH in young adults. Therefore, any ICH occurring in a young adult patient should immediately prompt a search for an underlying vascular malformation with either CTA or MRA. Furthermore, a high index of suspicion for an underlying vascular anomaly should also be entertained if there are no obvious risk factors for hemorrhage, such as trauma, hypertension, or anticoagulation, or if the location or appearance of the bleed is atypical. Although generally less

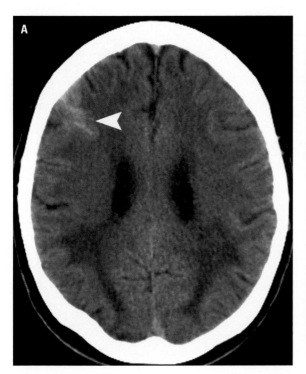
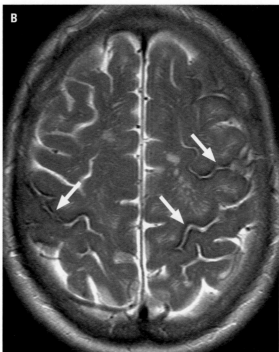

Figure 3.30. Spontaneous subarachnoid hemorrhage caused by amyloid angiopathy. **A:** Unenhanced axial CT image demonstrates isolated subarachnoid hemorrhage within right frontal lobe sulci *(arrowhead)*. Note also the confluent white matter hypodensity adjacent to the lateral ventricles, which is frequently seen in association with amyloid angiopathy. **B:** Axial T2WI in the same patient demonstrates areas of low-signal intensity in the cortex along the central and precentral sulci *(arrows)*, indicating superficial siderosis. (Images courtesy of Dr. John Grimme.)

accurate than DSA, CTA is still sensitive (roughly 90%) for detecting underlying secondary causes of cerebral hemorrhages, making it an excellent first-line screening tool.

The vascular anomalies that are most commonly responsible for clinically significant hemorrhages include AVMs, cavernous malformations (CMs), aneurysms, and dural arteriovenous fistulas (dAVFs).

Arteriovenous Malformations

AVMs are rare developmental lesions characterized by an abnormal communication between pial arteries and veins with no intervening capillary bed. The site of the anomalous connection is known as the central nidus, which may range in size from microscopic to several centimeters and may drain into either the superficial or deep cerebral venous system. The estimated annual incidence of cerebral AVMs is less than 0.1%, and the risk of hemorrhage from an AVM is approximately 3% to 4% per year.

On unenhanced CT, smaller AVMs may be difficult or impossible to appreciate, particularly when

they are associated with large hematomas. Larger AVMs usually demonstrate enlarged, isodense to hyperdense feeding arteries or draining veins in the vicinity of the hematoma (Fig. 3.31). Calcifications (which occur in up to 30%) or atrophy of the neighboring tissues may be clues to the presence of an AVM. On spin-echo MR sequences, the AVM nidus may be apparent as a mass of tightly packed, serpiginous flow voids adjacent to the hematoma. Areas of high signal may be seen in vessels that are thrombosed or demonstrate slow or turbulent flow.

CTA and MRA are particularly useful for visualizing the AVM nidus, feeding arteries, and draining veins (Fig. 3.31); however, complete characterization of the lesions for purposes of treatment planning usually requires conventional DSA. Up to 20% of AVMs are associated with saccular aneurysms, which may arise from the feeding pedicle, within the nidus, from draining veins, or from arteries remote from the AVM.

Rarely, hemorrhagic AVMs may be occult on CTA, MRA, and conventional DSA because of

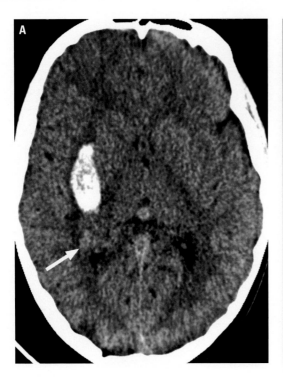

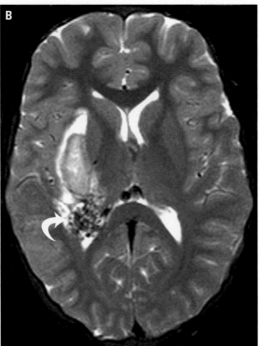

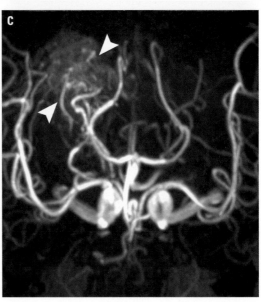

Figure 3.31. Hemorrhage caused by ruptured arteriovenous malformation. **A:** Unenhanced axial CT image in a pediatric patient demonstrates a hematoma adjacent to the right basal ganglia. There is a subtle periatrial hyperdense posterior to the hematoma *(arrow)*, which could be easily overlooked. **B:** Axial T2WI demonstrates a mass of multiple flow voids in this region *(curved arrow)*, representing the nidus of the AVM. **C:** MIP reconstruction from a 3D TOF-MRA viewed craniocaudally demonstrate the AVM nidus *(arrowheads)*, which is supplied primarily by branches of the right MCA.

compression of the AVM by the hematoma. In cases in which there is a high index of suspicion for an occult vascular malformation, follow-up angiography should be performed when hematoma has become resorbed.

Cavernous Malformations

Cavernomas or CMs are low-flow vascular lesions consisting of closely apposed, sinusoidal cavities lined by a single layer of endothelium and separated by a collagenous matrix lacking other vascular wall elements. They are more common than AVMs, occurring in 0.2% to 0.4% of the population. Both sporadic and familial forms occur, and patients with familial CMs typically harbor multiple lesions. The risk of hemorrhage from sporadic CMs ranges from 0.4% to 3.1% per year, whereas the risk of hemorrhage for familial CMs is between 4.3% and 6.5% per year. Patients may come to attention because of acute hemorrhage, headache, or seizure, but many CMs are identified incidentally on imaging studies performed for unrelated reasons.

Unless they have recently hemorrhaged, CMs may be difficult to appreciate on CT, particularly when they are small. They may appear as round or ovoid areas demonstrating slight hyperdensity (because of mineralization or blood products) and can occasionally be mistaken for acute hemorrhages (Fig. 3.32). Most CMs are less than 1 cm in diameter, but they can grow to several centimeters in size. On MR, CMs characteristically demonstrate a mixed signal intensity core containing hyperintense regions on both T1WI and T2WI, and a low-signal rim made up of hemosiderin (Fig. 3.31). CMs are generally angiographically occult lesions and therefore are not usually visible on CTA, MRA, or conventional angiography. In the setting of acute hemorrhage, it may be impossible to identify a CM within the hematoma because of compression or obliteration of the lesion. The presence of a nearby developmental venous anomaly (DVA) is a helpful clue

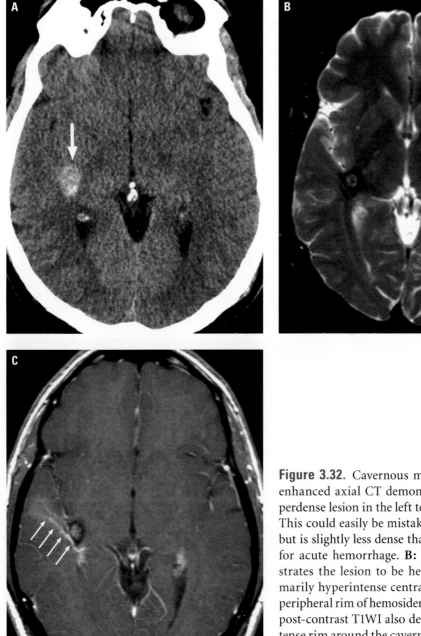

Figure 3.32. Cavernous malformation. **A:** Unenhanced axial CT demonstrates an ovoid, hyperdense lesion in the left temporal lobe *(arrow)*. This could easily be mistaken for an acute bleed but is slightly less dense than would be expected for acute hemorrhage. **B:** Axial T2WI demonstrates the lesion to be heterogeneous but primarily hyperintense centrally with a low-signal peripheral rim of hemosiderin. **C:** Corresponding post-contrast T1WI also demonstrates a hypointense rim around the cavernoma. In addition, the enhancing transcerebral vein of a nearby developmental venous anomaly *(small arrows)* is evident posterolateral to the malformation.

regarding the presence of an underlying CM. DVAs are congenital anatomic variants representing anomalous venous drainage of an area of the brain. They are most evident on contrast-enhanced T1WI or SWI, which characteristically demonstrate a cluster of small abnormal medullary veins (often referred to as a caput medusae) that drain via a larger transcerebral vein into a cortical vein, venous sinus, ependymal vein, or deep cerebral vein (Fig. 3.32). DVAs are more likely to be associated with sporadic CMs than familial CMs.

Aneurysmal Subarachnoid Hemorrhage

Approximately 85% of cases of nontraumatic SAH are caused by rupture of an intracranial aneurysm. These aneurysmal hemorrhages are associated with extremely poor outcomes, with roughly 50% of patients dying and more than 40% of survivors requiring long-term dependent care. Patients with aneurysmal SAH classically present with acute onset, severe headache ("thunderclap headache") that they often describe as being the worst headache of their lives. Additional signs and symptoms include nausea and vomiting, neck pain, photophobia, and decreased consciousness.

Most aneurysms are saccular and occur in predictable sites in the circle of Willis, usually at vessel bifurcations. The most common locations are the anterior communicating artery (AComA) (30% to 35%), the posterior communicating artery (PComA) (30% to 35%), the MCA bifurcation (20%), and the basilar artery (5%). Less common locations include the ICA artery terminus, the superior cerebellar artery, and the posterior inferior cerebellar artery (PICA). The prevalence of cerebral aneurysms in the general public is estimated to be around 2.3%, and the bleeding risk associated with previously unruptured aneurysms approximately 1% per year. The short-term risk of rebleeding from an untreated ruptured aneurysm is much higher, roughly 1% to 2% per day for the 3 to 4 weeks following initial rupture.

Unenhanced CT is the imaging modality of choice for suspected SAH with a reported sensitivity greater than 95% within the first 24 hours. As in cases of traumatic SAH, aneurysmal SAH appears as high-density material within the cortical sulci and cisterns. Intraventricular extension of hemorrhage and resultant hydrocephalus are common. SAH because of aneurysm rupture is typically diffuse, which often makes it impossible to localize the source of bleeding on a noncontrasted study. In some cases, the presence of a more prominent or focal clot may suggest an aneurysm's location. Aneurysms arising at the AComA tend to bleed into the anterior interhemispheric fissure, into the septum pellucidum, and into the frontal horns of the lateral ventricles (Fig. 3.33). MCA aneurysms tend to involve the ipsilateral Sylvian fissure (Fig. 3.34). PComA and basilar artery aneurysms tend to be more diffuse or localized to the basilar cisterns (Fig. 3.35).

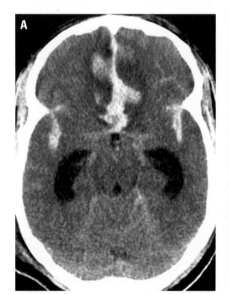 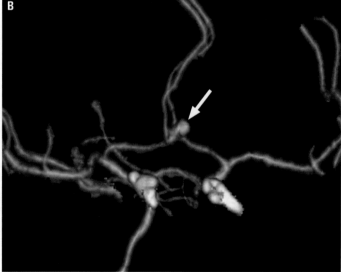

Figure 3.33. Subarachnoid hemorrhage secondary to ruptured AComA aneurysm. **A:** Unenhanced axial CT demonstrates diffuse SAH, which is predominantly localized to the interhemispheric fissure. There is marked dilatation of the temporal horns indicating hydrocephalus. **B:** Right anterior oblique view from a 3D surface shaded CTA reconstruction demonstrates the saccular aneurysm arising from the AComA *(arrow)*.

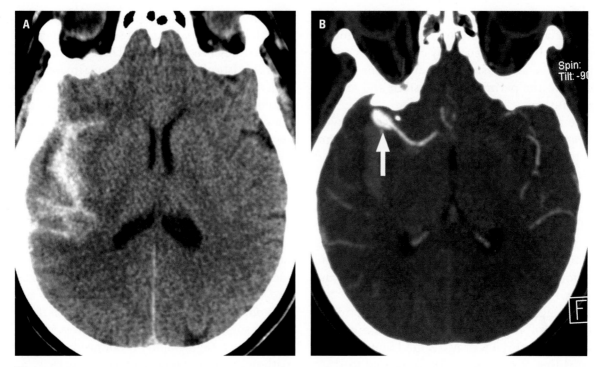

Figure 3.34. Subarachnoid hemorrhage secondary to ruptured MCA aneurysm. **A:** Unenhanced axial CT image demonstrates subarachnoid hemorrhage primarily localized to the right Sylvian fissure. **B:** Axial thin MIP image from a CTA demonstrates a saccular aneurysm arising from the right MCA bifurcation *(arrow)*.

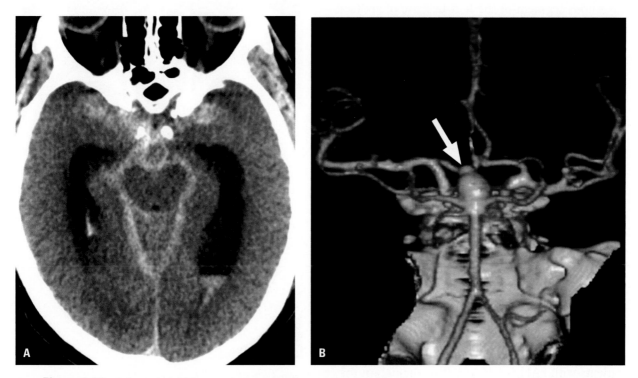

Figure 3.35. Subarachnoid hemorrhage secondary to ruptured basilar artery aneurysm. **A:** Unenhanced axial CT image demonstrates diffuse SAH filling the basilar cisterns. Blood is also present in the left lateral ventricle and there is ventricular enlargement. **B:** Posterior view from a 3D surface shaded CTA reconstruction demonstrates the lobulated, saccular aneurysm arising from the tip of the basilar artery *(arrow)*.

Of note, patients with PComA aneurysms may alternatively present with an isolated oculomotor nerve (CN III) palsy caused by compression on the nerve by the aneurysm. PICA aneurysms tend to bleed into the perimedullary cistern and around the brainstem.

The sensitivity of CT for SAH decreases with increasing time elapsed from the bleeding event, dropping to 74% at 3 days, 50% at 1 week, 30% at 2 weeks, and close to 0% at 3 weeks. Because of this, it is standard for lumbar puncture to be performed after a negative head CT in patients with suspected SAH. MR may also be more sensitive than CT for the detection of subacute SAH, with one study reporting sensitivities of 100% for $T2^{*}$-weighted imaging and 87% for FLAIR imaging performed between 4 and 14 days.

Although DSA remains the gold standard for detection of ruptured aneurysms, noninvasive assessment with CTA or MRA are frequently performed first (Figs. 3.33–3.35). Compared to DSA, CTA has a reported sensitivity of 96% to 98%, but the sensitivity is slightly lower for aneurysms smaller than 3 mm (90% to 94%). CTA is also less sensitive for aneurysms arising at the skull base or in the cavernous segment of the ICA because of artifacts caused by adjacent bone.

Three-dimensional time-of-flight (TOF) MRA is probably slightly less sensitive than CTA for aneurysm detection. In one meta-analysis, the estimated sensitivity and specificity of TOF-MRA at magnetic field strengths up to 1.5 T were reported to be 84% to 90% and 91% to 97%, respectively. Notably, although the sensitivity of MRA for detecting aneurysms larger than 3 mm was very high (94%), the sensitivity dropped dramatically for those smaller than 3 mm (38%). The lower sensitivity of current TOF-MRA techniques compared to CTA is probably caused by a combination of factors including lower spatial resolution, sensitivity to patient motion, and spin dephasing. For patients with suspected aneurysmal SAH, negative CTA or MRA should be followed up with a DSA.

Roughly 15% to 20% of patients with spontaneous SAH will have negative results on both noninvasive and conventional angiography. In up to 5% of patients with SAH, a false negative angiogram may occur as a result of transient aneurysm thrombosis, severe vasospasm, or inadequate angiographic technique, but most angiographically negative cases of SAH are caused by an etiology other than aneurysm rupture. Approximately 10% of cases of spontaneous SAH fall into the category of so-called nonaneurysmal perimesencephalic SAH. These hemorrhages are characteristically confined to the perimesencephalic cisterns anterior to the brainstem (Fig. 3.36). Their etiology is unknown, but it has been suggested that they may be caused by venous bleeding. Furthermore, patients with nonaneurysmal perimesencephalic SAH do not appear to be at risk for rebleeding and tend to have excellent outcomes compared to patients with aneurysmal SAH.

Whether spontaneous, angiographically negative SAHs require repeat angiography is controversial. Because there is small risk of aneurysms being missed on initial angiography, many centers, including our own, routinely perform a repeat CTA or DSA in all of these patients 1 to 2 weeks later to rule out previously occult aneurysms. On the other hand, some feel that repeat imaging (including noninvasive angiography) is not needed in patients with perimesencephalic pattern hemorrhage and a technically adequate negative angiogram.

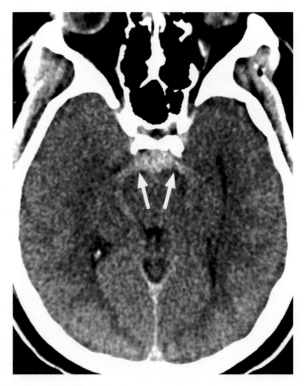

Figure 3.36. Nonaneurysmal perimesencephalic subarachnoid hemorrhage. Unenhanced axial CT image demonstrates SAH predominantly confined to the cisterns anterior to the brainstem *(arrows)*. Initial and repeat angiography in this patient was negative.

Dural Arteriovenous Fistulas and Carotid-Cavernous Fistulas

dAVFs are arteriovenous shunt lesions characterized by an abnormal direct connection between a meningeal artery and a meningeal vein or dural venous sinus. They account for approximately 10% to 15% of all intracranial vascular malformations. Development of a dAVF is occasionally associated with an antecedent event, such as trauma, prior venous thrombosis, or craniotomy, but most are idiopathic. Arteriovenous shunting induces venous hypertension, which may lead to generalized symptoms related to intracranial hypertension or more localized symptoms such as pulsatile tinnitus or symptoms related to focal brain edema. These symptoms are usually subacute or slowly progressive, but patients may present acutely with spontaneous ICH. Grading of dAVFs is based on the location and direction (antegrade or retrograde) of venous drainage, with higher grade dAVFs demonstrating predominantly retrograde drainage into cortical veins, which increases the risk for hemorrhage.

Hemorrhage caused by dAVFs may be intraparenchymal, subarachnoid, subdural, and/or epidural in location. Patients without hemorrhage may demonstrate an area of parenchymal edema or no parenchymal abnormalities at all. Direct evidence of a dAVF is generally not evident on unenhanced CT, and the definitive diagnosis usually requires CTA, MRA, or in many cases catheter angiography. Findings suggestive of a dAVF on CTA or contrast-enhanced CT include abnormally enlarged feeding meningeal arteries, enlarged or occluded dural venous sinuses often demonstrating shaggy margins, enlarged cortical draining veins, or prominent transosseous vessels. MRI and MRA/MRV may demonstrate similar imaging findings (Fig. 3.37). Dynamic CTA or MRA may be particularly useful for demonstrating arteriovenous shunting.

Warranting special mention are carotid-cavernous fistulas (CCFs), which are a subtype of intracranial arteriovenous fistulas. Because of their restricted anatomical boundaries, CCFs rarely cause hemorrhage but rather present with a fairly narrow range of symptoms and signs. Symptoms are usually limited to a cavernous sinus/orbital syndrome, manifesting as a combination of orbital pain, proptosis, chemosis, opthalmoplegia and orbital bruit, and later visual failure because of secondary glaucoma. CCFs are generally classified as direct (high flow)

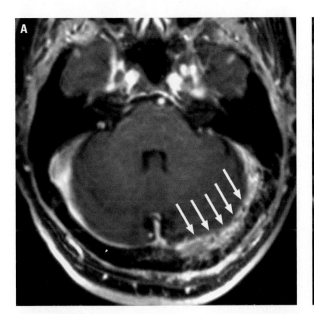 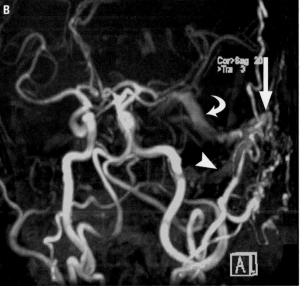

Figure 3.37. Dural arteriovenous fistula. **A:** Axial post-contrast T1WI in a patient with pulsatile tinnitus demonstrates an enlarged, heterogeneously enhancing left transverse sinus with shaggy margins *(small arrows)*. Note also the prominent, enhancing transosseous vessels adjacent to the sinus. **B:** Left anterior oblique MIP projection from a 3D TOF-MRA demonstrates the fistula *(large arrow)* supplied by meningeal branches of the external carotid artery. There is abnormal flow-related enhancement in the left sigmoid sinus *(arrowhead)* and transverse sinus *(curved arrow)* as a result of arteriovenous shunting.

or indirect (low flow). Direct CCFs result is usually the result of trauma or rupture of an intracavernous carotid aneurysm leading to direct communication between the ICA and the cavernous sinus. These CCFs are more likely to present acutely with prominent signs. Indirect CCFs represent abnormal communications between dural branches of the internal or external carotid arteries and the cavernous sinus. Symptoms of indirect CCFs typically evolve over a more prolonged period.

Indirect imaging findings of CCFs include proptosis, stranding of the retrobulbar fat, scleral thickening, and enlargement of the extraocular muscles and the superior ophthalmic vein (Fig. 3.38). On MRI, the cavernous sinus may demonstrate multiple flow voids. TOF MRA may demonstrate abnormal flow-related signal within the cavernous sinus and other adjoining venous structures including the superior ophthalmic vein and inferior petrosal sinus (Fig. 3.38). Time-resolved angiographic techniques

will demonstrate early filling of the cavernous sinus. Patients with suspected direct CCFs should proceed to DSA for confirmation and potential treatment given the risk for permanent vision loss.

HYDROCEPHALUS AND ASSOCIATED CONDITIONS

Hydrocephalus

Hydrocephalus is defined as an active distension of the ventricular system resulting from inadequate passage of CSF from its point of production in the ventricles to its point of absorption into the systemic circulation. Traditionally, hydrocephalus has been divided into two types: "communicating" and "noncommunicating." In communicating hydrocephalus, the ventricular system communicates with the subarachnoid space distal to the outlet foramina of

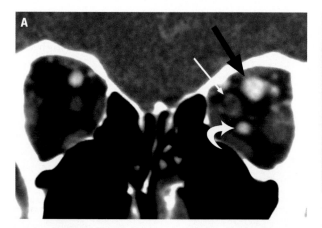

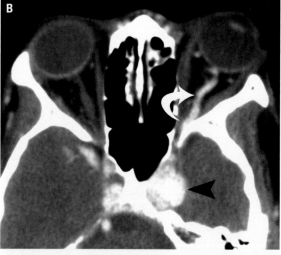

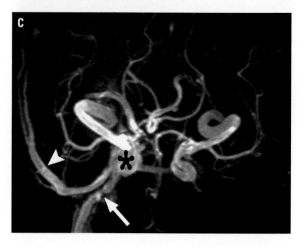

Figure 3.38. Direct cavernous-carotid fistulas. **A:** Coronal post-contrast CT image through the orbits demonstrates enlargement of the left superior *(black arrow)* and inferior *(curved arrow)* ophthalmic veins. The extraocular muscles in the left orbit are also enlarged and there is enhancement of the left optic nerve sheath *(thin white arrow)*. **B:** Axial CT image in the same patient again demonstrates enlargement of the left inferior ophthalmic vein *(curved arrow)*. The left globe is proptotic. The left cavernous sinus *(black arrowhead)* is enlarged and demonstrates a convex lateral margin. **C:** Craniocaudal projection MIP projection from a 3D TOF-MRA of the head in a different patient demonstrates abnormal flow-related enhancement within an enlarged right cavernous sinus *(asterisk)* and retrograde flow within the superior ophthalmic vein *(large white arrow)* and superficial middle cerebral vein *(white arrowhead)*. A small amount of intercavernous sinus flow is also present.

the fourth ventricle, with ventricular enlargement usually being the result of obstruction to CSF flow at the basal cisterns or impaired CSF resorption at the level of the arachnoid villi. Common etiologies include meningitis, SAH, and leptomeningeal carcinomatosis. Communicating hydrocephalus can also be caused by CSF overproduction by a choroid plexus tumor, which is the only truly nonobstructive cause of hydrocephalus.

In noncommunicating hydrocephalus, part of the ventricular system is isolated from the rest of the ventricular system or the subarachnoid space caused by obstruction proximal to the outlet foramina of the fourth ventricle. The most common causes for noncommunicating hydrocephalus are congenital aqueductal stenosis, intraventricular tumors and hemorrhage, and intra- or extra-axial masses compressing the outflow tracts of the ventricles.

Signs and symptoms of hydrocephalus are caused by the accompanying increase in intracranial pressure and may present acutely or more insidiously. Patients may present with headaches, nausea and vomiting, alterations in consciousness and behavior, papilledema, or oculomotor palsies. Infants with hydrocephalus may show an increasing head circumference and bulging fontanelles. CT is usually performed initially to evaluate suspected increased intracranial pressure and generally suffices to confirm the diagnosis of hydrocephalus. It is important to keep in mind that ventriculomegaly (defined simply as greater than expected ventricular size) alone is not sufficient to diagnose hydrocephalus because patients can have enlarged ventricles on imaging without elevated intracranial pressure (e.g., in patients with severe brain atrophy). In most cases, hydrocephalus can be distinguished from other causes of ventriculomegaly on the basis of associated effacement of the cortical sulci and other extra-axial CSF-containing spaces.

The imaging findings in obstructive forms of hydrocephalus vary with the site, completeness, and duration of obstruction. Lesions causing obstruction at the level of the foramen of Monro, including colloid cysts and anterior third ventricular tumors, result in enlargement of one or both of the lateral ventricles (Fig. 3.39). Early on, prominence of the temporal horns of the lateral ventricles is an important sign of obstruction when the remainder of the lateral ventricles have not yet enlarged. With continued obstruction, the frontal horns become more prominent and the angle between them

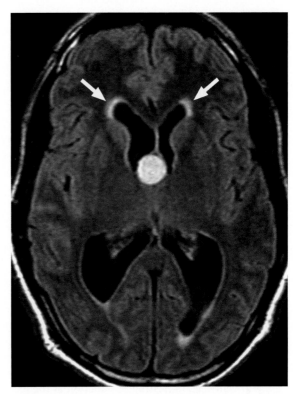

Figure 3.39. Obstructive hydrocephalus secondary to a colloid cyst. Axial FLAIR image demonstrate enlargement of the lateral ventricles. There is a circumscribed hyperintense mass centered between the foramina of Monro, compatible with a colloid cyst. These are classically hyperintense on T1-weighted and FLAIR imaging and hyperdense on unenhanced CT. There is abnormal hyperintensity along the frontal horns of the lateral ventricles indicating transependymal CSF flow *(arrows).*

(the so-called ventricular angle) becomes narrowed. Eventually, the entire ventricle becomes enlarged. The presence of interstitial edema around the walls of the ventricles indicates transependymal flow of CSF and is a sign of an acute decompensation of CSF flow. Interstitial edema appears as a halo of low density on CT or high-signal intensity on T2-weighted or FLAIR sequences surrounding the lateral ventricles and preferentially involves the white matter around the frontal and occipital horns (Figs. 3.39 and 3.40).

Obstruction at or near the cerebral aqueduct of Sylvius—which may be caused by congenital aqueductal stenosis or a tectal region tumor—causes triventricular enlargement of the lateral and third ventricles (Fig. 3.40). In cases of hydrocephalus secondary to extraventricular obstruction (i.e., communicating hydrocephalus), panventricular enlargement

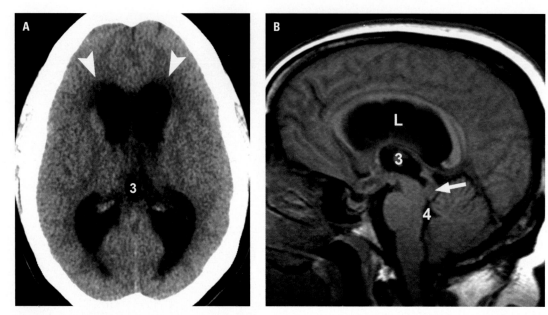

Figure 3.40. Noncommunicating hydrocephalus. **A:** Unenhanced axial CT image demonstrates triventricular enlargement of the lateral and third *(3)* ventricles. Hypodensity along the frontal horns of the lateral ventricles indicates transependymal CSF flow *(arrowheads)*. **B:** Unenhanced midsagittal T1WI again demonstrates lateral *(L)* and third *(3)* ventricular enlargement with a normal sized fourth *(4)* ventricle, indicating obstruction at the level of the cerebral aqueduct of Sylvius. There is a mass obstructing the aqueduct *(arrow)*, which in this case proved to be sarcoidosis (neurosarcoidosis).

may occur. Frequently, however, the fourth ventricle can appear normal or only minimally enlarged, often making it difficult to distinguish communicating hydrocephalus from aqueductal obstruction.

Complications of Cerebrospinal Fluid Shunts

CSF shunting procedures are commonly performed to treat hydrocephalus and represent roughly half of all neurosurgical procedures in the pediatric population. The most frequently used type of shunt is the ventriculoperitoneal (VP) shunt, which diverts CSF from the ventricles into the peritoneal cavity where it is subsequently resorbed into the systemic circulation. Modern VP shunts consist of three components: a proximal ventriculostomy catheter, a shunt valve to regulate CSF flow, and a distal peritoneal catheter. The shunt components are completely internalized and the catheters are typically impregnated with radiopaque material to facilitate visualization radiographically.

Shunt failure is an extremely common complication of CSF shunting, particularly in patients younger than 6 months of age, and are most often caused by a mechanical malfunction or shunt

infection. Shunt malfunctions usually occur in the first 6 months following insertion, and the overall failure rate is approximately 30% to 40% at 1 year and 50% at 2 years. Shunt obstruction accounts for most cases of shunt failure and typically presents with signs of increased intracranial pressure. The proximal ventricular catheter is the most common site of obstruction, which may be the result of plugging of the catheter by brain parenchyma, proteinaceous material, choroid plexus, or tumor cells, but blockages can occur at any point along the shunt system. Obstructions at the distal end of the shunt system are typically caused by adhesions or encystment in the peritoneum.

Radiologic investigation of suspected shunt malfunction generally includes an unenhanced head CT to assess for changes in ventricular size or intraventricular catheter position and plain radiographs covering the entire course of the shunt to identify catheter disconnections, kinks, breaks, or distal migration. Increasing ventricular size compared with baseline evaluations is a reliable indicator of an obstructive shunt malfunction; however, shunt malfunction cannot be excluded in the absence of ventricular enlargement because scarring around the ventricular walls may prohibit ventricle expansion in some patients. Furthermore, because some shunted patients continue to show ventriculomegaly even following successful shunting, it may be impossible to determine on the basis of a single CT examination without comparison examinations whether ventricular enlargement represents acute hydrocephalus because of shunt failure. Serial imaging may be required in these instances.

Shunt disconnections and fracture are additional causes of shunt malfunction. Disconnection of shunt components occurs at the connection points between the shunt tubing and the valve and will be apparent as gaps between the two components. Occasionally, shunt systems can have radiolucent connectors that may mimic disconnections, and having previous shunt series available for comparison can be invaluable for ruling out the catheter disconnections in these instances. CT may also be helpful in demonstrating a collection of CSF around the site of disconnection.

Fracture of distal shunt tubing is typically a late complication occurring many years after placement (Fig. 3.41). The most common sites for shunt fracture are in the lower neck near the clavicle or

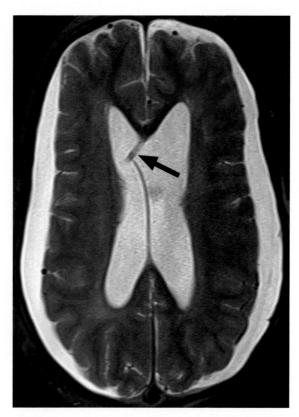

Figure 3.42. Bilateral postshunt subdurals. Axial T2WI obtained shortly following shunt placement demonstrates the development of bilateral subdural fluid collections, in this case subacute subdural hematomas. The tip of the proximal catheter can be seen in the right lateral ventricle *(arrow)*.

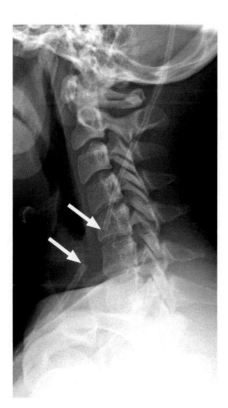

Figure 3.41. Ventriculoperitoneal shunt catheter fracture. Lateral radiograph of the cervical spine demonstrates a fractured and distracted distal shunt catheter *(arrows)* in a patient with shunt malfunction.

over the lower ribs, where the catheter is most likely to be repeatedly flexed. Frequently, there is a large gap between the disconnected catheter segments because of migration of the distal segment, which occasionally may reside entirely within the peritoneum. Calcification of the distal catheter is often evident in chronically indwelling catheters and is another indicator of potential shunt malfunction.

A less common cause of shunt failure is overshunting, which occurs when a shunt's valve is set to remove more fluid than necessary for a particular patient. Early rapid reduction in ventricular size can cause collapse of the brain and accumulation of extra-axial fluid around the brain such as subdural hygromas or hematomas (Fig. 3.42).

When the rate of CSF overdrainage is slower, patients may present in a delayed fashion with the so-called slit ventricle syndrome, which manifests as symptoms of shunt malfunction with small ventricles on imaging. The syndrome usually occurs

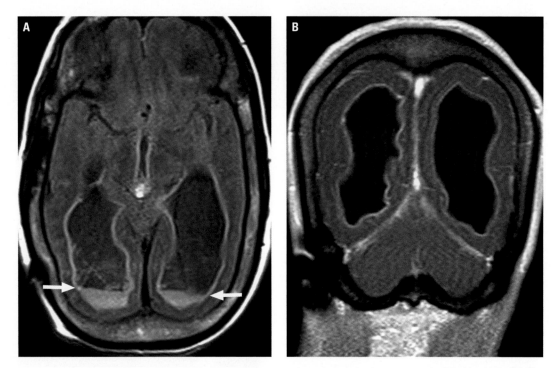

Figure 3.43. Shunt infection causing ventriculitis. **A:** Axial FLAIR image demonstrates fluid-debris levels in the lateral ventricles *(arrows)* and abnormal ependymal high signal. **B:** Coronal post-contrast T1WI demonstrates abnormal ependymal enhancement along the walls of the lateral ventricles.

in patients who have had shunts in place for several years. Symptoms of slit ventricle syndrome, which include headache, nausea and vomiting, or other signs of increased intracranial pressure, are usually repetitive or cyclical and are commonly postural in nature, with improvement in symptoms resulting from supine positioning. Although slit ventricle syndrome is uncommon, occurring in only 0.9% to 3.3% of shunted patients, it accounts for a disproportionately high number of shunt revisions.

Shunt infections occur at a rate of 5% to 10% and usually occur during the perioperative period within the first 2 months following placement. Patients present with symptoms of meningitis and/or ventriculitis (Fig. 3.43), the imaging findings of which are discussed subsequently.

INFECTIOUS AND INFLAMMATORY INTRACRANIAL EMERGENCIES

Bacterial Meningitis and Its Complications

Meningitis is defined as inflammation of the membranes surrounding the brain and spinal cord and is typically divided into bacterial and aseptic forms.

Bacterial meningitis occurs with an overall incidence of 2 to 10 per 100,000 individuals annually in the United States and most frequently affects neonates and infants younger than 2 years of age. Even in the modern era of widespread antibiotic use, bacterial meningitis is still associated with high rates of morbidity and mortality. *Streptococcus pneumoniae* and *Neisseria meningitidis* are currently the most common causes of bacterial meningitis, accounting for approximately 50% and 25% of meningitis cases in the United States, respectively.

Imaging is not required for the evaluation or management of uncomplicated cases of bacterial meningitis because diagnosis is typically based on clinical examination and CSF analysis. The classically described triad of fever, neck stiffness, and altered mental status is present in only approximately 25% to 40% of patients with acute bacterial meningitis. Therefore, there should be a low threshold for performing a lumbar puncture (LP) if meningitis is suspected clinically, and imaging may be requested to exclude increased intracranial pressure prior to an LP. In general, CT scans do not need to be performed before an LP unless there are clinical features indicative of impending brain herniation (seizures, a focal neurologic deficit, papilledema, decreased level of consciousness) or a patient has certain factors that predispose to herniation (old age, history of preexisting CNS disease, immunocompromised state). Absence of these criteria have a 97% negative predictive value for a normal head CT. Signs of raised intracranial pressure on CT include downward tonsillar herniation through the foramen magnum, effacement of the basilar cisterns, and effacement of the ventricles and cortical sulci.

Imaging is also indicated to rule out potential complications of meningitis, including cerebritis, brain abscess, subdural empyema, ventriculitis, venous thrombosis, hydrocephalus, or cerebral infarction. In uncomplicated cases of meningitis, CT scans, either with or without contrast, will usually be normal. FLAIR MR images may demonstrate abnormally high-signal intensity CSF in the subarachnoid spaces, owing to increased fluid protein concentrations (Fig. 3.44). This is a nonspecific finding, however, because similar CSF hyperintensity can be seen in patients with SAH or leptomeningeal carcinomatosis. Contrast-enhanced MRI may show focal or diffuse pial enhancement, but this finding will only be present in approximately 50% of patients with

meningitis. In some instances, imaging can reveal an underlying source of meningitis, such as a potential CSF leak or an infection of the paranasal sinuses, mastoids, or middle ear, which might prompt consultation with a neurosurgeon or otolaryngologist.

Cerebritis and Brain Abscess

Cerebritis and brain abscess are uncommon complications of bacterial meningitis and are most commonly caused by contiguous spread of infection originating in the pharynx, middle ear, mastoids, or paranasal sinuses. Abscesses may also occur as a result of hematogenous dissemination (septic emboli) from distant infectious processes, including endocarditis or chronic pyogenic lung disease. Intracardiac shunts and pulmonary vascular malformations (common in patients with hereditary hemorrhagic telangiectasia) also predispose patients to developing hematogenous abscesses. Brain abscesses are usually centered at gray–white junctions and occur most commonly in the frontal and temporal lobes.

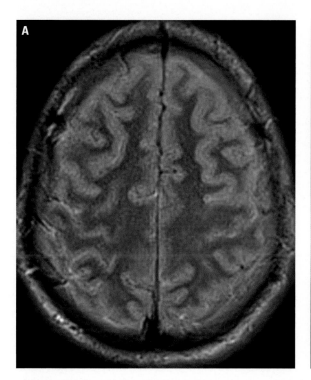
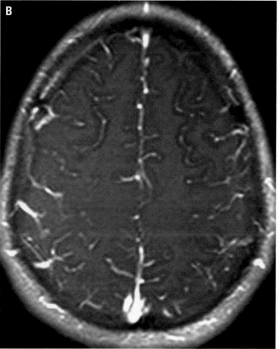

Figure 3.44. MR findings in uncomplicated meningitis. **A:** Axial FLAIR image demonstrates diffusely abnormal subarachnoid CSF hyperintensity in the cortical sulci, making this image look more like a T2WI. CSF should normally demonstrate low-signal intensity on FLAIR images. **B:** The corresponding post-contrast T1-weighted demonstrates diffuse leptomeningeal enhancement.

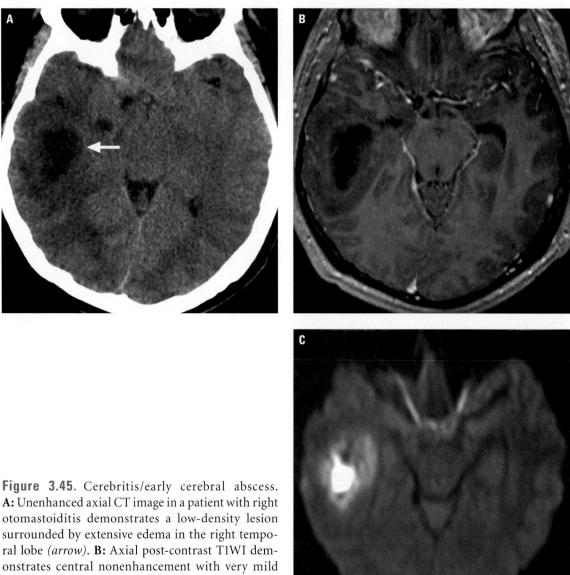

Figure 3.45. Cerebritis/early cerebral abscess. **A:** Unenhanced axial CT image in a patient with right otomastoiditis demonstrates a low-density lesion surrounded by extensive edema in the right temporal lobe *(arrow)*. **B:** Axial post-contrast T1WI demonstrates central nonenhancement with very mild peripheral enhancement suggesting a relatively immature capsule. **C:** On the diffusion-weighted image, the central portion of the abscess demonstrates high-signal intensity, indicating restricted pus.

In the early stages of cerebral abscess formation, a focal area of cerebritis develops, which on unenhanced CT appears as a subtle area of low density with mild mass effect, reflecting edema. On MRI, the lesion will demonstrate low-signal intensity on T1WI and high-signal intensity on T2-weighted and FLAIR images. Contrast enhancement is usually absent or minimal early on.

In the later stages of cerebritis and early abscess formation, there is progressive necrosis of tissue, which is reflected by increasing central hypodensity on CT (Fig. 3.45). On MRI, evidence of early capsule formation will become evident, typically by 2 weeks, with the lesion becoming better demarcated. On T1WI, the lesion will demonstrate low-signal intensity centrally with an isointense to slightly hyperintense rim, whereas on T2WI, the central area will be hyperintense and surrounded by a hypointense rim (Fig. 3.46). Surrounding vasogenic edema is typical. Contrast-enhanced images demonstrate enhancement of the peripheral rim, which is generally mild and irregular early on (Fig. 3.45) and becomes progressively more intense and well-defined as the capsule matures (Fig. 3.46). The capsule may be thicker on its lateral aspect and thinner medially, likely owing to the greater degree of vascularity

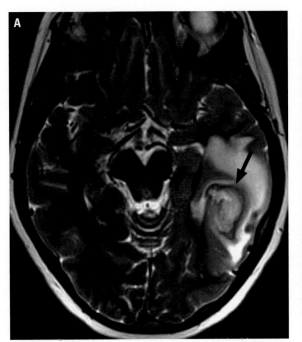 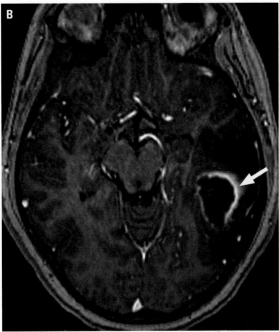

Figure 3.46. Cerebral abscess. **A:** Axial T2WI demonstrates a heterogeneous fluid collection in the left temporal lobe with surrounding vasogenic edema. The collection demonstrates a hypointense capsule, particularly anteriorly and laterally *(black arrow).* **B:** Corresponding post-contrast T1WI demonstrates peripheral enhancement, which is thicker along the lateral (cortical) site of the abscess, owing to the greater cortical blood supply.

where the abscess capsule abuts the cortex. In most pyogenic abscesses, DWI demonstrates restricted diffusion within the central necrotic regions, a finding that helps to distinguish abscesses from necrotic tumors (Fig. 3.45). Not all abscesses follow this rule, however, because fungal and tuberculous abscesses may show low signal on DWI.

Subdural Effusion and Abscess

Both sterile and infected extra-axial fluid collections may develop in patients with acute bacterial meningitis. Sterile subdural effusions are seen in up to a third of patients with meningitis. They most commonly occur in infants younger than the age of 2 years and are most frequently associated with meningitis caused by pneumococcus and *Haemophilus influenzae*. Effusions typically are large and bilateral and occur predominantly over the frontal and temporal lobes. They are isodense to CSF on CT and are isointense to CSF on T1WI and T2WI. On FLAIR images, subdural effusions may be slightly higher in signal compared to CSF because they may contain serosanguinous fluid.

Sterile effusions typically resolve spontaneously, but up to 15% become infected, resulting in development of a subdural empyema. Most empyemas are associated with sinus infections, with frontal sinusitis accounting for 50% to 80% of cases. On CT, subdural empyemas are isodense to slightly hyperdense relative to CSF and demonstrate peripheral enhancement following contrast administration (Fig. 3.47). Small subdural fluid collections can be extremely difficult to detect on CT, making MRI the imaging modality of choice for detecting and defining the extent of subdural empyemas. On MRI, empyemas may resemble CSF on T2WI but are typically of higher signal intensity than CSF on T1-weighted and FLAIR images (Fig. 3.48). On contrast-enhanced T1WI, empyemas demonstrate a peripheral rim of enhancement, which is usually more pronounced along its interface with the inner table of the skull.

It can be difficult to distinguish subdural empyemas from effusions because sterile effusions can also occasionally demonstrate peripheral enhancement on contrast-enhanced MRI. The distinction is important to make, however, because empyemas typically require surgical evacuation.

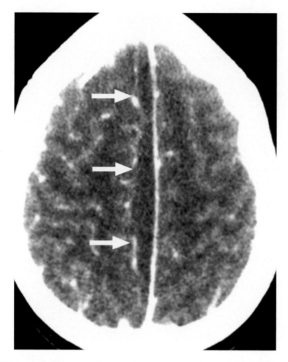

Figure 3.47. Subdural empyema. Axial post-contrast CT image in a child with meningitis demonstrates a subdural fluid collection *(arrows)* along the falx, which is hyperdense relative to CSF. The collection demonstrates peripheral enhancement that is more pronounced along the falcine (dural) side.

Thicker and more pronounced rim enhancement tends to favor empyema over effusion. DWI can also be useful in distinguishing between subdural empyemas and effusions because empyemas may demonstrate high signal and restricted diffusion, whereas sterile effusions will demonstrate ADC values similar to CSF (Fig. 3.49).

Ventriculitis

Ventriculitis is an uncommon but significant complication of meningitis. It occurs most frequently in infants and is usually caused by gram-negative bacterial infections. In most cases, pyogenic ventriculitis is a result of severe meningitis affecting the basal cisterns or of rupture of a cerebral abscess directly into a ventricle (Fig. 3.50). In addition, ventriculitis occurs as a complication of ventricular shunt catheters (Fig. 3.43).

On unenhanced CT and MRI, debris levels and hydrocephalus are the most common findings in patients with ventriculitis. MRI may additionally demonstrate hyperintense periventricular signal on T2-weighted and FLAIR images and ependymal enhancement on T1WI following contrast

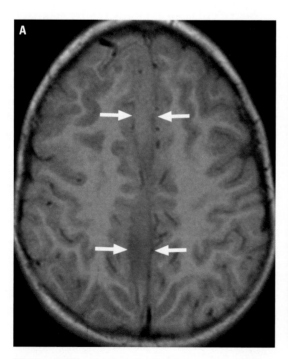
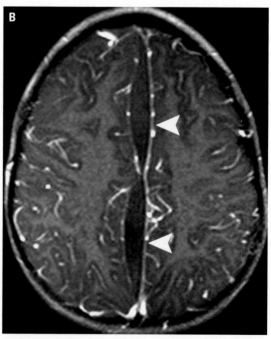

Figure 3.48. Subdural empyema. **A:** Unenhanced axial T1WI demonstrates a bilobed subdural fluid collection along the falx *(arrows)*, which is relatively isointense to the adjacent gray matter. **B:** Corresponding post-contrast T1WI demonstrates peripheral enhancement that is slightly thicker on the side abutting the dura *(arrowheads)*.

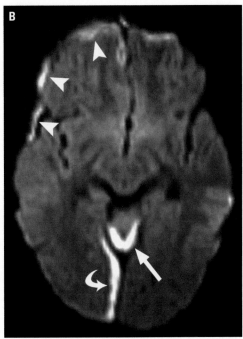
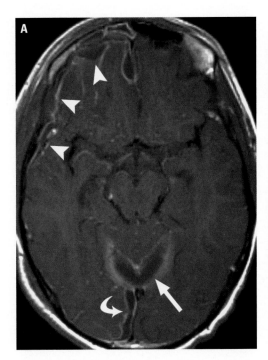

Figure 3.49. Subdural empyemas on DWI. **A:** Axial post-contrast T1WI demonstrates multiple peripherally enhancing subdural fluid collections adjacent to the frontal lobes *(arrowheads)*, tentorium *(straight arrow)*, and falx *(curved arrow)*. **B:** On the corresponding DWI image, these collections demonstrate high-signal intensity, reflecting restricted diffusion.

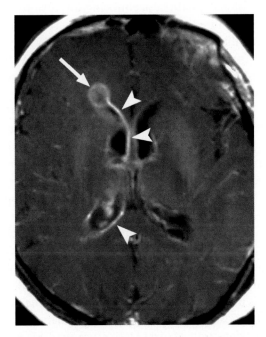

Figure 3.50. Cerebral abscess and ventriculitis. Axial post-contrast T1WI demonstrates a rim enhancing fluid collection adjacent to the right lateral ventricle compatible with a periventricular abscess *(arrow)*. There is also marked ependymal enhancement predominantly along the walls of the right lateral ventricle *(arrowheads)* indicating ventriculitis, which was likely caused by abscess rupture into the ventricle.

administration. On DWI, the intraventricular debris characteristically demonstrates reduced diffusion, presumably reflecting the presence of pus (Fig. 3.51). In the later stages of ventriculitis, intraventricular septations may develop.

Epidural Abscess

Epidural abscesses are typically caused by contiguous spread of infection from adjacent structures such as the paranasal sinuses or mastoids. These collections reside in the potential space between the dura and the inner table of the skull, and the thick inelastic dura acts as a barrier protecting the underlying brain from concomitant involvement. As a result, epidural abscesses tend to present with a more prolonged and insidious clinical course than subdural empyemas (usually over the course of several weeks to months). Early on, patients may complain only of fever or headache; other neurologic symptoms do not develop until the infection has breached the dura into the subdural space.

As is the case with subdural empyemas, MRI is the most sensitive imaging modality for detecting

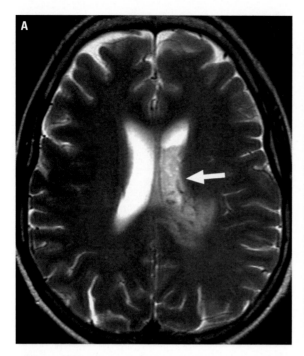
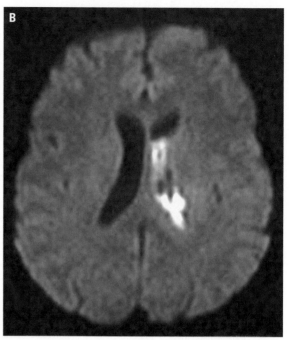

Figure 3.51. Ventriculitis on DWI. **A:** Axial T2WI demonstrates debris in the left lateral ventricle *(arrow)*, which is of lower signal intensity than normal CSF. There is also edema in the adjacent periventricular white matter. **B:** Corresponding DWI image demonstrates the intraventricular debris to have restricted diffusion, likely caused by its purulent nature. (Images courtesy of Dr. John Grimme.)

epidural abscesses. The signal characteristics of epidural abscesses are similar to those of subdural empyemas on T1-weighted, T2-weighted, and FLAIR images, but unlike subdural empyemas, epidural abscesses classically have a biconvex shape and can extend across the midline. On post-contrast scans, there is marked peripheral enhancement that is often thicker than that observed in subdural empyemas, particularly along the inner (or dural) side of the collection. The adjacent brain parenchyma is often normal in appearance, in contrast to subdural empyemas. Diffusion weighted imaging is less helpful for characterizing epidural abscesses than it is for subdural collections because epidural abscesses tend to show lower signal intensity on DWI. This is presumably caused by the longer clinical course associated with epidural abscesses, which allows time for pus within the abscess to become less viscous.

Viral Encephalitis

Herpes Encephalitis

More than 100 viruses have been associated with acute CNS infections. Among these viruses, herpes simplex virus (HSV) remains the most common

cause of encephalitis, accounting for 10% to 20% of cases. More than 90% of cases of herpes simplex encephalitis are caused by HSV type 1 (HSV-1), with most of the remainder being caused by HSV type 2 (HSV-2). HSV encephalitis is primarily a disease of the children and the elderly but can occur at any age. The disease may occur as a result of reactivation of latent viral infection or be the consequence of a primary infection. HSV causes a hemorrhagic, necrotizing encephalitis with a predilection for involvement of the anterior and medial temporal lobes and the orbital frontal lobes. Other extratemporal sites, including the cingulate gyrus, limbic system, brainstem, thalami, and parietal and occipital lobes, can also become involved, and approximately 15% of patients will have pure extratemporal involvement. Although the disease is often bilateral, one side is usually more severely affected than the other.

Diagnosis is made by polymerase chain reaction (PCR) detection of viral DNA from the CSF, which has reported sensitivities and specificities of up to 98%. Mortality exceeds 70% in untreated patients, and surviving patients are commonly left with long-term disabilities, usually as a result of hemorrhagic necrosis of a dominant temporal lobe. Therapy is most effective when it is initiated prior to the development of hemorrhagic necrosis or significant deterioration of consciousness. Therefore, imaging findings suggestive of HSV encephalitis should prompt immediate initiation of antiviral therapy even if confirmatory testing has yet to be performed.

CT imaging is initially normal in up to 25% of patients with HSV encephalitis and may only become positive after the second week. CT findings include hypodensities and mild mass effect in the temporal lobes (Fig. 3.52). Hemorrhage is highly suggestive of HSV encephalitis but usually occurs late in the disease course. Similarly, parenchymal or meningeal enhancement is rarely seen on CT prior to the second week of clinical symptoms.

MRI is more sensitive than CT to early changes of HSV encephalitis. Early in the disease, DWI demonstrates restricted diffusion in the affected areas, indicating development of cytotoxic edema (Fig. 3.52). On T2 and FLAIR imaging, cortical hyperintensity and swelling develop within the first 48 hours. Gadolinium-enhanced T1WI show patchy gyral or leptomeningeal enhancement in up to 50% of patients, and gradient echo T2WI or susceptibility-weighted images are useful for detecting areas of hemorrhage, which will appear as areas of signal void.

Other Viral Causes of Encephalitis

Over the last century, several newly recognized nonherpetic viruses, mostly arboviruses, have been implicated in outbreaks of viral encephalitis. Arbovirus infections are transmitted to humans through the bite of an infected arthropod and are primarily caused by members of the Flaviviridae, Togaviridae, and Bunyaviridae families of viruses.

Japanese encephalitis is a mosquito-borne flaviviral infection, primarily affecting children, and endemic to Southeast Asia. MRI in patients with Japanese encephalitis typically demonstrates hyperintense or mixed-intensity lesions in the thalami on T2WI. Basal ganglia, brainstem, cerebellar, and cortical involvement may also be seen. Thalamic lesions can be hemorrhagic as well.

St. Louis encephalitis, which is also caused by a flavivirus, is a common cause of encephalitis epidemics in the eastern and central portions of the United States. Most patients are tremulous, which is a characteristic feature of the disease. Isolated T2-weighted hyperintensity limited to the substantia nigra has been reported in St. Louis encephalitis but similar findings has also been reported in Japanese encephalitis.

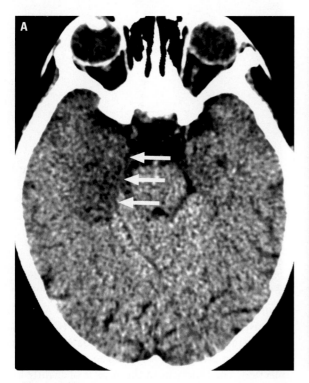 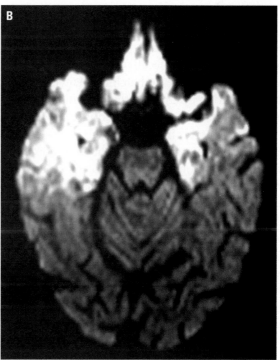

Figure 3.52. Herpes simplex virus encephalitis. **A:** Unenhanced axial CT image demonstrates decreased density in the right medial temporal lobe *(arrows)*. **B:** Axial DWI image in the same patient demonstrates reduced diffusion in the right temporal lobe, medial left temporal lobe, and inferior frontal lobes.

West Nile virus is another flavivirus that is closely related phylogenetically and antigenetically to the viruses responsible for Japanese encephalitis and St. Louis encephalitis. The imaging features of West Nile virus overlap those of Japanese encephalitis and include areas of increased signal intensity on T2-weighted, FLAIR, and, in many cases, DWI in the thalami, basal ganglia, and midbrain. Cortical involvement in the mesial temporal structures, which is more suggestive of herpes simplex encephalitis, is also common in West Nile virus encephalitis. Substantia nigra involvement, similar to that seen in Japanese and St. Louis encephalitis has also been reported. West Nile virus can also cause poliomyelitis-like or Guillain-Barré–like syndromes of the spine characterized by acute onset flaccid paralysis. Spinal MRI in these cases may show abnormalities in the ventral spinal horns and/or enhancement of the conus medullaris and the cauda equina.

Neurocysticercosis

Cysticercosis refers to infection by the larval form of the pork tapeworm, *Taenia solium*. It is the most common parasitic CNS infection worldwide and is becoming increasingly commonplace in the United States and other developed countries because of influx of migrants from countries where the disease is highly endemic. Infection occurs as a result of ingestion of eggs in fecally contaminated foods. Once ingested, the larvae hatch and enter the systemic circulation by crossing the intestinal mucosa. They subsequently become lodged in capillaries—primarily in the brain and muscle tissue—where they develop into mature cysts. The most common clinical presentations of neurocysticercosis are seizures and headaches, and diagnosis can be confirmed through serum or CSF analysis.

Intracranial neurocysticercosis can be classified as subarachnoid, parenchymal, or intraventricular. Parenchymal cysticercosis, which most commonly affects tissues at the gray–white matter junctions, is the second most common form of neurocysticercosis behind the subarachnoid form, but some have suggested that intraparenchymal lesions of cysticercosis actually represent subarachnoid cysts located in deep sulci or in perivascular spaces. The imaging features of cysticercosis are further dependent on the stage of cyst formation, which can be divided into (1) noncystic, (2) vesicular, (3) colloidal vesicular, (4) granular nodular, and (5) calcified nodular phases. The noncystic form is generally asymptomatic with negative imaging findings.

In the vesicular stage, well-circumscribed cysts typically measuring 5 to 20 mm in diameter are seen in the subarachnoid spaces, ventricles, or brain parenchyma. In roughly half of cases, a 2 to 4 mm nodule (the scolex) can be seen along the wall of the cyst. Although the cysts can be seen on CT, MR is the imaging modality of choice because it provides better delineation of cysts. In particular, high-resolution T2-weighted sequences are ideal for demonstrating cysts in the ventricles and subarachnoid spaces (Fig. 3.53). Although the cyst walls do not enhance, the scolex may show some enhancement on contrast-enhanced T1WI. Little or no edema surrounds the cysts in the vesicular stage.

The colloidal vesicular stage occurs as the larva dies and begins to degenerate. As the scolex dis-

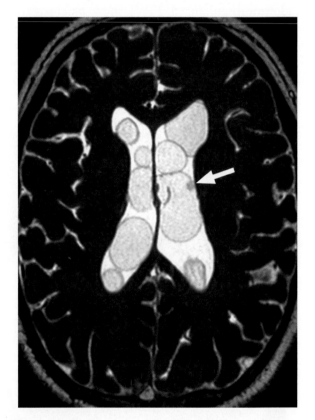

Figure 3.53. Intraventricular cysticercosis. Axial constructive interference in the steady state (CISS) image demonstrates multiple cysts in the lateral ventricles representing cysticercal cysts in the vesicular stage of infection. The fluid within the cysts is of slightly lower signal intensity than CSF. There is a small nodule along the wall of one of the cysts, likely representing a scolex *(arrow)*.

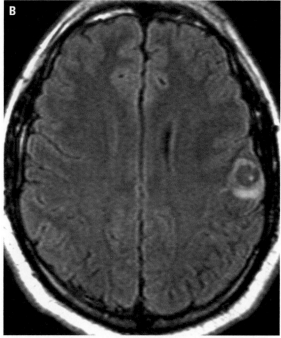

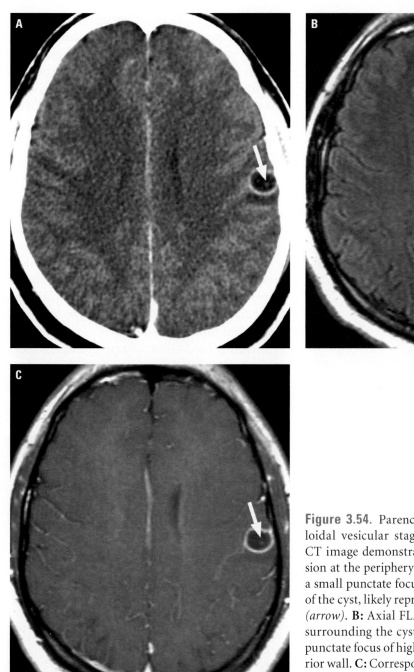

Figure 3.54. Parenchymal cysticercosis in the colloidal vesicular stage. **A:** Axial contrast-enhanced CT image demonstrates a cystic, rim-enhancing lesion at the periphery of the left frontal lobe. There is a small punctate focus of enhancement near the wall of the cyst, likely representing the degenerating scolex *(arrow)*. **B:** Axial FLAIR image demonstrates edema surrounding the cyst. The scolex appears as a small punctate focus of high-signal intensity near the posterior wall. **C:** Corresponding post-contrast T1WI again demonstrates enhancement along the periphery of the cyst and of the scolex *(arrow)*.

integrates during this stage, there is a marked inflammatory response around the cyst, appearing as edema and enhancement of the cyst rim (Fig. 3.54). The contents of the cyst may become hyperintense relative to CSF on T1WI and FLAIR images. When multiple cysts are grouped together with an appearance similar to a cluster of grapes in the vesicular and colloidal vesicular stages, the term racemose cysticercosis is used (Fig. 3.55). In the granular nodular

stage, the cyst begins to retract eventually forming a granulomatous nodule, which eventually calcifies. The imaging features at this stage are similar to those of the previous stage with thicker ring enhancement. Seizures in patients with neurocysticercosis are usually the result of perilesional inflammation occurring in the colloidal and granular stages.

Development of parenchymal calcifications represents the nonactive, end stage of the disease.

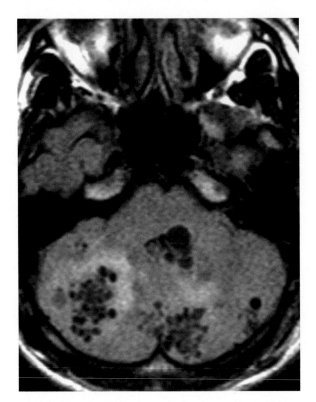

Figure 3.55. Racemose cysticercosis. Axial FLAIR image through the posterior fossa demonstrates multiple clustered cysts within the cerebellar hemispheres, with an appearance similar to bunches of grapes.

In this stage, unenhanced CT will demonstrate punctate parenchymal calcifications without significant surrounding edema or mass effect (Fig. 3.56). On MRI, the nodules will appear hypointense on conventional pulse sequences, usually without surrounding edema or enhancement.

Occasionally, patients with cysticercosis can develop meningitis—which may be evident as focal sulcal or cisternal enhancement—or vasculitis with resultant infarctions. In the latter case, noninvasive imaging with MRA may demonstrate focal segmental narrowing or beading of the intracranial arteries.

Acute Disseminated Encephalomyelitis

Acute disseminated encephalomyelitis (ADEM) is an inflammatory demyelinating disease of the CNS that is usually associated with a prior viral illness or vaccination. It most commonly affects children, with a mean age at presentation of 5 to 8 years, but the disease can affect patients at any age. ADEM

presents with rapid onset encephalopathy accompanied by multifocal neurologic disturbances and is often preceded by a prodromal phase of fever, malaise, headache, nausea, and vomiting beginning days to weeks after a preceding infectious episode or vaccination. Neurologic symptoms of ADEM include unilateral or bilateral pyramidal signs, acute hemiplegia, ataxia, CN palsies, visual loss caused by optic neuritis, seizures, impaired speech, paresthesias, signs of spinal cord involvement, and alterations in mental status ranging from lethargy to coma. With appropriate treatment (steroids, IV immunoglobulin [IVIg], and/or plasmapheresis), symptoms usually resolve over the course of several weeks. Although ADEM is classically considered a monophasic disorder, recurrent and multiphasic forms are described, and up to 28% of patients initially diagnosed with ADEM go on to with a diagnosis of multiple sclerosis.

Imaging in ADEM characteristically reveals multiple bilateral, asymmetric brain lesions involving gray and white matter. White matter lesions are

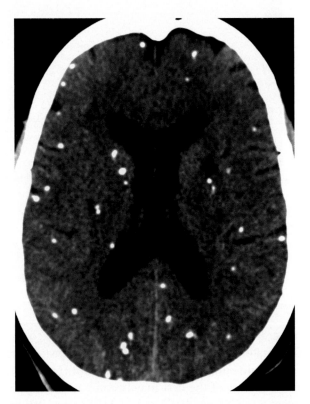

Figure 3.56. Calcified cysticercosis. Unenhanced axial CT image demonstrates numerous punctate parenchymal calcifications throughout both hemispheres, consisted with calcified cysts. The calcifications lack surrounding edema or mass effect.

more often subcortical than periventricular and may involve the overlying cortex. Deep gray matter involvement is seen in approximately 30% of cases. Unenhanced CT is often normal but may demonstrate larger lesions that will appear hypodense without significant mass effect. On MRI, the lesions of ADEM are hypointense on T1WI, hyperintense on T2-weighted and FLAIR images, and often demonstrate indistinct margins (Fig. 3.57). Contrast enhancement in ADEM lesions is variable and ranges from absent to solid or ring enhancement. Approximately 30% of patients with ADEM also have spinal cord lesions by imaging.

Rarely, patients may present with a more fulminant picture characterized by tissue necrosis and/or hemorrhage. In these cases, the disease is referred to as acute hemorrhagic encephalomyelitis (AHEM) or acute necrotizing encephalopathy of childhood (ANEC). Lesions of AHEM and ANEC are generally larger and show greater edema and mass effect than those of classic ADEM. Hemorrhage may also be evident in the lesions. ANEC is seen primarily in children of East Asian descent and is associated with influenza A and human herpesvirus-6 infections. It characteristically involves the bilateral

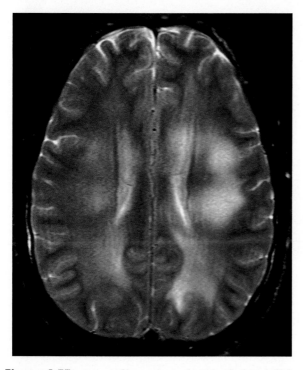

Figure 3.57. Acute disseminated encephalomyelitis. Axial T2WI demonstrates multiple, hyperintense, bilateral, asymmetric white matter lesions that have indistinct borders. The lesions cause little or no mass effect.

thalami and frequently also causes lesions in the brainstem tegmentum, supratentorial white matter, and cerebellum.

Opportunistic Central Nervous System Infections

Toxoplasmosis

Cerebral toxoplasmosis is the most common CNS opportunistic infection and cause of intracranial mass lesions in patients with acquired immune deficiency syndrome (AIDS). It is caused by the obligate intracellular protozoan—*Toxoplasma gondii*—which exists in three forms: oocysts, tachyzoites, and bradyzoites. Humans are usually infected when they ingest oocysts on contaminated vegetables or uncooked meats. The ingested oocytes transform into tachyzoites, which disseminate hematogenously primarily to the CNS, where they convert to bradyzoites or tissue cysts. Asymptomatic infection by *T. gondii* in immunocompetent individuals is extremely common, and it is estimated that up to 70% of the US population demonstrates seropositivity for the organism. In immunocompromised patients, cerebral toxoplasmosis is caused primarily by reactivation of latent *T. gondii* infection, which typically occurs when the CD4 count falls lower than 100 cells per μL. The incidence of cerebral toxoplasmosis in the HIV-positive population has declined significantly with the widespread use of highly active antiretroviral therapy (HAART), but the infection remains a significant cause of morbidity in AIDS patients.

Headache is the most common symptom of cerebral toxoplasmosis, but patients also present with fevers, altered mental status, or focal neurologic deficits. Unenhanced CT typically demonstrates multiple areas of hypoattenuation in the basal ganglia, thalami, and gray–white junctions of the cerebral hemispheres (Fig. 3.58). Solitary lesions are seen in only 14% of cases. On MRI, the lesions are typically of low to intermediate signal intensity on T2WI and low-signal intensity on T1WI. Most lesions measure 1 to 3 cm in diameter, and they generally demonstrate marked surrounding vasogenic edema. Following contrast administration, nodular or ring enhancement is the norm. A characteristic feature of toxoplasmosis is the so-called target sign, which refers to the presence of a small eccentric,

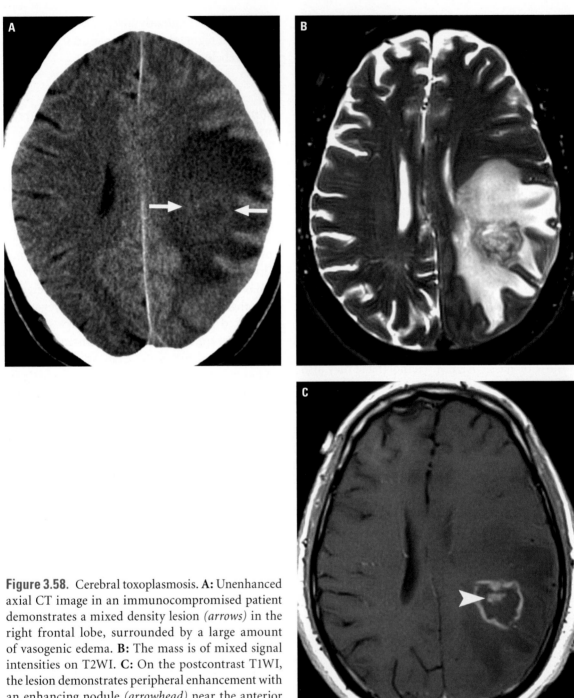

Figure 3.58. Cerebral toxoplasmosis. **A:** Unenhanced axial CT image in an immunocompromised patient demonstrates a mixed density lesion *(arrows)* in the right frontal lobe, surrounded by a large amount of vasogenic edema. **B:** The mass is of mixed signal intensities on T2WI. **C:** On the postcontrast T1WI, the lesion demonstrates peripheral enhancement with an enhancing nodule *(arrowhead)* near the anterior wall. This is an example of the "target sign," which is relatively specific for toxoplasmosis.

enhancing nodule along the enhancing rim (Fig. 3.58). This feature is reported to be highly specific for toxoplasmosis but is present in only approximately 30% of cases.

The primary differential consideration in HIV-positive patients is CNS lymphoma, which can appear virtually identical on CT and MRI.

Hemorrhage within a lesion favors toxoplasmosis because hemorrhage is rare in untreated lymphoma, whereas lymphoma tends to abut ependymal surfaces with greater frequency than toxoplasmosis. In addition, toxoplasmosis demonstrates decreased regional cerebral blood volume (rCBV) on perfusion-weighted MRI compared to lymphoma. Thallium-201 single photon emission computed tomography (SPECT) or fluorodeoxyglucose (FDG) positron emission tomography (PET) may be useful in differentiating toxoplasmosis from CNS lymphoma because lesions of toxoplasmosis are not radiotracer avid on either modality. With appropriate antibiotic therapy, toxoplasmosis lesions generally resolve within 3 to 6 weeks.

Cryptococcosis

Cryptococcus neoformans is the most common fungal CNS infection both in the general population and in immunocompromised hosts. *Cryptococcus* is an encapsulated yeastlike fungus commonly found in soil. The CNS and the lung are the two primary sites of infection with *Cryptococcus*, and most cases of CNS involvement are caused by hematogenous dissemination from a pulmonary source. CNS cryptococcosis typically presents with nonspecific signs of meningitis or meningoencephalitis, including headaches, fever, lethargy, nausea, vomiting, and memory loss. The diagnosis can be confirmed by demonstrating encapsulated yeast cells on direct microscopic examination of the CSF with India ink, positive CSF cultures for *C. neoformans*, or detection of the cryptococcal capsular polysaccharide antigen within the CSF. Blood cultures and serum cryptococcal antigen tests may also be positive.

The imaging manifestations of cryptococcal CNS infection are varied and include findings of meningoencephalitis, gelatinous pseudocysts in the basal ganglia, and parenchymal or intraventricular miliary nodules/cryptococcomas. Hydrocephalus is the most common radiologic abnormality and is seen in roughly half of patients with cryptococcal meningitis. Meningoencephalitis will typically appear as areas of cortical and subcortical hyperintensity on T2-weighted and FLAIR images with associated leptomeningeal and occasional parenchymal enhancement.

Gelatinous pseudocysts are characteristic of *Cryptococcus*, and the finding of multiple dilated perivascular spaces in an immunosuppressed patient should be considered highly suspicious for cryptococcal infection. These pseudocysts are caused by extension of infection from the basal cisterns into the brain via the perivascular spaces, resulting in enlargement of these spaces because

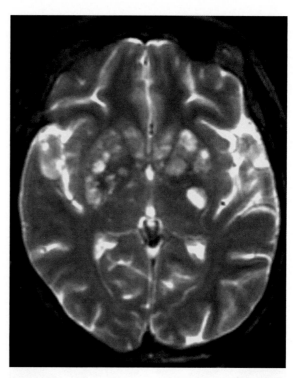

Figure 3.59. Cryptococcal meningitis gelatinous pseudocysts. Axial T2WI demonstrates multiple circumscribed high-signal intensity lesions in the basal ganglia. These pseudocysts represent extension of infection from the basal cisterns into the perivascular spaces, resulting in enlargement of these spaces due to deposition of gelatinous capsular material.

of deposition of gelatinous capsular material. Gelatinous pseudocysts appear as rapidly enlarging, well-demarcated, nonenhancing cystic lesions or dilated perivascular spaces in the basal ganglia and deep white matter, which are of low density on CT, and signal similar to CSF on T1-weighted and T2-weighted MR images (Fig. 3.59). On FLAIR images, the cysts are often hyperintense relative to CSF.

Cryptococcomas are enhancing nodular or masslike granulomatous lesions located in the brain parenchyma or along the ependymal surfaces of the choroid plexus. Parenchymal cryptococcomas are most commonly found in the basal ganglia, thalami, and cerebellum. They range in size from a few millimeters to several centimeters, are usually hyperintense on T2-weighted and FLAIR images, and demonstrate surrounding edema. Solid or rim enhancement is typical (Fig. 3.60), although nonenhancing cryptococcomas have been reported.

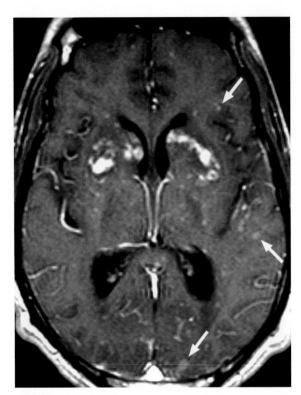

Figure 3.60. Cryptococcal meningitis with cryptococcomas. Axial post-contrast T1WI in a patient with cryptococcal meningitis demonstrates multiple enhancing lesions in the basal ganglia and is scattered throughout the cerebral hemispheres *(arrows)* consistent with cryptococcomas. The basal ganglia lesions are usually hyperintense on T2WI similar to gelatinous pseudocysts, but enhancement of cryptococcomas allows the two entities to be distinguished on imaging.

Invasive Aspergillus

Invasive aspergillosis, most commonly caused by the organism *Aspergillus fumigatus*, is a fungal infection affecting immunosuppressed patients, particularly following bone marrow transplantation. *Aspergillus* species are found ubiquitously in soil, plants, and decaying matter, and primary infections result from inhalation of the spores. Intracranial aspergillosis is usually the result of hematogenous spread from the lungs or direct invasion from the paranasal sinuses. The organisms tend to be angioinvasive and may cause vascular thrombosis and hemorrhagic infarcts. Mortality associated with invasive CNS aspergillosis is as high as 70%, but patients do survive with early, aggressive surgical and antifungal treatment.

Three imaging patterns are described for cerebral aspergillosis. The first pattern is that of multiple ring enhancing lesions consistent with cerebral abscesses. Like pyogenic abscesses, these fungal abscesses are predominantly located at gray–white junctions and demonstrate a hypointense rim on T2-weighted MR images. Fungal abscesses tend to have scalloped outer walls with intracavitary projections. The intensity of ring enhancement can be variable, however, and enhancement may even be absent in severely immunosuppressed patients who are unable to mount an adequate host immune response. On DWI, the walls of fungal abscesses show restricted diffusion, whereas the core portions of the abscesses do not, which may help to distinguish them from bacterial abscesses (Fig. 3.61).

The second pattern seen in cerebral aspergillosis is multiple infarcts that, like other ischemic infarcts, are hypodense on CT and hyperintense on T2-weighted and DWI images. Infarcts are commonly cortico-subcortical or involve the basal ganglia and thalami. Callosal lesions may also be observed, presumably because of angioinvasion of medial lenticulostriate arteries and perforating pericallosal branches supplying the corpus callosum. Hemorrhage occurs in approximately 25% of infarcts and abscesses caused by *Aspergillus*. Therefore, when a hemorrhagic lesion is seen in an immunocompromised patient, the specter of invasive aspergillosis should be raised.

The final pattern of intracranial aspergillosis is that of dural or cavernous enhancement or CST adjacent to diseased paranasal sinuses, presumably reflecting direct spread from primary sinonasal *Aspergillus* infection.

Progressive Multifocal Leukoencephalopathy

Progressive multifocal leukoencephalopathy (PML) is a progressive demyelinating disease caused by the John Cunningham (JC) virus, a DNA papovavirus that directly infects oligodendrocytes. PML can be seen as a complication of various immunocompromised states, but the greatest risk occurs in HIV-infected patients with CD4 counts between 50 and 100 cells per μL. Patients typically present with a progressive neurologic decline, manifested by cognitive impairment, changes in mental status, and personality changes. Focal neurologic deficits and seizures also occur. Diagnosis is generally made with PCR testing of CSF. Left untreated, PML has a 1-year mortality of nearly 90%.

On unenhanced CT, PML classically causes multifocal asymmetric areas of decreased attenuation in the periventricular and subcortical

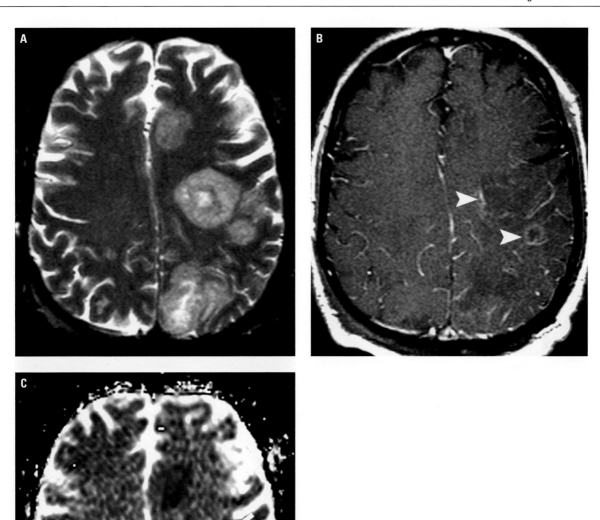

Figure 3.61. Cerebral aspergillosis. **A:** Axial T2WI in an immunocompromised patient demonstrates multiple parenchymal lesions with surrounding edema. **B:** On the post-contrast T1WI, some of the lesions demonstrate very mild peripheral enhancement *(arrowheads)*. **C:** Corresponding ADC map shows that the more centrally located lesion has reduced diffusion along its periphery and increased perfusion centrally, which is not typical of pyogenic abscesses.

white matter, frequently involving the subcortical U-fibers. Occasionally, patients may present with a solitary white matter lesion. The lesions are hypointense on T1WI and hyperintense on T2-weighted MR images. Mass effect is usually minimal, and there is usually no or little enhancement (Fig. 3.62). When present, enhancement in lesions of PML is peripheral and usually mild. It has been suggested that enhancement reflects some preserved ability to mount an immune response to the infection, and a few studies have reported the presence of enhancement to be associated with improved survival. Hemorrhage is not common in PML. DWI may demonstrate reduced diffusion in the periphery of PML lesions, presumably indicating the zone of active demyelination.

The chief radiographic differential for PML is primary HIV encephalitis, which tends to be more

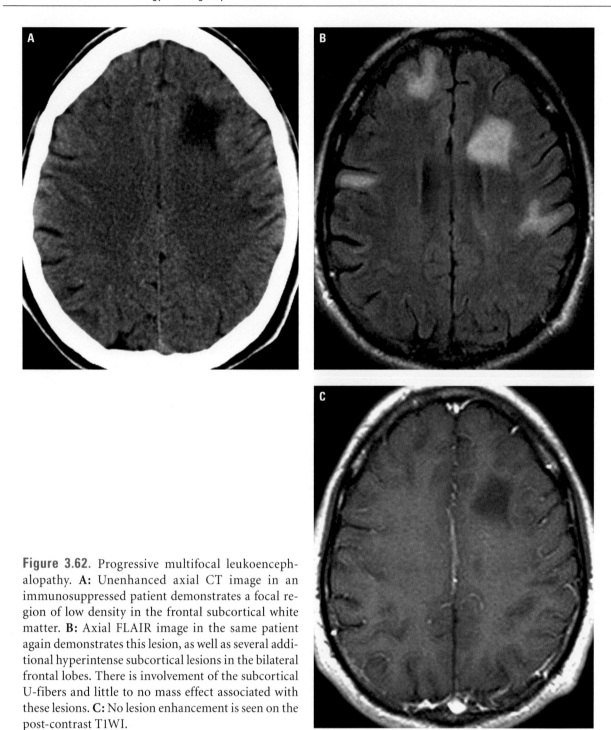

Figure 3.62. Progressive multifocal leukoencephalopathy. **A:** Unenhanced axial CT image in an immunosuppressed patient demonstrates a focal region of low density in the frontal subcortical white matter. **B:** Axial FLAIR image in the same patient again demonstrates this lesion, as well as several additional hyperintense subcortical lesions in the bilateral frontal lobes. There is involvement of the subcortical U-fibers and little to no mass effect associated with these lesions. **C:** No lesion enhancement is seen on the post-contrast T1WI.

symmetric and primarily involves the periventricular and deep white matter while sparing the subcortical U-fibers.

Tuberculosis

Tuberculosis has seen a resurgence that has corresponded to the spread of HIV worldwide. Both children and HIV-infected patients are at risk for developing CNS tuberculosis, and additional risk factors include alcoholism, malignancy, and use of immunosuppressive agents. Roughly 5% to 9% of patients with AIDS develop tuberculosis, and of these patients, up to 18% develop CNS tuberculosis. Most cases of CNS tuberculosis manifest as meningitis and are caused by hematogenous dissemination of *Mycobacterium tuberculosis*.

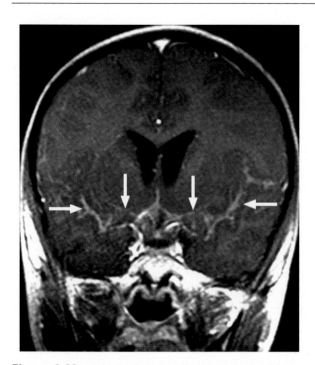

Figure 3.63. Tuberculous meningitis. Coronal post-contrast T1WI demonstrates leptomeningeal enhancement in the basilar cisterns and along the Sylvian fissures *(arrows)*, which is a classic distribution for tuberculous meningitis.

Hydrocephalus is the most common imaging finding in patients with CNS tuberculosis, being present in approximately 50% of patients. Diffuse meningeal enhancement on contrast-enhanced CT or MRI is seen almost as frequently and predominantly involves the basilar cisterns (Fig. 3.63). Noncontrasted CT may demonstrate obliteration of the basilar cisterns because of the presence of a thick inflammatory exudate. The most serious consequence of tuberculous meningitis is the development of vasculitis in the vessels of the circle of Willis, the vertebrobasilar system, and the perforating branches of the middle cerebral artery, resulting in infarctions in the territories supplied by these vessels (Fig. 3.64). These infarcts most commonly affect the basal ganglia and internal capsules.

Less common manifestations of CNS tuberculosis include focal cerebritis, intracranial tuberculomas, and tuberculous brain abscesses. Tuberculomas are granulomatous lesions consisting of epithelioid cells, giant cells, and lymphocytes around a variable-sized central area of caseating necrosis containing occasional bacilli. These lesions are primarily supratentorial and centered at corticomedullary junctions in adults but are more commonly infratentorial in

children. In 30% of patients, multiple tuberculomas will be present. Tuberculomas are isodense to hypodense relative to normal adjacent brain parenchyma on unenhanced CT. On MR, they are hypointense relative to adjacent parenchyma on T1WI and demonstrate signal intensity varying from hypointense to hyperintense on T2WI depending on whether the center of the lesion has liquefied. Contrast-enhanced studies demonstrate solid or rim enhancement. When the tuberculomas liquefy centrally, they demonstrate central hyperintensity on T2WI and peripheral enhancement, making them indistinguishable from other rim-enhancing lesions such as toxoplasmosis.

Tuberculous abscesses occur in less than 10% of patients with CNS tuberculosis and are seen more commonly in HIV-infected patients. Tuberculous abscesses differ from tuberculomas in that the central cores of abscesses contain larger concentrations of tubercle bacilli and the walls lack the giant cell epithelioid granulomatous reaction of tuberculomas. Abscesses are often larger than tuberculomas, have thinner walls, and are more likely to be solitary. On both CT and MRI, tuberculous abscesses

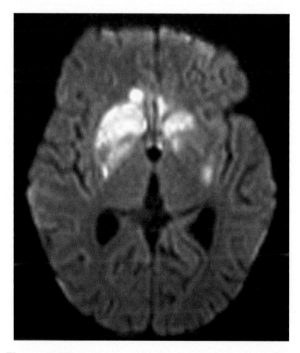

Figure 3.64. Infarcts caused by tuberculous meningitis. Axial DWI image in the same patient shown in Figure 3.63 demonstrates multiple areas of restricted diffusion in the basal ganglia, representing infarcts secondary to vasculitis of the lenticulostriate perforators caused by the basilar meningitis.

are similar in appearance to other types of abscesses, and like pyogenic abscesses, they can show restricted diffusion centrally.

Immune Reconstitution Inflammatory Syndrome

Brief mention should be made of immune reconstitution inflammatory syndrome (IRIS), an entity that only became recognized following the introduction of HAART. The syndrome usually occurs in the initial weeks to months following initiation of HAART, and patients present with paradoxical worsening of their clinical status despite a rising CD4 count and decreasing viral load. IRIS is believed to be the result of rapid restoration of the previously suppressed immune system, which subsequently mounts a dysregulated inflammatory response to latent organisms or their antigens. Between 15% and 25% of patients receiving HAART develop IRIS in the first few months of therapy, and mortality associated with IRIS approaches 4%. IRIS is particularly common in those with a history of cytomegalovirus retinitis, cryptococcal meningitis, and tuberculosis, and in those with low CD4 cell counts prior to initiation of HAART. The diagnosis of IRIS requires the exclusion of a newly acquired infection or progression of a newly diagnosed opportunistic infection.

The imaging manifestations of IRIS in the CNS are highly variable and depend on the underlying pathogen to which the immune response is being mounted. Cases of IRIS can demonstrate imaging features of specific opportunistic infections, but the findings may be somewhat atypical. For example, PML lesions in the setting of IRIS can show prominent enhancement and mass effect that is unusual in cases of classic PML in the absence of HAART.

MISCELLANEOUS INTRACRANIAL EMERGENCIES

Emergencies Related to Toxic Exposures

Conditions Related to Chronic Ethanol Abuse
Chronic ethanol abuse is associated with several characteristic CNS disorders that may be imaged on an emergent basis, including Wernicke encephalopathy and osmotic myelinolysis. Wernicke encephalopathy is a condition associated with poor nutritional intake (specifically thiamine deficiency), which is a frequent consequence of chronic alcoholism. Acute symptoms of Wernicke encephalopathy include nystagmus, abducens and conjugate gaze palsies, ataxia, and confusion.

CT is usually normal or only demonstrates cerebral and cerebellar atrophy. In some cases, hypodensity may be evident in the periaqueductal gray matter and medial thalami. MRI is the imaging modality of choice in patients with Wernicke encephalopathy. Characteristic findings of Wernicke encephalopathy include high-signal intensity on T2-weighted and FLAIR images in mamillary bodies, along the walls of the third ventricle, and in the periaqueductal gray matter (Fig. 3.65). Enhancement of the mamillary bodies on T1WI following contrast administration is virtually pathognomonic of the condition, but it is important to keep in mind that absence of imaging abnormalities does not exclude the diagnosis of Wernicke encephalopathy.

Osmotic myelinolysis is another condition associated with chronic alcoholism and other malnourished states. Rapid correction of hyponatremia is the most common cause of the disorder, which manifests with confusion, horizontal gaze paralysis, spastic quadriplegia, or seizures developing a few days after sodium correction. Central pontine myelinolysis is the most common imaging finding and is characterized by hypodensity on CT or T2-hyperintensity on MRI in the central portions of the pons, typically sparing the corticospinal tracts early on (Fig. 3.66). Extrapontine involvement of regions including the thalami, basal ganglia, cerebral white matter, and lateral geniculate bodies is also common in osmotic myelinolysis.

Carbon Monoxide Poisoning

Carbon monoxide (CO) poisoning is the most frequent cause of accidental poisoning in the developed world. CO competitively binds to iron in the porphyrin ring of hemoglobin with an affinity roughly 250 times greater than that of oxygen, resulting in a reduction of the oxygen-carrying capacity of the blood and tissue hypoxia. Common causes of CO poisoning include faulty furnaces, inadequately ventilated heating sources, and engine exhaust.

Symptoms of CO poisoning are nonspecific and include headache, nausea, vomiting, myalgia,

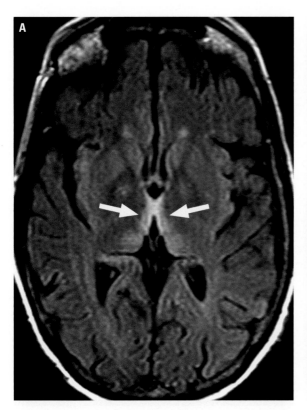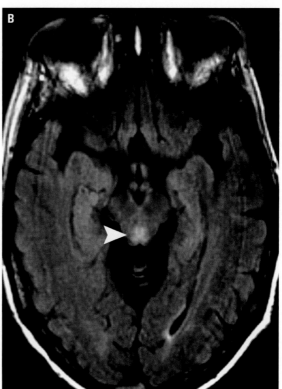

Figure 3.65. Wernicke encephalopathy. **A and B:** Axial FLAIR images in a chronic alcoholic patient demonstrate symmetric abnormal hyperintensity along the walls of the third ventricle (*arrows* in **A**) and in the periaqueductal gray matter (*arrowhead* in **B**).

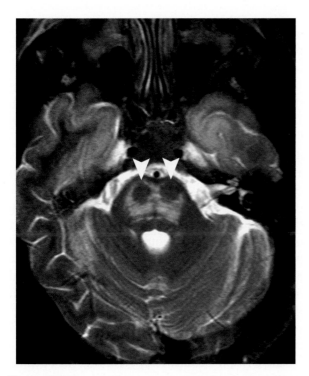

Figure 3.66. Central pontine myelinolysis. Axial T2WI demonstrates high-signal intensity in the central pons with sparing of the corticospinal tracts (*arrowheads*).

dizziness, and cognitive impairment. Severe poisoning may result in seizures, loss of consciousness, or death. On physical examination, patients may demonstrate cherry red lips and mucosa, cyanosis, or retinal hemorrhages, and suspected CO poisoning can be confirmed with blood carboxyhemoglobin levels.

CT in patients with acute CO poisoning demonstrates symmetric hypodensity in the basal ganglia, with preferential involvement of the globi pallidi. On MRI, these regions demonstrate low-signal intensity on T1WI, high-signal intensity on T2-weighted and FLAIR images, and restricted diffusion on DWI (Fig. 3.67). Additionally, less common areas of involvement include the substantia nigra, the thalami, the hippocampi, and the cerebral cortex.

A small percentage of patients with CO poisoning develop a delayed leukoencephalopathy identical to that seen in patients with hypoxic-ischemic brain injury (see previous text). Characteristic brain imaging findings include bilateral, symmetric, confluent areas of low density on CT and high-signal intensity on T2WI and FLAIR images in the periventricular

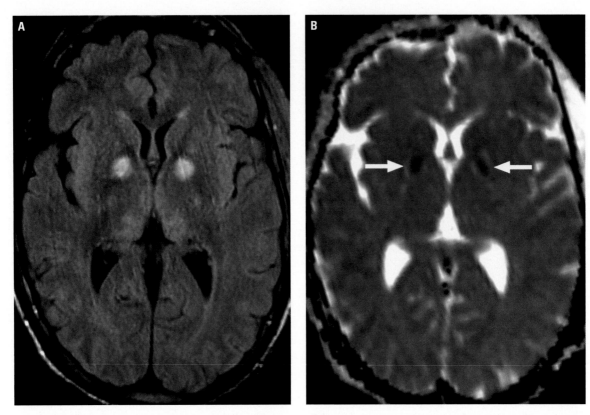

Figure 3.67. Carbon monoxide poisoning. **A:** Axial FLAIR image in a patient exposed to carbon monoxide demonstrates symmetric abnormal hyperintensity centered in the globi pallidi. **B:** The corresponding ADC map demonstrates low signal in these regions *(arrows)*, reflecting restricted diffusion.

white matter and centrum semiovale. These areas typically show reduced diffusion on DWI.

Pituitary Apoplexy

Pituitary adenomas are extremely common in the general population, with an estimated prevalence of approximately 17%. These tumors may come to attention as a result of excessive hormone secretion or because of mass effect on adjacent structures, but frequently they are asymptomatic incidental findings on brain MRI. In rare instances, pituitary adenomas can hemorrhage and rapidly enlarge, resulting in a potentially life-threatening condition known as pituitary apoplexy. Pituitary apoplexy is characterized clinically by the sudden onset of headache, bitemporal hemianopsia, ophthalmoplegia, and pituitary dysfunction—with or without alterations in consciousness. Several predisposing conditions have been described, including bromocriptine therapy, pregnancy, hypertension, radiotherapy, anticoagulation, and prior LP, but most cases

occur without a known risk factor. Less commonly, pituitary apoplexy is the result of pituitary gland infarction without a preexisting tumor.

CT in cases of pituitary apoplexy may demonstrate a hemorrhagic mass in the suprasellar cistern. There may also be sellar enlargement if there is an underlying macroadenoma. MRI is the imaging modality of choice in patients with suspected pituitary apoplexy. Sagittal MR images will demonstrate an enlarged, superiorly convex pituitary gland extending into the suprasellar cistern and compressing the optic chiasm. The gland may be hyperintense on unenhanced T1-weighted sequences and/or hypointense on T2-weighted sequences, reflecting the presence of hemoglobin breakdown products, and may demonstrate a blood/fluid level (Fig. 3.68). Patients with pituitary apoplexy occasionally develop noncommunicating hydrocephalus caused by compression of the anterior third ventricle.

There is some controversy regarding the optimal treatment of patients presenting with pituitary apoplexy, but patients presenting with severe visual defects generally require early surgery to relieve

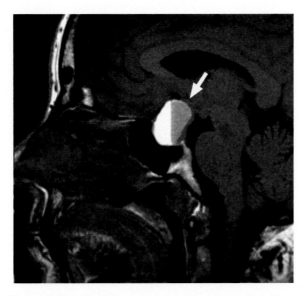

Figure 3.68. Pituitary apoplexy. Unenhanced midsagittal T1WI demonstrates a cystic sellar and suprasellar mass with a fluid–fluid level compressing the optic chiasm *(arrow)*. High-signal intensity material in the cyst reflects blood products.

compression on the optic chiasm and to prevent permanent vision loss. Patients without visual loss or alterations in consciousness may be treated conservatively.

SUGGESTED READINGS

1. Devuyst G, Bogousslavsky J, Meuli R, et al. Stroke or transient ischemic attacks with basilar artery stenosis or occlusion: clinical patterns and outcome. *Arch Neurol.* 2002;59(4):567–573.

2. Ebright JR, Pace MT, Niazi AF. Septic thrombosis of the cavernous sinuses. *Arch Intern Med.* 2001;161(22):2671–2676.

3. Fischbein NJ, Wijman CA. Nontraumatic intracranial hemorrhage. *Neuroimaging Clin N Am.* 2010;20(4):469–492.

4. Foerster BR, Thurnher MM, Malani PN, et al. Intracranial infections: clinical and imaging characteristics. *Acta Radiol.* 2007;48(8):875–893.

5. Goeser CD, McLeary MS, Young LW. Diagnostic imaging of ventriculoperitoneal shunt malfunctions and complications. *Radiographics.* 1998;18(3):635–651.

6. Hacein-Bey L, Provenzale JM. Current imaging assessment and treatment of intracranial aneurysms. *AJR Am J Roentgenol.* 2011;196(1):32–44.

7. Huang BY, Castillo M. Hypoxic-ischemic brain injury: imaging findings from birth to adulthood. *Radiographics.* 2008;28(2):417–439.

8. Kimura-Hayama ET, Higuera JA, Corona-Cedillo R, et al. Neurocysticercosis: radiologic-pathologic correlation. *Radiographics.* 2010;30(6):1705–1719.

9. Kloska SP, Wintermark M, Engelhorn T, et al. Acute stroke magnetic resonance imaging: current status and future perspective. *Neuroradiology.* 2010;52(3):189–201.

10. Leach JL, Fortuna RB, Jones BV, et al. Imaging of cerebral venous thrombosis: current techniques, spectrum of findings, and diagnostic pitfalls. *Radiographics.* 2006;26(suppl 1):S19–S43.

11. Narvid J, Do HM, Blevins NH, et al. CT angiography as a screening tool for dural arteriovenous fistula in patients with pulsatile tinnitus: feasibility and test characteristics. *AJNR Am J Neuroradiol.* 2011;32(3):446–453.

12. Petrovic BD, Nemeth AJ, McComb EN, et al. Posterior reversible encephalopathy syndrome and venous thrombosis. *Radiol Clin North Am.* 2011;49(1):63–80.

13. Rekate HL. A contemporary definition and classification of hydrocephalus. *Semin Pediatr Neurol.* 2009;16(1):9–15.

14. Rossi A. Imaging of acute disseminated encephalomyelitis. *Neuroimaging Clin N Am.* 2008;18(1):149–161, ix.

15. Schaefer PW, Copen WA, Lev MH, et al. Diffusion-weighted imaging in acute stroke. *Neuroimaging Clin N Am.* 2005;15(3):503–530, ix–x.

16. Sener RN. Acute carbon monoxide poisoning: diffusion MR imaging findings. *AJNR Am J Neuroradiol.* 2003;24(7):1475–1477.

17. Smith AB, Smirniotopoulos JG, Rushing EJ. From the archives of the AFIP: central nervous system infections associated with human immunodeficiency virus infection: radiologic-pathologic correlation. *Radiographics.* 2008;28(7):2033–2058.

18. Spampinato MV, Castillo M, Rojas R, et al. Magnetic resonance imaging findings in substance abuse: alcohol and alcoholism and syndromes associated with alcohol abuse. *Top Magn Reson Imaging.* 2005;16(3):223–230.

19. Tatter SB, Crowell RM, Ogilvy CS. Aneurysmal and microaneurysmal "angiogram-negative" subarachnoid hemorrhage. *Neurosurgery.* 1995;37(1):48–55.

20. Turgut M, Ozsunar Y, Basak S, et al. Pituitary apoplexy: an overview of 186 cases published during the last century. *Acta Neurochir (Wien).* 2010;152(5):749–761.

CHAPTER 4

Imaging Maxillofacial Trauma

Mark P. Bernstein ■ Alexander B. Baxter ■ John H. Harris Jr.

INTRODUCTION

Epidemiology

Facial fractures account for a large proportion of emergency room visits and 2% of all hospital admissions. Significant facial injuries are clinically occult in more than half of all intubated multitrauma patients. Mechanisms include motor vehicle collisions (MVCs), assault, falls, sports injuries, and civilian warfare. Together, MVCs and assault account for more than 80% of all injuries and commonly involve young adult males and alcohol use. A recent decline in MVC-related maxillofacial trauma appears to reflect improved automobile safety as a result of airbags, mandatory seatbelt laws, and improved road conditions.

Clinical Issues

The face protects the skull from frontal injury; supports the organs of sight, smell, taste, and hearing; and serves as the point of entry for oxygen, water, and nutrients.

The first aim of the physician caring for a patient with acute facial trauma is to preserve life. Initial management of any trauma patient is aimed at ensuring that airway, breathing, and circulation are maintained. In acute facial injury, pharyngeal hemorrhage, bone fragments, and loss of hyomandibular support with posterior displacement of the tongue can all compromise the airway. Laryngeal injury may be initially occult with subsequent precipitous airway compromise. Hoarseness and stridor are clues to its presence.

Circulation to the face is via branches of the external and internal carotid arteries. Injuries to these vessels are common and may result in a rapidly expanding hematoma or profuse arterial bleeding. In closed injuries, bleeding is controlled by packing or balloon tamponade using a Foley catheter. Angioembolization may be required when packing fails, typically from bleeding maxillary and palatine arteries in association with midface fractures and in penetrating trauma with vascular injury.

Once the patient is stabilized, clinical attention in the setting of facial trauma can be directed to restore form and function with preservation of vision, smell, taste and speech, and finally minimizing cosmetic deformity.

Biomechanics and Associated Life-Threatening Injuries

Direction and magnitude of an impacting force determines the pattern and severity of maxillofacial fractures. For example, the nose, mandibular body, and zygoma are typically injured in assault because of their prominent positions on the face and the relatively small amount of energy transferred in a strike or a punch. MVC, falls and other high-velocity injuries result in more complex, midfacial fractures. A collision of 30 miles per hour exceeds the tolerance of most facial bones (Fig. 4.1A).

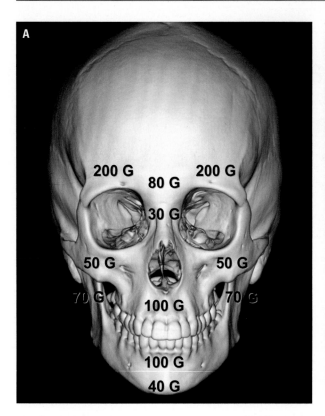

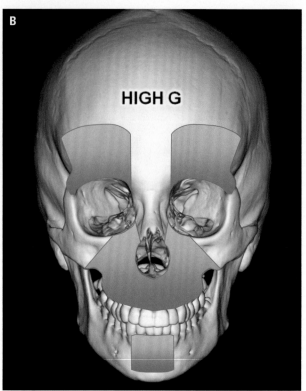

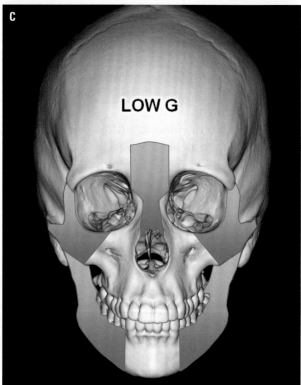

Figure 4.1. Biomechanics of the facial skeleton. **A:** Maximum tolerable impact forces. (Modified from Swearingen JJ. *Tolerances of the Human Face to Crash Impact.* Oklahoma City, OK: Civil Aeromedical Research Institute; 1965.) **B:** High G-force facial injuries: minor injuries 32%, major injuries 51%, death 15%. **C:** Low G-force facial injuries: minor injuries 30%, major injuries 21%, death 3%. (Modified from Luce EA. Maxillofacial trauma. *Curr Probl Surg.* 1984;21(2):1–68.)

Luce et al. studied injuries associated with major facial fractures in 1,020 patients and grouped them into high and low G-force mechanisms. Life-threatening injuries included intra-abdominal injury requiring surgery, pneumothorax, chest trauma requiring ventilator support, and severe closed head injury. Twenty-one percent of patients with low G-force facial trauma had one or more of these associated injuries compared with 50% in patients with high G-force mechanisms (Figs. 4.1B, 4.1C). Mortality in the latter group was 12%.

Mulligan et al. investigated the relationship between facial fractures, cervical spine injuries, and head injuries in 1.3 million trauma patients between 2002 and 2006. Nine percent sustained one or more facial fractures. The 6.7% of facial fracture patients had concomitant cervical spine injury, and 61.8% had associated head injury. Almost 5% suffered injuries to all three areas.

Cole et al., in a study of 247 victims of facial gunshot wounds, found associated cervical spine injury in 8% and head injury in 17%.

IMAGING

Imaging in facial trauma aims to define the number and locations of facial fractures and to identify injuries that could compromise the airway, vision, mastication, lacrimal system, and sinus function. Individual fractures should be listed and associated soft tissue injuries described with attention to these areas. If possible, bony findings should be summarized in one of several typical fracture patterns.

Imaging in most emergency departments for significant facial trauma begins with computed tomography (CT) scanning. Helical CT and, more recently, multidetector CT (MDCT) have supplanted plain radiography and have revolutionized the imaging of the maxillofacial trauma. CT is more cost efficient and more rapidly performed than radiographs of the face and mandible. MDCT is now considered the optimal imaging modality, particularly in the polytrauma setting because it allows safe and rapid image data acquisition and multiplanar reconstruction without patient manipulation. MDCT accurately depicts both bony and soft tissue injury. Submillimeter slice thickness permits exquisite multiplanar reformations (MPRs) and

three-dimensional (3D) reconstructions. Fracture fragment displacement and rotation are easily determined and fracture patterns may be readily classified and assessed for stability. Volume reformations from helical and MDCT datasets enhance diagnostic accuracy and allow the surgeon to better plan operative repair by depicting complex injuries in three dimensions.

Magnetic resonance imaging (MRI) can be a useful adjunct in patients with cranial nerve deficits not explained by CT, evaluation of incidentally discovered masses, and suspected vascular dissection. Its advantages include multiplanar imaging, excellent soft tissue contrast, and lack of ionizing radiation. The practical limitations of long scan times, limited patient access, poor evaluation of bone and contraindication in patients with pacemakers, some aneurysm clips, and ocular metallic foreign bodies prevent its primary application in the emergency setting.

Multidetector Computed Tomography Technique

At Bellevue Hospital, patients with direct facial injury and suspected maxillofacial fractures are scanned from the hyoid through the top of the frontal sinuses. Acquisitions using 64-MDCT with 0.625-mm detector width and 0.4 mm overlapping sections allow high-quality MPRs to be generated and evaluated at the workstation. The 2 mm thick images in three planes oriented parallel and perpendicular to the hard palate provide symmetrical images for interpretation (Figs. 4.2A–4.2D). Reconstructions in bone and soft tissue algorithm and specialized reformations may be generated depending on the presence and type of fractures. For example, oblique sagittal reformations along the plane of the optic nerve elegantly characterize orbital floor fractures with respect to depression, orbital depth, and relation to the inferior rectus muscle (Fig. 4.2E). Panoramic or oblique sagittal planes optimize evaluation of mandibular angle and ramus fractures (Fig. 4.2F). The 3D reconstructions can be oriented in any plane and are often acquired in patients with complex injuries as an aid to surgical planning (Fig. 4.2G).

The multitrauma patient requires a comprehensive examination to evaluate multiple body regions

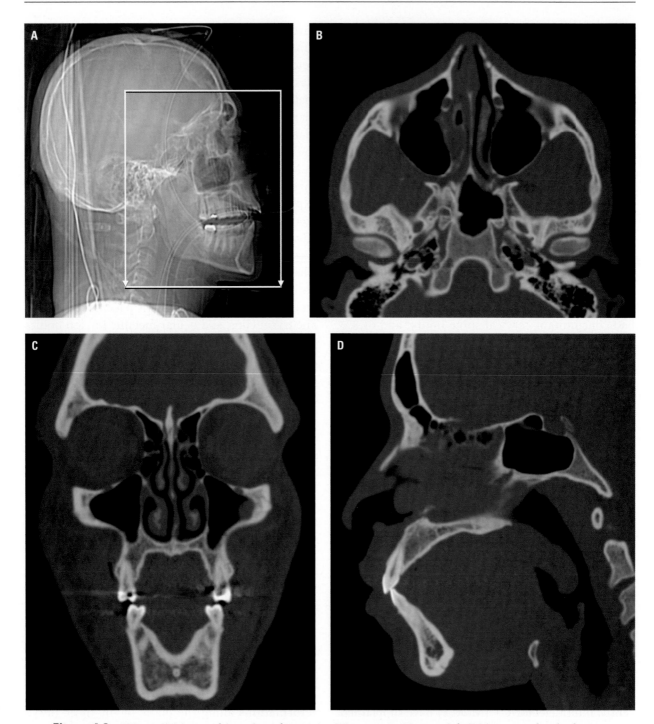

Figure 4.2. CT acquisition and imaging planes. **A:** CT scout. **B:** Transaxial CT image at level of zygomatic arches. **C:** Coronal CT reformation through the mid-orbits and maxillary sinuses. **D:** Midsagittal CT reformation. *(continued)*

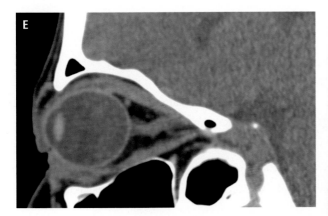

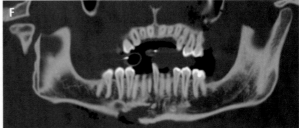

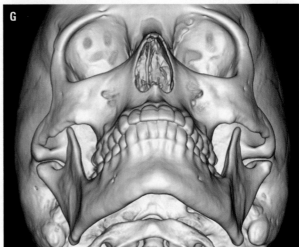

Figure 4.2. *(continued)* **E:** Oblique sagittal reformation along the plane of the optic nerve. **F:** Curved reformat panoramic CT simulates the Panorex radiograph. **G:** 3D CT reconstruction in Water's projection.

in a single visit to the CT suite. With current technology, scanning of the head, face, and cervical spine may be acquired as a single acquisition and no longer requires patient repositioning for direct coronal plane imaging.

FACIAL FRACTURES

Facial fracture complexes are classified by location and pattern: nasal, naso-orbito-ethmoid (NOE), frontal sinus, orbital, zygomatic, maxillary, and mandibular. Manson et al. have proposed further categorizing each area by the energy of the injury, namely low, moderate, and high energy. Low-energy injuries show little or no comminution or displacement. Moderate-energy injuries, the most common, demonstrate mild to marked displacement, whereas high energy is reserved for cases of severe fragmentation, displacement, and instability. Impact energy subclassifications dictate management from simple closed reduction to wide exposure open reduction and internal fixation.

NASAL FRACTURES

Anatomy

The upper third of the nose is supported by a bony skeleton consisting of the nasal bones proper, the frontal process of the maxilla, and the nasal process of the frontal bone. The middle and lower thirds are composed of the upper lateral and lower alar cartilages, respectively. The anterior nasal septum is cartilaginous. The posterior perpendicular plate of ethmoid, vomer, nasal crest of maxilla, and nasal crest of the palatine bone form the bony nasal septum (Fig. 4.3).

Injuries

Nasal bone fractures are common and account for half of all facial fractures. Most of these involve the distal third because this represents the most prominent projection of the facial skeleton. Peak incidence is in the second to third decades, with

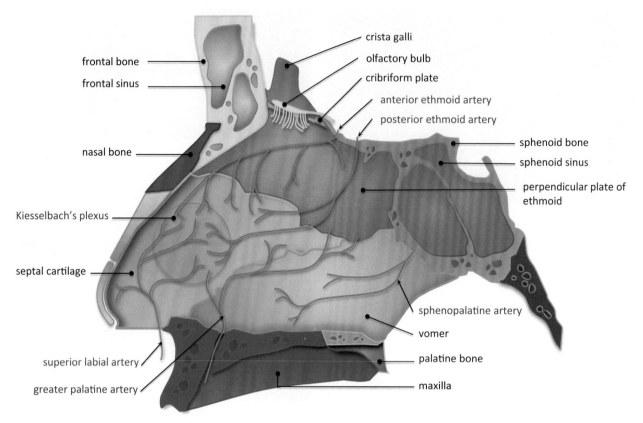

Figure 4.3. Nasal bone anatomy.

injuries twice as common among men. Potential sequelae include nasal obstruction, cosmetic deformity, and cerebrospinal fluid (CSF) leak. Septal hematoma, if unrecognized, may result in later ischemic septal necrosis and "saddle nose" deformity.

Nasal injuries are classified by the energy and direction of the impact force. Lateral force from assault is the most common mechanism and causes contralateral displacement of the nasal bones and frontal processes of the maxilla. In low-velocity injuries, detachment of the nasal septal cartilage from the vomer may accompany the fracture. High-velocity injuries and frontal impacts result in central, comminuted, septal fractures. Inferior forces typically cause an isolated septal injury. The nasal bones are most resistant to frontal impact; once the force is great enough to fracture the upper nasal bones, the delicate ethmoid air cells behind them offer little resistance to further impaction and allow the nasal bones to telescope into the deep face. This fracture pattern usually also involves the medial orbital walls and is referred to as an NOE fracture.

Epistaxis is a serious complication of nasal fractures. Even minor trauma can result in hemorrhage from Kiesselbach's plexus (Fig. 4.3), a robust vascular network that supplies the nose. Severe bleeding is usually caused by injuries to the anterior ethmoid artery branch of the ophthalmic artery (anterior bleeding) and to the sphenopalatine artery branches (posterior bleeding).

Imaging

CT analysis aids operative management of severe nasal bone fractures and identifies associated facial soft tissue and bony injuries. Fractures are described as unilateral or bilateral, simple or comminuted, displaced or undisplaced, impacted or non-impacted, and with or without nasal septal involvement. A proposed classification scheme is illustrated in Figure 4.4. Posterior packing with balloon tamponade may be seen as treatment for epistaxis (Fig. 4.5). Septal involvement can complicate nasal bone realignment and should be specifically addressed in

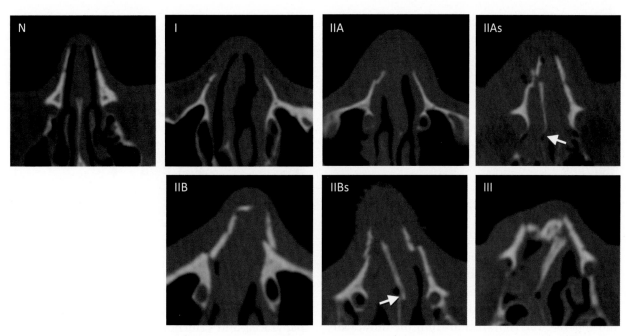

Figure 4.4. Nasal bone fractures—classification. *(N)* Normal. *(I)* Simple, undisplaced. *(IIA)* Simple, displaced, unilateral without telescoping. *(IIAs)* Simple, displaced, unilateral with septal fracture *(arrow)*. *(IIB)* Simple, displaced, bilateral. *(IIBs)* Simple, displaced, bilateral with septal fracture *(arrow)*. *(III)* Comminuted with telescoping.

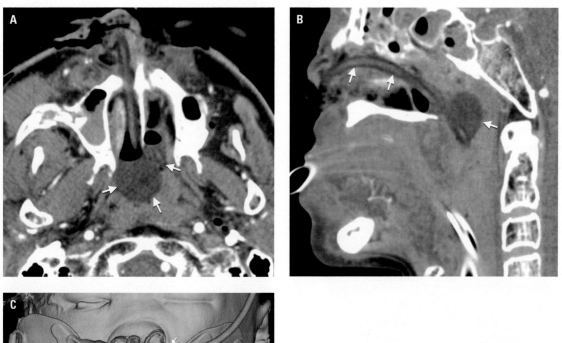

Figure 4.5. Posterior nasal packing with Foley balloon tamponade. Transaxial **(A)** CT reformation show bilateral transnasal Foley catheters with balloons inflated (greater on the right; *arrows*). Right parasagittal CT reformation **(B)** shows Foley and balloon posterior to the hard palate *(arrows)*. 3D reconstruction **(C)** shows bilaterally placed nasal catheters *(arrows)*.

the radiology report. Generally, nasal fractures with associated septal fracture, significant dislocation, or severe concomitant soft tissue injury require open repair, whereas most others can be treated with closed reduction.

NASO-ORBITO-ETHMOID FRACTURES

Anatomy

The NOE region refers to the space between the eyes or interorbital space. The interorbital space represents the confluence of the bony nose, orbit, maxilla, and cranium. It is bound laterally by the thin medial orbital walls and posteriorly by the sphenoid sinus. The cribriform plate and the medial floor of the anterior cranial fossa define its superior margin and separate the NOE region from the dura, CSF, and brain. Inferior margin is the lower border of the ethmoid air cells (Fig. 4.6). The frontal process of maxilla, nasal process of the frontal bone, and thick proximal nasal bones comprise the anterior border of the interorbital space. Together, these form the relatively strong central facial "pillar." Important soft tissue structures of the interorbital space include the olfactory nerves, lacrimal sac, nasolacrimal duct, ethmoid vessels, and the medial canthal ligaments.

Injuries

NOE injuries result from direct anterior impact to the upper nasal bridge and are characterized by fracture of the nasal bones, nasal septum, frontal

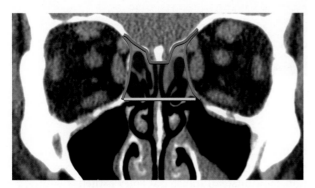

Figure 4.6. Naso-orbito-ethmoid (NOE) regional anatomy. Coronal CT reformation shows the interorbital space *(shaded green)* defined by medial orbital walls *(lateral margins; blue)*, cribriform plate *(superior margin; red)*, and lower border of the ethmoid sinuses *(inferior margin; yellow)*.

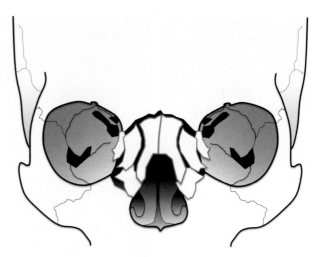

Figure 4.7. Naso-orbito-ethmoid (NOE) injury.

process of the maxilla, ethmoid bones (lamina papyracea and cribriform plate), lacrimal bones, and frontal sinus (Fig. 4.7). They may be associated with other facial fractures and remote multisystem trauma. NOE fractures have been classified by Gruss who grouped them by extent of injury, displacement, orbital involvement, and associated facial fractures (Table 4.1).

Type 1 fractures detach the frontal process of maxilla, displacing the fragments posteriorly and laterally without severe comminution. Type 2

TABLE 4.1	Classification of Naso-Orbital-Ethmoid Injuries
Type 1	Isolated bony NOE injury
Type 2	Bony NOE and central maxilla
2a	Central maxilla only
2b	Central and one lateral maxilla
2c	Central and bilateral lateral maxillae
Type 3	Extended NOE injury
3a	Superiorly—craniofacial injuries
3b	Laterally—with LeFort II and III fractures
Type 4	NOE injury with orbital displacement
4a	With oculo-orbital displacement
4b	With orbital dystopia
Type 5	NOE injury with bone loss

From Gruss JS. Naso-ethmoid-orbital fractures: classification and role of primary bone grafting. *Plast Reconstr Surg.* 1985; 75(3):303–317.

fractures are more severely comminuted and impacted through the interorbital space, shattering the nasomaxillary buttress (discussed with maxillary fractures subsequently), and surround the piriform aperture. Subtypes a–c describe the integrity of the zygomaticomaxillary buttresses, from intact to unilateral to bilateral involvement, respectively. Type 3 fractures occur in conjunction with more extensive craniofacial injuries and reflect superolateral extension, including cribriform plate disruption with intracranial involvement and dural violation (superior extension), or LeFort II and III fractures (lateral extension). Type 4 injuries include varying degrees of orbital detachment and displacement; whereas type 5 injuries are associated with significant bone destruction or loss, potentially complicating reconstructive strategies.

The medial and lateral canthal ligaments support the globe and keep the eyelid apposed to it. Fracture through the inferomedial orbital rim suggests injury to both the medial canthal ligament and lacrimal apparatus. Patients present with nasal and periorbital ecchymosis, depression of the nasal bridge, telecanthus, enophthalmos, and a shortened palpebral fissure.

The junction of the frontal process of maxilla and the inferomedial orbital rim make up the bony anchor of the medial canthal ligament. In the setting of NOE fracture, this bony anchor is referred to as the "central" fragment and may be either intact or comminuted or fractured through the medial canthal ligament insertion site. Markowitz et al. have devised a classification system to address its integrity and dictate optimal repair (Fig. 4.8) (Table 4.2).

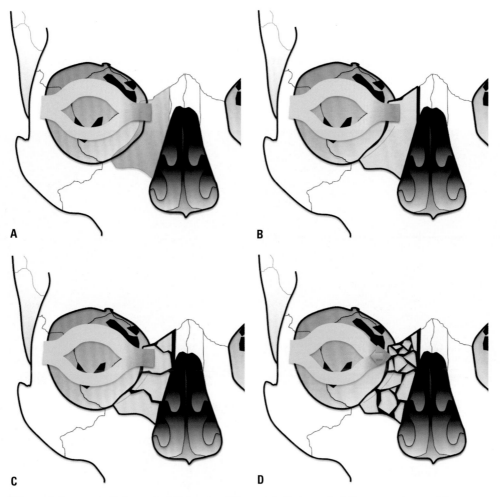

Figure 4.8. A: Medial canthal ligament injury. Medial canthal ligament *(orange)* is shown anchored to the bony "central fragment." The central fragment lies at the junction of the frontal process of maxilla and inferomedial orbital rim. **B, C, and D:** Medial canthal ligament injury. Manson classification.

TABLE 4.2	**Classification of Central Fragment (the Bone Bearing the Medial Canthal Ligament Insertion) Injury, and Incidence**		
		Unilateral	Bilateral
Type I	Single segment	50%	13%
Type II	Comminuted	44%	85%
Type III	Comminuted into canthal insertion	6%	2%

From Markowitz BL, Manson PN, Sargent L, et al. Management of the medial canthal tendon in nasoethmoid orbital fractures: the importance of the central fragment in classification and treatment. *Plast Reconstr Surg.* 1991;87(5):843–853.

Imaging

CT shows impaction of the intraorbital contents with posterior telescoping of ethmoid air cells, nasal septal buckling, and intrasinus hemorrhage. Inferomedial orbital rim fracture with displacement of the central fragment indicates medial canthal ligament involvement (Fig. 4.9). Injuries may be unilateral or bilateral and of variable comminution depending on impact energy.

Low-energy injuries are exclusively unilateral with a single displaced inferomedial orbital rim fracture fragment. Moderate-energy NOE fractures are more common and are characterized by several fractures of the inferomedial orbital rim without fragmentation of the bony medial canthal ligament insertion. High-energy injuries disrupt the medial canthal ligament anchor and require more complex surgical repair. NOE fractures are often associated with LeFort II and III injuries and close attention should be paid to the pterygoid plates.

Clinical consequences include telecanthus, enophthalmos, ptosis, and lacrimal system obstruction. Associated cribriform plate fracture may result in anosmia, CSF leak, and pneumocephalus (Fig. 4.10). The latter can evolve into tension pneumocephalus after cardiopulmonary resuscitation efforts. Disruption of the sinus roof predisposes to intracranial nasogastric tube and Foley catheter (for control of posterior nasal bleeding) malposition (Fig. 4.11).

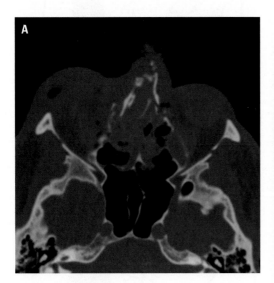

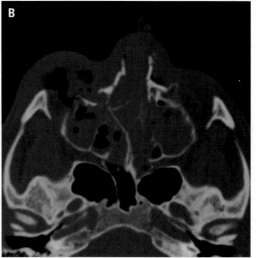

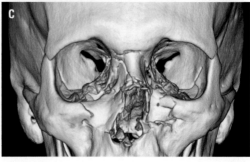

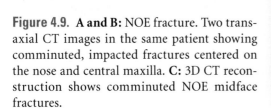

Figure 4.9. A and B: NOE fracture. Two transaxial CT images in the same patient showing comminuted, impacted fractures centered on the nose and central maxilla. **C:** 3D CT reconstruction shows comminuted NOE midface fractures.

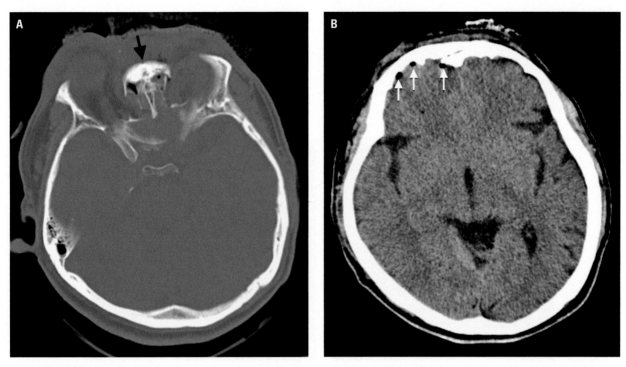

Figure 4.10. A and B: NOE fracture. **A:** Transaxial CT image shows comminuted and impacted NOE fractures at the level of the upper nasal bridge *(black arrow)*. Pneumocephalus *(white arrows* in **B)** from fracture of the cribriform plate.

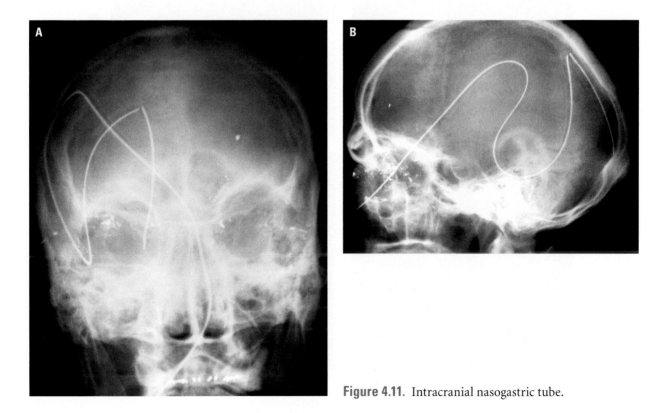

Figure 4.11. Intracranial nasogastric tube.

NASOLACRIMAL INJURIES

Anatomy

The nasolacrimal fossa and canal make up the bony lacrimal excretory system. The fossa originates in the medial orbital wall and is made up of the thick anterior lacrimal crest of the frontal process of the maxilla and the posterior lacrimal crest of the lacrimal bone. The nasolacrimal canal descends into the thinner nasal portion of the maxilla, terminating beneath the inferior turbinate (Fig. 4.12).

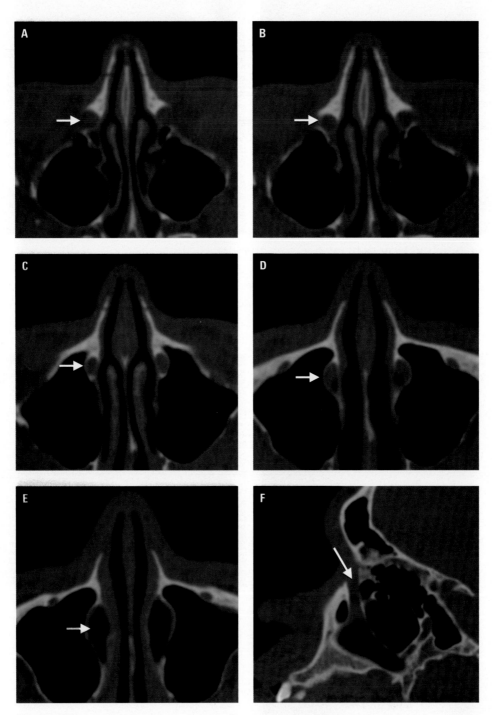

Figure 4.12. Nasolacrimal fossa and canal anatomy. Nasolacrimal fossa originates in the medial orbital wall *(arrow)* (**A**) and lies behind the thick anterior lacrimal crest of the frontal process of maxilla *(arrow)* (**B**). The nasolacrimal canal descends into the thin nasal portion of maxilla *(arrow)* (**C and D**) and terminates below the inferior turbinate *(arrow)* (**E**). Sagittal CT reformation (**F**) shows the entire course *(arrow)*.

The lacrimal drainage system, consisting of the nasolacrimal sac and duct, is protected within the bony fossa and canal, respectively.

Injuries and Imaging

Nasolacrimal injuries are anticipated with NOE fractures, but can occur in other injuries as well. Symptomatic lacrimal obstruction (epiphora and dacryocystitis) has been reported in 0.2% of nasal fractures, 4% of LeFort II and III fractures, and 21% of NOE fractures.

Unger studied the CT appearance of nasolacrimal injuries in 25 patients and found that all nasolacrimal fractures were associated with other facial fractures. Fractures limited to the stronger nasolacrimal fossa were less common than injuries combined with the fragile nasolacrimal canal. Canal fractures are mostly comminuted (Fig. 4.13) whereas fossa fractures are mostly avulsions in which the fossa remains intact but is separated from its normal attachments. The sac and duct normally contain either air or fluid and duct obstruction must be diagnosed clinically.

FRONTAL SINUS FRACTURES

Anatomy

Frontal sinus anatomy is variable—10% have a unilateral sinus, 5% a rudimentary sinus, and 4% have no sinus (Fig. 4.14). The anterior sinus wall is much thicker and stronger than the posterior wall and can tolerate up to 2,200 lb of force before fracturing. The dura and frontal lobes are immediately posterior to the sinus; the orbital roof is inferior and lateral. Inferomedially, the frontal sinus drains into the middle nasal meatus via the nasofrontal duct more commonly referred to as the nasofrontal outflow tract (NFOT) (Fig. 4.15).

Injuries

Frontal sinus fractures account for 5% to 15% of all craniomaxillofacial fractures and result from anterior upper facial impact. Frontal sinus fracture indicates high G-forces that propel the head and cervical spine into extension, often with severe associated intracranial injury and facial fractures. Management decisions depend on fracture type, neurologic status, CSF leak, posterior table fracture pattern, and NFOT injury.

NFOT integrity is the most critical determinant and a reliable sign of high energy transfer. Patients with frontal sinus fractures and NFOT injury have two to three times as many associated facial fractures, most commonly orbital roof and NOE fractures than patients with frontal sinus fracture alone. The incidence of cerebral injury with frontal sinus fracture rises from significant (31%) to striking (76%) when the NFOT is involved. Patients suffering frontal sinus fractures have a 25% overall mortality and frequently present in shock (52%) or coma (42%). Table 4.3 summarizes associated injuries based on integrity of the NFOT in 857 patients with frontal sinus fractures.

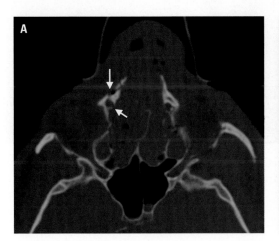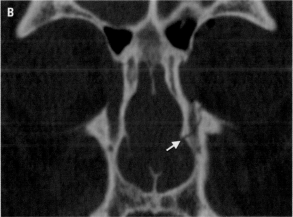

Figure 4.13. Nasolacrimal injuries. Transaxial CT image shows comminuted fractures across the right nasolacrimal fossa (*arrows*).

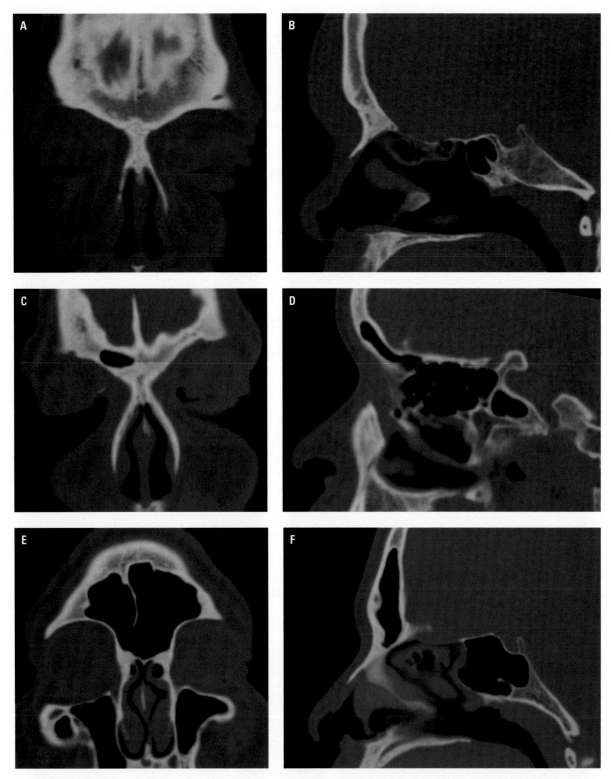

Figure 4.14. Frontal sinus variability. Coronal and sagittal CT reformations in patients with no frontal sinus (**A and B**), small unilateral frontal sinus (**C and D**), and larger bilateral frontal sinuses (**E and F**).

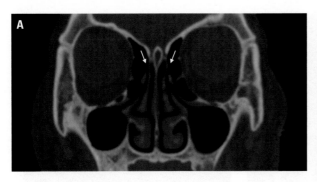

Figure 4.15. NFOT anatomy. **A:** Coronal CT reformation show the normal nasofrontal outflow tracts bilaterally *(arrows)*. **B:** Sagittal CT reformation depicts the outflow tract draining the frontal sinus (FS) in a different patient *(arrowheads)*.

Imaging

Frontal sinus fractures may involve the anterior table, the posterior table, or both (Figs. 4.16, 4.17). One-third are limited to the anterior table and half involve both anterior and posterior tables. Separation of fracture fragments by more than one table

TABLE 4.3	Associated Injuries in Frontal Sinus Fractures	
Injury	**NFOT Intact**	**NFOT Injury**
Intracranial	31%	76%
NOE	12%	31%
Orbital roof	13%	40%
Orbital wall	7%	13%
Orbital floor	2%	7%
Zygoma	8%	18%
LeFort	2%	17%
Mandible	3%	5%
Cervical spine	7%	14%
Upper extremity fracture	15%	25%
Lower extremity fracture	13%	23%
Pneumothorax	12%	24%
Abdominal	7%	13%

NFOT, nasofrontal outflow tract; NOE, naso-orbitoid-ethmoid. From Stanwix MG, Nam AJ, Manson PN, et al. Critical computed tomographic diagnostic criteria for frontal sinus fractures. *J Oral Maxillofac Surg.* 2010;68(11):2714–2722.

width constitutes displacement. NFOT injury occurs in 70% of cases (Table 4.4) and is indicated by (1) anatomic outflow tract obstruction, (2) frontal sinus floor fracture, and (3) medial anterior table fracture. A fracture fragment partially or entirely within the tract indicates outflow tract obstruction. Any of these features permits diagnosis of NFOT injury. MPRs aids in identification of the NFOT and are often necessary for comprehensive assessment (Fig. 4.18).

Isolated and undisplaced anterior table fractures require no operative fixation. Displaced posterior table fractures indicate that the dura has been breached and there is potential contiguity between the sinus and brain. Ninety-eight percent of displaced posterior table fractures are associated with NFOT injuries. Posterior table injuries require sinus obliteration or cranialization to prevent mucocele or mucopyocele formation. Cranialization is also necessary for persistent CSF leak and involves the stripping of mucosa, obliteration of the nasofrontal duct, and removal of posterior table fragments (Fig. 4.19). Complications of posterior table fractures can be life threatening and include meningitis, encephalitis, brain abscess, and cavernous sinus thrombosis.

ORBITAL TRAUMA

Anatomy

The orbit comprises seven bones: frontal, zygoma, maxilla, lacrimal, ethmoid, sphenoid, and palatine (Fig. 4.20). It is more practical, however, to consider the bony orbit as a square pyramid lying on

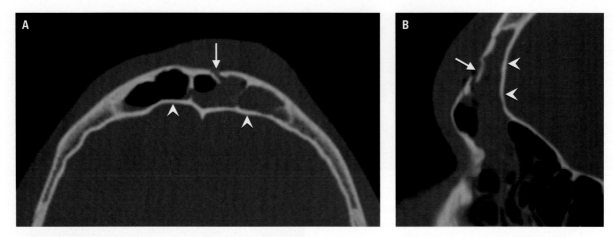

Figure 4.16. A,B: Frontal sinus fractures. Transaxial **(A)** and sagittal CT reformation **(B)** show fracture of the anterior table of the frontal sinus *(arrows)*, with partial sinus opacification with hemorrhage. The posterior table is intact *(arrowheads)*.

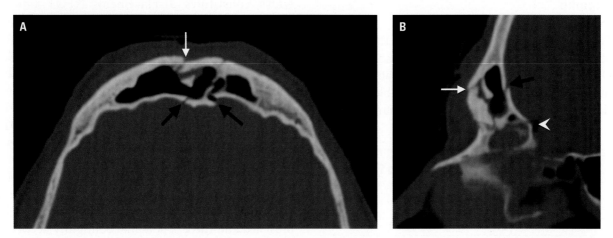

Figure 4.17. A and B: Frontal sinus fractures. Transaxial **(A)** and sagittal CT reformation **(B)** show fracture of the anterior table *(white arrow)* and posterior table *(black arrow)* of the frontal sinus. Pneumocephalus is present *(arrowhead)*.

TABLE 4.4	**Frontal Sinus Fracture Distribution and Incidence of Nasofrontal Outflow Tract Injury**			
Fracture Pattern	**NFOT Intact**	**NFOT Injury**	**Total**	**%**
Anterior wall, undisplaced	152	33	185	38.3
Anterior wall, displaced	35	108	143	
Posterior wall, undisplaced	14	17	31	6.9
Posterior wall, displaced	2	26	28	
Both walls, undisplaced	43	98	141	54.8
Both walls, displaced	5	324	329	
	251 (29.3%)	606 (70.7%)	857	

From Rodriguez ED, Stanwix MG, Nam AJ, et al. Twenty-six-year experience treating frontal sinus fractures: a novel algorithm based on anatomical fracture pattern and failure of conventional techniques. *Plast Reconstr Surg.* 2008;122(6):1850–1866.

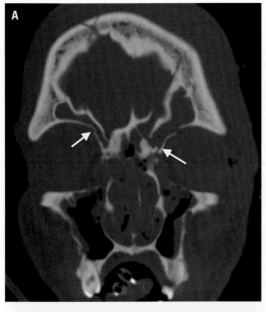

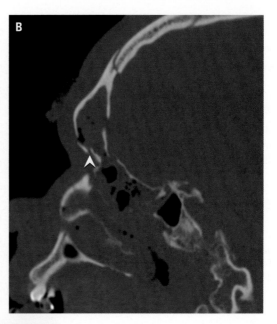

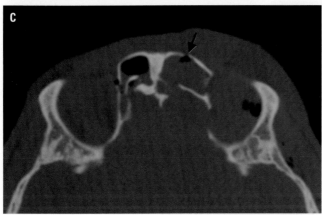

Figure 4.18. Nasofrontal outflow tract injury. Any one of the following features indicate NFOT injury: **A:** Anatomic outflow tract obstruction seen on coronal CT reformation with fracture fragments projecting into the outflow tract *(arrows)*. **B:** Frontal sinus floor fracture *(arrowhead)* seen on sagittal CT reformation. **C:** Medial anterior table fracture *(arrows)* seen on transaxial CT image.

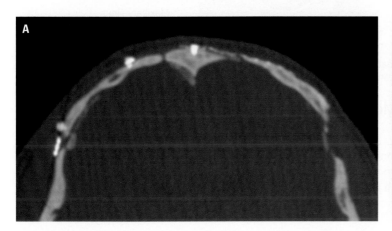

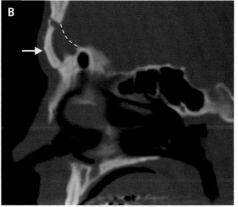

Figure 4.19. Cranialization after frontal sinus fractures of the anterior and posterior tables. **A:** Transaxial CT image shows reconstruction of anterior table with mesh and fixation screws. **B:** Sagittal CT reformation shows anterior reconstruction *(arrow)* and lack of posterior table *(dotted line)*; the former frontal sinus is now "cranialized."

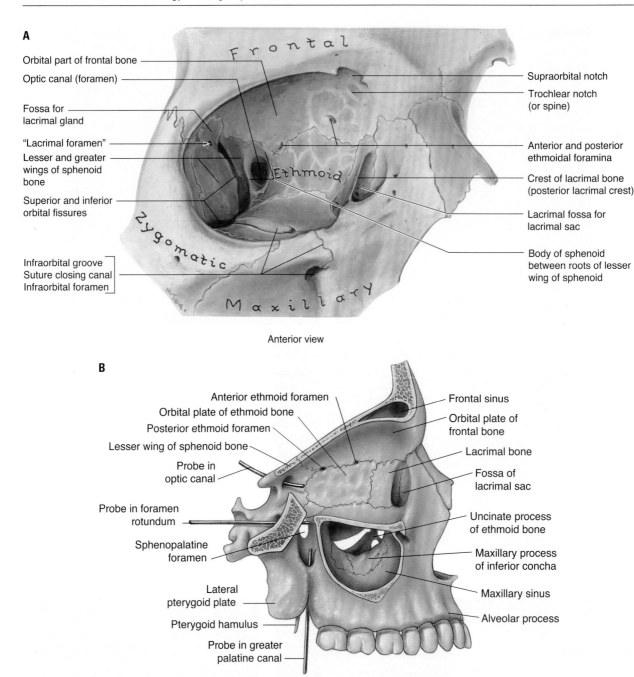

Figure 4.20. Bony orbit anatomy. A: Frontal view. B: Medial view (Panel A from Moore KL, Dalley AF II. *Clinical Oriented Anatomy.* 4th ed. Baltimore, MD: Lippincott Williams & Wilkins; 1999, with permission. Panel B from Anatomical Chart Co., with permission).

its side and bounded by a medial wall, orbital floor, lateral wall, and orbital roof (Fig. 4.21). The strong orbital rim serves to protect the thinner orbital walls.

The medial orbital walls are parallel to each other and separated by the paired ethmoid sinuses. Their anterior margin forms the thick nasolacrimal fossa, which is bounded by the anterior and posterior lacrimal crests, and houses the nasolacrimal sac. The greater portion of the medial wall comprises the lamina papyracea (Fig. 4.20B), so named on account of its paper-thin and delicate structure.

The orbital floor is made up of portions of the zygoma, maxilla, and palatine bones. It is the shortest of the four walls and terminates at the posterior margin of the maxilla rather than at the orbital apex. The orbital floor is also the roof of the maxillary sinus. Within the orbital floor, the infraorbital groove and canal transmit the infraorbital nerve (CN V$_2$), the infraorbital artery, and the infraorbital vein. Like the medial wall, the orbital floor is extremely thin—especially the portion medial to the infraorbital nerve—and is prone to fracture.

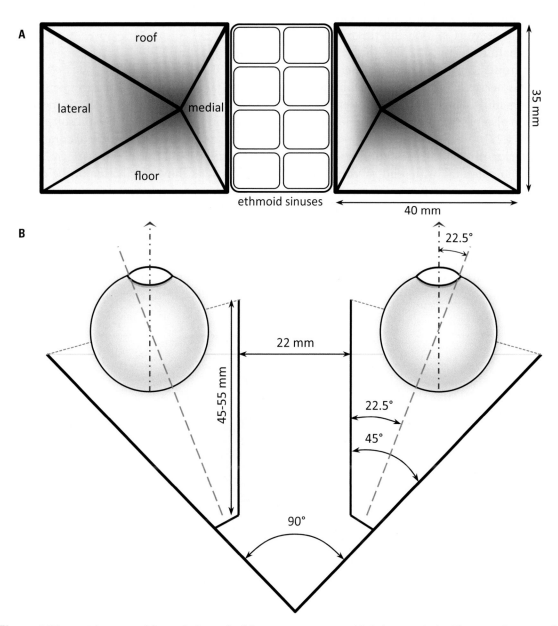

Figure 4.21. A: Diagram of frontal view of orbits as square pyramids lying on their sides. **B:** Diagram of horizontal section through the orbits. Medial walls are parallel, separated by ethmoid sinuses. Lateral walls diverge 45 degrees from midline. Orbital axis bisects the bony orbit at 22.5 degrees.

The greater wing of the sphenoid and the zygoma join to form the lateral orbital wall. It is the thickest of the four walls. The superiorly convex orbital roof is mainly composed of the relatively strong frontal bone with a small contribution from the lesser wing of sphenoid. It forms the lateral floor of the anterior cranial fossa.

The optic canal and superior orbital fissure connect the orbital apex to the intracranial cavity. The optic canal is 8 to 12 mm long and contains the optic nerve (CN II) and the ophthalmic artery. The superior orbital fissure communicates with the middle cranial fossa; separates the greater and lesser wings of the sphenoid; and transmits the superior and inferior divisions of the oculomotor nerve (CN III), the trochlear nerve (CN IV), the three branches of the ophthalmic nerve (CN V$_1$) (the nasociliary nerve, the frontal nerve, the lacrimal nerve), and the abducens nerve (CN VI). The orbital branch of the middle meningeal artery and the superior ophthalmic vein also pass through the superior orbital fissure (Fig. 4.22).

The inferior orbital fissure separates the orbital floor and lateral wall and is contiguous with the pterygopalatine fossa. Crossing the inferior orbital fissure are the infraorbital nerve (CN V$_2$), the zygomatic nerve (CN V$_2$), and the ascending branches from the pterygopalatine ganglion. Orbital apex injury indicates high energy transfer, often with severe associated facial and intracranial injuries.

Injuries

Orbital fractures may be isolated or associated with a more complex fracture pattern. Approximately 70% of patients with orbital fractures have concomitant injuries and up to 30% have associated ocular injuries. Ophthalmologic exam is essential and should be performed at initial evaluation.

Traumatic optic neuropathy (TON) affects 5% of patients with severe facial trauma. Symptoms range from diminished color perception to complete vision loss. Globe or optic nerve injury may be direct, via bone fragments for example, or indirect. Recovery for those presenting with blindness is unlikely.

Imaging

Transaxial and coronal CT images demonstrate paranasal sinus hemorrhage, orbital and facial fractures, and any associated orbital soft tissue injury. Coronal reconstructions allow accurate evaluation of the thin orbital floor (Figs. 4.2C, 4.23A). Sagittal reformations show the incline of the orbital floor, the anteroposterior extent and the depth of any defect and are useful for surgical planning. Because the orbital axis is oblique, reconstructions parallel to the optic nerve are optimal (Figs. 4.2D, 4.23D). The globe, lens, optic nerve, and extraocular muscles are best evaluated using soft tissue windows and reconstruction algorithm (Figs. 4.23B, 4.23D).

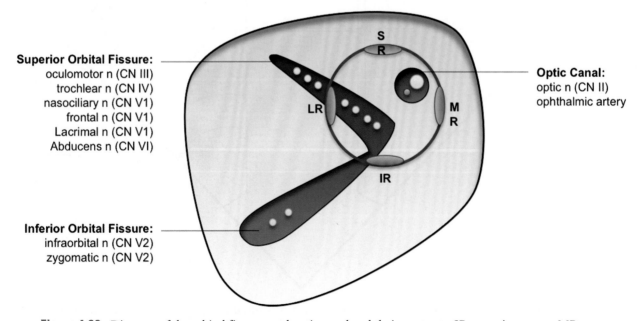

Superior Orbital Fissure:
oculomotor n (CN III)
trochlear n (CN IV)
nasociliary n (CN V1)
frontal n (CN V1)
Lacrimal n (CN V1)
Abducens n (CN VI)

Optic Canal:
optic n (CN II)
ophthalmic artery

Inferior Orbital Fissure:
infraorbital n (CN V2)
zygomatic n (CN V2)

Figure 4.22. Diagram of the orbital fissures and optic canal and their contents. SR, superior rectus; MR, medial rectus; IR, inferior rectus; and LR, lateral rectus.

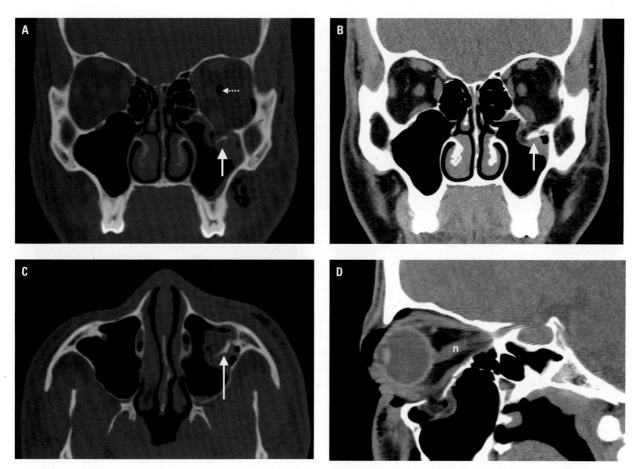

Figure 4.23. Orbital floor blow-out fracture. Coronal CT reformation in bone (**A**) and soft tissue (**B**) windows shows fracture of the left orbital floor *(arrows)*. Small amount of orbital fat herniates across the floor defect. Orbital emphysema from maxillary sinus air escaping into the orbit *(small dotted arrow)*. Transaxial CT image (**C**) shows the "free fragment" sign *(long arrow)*. Oblique sagittal CT reformation (**D**) along the plane of the optic nerve *(n)* optimally shows the anteroposterior extent of the fracture for surgical planning.

BLOW-OUT FRACTURES

The term "blow-out" fracture was coined in 1957 by Smith and Regan to describe an orbital floor fracture with inferior rectus muscle entrapment. This injury results from blunt trauma with sudden increase in intraorbital pressure, orbital wall fracture, and displacement of the bony fragment away from the orbit (Figs. 4.23, 4.24). Unrepaired, the resultant increase in orbital volume can lead to functional and cosmetic problems.

Blow-out fractures are designated as "pure" if the orbital rim remains intact. Fracture may occur with or without herniation of intraorbital fat or extraocular muscles. Large floor defects allow the globe to sink posteriorly and inferiorly, known as enophthalmos. Herniated orbital rectus muscles may become entrapped on a free edge of the floor

or medial wall causing diplopia. Because the medial and inferior orbital walls communicate with the ethmoid and maxillary sinuses, orbital emphysema is frequently associated with blow-out fractures.

The mechanism of injury responsible for the blow-out fracture has been the subject of some debate. Three main proposals exist: the hydraulic theory, the bone conduction theory, and the globe-to-wall theory.

Smith and Regan created orbital floor blow-out fractures by striking a hurling ball placed over the orbital rim of cadaver skulls with a hammer, leaving the orbital rim intact. The transmitted force was said to cause compression of the intraorbital contents, applying outward pressure on the orbital walls. This hydraulic force would cause the weakest wall to fracture.

The bone conduction theory states that direct impact to the inferior orbital rim would cause the

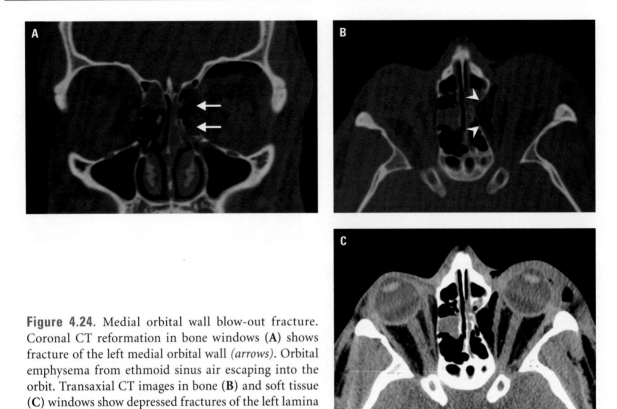

Figure 4.24. Medial orbital wall blow-out fracture. Coronal CT reformation in bone windows (**A**) shows fracture of the left medial orbital wall *(arrows)*. Orbital emphysema from ethmoid sinus air escaping into the orbit. Transaxial CT images in bone (**B**) and soft tissue (**C**) windows show depressed fractures of the left lamina papyracea of the medial orbital wall.

thin orbital floor to fracture. This energy transmission was shown using high-speed cineradiography in 1974 by Fujino et al. where elastic motion of the inferior orbital rim propagated to buckle and crack the orbital floor while the rim returned to its normal position. This theory does not explain, however, the commonly seen medial orbital blow-out fracture.

The globe-to-wall theory, first proposed by Pfeiffer in 1943, suggests that retropulsion of an impacted globe could strike the orbital floor or medial wall, causing fracture by direct globe-to-wall contact. Erling et al. have added support to this theory using CT imaging of the fracture defects resembling the size and shape or "footprints" of the globe (Fig. 4.25).

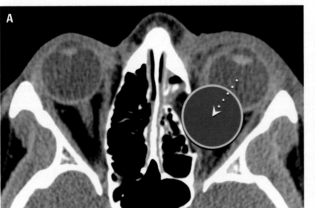
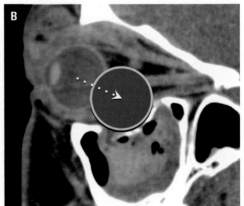

Figure 4.25. Globe-to-wall theory. Fracture of the medial orbital wall (**A**) and orbital floor (**B**) may be caused by direct impact of retropulsed globe *(circles)* creating fracture defects resembling the "footprints" of the globe.

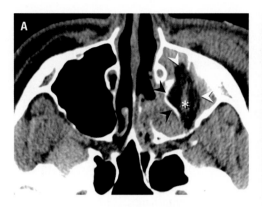
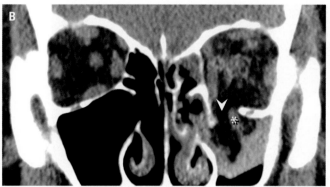

Figure 4.26. Orbital floor blow-out fracture. Herniation of orbital fat *(white arrowheads)* and the inferior rectus muscle *(asterisk)* into the left maxillary sinus from large orbital floor fracture on transaxial (**A**) and coronal CT reformation (**B**). "Free fragment" sign in maxillary sinus *(black arrowheads)*.

It is very likely that all three theories play a role because one type does not preclude another from either existing. In fact, a broad impact to the entire orbital rim by an object larger than the orbit best supports the hydraulic theory, whereas a direct focal blow to the inferior rim could certainly result in buckling of the orbital floor. Finally, with a direct globe impact, the globe-to-wall contact theory can explain many of the resultant CT findings.

Transverse CT images reveal a free fragment in the maxillary sinus with depressed or displaced orbital floor fractures known as the "free fragment" sign (Figs. 4.23C, 4.26A). Coronal CT reformations readily reveal the orbital floor fracture and can identify herniation (Fig. 4.26B). The diagnosis of entrapment may be suspected on CT by kinking of the muscle (Fig. 4.27A) or isolation of the inferior rectus muscle by a trapdoor floor fracture, more commonly seen in children and is a surgical emergency (Fig. 4.27B).

In the acute setting, hemorrhage into the adjacent sinus (maxillary for floor blow-out fractures, and ethmoid for medial blow-out fractures) is present; the lack of hemorrhage indicates a remote injury (Fig. 4.28).

BLOW-IN FRACTURES

The blow-in fracture refers to an orbital fracture with an inwardly displaced orbital fragment, decreased orbital volume, and associated proptosis. Like blow-out fractures, these are termed "pure" if the orbital rim is intact (very uncommon), or "impure" if the rim is fractured. This injury results from high energy transfer and is rarely isolated (Table 4.5).

Fractures of the orbital rim typically occur at sutural junctions and are classified as superior, inferolateral, and inferomedial. Blow-in fractures of the superior orbital rim are usually associated with frontal sinus fractures and severe head injuries (Figs. 4.29, 4.30). Inferolateral rim blow-in fractures

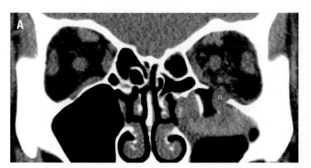
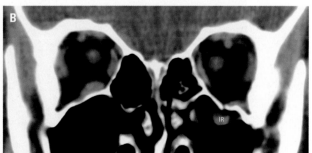

Figure 4.27. Orbital floor blow-out fracture with entrapment. **A:** Coronal CT reformation with thickened inferior rectus (IR) muscle abutting the free edge of the orbital floor fracture fragment, raising concern for entrapment. **B:** Coronal CT reformation shows isolation of the inferior rectus (IR) muscle in the maxillary sinus by a trapdoor orbital floor fracture—a surgical emergency to prevent muscle ischemia.

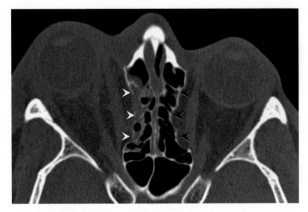

Figure 4.28. Medial orbital wall blow-out fractures. Transaxial CT image shows bilateral medial orbital wall fractures, acute on the right *(white arrowheads)* with adjacent intrasinus hemorrhage as compared to remote on the left *(black arrowheads)* lacking intrasinus hemorrhage.

TABLE	4.5	Injuries Associated with Blow-In Fractures of the Orbit	
Injury			**Incidence (%)**
Ocular injury	Globe rupture		12
	Optic nerve injury		2
	Superior orbital fissure syndrome		10
Other facial fractures			73
Head injury			44

From Antonyshyn O, Gruss JS, Kassel EE. Blow-in fractures of the orbit. *Plast Reconstr Surg.* 1989;84(1):10–20.

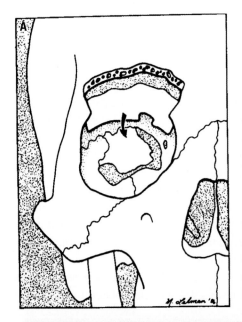

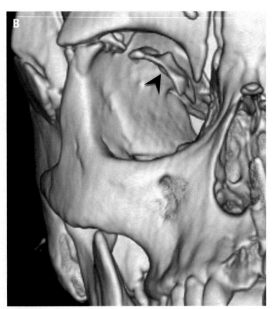

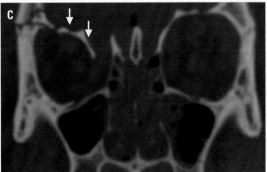

Figure 4.29. Superior orbital rim blow-in fracture. Illustration **(A)** and 3D CT reconstruction **(B)** show fracture of the superior orbital rim and internally depressed orbital roof fracture fragment *(arrowhead)*. **C:** Coronal CT reformation shows depression of orbital roof fracture fragment into the orbit *(arrows)* (Panel A from Antonyshyn OM, Gruss JS, Kassel EE. Blow-in fractures of the orbit. *Plast Reconstr Surg.* 1989;84(1):10–20, with permission).

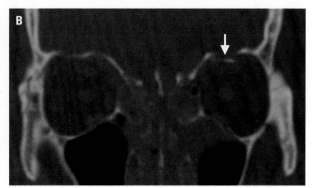

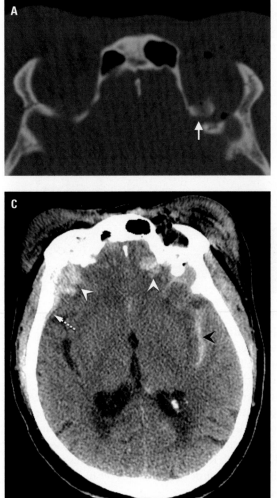

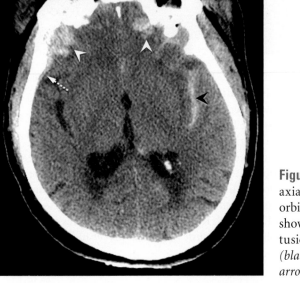

Figure 4.30. Blow-in fracture of the orbital roof. Transaxial (**A**) and coronal CT reformation (**B**) show depressed orbital roof fracture fragment *(arrows)*. **C:** CT head image shows associated intracranial injuries with frontal contusions *(white arrowheads)*, subarachnoid hemorrhage *(black arrowheads)*, and thin subdural hematoma *(dashed arrow)*.

show medial displacement of the zygoma separated at the zygomaticofrontal and zygomaticomaxillary sutures (Fig. 4.31). Inferomedial fractures occur as the medial orbital rim is laterally displaced from the nasofrontal and zygomaticomaxillary sutures, as may be seen with an NOE fracture (Fig. 4.32).

Inwardly displaced fracture fragments may also impinge on the intraorbital soft tissues. Fractures extending to the orbital apex may injure the optic nerve in several ways, including direct penetration by bony fragments, hemorrhage into the sheath, avulsion from the posterior globe, and ischemia from increased intraorbital pressure. Ocular injuries are reported in 14% to 29% of cases of orbital blow-in fractures.

Associated injuries are common, including NOE, zygomaticomaxillary complex (ZMC) fractures, and LeFort II and III fractures. Soft tissue injury to the globe, optic nerve, extraocular muscles, and, in particular, the brain should be sought. On CT, transaxial images are best for assessing proptosis as well as medial and lateral orbital fractures (Fig. 4.31C). Coronal and sagittal MPRs show superior orbital rim and orbital roof fractures to advantage (Figs. 4.29C, 4.30B).

BLOW-UP FRACTURES

Essentially a superior blow-out fracture, the blow-up fracture causes cranial displacement of the orbital roof, increasing orbital volume. Fractures typically involve the superior orbital rim, and intracranial injury should be suspected. The blow-up fracture is

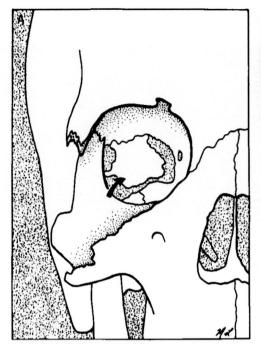

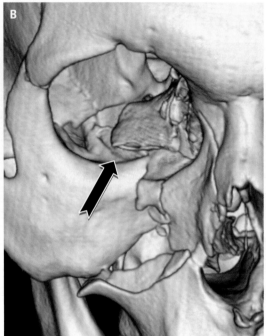

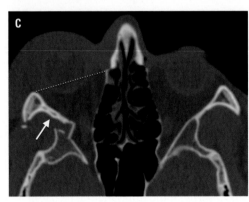

Figure 4.31. Inferolateral rim blow-in fracture. **A:** Illustration and 3D CT reconstruction (**B**) show inferolateral blow-in fractures *(black arrows)*. **C:** Transaxial CT shows medially displaced lateral orbital wall fractures *(white arrow)* causing decreased intraorbital volume and traumatic exophthalmos with more than 50% of the globe beyond a line between medial and lateral orbital rims *(dotted line)* (Panel A from Antonyshyn OM, Gruss JS, Kassel EE. Blow-in fractures of the orbit. *Plast Reconstr Surg.* 1989;84(1):10–20, with permission).

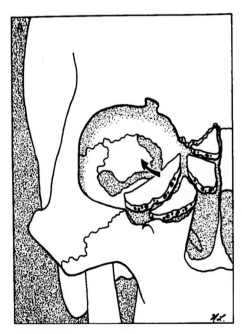

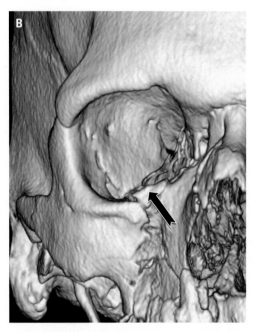

Figure 4.32. Inferomedial rim blow-in fracture. **A:** Illustration and 3D CT reconstruction (**B**) show inferomedial orbital rim blow-in fractures *(black arrows)* (Panel A from Antonyshyn OM, Gruss JS, Kassel EE. Blow-in fractures of the orbit. *Plast Reconstr Surg.* 1989;84(1):10–20, with permission).

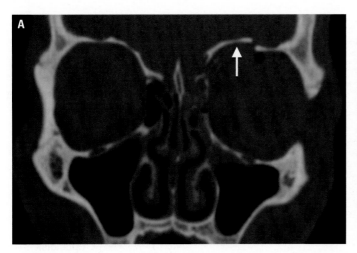
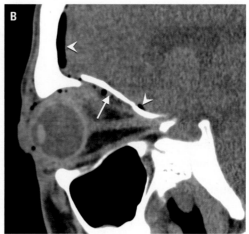

Figure 4.33. Blow-up fracture. Coronal (**A**) and oblique sagittal (**B**) CT reformations show cranially displaced orbital roof fracture *(arrows)* with pneumocephalus *(arrowheads)*.

more likely to be isolated to the orbital roof when a large frontal sinus is present. Coronal CT MPRs best delineate fracture location, extent, and displacement, as well as associated intracranial injury (Fig. 4.33).

GLOBE INJURY

Ocular injuries are common, making up 3% of visits to US emergency rooms. The clinical assessment of visual acuity and ocular mobility are crucial in the trauma patient and should be performed at the earliest possible opportunity. Emergent surgical management is indicated for intraorbital or intraocular foreign bodies, direct ocular injury, intraorbital compressive hematoma, or muscle entrapment. CT assesses the integrity of the bony orbit and any injury to the orbital soft tissues. Although MRI is more sensitive to subtle injuries of the globe and optic nerve, it can only be performed after intracranial and intraorbital ferromagnetic foreign bodies have been excluded on CT.

Anatomy

The normal globe is largely spherical with a diameter of 24 mm with a bulge corresponding to the anterior segment. The lens is anchored to the sclera by radially oriented zonular fibers, and separates the anterior segment from the posterior segment of the globe. The small anterior segment is subdivided by the iris into anterior and posterior chambers. Aqueous humor fills the anterior segment, whereas the vitreous humor occupies the posterior segment (Fig. 4.34).

Normally, half the globe lies behind a line drawn between the anterior margin of the lateral and medial walls on transaxial CT in the mid-orbital plane. In exophthalmos, more than half the globe lies anterior to this line. In the setting of trauma, the position of the globe within the orbit should be carefully examined. Traumatic exophthalmos is seen with orbital injuries that decrease orbital volume such as blow-in fractures (Fig. 4.31C), retrobulbar hematomas, and foreign bodies. Enophthalmos can be seen in injuries that increase orbital volume such as blow-out fractures.

Intraorbital Foreign Bodies

Localization of any intraocular or intraorbital foreign body is critically important in the trauma setting. CT is considered the gold standard for this purpose and can determine whether a foreign body is intraocular (Fig. 4.35), extraocular (Figs. 4.36, 4.37), or intrascleral. Size and density determine foreign body detectability on CT. Metallic foreign bodies smaller than 1 mm can be detected by CT, aided by the associated streak artifacts produced. Dry wood and plastic are hypodense on CT, similar to air and fat, respectively. Geometric margins are clues to wood foreign bodies so they are not mistaken for air. A major concern is whether an intraorbital foreign body is displaced into, or could migrate to the cranial vault with increased morbidity and mortality.

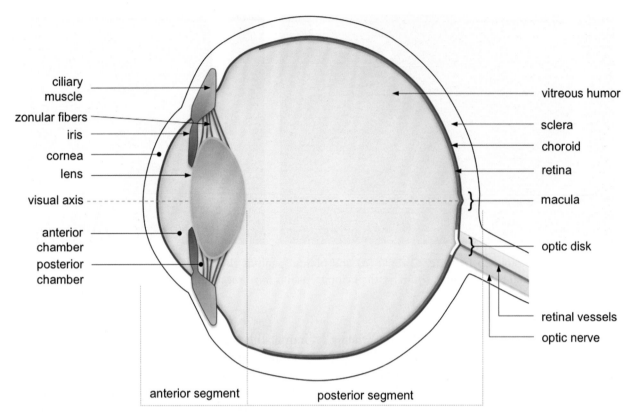

Figure 4.34. Globe anatomy.

Globe Rupture

Globe rupture, also referred to as open-globe injury, results from extrusion of the vitreous following perforation of the sclera, facilitated by the pressure gradient between intraocular (15 mm Hg) and intraorbital (5 mm Hg) compartments. Globe

rupture is seen on CT as an abnormal globe contour, particularly posterior flattening, and has been referred to as the "flat tire" or "mushroom" sign (Fig. 4.38). Intraocular air and intraocular foreign bodies are also signs of an open-globe injury. Globe hemorrhage may be intravitreous (Fig. 4.39) or subscleral or subretinal (Fig. 4.40) in location.

Anterior Chamber Injuries

Corneal lacerations and traumatic hyphema are anterior chamber injuries; and although best evaluated by direct inspection, it may be visible on CT. Corneal lacerations often result from penetrating injuries and result in a flattening of the anterior chamber. Traumatic hyphema may be seen as high attenuation blood within the anterior chamber in front of the iris. When upright, a blood-fluid level is readily seen.

Lens Injury

Injuries of the lens include dislocation, subluxation, and traumatic cataract. With complete dislocation, the lens lies along the dependent retina

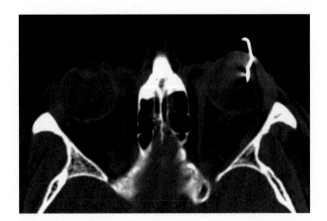

Figure 4.35. Intraocular foreign body. Transaxial CT images in a construction worker who sustained a staple gun injury with the staple penetrating the left globe.

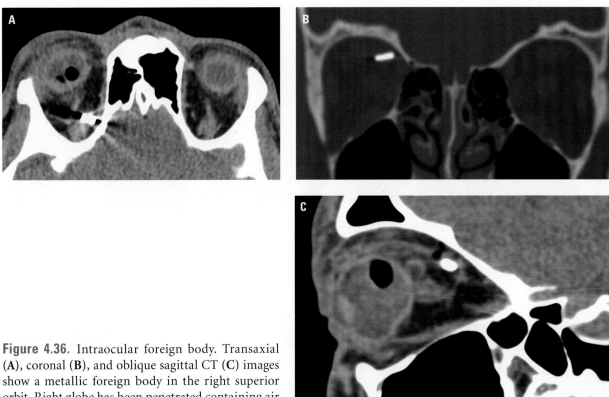

Figure 4.36. Intraocular foreign body. Transaxial (**A**), coronal (**B**), and oblique sagittal CT (**C**) images show a metallic foreign body in the right superior orbit. Right globe has been penetrated containing air and small amount of hemorrhage.

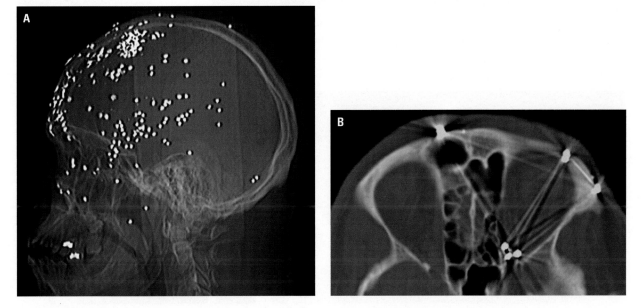

Figure 4.37. Intraorbital foreign bodies. Scout (**A**) and transaxial CT (**B**) images post shotgun injury with numerous pellets to the patient's head and face with three pellets at the left orbital apex.

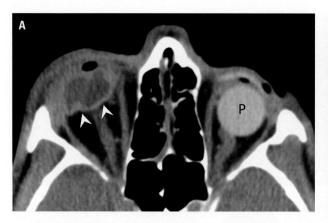
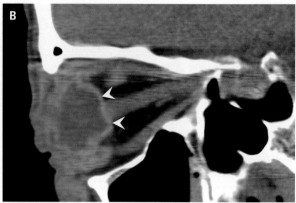

Figure 4.38. Globe rupture. Transaxial (**A**) and oblique sagittal CT reformation (**B**) of patient who sustained acute right globe rupture in an altercation. Note the posterior flattening of the globe referred to as the "flat tire" sign *(arrowheads)*. Left globe prosthesis *(P)* from prior left globe rupture in an altercation. Patient is now blind.

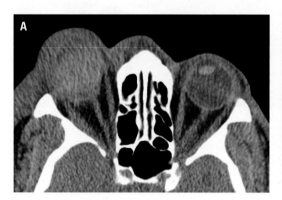
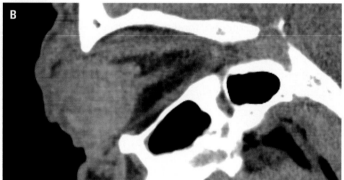

Figure 4.39. Globe hemorrhage. Transaxial (**A**) and oblique sagittal CT reformation (**B**) show right periorbital swelling with hyperdense globe representing intravitreous globe hemorrhage.

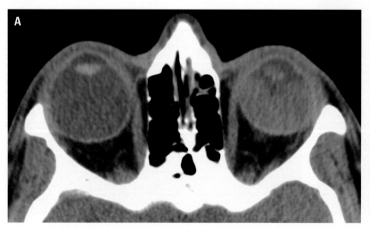
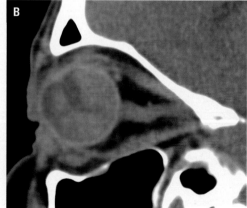

Figure 4.40. Globe hemorrhage. Transaxial (**A**) and oblique sagittal CT reformation (**B**) show left subretinal hemorrhage and lens subluxation.

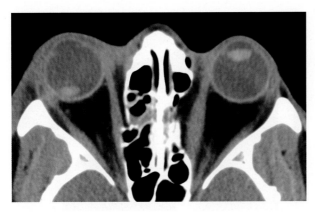

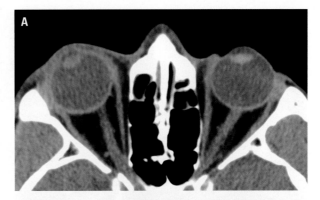

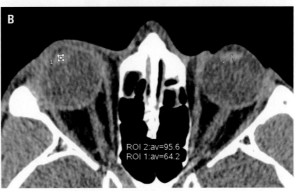

Figure 4.41. Lens dislocation. Transaxial CT image shows dislocation of the right lens, lying dependently within the globe. Old left medial orbital fracture is present.

(Fig. 4.41). When the zonular fibers supporting the lens are only partially torn, the lens may only be subluxed and can appear vertically oriented, supported anteriorly on one side (Fig. 4.42). Traumatic cataract results from acute lenticular

Figure 4.43. Traumatic cataract. Transaxial CT image (**A**) shows a relatively hypodense right lens on the injured side. Density measurements (**B**) show more than 30 Hounsfield unit (HU) difference between the right and left lenses, diagnostic of a right traumatic cataract.

edema. On CT, the affected lens is hypodense relative to the uninjured contralateral one (Fig. 4.43).

Optic Nerve Injury

TON may be caused by direct or indirect optic nerve injury. Direct injuries are uncommon; usually the result of a displaced bone fragment or foreign body that penetrates the optic nerve and close attention should be paid to the orbital apex and optic canal. More commonly, optic neuropathy is caused by global compression or ischemia of the optic nerve from intraorbital hematoma and attendant-increased intraorbital pressure. Retrobulbar hemorrhage encircles the insertion of the optic nerve (Fig. 4.44) and may cause vision loss by compression and occlusion of the central retinal artery. If CT does not reveal the etiology for a patient with optic nerve injury and there are no contraindications to MRI, high-resolution T2-weighted images are best able to identify signal changes in the nerve.

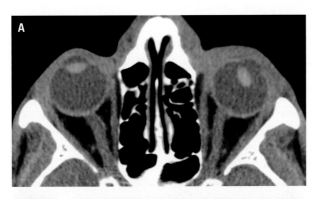

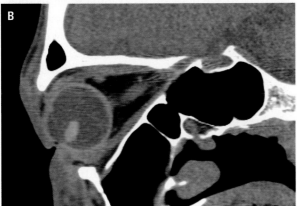

Figure 4.42. Lens subluxation. Transaxial (**A**) and oblique sagittal CT reformation (**B**) show subluxation of the left lens, with the superolateral zonular fibers torn.

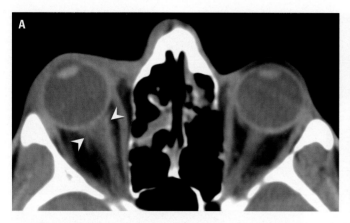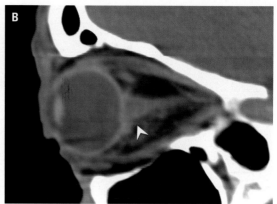

Figure 4.44. Retrobulbar hematoma. Transaxial (**A**) and oblique sagittal CT reformation (**B**) show hemorrhage at the insertion of the right optic nerve *(arrowheads)*. Note the normal, distinct, insertion on the left.

ZYGOMA FRACTURES

Anatomy

The zygoma forms the malar eminence and defines the anterolateral cheek projection. It is a thick, strong bone and forms the core of the zygomaticomaxillary vertical buttress. The zygoma is attached to the facial skeleton at several sutures and these are prone to fracture: the frontal bone (zygomaticofrontal suture), the maxilla (zygomaticomaxillary suture), the arch of the temporal bone (zygomaticotemporal suture), and the greater wing of sphenoid (zygomaticosphenoid suture) (Fig. 4.45). Because the zygoma forms a portion of the lateral orbital wall and floor, orbital fractures are a frequent component of zygoma fractures. Additionally, fracture across the infraorbital canal may injure the infraorbital nerve with consequent malar paresthesia.

The temporoparietal fascia and the origin of the masseter muscle attach to the zygoma, and tension caused by contraction of the masseter causes deformation and rotation of the fractured zygomatic arch.

Fractures

The term *zygomaticomaxillary complex* (ZMC) fracture replaces the former misnomer "tripod" and "tetrapod" terms. The fracture complex is a spectrum of injuries classified by impact energy. Low-energy injuries lead to isolated arch fractures (Fig. 4.46). Moderate-energy forces produce the classic ZMC pattern, which results from an anterolateral impact to the cheek. The zygoma is separated from the face along its sutural attachments, but the relatively strong body of the zygoma remains intact (Fig. 4.47). High-energy impacts produce comminution (Fig. 4.48) and are often associated with other craniofacial fractures.

Some surgeons refer to these injuries as orbitozygomatic fractures stressing the importance of associated orbital involvement. Lateral orbital fractures may be displaced into the orbit, reducing orbital volume and produce acute traumatic exophthalmos (Fig. 4.31C). Alternatively, lateral displacement of the lateral orbital wall and fractures of the orbital floor result in orbital volume expansion with resultant enophthalmos.

Clinically, patients exhibit periorbital swelling, ecchymosis, palpable step-off deformities along the lateral and inferior orbital rims, infraorbital numbness, abnormal globe position, and trismus.

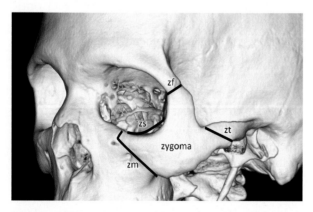

Figure 4.45. Zygoma anatomy. Four attachments of the zygoma are the frontal bone (*zf*, zygomaticofrontal suture), the temporal bone (*zt*, zygomaticotemporal suture), the maxilla (*zm*, zygomaticomaxillary suture), and the sphenoid (*zs*, zygomaticosphenoid suture).

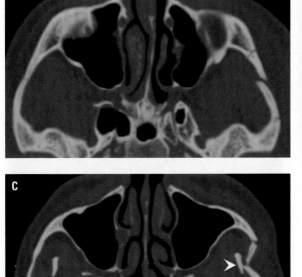

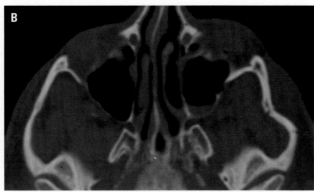

Figure 4.46. Zygomatic arch fractures. Transaxial CT images showing comminuted, nondepressed left zygomatic arch fracture (**A**); comminuted, depressed left zygomatic arch fracture (**B**); and comminuted, depressed left arch fracture abutting the coronoid process of the mandible *(arrowhead* in **C**). (Part C from Mehta N, Butala P, Bernstein MP. The imaging of maxillofacial trauma and its pertinence to surgical intervention. *Radiol Clin North Am.* 2012;50(1):43–57, with permission).

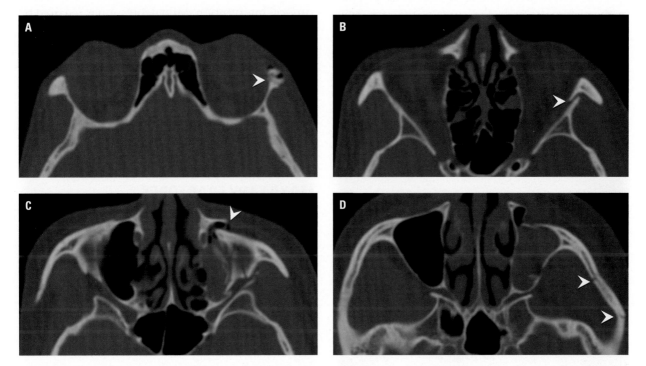

Figure 4.47. ZMC fracture. Serial transaxial CT images show fractures of the zygomaticofrontal suture (**A**), the lateral orbital wall (zygomaticosphenoid suture) (**B**), the maxilla (zygomaticomaxillary suture) (**C**), and the zygomatic arch (zygomaticotemporal suture) (**D**). *(continued)*

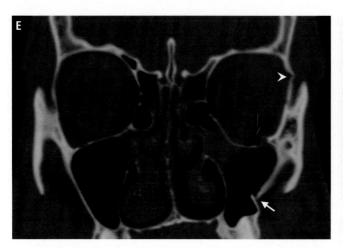
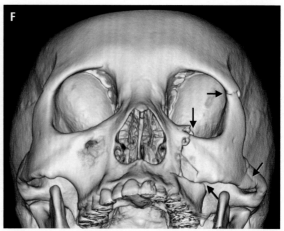

Figure 4.47. *(continued)* Coronal CT reformation (**E**) shows fractures at the ZF suture *(arrowhead)*, the orbital floor (ZS suture, *black arrow*), and maxilla (ZM suture, *white arrow*). **F:** 3D CT reconstruction in Waters' projection shows the classic ZMC fracture pattern.

Imaging

Transverse, coronal, oblique sagittal, and 3D CT images elegantly display ZMC fractures (Figs. 4.47, 4.48). Transverse imaging is ideally suited to identify the direction and displacement of lateral orbital wall fractures. Careful attention should also be paid to the zygomatic arch. Fractures of the arch may be subtle, but any acute angulation in the presence of other ZMC fracture lines or swelling should be regarded as an undisplaced arch fracture. Coronal reformations are essential for orbital floor evaluation, a component of all classic ZMC fractures by definition (Fig. 4.47E). Coronal images also best display fracture at the zygomaticofrontal suture. Oblique sagittal imaging is particularly useful in evaluation of orbital floor fracture depth and depression (Fig. 4.23D). 3D reconstructions allow the surgeon to understand the degree of displacement and rotation and aid in surgical planning.

Nondepressed isolated arch fractures require no surgical intervention. Mild depression is repaired by a simple surgical elevation procedure. Comminuted fractures are frequently deformed by pull from the masseter and require open reduction. Severe collapse and depression of the arch may impede normal motion of the coronoid process of the mandible as it rotates upward, preventing closure of the mouth (Fig. 4.46C).

MAXILLARY FRACTURES

Anatomy

The paired maxillae occupy the central midface, house the upper teeth by way of the alveolus, and attach to the zygomatic bones laterally. Along with the portions of the frontal, pterygoid, and zygomatic bones, they form buttresses that support the integrity of the midface. The strongest buttresses are vertically oriented, developed as a response to the actions of the muscles of mastication. The weaker, horizontal buttresses provide secondary support and play an important role in resistance to trauma.

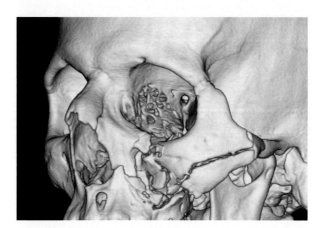

Figure 4.48. ZMC fracture. 3D CT reconstruction shows a higher energy ZMC fracture with comminution of the zygoma body in addition to fracture across the sutures.

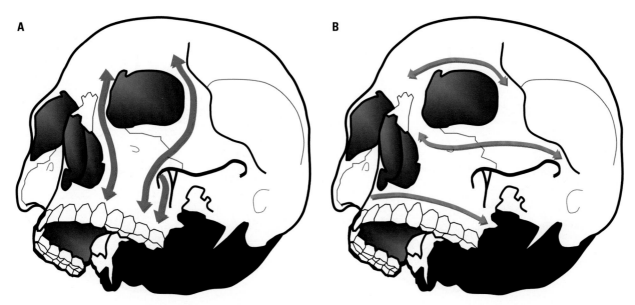

Figure 4.49. Maxillary buttresses. **A:** Vertical buttresses are represented by *thick red arrows*. From medial to lateral, these are the nasofrontal, zygomatic, and pterygomaxillary buttresses. **B:** Horizontal buttresses are represented by *thinner orange arrows*.

The three vertical buttresses of the maxilla are outlined in Figure 4.49. From medial to lateral, they are the nasofrontal, zygomatic, and pterygomaxillary buttresses. The nasomaxillary (also referred to as the nasofrontal or medial) buttress lies along the lateral nasal margin. It extends caudally to the anteromedial maxillary alveolus, and cranially along the medial orbital rim to the medial frontal bone. The lateral zygomatic buttress extends along the lateral orbital margin from the frontal bone caudally to the maxillary alveolus above the first molar. A lateral projection of the zygomaticomaxillary buttress extends to the zygomatic arch. The posterior pterygomaxillary buttress extends vertically from the posterior maxillary alveolus to the cranial base via the pterygoid plates of the sphenoid bone.

The horizontal buttress system includes the supraorbital and infraorbital rims, the inferior nasal aperture, the alveolus, and the palate, each of which provide support to the face by cross-linking the vertical buttresses. Together, they form a bony framework that encloses and protects the orbit, nasal cavity, and oral cavity.

LEFORT FRACTURES

In 1901, Rene LeFort described the "great lines of weakness of the face" after inflicting blows to cadaver heads. His initial descriptions outlined symmetric midface fracture patterns, all of which involved the pterygoid plates. In clinical practice, most midface fractures are asymmetric, and each side can be described as a separate hemi-LeFort fracture to simplify communication between radiologists and surgeons.

The horizontal LeFort I fracture results from direct frontal impact to the upper jaw and separates the palate and maxillary alveolus from the remainder of the facial skeleton. LeFort I fractures traverse the floor of the maxillary sinus, piriform apertures, and lower nasal septum, extending posteriorly through the pterygoid plates (Fig. 4.50A). Clinically, they result in malocclusion with a free-floating hard palate.

The LeFort II fracture is an oblique coronal fracture tilted anteriorly from inferior to posterior. It results from a direct frontal impact to the central midface and separates the nasal walls, cavity, and hard palate from the orbits and cranium. The fracture crosses the zygomaticomaxillary sutures, disrupts the inferomedial orbital rims, and separates the upper nasal bones from the frontal bone (Fig. 4.50B). As in all LeFort fractures, it involves the pterygoid plates posteriorly.

The LeFort III fracture represents complete craniofacial disjunction, separating the entire facial skeleton from the cranium by fracturing the nasofrontal suture, the medial and lateral orbital walls, and separating the zygomaticofrontal sutures and

A

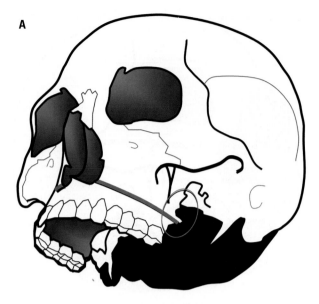

B

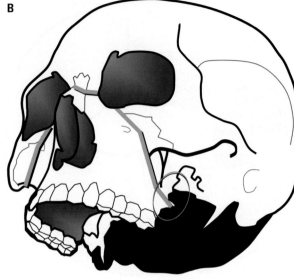

C

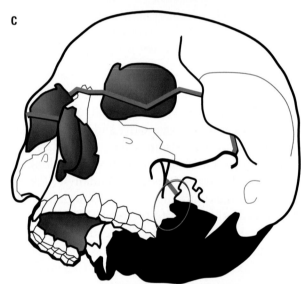

Figure 4.50. LeFort maxillary fracture patterns. **A:** LeFort I *(blue lines)* fracture is horizontal, above the alveolus, traversing the floor of the maxillary sinus, piriform apertures, and lower nasal septum, terminating through the pterygoid plates *(oval)*. **B:** LeFort II *(green lines)* fracture is "pyramidal" crossing the zygomaticomaxillary sutures, fracturing the inferior orbital rims medially, and traversing the nasofrontal junction. Posteriorly, the fracture involves the pterygoid plates *(oval)*. **C:** LeFort III *(red lines)* fracture is horizontal, fracturing the nasofrontal suture, crossing the medial and lateral orbital walls, separating the zygomaticofrontal sutures and zygomatic arches, and terminating through the pterygoid plates *(oval)*.

zygomatic arches as well as the pterygoid plates (Fig. 4.50C).

LeFort fractures typically disrupt the facial buttresses and comminute the more fragile posterior bones, causing both functional impairment and cosmetic deformities. NOE, zygomatic, mandibular, and cranial fractures are commonly associated injuries.

The surgical approach necessary to correct these injuries is complex. Portions of the facial skeleton may be displaced posteriorly, compressed vertically, and widened laterally, all of which can disrupt function. Concurrent fractures of the hard palate, dentoalveolar units, and mandible will result in malocclusion. The degree of comminution is another important factor because severe comminution may preclude adequate restoration of facial anatomy,

thus necessitating supplemental bone grafting. Reduction of fractures involving the orbital apex and anterior skull base risk optic nerve and carotid artery injury. As surgical repair for LeFort fractures entails significant manual force, it is important for the surgeon to know how close the fracture line approaches the orbital apex and carotid canal so that a more gentle reduction technique can be employed.

Imaging

The hallmark of LeFort maxillary injuries is fracture of the pterygoid plates (Fig. 4.51). Although each LeFort fracture pattern shares this common feature, each also has a unique fracture, allowing for specific

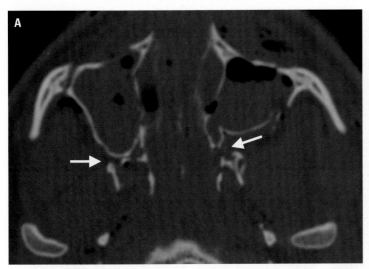
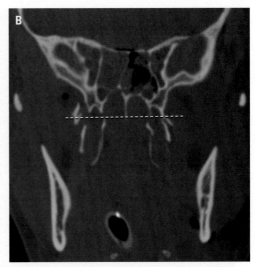

Figure 4.51. LeFort fractures—pterygoid plates. Transaxial CT (**A**) shows bilateral fractures of the pterygoid plates *(arrows)*. Coronal CT reformation (**B**) optimally shows the pterygoid plate fractures *(dashed line)*—the hallmark of LeFort fractures.

identification. LeFort I fractures involve the lateral piriform aperture. LeFort II fractures involve the inferior orbital rim. LeFort III fractures involve the lateral orbital wall and zygomatic arch.

Approaching the CT of a patient with midfacial fractures is algorithmic. One first assesses the integrity of the pterygoid plates to include or exclude a LeFort fracture. If the pterygoid plates are fractured, then the LeFort fracture pattern type is determined by identifying each pattern's unique feature: lateral piriform aperture fracture (LeFort I) (Fig. 4.52), inferior orbital rim fracture (LeFort II) (Fig. 4.53), and lateral orbital wall and zygomatic arch fractures (LeFort III) (Fig. 4.54). Because these injury patterns are rarely symmetric, evaluating each side independently is appropriate. More than one LeFort fracture pattern may be present on either side, and all three patterns may coexist in a single patient (Fig. 4.55).

The palate serves as one of the principle guides for restoring preinjury facial width and hard palate

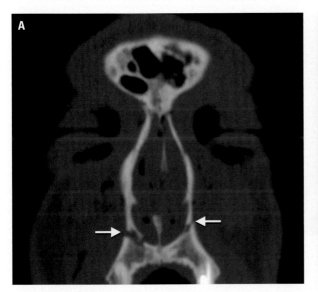
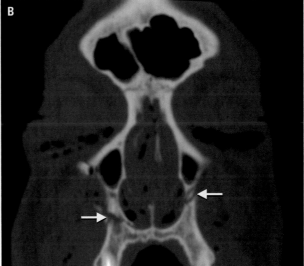

Figure 4.52. LeFort I fractures. Consecutive coronal CT reformations (**A and B**) show bilateral fractures through the lateral piriform apertures *(arrows)*, a feature unique to LeFort I fractures. *(continued)*

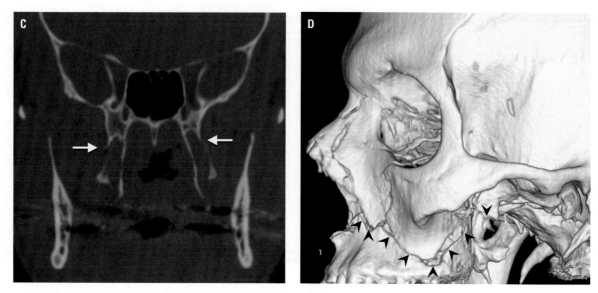

Figure 4.52. *(continued)* **C:** Coronal CT reformation through the pterygoid plates shows bilateral fractures *(arrows)*. **D:** 3D CT reconstruction in lateral projection with mandible removed shows LeFort I fracture plane from the lateral piriform aperture anteriorly to the pterygoid plate posteriorly *(arrowheads)*.

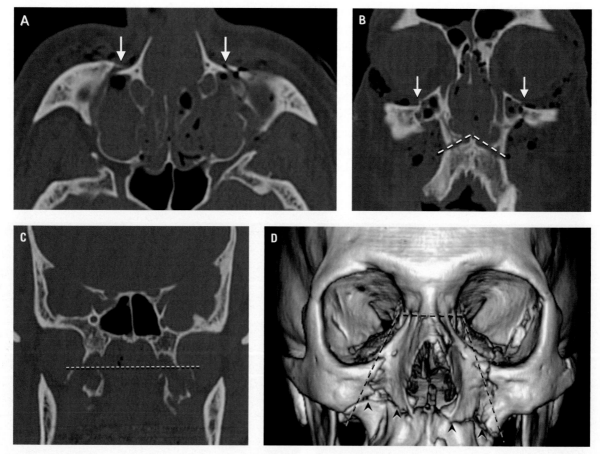

Figure 4.53. LeFort II fractures. Transaxial **(A)** and coronal CT reformation **(B)** show bilateral inferior orbital rim fractures *(arrows)*, a feature unique to LeFort II fractures. Fractures across the lateral piriform apertures *(dashed line)* represent concurrent bilateral LeFort I fractures. **C:** Coronal CT reformation shows bilateral pterygoid plate fractures *(thin dashed line)*, requisites for LeFort fractures. **D:** 3D CT reconstruction shows bilateral LeFort I *(arrowheads)* and bilateral LeFort II patterns *(green dashed line)*.

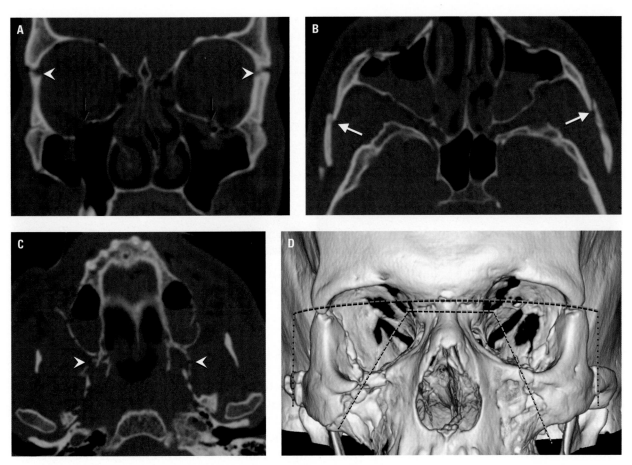

Figure 4.54. LeFort III fractures. Coronal CT reformation (**A**) shows bilateral lateral orbital wall/zygomaticofrontal suture fractures *(arrowheads)*, a feature unique to LeFort II fractures. Fractures across the orbital floors *(black arrows)* represent concurrent bilateral LeFort II fractures. **B:** Transaxial CT image shows bilateral zygomatic arch fractures *(white arrows)*, also a requirement for LeFort III fracture pattern. **C:** Transaxial CT image shows bilateral pterygoid plate fractures *(arrowheads)*. **D:** 3D CT reconstruction shows bilateral LeFort III fracture pattern *(red dashed line)*, as well as pyramidal bilateral LeFort II fracture pattern *(green dashed line)*.

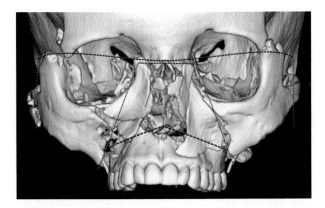

Figure 4.55. LeFort fractures. 3D CT reconstruction shows bilateral LeFort I *(blue dashed line)*, bilateral LeFort II *(green dashed line)*, and bilateral LeFort III *(red dashed line)* fractures in a single patient.

fractures are invariably present with LeFort injuries, most commonly with asymmetric LeFort fracture patterns and panfacial fractures. They are typically sagittally oriented and diagnosis is best made on axial images and coronal reformations (Fig. 4.56). Palatal fractures reflect high-energy injuries and, if unrecognized and untreated, will result in malocclusion.

MANDIBULAR FRACTURES

Anatomy

The mandible is the strongest of the facial bones. It is a horseshoe-shaped bone with an anterior horizontal component and two posterior vertical

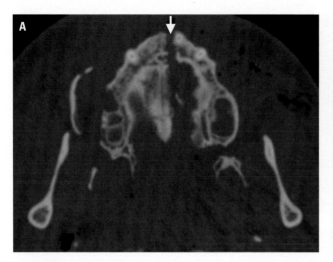
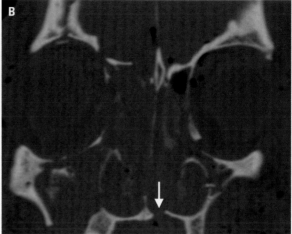

Figure 4.56. Hard palate fractures. Transaxial (**A**) and coronal CT reformation (**B**) show sagittal split hard palate fracture *(arrows)* in a patient suffering a panfacial smash.

struts that contribute to the facial buttress system (Fig. 4.57). From medial to lateral, the horizontal component comprises the mandibular symphysis, parasymphysis, and body. The angle of the mandible connects the horizontal and vertical portions on each side. Each posterior vertical strut comprises the ramus, which splits superiorly into the coronoid process anteriorly and the condyle posteriorly, separated by the sigmoid notch. The condyle articulates with the glenoid fossa via a mobile cartilaginous disc within the temporomandibular joint (TMJ) capsule. The TMJs represent the only mobile segments of the facial skeleton and are complex synovial joints permitting hinge, translation, and rotational movements. Other key anatomic features of the mandible include the mandibular teeth, the inferior alveolar nerve within the inferior alveolar nerve canal, and the attachments of the muscles of mastication: the masseter, temporalis, and medial and lateral pterygoid muscles (Fig. 4.58).

The muscles of mastication are all innervated by the mandibular branch of the trigeminal nerve (CN V_3). The masseter originates on the zygomatic arch and inserts on the lower lateral ramus. The temporalis originates at the temporalis fossa inserting upon the coronoid process and anterior ramus. The medial pterygoid arises from the medial aspect of the lateral pterygoid plate to insert on the medial aspect of the mandibular angle. These three muscles act on the posterior mandible to close the mouth. The lateral pterygoid muscle originates from the lat-

Figure 4.57. Mandible anatomy. (From Anatomical Chart Co., with permission.)

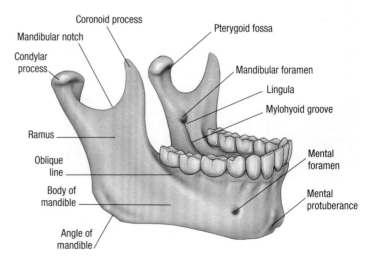

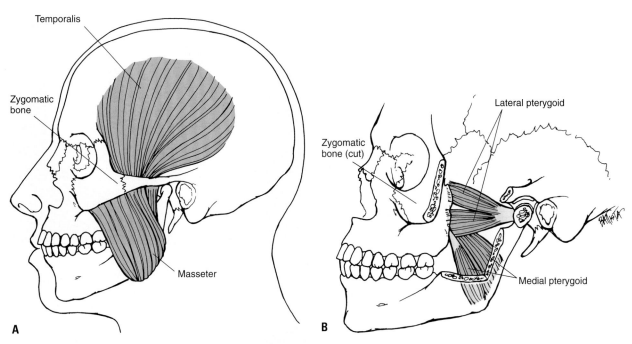

Figure 4.58. Muscles of mastication. (From Oatis, CA. *Kinesiology: The Mechanics and Pathomechanics of Human Movement*. Baltimore, MD: Lippincott Williams & Wilkins; 2004, with permission.)

eral aspect of the lateral pterygoid plate and inserts on the condyle. The lateral pterygoid muscle helps open the mouth. The suprahyoid muscles (digastric, geniohyoid, and genioglossus) elevate the hyoid and tongue base during swallowing and assist in opening the mouth.

Fractures

Mandible fractures make up a large proportion of all facial fractures and were formerly most frequently seen in MVCs. Because of the introduction of the airbag, assault is now the primary cause.

Mandible fractures are classified by anatomic location and described as symphyseal, parasymphyseal, body, alveolar, angle, ramus, coronoid, and condylar. Condylar fractures are subdivided into high and low (cranial and caudal, respectively) and whether they are displaced, dislocated, or intracapsular. Intracapsular fractures are managed conservatively, whereas extracapsular fractures require surgical repair. Low extracapsular condylar fractures may benefit from an endoscopic approach; however, open reduction is necessary for high condylar fractures.

Mandibular angle and body fractures are described as favorable or unfavorable in the horizontal and vertical planes according to the effect of muscle action on the fracture fragments (Fig. 4.59). The masseter and temporalis muscles attached to the ramus pull the proximal segment upward, whereas the medial pterygoid pulls it medially. The suprahyoid muscles pull the symphysis inferiorly and posteriorly. When the fractures are horizontally and vertically unfavorable, the fragments are displaced. Conversely, the same muscular actions reduce the fragments in horizontally and vertically favorable fractures.

Because the mandible forms a ring-like structure with its attachment to the skull base, a second mandibular fracture is present in at least 50% of cases and should be sought in all patients. Most commonly, a parasymphyseal fracture is associated with a contralateral condylar fracture (Fig. 4.60). A flail mandible refers to a symphyseal fracture with bilateral condylar fractures (Fig. 4.61) and represents a surgical challenge to restore preinjury facial width and height. The muscles of mastication influence fracture displacement and, in turn, stability (Figs. 4.59B, 4.59C).

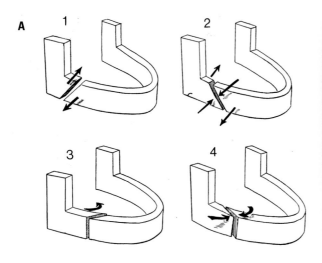

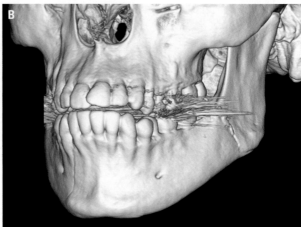

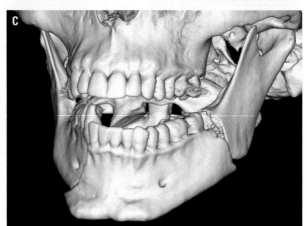

Figure 4.59. Favorable and unfavorable mandible fracture orientation. The direction of force from the muscles of mastication acting on the mandible across a fracture may distract fracture fragments (unfavorable) or reduce fracture fragments (favorable). 3D CT reconstructions show favorable (**B**) and unfavorable (**C**) double mandible fractures.

Fractures through the alveolus and tooth socket represent are considered open (Fig. 4.62). A lucent socket indicates acute tooth loss and should prompt investigation of the aerodigestive system for aspirated or ingested tooth fragments (Fig. 4.63).

Imaging

CT imaging, particularly MDCT, has replaced conventional radiography of the mandible and represents the best imaging tool in the evaluation of maxillofacial trauma. Single-slice helical CT was found to have 100% sensitivity for mandibular fractures, where panoramic radiography was only 86% sensitive. Although CT is optimal for identifying fractures of the symphysis—the rami and condyles—dental root fractures are best seen on panoramic radiography.

In the emergency setting, CT of face and mandible is obtained in a single acquisition from the hyoid to the top of the frontal sinuses with coronal and sagittal reformations. Complete evaluation ensures that clinically suspected co-existing mandibular and facial injuries can be efficiently diagnosed in a single visit and in a single scan.

MDCT evaluation of the mandible with MPRs provides an excellent tool for determining fracture location, displacement, and comminution (Fig. 4.60). Coronal and oblique sagittal reformations are ideal for diagnosis of ramus and condylar fractures (Fig. 4.61B). Condylar fractures typically show anteromedial displacement of the condylar head fragment secondary to the actions of the medial pterygoid muscle (Fig. 4.64). Unfavorable mandibular angle and body fractures are readily seen as the muscles of mastication distract the fracture fragments

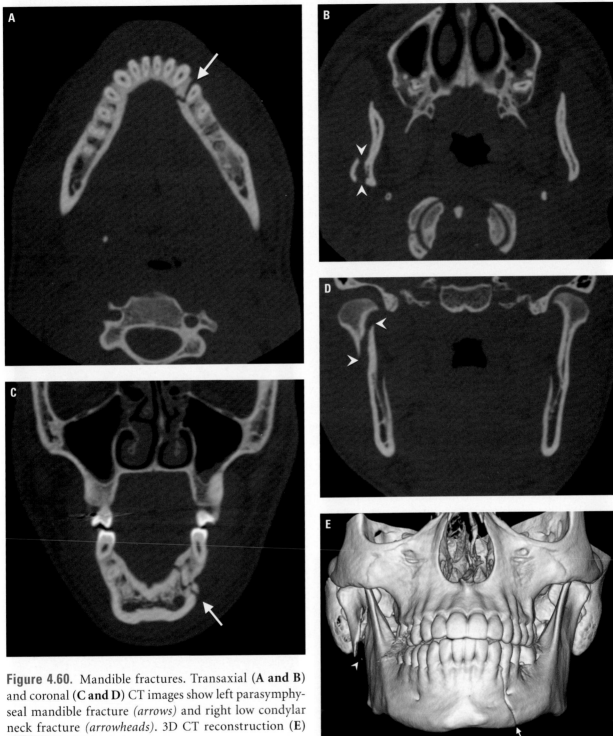

Figure 4.60. Mandible fractures. Transaxial (**A and B**) and coronal (**C and D**) CT images show left parasymphyseal mandible fracture *(arrows)* and right low condylar neck fracture *(arrowheads)*. 3D CT reconstruction (**E**) elegantly shows both fractures.

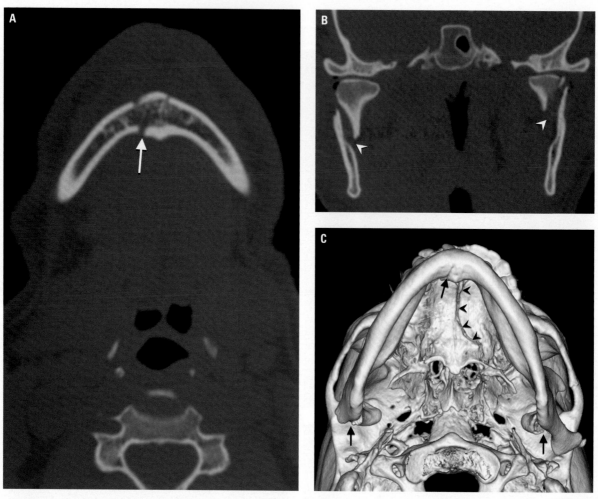

Figure 4.61. Flail mandible. **A:** Transaxial CT image shows a symphyseal mandible fracture *(white arrows)*. **B:** Coronal CT reformation shows bilateral condylar neck fractures *(white arrowheads)*. Together, these injuries constitute a flail mandible. **C:** 3D CT reconstruction in submentovertex orientation shows the flail mandible *(black arrows)*, as well as a sagittal split palatal fracture *(black arrowheads)*.

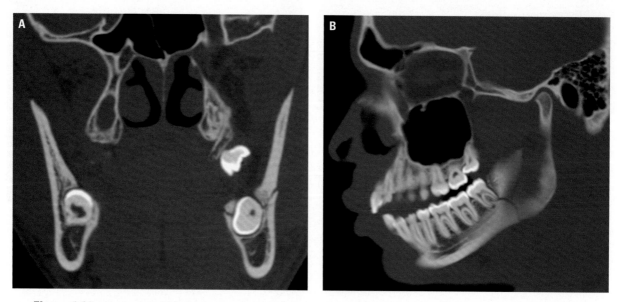

Figure 4.62. Open mandible fractures. **A:** Coronal CT reformation shows fracture line crossing a left molar tooth and socket, representing an open fracture. **B:** Oblique sagittal CT reformation in a different patient shows an open fracture involving the tooth socket.

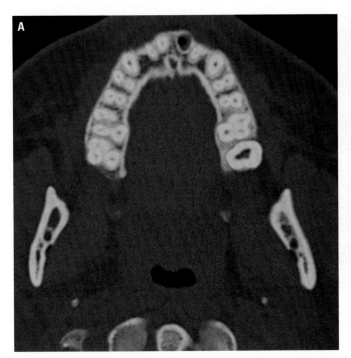

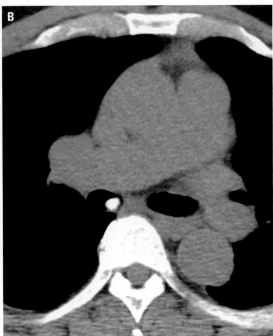

Figure 4.63. Missing tooth. **A:** Transaxial CT image shows gas and fluid in the left maxillary central incisor socket, compatible with acute tooth loss. **B:** Transaxial CT through the chest shows aspirated tooth in the right mainstem bronchus.

(Fig. 4.59C). However, favorable angle and body fractures are aligned and reduced by the muscular forces. On CT, favorable fractures may be difficult to identify and require careful review in all three planes for diagnosis. Proper window and level setting is essential so cortical bone is not

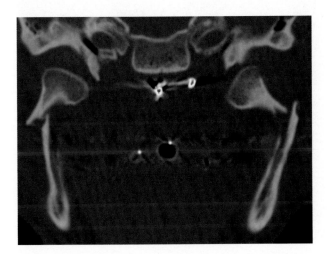

Figure 4.64. Gunshot wound to the mandible with bilateral condylar neck fractures. Note medial pull of condylar heads by the medial pterygoid muscles.

too bright, but rather slightly grey, and fracture planes may be identified.

Three-dimensional reconstructions are particularly helpful in treatment planning of comminuted and displaced fractures and dislocations, and in our experience play an important role in assessing chipped and fractured teeth. Curved coronal CT reformations simulate the panoramic radiograph and are well suited for complex mandibular fractures including the flail mandible (Fig. 4.65).

PANFACIAL FRACTURES

Fractures

Panfacial fractures or facial smash injuries involve simultaneous, severe, high-energy trauma to multiple regions. Some authors organize their description of fractures as mandible, midface, and upper facial bones. Others specify LeFort, calvarial and mandibular fractures (Fig. 4.66A).

Panfacial fractures are often accompanied by multisystem trauma, and a trauma team

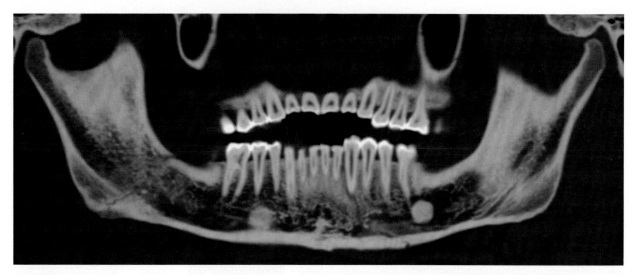

Figure 4.65. Mandible fractures. Curved panoramic CT reformation shows right angle and left parasymphyseal fractures.

approach is vital. Clinical sequelae include malocclusion, "dish face" deformity, enophthalmos, diplopia, CSF leak, and significant soft tissue injury with major distortions of facial width, height, and projection. High-resolution MDCT, along with improved rigid fixation systems, bone graft harvesting, and surgical exposure techniques have helped improve the restoration of form and function of the panfacial fracture patient (Fig. 4.66B).

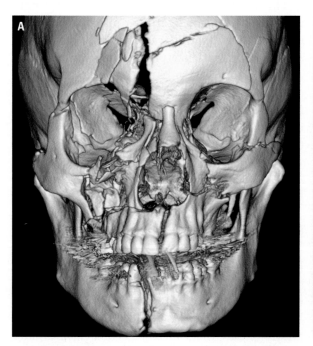
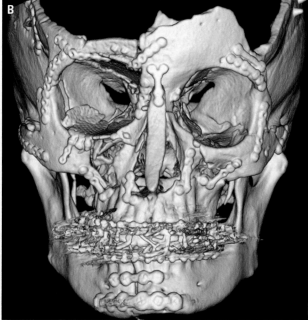

Figure 4.66. Panfacial smash. 3D CT reconstructions at presentation (**A**) and postreduction (**B**) in patient sustaining calvarial, LeFort, and mandibular fractures. Note the placement of miniplates along the vertical and horizontal buttresses to reconstruct the panfacial smash.

SUGGESTED READINGS

1. Manson PN, Markowitz B, Mirvis S, et al. Toward CT-based facial fracture treatment. *Plast Reconstr Surg.* 1990;85(2):202–212.
2. Stanwix MG, Nam AJ, Manson PN, et al. Critical computed tomographic diagnostic criteria for frontal sinus fractures. *J Oral Maxillofac Surg.* 2010;68(11):2714–2722.
3. Kubal WS. Imaging of orbital trauma. *Radiographics.* 2008;28(6):1729–1739.
4. Rhea JT, Novelline RA. How to simplify the CT diagnosis of Le Fort fractures. *AJR Am J Roentgenol.* 2005;184(5):1700–1705.
5. Sun JK, LeMay DR. Imaging of facial trauma. *Neuroimaging Clin N Am.* 2002;12(2):295–309.
6. Leipziger LS, Manson PN. Nasoethmoid orbital fractures. Current concepts and management principles. *Clin Plast Surg.* 1992;19(1):167–193.
7. Rohrich RJ, Hollier LH. Management of frontal sinus fractures. Changing concepts. *Clin Plast Surg.* 1992;19(1):219–232.
8. Harris L, Marano GD, McCorkle D. Nasofrontal duct: CT in frontal sinus trauma. *Radiology.* 1987;165(1):195–198.
9. Lawrason JN, Novelline RA. Diagnostic imaging of facial trauma. In: Mirvis SE, Young JWR, eds. *Diagnostic Imaging in Trauma and Critical Care.* Baltimore, MD: Lippincott Williams & Wilkins; 1992:243–290.
10. Rhea JT, Rao PM, Novelline RA. Helical CT and three-dimensional CT of facial and orbital injury. *Radiol Clin North Am.* 1999;37(3):489–513.
11. Le Fort R. Etude experimentale sur les fractures de la machoire supérieure. *Rev Chir de Paris.* 1901;23: 208–227, 360–379, 479–507.
12. Avery LL, Susarla SM, Novelline RA. Multidetector and three-dimensional CT evaluation of the patient with maxillofacial injury. *Radiol Clin North Am.* 2011;49(1):183–203.
13. Fraioli RE, Branstetter BF IV, Deleyiannis FW. Facial fractures: beyond Le Fort. *Otolaryngol Clin North Am.* 2008;41(1):51–76.
14. Go JL, Vu VN, Lee KJ, et al. Orbital trauma. *Neuroimaging Clin N Am.* 2002;12(2):311–324.

CHAPTER 5

Cervical Spine Injuries

Richard H. Daffner ■ John H. Harris Jr.

GENERAL CONSIDERATIONS

Vertebral fractures and dislocations have, over the course of human history, evoked the greatest degree of fear of any types of injuries. Spinal injuries can produce the most devastating of insults and result in a gamut of abnormalities ranging from mild pain and discomfort to severe paralysis and even death. Although technology has improved to allow more rapid and accurate diagnoses, the physician who is confronted with a spine-injured patient often feels incapable of interpreting the imaging studies that would delineate the full extent of injury.

This chapter presents the systematic approach to the diagnosis of vertebral trauma that we and our colleagues use for the interpretation of images (radiographs, computed tomography [CT] scans, and magnetic resonance [MR] images) of patients suspected of having vertebral injury. Furthermore, it will discuss, in depth, several concepts that we have developed—namely, that vertebral injuries occur in a predictable pattern, and that the imaging findings for injuries caused by the same mechanism are identical no matter where they are encountered within the vertebral column. We should state at the outset that although the principles and imaging findings described here are in the cervical region, the concepts apply throughout the vertebral column.

As recently as a decade ago, radiography was the mainstay for diagnosing vertebral injuries. Radiographs were supplemented by CT when an abnor-mality was found. Occasionally, if the patient had neurologic findings, magnetic resonance imaging (MRI) was also used. Advances in medical imaging have now given the referring physician and the radiologist many options evaluating patients with suspected vertebral injury. Among these advances is multiplanar CT that produces detailed images in a relatively short period. As a result, the protocols for studying these patients have been drastically altered. At the same time, however, the imaging of patients for suspected spine trauma has also become one of the most controversial topics across many specialty lines over the same period. This controversy has engendered several questions. Which patients need imaging? Are there certain clinical and historical factors that can identify those trauma patients who are at high risk or low risk for vertebral injury? Once imaging is indicated, which modality should be used? Should CT be the method of choice? Is there still a role for radiography? To answer these questions, several factors including ease of performance, efficacy of making a diagnosis, time required for the study, cost, and radiation exposure influence the selection of the appropriate imaging study and need to be considered.

Additionally, several disparate factors will influence the decision to image. These include the mechanism of injury (MOI), the age and physical condition of the patient, the ability of the medical staff and the diagnostic capability of the institution to provide initial definitive evaluation and management, and the ever-present specter of medicolegal concerns. The last factor is supported by several studies that showed that as many as one-third of all cervical spine imaging examinations were obtained because of potential "medicolegal consequences."

INCIDENCE

The incidence of cervical injuries is extremely variable depending on the patient populations studied. The reported incidence of blunt traumatic cervical spine injury has been variously reported as low as 1.7% and as high as 5.9%. Of 292 pediatric patients ranging from 5 months to 17 years of age (mean age, 10 years), the incidence of acute cervical spine injury was 0.7%. Contrary to the incidence of cervical spine injury in the pediatric age group, there is around 24% incidence of cervical spine fractures in patients older than 65 years of age. Again, population studied influences the results.

Finally, we must emphasize the importance of "combined injuries" of the cervical spine. *Combined* refers to concomitant acute cervical spine injuries at more than one level. The second (or third) concomitant injury may be proximate (involving adjacent vertebrae to the primary injury) or remote (more than one segment removed either proximally or distally from the primary injury) and may be obvious on radiographs or so subtle as to be visible only by CT. In many instances, the noncontiguous injury may be in the thoracic or lumbar regions. In our experience, 25% of patients with one vertebral injury have another, often, noncontiguous level involved.

INDICATIONS

The cost of health care is in the spotlight daily and the public and third-party payers are attempting to cut those costs. This has necessitated reevaluating of the indications for performing various modalities of diagnostic imaging. To this end, the American College of Radiology (ACR) has attempted to address these issues in their ACR Appropriateness Criteria. It is not surprising, therefore, that one of the "hot button topics" in trauma care relates to the imaging of possible vertebral injuries. Trauma patients, consequently, are of great concern not only to the physicians who treat them but also to the hospital administrators

seeking ways to maintain hospital income as well as to third-party health care providers whose goals are cost containment. The emergency physician and trauma surgeon are often caught between protocol-driven requirements to obtain (cervical) imaging, coupled with the fear of malpractice litigation of missing an injury, and the pressures of medical cost containment.

Most trauma centers follow a series of protocols that are aimed at efficiently identifying all the abnormalities in critically injured patients. Sometimes, these protocols are followed religiously, without any careful thought about the individual patient, the mechanism, and the risk of particular injuries. These protocols have been developed by trauma surgeons and, for the most part, have proven effective. A significant amount of cervical imaging is performed solely because the patient arrives at the hospital wearing a cervical collar, applied by paramedical personnel as standard operating procedure regardless of the history of the injury. We have seen many patients with no cervical injury who were imaged for this reason.

Conservative estimates in the literature that indicate that more than a million blunt trauma patients who have the potential for cervical spine injuries are seen in emergency departments (EDs) in the United States annually. Numbers such as these make it imperative that we have a reliable method of properly screening patients to ensure that those who need imaging have it, and to exclude those who do not.

Calls for cost containment by the federal government and health insurers began in the late 1980s. Several investigators looked for ways to decrease the number of imaging studies being performed, particularly on patients seen in the emergency setting. Two early studies by emergency physicians resulted in the so-called Ottawa Rules for reducing the number of ankle and knee radiographs following injury, respectively. Radiologists also began seeking ways to reduce the number of imaging examinations in trauma patients. One of the first studies was by Mirvis and colleagues in 1989, who found that protocol-driven imaging was not only time-consuming and expensive, but also resulted in the unnecessary expenditure of hundreds of thousands of dollars (in 1989). Their group found that 34% of the patients imaged were mentally alert and without symptoms referable to the cervical region. They recommended that radiologists work closely with trauma surgeons to develop more rational methods for determining risk of injury in an effort to improve efficacy and reduce costs. And thus began a series of investigations that continue to this day designed to assess risk factors and assure that only patients needing imaging are studied.

Vandemark published the first report on risk-based indications for cervical spine imaging in 1990. He listed 10 criteria that would identify patients at high risk for having a cervical injury: high-velocity blunt trauma, generally from a motor vehicle crash (MVC); presence of multiple fractures (large bones); presence of pain, spasm, or deformity of the cervical spine; altered mental status from alcohol and/or drugs or the injury itself (Glasgow Coma Scale [GCS] <15); drowning, immersion, or diving accident; fall greater than 10 ft (3 m); head or severe facial injury; known thoracic or lumbar fracture; rigid spine disease (diffuse idiopathic skeletal hyperostosis [DISH] or ankylosing spondylitis); and any conscious patient who complains of paresthesias or burning in the extremities. If a trauma patient had only one of these criteria present, that patient was deemed to be at high risk for a cervical injury and, thus, imaging (radiography at that time) was needed.

A decade later, because CT was being used more frequently for screening for cervical injury in trauma patients, Hanson and colleagues published a slightly different set of indications of high risk criteria (HRC) using mechanistic and clinical parameters. These included high speed, defined as 35 mph (50 kph) or greater, a death at the crash scene, and a fall of greater than 10 ft. Clinical criteria similar to Vandemark's included closed head injury; neurologic symptoms referable to the cervical region, neck pain or tenderness, and pelvic or multiple extremity fractures.

Two additional large studies were designed to identify factors that would indicate *low* probability of cervical injury. The first of these was the National Emergency X-Radiography Utilization Study (NEXUS) that reviewed the data from 34,000 patients seen at multiple US trauma centers. The NEXUS investigators found that there were five clinical signs that would indicate low risk of cervical injury (NEXUS Low-Risk Criteria [NLC]): *n*ormal alertness, *no* intoxication, *no* midline tenderness, *no* focal neurologic deficits, and *no* painful distracting injuries. We refer to these as the *5 No's*.

The second study was performed by the same group of Canadian researchers who formulated the "Ottawa Rules" for ankle and knee injuries. They examined data from 8,924 patients in 10 large Canadian trauma centers. They applied their findings only to patients who were alert (GCS 15) and clinically stable, with no severe distracting injuries. Their study resulted in the Canadian C-spine rule (CCR), which relies on the answers to three questions relating to the traumatic incident and to the victim: (1) Are there any high-risk factors that mandate imaging? (2) Are there any low-risk factors that will allow the safe assessment of the cervical range of motion? (3) Can the patient actively rotate the head 45 degree to the left and right? They identified three high-risk factors: age older than 65 years, a factor not included in the other criteria; the presence of paresthesias in the extremities; and a "dangerous MOI," defined as a fall of greater than 3 ft (1 m) or five stairs, axial loading to the head, diving accident, high-speed MVC (>60 mph [100 km/h]), MVC with rollover or ejection of the victims, crash of any form of motorized recreational vehicle (motorcycle, snowmobile, water craft), or any bicycle collision.

The CCR go further in defining low-risk factors. These include the history of a "simple" or rear-end MVC. This is a crash in which the victim's vehicle was not hit by a large vehicle (truck or bus), was not struck by a high-speed vehicle, was not pushed into oncoming traffic, did not involve a rollover, and in which the impact was so slight that the air bags did not deploy. Additional low-risk factors included history of the victim being ambulatory at any time, sitting in the ED, delayed onset of neck pain, and absence of midline cervical tenderness.

The Canadian rules state that if high-risk factors are present, imaging is indicated; if absent, an assessment for a range of motion (flexion, extension, 45 degree rotation to each side) should be performed. If low-risk factors are absent, imaging need not be performed; if present, there should be an assessment for motion. If motion is normal, imaging is not indicated; if abnormal, imaging should be performed.

How effective is the CCR? Stiell and colleagues found that if their criteria were applied to the 8,924 patients in their study, only four fractures would have been missed. A closer assessment showed that each of these injuries were considered to be of a "minor" nature, meaning they produced no neurologic deficits and were mechanically stable. Furthermore, when they compared the CCR with the NEXUS low-risk criteria in alert and stable patients, they found that the CCR was superior in both sensitivity and specificity for ruling out cervical injury. They concluded that by using the CCR, they could eliminate up to 25% of the imaging that was performed for suspected cervical injury.

The ACR began developing Appropriateness Criteria in 1993 as a guide for clinicians and radiologists to provide "the right examination, for the right reasons, performed the right way." Each panel consisted of radiologists considered expert in their particular discipline as well as several non-radiologists. The musculoskeletal panel includes an orthopedic surgeon and an emergency medicine physician. Each panel conducts a literature review on the topic of study and produces a document that is based on the evidence in the peer review literature as well as on their own personal experience. The Expert Panel on Musculoskeletal Imaging formulated the latest document on appropriate imaging for patients with suspected vertebral trauma in conjunction with their counterparts in neuroradiology. Their findings are published on the ACR website (http://www.acr.org) as well as

in the *Journal of the American College of Radiology* (JACR). The document concurs that adult patients who satisfy any of the low-risk criteria (as outlined previously) need no imaging.

Finally, in recent years, Goergen and colleagues in Australia have integrated the conclusions from the studies mentioned earlier and have proposed a pre-imaging cervical spine injury risk stratification algorithm. Their algorithm begins with the five NEXUS criteria. If all are negative, no imaging is required. If any of the NCL criteria are present, they determine whether or not the patient needs a cranial CT examination. If not, they recommend cervical radiography. If, however, the patient requires cranial CT, they apply Hanson's HRC. Again, if none of these are present, they recommend cervical radiography; if any of the criteria are present, they recommend cervical CT. We take issue with the use of radiography instead of CT as the first modality of imaging for reasons that will be discussed subsequently. Figure 5.1 shows our modification of Goergen's algorithm.

Table 5.1 lists the various high- and low-risk criteria used to determine if cervical imaging is indicated for trauma.

In summary, the following are the specific circumstances under which cervical imaging should be performed following blunt trauma in the

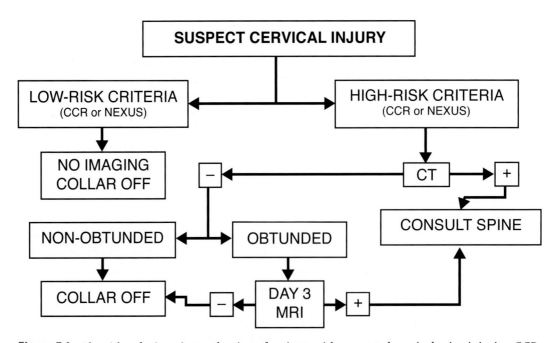

Figure 5.1. Algorithm for imaging evaluation of patients with suspected cervical spine injuries. CCR, Canadian C-spine rule; NEXUS, National Emergency X-Radiography Utilization Study; CT, computed tomography; MRI, magnetic resonance imaging.

TABLE 5.1	Risk Criteria For Spine Injury

High Risk

- Altered mental status
- Multiple fractures
- Drowning or diving accident
- Significant head or facial injury
- Age >65 years
- "Dangerous mechanism"
  - Axial load to head
  - Fall from >1 m
  - High-speed MVC (>60 mph)
  - MVC with large vehicle
  - MVC with rollover, ejection
  - Pedestrian or bicyclist struck by vehicle
  - Crash from motorized recreation vehicle
- Paresthesias in extremities
- Rigid spine disease
  - Ankylosing spondylitis
  - DISH

Low Risk

- Canadian C-spine rule (no imaging)
  - Absence of high-risk factors
  - Low-risk factors that allow safe assessment of range of motion
    - Simple rear-end MVC
    - Sitting in ED
    - Ambulatory at any time
    - Delayed onset of neck pain
    - Absent midline cervical tenderness
  - Able to rotate neck 45 degrees left and right
- NEXUS criteria
  - No midline tenderness
  - No focal neurologic deficits
  - No intoxication or indication of brain injury
  - No painful distracting injuries
  - Normal alertness

DISH, diffuse idiopathic skeletal hyperostosis; ED, emergency department; MVC, motor vehicle crash; NEXUS, National Emergency X-Radiography Utilization Study.

presence of any one or more of the following clinical conditions:

- Hemodynamic instability
- Unconsciousness
- Altered mental status of whatever etiology, including the inebriated patient who falls from standing

- Major craniofacial trauma
- Myelopathy, radiculopathy
- Major blunt trauma to the neck
- Focal cervical pain and tenderness, particularly posterior and midline
- Painful limitation of cervical spine motion
- Proximate "distracting" injury, for example, concomitant upper rib fracture, sternal fracture, shoulder girdle dislocation, fracture, or fracture-dislocation
- Major remote "distracting" injuries, for example, multiple rib fractures, major blunt abdominal trauma, and pelvic ring disruption

Isolated remote major injuries—for example, acetabular fracture, dislocated hip, fracture-dislocation of the ankle, Lisfranc fracture-dislocation—sustained in a fall or MVC capable of also producing cervical spine injuries should not be considered "distracting" injuries requiring automatic cervical spine imaging in an alert, communicative patient without cervical spine signs and symptoms.

If the patient has not sustained one of the injuries listed earlier or does not meet other high-risk criteria, imaging should not be performed.

Two other exceptions need to be mentioned. Cervical spine imaging is not indicated in patients with gunshot wounds to the cranium. In this context, it is essential to note that this distinction is restricted to gunshot (but not shotgun) wounds to the cranium (not to the face or the face and head). Patients with isolated mandibular fractures are reported to have virtually no concomitant cervical spine fractures need not be examined. Patients with other severe midface fractures should be studied.

IMAGING

Radiography

Radiography was used extensively and relied upon in the past to screen patients and to make an initial diagnosis. Multiplanar imaging was then used to confirm the initial impression and to outline the extent of damage. However, as CT and MR technology improved, radiography now has a "backseat." However, despite the many advantages of CT, it is often necessary, in many instances, to refer to radiographs for guidance, especially for operative planning. In addition, there are still many places in the world where CT is not readily available and trauma physicians still must use radiography. For this reason, we feel there is still a role for radiography and include it in this discussion.

Techniques

Is there a "routine" series of radiographs for examining a patient with a suspected acute vertebral injury? This question is frequently asked of radiologists by our surgical colleagues. There are differing opinions of which views should be routine. The following discussion reflects our practices at large urban trauma centers that deal in significant numbers of spine injuries.

Once it has been determined that a patient needs cervical radiography, what is the least number of views required to ensure that a significant injury is not present? Most investigators agree that the absolute minimal radiographic views are the supine lateral, the anteroposterior (AP), and, where possible, the atlantoaxial (odontoid). To a great extent, the ACR Appropriateness Criteria also agrees with this premise. However, our collective experience has shown that the average trauma patient is quite large (in excess of 100 kg [220 lb]). These patients are extremely difficult to completely evaluate the cervicothoracic junction on lateral radiographs. In most instances, the supine ("trauma") oblique views can adequately demonstrate this region. We agree with advocates of the three-view cervical series that the supine oblique views generally do not provide significant additional information about injuries. However, the ability of the supine oblique views to adequately demonstrate the cervicothoracic junction in most patients justifies its use. Our collective experience has shown that the combination of a normal AP and normal bilateral supine oblique radiographs is sufficient to adequately evaluate the cervicothoracic junction. Of course, if the patient is able to undergo cervical CT, this issue is moot.

The most important cervical projection is the lateral. Gehweiler and colleagues observed at least two-thirds of significant pathology can be detected on this view. However, the surgeon and the radiologist should not rely solely on the lateral view to clear the cervical region in a trauma patient. The hazards of this practice are illustrated in Figure 5.2. From

a practical standpoint, however, the presence of life-threatening injury often dictates that the patient be taken immediately to surgery before a complete cervical series can be obtained. *The treatment of life-threatening injuries always precludes obtaining a complete series of radiographs.* Once again, the speed of modern multiplanar CT renders this point moot in most instances.

In our institutions, all radiographs of the spine are obtained with the patient in a supine position. We do not turn the patient for lateral views or oblique views. A portable x-ray unit usually is adequate. Ambulatory patients may be studied in the upright position. All images are processed and displayed on our digital imaging system, where it is often possible to electronically compensate for overexposure or underexposure.

The lateral view is obtained by means of a horizontal beam with a grid cassette. Forty-inch focal film distance is used and the cassette is placed adjacent to the patient's head as close to the shoulders as possible. Gentle traction may be placed on the shoulders to facilitate imaging of C7. *Under no circumstances should traction be applied to the head.* It may be impossible to place traction on the upper limbs in patients with upper limb fractures. Additional views with the "swimmer's" technique may be necessary for complete imaging of the lower cervical region. If, despite all these efforts it is still impossible to see C7 and T1 in muscular or obese patients, CT with sagittal reconstruction will be necessary to clear this area. In most instances, however, the supine oblique views will be sufficient to demonstrate this region.

Once an adequate lateral radiograph has been obtained, the x-ray tube is placed in an upright position with 20 degrees of cranial angulation. The central beam is directed at the cricoid cartilage (C6). The cassette is placed under the backboard on which the patient is lying. Again, a 40-inch focal film distance is used.

The atlantoaxial region is obtained with the patient's mouth open when possible. This projection, along with the swimmer view, is the most frequently repeated view. This view can be delayed until the patient is able to fully cooperate. It may be necessary on occasion to remove the anterior portion of the cervical collar in which the patient has arrived. To prevent motion, sandbags should be placed at either side of the patient's head and secured with a generous amount of tape; alternatively, an assistant can

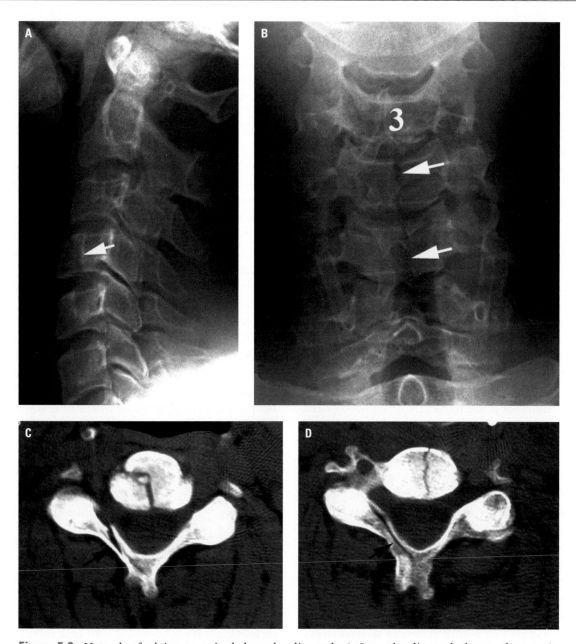

Figure 5.2. Hazards of relying on a single lateral radiograph. **A:** Lateral radiograph shows a fracture in the body of C4 *(arrow)*. **B:** Frontal radiograph shows fractures in C4 and C5 *(arrows)*. **C** and **D:** Axial CT images show the vertebral body fractures seen in **B**. However, there are also fractures in the lamina on the right *(arrows)*.

hold the head. Angled views for demonstrating the arches of C1 may also be necessary.

The supine or "trauma" oblique view was developed independently at approximately the same time by Gehweiler and colleagues and Abel. For this projection, the cassette is placed flat on the table adjacent to the patient's head and neck. The patient remains *supine* on the table. The x-ray tube is angled 30 to 40 degrees off the horizontal with

a 15-degree cranial tilt of the tube. This cranial tilt throws the shoulders off the spine and assures that the cervicothoracic junction is demonstrable in most patients, even those with heavy shoulders. The resulting images from this technique show distortion because of the angulation. Nevertheless, the vertebral bodies, pedicles, articular pillars, and laminae are adequately demonstrated. In addition, the posterior arch of the atlas is usually visible. A pair of these oblique radiographs essentially represents two views of the same region at approximately 90 degrees to each other, preserving the cardinal principle of radiographic diagnosis—to examine an injured part with two views at 90 degrees. As mentioned earlier, a diagnosis in the lower cervical region can be made with confidence by means of a combination of the AP view and both supine oblique views.

Advocates of lateral flexion and extension radiography have recommended these studies be performed to determine whether a cervical spine injury demonstrated by radiography or by CT is "stable." Knowledge of the pathophysiology of the cervical spine injury as reflected by the radiologic appearance of the injury, coupled by the neurologic status of the patient, should provide reasonable evidence of mechanical and/or neurologic stability. Further, mechanical instability is readily established or confirmed by CT and neurologic instability by MRI. Neither of these modalities requires motion of the cervical spine that could, in the presence of a mechanically or neurologically unstable injury, cause or aggravate spinal cord injury. We will address the issue of stability later in this chapter.

In addition, these same advocates feel that lateral flexion and extension radiographs should be reserved for patients in whom anterior subluxation (hyperflexion sprain) is suggested by the MOI (rear-end MVC) by focal posterior cervical midline pain and tenderness, by equivocal neutral lateral cervical spine radiograph, or by the concerns of the attending physician. Although some hospitals use these views routinely, we use active flexion and extension views on a limited basis. Our experience has shown these views to be of limited value in the evaluation of patients with acute trauma, usually because of muscle spasm or the inability of the patient to cooperate for an adequate study. Flexion and extension views should be reserved for patients who have minor degrees of anterolisthesis or retrolisthesis. In most cases, the cause of the listhesis is degenerative disk disease at the same level.

Flexion and extension radiography is a *hands-off* examination for the radiologist and the technologist. *Under no circumstances should the patient's head be passively moved for this study.* A mentally alert patient is instructed to flex and extend to the point of discomfort only. A physician should be present to supervise, primarily to tell the patient to stop moving if he or she experiences pain. In all our years of experience in ED radiology at Level I trauma centers, we know of no alert patient who has injured himself or herself performing these movements. Furthermore, there is no report in the literature of the development of significant injury when these studies are performed as described earlier. Finally, if it is absolutely necessary to determine the integrity of the cervical ligaments, MRI is the procedure of choice.

There are certain pitfalls and limitations to cervical radiography, not the least of which are the cumbersome nature of the procedure and the time needed to obtain a satisfactory examination. If it is necessary to repeat views that occurred in 79% of patients in one study, this adds to the time. Furthermore, we concur with numerous authors who have found that cervical radiographs cannot always be relied on solely to make a diagnosis. For these reasons, in our institution's CT has replaced radiographs because of the ability of the CT examination to find more fractures in a fraction of the time a radiographic study requires. Adequate radiographic visualization of the cervicothoracic junction is frequently difficult. Muscular or obese patients present special diagnostic problems. Failing to adequately demonstrate the cervicothoracic junction presents the hazard of missing an occult fracture or dislocation (Fig. 5.3).

What about children? Radiographic examination of the cervical spine in children need not be as extensive as in adults because children do not suffer the same types of injuries that adults do. Cervical radiographs in children with suspected vertebral injury tend to fall into two categories—normal or grossly abnormal. The subtle radiographic changes found in adults are rarely present in children. Injuries commonly found in children include occipitoatlantal disruptions, atlantoaxial rotary subluxation or fixation, and occasional physeal injuries. Therefore, our institutions limit the pediatric cervical radiographic examination to lateral, AP, and open-mouth views. We do not obtain flexion or extension views on these patients. *Children younger than the age of 16 years do not need CT; radiography is adequate. Those older than the age of 16 years should be studied the same way as adults, primarily with CT.*

In infants and very young children, it is usually impossible to obtain a diagnostically useful

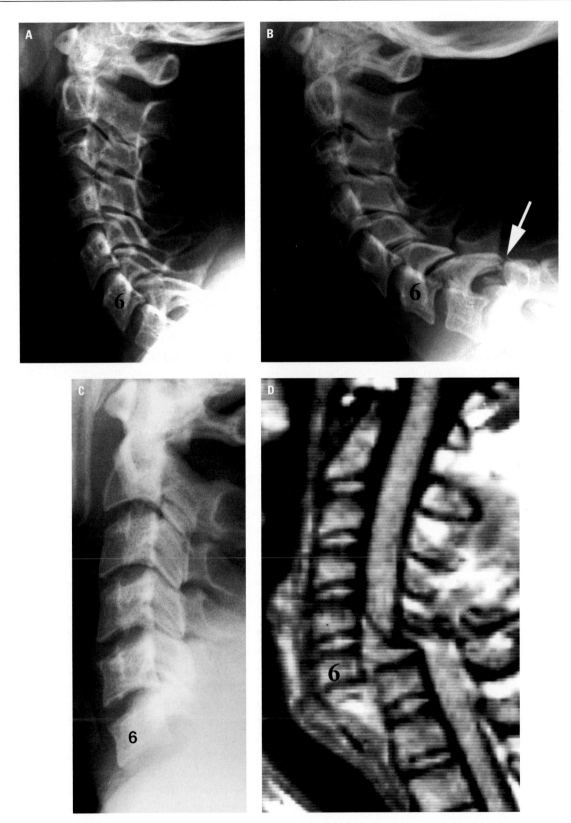

Figure 5.3. Incomplete visualization hazard. **A:** Lateral radiograph shows no fractures in the first 7 vertebrae. The bottom of C7 is not shown. **B:** Lateral radiograph repeated with traction on the arms shows dislocation of C7 on T1 with perching of the facets *(arrow)*. **C:** Lateral radiograph in another patient shows no abnormalities in the six cervical vertebrae shown. **D:** T2-weighted sagittal MR image shows complete dislocation of C6 on C7 with severing of the spinal cord.

open-mouth projection and, in that circumstance, the radiographic assessment of the cervicocranium must be made on the basis of the lateral (including contact lateral) examination alone. As in the adult population, the lateral radiograph of the pediatric cervical spine must include from the base of the skull through the cervicothoracic junction. Similarly, as with adults, the contour of the prevertebral soft tissues is invaluable in assessing the cervicocranium. However, unique to infants and young children are the physiologic pseudomass and physiologic pseudosubluxation of C2 and of C3. These two phenomena will be described in detail later in the chapter.

Clearing the cervical spine in infants and very young children, particularly those who arrive in the emergency center in cervical immobilization, is a common problem because although the vertebrae may be normally aligned and intact on the lateral radiograph, the retropharyngeal soft tissue shadow frequently appears abnormal. This soft tissue observation assumes greater significance because the child is usually screaming and it is impossible to time the lateral radiographic exposure to coincide with inspiration because of patient tachypnea. Furthermore, attending physicians are usually loath to remove the cervical immobilization to do a physical examination of the cervical spine for fear of causing damage to the cervical cord in the presence of a "radiographically unrecognized, unstable cervical spine injury."

In this scenario, the cervical spine can be successfully assessed by remembering three salient facts. First, the incidence of cervical spine injury in pediatric patients is reported as being less than 1%; second, the likelihood of a radiographically unrecognized mechanically unstable cervical spine injury is exceedingly rare; and third, it is common knowledge that infants and very young patients demonstrate, for example, pyarthrosis or osteomyelitis of the lower extremity by failing to use that extremity. Under the clinical and radiographic circumstances described earlier, Swischuk advocates having a physician or nurse gently hold the patient's head in neutral position while the cervical spine immobilization is removed. Simultaneously, the infant's head is released by the nurse or physician. In the absence of a cervical spine injury, the infant, happy to be free of the immobilization, will voluntarily look around the room by moving the head and cervical spine, thereby clinically clearing the cervical spine. Conversely, in the rare instance of

radiographically unrecognized cervical spine injury, the infant will not move the head or neck because of pain and muscle spasm. In that instance, immobilization should be reestablished and the patient sent for MR examination of the cervical spine.

Computed Tomography

CT is now the imaging modality of choice for examination of the cervical spine. Although the technology was developed in the 1970s, cervical CT was initially reserved for the following situations: equivocal conventional radiographic examination, inability to clear the cervicocranium and/or the cervicothoracic junction clinically or by conventional radiography, all fractures involving the spinal canal, and all fracture-dislocations. In the 1990s, however, investigators began recognizing the value of using CT as a primary tool for identifying cervical fractures. Borock and colleagues, in 1991, using CT as an adjunct to the three-radiograph cervical spine series for indications similar to those cited earlier found that CT demonstrated 98% of injuries. Furthermore, the combination of the radiographic study and CT detected 100% of cervical spine injuries.

Shortly thereafter, Blacksin and Lee recommend CT for evaluation of the cervicocranium in patients in whom the open-mouth projection is not possible. Another study found that CT of the cervicocranium as a caudal extension of head CT in pediatric patients less than 6 years of age to be diagnostic in 91% of examinations compared with only 9% of open-mouth projections of the same patient population, and they recommend CT of the cervicocranium as part of the initial radiographic evaluation of the upper cervical spine in young pediatric patients. Throughout the remainder of the 1990s and early years of the new millennium, there were increasing numbers of papers recommending CT be performed instead of radiography.

CT was shown to not only be effective in demonstrating fractures, it could do so in as much as half the time as that required for a conventional radiographic study. And time to a trauma surgeon is golden. During the same period, the technology changed, first with helical CT and then with multidetector scanning. Both of those technology advances reduced the time necessary to perform a CT examination of the cervical spine.

Today, multidetector CT (MDCT) using 16-, 64-, and sometimes 256-detectors reduces the time of scan to mere seconds, significantly reducing motion artifacts. In addition to the rapid scan time, MDCT allows for excellent multiplanar and three-dimensional (3D) reconstruction has resulted in improved diagnoses of vertebral injuries.

Vertebral CT is easy to perform. In our trauma centers, we routinely obtain the cervical scan at the same time the patient undergoes a cranial scan. The cervical images are reconstructed from the data set at a thinner slice thickness than that for the brain. Summers and Galli have shown, using the Visible Human database (Visible Human Project, National Library of Medicine), that conventional CT with 5-mm cut intervals missed as many as 75% of cervical spine fractures and that 3-mm cut intervals demonstrated 100% of all but the smallest fractures. Other authors recommend cut intervals of 1.5 to 2.0 mm through the cervicocranium and 3-mm intervals through the lower cervical and cervicothoracic spine.

Our standard procedure on our 64-slice MDCT for a cervical scan is to obtain contiguous 2 mm slices from the skull base to the bottom of T1 or T2. Two-millimeter axial images are reconstructed from the data in both bone and soft tissue windows (Fig. 5.4). In addition, sagittal and coronal multiplanar images are also reconstructed from

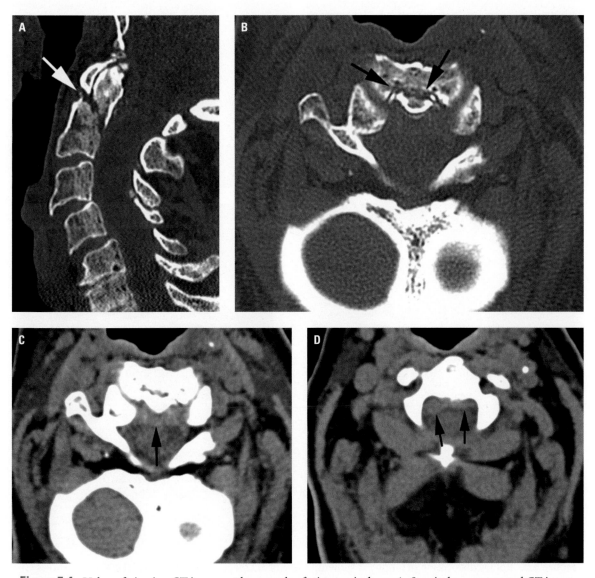

Figure 5.4. Value of viewing CT images at bone and soft tissue windows. **A:** Saggital reconstructed CT image shows a dens fracture *(arrow)* with slight retrolisthesis. **B:** Axial image at bone window shows the fracture *(arrows)*. **C** and **D:** Axial images at soft tissue window shows an associated epidural hematoma *(arrows)*.

the data set. We find the sagittal reconstructed image is most useful for a macroscopic evaluation of all levels of the spine. If necessary, the data set can be revisited to reconstruct 1 mm slices for small fractures. However, we rarely find this necessary. We do not routinely use intravenous contrast enhancement unless a CT angiogram is ordered.

The 3D volumetric CT reformation is infrequently used in the initial evaluation of acute blunt spinal trauma. The value of 3D CT is derived largely from the display of spatial relationships of the vertebra and of fragment alignment for treatment planning and teaching purposes. We have found it most useful for demonstrating atlantoaxial dislocations (Fig. 5.5).

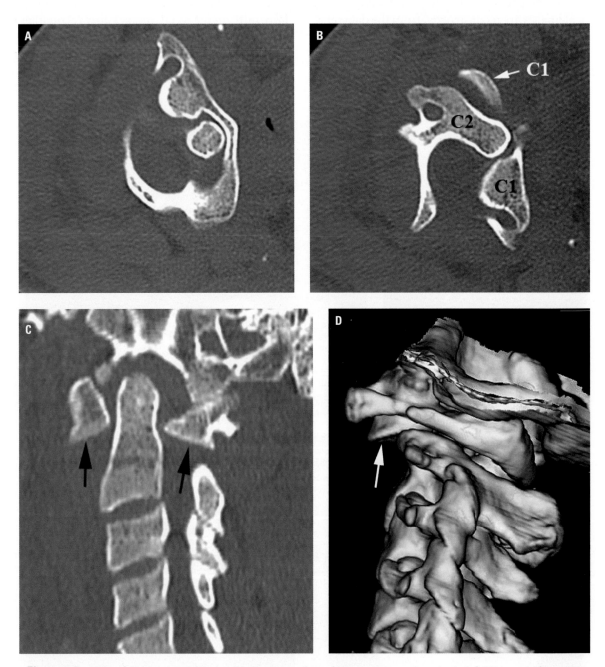

Figure 5.5. Rotary dislocation of C1 on C2 showing value of 3D reconstruction. **A:** Axial CT image shows C1 rotated to the left. **B:** Axial image slightly lower shows the degree of rotation of C1 on C2. **C:** Sagittal reconstructed image shows the dislocated inferior facets of the lateral masses of C1 *(arrows)*. **D:** 3D reconstructed image adds perspective to the dislocated facet *(arrow)*.

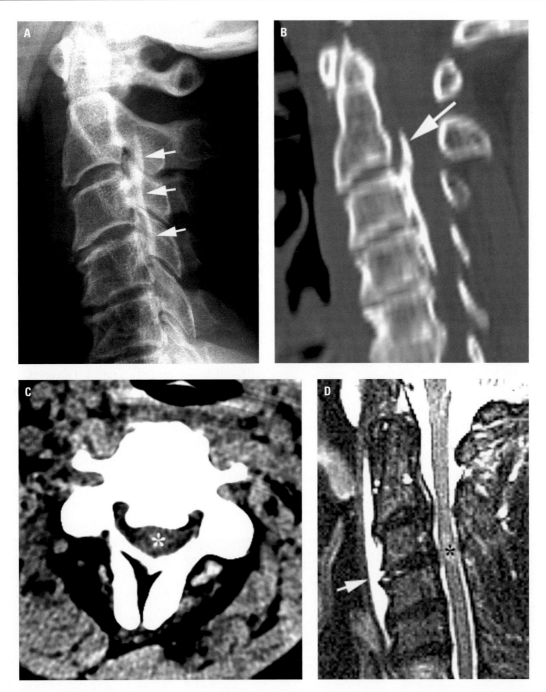

Figure 5.6. Ossification of the posterior longitudinal ligament (OPLL) with cord injury. **A:** Lateral radiograph shows the dense ossification of the posterior longitudinal ligament *(arrows)*. **B:** Sagittal reconstructed CT image shows the extent of canal compromise *(arrow)*. **C:** Axial image at soft tissue window shows compression of the thecal sac *(asterisk)*. **D:** Sagittal Short Tau Inversion Recovery (STIR) image shows central cord edema *(asterisk)*. Note the fluid collection anteriorly *(arrow)*.

Scout views are obtained to determine the level of the scan. In the cervical region, they are performed in the lateral position. Enlarged scout images are displayed with and without level annotations.

CT provides detailed information about the *extent* of injury. In addition to being the best method for demonstrating canal (Fig. 5.6) or intervertebral foramen encroachment (Fig. 5.7), it is also useful for identifying fractures of the laminae, pedicles, and

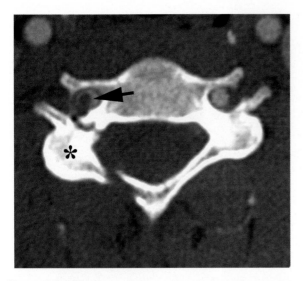

Figure 5.7. Transverse foramen involvement in a patient with fractures of the pedicle and lamina. Axial image shows rotation of the right articular pillar *(asterisk)*. Note the hematoma in the right vertebral artery *(arrow)* compared with the normal left artery.

articular pillars. It is especially useful for showing fractures that accompany perched or locked facets (Fig. 5.8).

Most imaging in the United States is performed by digital means using picture archiving and computer storage (PACS). This sophisticated computer technology allows us to manipulate data to improve images, giving us the ability to darken or lighten images or to shift data to improve demonstration of certain areas. This has become particularly useful when reviewing images on patients who are not lying perfectly straight in the CT gantry (Fig. 5.9).

CT has enabled us to evaluate two regions that posed significantly difficult diagnostic problems in the past—the craniovertebral and the cervicothoracic junctions. The reasons for this difficulty related to the inability of the open-mouth and the lateral radiographs to adequately demonstrate the craniocervical junction. The cervicothoracic junction posed additional difficulties because of patient size and the frequent overlap of shoulders over the area. Craniocervical junction fractures, specifically of the occipital condyles were once considered rare. Cervicothoracic junction fractures are notoriously difficult to see on radiographs. However, CT demonstrates these areas not only on axial views but also on the sagittal and coronal multiplanar reconstructed images.

CT angiography (CTA) is a useful adjunct to cervical CT, used primarily for patients with fractures that involve the transverse foramina and who

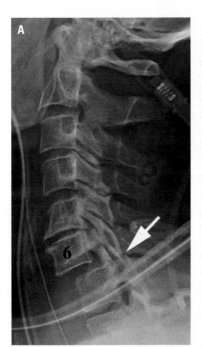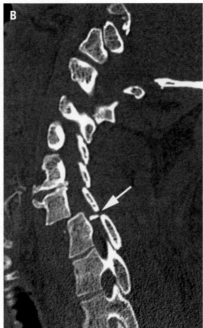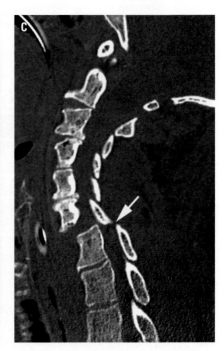

Figure 5.8. Bilateral facet lock C6-C7. **A:** Lateral radiograph shows anterolisthesis of C6 with malalignment of the facets *(arrow)*. **B** and **C:** Sagittal reconstructed images show the point of locking *(arrows)*.

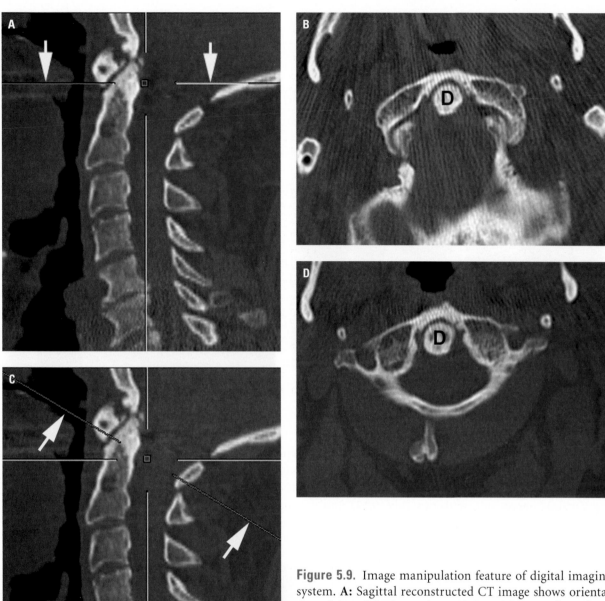

Figure 5.9. Image manipulation feature of digital imaging system. **A:** Sagittal reconstructed CT image shows orientation of the original scan *(arrows)*. **B:** Axial image through C1 and the tip of the dens *(D)* at the level shown in **A. C:** Sagittal image shows a shift of the orientation line *(arrows)* following manipulation. **D:** Axial image now shows the entirety of C1. (From Daffner RH. *Imaging of Vertebral Trauma.* 3rd ed. Cambridge, United Kingdom: Cambridge University Press; 2011, with permission.)

are suspected of having injury or occlusion to the vertebral artery. It is also useful for patients with penetrating injuries to the neck to determine the integrity of the carotid arteries. These studies are obtained separately from the routine cervical scan. Typically, the study is performed from the level of the orbits to the aortic arch (as determined from an AP scout view). A 100 mL of nonionic contrast is injected intravenously at a rate of 3.5 to 4 mL/sec. Scanning at 2 mm intervals starts 12 to 18 seconds after the injection begins and the images are reconstructed at 1 mm. In addition, sagittal and coronal, as well as 3D volumetric reconstruction, is performed for interpretation (Fig. 5.10).

In many institutions, CT may be combined with myelography to evaluate traumatic encroachment

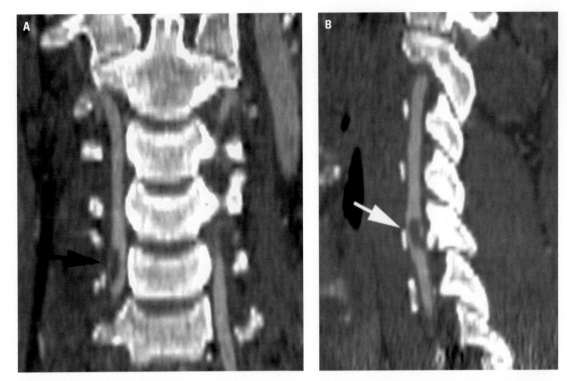

Figure 5.10. CT angiogram showing a clot in the vertebral artery on the right *(arrows)*. **A:** Coronal, **(B)** sagittal reconstructed images. Same patient as in Figure 5.7.

of the subarachnoid space and spinal cord by bone fragments or herniated intervertebral disk fragments (Fig. 5.11). CT myelography is also useful for studying cervical nerve root avulsions (Fig. 5.12) and, on occasion, posttraumatic cystic myelopathy. As a rule, MRI is preferred for those indications; however, CT myelography is performed because MRI is either unavailable, the patient is too unstable, or the patient has a contraindication such as a cardiac pacemaker.

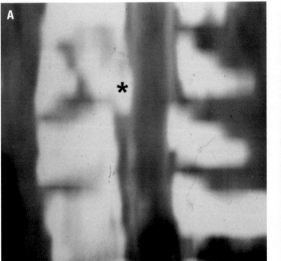
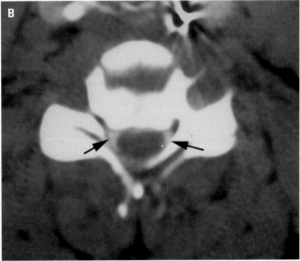

Figure 5.11. CT myelogram in a patient with a burst fracture. **A:** Sagittal reconstructed image shows a displaced bone fragment *(asterisk)* in the vertebral canal. **B:** Axial image shows effacement of the column of contrast *(arrows)* by the fragment. (From Daffner RH. *Imaging of Vertebral Trauma.* 3rd ed. Cambridge, United Kingdom: Cambridge University Press; 2011, with permission.)

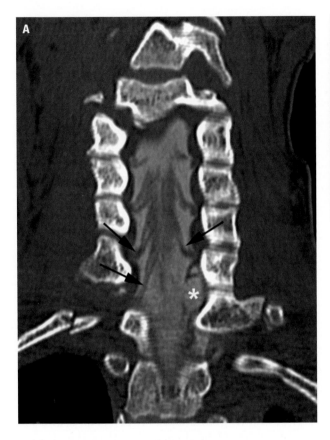

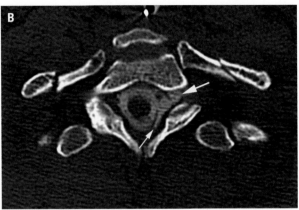

Figure 5.12. CT myelogram snowing nerve root avulsion. A: Coronal reconstructed image shows contrast filling the sheath of the avulsed nerve root on the left *(asterisk)*. Note the appearance of the normal roots *(arrows)*. B: Axial image shows filling of the nerve sheath on the left *(large arrow)* and extravasation of contrast into the epidural space *(small arrow)*. (From Daffner RH. *Imaging of Vertebral Trauma*. 3rd ed. Cambridge, United Kingdom: Cambridge University Press; 2011, with permission.)

CT has several pitfalls and limitations. Patient-related problems result primarily from motion, patient size, and artifacts caused by dental fillings and metallic implants. Motion produces blurred images and engenders the possibility of a missed diagnosis. Motion can also disrupt multiplanar reconstructions, in many instances, simulating a fracture. Fortunately, motion artifacts are easily identified on the axial images. On sagittal and coronal reconstructed images, the artifact frequently produces a linear shift in data in the surrounding tissues. When in doubt, repeating scan, referral to the scout view, or to radiographs may solve the dilemma.

The patient's weight and size are also sources of artifacts. Most modern CT machines have a patient weight limit of 400 to 450 lb because the table must project into the gantry for the examination. Large patients frequently contact the ring of the scanner and this produces streak artifacts that can hide underlying pathology. Dental fillings or other metallic implants (e.g., joint replacements, rods, hooks, screws, plates, vascular clips, bullet fragments) produce streak artifacts that severely compromise the CT image. Many of the new scanners have metal-supression software that can reduce

these artifacts. Furthermore, changing the window setting on the viewing monitor may alleviate some of these problems.

There are three technical pitfalls that can compromise the information being obtained from the CT examination. These are the partial volume averaging effect, poor level calibration, and fractures in the plane of the scan. The partial volume-averaging effect is a well-known CT phenomenon. Normally, CT results in an image that represents an average of the radiographic densities of all structures contained within that section of tissue. Any normal structure that is not completely located within that plane may be distorted or totally discarded from the final image.

Fractures are usually seen on more than one cross-section. It is possible, however, particularly when imaging thin structures such as the laminae or posterior arch of C1, that a fracture is demonstrated on one view only. Furthermore, normal overlap of structures from adjacent vertebrae occurs, lines of interruption will be apparent in the bony shadow, which could be misinterpreted as fractures. This is most often a problem in the cervical region because of the small size of adjacent vertebrae.

On some older CT machines, an annotation discrepancy on the scout view can result in erroneous information being obtained about the level of injury. This, generally, does not present a significant problem when knowledge of anatomy (dens, ribs, sacrum) is used to determine the levels of fracture.

Fractures that are oriented in the horizontal plane, particularly of the dens or body of C2, may not always be demonstrated by CT. We can overcome this pitfall by tilting the gantry to place the fracture out of the plane of the scan. In some cases, however, it will be necessary to resort to reviewing the scout view or to radiography to identify the fracture.

Magnetic Resonance Imaging

MRI is an indispensable tool for diagnosing of a broad spectrum of vertebral and spinal cord pathology as well as the sequelae of trauma. Although radiography and CT reveal important details about fractures and abnormal alignment, MRI is unique in its depiction of all aspects of intrinsic spinal cord injury, fractures (overt and occult), and ligament injuries. Spinal cord compression by bone fragments, disk herniation, and epidural or subdural hematomas can also be diagnosed. Serial examinations can also reveal the onset of posttraumatic progressive myelopathy secondary to hemorrhagic cord contusion. Furthermore, refinement of MR angiography (MRA) has provided adjunctive information about vertebral artery dissection or occlusion. Finally, we are using MRI to "clear" the spine in patients who remain comatose for 48 hours.

MRI is also recommended in patients with acute traumatic radiculopathy such as occurs in scapulothoracic dissociation. Although the root avulsion may not always be demonstrated, secondary signs of avulsion such as pseudomeningocele or contralateral displacement of the cervical cord may be found.

Another benefit of MRI, when supplementing spinal CT, is significantly reducing the need for myelography. The risks associated with myelography are increased in the setting of acute trauma. We now reserve (CT) myelography for cases in which MRI is contraindicated, where the patient is hemodynamically unstable, where the technical challenges of the MR examination result in suboptimal image quality, or for parts of the world where MRI is unavailable.

A discussion of MR technique requires both an understanding of the logistics involved in the scanning of acutely injured patients in a safe manner and knowledge of the appropriate pulse sequences to achieve diagnostic efficacy.

Patient safety during MRI is a major concern. The MRI suite should have the capacity for video and audio observation of the patient. Verbal interaction is desirable for patients able to speak. For those who cannot communicate because of anesthesia, sedation, or the nature of their injury, physiologic monitoring is imperative to assure that hemodynamic stability is maintained. Nursing personnel should be allowed to stay in the MR suite close to the patient.

The Safety Committee of the International Society of Magnetic Resonance as well as the ACR and the American Society of Neuroradiology have made recommendations regarding patient safety during MR studies. MRI facilities that have been accredited by the ACR follow these guidelines. Monitoring is strongly recommended for sedated as well as alert patients. Electrocardiographic, blood pressure, and blood oxygenation by pulse oximeter monitoring should also be performed, and the readings should be displayed within the control room. Care must be taken to prevent thermal injury on monitored patients by avoiding coiled or looped wires in which electrical current can be induced. This is particularly important in patients with sensory deficits who cannot feel the heat.

Patients with a known history of metalworking, surgical prosthesis implantation, or shrapnel/bullet wound should be carefully screened with radiographs before undergoing an MR examination. Any potentially retained or implanted metallic object must be either proved MR compatible using available resources (http://www.imrser. org) or visualized using radiography, and should be remote from vital structures. Ferromagnetic metallic objects in close association to sensitive structures can have disastrous complications when exposed to the strong magnetic fields of the MRI magnet because of local motion or thermal effects.

One of the advantages of MRI is the availability of an almost limitless menu of scanning parameters. A discussion of the specific scanning sequences is beyond the scope of this chapter. However, a few words on them is appropriate. Short TR spin echo sequences have remained essential components of the examination to show the alignment of the vertebral axis in the midsagittal plane and to assess and the external morphology of the spinal cord. These sequences are also useful for demonstrating alteration of vertebral body marrow signal because of compression fractures and can reveal signal abnormalities that indicate hemorrhage, particularly in the subacute time frame. This is also particularly useful for finding additional "occult" injuries (Fig. 5.13). Acute hemorrhage is best demonstrated on either T2-weighted gradient echo sequences or fast or turbo spin echo T2-weighted sequences. In general, these sequences achieve a 50% to 70% decrease in time of study, with a consequent reduction of motion artifacts. Although fast spin echo sequences are slightly less sensitive to the magnetic susceptibility effects of acute hemorrhage, they help to minimize artifact that can occur when metallic fixation devices are present. A gradient echo sequence in a complementary (usually axial) plane is a practical option to improve sensitivity to hemorrhage.

Short Tau Inversion Recovery (STIR) is a fat suppression technique where the signal of fat is zero. In comparison to conventional spin echo, fat signal is darkened. Body fluids have both a long T1 and a long T2. Consequently, STIR is extremely sensitive for detection of edema.

We use the following scanning parameters for cervical spine injury:

■ Sagittal T1-weighted spin echo
■ Sagittal turbo T2-weighted spin echo
■ Sagittal STIR
■ Axial T1-weighted spin echo
■ Axial gradient echo (GRE)

As with any diagnostic study, there are pitfalls for MRI. First and foremost is the patient who is too hemodynamically unstable to allow scanning. Second are patients with implanted devices such as pacemakers, defibrillators, cochlear implants, as well as patients with ferromagnetic foreign bodies.

Patient Condition and Cervical Spine Imaging

The applications of the various imaging modalities to the evaluation of patients suspected of having sustained blunt cervical spine trauma is governed by the condition of the patient. Patients with suspected cervical spine injury may be assigned to one of four classes based on clinical

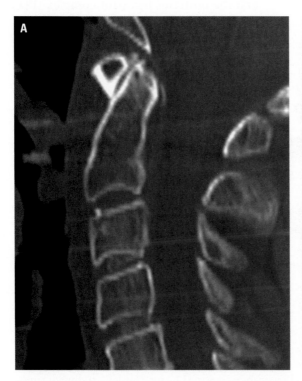
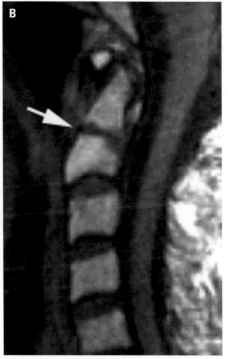

Figure 5.13. Radiographically occult dens fracture demonstrated by MRI. **A:** Sagittal reconstructed CT image is normal. **B:** T1-weighted sagittal MR image shows a horizontal fracture through the dens. This fracture was in the plane of the CT scan and could not be demonstrated.

status as follows: (1) clinically stable without cervical neurologic deficit, (2) clinically stable with cervical neurologic deficit, (3) clinically unstable but neurologically intact (multiple trauma, polytrauma), and (4) clinically unstable with neurologic deficit. Patients in the first category should be screened using the Canadian rules. If the patient is alert and there are no high-risk parameters, no imaging needs to be performed if the patient can actively flex and extend and rotate his or her neck. Patients in all other categories should undergo cervical CT. Those with neurologic deficits should also undergo cervical MRI as soon as practicable.

RADIOGRAPHIC ANATOMY

No discussion of this type would be complete without a brief review of the anatomic structures contributing to the overall physiology and stability of the cervical spine. The mechanical stability of the entire spine with the exception of the cervicocranium is maintained by both ligamentous and osseous structures.

The ligamentous structures of the cervicocranium include, in addition to the occipitoatlantal and atlantoaxial articular joint capsules, from anterior to posterior, the upward extension of the anterior

longitudinal ligament (ALL), which is the atlantoaxial ligament (from C2 to C1) and its further upward extension, the anterior atlantooccipital membrane (from the anterior arch of C1 to the anterior margin of the foramen magnum), the dentate ligament (apical ligament of the dens), the cruciform ligament and the upward extension of the posterior longitudinal ligament, the tectorial membrane (Fig. 5.14A), the alar "check" ligaments that extend from the tip of the dens to the occipital condyles, and the transverse atlantal ligament (the horizontal fibers of the cruciform ligament) (Fig. 5.14B). The transverse atlantal ligament extends between the lateral masses of C1 and, passing posterior to the dens, articulates with the dens by a true synovial joint. The transverse atlantal ligament maintains the normal relationship between the dens and the anterior tubercle of C1, that is, the anterior atlantodental interval (AADI). Within the cervicocranium, mechanical stability is maintained by the very dense ligaments identified earlier. The cervicocranial skeleton contributes very little to structural stability, there being no skeletal structures comparable to the articular masses of the lower segments.

The ligaments of the lower cervical spine include the ALL, the posterior longitudinal ligament (PLL), and the posterior ligament complex (PLC), which includes the capsule of the apophyseal joints, the ligamentum flavum (the yellow ligament), and the

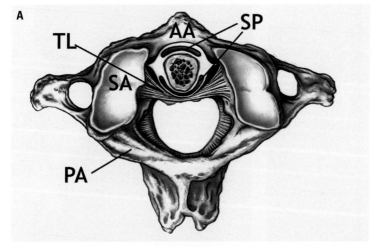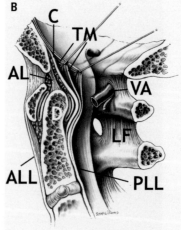

Figure 5.14. Occipitoatlantoaxial ligaments. **A:** Atlantoaxial joint from above. AA, anterior arch of atlas; PA, posterior arch of atlas; SA, superior articular facet of atlas; SP, synovial pads; TL, transverse ligament. **B:** Sagittal section of craniovertebral junction. AL, apical ligament of dens; ALL, anterior longitudinal ligament; C, cruciform ligament; LF, ligamentum flavum; PLL, posterior longitudinal ligament; TM, tectorial membrane; VA, vertebral artery. (From Daffner RH. *Imaging of Vertebral Trauma.* 3rd ed. Cambridge, United Kingdom: Cambridge University Press; 2011, with permission.)

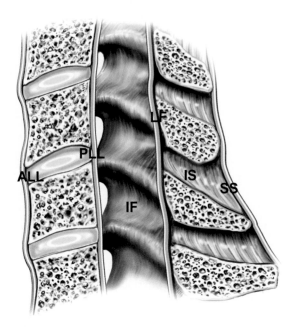

Figure 5.15. Schematic view of vertebral ligaments. ALL, anterior longitudinal ligament; IF, interfacetal ligament; IS, interspinous ligament; LF, ligamentum flavum; PLL, posterior longitudinal ligament; SS, supraspinous ligament.

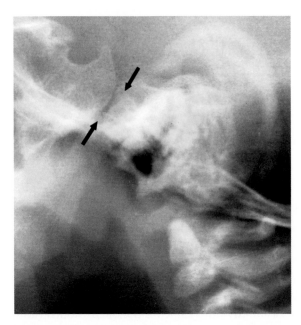

Figure 5.16. Normal spheno-occipital synchondrosis *(arrows)*.

course, on sagittal reconstructed cervical images of adults and children (Fig. 5.17). The relevance of the basion is its role in the recognition of occipitoatlantal dissociation, which is discussed subsequently.

The convex occipital condyles articulate with the medially oriented, biconcave superior articular

interspinous and supraspinous ligaments (Fig. 5.15), as well as the intervertebral disks. The skeletal contribution to mechanical stability derives from the normal anatomic relationship of the articular masses as they form the apophyseal (interfacetal) joints.

The cervicocranium differs greatly anatomically, morphologically, and physiologically from the lower cervical spine. Thus, the radiographic anatomy of each is presented separately.

Cervicocranium

The skeletal components of the cervicocranium include the margins of the foramen magnum, the occipital condyles, and the atlas and axis vertebrae. The clivus is formed by fusion of the posterior portion of the body of the sphenoid with the basilar portion of the occipital bone at the sphenoccipital synchondrosis (Fig. 5.16). The synchondrosis may normally remain visible on radiographs and sagittal CT images until early adulthood and should not be misinterpreted as a fracture. The tip of the clivus, the basion, is a very important radiologic landmark visible on virtually all lateral radiographs, and, of

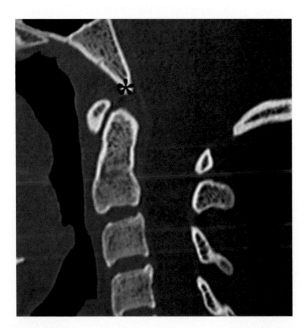

Figure 5.17. Sagittal reconstructed CT image showing the normal basion *(asterisk)* at the tip of the clivus. This structure is much easier to see on CT than on lateral radiographs.

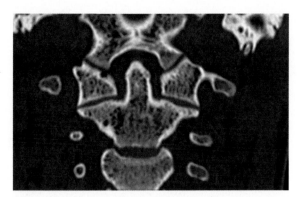

Figure 5.18. Normal occipitoatlantal junction as shown on coronal reconstructed CT image.

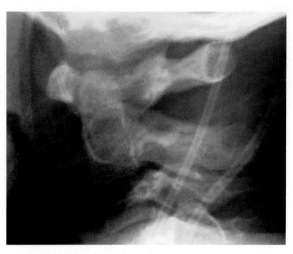

Figure 5.20. Normal craniocervical junction of a 5-year-old child. Note the physiologic pseudosubluxation of C2 with respect to C3.

surfaces of the lateral masses of C1 (Fig. 5.18). Whereas the occipitoatlantal articulation is occasionally not visible on the open-mouth radiograph of the atlantoaxial articulation, it is clearly demonstrated by panoramic zonography (Fig. 5.19) and by multiplanar CT (see Fig. 5.18). In infants and young children, the occipital condyles may normally be visible on the lateral cervical spine radiograph (Fig. 5.20) because the condyles are not yet obscured by the physiologically underdeveloped mastoid processes and lateral masses of C1. However, it is very important to realize that the occipitoatlantal articulation is not normally visible on the lateral radiograph of adolescents or adults because of the overlap of the mastoids. This is one reason occipital condyle fractures (as well as lateral mass fractures of C1) were considered rare in the days before CT began being used as the main screening tool.

The atlas vertebra (C1) (Fig. 5.21) is a ring-like bone with an anterior arch (and tubercle), bilaterally large lateral masses from which arise the short transverse processes, and a posterior arch (and tubercle).

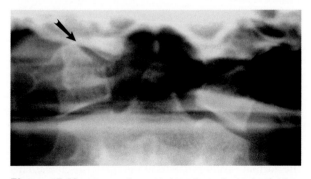

Figure 5.19. Normal occipitoatlantal articulation (*arrows*) as shown by panoramic zonography.

C1 differs from all other vertebrae in that it does not have a body. C1 articulates with the dens through the interposed true synovial joint. From a purely semantic standpoint, *C1 is the only vertebra with lateral masses.* The analogs in the other cervical vertebrae are the articular pillars (see the following texts). Anomalies, such as failure of fusion of the posterior or anterior arches, or partial or complete agenesis of the posterior arch of the atlas occur. Of these, failure of fusion of the posterior arch is the most common. It can be recognized on a lateral radiograph as absence of the spinolaminar line (see below) at C1, and as a cleft in the arch on an axial CT image (Fig. 5.22). This anomaly has smooth, rounded borders that do not fit together like pieces of a jigsaw puzzle, the way fractures would. When encountered, the finding should be mentioned in the report on the study as a normal variant. Anomalies of the ring of C1 usually result in hypertrophy of the anterior arch, a response to increased stress placed on that structure.

Like the atlas (C1), the axis (C2) is morphologically distinct from all other vertebrae in the upward extension of its body into the dens and by the absence of clearly defined pedicles (Fig. 5.23).

In approximately 20% of patients younger than the age of 8 years, the anterior arch of the atlas appears to lie above the tip of the dens (Figs. 5.24 and 5.25). This is partly because of the physiologic laxity of the cervicocranial soft tissues and partly because the tip of the dens is not ossified in infants and young children. This normal relationship should

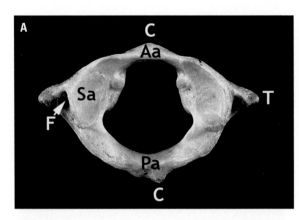

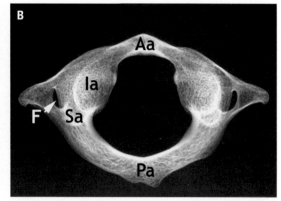

Figure 5.21. Atlas vertebra as viewed from above. **A:** Anatomic specimen. **B:** Radiograph. Aa, anterior arch; C, central tubercles; F, transverse foramen; IA, inferior articular facet; Pa, posterior arch; Sa, superior articular facet; T, transverse process. (From Daffner RH. *Imaging of Vertebral Trauma.* 3rd ed. Cambridge, United Kingdom: Cambridge University Press; 2011, with permission.)

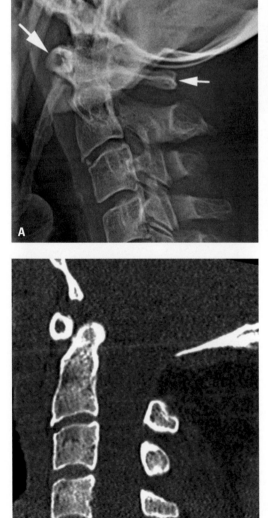

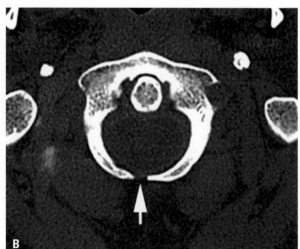

Figure 5.22. Failure of fusion of posterior arch of atlas. **A:** Lateral radiograph shows absence of the spinolaminar line of the atlas *(small arrow)* and hypertrophy of the anterior arch *(large arrow)*. **B:** Axial CT image shows the cleft in the posterior arch *(arrow)*. **C:** Sagittal midline CT image shows no posterior arch.

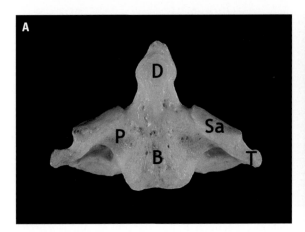

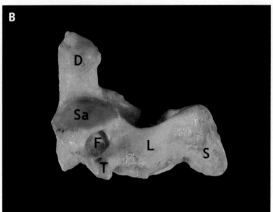

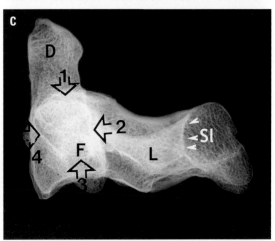

Figure 5.23. Axis vertebra. **A:** Frontal view of specimen. **B:** Lateral view. B, body; D, dens; F, transverse foramen; L, lamina; P, pedicle, Sa, superior articular facet; T, transverse process. **C:** Lateral radiograph showing Harris' ring. *(1)* Superior articular facet; *(2)* posterior body line; *(3)* transverse foramen *(T)*; *(4)* anterior body line. D, dens; Sl, spinolaminar line *(arrowheads)*. (From Daffner RH. *Imaging of Vertebral Trauma.* 3rd ed. Cambridge, United Kingdom: Cambridge University Press; 2011, with permission.)

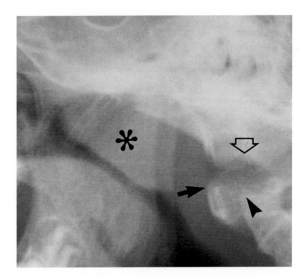

Figure 5.24. Lateral radiograph of the craniovertebral junction in an infant showing the superior margin of the anterior tubercle of C1 *(arrow)* rostral to the tip of the dens *(arrow head)* and the occipital condyles *(open arrow)*. The lobulated mass *(asterisk)* is adenoidal tissue.

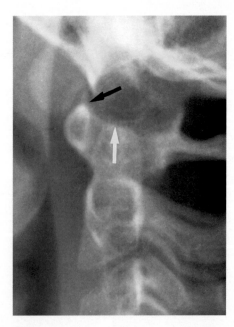

Figure 5.25. Nine-year-old child in whom the superior portion of the anterior tubercle of C1 *(black arrow)* is normal rostral to the tip of the dens *(white arrow)*.

not be misinterpreted as atlantoaxial dislocation or subluxation.

The axis vertebra (C2) arises from several separate ossification centers (Fig. 5.26), some of which have radiographic relevance. During infancy and before the apophysis of the tip of the dens ossifies, the rostral-most portion of the dens has a V-shaped configuration on the AP radiograph (Fig. 5.27A). Should the terminal apophysis fail to unite, the resultant separate ossicle is called the os terminale (Figs. 5.27B and C).

The subchondral (subdental) synchondrosis lies between the base of the dens and the axis body and appears as a normal horizontal lucent defect in the axis body on the lateral radiograph of the cervicocranium of infants and young children (Fig. 5.28). This synchondrosis, like others of the axis, fuses between the 3rd and 6th years of life. The subchondral synchondrosis may persist as a pair of thin, sclerotic parallel densities that are the "scar" of the synchondrosis that should not be misinterpreted as an incomplete or impacted fracture.

The neurocentral synchondrosis (see Fig. 5.26) is usually seen only on oblique projections of the pediatric cervical spine. This synchondrosis, clearly depicted by CT (Fig. 5.29), should be distinguished from acute fractures by its location and imaging

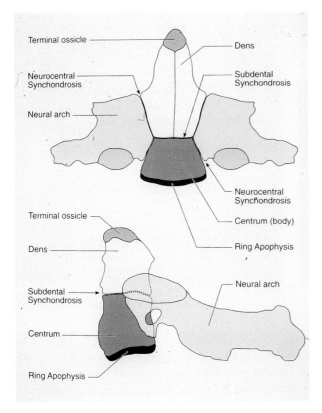

Figure 5.26. Axis ossification centers and synchondroses. (From Daffner RH. *Imaging of Vertebral Trauma*. 3rd ed. Cambridge, United Kingdom: Cambridge University Press; 2011, with permission.)

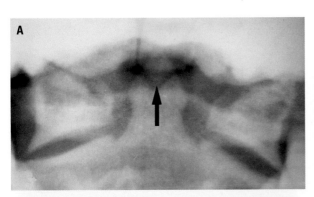
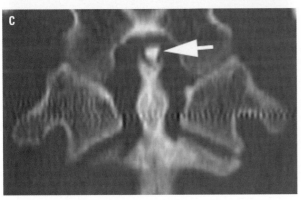
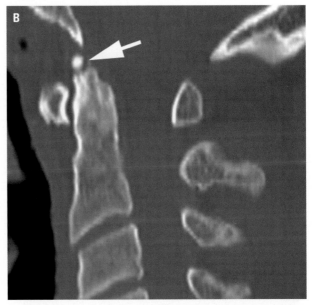

Figure 5.27. V-shaped dens tip with accessory ossicle. **A:** Open-mouth radiograph shows the V-shaped dens containing the accessory ossicle *(arrow)*. **B:** Sagittal and **(C)** coronal reconstructed CT images show terminal ossicle *(arrows)*.

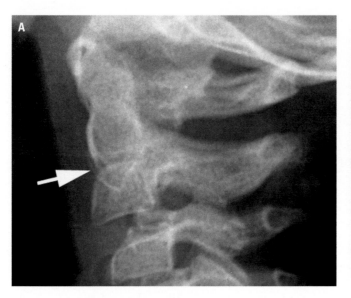
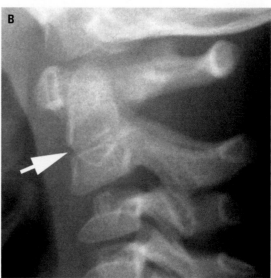

Figure 5.28. Subdental synchondrosis *(arrows)* in two infants. This is a normal finding.

characteristics. Further, *acute fractures of the axis body are extremely rare in infants and young children.* To reiterate, neither the subchondral nor the neurocentral synchondroses should be mistaken for a fracture.

The distance between the anterior surface of the dens and the posterior surface of the atlas tubercle is the AADI, also called the predental space. In infants and children, until the age of approximately 8 years, the AADI varies in width with flexion and extension but it usually does not exceed 5 mm. Additionally, in infants and young children, it is common for the AADI to have a V-configuration in neutral and flexion lateral projections (Fig. 5.30). In extension, the contiguous surfaces of the AADI become congruous. This change in configuration of the AADI is caused by the physiologic laxity

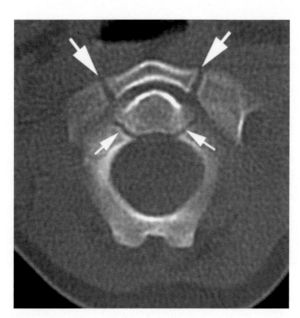

Figure 5.29. Normal neurocentral synchondroses of C1 *(large arrows)* and C2 *(small arrows).*

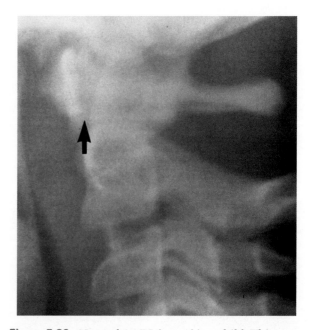

Figure 5.30. Normal AADI *(arrow)* in a child. This space should never exceed 5 mm. The V-shaped predental space is a normal variant, found in approximately 15% of individuals.

of the transverse atlantal ligament normal in patients of this age. In adults, because of the maturity of the transverse atlantal ligament, the AADI remains constant during flexion and extension (Fig. 5.31) and does not normally exceed 3 mm with a 40-cm target-radiograph distance. The most common cause of widening of this interval in adults is rheumatoid arthritis (Fig. 5.32).

The frontal and lateral projections of the atlantoaxial articulation provide different but equally useful information. The frontal (open-mouth) projection (Fig. 5.33A) shows the normal atlantoaxial relationship in the coronal plane, where, traditionally, the important findings are the lateral atlantodental interval, the configuration of the

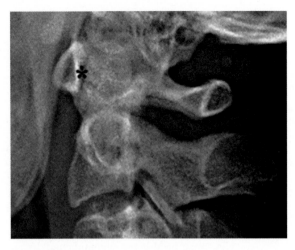

Figure 5.31. Normal AADI *(asterisk)* in an adult. This space should never exceed 3 mm.

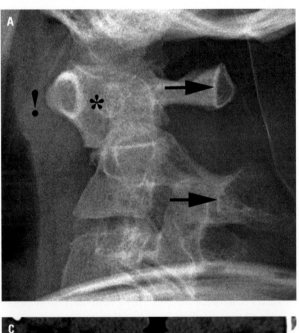

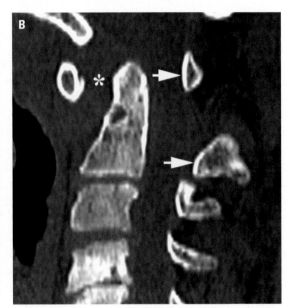

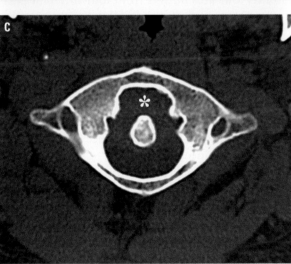

Figure 5.32. Wide AADI *(asterisk)* in a patient with rheumatoid arthritis. **A:** Lateral radiograph shows, in addition to the wide predental space, a shift in the alignment of the spinolaminar line *(arrows)*. Note the prevertebral soft tissue swelling *(!)* caused by pannus proliferation. **B:** Sagittal reconstructed and **(C)** axial CT images show the same findings.

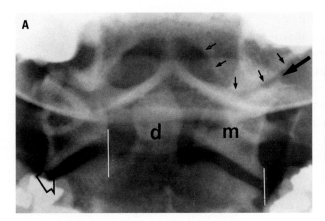 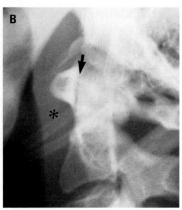

Figure 5.33. Normal craniocervical junction in an adult. **A:** A properly positioned open-mouth view must include the occipital condyles *(small arrows)*, the occipitoatlantal articulation *(large solid arrow)*, the lateral masses of C1 *(m)*, the dens *(d)*, the atlantoaxial joint spaces *(open arrow)*, and the superior portion of the axis body. The space between the dens and the lateral mass of C1 is the lateral atlantodental interval, which may vary in width. Normally, the corners of the contiguous facets of C1 and C2 should be on the same vertical plane plus or minus 2 mm *(white lines)*. **B:** Lateral radiograph shows a normal AADI *(arrow)*. The prevertebral soft tissue shadow *(asterisk)* is normal.

lateral masses of C1, the relationship of the lateral margins of the contiguous facets of C1 and C2, and the position of the bifid spinous process of C2. However, if the open-mouth projection does not include the occipital condyles and the occipitoatlantal articulation, it is an inadequate study and therefore precludes clearing of the cervicocranium radiographically. This issue is moot when CT is used as the prime screening imaging modality.

The lateral projection (Fig. 5.34) shows the normal relationship of the basion to the *posterior axial line* (PAL), the upward extension of the posterior cortex of the axis body. This line allows is critical for identifying disruptions of the occipitoatlantal joint, using two simple measurements. The *basion–axial interval (BAI)* is the distance between the PAL and the basion (Figs. 5.34A and B), and should not be less than 6 mm or not more than 12 mm in adults or children. The measurement is the same on radiographs as well as on saggital reconstructed CT images. The BAI is reliable, even in the presence of anomalies of the posterior elements of the atlas and axis, inclination of the dens, and variations in the slope of the clivus. It is not affected by flexion or extension.

A second measurement, the *basion–dens interval*, is the distance between the basion and the tip of the dens (Figs. 5.34C and D). Conveniently, the maximum distance in adults and children older

than the age of 13 years is also 12 mm. Unfortunately, the basion–dens interval measurement is not accurate in children younger than 13 years of age because of incomplete ossification and fusion of the dens. This measurement is also valid on both radiographs as well as on sagittal reconstructed CT images.

There is another important landmark on the lateral radiograph referred to as *Harris' ring*. This "ring" appearance is not from an actual structure. It results from the overlap of the images of several portions of the body of the axis. The ring is the result of the phenomenon of *subjective contours* and each of its four arcs derives from four different parts of C2. The upper arc represents the superior articular facets, the anterior arc represents the anterior body cortex and the pedicle, the inferior arc represents the lower margin of the transverse foramen, and the posterior arc represents the posterior vertebral body line (PVL) (Fig. 5.35). Harris' ring can only be seen on radiographs and not on CT images because the contours are perceived (hence subjective) rather than based on a real structure.

There is a final relationship regarding the axis to its mates that had greater importance in the diagnosis of occult cervical fractures in the days before CT was the main screening modality. This was originally described by Smoker, who noted that the AP width of the body of C2 should be the same as C3.

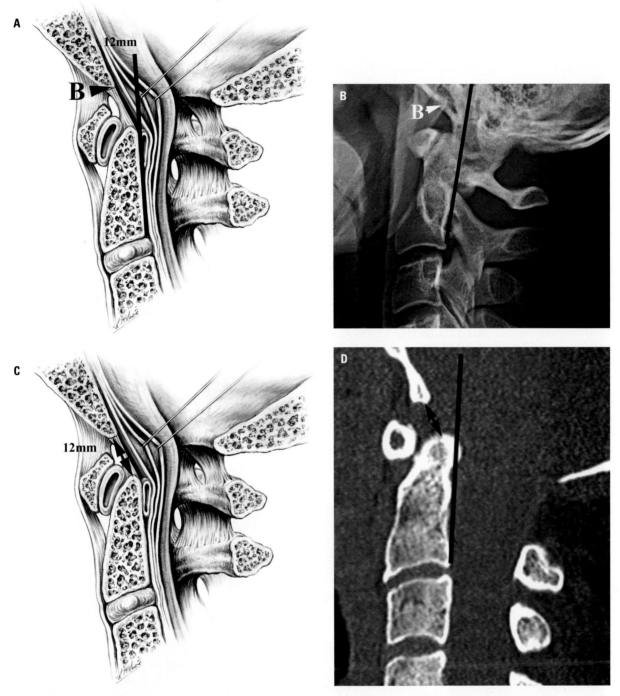

Figure 5.34. Dens–basion line. Normally, the basion (*B*) should be not less than 6 mm nor more than 12 mm in front of a line along the posterior body of C2. **A:** Drawing. **B:** Lateral radiograph. **C** and **D:** Dens–basion interval. The tip of the dens should be no further than 12 mm from the basion. **C:** Drawing. **D:** Sagittal CT image. These measurements are valid on radiographs as well as on CT images.

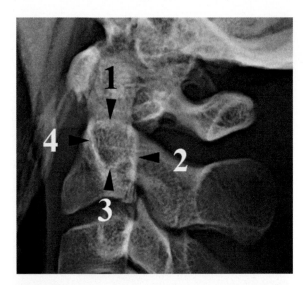

Figure 5.35. Harris' ring. Lateral radiograph showing the four components of the "ring": *(1)* superior articular facet; *(2)* posterior body line; *(3)* inferior margin of transverse foramen; *(4)* anterior body line. (From Daffner RH. *Imaging of Vertebral Trauma.* 3rd ed. Cambridge, United Kingdom: Cambridge University Press; 2011, with permission.)

She observed that subtle fractures of the body of C2 frequently widened the vertebra and she called the sign the "fat C2" sign. The use of CT to routinely screen for cervical injuries has relegated this sign to a historic curiosity.

The atlantoaxial joint permits flexion, extension, rotation, vertical approximation, and lateral bending (gliding). The maximum allowable motion in flexion and extension at that level is about 20 degrees, the maximum allowable rotation is 45 degrees, and the maximum allowable lateral flexion is 5 degrees. Interestingly, the fact that motion occurs along all three (X, Y, and Z) axes accounts for the predominance of cervical injuries at this level in the elderly. The reason for this is the fact that the C0-C2 region remains the most mobile portion of the cervical spine as aging produces arthritis at lower levels.

Both rotation and lateral bending (lateral tilt of the head with respect to the cervical spine) physiologically produce asymmetry of the lateral masses of C1 with respect to the dens as well as asymmetry between articulating surfaces of the lateral masses of C1 and C2. Additionally, extreme rotation of C1 on C2 results in narrowing or loss of the C1-C2 joint space (vertical approximation). These changes may be observed on radiographs as well as on coronal reconstructed CT images. Thus, asymmetry of the lateral masses of C1 may be normal and, in the absence of an appropriate history or physical finding, must be recognized as physiologic and not be misinterpreted as either torticollis or atlantoaxial rotary dissociation.

The lower cervical vertebrae (Fig. 5.36) are all morphologically similar, differing only slightly in size or

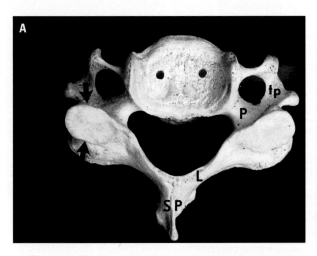

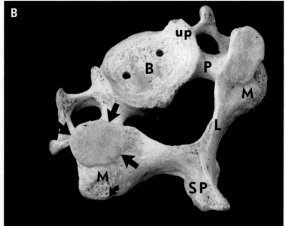

Figure 5.36. Normal adult cervical vertebra seen from above (**A**) and from a slightly oblique superior position (**B**). The articular masses *(pillars) (M)* are posterior and lateral to the body (**B**); the pedicles *(P)* connect the body to the articular masses; the laminae *(L)* arise from the articular masses and pass posteromedially to fuse, forming the spinous process *(SP).* Both the pedicles and laminae have a 45 degree relationship to the body and a 90 degree relationship to each other. The uncinate process *(up)* is an upward extension of the lateral aspect of the superior end plate. The transverse process *(tp)* arises from both the body and the pedicle and contains the transverse foramen, through which the vertebral artery passes from C6 upward. The smooth surface *(straight arrows)* atop the articular mass is the superior articular facet. The *curved arrow* indicates the posterior margin of the inferior articular facet.

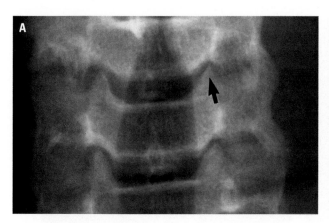

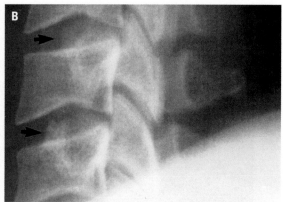

Figure 5.37. Normal uncinate processes *(arrows)* forming the joints of Luschka. **A:** Frontal radiograph. **B:** Lateral radiograph.

configuration. All of the lower cervical vertebrae have a body as their principal and largest component. The uncinate process, an upward extension of the lateral aspect of the superior end plate, develops after puberty and articulates with the contiguous suprajacent vertebral body to form the joint of Luschka (Fig. 5.37). Osteophytes along these joints result in horizontal lucencies along the vertebral bodies on radiographs, suggesting fractures (Fig. 5.38). Fortunately, cervical fractures do not occur along this plane (unlike Chance-type fractures in the thoracolumbar region).

This phenomenon is not found on CT images. The pedicles, which extend posterolaterally from each side of the vertebral body, connect the body to the dense articular masses more commonly called the *articular pillars.* This latter term is preferred to distinguish these structures from the lateral masses of C1. Transverse processes arise from the lateral aspect of the vertebral body and the junction of the pedicle and articular mass. The transverse process contains the transverse foramen for transmission of the vertebral artery from C6 cephalad.

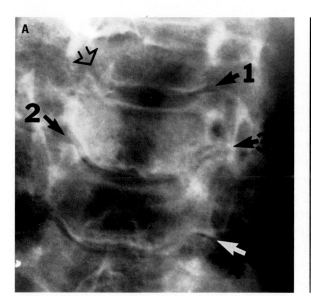

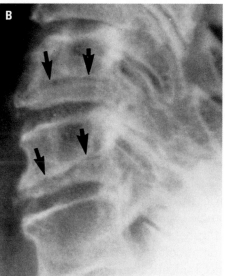

Figure 5.38. Degenerative changes along the Luschka joints. **A:** Frontal radiograph shows a relatively normal Luschka joint *(open arrow).* There are progressively severe changes of spondylosis at the other joints *(1, 2, 3, 4).* These changes include narrowing of the joint spaces, spur formation, and reactive sclerosis. **B:** Lateral radiograph shows the sclerotic margins of the uncinate processes *(arrows)* producing a lucency (Mach band) suggesting fractures. Horizontal Chance-type fractures do not occur in the cervical region.

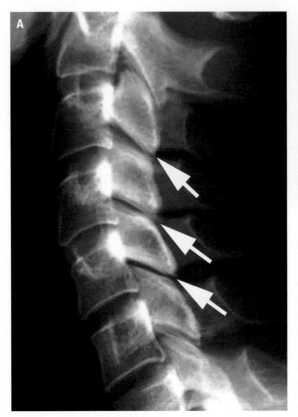

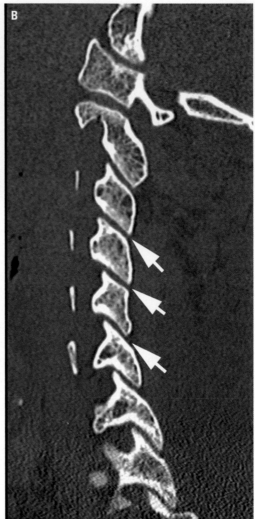

Figure 5.39. Normal facet joints *(arrows)* overlap one another like shingles on a roof (imbrication). **A:** Lateral radiograph. **B:** Sagittal reconstructed CT image.

Each articular pillar has a superior and inferior articulating facet. The inferior and superior facets of contiguous vertebrae constitute an interfacetal (facetal or apophyseal) joint (Fig. 5.39). The inferior facet of the segment above anatomically lies above and posterior to the superior facet of the segment below. The plane of inclination of the interfacetal joints varies throughout the spine but the cervical spine is angled approximately 35 degrees caudally. The arrangement of these joints resembles the shingles on a roof, a term called *imbrication*. This appearance is identical on radiographs or on sagittal CT images. On axial CT and MR images, however, the interfacetal joints resemble a hamburger bun, with the flat portions articulating (Fig. 5.40). Facet dislocations and locking disturb this relationship and produce the *"reverse hamburger bun sign"* (Fig. 5.41). The laminae extend obliquely me-

dially and posteriorly from the articular masses to fuse in the midline to form the spinolaminar line and spinous process. Together, the pedicles, articular pillars, and laminae form the posterior (neural) arch. The vertebrae are separated by the intervertebral disk.

The ring apophyses become radiographically visible about the 16th year and fuse to the vertebral bodies at approximately age 25 years. During this interval, the nonunited apophyses may resemble avulsion fractures. Knowledge of the presence of these centers, the ages of their appearance and fusion, and their uniform appearance with round smooth margins in multiple vertebral bodies identifies these as normal structures (Fig. 5.42).

The three-column concept of the spine (Fig. 5.43) is very important to understanding the reciprocal

A

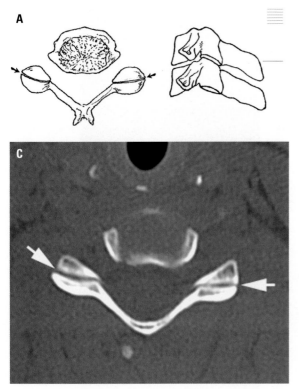

C

B

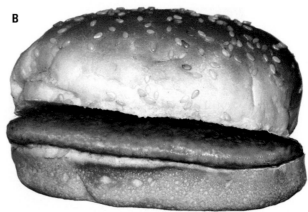

Figure 5.40. Normal facet joints *(arrows)* on axial CT fit together like a hamburger bun ("hamburger bun sign"). **A:** Drawing; **B:** Hamburger; **C:** Axial CT. (From Daffner SD, Daffner RH. Computed tomography diagnosis of facet dislocations: the "hamburger bun" and "reverse hamburger bun" signs. *J Emerg Med*. 2002;23:387–394, with permission.)

A

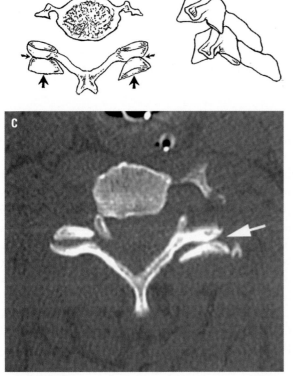

C

B

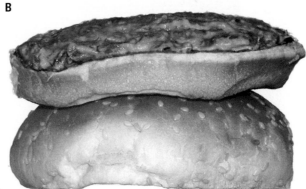

Figure 5.41. Facet dislocation and locking produces the "reverse hamburger bun sign", where the rounded exteriors of the facets articulate. **A:** Drawing; **B:** "Reverse" hamburger; **C:** Axial CT image showing unilateral facet locking on the left *(arrow)* showing the "reverse hamburger bun sign." (From Daffner SD, Daffner RH. Computed tomography diagnosis of facet dislocations: the "hamburger bun" and "reverse hamburger bun" signs. *J Emerg Med*. 2002;23: 387–394, with permission.)

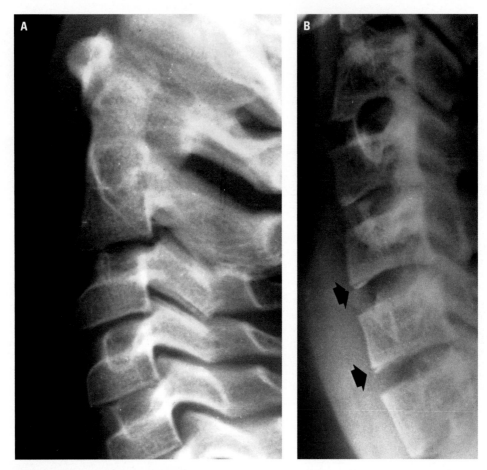

Figure 5.42. Normal ring apophyses. **A:** Lateral radiograph in a 9-year-old shows curved margins of the anterior aspect of the superior end plates of the lower vertebrae, representing nonossified ring apophyses. **B:** Lateral radiograph of an adolescent shows the inferior end plate apophyses *(arrows)*. It is not uncommon to find ununited ring apophyses in adults.

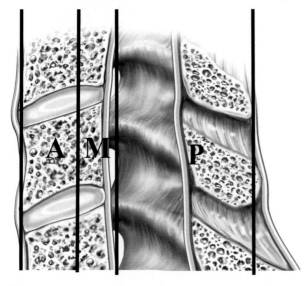

Figure 5.43. Three-column concept of the spine according to Denis. *A* = anterior column; *M* = middle column; *P* = posterior column.

movements of the spine that occur during both normal and pathologic flexion and extension—particularly in the cervical and lumbar areas—and in the concept of spinal stability. The anterior longitudinal ligament, the annulus, and the anterior two-thirds of the vertebral body and disk constitute the anterior column; the posterior third of the body and disk, the posterior annulus, and the posterior longitudinal ligament constitute the middle column; and everything posterior to that constitutes the posterior column.

The lateral radiograph or sagittal reconstructed CT image of the cervical spine (Fig. 5.44) provides the most comprehensive overview of cervical spine skeletal and soft tissue anatomy (and pathology). The cervical spine is normally lordotic, although approximately 17% of all adults have some degree of straightening or reversal of cervical lordosis. Normal cervical lordosis may be voluntarily

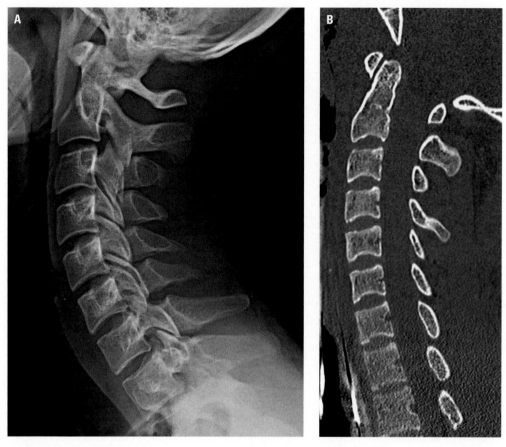

Figure 5.44. Normal cervical curvature. **A:** Lateral radiograph; **(B)** Sagittal reconstructed CT image.

reversed by assuming the "military" or "West Point" position, with the neck severely flexed so that the chin rests on the chest (Fig. 5.45A), by muscle spasm, in supine posture, or by the application of a rigid cervical collar (Fig. 5.45B). These findings may be encountered on CT examinations as well. Reversal of cervical lordosis most commonly occurs in such a way that the posterior cortical margins of the vertebral bodies appear as a smooth, continuous, uninterrupted kyphotic curve throughout the cervical spine (Fig. 5.45B) or as though each cervical segment has individually rotated and translated anteriorly as an independent segment with respect to its adjacent segments. In this event, there is a distinct anterior offset of the posterior cortical margin of each vertebral body with respect to that of each adjacent vertebral body. Such "displacement" is normal, and, even in the neutral lateral projection, it has been demonstrated that up to 3.5 mm of anterior "offset" or "step-off" from one vertebral body to the next (Fig. 5.46) is within normal limits. In these instances, the spinolaminar line

will align normally. Degenerative spondylosis is another cause of malalignment. In these instances, there will be associated narrowing of the disk space and the interfacetal joints. The point being made is that minor anterior (or posterior) displacement of one vertebra with respect to its subjacent member, alone and without any other collaborating sign, is not sufficient evidence to make the radiologic diagnosis of an acute cervical spine injury, that is, subluxation.

Another important imaging finding is the appearance of the PVL. This line, representing the posterior border of the vertebral body, should be solid and uninterrupted. In the lower thoracic and lumbar regions, this line is interrupted in the center by a nutrient foramen. Any displacement, rotation, interruption, angulation, or absence of the PVL is abnormal, and the cause should be sought (Fig. 5.47). CT usually shows the cause of this abnormality.

Finally, two other important relationships on the lateral radiograph or the sagittal reconstructed

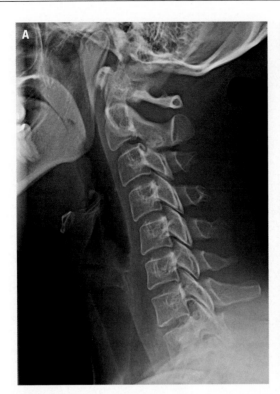
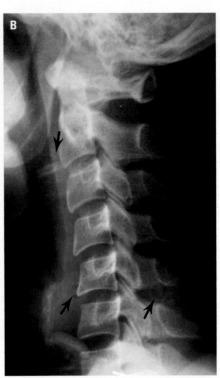

Figure 5.45. Alignment "abnormalities" caused by posture. **A:** Physiologic reversal of lordosis from the "military" posture. Note the position of the mandible in its relationship to the spine, indicating that the patient has assumed the chin-on-chest posture. **B:** Reversal of lordosis caused by an immobilization collar. The snaps are visible *(arrows)*. In both instances, there is a smooth, contiuous, uninterrupted reversal of lordosis, and the spinolaminar line is normal.

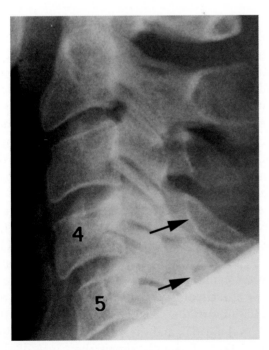

Figure 5.46. Minor offset. The anterior position of C4 with respect to C5 is physiologic and should not be interpreted as pathologic subluxation. The spinolaminar line *(arrows)* is normal.

CT images are the width of the disk spaces and the width of the spaces between the spinous processes—the interlaminar or interspinous distances. Disk space narrowing is the normal expected appearance in patients with degenerative spondylosis. Disk space narrowing may also occur as the result of flexion injuries. However, as with several of the other findings mentioned earlier, there are generally other signs of injury. A wide disk space, particularly in elderly patients, should raise your suspicions that there may have been an extension injury (Fig. 5.48).

The interlaminar distances should be uniform and not vary by more than 2 mm from level to level. Injuries, such as a hyperflexion sprain, that disrupt the posterior ligamentous structures produce widening of this distance (Fig. 5.49). One caveat, however, is a fairly common anomaly of the spinous process of C3, which may be horizontal and have associated widening of the interlaminar space (Fig. 5.50). In this instance, like the other variants mentioned earlier, there will be no other signs of a flexion injury (anterolisthesis, wide interfacetal joints).

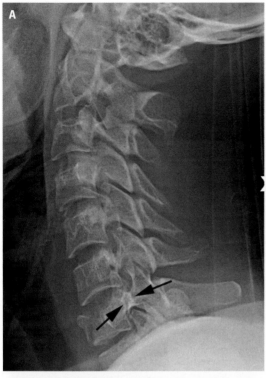

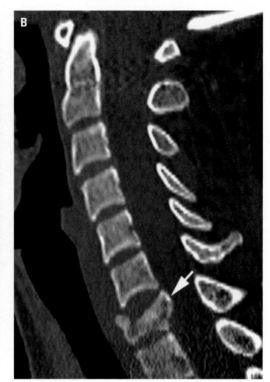

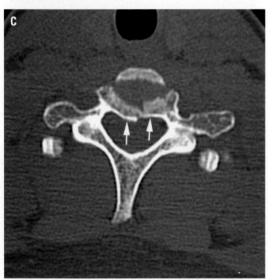

Figure 5.47. Abnormal PVL because of a burst fracture of C7. **A:** Lateral radiograph shows compression of the superior surface of the body of C7 and duplication of the upper portion of the PVL *(arrows)*. **B:** Sagittal reconstructed CT image shows a bone fragment displaced into the vertebral canal *(arrow)*. **C:** Axial CT image shows that the sagittal fracture resulted in retropulsion of a bone fragment into the vertebral canal producing the double PVL *(arrows)*.

Finally, no discussion of the lateral radiograph would be complete without mention of the soft tissues. In the days when radiography was the main screening modality for suspected cervical injuries, these findings had a greater significance. However, today, cervical spine CT has relegated these findings to a secondary role. Still, they are important to be aware of.

The *retropharyngeal space* is a potential space that becomes visible only when it is distended with fluid. It is measured from the anteroinferior aspect of the body of C2 to the posterior aspect of the pharyngeal air column and should never exceed 7 mm in adults and children. This distance can be directly measured from a sagittal reconstructed CT image. Injuries in this region produce widening of this space even in the absence of more obvious skeletal abnormalities (Fig. 5.51). We have observed that the contour of the soft tissue changes are as important as the actual measurements and convex bowing away from the craniovertebral junction is a finding

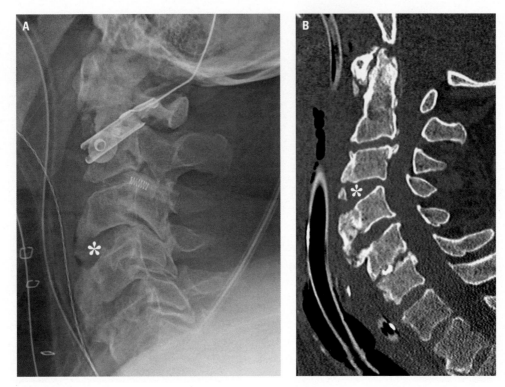

Figure 5.48. Wide disk space *(asterisk)* in a patient with an extension dislocation at C3-C4. **A:** Lateral radiograph. **B:** Sagittal reconstructed CT image.

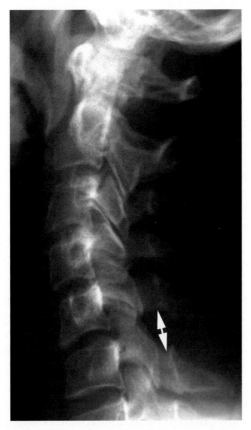

Figure 5.49. Hyperflexion sprain C5-C6 has resulted in widening of the interlaminar distance *(double arrow)*.

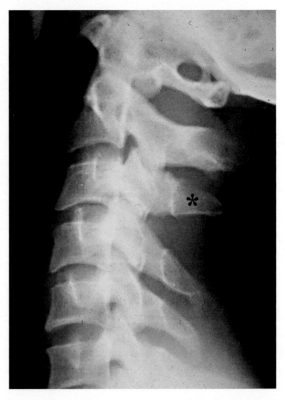

Figure 5.50. Anomalous contour of the spinous process of C3 *(asterisk)* has resulted in widening of the interlaminar distance between C3 and C4. The facet joints are normal, as is the alignment of the vertebral bodies.

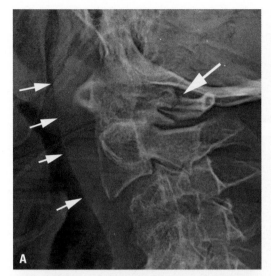

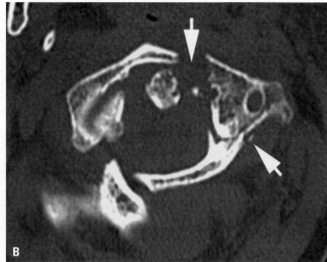

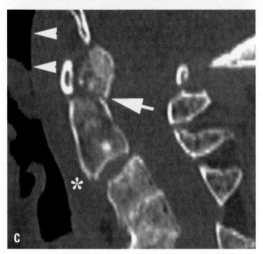

Figure 5.51. Retropharyngeal soft tissue widening in a patient with fractures of C1 and C2. **A:** Lateral radiograph shows fractures of the posterior arch of the atlas *(large arrow)*. There is retropharyngeal soft tissue swelling with a convex contour *(small arrows)* caused by hemorrhage. **B:** Axial CT image shows fractures through the anterior and posterior arches of C1 *(arrows)*. **C:** Sagittal reconstructed CT image shows a dens fracture *(arrow)*, retropharyngeal soft tissue swelling *(asterisk)*, and a convex contour to the abnormal soft tissues *(arrowheads)*. (From Daffner RH. *Imaging of Vertebral Trauma*. 3rd ed. Cambridge, United Kingdom: Cambridge University Press; 2011, with permission.)

to be sought in addition to the width (Fig. 5.51). The retropharyngeal fascia extends uninterrupted from the posterior pharynx to the mediastinum, and as such serve as a potential conduit for fluid in either direction from the neck to the thorax. Thus, facial or aortic injuries, as well as infections, can widen this space. *As a rule, massive widening is not caused by cervical injury.*

Injury to the craniovertebral junction frequently produces a prevertebral hematoma that appears as a soft tissue mass anterior to C1 and C2 (Fig. 5.52). This sign is a reliable indicator of injury only when the history supports that diagnosis and other radiographic findings are lacking. Again, we emphasize that the *contour* of the soft tissues is more important than the actual measurements.

The *retrotracheal space* is measured from the anteroinferior aspect of the body of C6 to the posterior tracheal wall (or shadow of the endotracheal tube), and should never exceed 14 mm in children or 22 mm in adults. As with widening of the retropharyngeal space, retrotracheal space widening accompanies severe disruptive injuries. This sign has largely been rendered obsolete by CT.

The *prevertebral fat stripe* courses caudally along the anterior surfaces of the vertebral bodies from C2 through C6. This thin band of fatty tissue, which is sometimes difficult to see, parallels the anterior longitudinal ligament to the level of C6, where it gradually deviates anteriorly and inferiorly toward the base of the neck. Displacement of this line from its normal location was once considered a reliable indicator that an underlying injury has produced a hematoma. Like the retropharyngeal space, cervical CT has rendered this sign a historic curiosity.

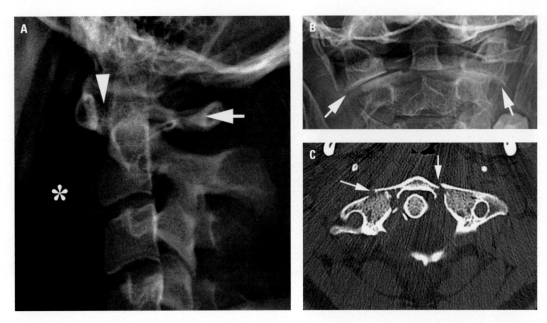

Figure 5.52. Craniovertebral hematoma caused by Jefferson fracture. **A:** Lateral radiograph shows prevertebral soft tissue swelling *(asterisk)*, widening of the predental space *(arrowhead)*, and anterolisthesis of the atlas on the axis *(arrow)*. **B:** Open-mouth view shows offset of the lateral masses of C1 on C2 *(arrows)*. There is widening of the spaces between the dens and the lateral masses of C1. **C:** Axial CT image shows comminuted fractures of both sides of the anterior arch of the atlas *(arrows)* as well as a wide atlantoaxial dens interval. (From Daffner RH. *Imaging of Vertebral Trauma.* 3rd ed. Cambridge, United Kingdom: Cambridge University Press; 2011, with permission.)

On the frontal radiograph of the lower cervical spine (Fig. 5.53), the vertebral bodies constitute the middle third of the radiographic image and are identified by superior and inferior end plates. The uncinate processes and Luschka joints are defined and described earlier (see Fig. 5.37). The posteriorly situated laminae, defined by their cortical margins, and the midline spinous processes are visible through the vertebral bodies. The spinous processes are normally variable in their size and configuration. The interspinous (interlaminar) distances are narrower between C4 and C6, reflective of the apex of the concavity of the cervical lordosis. Again, these distances should not be more than 2 mm different, level to level. The pedicles, being obliquely posteriorly oriented between the vertebral bodies and articular masses, may be variably visible, extending laterally from the middle third of the lateral margin of the vertebral bodies. The transverse distance between them should not vary by more than 2 mm from level to level. The articular pillars of the cervical vertebrae are lateral to the vertebral bodies and this anatomy is represented as the seemingly intact column of bone with smoothly undulating lateral margins seen lateral to the vertebral bodies. The plane of inclination of the interfacetal joints being 35 degrees to the coronal plane renders the joint spaces invisible to the x-ray beam. "Lateral column" is the term ascribed to the radiographic optical illusion of the superimposed articular masses as seen in the AP projection of the cervical spine. Coronal CT reconstructed images will show the individual interfacetal joints.

The tracheal air column produces a sharply demarcated lucency superimposed on the midline of the middle and lower cervical vertebrae (Fig. 5.53). The proximal margins of the air column converge symmetrically into the subglottic area.

We have mentioned several important measurements in the previous discussion. Most of them relate to 2 mm as the maximum difference between different structures. We refer to these as the "Rules of twos," which are summarized subsequently:

2 mm is the normal upper limit for differences for

- interlaminar (interspinous) space,
- interpedicle distance (transverse or vertical),
- unilateral or bilateral atlantoaxial offset, and
- interfacetal joint width.

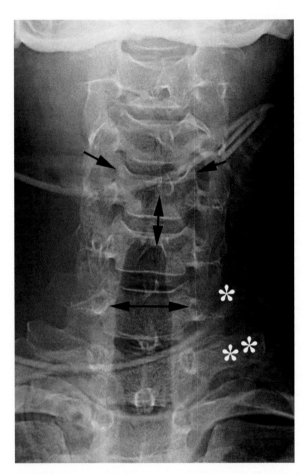

Figure 5.53. Normal AP cervical radiograph. Note the uncinate processes *(single arrows)*, the normal interspinous distance *(vertical double arrow)*, and the normal interpedicle distance *(horizontal double arrow)*. The transverse process of C7 *(asterisk)* points caudal; that of T1 *(double asterisk)* points rostral.

RADIOGRAPHIC MANIFESTATIONS OF TRAUMA: CLASSIFICATION AND THE ABC'S OF DIAGNOSIS

Vertebral injuries have been defined using many classifications. Indeed, many surgeons find that using a classification system based on mechanisms is beneficial in planning surgical reduction and stabilization. An understanding of the mechanisms and the pathophysiology of injury is essential to the interpretation of the imaging manifestations of spinal (cervical) trauma. Many classifications are used to define vertebral injuries. The MOI is the "common property or character" that serves as the basis for grouping of these spine injuries into classes (families). This mechanistic approach to classifying

cervical spine injuries is not new, having been the basis for many other attempts at classification of acute cervical spine injuries.

There are several important facts that are shared by all classifications. First and foremost, it is important to recognize that *vertebral fractures, like those of the peripheral skeleton, occur in predictable and reproducible patterns.* These patterns are the direct result of the kind of force applied to the affected bone. Furthermore, the same force applied to the cervical, thoracic, or lumbar column produces injuries that have a remarkably similar appearance.

Biomechanical studies and autopsy or cadaver experiments have established the fundamental relationship between primary mechanisms of injury and injury patterns that are characteristic of the families of acute injuries of the (cervical) spine. According to Fielding, "the MOI is of major importance in the complete understanding of spine trauma." There are essentially four primary mechanisms of injury: flexion, extension, rotary or torque, and shearing. With the exception of atlantoaxial rotary subluxation and fixation, rotary and shearing injuries occur primarily in the thoracic and lumbar regions. Secondary injuring mechanisms include vertical comprehension (axial load), lateral flexion, or a combination of these forces (simultaneous flexion and rotation or simultaneous extension and rotation, for example). Furthermore, pure or predominant vector forces may be further modified by simultaneous lateral flexion or shear forces, which helps to explain variations of the radiographic appearance of typical acute spine injuries.

Each primary and secondary mechanism has been shown to produce injuries characteristic of each vector force or combination of forces. Furthermore, these injuries may occur as either isolated events or in combination with one another. The incident force, the position of the victim at the time of injury, and the victim's velocity, in turn, determine the severity and extent of the damage produced by any one mechanism. In addition, the patient's age will also influence the type and location of the injury. The reason for this is that as we age, the cervical spine becomes less flexible, with the greatest allowable motion occurring at C1-C2. Nor surprisingly, patients older than the age of 65 years suffer most of their injuries in this region, as compared to younger patients, where the bulk of injuries are at C4-C6. Each mechanism produces a pattern of recognizable imaging signs in a spectrum extending from mild soft tissue damage to severe skeletal and ligamentous disruption. The findings are so consistent from injury to injury that we refer to these patterns as the "fingerprints" of the injury. The fingerprints primary flexion and extension injuries will be enumerated subsequently.

For a classification of cervical spine injuries to have clinical value, it must be practical, that is, relevant to the mainstream of clinical practice, be based on accepted and logical concepts understood by all involved in the management of the patient, and employ widely accepted terminology that permits unambiguous communication concerning any specific injury. The classification based on the MOI we find useful meets these prerequisites. In addition, this classification embodies (1) the physical concept of reciprocal motion (i.e., in flexion, the anterior column of the spine is compressed whereas the posterior column is reciprocally distracted), (2) the fundamental principle that different injuries ("families of injuries") may be caused by the same mechanism, and (3) the general principle of a direct relationship between the magnitude of force of the MOI and the severity and/or magnitude of the injury itself. These same principles apply to injuries of the peripheral skeleton as well.

Finally, any classification of injuries would not be useful unless a careful search for different imaging signs was used in interpreting studies of the spine. Those signs should apply to radiographs, CT, and MRI studies alike. We use a logical system that we call the *ABC'S* for evaluating studies in patients suspected of having sustained vertebral trauma:

- *A*—Alignment and anatomy abnormalities
- *B*—Bony integrity abnormalities
- *C*—Cartilage (joint) space abnormalities
- *S*—Soft tissue abnormalities

Many of the parameters used to identify the abnormalities listed earlier have already been described and illustrated and need not be repeated here. The findings will be emphasized as we discuss specific injuries. However, the following is a summary of each of the abnormalities that may occur under each category:

Alignment and anatomy abnormalities:

- Anterior or posterior vertebral body line disruption
- Spinolaminar line disruption
- Jumped and/or locked facets
- Spinous process rotation
- Interlaminar (interspinous) space widening
- Interpedicle distance widening

- Predental space widening
- Acute kyphotic angulation
- Loss of lordosis
- Torticollis

Bony integrity abnormalities:

- Obvious fracture
- Harris' ring disruption
- "Fat C2" sign
- Interpedicle distance widening
- PVL disruption

Cartilage (joint) space abnormalities:

- Wide predental space
- Disk space widening or narrowing
- Interfacetal joint widening
- "Naked" facets
- Interlaminar (interspinous) space narrowing
- Abnormal dens–basion line

Soft tissue abnormalities:

- Retropharyngeal space widening and convexity
- Retrotracheal space widening
- Prevertebral stripe displacement
- Mass in craniocervical junction
- Laryngeal or tracheal deviation

Acute Traumatic Injuries of the Cervical Spine

Hyperflexion

Hyperflexion injuries are caused by a pure or predominant forward rotation and/or translation (displacement) of a cervical vertebra in the sagittal plane. Flexion injuries are the result of simultaneous compression of the anterior and distraction of the posterior columns of the spine—conditions that should be patently obvious during hyperflexion. Injuries in this group may be purely soft tissue, purely osseous, or a combination.

Hyperflexion Sprain (Anterior Subluxation)

Hyperflexion sprain with resultant anterior subluxation is the flexion component of the "whiplash" injury. The most common MOI is abrupt deceleration in a relatively low-speed MVC, such as in "rear-ending" a stopped car. In this situation, on impact, flexion occurs in the driver of the moving vehicle. The opposite mechanism occurs to the victim in the stopped vehicle. In this situation, the victim's neck and head are thrown first into extension and then into flexion.

Hyperflexion sprain is defined as disruption of the posterior ligament complex, which includes the supraspinous and interspinous ligaments, the ligamentum flavum, the capsule of the apophyseal joints, the posterior longitudinal ligament, and a minor tear of the annulus posteriorly, with varying degrees of extension into the posterior aspect of the disk. Most of the annulus, the disk, and the anterior longitudinal ligament remain intact. Although this is a purely soft tissue injury, hyperflexion sprain is clinically significant because of the morbidity associated being between a 20% to 50% incidence of failure of ligamentous healing, producing "delayed instability."

Hyperflexion injuries are characterized from an imaging standpoint by an abrupt kyphotic angulation at the level of the ligamentous injury. The findings may be seen on radiographs as well as on sagittal reconstructed CT images. The interlaminar or interspinous space is inappropriately widened ("fanning"), the inferior facets of the involved vertebra move upward and forward with respect to the contiguous facets of the subjacent vertebra, and the disk space is widened posteriorly and narrowed anteriorly. The involved vertebra either rotates anteriorly, pivoting on the anteroinferior corner of its body, or is displaced (translated) slightly anteriorly (Figs. 5.54 and 5.55).

It is essential to be aware that hyperflexion sprains may also occur without anterior translation of the subluxed vertebra, but when this is present, it is typically less than 3 mm. This measurement helps distinguish hyperflexion sprain from unilateral interfacetal dislocation (UID), bilateral

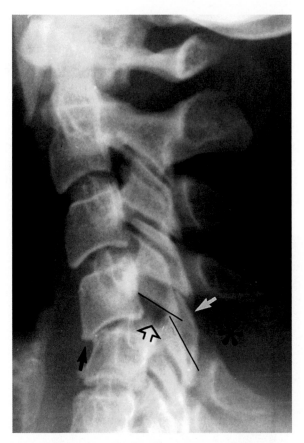

Figure 5.54. Hyperflexion sprain (anterior subluxation). Lateral radiograph shows widening of the interlaminar space *(asterisk)*, partial uncovering of the superior facets of the subjacent vertebra *(white arrow)*, and incongruity of the contiguous facets *(black lines)*. In addition, there is anterolisthesis *(black arrow)* and widening of the space between the posterior cortex of the subluxed vertebral body and articular process of the subjacent vertebra *(open arrow)*. The anterolisthesis is less than that found as a result of UID.

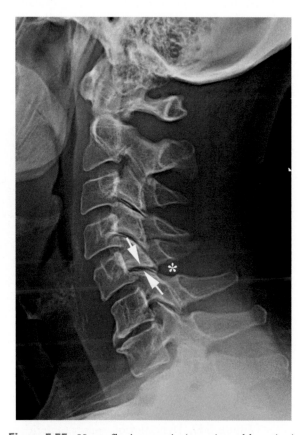

Figure 5.55. Hyperflexion sprain (anterior subluxation). Lateral radiograph shows widening of the interlaminar distance *(asterisk)* as well as wide interfacet joints at C5-C6 *(arrows)*.

interfacetal dislocation (BID), and pedicolaminar fracture-separation (PLF-S) on the lateral radiograph, where the degree of translation is greater. Of course, these distinctions are also more apparent on CT studies.

The essential imaging findings of anterior subluxation on the lateral cervical radiograph or sagittal reconstructed CT are found at the apophyseal joints because of the effect of hyperflexion on the joints. These signs include (1) partial uncovering of the subjacent superior facets and (2) incongruity of the contiguous facets of the affected apophyseal joints and widening of the interlaminar (interspinous) distance. The importance of this observation is shown in Figure 5.56, in which there is no kyphotic angulation and "fanning" is equivocal on the initial neutral radiograph. However, the inferior portion of the subjacent superior facet is uncovered and the contiguous facets of C5 and C6 are not congruous. Although subtle, these findings are real when compared to the normal apophyseal joints at the other levels. Another finding that occurs with anterior subluxation is disruption of the spinolaminar line. The degree of anterolisthesis parallels the amount of anterior translation.

In the past, flexion and extension lateral radiographs were used to make the diagnosis of hyperflexion sprain. However, it has been our experience

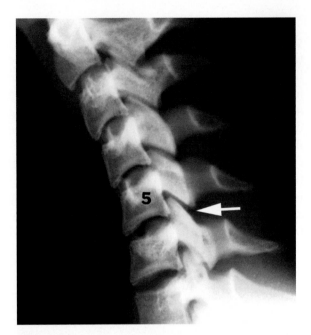

Figure 5.56. Subtle hyperflexion sprain (anterior subluxation). There is reversal of lordosis as well as widening of the interfacetal joints at C5-C6 *(arrow)*.

that these studies are often negative in the acute stage because of muscle spasm or the patient's inability to cooperate. Today, if the diagnosis is suspected from either radiographs or CT, MRI should be performed (Fig. 5.57).

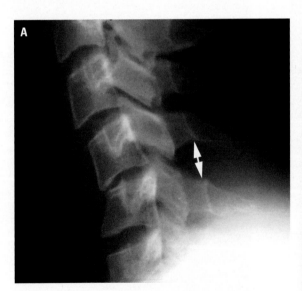

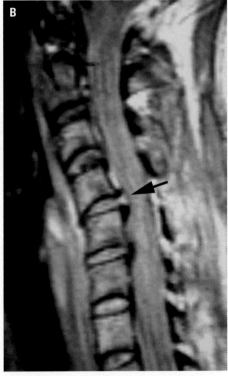

Figure 5.57. Hyperflexion sprain (anterior subluxation). **A:** Lateral radiograph shows widening of the interlaminar space *(double arrow)*. **B:** T2-weighted sagittal MRI image shows rupture of the posterior longitudinal ligament and disk herniation *(arrow)* at C4-C5.

White and Punjabi have defined "clinical instability" as "the loss of the ability of the spine under physiologic loads to maintain its pattern . . . so that there is no initial or additional neurologic deficit, no major deformity, and no incapacitating pain." As shown in Figure 5.58, if the sagittal angulation of the subluxated vertebra exceeds the normal 11 degrees, it is reasonable to assume that the posterior ligament complex is torn. Because the incidence of "delayed instability" (Figs. 5.59 and 5.60) is so high, the usual treatment of choice for hyperflexion sprain is posterior spinal fusion.

The signs of interfacetal joint subluxation and kyphotic angulation (Fig. 5.61A) must be distinguished from the smooth, continuous, uninterrupted physiologic reversal of cervical lordosis of the military position (Fig. 5.61B), recumbency (Fig. 5.61C), or muscle spasm (Fig. 5.61D). In each of these situations, the spinolaminar line is normal.

Although the importance of incongruity of the contiguous surfaces of the apophyseal joints to hyperflexion sprain has been emphasized, the most common etiology of anterior translation of a cervical vertebra is severe degenerative disease with marked apophyseal joint and disk space narrowing. As a rule, the apophyseal joints remain

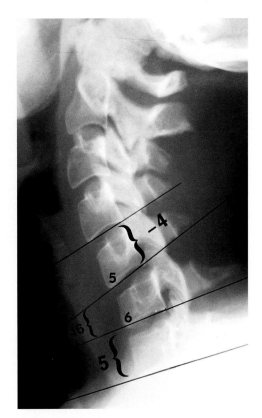

Figure 5.58. Hyperflexion sprain (anterior subluxation) of C5-C6 demonstrating "clinical instability" because of the angle of the interspace at the involved level exceeding 11 degrees.

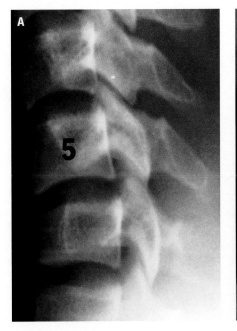
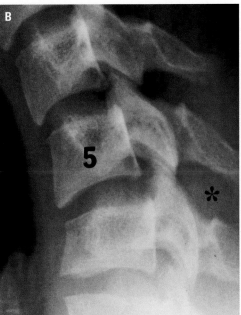

Figure 5.59. Hyperflexion sprain (anterior subluxation) demonstrating delayed instability. **A:** Initial lateral radiograph shows slight widening of the interlaminar distance at C5-C6 and kyphotic angulation. **B:** Four months later shows further angulation and interlaminar widening (*asterisk*), indicating injury to the posterior ligament complex.

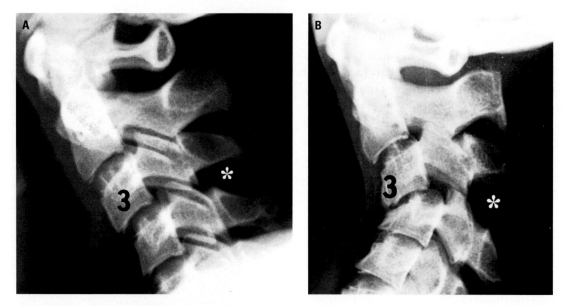

Figure 5.60. Hyperflexion sprain (anterior subluxation) demonstrating delayed instability. **A:** Initial radiograph at time of injury shows kyphotic angulation at C3-C4 and minimal widening of the interlaminar distance *(asterisk)*. **B:** Six weeks later there is exaggeration of the findings with further widening of the interlaminar distance *(asterisk)*. Note the compression deformity of C4.

congruent and the subluxation occurs as a result of loss of cartilage. Furthermore, the subluxation is usually either fixed on flexion and extension radiographs, or is associated with less than 2 mm of motion.

Bilateral Interfacetal Dislocation

BID occurs at both interfacetal joints at the same level. This injury may occur at any level from C2-C3 through C7-T1. As the result of severe hyperflexion, all the ligamentous structures

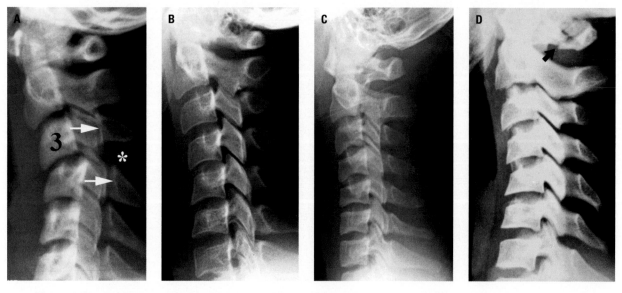

Figure 5.61. Comparison of hyperflexion sprain (**A**) with "military posture" (**B**) reversal of lordosis because of recumbancy (**C**) and effect of muscle spasm (**D**). In the hyperflexion sprain (**A**), there is widening of the interlaminar distance *(asterisk)* and disruption of the spinolaminar line *(arrows)* because of slight anterolisthesis of C3 on C4. In **B and D**, these abnormalities are not present.

of the anterior, middle, and posterior columns are disrupted, and the articular pillars of the involved vertebra are displaced superiorly and anteriorly over the superior articular processes of the subjacent vertebra. The dislocated articular masses come to rest in the inferior portion of the corresponding intervertebral foramen, anterior to the superior articular processes of the subjacent vertebra. Typically, in BID, the anterior displacement of the involved vertebra is approximately 50% of the AP diameter of the dislocated vertebral body, (Fig. 5.62) and thus is considerably greater

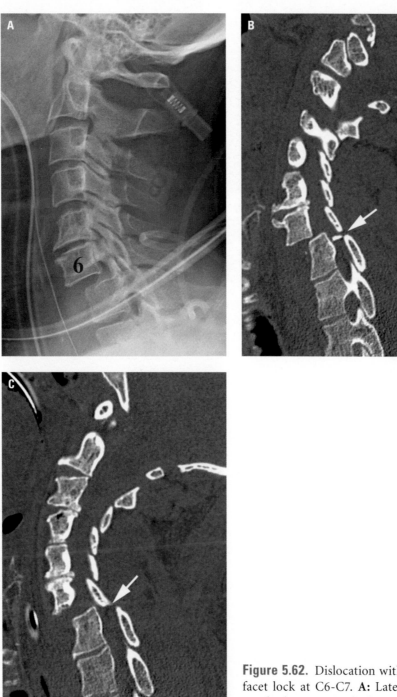

Figure 5.62. Dislocation with bilateral facet lock at C6-C7. **A:** Lateral radiograph shows anterolisthesis of C6 on C7. **B** and **C:** Saggital reconstructed CT images show the locked facets *(arrows)*.

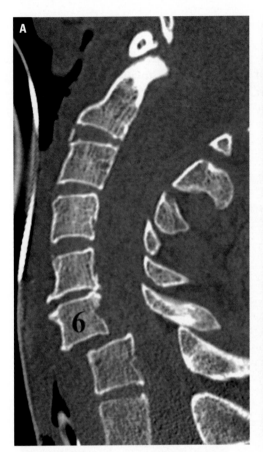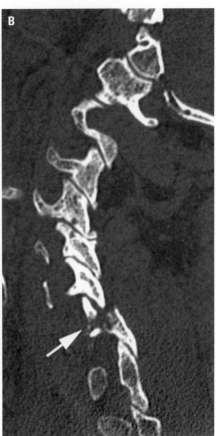

Figure 5.63. Dislocation with posterior facet/pillar fracture. **A:** Sagittal reconstructed CT image shows anterior dislocation of C6 on C7. **B:** Saggital image on the right shows a fracture of the articular pillar and facet of C7 *(arrow)* with locking of the inferior facet of C6 on the fractured pillar.

than the anterior displacement seen with either hyperflexion sprain or UID.

Although BID is considered a pure soft tissue injury, small fractures may arise from the articular processes at the site of dislocation. These fracture fragments are usually of no clinical significance, considering the magnitude of the ligamentous injury. Uncommonly, when the causative force is of sufficient magnitude, a major posterior column fracture may occur with BID (Fig. 5.63).

BID is sometimes imprecisely and inappropriately referred to as "bilateral locked" vertebra, thereby conveying that it is a stable injury, when nothing could be further from reality. The ligamentous and skeletal pathophysiology of BID described earlier renders the injury mechanically unstable, and the associated myelopathy indicates neurologic instability (Fig. 5.64). MRI should be performed for all patients with evidence of BID

to assess the nature and extent of the spinal cord injury as well as associated disk and ligamentous injury (Fig. 5.65).

In children, and less commonly in adults, BID may be the result of a distracting MOI (Fig. 5.66). As a result, the degree of anterior translation of the dislocated vertebra is considerably less than with the pure hyperflexion mechanism.

"Perched" vertebra is a term applied to an incomplete BID in which the articular pillars of the involved vertebra come to rest atop the superior articular processes of the subjacent vertebra. The perched vertebra may be conceptualized as being midway between hyperflexion sprain and BID. On a lateral radiograph, the perched vertebra may be recognized primarily by "fanning" and anterior translation of the involved segment. On frontal radiographs, the interspinous distance at the level of the injury is increased, indicating a flexion injury.

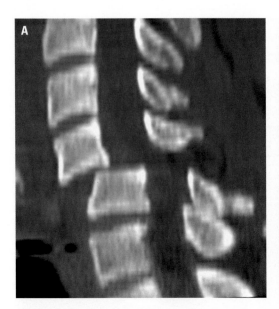

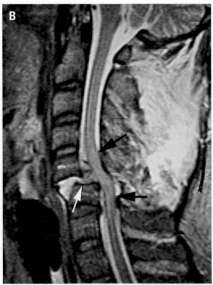

Figure 5.64. Dislocation with bilateral facet lock. **A:** Sagittal reconstructed image shows anterior dislocation of C5 on C6. **B:** Saggital STIR MR image shows the anterolisthesis as well as rupture of the posterior longitudinal ligament *(white arrow)*. Note the swollen, edematous spinal cord *(black arrows)*.

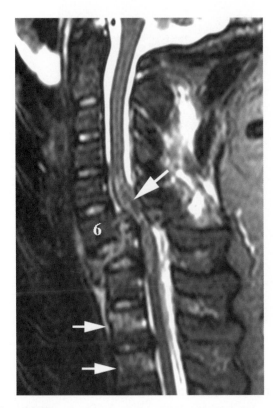

Figure 5.65. Cord injury because of cervical dislocation. Sagittal STIR image shows anterolisthesis as well as hemorrhage and surrounding edema in the spinal cord *(large arrow)*. In addition, there are signal changes indicating microfractures in the bodies of T1 and T2 *(small arrows)*.

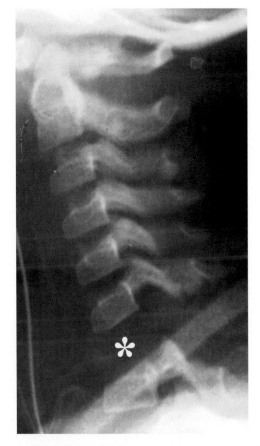

Figure 5.66. Distraction type of dislocation in a child. Note the wide disk space *(asterisk)*.

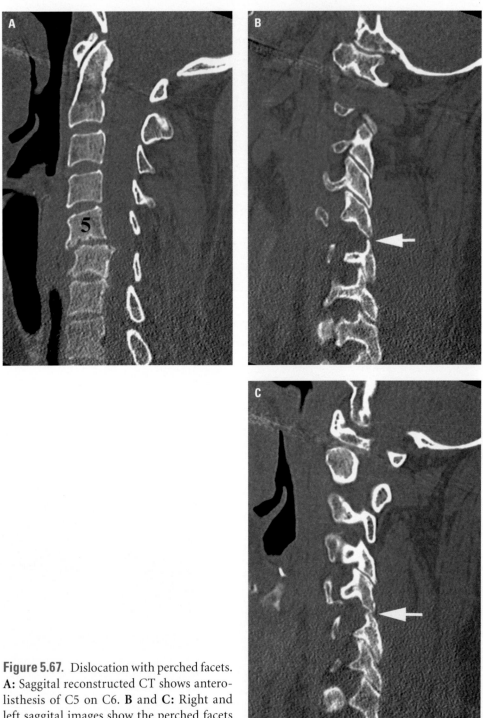

Figure 5.67. Dislocation with perched facets. **A:** Saggital reconstructed CT shows antero-listhesis of C5 on C6. **B** and **C:** Right and left saggital images show the perched facets *(arrows).*

Generally, the findings are apparent on sagittal CT reconstructions (Fig 5.67). On axial images, there is reversal of the contours of the facets to produce the "reverse hamburger bun" sign (Fig. 5.68). The perched vertebra is mechanically unstable but may not be associated with a neurologic deficit.

Wedge (Compression) Fracture

The Wedge fracture (Fig. 5.69) is caused by mechanical compression of one vertebra between adjacent vertebrae during flexion. The simple wedge fracture is characterized radiographically by an impaction fracture of the superior end plate

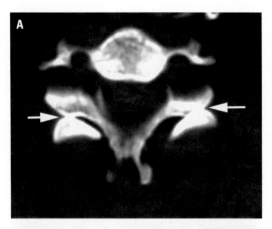

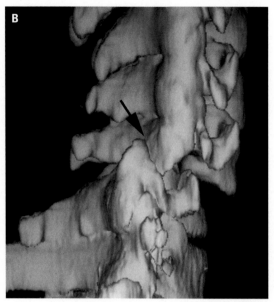

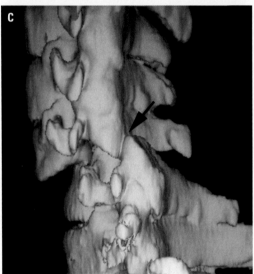

Figure 5.68. Dislocation with bilateral facet lock. **A:** Axial CT image shows a classic "reverse hamburger bun sign" *(arrows)*. **B** and **C:** 3D reconstructed images show the locked facets *(arrows)*.

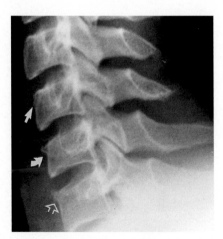

Figure 5.69. Simple wedge (compression fractures of C5, C6, and C7, each with different radiographic features. At C5, there is disruption of the anterosuperior cortex *(straight arrow)*. At C6, there is a "step-off" deformity and slight impaction *(curved arrow)*. At C7, there are similar but less severe changes *(open arrow)*. These fractures are called "simple" because the posterior cortex is intact.

of the involved vertebral body whereas the inferior end plate remains intact. Compression and impaction of the superior end plate are greatest anteriorly, resulting in the "wedge" configuration of the vertebral body. The findings are readily apparent on CT (Fig. 5.70). Signs of disruption of the posterior ligament complex may also be present. In this instance, on the frontal projection, the interspinous distance is increased as one would expect with a flexion injury and disruption of the posterior ligament complex. The vertebral body appears otherwise intact. Specifically, the absence of a vertical fracture of the vertebral body helps distinguish the wedge fracture from the burst fracture. Despite these findings, the wedge fracture is considered mechanically stable because the apophyseal joints and ligamentous structures of the anterior column are maintained. Furthermore, the wedge fracture is typically neurologically stable.

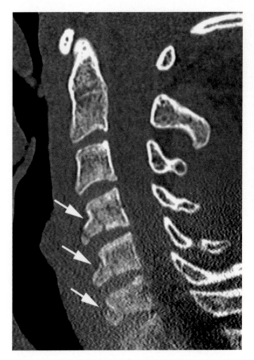

Figure 5.70. CT appearance of simple wedge fractures of C4-C6 *(arrows)*. The posterior cortex is intact.

Clay Shoveler's (Coal Shoveler's) Fracture

The clay shoveler's fracture (Fig. 5.71) is an avulsion injury of the spinous process of C6, C7, or T1. The fracture results from abrupt flexion of the head and neck against the tensed ligaments of the posterior aspect of the neck, as would occur when attempting to throw a shovelful of clay out of a hole, the shovel would become stuck in the clay, causing the shoveler's head and neck to be jerked into violent flexion. Clay shoveler's fracture may occur in any violent type of hyperflexion injury in which the interspinous ligament remains intact, such as those incurred in football and power lifting. The fracture involves the spinous process itself or may extend into the posterior aspect of the lamina on one side or the other. The clay shoveler's fracture line has a characteristically obliquely horizontal orientation and location in the spinous process that is essentially perpendicular to the fibers of the interspinous ligament, characteristic of an avulsion fracture, of which this injury is an example. The clay shoveler's fracture is both mechanically and neurologically stable.

Flexion Teardrop Fracture

The flexion teardrop fracture, a variant of the burst fracture (see below), is one of the most devastating of all cervical injuries. This injury is actually a fracture-dislocation of one of the cervical vertebrae caused by a massive hyperflexion injury with associated axial loading of the cervical spine. It is commonly caused by diving into shallow water and striking the head on the bottom. Other etiologies are football and MVCs in which the victim is ejected.

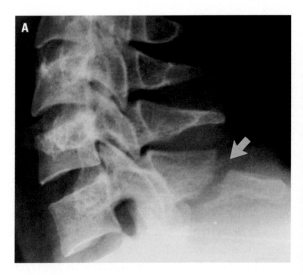

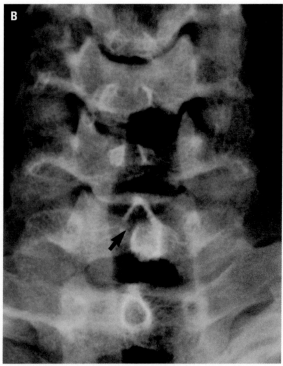

Figure 5.71. Clay shoveler fracture. **A:** Lateral radiograph shows the fractured spinous process *(arrow)*. **B:** Frontal radiograph shows a duplicate density of the spinous process *(arrow)*.

The injury, by definition, is associated with the acute anterior cervical cord syndrome consisting of instant complete quadriplegia and loss of pain, touch, and temperature sensations but with retention of posterior column sensations of position, motion, and vibration. The cord damage is secondary to the severe hyperkyphotic angulation at the level of the fracture-dislocation.

Pathophysiologically, the lesion is characterized by complete disruption of all the soft tissues at the level of injury, including the posterior ligament complex, the posterior longitudinal ligament, the intervertebral disk, the ALL, and the subluxation or dislocation of the interfacetal joints. The lateral radiograph shows the soft tissue and skeletal changes described earlier (Fig. 5.72). The injury derives its name from the characteristic triangular, displaced, separate fracture fragment that consists of the entire anteroinferior corner of the vertebral body that resembles a tear. Other radiographic signs include the flexed attitude of the involved vertebra and those above it, acute hyperkyphosis at the level of injury, prevertebral soft tissue swelling, and signs of disruption of the posterior ligament complex. CT shows that many of these injuries also have findings commonly encountered in burst fractures (Fig. 5.73).

Burst fractures

Burst fractures are another injury that result from severe flexion and axial loading. This mechanism produces comminuted fractures of the vertebral body in various configurations that range from stellate, coronal, and sagittal. Although most burst fractures occur in the thoracic and lumbar areas, two variations occur in the cervical region. The first is the flexion teardrop fracture discussed earlier. The second variety combines the findings of the teardrop fracture with retropulsion of bone fragments from the PVL into the vertebral canal. Typically, there is also widening of the interfacetal joints as well as

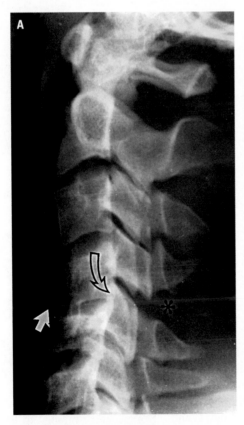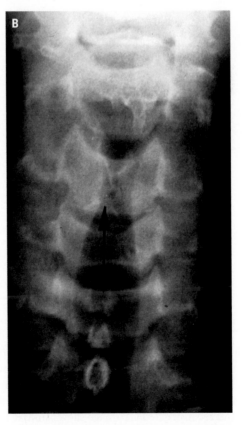

Figure 5.72. Flexion teardrop fracture. **A:** Lateral radiograph shows the teardrop fragment off the anteroinferior margin of C4 *(solid arrow)* and slight retrolisthesis of the body of C4 into the vertebral canal *(open curved arrow)*. The wide interlaminar distance *(asterisk)* identifies the mechanism as flexion. **B:** Frontal radiograph shows widening of the interspinous distance *(double arrow)*.

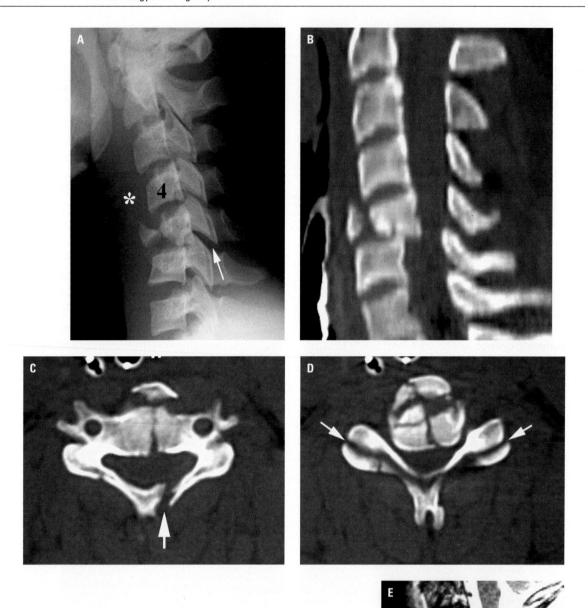

Figure 5.73. Flexion teardrop fracture. **A:** Lateral radiograph shows a large teardrop fragment from the anteroinferior margin of C5. There is retrolisthesis of C4 on C5 and widening of the facet joint *(arrow)*. Note the prevertebral soft tissue swelling *(asterisk)*. **B:** Sagittal reconstructed CT image shows similar findings. **C** and **D:** Axial CT images show that there is also burst pathology with involvement of the lamina of C5 on the right *(arrow* in **C**). Note the severe comminution of the body of C5 and widening of the facet joints *(arrows* in **D**). **E:** Sagittal STIR MR image shows cord hemorrhage *(arrow)* surrounded by a wide zone of edema.

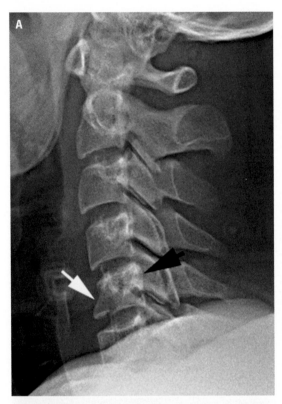

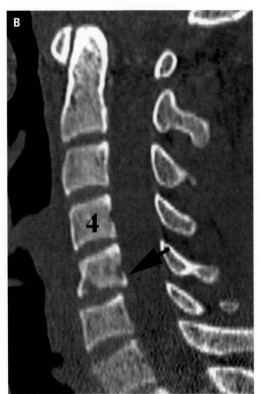

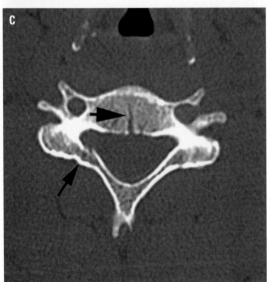

Figure 5.74. Burst fracture caused by axial loading. **A:** Lateral radiograph shows a fracture of the anteroinferior margin of the body of C4 *(white arrow).* Note bowing of the posterior body line *(black arrow).* **B:** Sagittal reconstructed CT image shows the canal encroachment *(arrow).* **C:** Axial CT image shows a sagittal fracture of the vertebral body *(large arrow)* as well as a laminar fracture on the right *(small arrow).* (From Daffner RH. *Imaging of Vertebral Trauma.* 3rd ed. Cambridge, United Kingdom: Cambridge University Press; 2011, with permission.)

widening of the interlaminar (interspinous) space (Fig. 5.74). Other findings include sagittal fractures and lamina fractures (sagittal cleavage fracture) (Fig. 5.75). Cervical burst fractures are more likely to occur as the result of pure axial loading. These injuries will be discussed subsequently under vertical compression injuries. Burst fractures, regardless of MOI, are unstable and are associated with severe neurological deficits.

Simultaneous Hyperflexion and Rotation
Unilateral Interfacetal Dislocation
UID is the injury produced by simultaneous hyperflexion and rotation. The dislocation occurs on the side opposite the direction of rotation and consists of anterior dislocation of one articular mass (and its inferior facet) with respect to the contiguous subjacent articular mass. In the process, the posterior ligament complex is disrupted. The dislocated

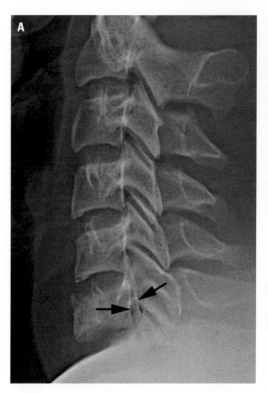

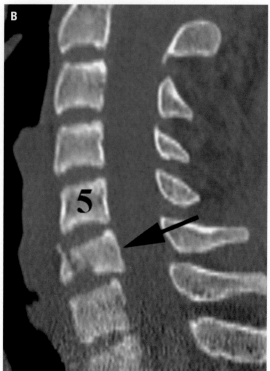

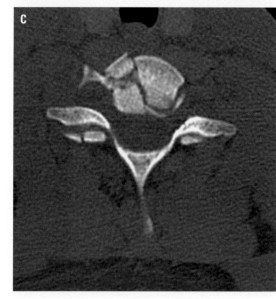

Figure 5.75. Burst fracture of C6. **A:** Lateral radiograph shows a compression deformity of the anterior superior body of C6. There is duplication of the posterior body line *(arrows)*. **B:** Sagittal reconstructed CT image shows retropulsion of a bone fragment into the vertebtral canal *(arrow)*. **C:** Axial CT image shows severe comminution of the vertebral body with canal encroachment by fragments. (From Daffner RH. *Imaging of Vertebral Trauma.* 3rd ed. Cambridge, United Kingdom: Cambridge University Press; 2011, with permission.)

articular pillar comes to rest in the intervertebral foramen anterior to the subjacent articular mass, where it is mechanically wedged in between the subjacent vertebral body anteriorly and the superior articular process posteriorly. The injury is appropriately referred to as the "locked" vertebra. CT has actually shown that most of these injuries are incomplete and the locking occurs as a result of the pillar of the superior vertebra impacting on the fractured

subjacent pillar (Fig. 5.76). UID is rarely associated with neurologic deficit, and when it is, the neurologic deficit is of nerve root distribution. Disruption of the posterior ligament complex and the disk, with either attenuation or actual disruption of the ALL, is intrinsic to UID. These findings inherently make the injury unstable. The ligamentous injuries are of little clinical significance because anterior and posterior fusion is the treatment of choice for UID.

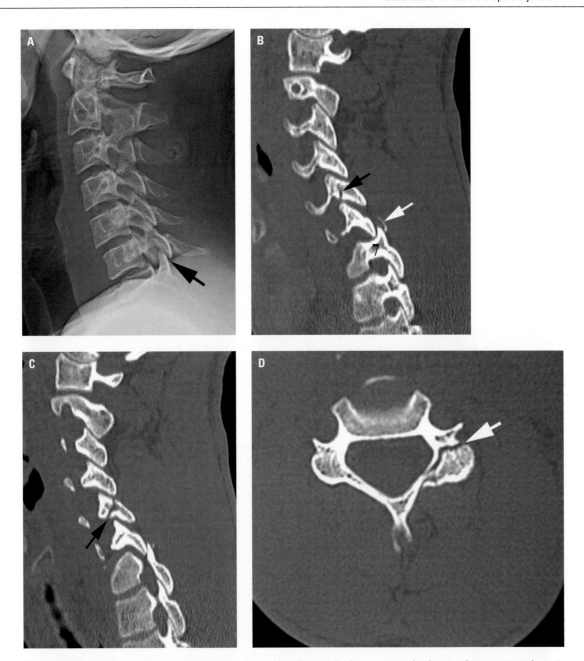

Figure 5.76. UID with locking C6-C7. **A:** Lateral radiograph shows anterolisthesis of C6 on C7. There is posterior facet lock *(arrow)*. **B** and **C:** Sagittal reconstructed CT images show a fracture of the superior facet of C7 with locking *(white arrow)*. There are pillar fractures of C6 on the same side *(black arrows)*. **D:** Axial CT image shows the articular pillar fracture on the left *(arrow)*. Note that the spinous process of C6 is rotated to the left—the side of the locked facet.

In the past, when radiography was the main screening modality for suspected cervical injuries, UID was frequently missed. Indeed, a review of depositions of radiologists and emergency medicine physicians who were sued for missing these injuries revealed that the defendants all thought the radiographs "looked funny." Fortunately, now that CT is used for screening, these injuries are infrequently missed. The radiographic signs of UID are the changes secondary to rotation and flexion at and above the level of dislocation. On the AP radiograph, the spinous processes at and above the level of dislocation are displaced from the midline to the side of dislocation. On the lateral projection, the dislocated vertebra is anteriorly displaced with respect to the subjacent vertebra a distance less than one-half the AP diameter of a vertebral body. The amount of anterior translation of UID is therefore less than occurs with bilateral dislocation but generally greater than that of hyperflexion sprain.

The rotational component of UID is evidenced by the lack of superimposition of the articular pillars at and above the dislocation. The posterior cortical margins of the articular masses on the side of dislocation lie anterior to those on the opposite side, which have rotated posteriorly. Consequently, the interfacetal joint spaces on the side of dislocation are superimposed on the vertebral bodies. At the level of the dislocation, the dislocated articular mass is usually identifiable, lying anterior to its contiguous subjacent articular mass. This, sometimes, can be seen as a "bowtie" appearance. On the opposite side, the inferior facet of the articular mass is subluxed with respect to its contiguous facet; that is, the inferior facet of the nondislocated articular mass is displaced upward and forward with respect to its contiguous facet but remains above and behind the facet below.

Additionally, rotation results in a decrease in the laminar space—the distance between the posterior cortical margin of the articular mass and the spinolaminar line—on the side opposite the dislocation. These findings are all seen in Figure 5.77.

CT has made the diagnosis of UID easier and readily demonstrates the displacement, rotation, locking, and any associated fractures (Figs. 5.75 and 5.78). Furthermore, the abnormalities at the pillar level also produce the "reverse hamburger bun" sign. CT also shows the reason that the spinous processes of the vertebrae above the lock are rotated toward the side of injury.

The "fingerprints" of hyperflexion injuries include the following:

- Compression (Fig. 5.69), fragmentation (Fig. 5.75), and burst fractures of the vertebral bodies (Figs. 5.74 and 5.75)
- Teardrop fragments of the anteroinferior margins of the vertebral bodies (Fig. 5.73)

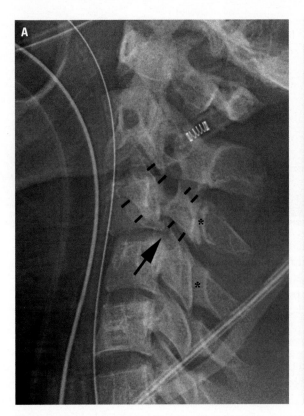 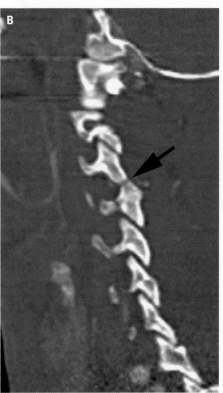

Figure 5.77. UID with locking C3-C4. **A:** Lateral radiograph shows anterolisthesis of C3 on C4. Note the locking of the facet *(arrow)*. There is also a well-defined "bowtie sign" *(dash lines)* as well as an abrupt change in the distance between the posterior margin of the articular pillar and the spinolaminar line at C3-C4 *(asterisk)*. **B:** Sagittal reconstructed CT image shows locking on a fractured facet *(arrow)*.

- Widening of the interlaminar or interspinous spaces (Fig. 5.55)
- Anterolisthesis (Figs. 5.62 and 5.77)
- Disruption of the PVL (Figs. 5.74 and 5.75)
- Jumped or locked facets (Figs. 5.67 and 5.78)
- Narrowing of the intervertebral disk spaces, usually above the level of involvement

Hyperextension Injuries
Hyperextension Dislocation

Hyperextension dislocation of the cervical spine was first described by Taylor and Blackwood in 1947. This injury, which has several variants, has been called several names: "hyperextension sprain" by Braakman and Penning and "hyperextension sprain (momentary dislocation) with fracture" by Gehweiler et al. Hyperextension dislocation is fundamentally a soft tissue injury involving the lower cervical segments caused by a force delivered to the face driving the head and neck into hyperextension.

The pathophysiology of hyperextension dislocation includes some degree of tearing of the longus colli and longus capitis muscles, complete tearing of the anterior longitudinal ligament and annulus, disruption of the intervertebral disk and annulus posteriorly, stripping of the posterior longitudinal

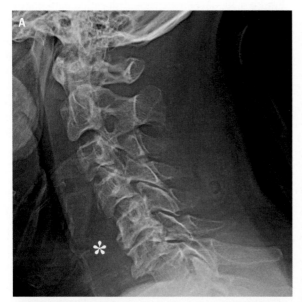
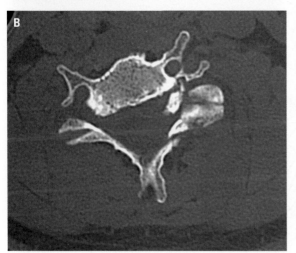
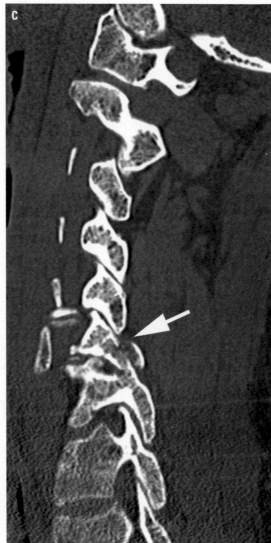

Figure 5.78. UID with locking C6-C7. **A:** Lateral radiograph shows anterolisthesis of C6 on C7. There is massive prevertebral soft tissue swelling *(asterisk)*. **B:** Axial CT image shows comminuted fractures of the articular pillar and facet on the left. Note the rotation of the spinous process to the left—the side of the locking. **C:** Sagittal reconstructed CT image shows the locked facet *(arrow)* on a fractured articular pillar.

ligament from the posterior cortical margin of the subjacent vertebral body, and disruption of the ligamentum flavum. As the involved vertebra is driven posteriorly, the spinal cord is compressed against the ligamentum flavum and the lamina of the subjacent vertebra, resulting in some degree of the acute central cervical spinal cord syndrome. This extensive soft tissue pathology is clearly delineated on the sagittal MR image (Fig. 5.79). In approximately two-thirds of patients with herniated disk, the anterior annulus is not disrupted and the intact Sharpey's fibers cause an avulsion fracture of the anterior aspect of the inferior end plate of the involved vertebra (Fig. 5.80).

The diagnosis of hyperextension dislocation is based on a constellation of clinical and imaging signs. Clinically, the patient with this injury should have evidence of lower facial trauma and some manifestation of the acute central cervical spinal cord syndrome, ranging from upper-extremity paresthesia to complete permanent quadriplegia.

From an imaging standpoint, hyperextension dislocation is a paradox because the momentary posterior displacement of the involved vertebra ("dislocation") may be completely reduced when the causative force is dissipated. Consequently, a dislocation may not be present on a lateral cervical radiograph or sagittal reconstructed CT. However, like all extension mechanisms, the hallmark of this injury is a wide disk space (Fig. 5.81). This finding is so specific, that its mere presence should

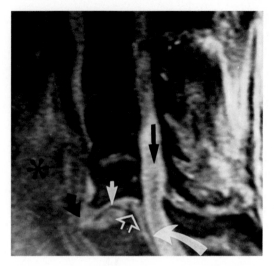

Figure 5.79. Hyperextension dislocation pathology demonstrated by MRI. Sagittal STIR image shows tear of the anterior longitudinal ligament *(curved black arrow)* and displacement of the involved vertebra with a torn posterior annulus *(open arrow)* as well as stripping and rupture of the posterior longitudinal ligament *(curved white arrow)*. The disk space is wide and shows hemorrhage within it *(short white arrow)*. There is also hemorrhage in the spinal cord *(black straight arrow)*. Note the significant prevertebral soft tissue swelling *(asterisk)*, as well as bright signal posteriorly indicating significant soft tissue injury.

raise your suspicions that an extension injury has occurred. Furthermore, a normal-appearing disk space in an elderly patient with severe neurologic compromise and extensive spondylosis should also be considered with suspicion. Additional

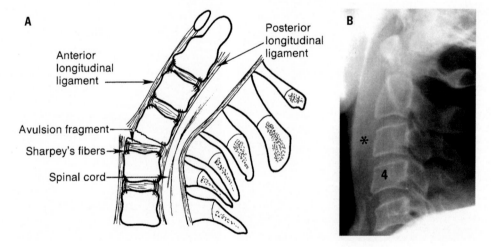

Figure 5.80. Hyperextension dislocation (sprain). **A:** Schematic representation demonstrating the etiology of the fracture fragment from the anteroinferior aspect of the involved vertebra. This avulsion is caused by intact Sharpey's fibers. **B:** Lateral radiograph showing normal alignment. Note the significant prevertebral soft tissue swelling *(asterisk)* as well as subtle widening of the C4-C5 disk space.

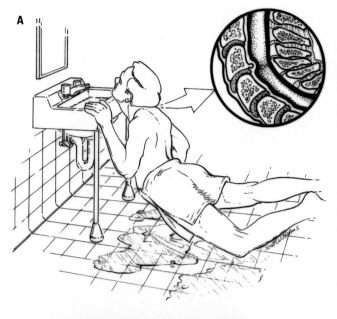

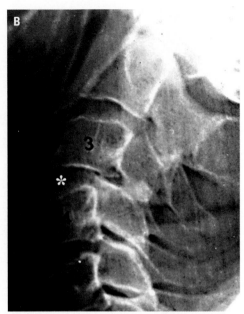

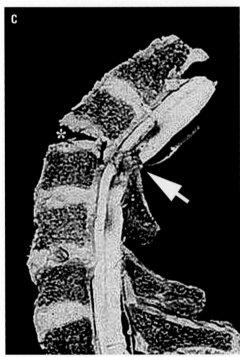

Figure 5.81. Hyperextension dislocation (sprain). **A:** Typical MOI in an elderly individual. This mechanism results in compression of the spinal cord by osteophytes or syndesmophytes and typically produces a central cord syndrome. **B:** Lateral radiograph shows widening of the C3 disk space and retrolisthesis of C3 on C4. **C:** Autopsy specimen from the same patient shows widening of the C3 disk space *(asterisk)* and hemorrhage in the spinal cord *(arrow)*. (From Daffner RH. *Imaging of Vertebral Trauma*. 3rd ed. Cambridge, United Kingdom: Cambridge University Press; 2011, with permission.)

imaging signs of hyperextension dislocation in adults include some degree of retrolisthesis, and on occasion normally aligned cervical vertebrae. In addition, there is usually diffuse prevertebral soft tissue swelling (Fig. 5.80), and an avulsion fracture of the anteroinferior margin of the involved vertebra characterized by a configuration in which its transverse dimension exceeds its vertical height (Fig. 5.82). Another less frequent sign is a vacuum defect in the involved disk (Fig. 5.83).

These findings may be observed on radiographs and saggital reconstructed CT images.

Hyperextension dislocation occasionally involves C2, where it may be confused with the extension teardrop fracture in the elderly. Each of these injuries is associated with an avulsion fracture of the vertebral body and the distinctive radiographic features of the avulsion fragment of each is important in the differential diagnosis. As described earlier, the transverse dimension of the avulsion fracture

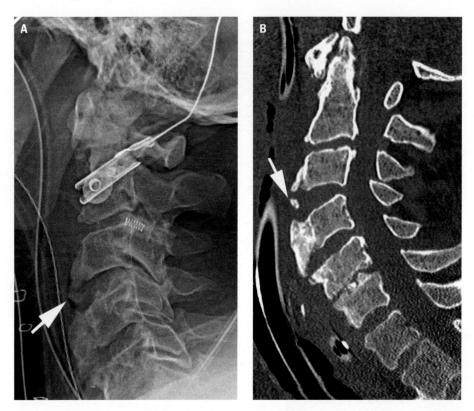

Figure 5.82. Hyperextension dislocation C3-C4. **A:** Lateral radiograph shows the avulsed fragment from the inferior margin of C3 *(arrow)*. Note that the horizontal length of the fragment exceeds its height. **B:** Sagittal reconstructed CT image shows a portion of the avulsed fragment *(arrow)* as well as widening of the disk space.

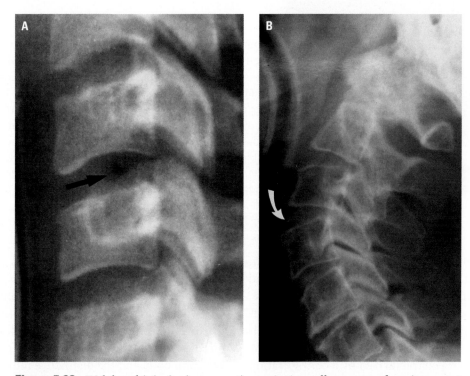

Figure 5.83. Disk bond injuries in two patients. **A:** A small amount of gas is present in the disk *(arrow)* without widening. **B:** There is widening of the disk with a small amount of gas at the anteroinferior margin of of the disk space *(curved arrow)*.

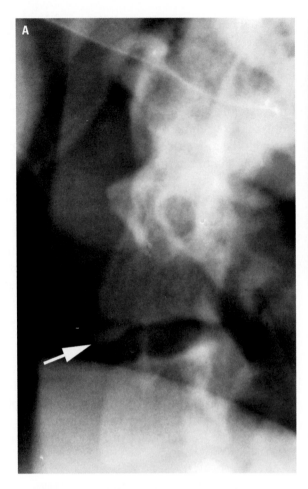

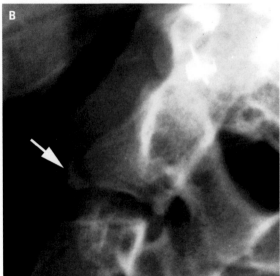

Figure 5.84. Comparison of the typical avulsion fractures from hyperextension dislocation (**A**) with that of the hyperextension teardrop fracture (**B**). In the hyperextension dislocation (**A**), the horizontal dimension of the fragment *(arrow)* exceeds its height. There is usually diffuse prevertebral soft tissue swelling. In the hyperextension tear drop fracture (**B**), the vertical height exceeds the horizontal length *(arrow)*. The soft tissue changes are focal and minimal.

of hyperextension dislocation exceeds its vertical height (Fig. 5.84A). Conversely, the vertical height of the extension teardrop fracture is either equal to or greater than its transverse dimension (Fig. 5.84B). Other important distinctions include diffuse prevertebral soft tissue swelling and the acute central cervical cord syndrome in the dislocation, as opposed to minimal focal prevertebral soft tissue swelling and uncommon neurologic deficit with the extension teardrop fracture.

The diffuse prevertebral soft tissue swelling found in hyperextension dislocation is caused by a hematoma contained in the retropharyngeal fascial space as a result of tearing of the longus colli and longus capitis muscles during hyperextension. Although observing soft tissue swelling was an important indicator of underlying injury in the days before CT was used primarily for screening for cervical injury, today, it is just an ancillary imaging finding on CT and/or MRI. Interestingly, in adolescents, the severity of the acute central cervical cord syndrome is less than in adults. The lesser prevertebral

soft tissue swelling and less severe myelopathy may both be indicative of the lesser magnitude of force required to avulse a nonunited ring apophysis than a fragment from an adult vertebral body. Therefore, the radiologic diagnosis of hyperextension dislocation in adolescent patients is based on the presence of a displaced ring apophysis and minor prevertebral soft tissue swelling (Fig. 5.85).

The "Taylor mechanism" is the development of the acute central cervical cord syndrome in an elderly patient following relatively minor trauma in which the neck moves only through physiologic hyperextension. The lateral cervical spine radiograph or sagittal CT image will show only spondylosis with posteriorly projecting osteophytes and without prevertebral soft tissue swelling. Taylor demonstrated that sufficiently large posteriorly projecting osteophytes can cause as much as 30% narrowing of the cervical canal during physiologic hyperextension, which is sufficient to produce cord compression and the acute central cervical cord syndrome.

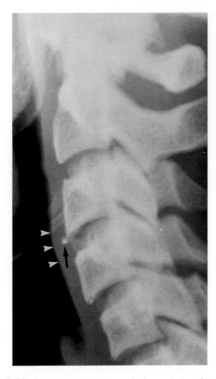

Figure 5.85. Hyperextension dislocation of C3 in an adolescent identified by avulsion of the inferior ring apophysis *(arrow)* of C3. Only focal soft tissue swelling *(arrowheads)* is present adjacent to the avulsed apophysis.

Hyperextension fractures occurring in patients with rigid spine disease (ankylosing spondylitis [Fig. 5.86] or diffuse idiopathic skeletal hyperostosis [DISH, Forestier disease][Fig. 5.87]) fractures the ossified anterior syndesmophytes and then either extends obliquely through the disk into the subjacent vertebral body or extends posteriorly through the disk space itself. In the latter situation, we often refer to the findings as the "broken DISH" (Fig. 5.88).

There is another variation of the hyperextension dislocation that may suggest a flexion mechanism on initial imaging studies. Instead of retrolisthesis, the severe hyperextension mechanism results in fractures to the articular pillars and vertebral arches. These produce anterolisthesis with *normal* interlaminar or interspinous spaces and *normal* spinolaminar lines (Fig 5.89). Fortunately, these injuries are rare.

Avulsion Fracture of the Anterior Arch of the Atlas

The avulsion fracture of the anterior arch of C1 is caused by traction on the intact fibers of the cephalad extension of the anterior longitudinal ligament and the longus colli muscles. This fracture

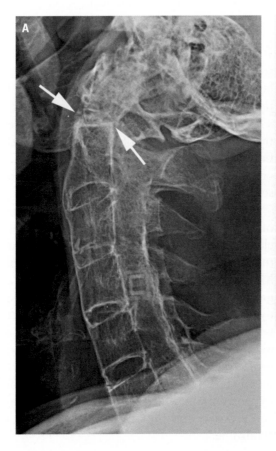

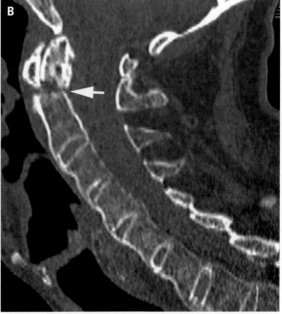

Figure 5.86. Hyperextension fracture *(arrows)* of the dens in a patient with ankylosing spondylitis. **A:** Lateral radiograph. **B:** Sagittal reconstructed CT.

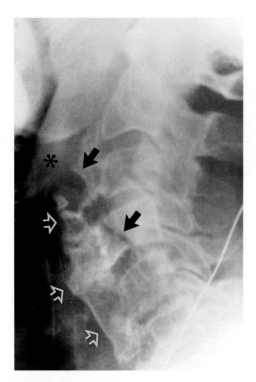

Figure 5.87. Hyperextension fracture in DISH *(open arrows)* ("broken DISH"). The fracture, which is accompanied by diffuse prevertebral soft tissue swelling *(asterisk)*, extends through the syndesmophyte, the disk space, and obliquely through the body of C4 *(arrows)*.

may involve the inferior pole of the anterior arch (Fig. 5.90A) or the midplane. The contiguous margins of the fracture line are irregular and noncorticated, and there is usually an associated cervicocranial hematoma. This fracture is easily distinguishable from the ununited secondary ossification center of the inferior pole of the tubercle because it lacks sclerotic margins and has a positive "jigsaw puzzle effect." The accessory ossification center has smooth margins and will not fit into the adjacent bone like a piece of a jigsaw puzzle. Furthermore, the ossification lacks prevertebral soft tissue swelling (Fig. 5.90B).

Isolated Fracture of the Posterior Arch of the Atlas

Isolated fractures of the posterior arch of C1 (Fig. 5.91) are caused by its compression between the occipital bone and the heavy spinous process of C2 during hyperextension. The only differential diagnosis concerning this fracture is the Jefferson bursting fracture of C1, which can easily be diagnosed by cervical CT. The typical Jefferson fracture involves the anterior arch and/or the lateral masses as well as the posterior arch. Furthermore, the isolated posterior arch fracture rarely produces prevertebral soft tissue swelling.

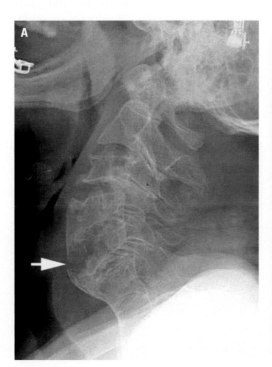

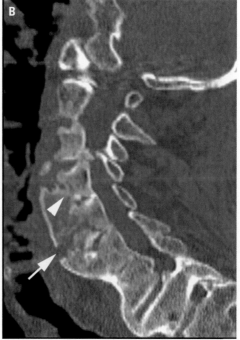

Figure 5.88. "Broken DISH." **A:** Lateral radiograph shows a break in the syndesmophyte chain anterior to C5 *(arrow)*. **B:** Sagittal reconstructed CT image shows the same fracture *(arrow)* as well as an additional fracture at C4 *(arrowhead)*.

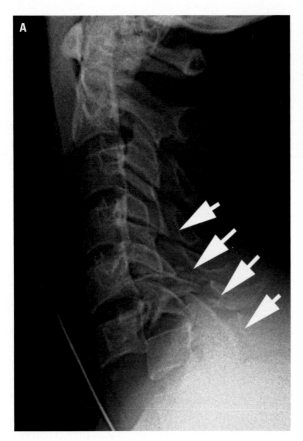

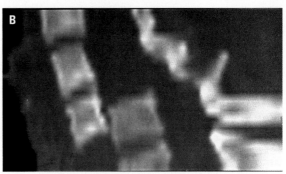

Figure 5.89. Hyperextension fracture-dislocation. **A:** Lateral radiograph and (**B**) sagittal reconstructed sagittal image show anterior dislocation of C6 on C7. Although this might suggest a flexion injury, the spinolaminar line remains intact (*arrows in* **A**). (From Daffner RH. *Imaging of Vertebral Trauma*. 3rd ed. Cambridge, United Kingdom: Cambridge University Press; 2011, with permission.)

Laminar Fracture

Isolated fractures of the laminae are rare, are caused by hyperextension, and may be associated with fracture of an adjacent spinous process. In these instances, CT shows that the laminar fracture extends into the spinous process. Laminar fractures are usually subtle and may be only visible by CT. Spinolaminar fractures secondary to gunshot wounds are usually obvious on the lateral radiograph. CT is crucial to assess the position of bone and bullet fragments with respect to the spinal canal.

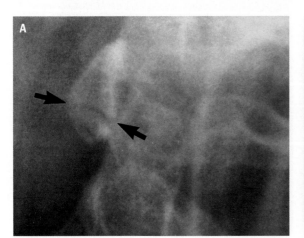

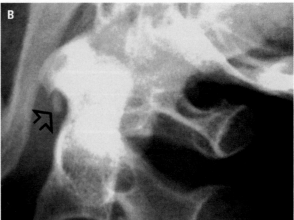

Figure 5.90. Acute avulsion fracture of the inferior pole *(arrows)* of the anterior tubercle of C1 (**A**). The characteristics of the fracture line clearly distinguish this acute injury from the developmentally nonunited secondary ossification center *(open arrow)* (**B**) at the same site.

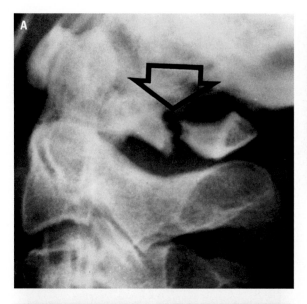

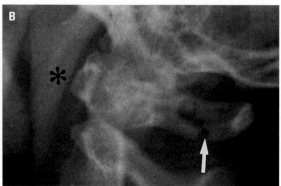

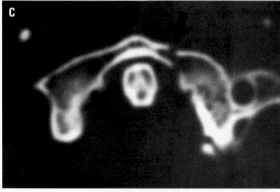

Figure 5.91. Posterior atlas arch fractures. **A:** Isolated fracture of the posterior arch of C1 *(open arrow)*. It is easy to understand from (**A**) how the thin posterior arch of C1 could be fractured by compression between the occiput and the mass of the spinous process of C2. The only differential diagnostic possibility is the Jefferson bursting fracture *(arrows* in **B** and **C**). Note the prevertebral soft tissue swelling in **B** *(asterisk)*.

Extension Teardrop Fracture

The extension teardrop fracture derives its name from its dominant MOI (hyperextension) and the resulting characteristic triangular fracture fragment. The latter is avulsed by the intact fibers of the anterior longitudinal ligament, which insert on the anteroinferior aspect of the vertebral body. In contradistinction to the separate fragment of hyperextension sprain (dislocation), *the vertical height of the extension teardrop fracture fragment is equal to or exceeds its transverse dimension* (Fig. 5.92). Clinically, the extension teardrop fracture, also in contrast to the hyperextension sprain, is not associated with a myelopathy. Although most of these injuries occur at C2, in younger patients this fracture may occur in the lower cervical spine and may be associated with massive diffuse prevertebral soft tissue swelling similar to that seen with hyperextension sprain. The presence of such diffuse prevertebral soft tissue swelling is a clue that the injury may, in fact, be more extensive, particularly when the patients have signs

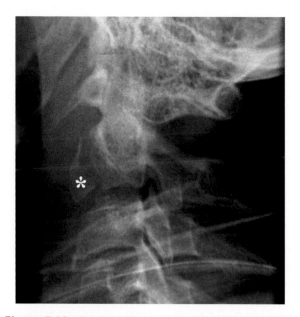

Figure 5.92. Hyperextension teardrop fracture of C2 *(asterisk)*. This fracture is unusual in that the vertical height exceeds the horizontal length. This patient was neurologically intact.

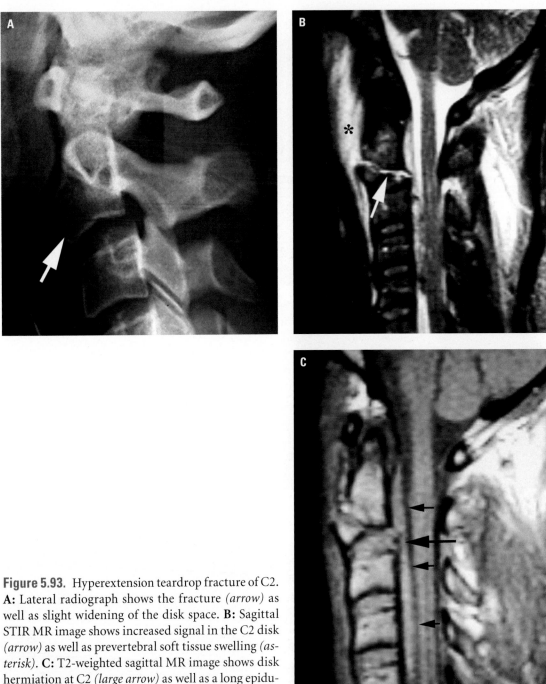

Figure 5.93. Hyperextension teardrop fracture of C2. **A:** Lateral radiograph shows the fracture *(arrow)* as well as slight widening of the disk space. **B:** Sagittal STIR MR image shows increased signal in the C2 disk *(arrow)* as well as prevertebral soft tissue swelling *(asterisk)*. **C:** T2-weighted sagittal MR image shows disk herniation at C2 *(large arrow)* as well as a long epidural hematoma *(short arrows)*. Surprisingly, the patient was neurologically intact.

of acute central cervical cord syndrome. In these instances, MRI is necessary to confirm the extent of injury (Fig. 5.93).

Traumatic Spondylolisthesis ("Hanged Man's" Fracture)
Traumatic spondylolisthesis (TS) derives the name "hanged man's fracture" from its presumed morphologic similarity to the cervical spine injury

associated with judicial hanging. However, radiologic and pathologic examination of the cervical spine of two subjects of judicial hanging found that neither subject sustained TS and that the cervical spine fractures were irrelevant to the cause of death.

The MOI of the hanged-man fracture is predominantly hyperextension. In most cases because

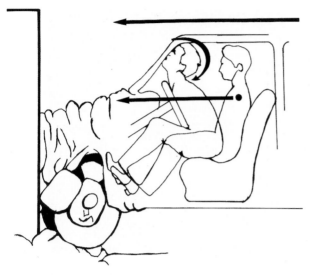

Figure 5.94. Mechanism of the hanged-man's fracture in an MVC. The unrestrained driver pitches forward, impaling the thorax on the steering wheel. If the face strikes the windshield before the vertex of the head, the head is forced backward in hyperextension to produce the cervical injury. (From Daffner RH. *Imaging of Vertebral Trauma*. 3rd ed. Cambridge, United Kingdom: Cambridge University Press; 2011, with permission.)

of MVCs, the victim impales his thorax on the steering wheel and the head is forced backward in extension (Fig. 5.94). Surgical and trauma literature frequently refer to this injury as a bilateral "pedicle" fracture of C2. Anatomically, the axis vertebra does not have a distinct pedicle as do the lower cervical vertebrae. The area of transition from the axis body to the base of the superior facet (Fig. 5.95) is the axis "pedicle." Classically, the hanged-man fracture is a bilateral fracture of the pars interarticularis of C2 (Fig. 5.96), that is, the part of the articular mass between the superior and inferior articular processes. In reality, CT has shown us that there are variations on the injury and fractures may indeed occur through the pars. However, in our experience, most involve portions of the posterior vertebral body, the articular pillars, or the anterior laminae (Fig. 5.97). For this reason, we prefer to refer to these injuries as hanged man type fractures so as to not offend the purists. These variants are also called "atypical" TS, in which one (unilateral) (Fig. 5.98) or both (bilateral) (Fig. 5.99) fractures occur in the coronal plane of the middle column of the axis body. The management of atypical hanged-man fractures is sufficiently different than that of the typical injury that the distinction is clinically relevant. Again, CT is critical for making the correct diagnosis.

The Effendi classification of hanged-man injuries is based on the degree of displacement of the axis body. In Type I injury, the axis body is minimally displaced and the C2-C3 disk space appears normal; in Type II, the axis body is displaced either anteriorly or posteriorly. With posterior displacement, the disk space is widened, indicating the hyperextension mechanism; Type III injury consists of the changes that characterize Type II injury plus a C2-C3 bilateral interfacetal dislocation. With the Type III injury, there is anterior

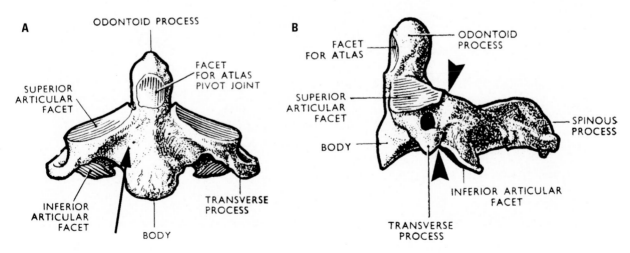

Figure 5.95. Schematic representation of the axis vertebra. **A:** The frontal perspective shows the axis pedicle *(long arrow)*. **B:** The lateral perspective shows the pars interarticularis *(arrowheads)*.

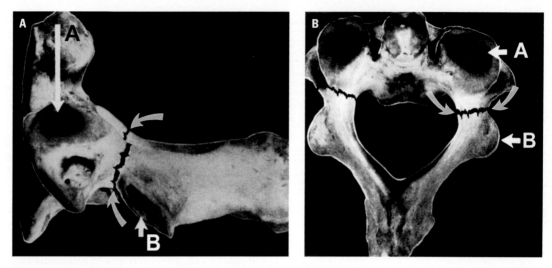

Figure 5.96. Schematic representation of TS in (**A**) lateral and (**B**) axial perspectives, showing the fracture through the pars interarticularis *(curved arrows)* between the superior (**A**) and inferior (**B**) articulating facets.

displacement of the posterior arch of the atlas, which maintains its normal anatomic relationship to the dens (Fig. 5.100).

Types I and II injuries are not associated with neurologic signs or symptoms. The reason for this is that the bilateral fractures result in autodecompression of the spinal cord. Type III is mechanically unstable because of the C2-C3 BID and has neurologic findings because of the associated spinal cord injury secondary to the displacement.

Simultaneous Hyperextension and Rotation

The combination of hyperextension and rotation causes either the pillar fracture or the pedicolaminar fracture-separation. Both of these injuries are now commonplace when CT is used as the main screening modality in injured patients.

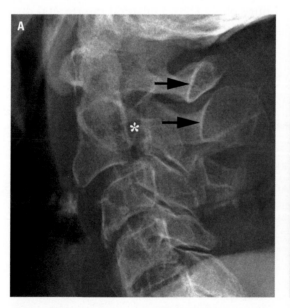
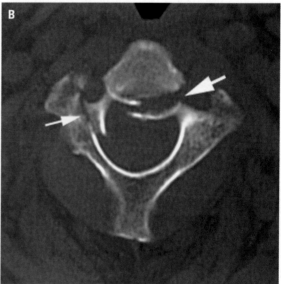

Figure 5.97. Hanged-man fracture. **A:** Lateral radiograph shows anterolisthesis of the body of C2 and duplication of the posterior body line *(asterisk)*. There is malalignment of the spinolaminar line *(arrows)*. **B:** Axial CT image shows fractures through the posterior body on the left *(large arrow)* and the pars on the right *(small arrow)*.

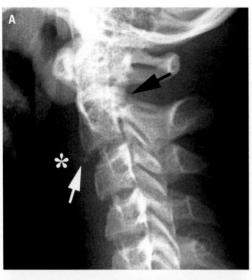

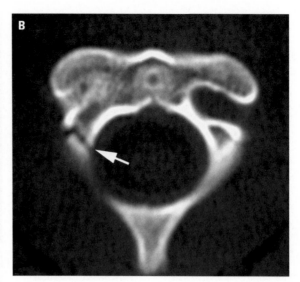

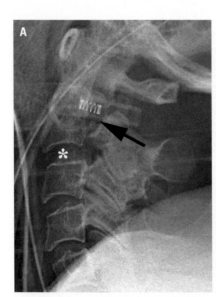

Figure 5.98. Unilateral hanged-man fracture. **A:** Lateral radiograph shows a fracture through the neural arch *(black arrow)*. There is also an avulsion fracture of the anteroinferior body of C2 *(white arrow)*. Note the prevertebral soft tissue swelling *(asterisk)*. **B** and **C:** Axial CT images show right-sided fractures *(arrows)*.

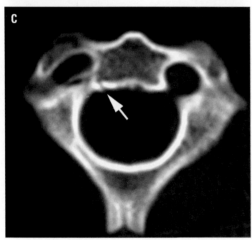

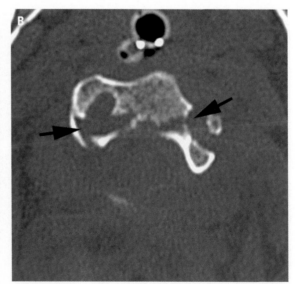

Figure 5.99. Hanged-man fracture. **A:** Lateral radiograph shows the fracture through the neural arch *(arrow)*. The C2 disk space is slightly widened. **B:** Axial CT image shows the bilateral fractures involving the transverse foramina.

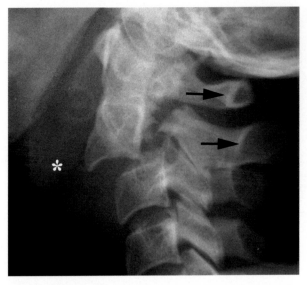

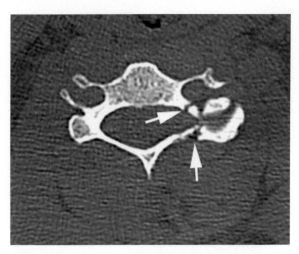

Figure 5.101. Comminuted articular pillar fracture (arrows).

Figure 5.100. Hanged-man fracture with dislocation (Effendi III). In addition to the anterolisthesis of the body of C2, the atlas remains in its normal anatomic position with disruption of the spinolaminar line (arrows). Note the prevertebral soft tissue swelling (asterisk).

Pillar Fractures

The pillar fracture is a unilateral vertical or oblique fracture of the articular mass caused by impaction by the ipsilateral adjacent articular mass during hyperextension and rotation. The fracture occurs on the side in the direction of rotation, that is, the side of lateral compression. Classically, the pillar fracture was thought to be confined to the articular mass, with the adjacent pedicle and lamina being intact. However, CT has shown that the pillar fracture usually extends anteriorly into the transverse process or posteriorly into the lamina (Fig. 5.101). CT has also shown that many of the unilateral locked facet injuries are associated with pillar fractures rather than with complete dislocation (Fig. 5.102). The pillar fracture is considered mechanically and neurologically stable. Acute neurologic findings or

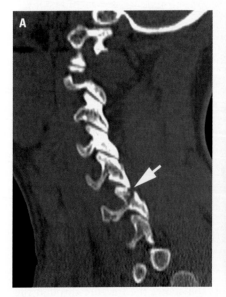

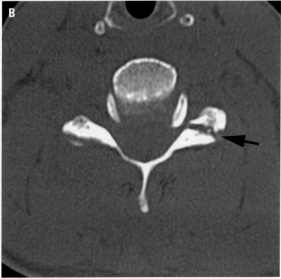

Figure 5.102. Articular pillar fracture in a patient with unilateral interfacet lock. **A:** sagittal reconstructed and (**B**) axial CT images show the fracture (arrows).

myelopathy do not occur with pillar fractures because the spinal canal remains intact and the cord is protected. However, in approximately 40% of patients, delayed local neuropathy may develop as a result of nerve root impingement or secondary degenerative osteoarthritis of the facet joint.

Radiographically, the findings are difficult to recognize. However, there are distinct abnormalities on frontal and lateral radiographs (Fig. 5.103). A lucent defect representing the articular mass fracture may be visible in the frontal projection. On the lateral radiograph, posterior displacement of the mass fragment produces lack of superimposition of the posterior cortical margins of the articular masses only at the level of the mass fracture. This finding has been called the "double outline" sign. CT now makes the diagnosis of articular pillar fractures much easier.

Pedicolaminar Fracture-Separation ("Floating Pillar")

Another lower cervical spine injury is characterized by ipsilateral pedicle and laminar fractures. The MOI is the result of simultaneous hyperextension and rotation with the fractures occurring on the side of rotation (impaction). This combination of injuries causes the articular mass to become a free-floating

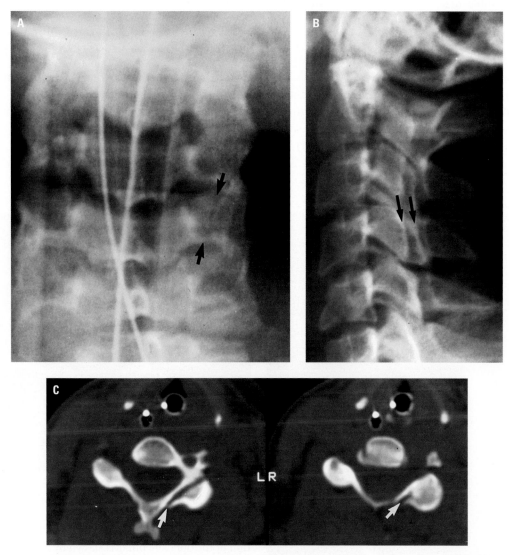

Figure 5.103. Pillar fracture extending into the lamina. **A:** Frontal radiograph shows a faint, oblique lucent defect *(arrows)* representing a fracture of the articular pillar at the level of C4. **B:** Lateral radiograph shows a double-outline sign *(arrows)*. **C:** Axial CT images shows the pillar fracture *(arrows)* extending obliquely posteriorly into the lamina, the medial cortex of which remains intact.

fragment, referred to as the "floating pillar." Shan-muganathan et al. refer to this same injury as "traumatic isolation of the cervical articular pillar" and suggest that it is the result of either hyperflexion and rotation or hyperflexion and distraction.

Four varieties of this injury occur:

Type I. Fracture-separation without displacement (disc intact)

Type II. Fracture-separation associated with rupture of disk and anterior longitudinal ligament

Type III. Fracture-separation associated with rupture of disk and anterior longitudinal ligament plus anterolisthesis of involved vertebra by approximately 3 mm

Type IV. Double-disk lesions; that is, fracture-separation with disruption of the disk above and below the involved vertebra

The pedicle fracture usually extends into the transverse process.

The imaging signs of the pedicolaminar fracture vary with the type of injury. A common feature of all varieties on the lateral radiograph is duplication and rotation of the involved pillar (Fig. 5.104). CT identifies the extent of involvement no matter what the type. Of the four, Types I and II rarely produce anterolisthesis. Types III and IV, on the other hand, do. Type IV injury is considered unstable, both mechanically and neurologically. Subluxation or frank dislocation of the contralateral interfacetal joint is also characteristic of Type IV injury and distinguishes it from Type III injury. Anterolisthesis of pedicolaminar fracture-separation must not be assumed to represent a hyperflexion injury such as unilateral or bilateral interfacetal dislocation or subluxation. The distinction between the anterolisthesis of pedicolaminar fracture-separation and the flexion-related injuries with anterolisthesis of the involved vertebra rests, very clearly, on recognition of the posterior element injury in the lateral column on the CT exam (Fig. 5.105).

The "fingerprints" of extension injuries include the following:

- Widening of the disk space below the level of injury (see Figs. 5.82 and 5.99)
- Triangular avulsion fractures of the anterosuperior lip of vertebral bodies
- Retrolisthesis (see Figs. 5.81 and 5.82.)
- Neural arch fractures (see Figs. 5.97 and 5.100)

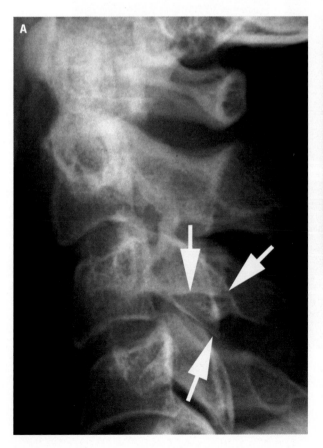

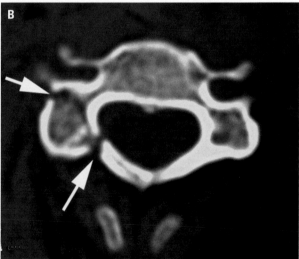

Figure 5.104. Pedicle-lamina fracture producing a "floating" pillar. **A:** Lateral radiograph shows elevation of a duplicated pillar image *(upper arrows)*. The normal position of the opposite pillar is shown by the *lower arrow*. **B:** Axial CT image shows fractures of the right pedicle and lamina *(arrows)* with rotation of the pillar, accounting for the "floating" appearance. (From Daffner RH. *Imaging of Vertebral Trauma*. 3rd ed. Cambridge, United Kingdom: Cambridge University Press; 2011, with permission.)

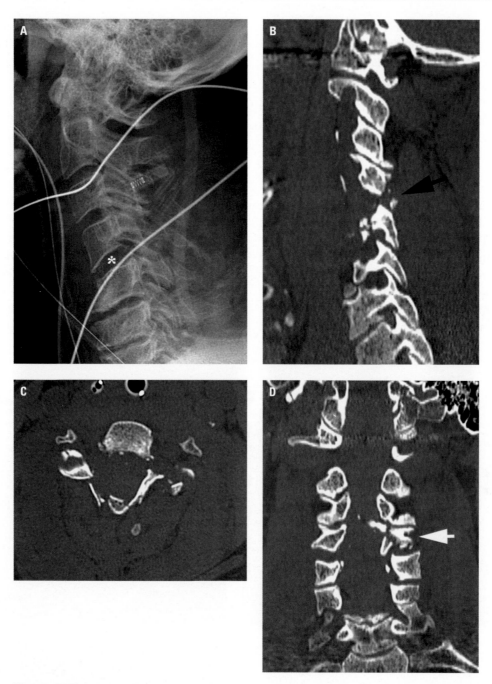

Figure 5.105. Pedicle-lamina fracture resembling a flexion injury. **A:** Lateral radiograph shows a wide C4 disk space. **B:** Sagittal reconstructed CT image shows a wide C4 facet joint with fractures of the pillar *(arrow)*. **C:** Axial CT image shows bilateral fractures of the posterior elements. **D:** Coronal reconstructed CT image shows a crushed pillar on the left *(arrow)* with displacement of bone fragments into the vertebral canal.

In the less common extension fracture-dislocation injury involving the articular pillars and vertebral arches, there are two fingerprints:

- Anterolisthesis with *normal* interlaminar or interspinous spaces
- *Normal* spinolaminar lines (see Fig. 5.89)

Lateral Flexion (Bending, Tilt)

Lateral tilt may occur as a predominant MOI in the cervicocranium, resulting in such injuries as unilateral fracture of an occipital condyle (Fig. 5.106), lateral mass of C1 (Fig. 5.107), eccentric fracture of the superior articular process of C2, or combinations of these injuries. These are discussed and illustrated in greater detail subsequently under cervicocranium. Lateral tilt may also modify a more dominant MOI, as in the instance of an eccentric Jefferson bursting fracture (Fig. 5.108). In the lower cervical spine, lateral tilt may result in the rare uncinate process fracture or the isolated pillar fracture, described earlier.

Vertical Compression (Axial Loading) Injuries

Vertical compression injuries occur only in areas of the spine that can be voluntarily straightened, that is, the cervical and lumbar regions. To produce this type of injury, the axial load force must be applied to the cervical (or lumbar) spine at the precise instant that the spine is straight. The axial load typically strikes the top of the head, with the force of the impact being transmitted through the base of the calvarium to the occipital condyles, through the lateral masses of C1 to the axis vertebra and, from there, to the lower cervical segments. Had the same force been applied with the neck flexed or extended, hyperflexion or hyperextension injuries,

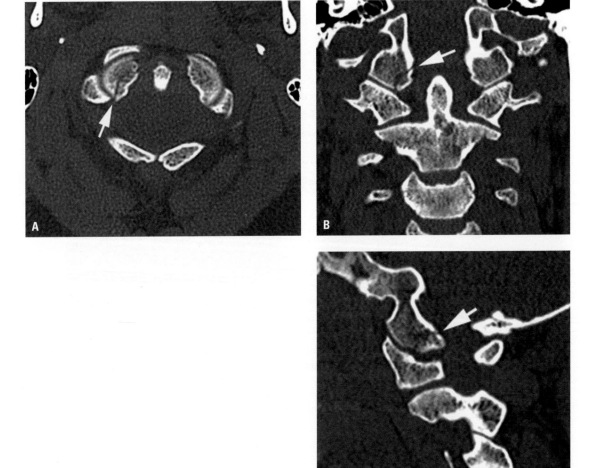

Figure 5.106. Type I occipital condyle fracture *(arrows)*. **A:** Axial, **(B)** coronal, and **(C)** sagittal reconstructed CT images.

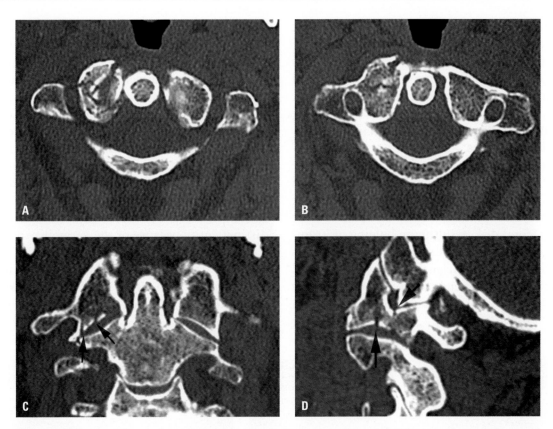

Figure 5.107. Lateral mass fracture on the right *(arrows).* **A** and **B**: axial, **(C)** coronal, and **(D)** sagittal reconstructed CT images.

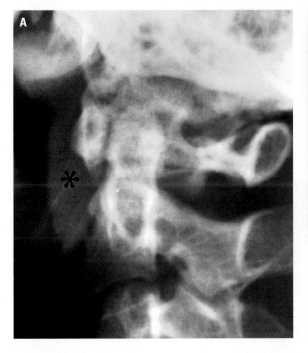

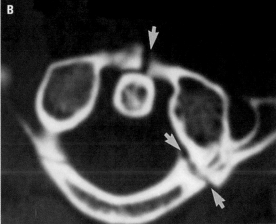

Figure 5.108. Eccentric Jefferson bursting fracture. **A:** Lateral radiograph shows prevertebral soft tissue swelling only *(asterisk).* **B:** Axial CT image shows fractures of the midline of the anterior arch as well as the posterior arch on the left *(arrows).*

respectively, would result. Pure vertical compression causes the Jefferson bursting fracture of the atlas or a variant of the burst fracture of the lower cervical spine. The Jefferson bursting fracture is discussed subsequently under cervicocranium.

Burst (Bursting, Dispersion, Axial-loading) Fracture, Lower Cervical Spine

The pathophysiology of the burst fracture of the lower cervical spine begins with the intervertebral disk. The compressive force transmitted to the lower cervical spine is initially dissipated in the intervertebral disk, resulting in bulging of its annulus. As the force persists and the annulus resists rupture, the liquid nucleus pulposus is imploded through the inferior end plate of the immediately superiorly adjacent vertebral body, causing an

abrupt increase in pressure within the body, which in turn is dissipated by exploding the vertebral body from within outward, resulting in dispersion of fragments in all directions, including posteriorly into the spinal canal.

The posterior fragments may impinge on the ventral surface of the cord to varying degrees. Consequently, the presenting neurologic signs may vary from minor transient paresthesia to complete quadriplegia. Although some authorities consider the burst fracture to be simply a variant of the flexion teardrop fracture, most consider it to be a distinct entity because of the variability of spinal cord injury.

The characteristic appearance of the burst fracture is illustrated in Figure 5.109. A vertical fracture line extending through the midportion of the

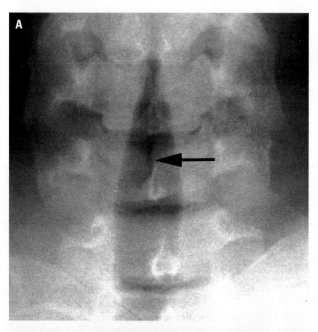

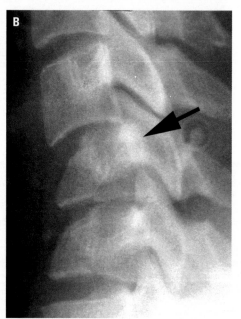

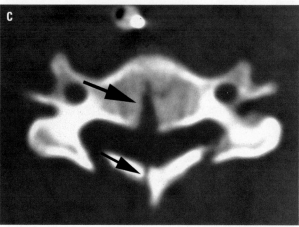

Figure 5.109. Burst fracture of C6. **A:** Frontal radiograph shows a sagittal fracture *(arrow)* through the body of C6. **B:** Lateral radiograph shows posterior bowing of the body of the vertebra *(arrow)*. **C:** Axial CT image shows the sagittal fractures through the body *(large arrow)* and lamina *(small arrow)*.

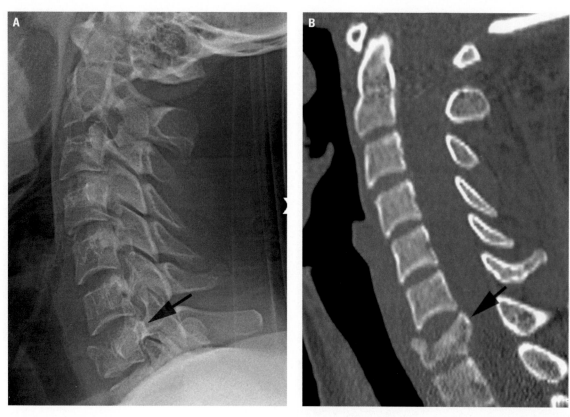

Figure 5.110. Burst fracture of C7. **A:** Lateral radiograph and **(B)** sagittal reconstructed CT image show compression of the vertebral body and retropulsion of a bone fragment from the posterior vertebral body *(arrows)*.

vertebral body, seen on the AP radiograph, distinguishes the burst fracture from the simple wedge fracture. Because each hemivertebral body fragment is laterally displaced, the superior Luschka joints widen and the inferior joints, logically, narrow. In some instances, a wide interpedicle distance may be seen. In order for the vertebra to appear widened in the frontal plane, the posterior arch must be also fractured. The posterior arch fracture is typically a minimally displaced laminar fracture that is usually not visible on radiographs but is clearly shown on CT (Fig. 5.109C).

On the lateral projection, the attitude of the cervical spine is essentially straight without hyperkyphotic angulation or other sign of hyperflexion. The involved vertebral body is comminuted, with fractures of each end plate and anterolisthesis of the anterior fragment and retrolisthesis of the posterior fragment (Fig. 5.110). One of the features that distinguish the burst fracture caused by pure axial compression from that caused by hyperflexion is the fact that the facet joints remain normally aligned in

the former injury and are typically widened in the latter (Fig. 5.111).

Injuries Caused by Diverse Mechanisms

Most cervical spine injuries can be grouped into families of injuries caused by a predominant MOI or by combinations of mechanisms of injury. Usually, one mechanism predominates. However, the reader should keep in mind that additional injuries may occur as a result of secondary impacts (such as occurs when a victim is ejected from a motor vehicle). In addition, there is a small group of injuries, typically in the cervicocranium, in which the pathology may be caused by as many as four diverse mechanisms of injury—flexion, extension, rotation, and shearing. We will now discuss some of the more common entities.

Occipitoatlantal Dissociation and Subluxation

Occipitoatlantal dissociation is a generic term that includes complete separation of the occipital condyle from the lateral masses of C1 (occipitoatlantal

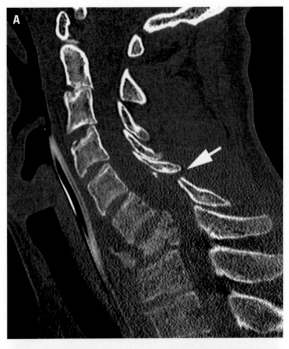

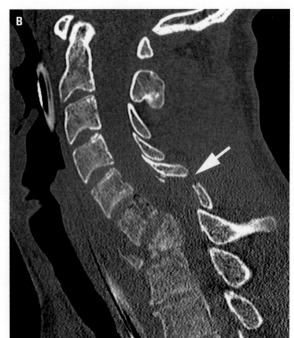

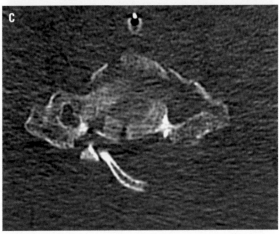

Figure 5.111. Hyperflexion burst fracture. **A** and **B:** sagittal reconstructed images of the right and left sides show typical burst fracture pathology in the vertebral body with perching of the facets *(arrows)*, typical of a hyperflexion injury. Compare with Figure 110. **C:** Axial CT image shows characteristic features of a burst fracture.

dislocation) and partial separation of the same articulation (occipitoatlantal subluxation). In the past, both of these injuries were considered to be uniformly fatal. However, we are encountering patients who survive the initial traumatic injury and are presented for imaging.

In occipitoatlantal dislocation, the skull may be displaced anteriorly by hyperflexion; rostrally by vertical distraction; anteriorly and rostrally by a combination of hyperflexion, shearing, and distraction; or, rarely, posteriorly by hyperextension. Of these, anterior occipitoatlantal dislocation is the most common. As mentioned earlier, most of these patients die at the scene of the accident. Conversely, occipitoatlantal *subluxation* is compatible with life.

Consequently, the accurate radiologic diagnosis of occipitoatlantal subluxation is essential for patient management.

The Powers (Fig. 5.112) and the "X" line methods (Fig. 5.113) were described as accurate detectors of anterior occipitoatlantal dissociation (Powers' ratio only) and both anterior and posterior occipitoatlantal dissociation (X line). Both methods proved cumbersome to perform and neither had application to distracted or anterior and distracted occipitoatlantal dissociation. Both have been replaced by the BAI, described subsequently. Interestingly, all three methods may be performed on sagittal CT reconstructed images as well as on lateral radiographs.

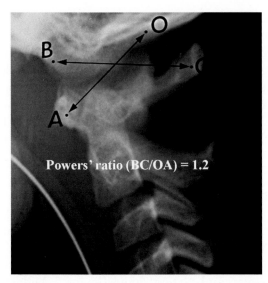

Figure 5.112. Occipitoatlantal dislocation. Powers' ratio of BC/OA is 1.2. Normal is less than 1.0. (From Daffner RH. *Imaging of Vertebral Trauma.* 3rd ed. Cambridge, United Kingdom: Cambridge University Press; 2011, with permission.)

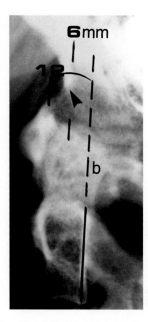

Figure 5.114. Normal BAI. In adults, the basion *(arrowhead)* should lie within 12 mm of the posterior axial line *(b)*.

The BAI measurements are based on review of 300 adult patients without radiographic evidence of acute cervical spine injury. That research established that in 96%, the basion normally lies within 12 mm anterior to an upward extension of

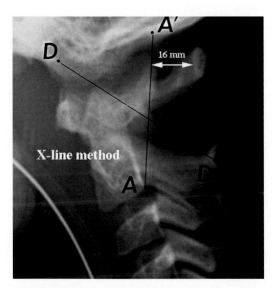

Figure 5.113. Occipitoatlantal dislocation. X-line (Lee) method. The descending line (**D to D'**) touches the tip of the dens and is normal; the ascending line (**A to A'**) is 16 mm anterior to the posterior arch of the atlas, which it should touch. Same patient as Figure 112. (From Daffner RH. *Imaging of Vertebral Trauma.* 3rd ed. Cambridge, United Kingdom: Cambridge University Press; 2011, with permission.)

the posterior cortical margin of the axis body (the posterior axial line) (Fig. 5.114) and that in 4%, the basion is normally less than 4 mm posterior to the posterior axial line. The relationship between the basion and the posterior axial line is the BAI. In the normal subjects in whom the basion lies posterior to the posterior axial line, the absence of prevertebral soft tissue swelling, reflective of the absence of a cervicocranial hematoma, confirmed this minor posterior location of the basion to be normal. In 35 adult patients in whom lateral flexion and extension cervical radiographs were obtained, the excursion of the basion did not exceed the normal parameters described earlier.

The distance between the basion and the tip of the dens, the basion–dental interval (BDI), measured in 200 patients without cervical spine injury, was between 3.5 and 12.5 mm with a 95% normal confidence rate. Consequently, we concluded that if the BDI is 12 mm or less, distracted occipitoatlantal dissociation does not exist.

The diagnosis of anterior occipitoatlantal dislocation is usually easy, the skull being frankly dislocated with respect to the lateral masses of C1 (Fig. 5.115). The diagnosis of anterior occipitoatlantal subluxation, on the other hand, may be much more difficult. However, an abnormal BAI and/or BDI in association with a nasopharyngeal mass (hematoma) is sufficient to establish the diagnosis

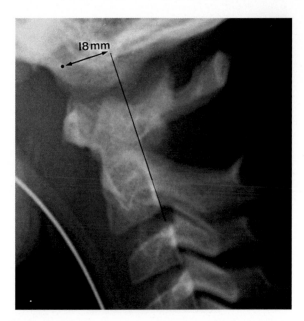

Figure 5.115. Occipitoatlantal dislocation. Same patient as Figure 112.

(Fig. 5.116). The occipitoatlantal space and the occipital condyles should also be visible in occipitoatlantal subluxation. The findings are identical on radiographs and sagittal reconstructed CT images (Fig. 5.117).

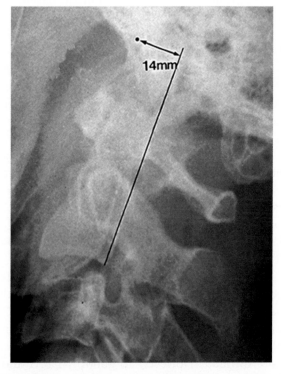

Figure 5.116. Occipitoatlantal subluxation. The basion is 14 mm in front of the posterior axial line.

Distracted occipitoatlantal dissociation in infants and young children is frequently associated with concomitant atlantoaxial dissociation (Fig. 5.118). In adults with pure distracted occipitoatlantal dislocation, the BDI exceeds 12 mm and is associated with a nasopharyngeal hematoma (Fig. 5.119). In simultaneous anterior and distracted occipitoatlantal subluxation, both the BDI and the BAI exceed 12 mm.

Dens Fractures

Dens fractures have been attributed to "hyperflexion," "hyperextension," "several complex forces including flexion and extension and probably rotation," "hyperflexion and hyperextension," and "lateral hyperflexion." Anderson and D'Alonzo described three types of dens fractures (Fig. 5.120). Type I was described as an avulsion fracture of the tip of the dens at the site of attachment of the alar "check" ligaments; Type II is a fracture at the base of the dens, confined to the dens itself; and Type III is not a fracture of the dens at all but is a fracture through the superior portion of the axis body.

Many authors, ourselves included, seriously questioned the existence of the Type I dens fracture. In Anderson and D'Alonzo's original paper, they reported having only two Type I dens fractures, one of which was "shown" to heal and the other was "shown" to go on to nonunion. Close examination of their original illustrations revealed that the fracture that was thought to heal, was, in fact, a Mach band caused by the overlap of the image of the occiput on the tip of the dens. The follow-up radiograph was positioned slightly differently without the overlap and hence the "fracture" was presumed to have "healed." The second example was a terminal ossicle, a normal variant that had all the characteristics of an accessory bone with round smooth margins. Consequently, if there was no Type I dens fracture, it seemed implausible to refer to the other types as II and III, so Gehweiler proposed the terms "high" and "low" for Types II and III, respectively.[8] These terms are in common practice today. In all likelihood, exceptions exist and we illustrate such a patient (Fig. 5.121).

Type II Dens Fracture

The Type II dens fracture, limited to the base of the odontoid process itself, is the most common axis fracture. This fracture is usually transversely

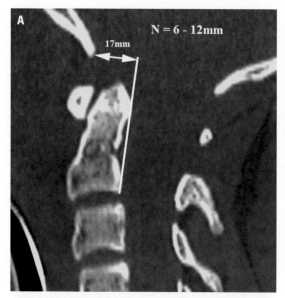

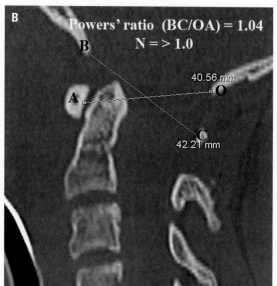

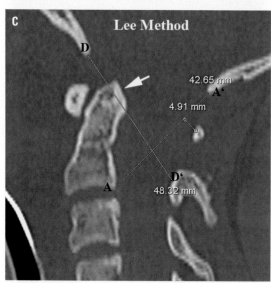

Figure 5.117. Occipitoatlantal dislocation. The same principles for diagnosis apply to using CT instead of radiography. CT allows landmarks to be found more readily and the measurements are more accurate. **A:** Harris' (BAI) method. **B:** Powers' ratio. **C:** X-line (Lee) method. (From Daffner RH. *Imaging of Vertebral Trauma.* 3rd ed. Cambridge, United Kingdom: Cambridge University Press; 2011, with permission.)

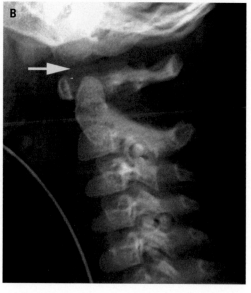

Figure 5.118. Vertical occipitoatlantal dislocation *(arrows)* in two children. Note the prevertebral soft tissue swelling *(asterisk)* in **A**.

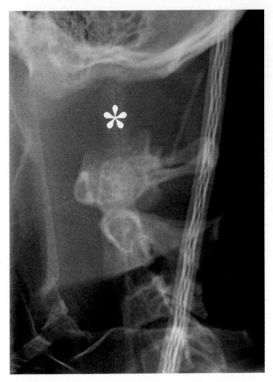

Figure 5.119. Vertical occipitoatlantal dislocation *(asterisk)* in an adult.

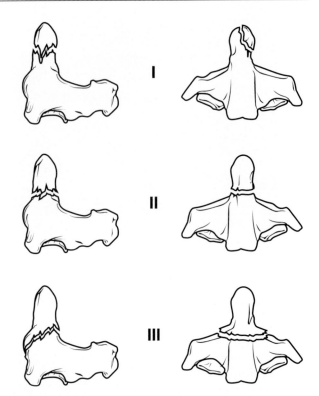

Figure 5.120. Anderson-D'Alonzo classification of dens fractures.

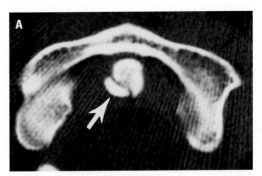

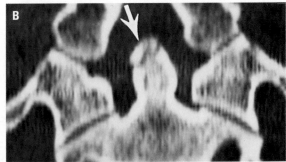

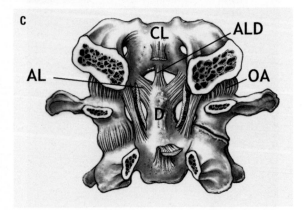

Figure 5.121. Type I dens fracture. **A:** Axial and (**B**) coronal reconstructed CT images show the fracture *(arrows)*. **C:** Deep ligaments of the craniovertebral junction. The Type I dens fracture results fron tension on the AL. AL, alar ligament; ALD, apical ligament of the dens; CL, cruciform ligament; D, dens; OA, occipitoatlantal joint ligament. (**C** from Daffner RH. *Imaging of Vertebral Trauma*. 3rd ed. Cambridge, United Kingdom: Cambridge University Press; 2011, with permission.)

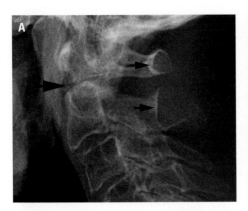 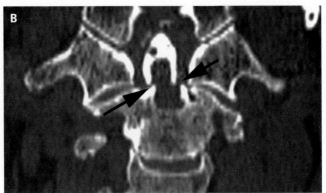

Figure 5.122. Type II dens fracture. **A:** Lateral radiograph shows fracture at the base of the dens *(large arrow)* as well as malalignment of the spinolaminar line *(small arrows)*. **B:** Coronal reconstructed CT image shows the fracture at the base of the dens *(arrows)* with right-sided displacement.

oriented, only extends above the level of the accessory ligaments when comminuted, and carries a 30% to 50% incidence of nonunion, particularly in the elderly, probably because the fracture occurs in an area with a high component of cortical bone. The highest incidence of nonunion is associated with dens fractures displaced 6 mm or greater. Type II dens fractures are frequently minimally displaced and, because of superimposition of the lateral masses of C1, may be extremely subtle on the lateral cervical radiograph. On modern CT examinations, these fractures are easily identified (Fig. 5.122). Because of its transverse orientation, Type II dens fracture may not always be recorded on axial CT images but is usually visible on reformatted images.

Type III Dens Fracture
The Type III fracture line occurs in the superior portion of the axis body and typically extends between the superior articular facets with an inferior convexity in the frontal projection and, in lateral projection, disrupts the axis (Harris') "ring." This "ring" is a really composite shadow involving the superior portion of the axis body on the lateral cervical radiograph. The anterior arc of the ring represents the anterior cortex of the axis "pedicle," that is, the area of bone between the body and that supporting the superior articular facet; the superior arc represents the cortical bone within the concavity between the superior articulating facet and the base of the dens; the posterior arc represents the posterior cortex of the axis body; and the inferior

arc is the lower margin of the transverse foramen (Fig. 5.123).

The Type III dens fracture may be severely displaced and obvious on the lateral cervical radiograph or CT (Fig. 5.124) or impacted and only slightly displaced (Fig. 5.125), resulting in the "fat axis body." Although the axis ring is disrupted in all Type III fractures, this observation is of relatively little importance when displacement of the fragments makes the fracture readily apparent. Minimally displaced Type III fractures, on the other hand, are very subtle and difficult to recognize on the lateral cervical radiograph. In these instances, disruption of the axis ring and recognition of abnormal soft tissue contour may be the only radiographic signs of the fracture. Fortunately, CT facilitates the diagnosis of both types of fracture. Because the Type III dens fracture occurs through the largely cancellous bone of the axis body, this fracture is not complicated by nonunion to the degree seen with the Type II fracture.

Mach bands caused by superimposition of the occiput or the inferior cortex of the posterior arch of C1 (Fig. 5.126) may simulate either a Type I or a Type II dens fracture on radiographs. Extension of the Mach lines beyond the dens or the axis body makes the distinction from acute fractures obvious. Mach bands are not an issue with CT studies.

Injuries of the Cervicocranium
The cervicocranium includes the occipital bone surrounding the foramen magnum, including the occipital condyles (sometimes referred to as C0)

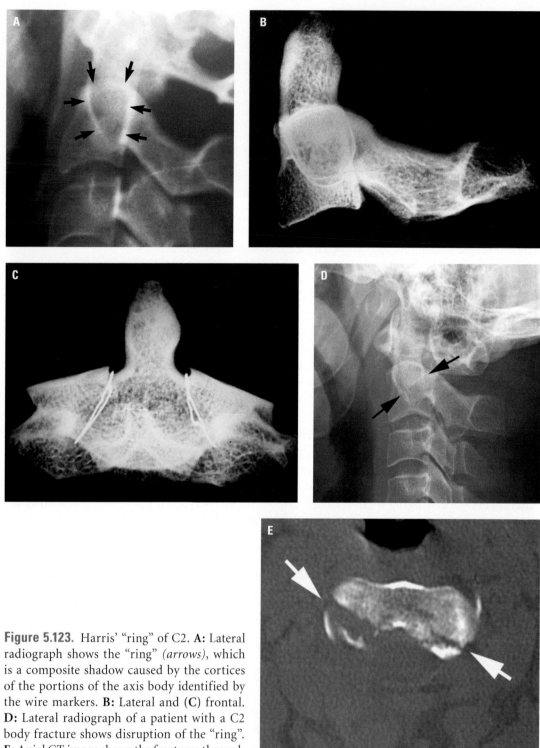

Figure 5.123. Harris' "ring" of C2. **A:** Lateral radiograph shows the "ring" *(arrows)*, which is a composite shadow caused by the cortices of the portions of the axis body identified by the wire markers. **B:** Lateral and **(C)** frontal. **D:** Lateral radiograph of a patient with a C2 body fracture shows disruption of the "ring". **E:** Axial CT image shows the fractures through the posterior body of C2 *(arrows)*.

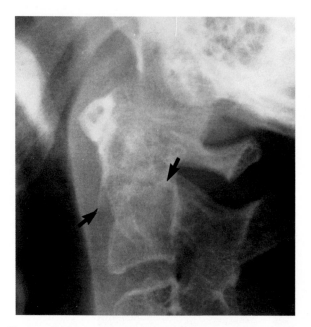

Figure 5.124. Type III dens fracture *(arrows)* with anterior displacement.

through the C2-C3 intervertebral disk. The cervicocranial injuries that comprise this group include the following:

- Occipitoatlantal dislocation and subluxation
- Occipital condylar fracture (OCF)
- Lateral mass C1 fracture
- Jefferson bursting fracture
- Anterior arch C1 fracture

- Dens fractures
- Traumatic spondylolisthesis

We have already discussed most of these injuries. We shall now elaborate on the remainder.

Occipital Condylar Fracture

Occipital condyle fractures were once considered rare. However, in the past two decades, increased use of CT for assessing patients suspected of cervical spine injury has shown that these injuries are not uncommon. OCF have been classified as Types I, II, and III. Type I is a pure axial loading fracture limited to the occipital condyle without displacement of fragments into the foramen magnum. The same impaction mechanism can produce the Jefferson bursting fracture of the atlas (see below). Although the alar "check" ligament may be detached from the fractured condyle, mechanical stability is preserved by the intact tectorial membrane and the contralateral alar ligament. Type I fracture may occur as an isolated injury (Fig. 5.127) or, because of the axial load, may occur in conjunction with a Jefferson bursting fracture (Fig. 5.128).

The Type II occipital condyle fracture is really a fracture of the basiocciput that extends from the occipital bone (Fig. 5.129). It results from a blow to the vertex and is stable because of the intact alar ligaments and pectoral membranes.

The Type III condyle fracture results from rotary and/or lateral bending and produces a small fragment from the medial surface of the condyle that is

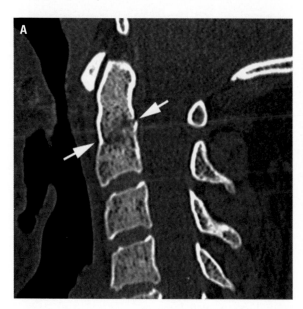

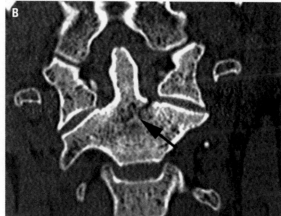

Figure 5.125. Nondisplaced Type III dens fracture *(arrows).* **A:** Sagittal and **(B)** coronal reconstructed CT images.

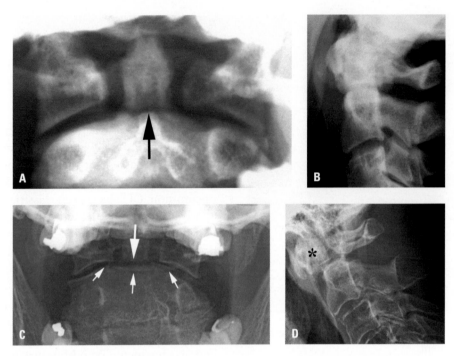

Figure 5.126. Mach band (**A** and **B**) vs. fracture (**C** and **D**) of the dens. **A:** Open-mouth radiograph shows a lucent line *(arrow)* across the base of the dens. **B:** Lateral radiograph shows no fracture. The soft tissues are normal. **C:** Open-mouth view shows a lucent line *(large arrow)* across the base of the dens. Note the image of the posterior arch of the atlas below *(small arrows)*. **D:** Lateral view shows a Type II dens fracture with anterior displacement *(asterisk)*.

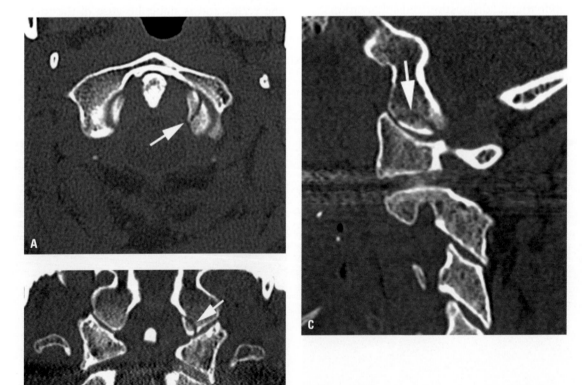

Figure 5.127. Type I occipital condyle fracture *(arrows)* on the left. **A:** Axial, (**B**) coronal, and (**C**) sagittal reconstructed images.

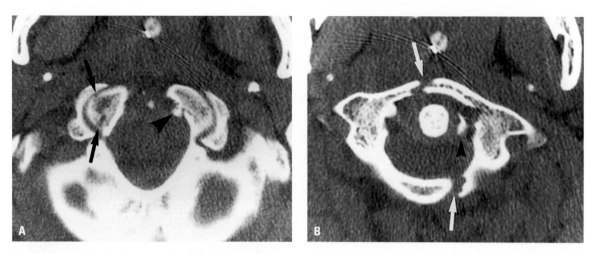

Figure 5.128. Right Type I and left Type III OCF associated with a Jefferson bursting fracture. **A:** Axial CT image shows a Type I occipital condyle fracture *(arrows)* on the right and a Type III *(arrowhead)* on the left avulsed by the alar "check" ligament. **B:** A more caudal axial image shows the Jefferson fracture *(arrows)*. The position of the avulsed fragment *(arrowhead)* to the left of the dens and arising from the left lateral mass of C1 indicates that the transverse atlantal ligament is intact but is no longer attached to the left lateral mass of C1.

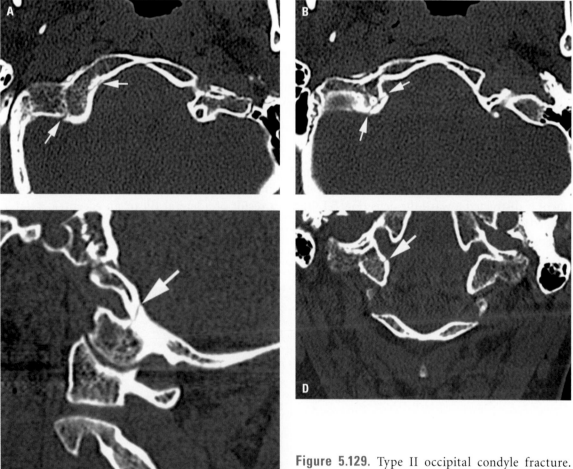

Figure 5.129. Type II occipital condyle fracture. **A** and **B:** Axial CT images show the fracture of the skull base extending toward the right occipital condyle *(arrows)*. **C:** Sagittal reconstructed. **D:** Axial CT images show the fracture in the right condyle *(arrows)*.

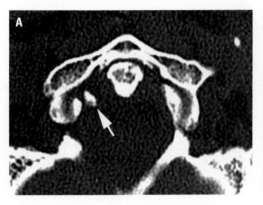

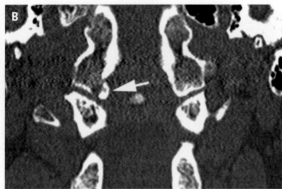

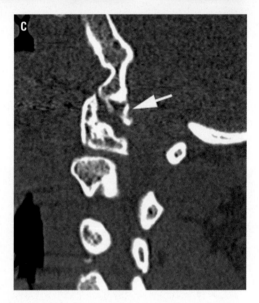

Figure 5.130. Type III occipital condyle fracture on the right. (**A**) axial, (**B**) coronal, and (**C**) sagittal reconstructed CT images show the fracture fragment *(arrows)* displaced into the foramen magnum.

avulsed by the intact alar ligament during rotation, lateral tilt, or a combination of the two. The separate fragment is distracted toward the dens (Fig. 5.130). The Type III injury is considered potentially unstable because of the avulsed alar ligament.

Lateral Mass C1 Fracture

Fractures of the lateral mass of C1 usually occur as a result of a lateral tilt or an eccentric axial loading MOI. The fracture may be limited to the lateral mass of C1 (Fig. 5.131) or, more commonly, occur in

Figure 5.131. Isolated lateral mass fracture on the right *(arrows)*.

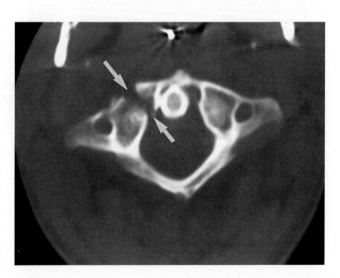

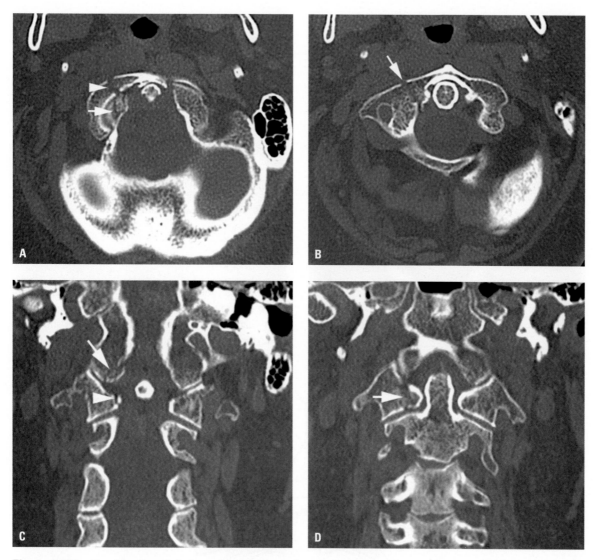

Figure 5.132. Combined occipital condyle and lateral mass fractures. **A:** Axial CT image shows the occipital condyle fracture on the right *(arrowhead)* and the lateral mass fracture *(arrow)*. **B:** Axial image slightly lower shows the lateral mass fracture to advantage *(arrow)*. **C:** Coronal reconstructed CT image shows the occipital condyle fracture *(arrow)* and the lateral mass fracture on the right *(arrowhead)*. **D:** Coronal image slightly posterior shows the lateral mass fracture to advantage *(arrow)*.

association with OCF (Fig. 5.132) and/or a fracture of the corresponding articular process of C2.

Jefferson Bursting Fracture

The Jefferson bursting fracture is the injury in the cervicocranium caused by a vertical compression (axial-loading) MOI at the precise instant that the cervical spine is straight—neither flexed nor extended. The causative force is transmitted from the vertex to the occipital condyles and hence to the lateral masses of C1. At this point, the force may be transmitted caudally through the lateral masses of C1 to the articular masses of C2 and from there

to the lower cervical spine, where the force is dissipated in the burst, bursting, dispersion fracture of the lower cervical spine.

Alternatively, should the causal force be dissipated in the lateral masses of C1, each lateral mass is driven laterally by the biconvex occipital condyles, which are nestled in the biconcave superior surfaces of the lateral masses of C1, resulting in fracture(s) of both the anterior and posterior arches of C1 (Fig. 5.133). Jefferson's original paper in 1920 identified two fracture sites in the anterior arch, one on each side of the anterior tubercle and two in the posterior arch, one fracture on each side (Fig. 5.134).

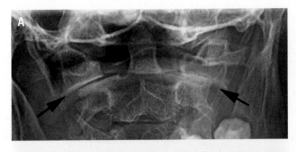

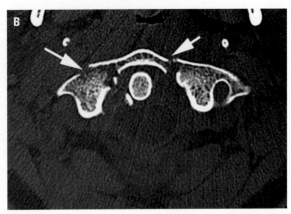

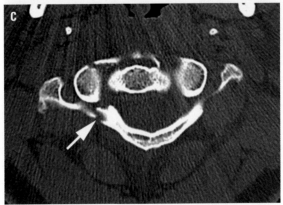

Figure 5.133. Jefferson bursting fracture. **A:** Open-mouth radiograph shows bilateral lateral atlantoaxial offset *(arrows)*. **B** and **C:** Axial CT images show the fractures of the anterior and posterior arches of C1 *(arrows)*.

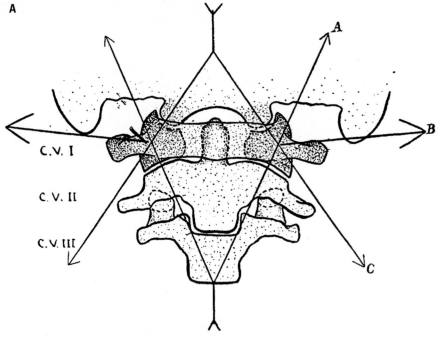

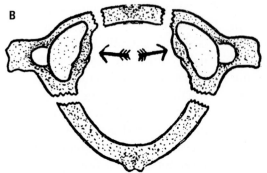

Figure 5.134. Jefferson bursting fracture as originally described by Jefferson. **A:** Schematic representation indicating the direction of axial-load vector forces. **B:** The atlas fracture sites. (From Jefferson G. Fracture of the atlas vertebra: report of four cases and a review of those previously recorded. *Br J Surg.* 1919–1920;7(27):407–422, with permission.)

CT has shown that the Jefferson fracture requires only one anterior and one posterior arch fracture. Because the atlas is a ring, a break in one portion of the ring should be accompanied by at least one other break. Furthermore, any combination of anterior and posterior arch fractures, with or without concomitant lateral mass fractures may occur.

Radiographically, on the open-mouth projection or on coronal reconstructed CT image, each lateral mass of C1 should be laterally displaced either symmetrically (Fig. 5.135) if the causative force is distributed equally to each condyle, or asymmetrically if the force is eccentrically applied to the vertex. The degree of displacement should exceed 3 mm as a minimum. Usually, the average displacement is 7 mm. There is one caveat when encountering unilateral or bilateral atlantoaxial offset of 2 mm or less. Patients with congenital anomalies of C1—failure of fusion of the anterior or posterior arches, partial or complete agenesis of the posterior arch—may have up to 2 mm of unilateral or bilateral offset. In most instances, the

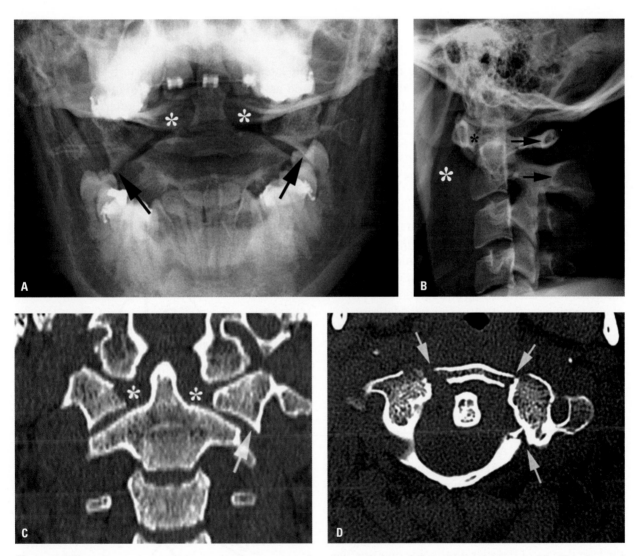

Figure 5.135. Jefferson bursting fracture. **A:** Open-mouth radiograph shows bilateral lateral atlantoaxial offset *(arrows)* as well as widening of the spaces between the dens and the lateral masses *(asterisks)*. **B:** Lateral radiograph shows massive prevertebral soft tissue swelling *(white asterisk)*, malalignment of the spinolaminar line *(arrows)*, and widening of the predental space *(black asterisk)*. **C:** Coronal reconstructed CT image shows the lateral atlantoaxial malalignment on the left *(arrow)* and widening of the spaces between the dens and the lateral masses *(asterisks)*. **D:** Axial CT image shows the fractures of the anterior and posterior arches of the atlas *(arrows)*.

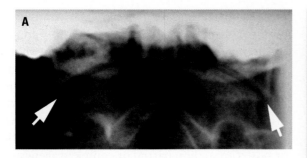

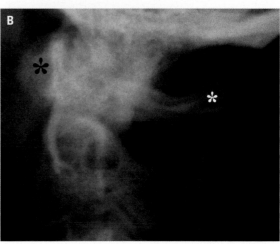

Figure 5.136. Arch anomaly. **A:** Open-mouth radiograph shows bilateral lateral atlantoaxial offset *(arrows)*. **B:** Lateral radiograph shows absence of the spinolaminar line *(white asterisk)* and hypertrophy of the anterior arch *(black asterisk)*.

anomaly is readily apparent on the radiographs (absent spinolaminar line of C1 and an associated hypertrophy of the anterior arch) (Fig. 5.136). On the lateral cervical spine radiograph, only the posterior arch fracture(s) are visible. Of course, axial as well as coronal and sagittal reconstructed CT images will show the full extent of the injuries.

Torticollis ("Wry Neck")

Acute nontraumatic torticollis occurs commonly in childhood and is of protean etiology, most frequently unknown. Torticollis is clinically manifested by simultaneous lateral tilting and rotation of the head. Both lateral tilting and rotation are physiologic motions at the atlantoaxial articulation.

Torticollis is usually self-limiting, with the clinical signs and symptoms disappearing in 4 to 5 days. This spontaneous resolution has been called atlantoaxial rotatory displacement by Fielding and Hawkins. When persistent, the condition is called atlantoaxial rotatory fixation and is caused by entrapment of the C1-C2 apophyseal joint capsule in the joint spaces. Atlantoaxial rotatory fixation usually requires surgical intervention.

The radiographic appearance of the atlantoaxial articulation in torticollis, then, simply reflects the physiologic changes at the C1-C2 level attributable to simultaneous rotation and lateral tilt. In rotation, the lateral mass of the atlas on the side opposite the direction of rotation moves anteriorly and assumes an oblique attitude toward the central x-ray beam. Consequently, this articular mass is increased in transverse diameter, and the space between the mass and the dens is diminished. Reciprocally, the oppo-

site lateral mass moves posteriorly during rotation and assumes a truncated configuration in frontal projection. The atlantodental interval on this side (the side of the direction of rotation) may be either unchanged or increased in width. This concept is schematically illustrated in Figure 5.137. In marked rotation, the joint space between the lateral mass of C1 and C2 may be obliterated as a result of the lateral mass of C1 rotating either anterior or posterior to

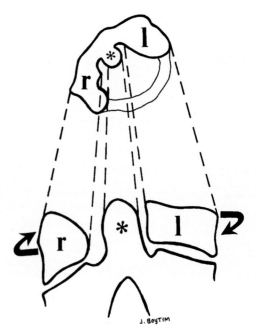

Figure 5.137. Illustration of the physiologic basis for the appearance of the atlantoaxial articulation because of rotation in the open-mouth projection.

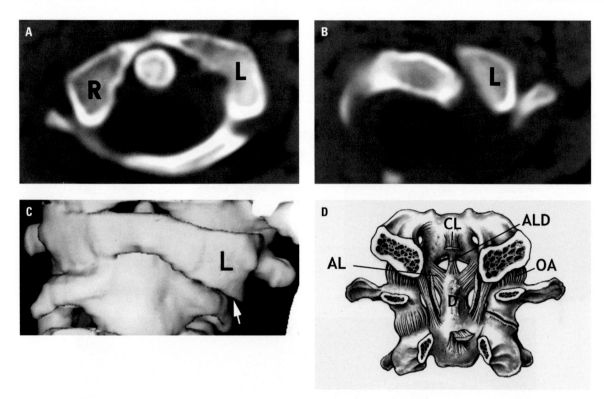

Figure 5.138. Atlantoaxial rotary displacement. **A:** Axial CT image shows anterior rotation of the left *(L)* and reciprocal posterior rotation of the right *(R)* lateral masses of C1, with respect to the dens. **B:** Axial image shows the relationship of the left lateral mass *(L)* with respect to the axis body. **C:** Frontal 3D image shows the left lateral mass *(L)* to be anteriorly displaced, and the right posteriorly displaced. **D:** Drawing of the deep ligamentous anatomy of the craniovertebral junction. AL, alar ligament; ALD, apical ligament of the dens; CL, cruciform ligament; D, dens; OA, occipitoatlantal joint. (**D,** from Daffner RH. *Imaging of Vertebral Trauma.* 3rd ed. Cambridge, United Kingdom: Cambridge University Press; 2011, with permission.)

its subjacent counterpart. The degree of rotation is easily demonstrated on axial CT images. Coronal and 3D reconstructed images will show whether or not locking of the articular processes has occurred (Fig. 5.138). It is possible to measure the angle of rotation. Under normal circumstances, the total allowable rotation is 45 degrees, 22.5 degrees in either direction. Of course, the most common cause of asymmetry between the dens and the lateral masses of the atlas is positional and simple rotation of the patient's head.

Miscellaneous Injuries
Combined Cervical Spine Injuries
Previously, we stated that it is not uncommon for concomitant multiple injuries of the cervical spine following blunt trauma. These are frequently the result of secondary impacts. The importance of an awareness of combined injuries is in the "satisfaction of search," in that the identification of one injury must not preclude diligent search for other injuries. The incidence of combined injuries is as high as 25% of cervical trauma. Furthermore, in our experience, as well as that of others, multiple noncontiguous injuries (cervical-thoracic, cervical-lumbar, and thoracic-lumbar) are encountered in 25% of patients with one spine injury. Combined cervical spine injuries may be the result of the same or different mechanisms and may occur in adjacent or remote cervical levels. This is one reason that we perform complete examinations of the spine with CT.

Acute Rupture, Transverse Atlantal Ligament
An AADI greater than 3 mm on the neutral lateral cervical spine radiograph in a patient with blunt cervical spine trauma indicates disruption of the transverse atlantal ligament. It must be remembered, however, that rheumatoid arthritis may widen the AADI because of erosion of the dens and/or attenuation of the transverse atlantal ligament.

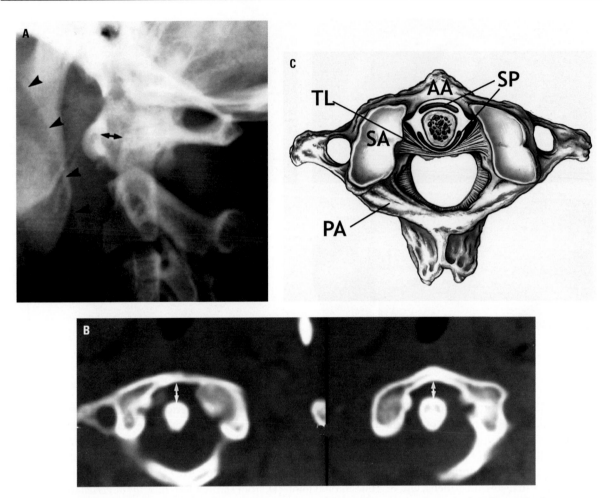

Figure 5.139. Acute traumatic rupture of the transverse atlantal ligament. **A:** Lateral radiograph shows an abnormal prevertebral soft tissue contour *(arrowheads)*. The AADI *(predental space)* is greater than 3 mm *(double arrow)*. **B:** Serial axial CT images show the wide predental space *(double arrows)*. **C:** Atlantoaxial joint seen from above. AA, anterior arch of atlas; PA, posterior arch of atlas; SA, superior articular facet of atlas; SP, synovial pads, TL, transverse atlantal ligament. (**C,** from Daffner RH. *Imaging of Vertebral Trauma.* 3rd ed. Cambridge, United Kingdom: Cambridge University Press; 2011, with permission.)

Isolated acute rupture of the transverse atlantal ligament is uncommon and may be the result of a hyperflexion, lateral tilt, or vertical compression MOI. On both lateral cervical radiograph and axial CT, the AADI is wide without fracture (Fig. 5.139). Transverse atlantal ligament rupture is much more commonly associated with the Jefferson fracture secondary to lateral displacement of the lateral mass of C1. The transverse atlantal ligament may be detached from the lateral mass of C1 by sagittally oriented fractures of the lateral mass.

Vertebral Artery Injury
Before 1995, sporadic case reports of vertebral artery injuries secondary to blunt cervical spine trauma appeared in the radiologic, trauma, and orthopedic literature. TS, burst fractures of the lower cervical spine, and cervical spine fracture-dislocations as well as severe hyperflexion and hyperextension injuries have been implicated in causing vertebral artery trauma. Vertebral artery injury has been described as common in the presence of transverse process fractures that involve the transverse foramen (Fig. 5.140). However, most vertebral artery injuries are "clinically occult," presumably because of collateral circulation provided through the circle of Willis. Before the advent of CTA or MRA, vertebral artery injury was considered rare primarily because unilateral vertebral injury is usually asymptomatic and vertebral arteriography was performed only because of signs and symptoms of massive cerebellar or brainstem injury.

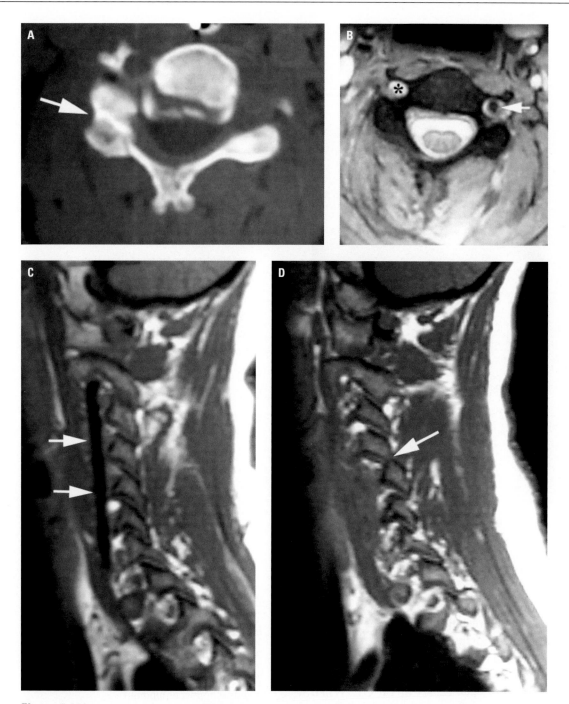

Figure 5.140. Unilateral facet dislocation with vertebral artery injury. **A:** Axial CT image shows the locked facet on the right *(arrow)*. **B:** STIR axial MR image shows the normal loss of signal *(black)* of the left vertebral artery *(arrow)*. There is no flow on the right *(asterisk)* and the vertebral artery appears white. **C:** Sagittal MR image of on the left shows the normal vertebral artery *(arrows)*. **D:** On the right, the vertebral artery is not seen. Note the locked facet *(arrow)*.

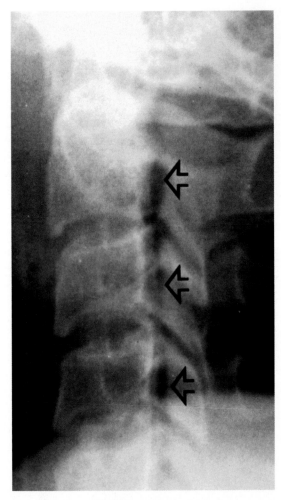

Figure 5.141. Traumatic pneumorrhachis. Lateral radiograph shows air *(open arrows)* in the anterior cervical subarachnoid space. The source of the air was a basilar skull fracture.

Traumatic Pneumorrhachis

Traumatic pneumorrhachis (air within the spinal canal) is rare and occurs when air enters the cervical subarachnoid space as seen on the lateral cervical spine radiograph (Fig. 5.141) or on CT. When it occurs, it is usually a sign of a basilar skull fracture that involves the sphenoid sinus or the mastoid air cells. There is a high risk of meningitis and a 16% mortality rate to pneumorrhachis.

Normal Variants, Anomalies, and Other Conditions That May Simulate Acute Injury

There are numerous variants and anomalies that are found on radiographs and CT studies of the cervical spine that, in the setting of acute blunt trauma, may

TABLE 5.2	Common Cervical Pseudofractures
Variants and Anomalies	

- True variants
  - Failure of fusion
  - Cleft sulcus of vertebral artery of atlas
  - Spur-like deformities of lateral masses of atlas
  - Accessory ossification centers
  - Synchondrosis at base of dens
  - Ununited ring apophysis
  - Os odontoideum
  - Nuchal ligament ossification
  - Vascular grooves
- Old or repetitive trauma
  - Os odointoideum
  - Accessory ossicles
  - Intercalary bones
  - Limbus deformity

Mach Bands

- Normal structures
  - Arch of atlas on dens
  - Posterior vertebral arches
  - Transverse processes
  - Uncinate processes
  - Articular pillars
  - Teeth on vertebrae
- Osteophytes
  - Uncinate spurs
  - Disc margin spurs
- Soft tissues

Extraneous Materials

- Immobilization collars
- Clothing
- Life-support equipment

Old Fractures

Motion Artifacts

be problematic in their interpretation (Table 5.2). A comprehensive discussion is beyond the scope of this book, but some principles of identifying these entities will be made. The reader is referred to the chapter on Normal Variants and Pseudofractures in Daffner's *Imaging of Vertebral Trauma*, 3rd edition or to the encyclopedic work by Keats and Anderson for comprehensive coverage of normal variants and congenital anomalies that may simulate acute injury.

There are four groups of findings that may be misinterpreted as cervical fractures:

■ Normal variants and anomalies
■ Mach bands
■ Overlapping extraneous materials
■ Old fractures

Some of these have already been mentioned in this chapter. However, a few general comments regarding pseudofractures are in order. Most acute fractures have well-defined irregular margins that will fit together like pieces of a jigsaw puzzle (Fig. 5.142). This principle is reliable even when the

fracture fragments are displaced. When this has occurred, it is possible to mentally move the fragments together. Ununited old fractures or accessory ossicles have smooth, round margins, and do not have the "jigsaw puzzle effect" (Fig. 5.143).

Similarly, lucent lines caused by failure of fusion of a vertebral arch have well-defined sclerotic, usually smooth margins (Fig. 5.144). CT scanning has introduced a whole new family of pseudofractures—vascular grooves. These may be recognized by having sclerotic margins as well as a serpentine course (Fig. 5.145). In addition, when one is unsure whether such a lucency is vascular or a fracture, referring to the sagittal and coronal reconstructed images will show that the line in question is clearly a vessel (Fig. 5.146).

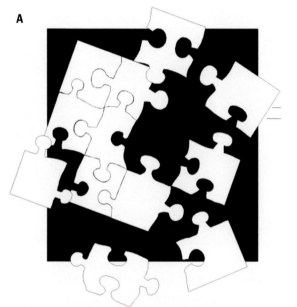

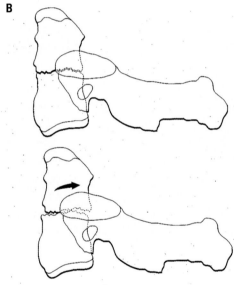

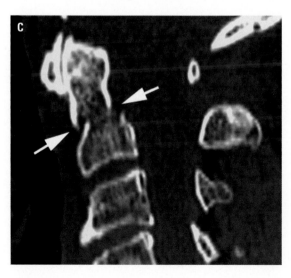

Figure 5.142. Jigsaw puzzle effect. A: Drawing of a jigsaw puzzle. Each piece fits precisely into its designated space regardless of its position. B: Drawing of a dens fracture showing that the fracture fragments, even if displaced, will fit together like pieces of a jigsaw puzzle. C: Sagittal reconstructed CT image shows a dens fracture (arrows) with slight anterior displacement. The fracture fragments can be mentally moved back into place. Accessory ossicles will not fit perfectly. (From Daffner RH. *Imaging of Vertebral Trauma*. 3rd ed. Cambridge, United Kingdom: Cambridge University Press; 2011, with permission.)

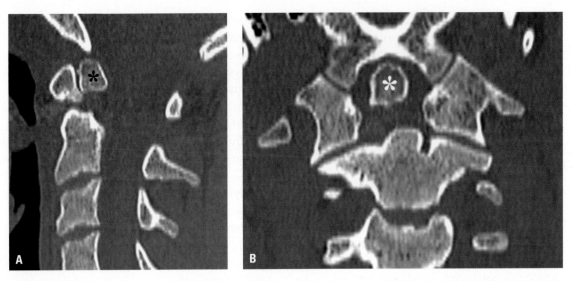

Figure 5.143. Os odontoideum. **A:** Sagittal and **(B)** coronal reconstructed CT images shows the os *(asterisk)* above the stump of the dens. The pieces will not fit together like a jigsaw puzzle. Compare with Figure 5.142C.

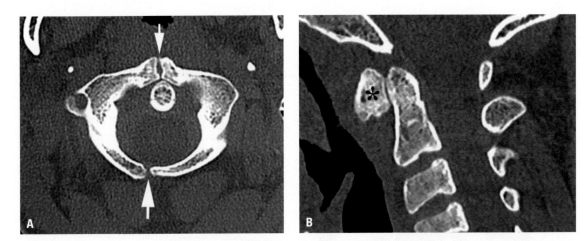

Figure 5.144. Failure of fusion of the arches of C1. **A:** Axial CT image shows the clefts in the anterior *(small arrow)* and posterior *(large arrow)* arches. **B:** Sagittal reconstructed CT image shows hypertrophy of the anterior arch *(asterisk)*. Hypertrophy is commonly found with anomalies of the atlas ring.

Figure 5.145. Vascular grooves *(arrows)* in a vertebral body. Note the serpentine pattern and sclerotic borders.

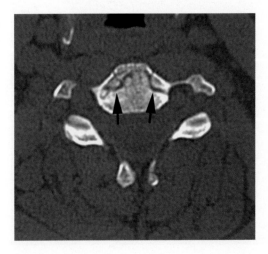

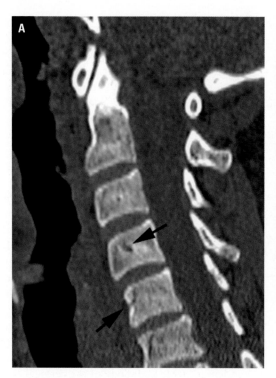

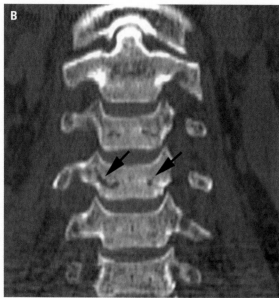

Figure 5.146. Coronal and sagittal reconstructed CT images of the same patient as Figure 5.145 show the tubular nature of the vessels *(arrows)*.

SUGGESTED READINGS

1. American College of Radiology. Suspected spine trauma. ACR Appropriateness Criteria. 2011. American college of Radiology Web site. http://www.acr.org/SecondaryMainMenuCategories/quality_safety/app_criteria/pdf/ExpertPanelonNeurologicImaging/SpineTraumaUpdateinProgressDoc13.aspx. Accessed 2012.

2. Clark WM, Gehweiler JA Jr, Laib R. Twelve significant signs of cervical spine trauma. *Skeletal Radiol.* 1979;3(4):201–205.

3. Como JJ, Diaz JJ, Dunham CM, et al. Practice management guidelines for identification of cervical spine injuries following trauma: update from the Eastern Association for the Surgery of Trauma Practice Management Guidelines Committee. *J Trauma.* 2009;67(3):651–659.

4. Daffner RH. Pseudofracture of the dens: Mach bands. *AJR Am J Roentgenol.* 1977;128(4):607–612.

5. Daffner RH, Goldberg AL, Evans TC, et al. Cervical vertebral injuries in the elderly: a ten year study. *Emerg Radiol.* 1998;5(1):38–42.

6. Daffner RH. *Imaging of Vertebral Trauma.* 3rd ed. Cambridge, United Kingdom: Cambridge University Press; 2011.

7. Effendi B, Roy D, Cornish D, et al. Fractures of the ring of the axis. A classification based on the analysis of 131 cases. *J Bone Joint Surg Br.* 1981;63-B(3):319–327.

8. Gehweiler JA Jr, Osborne RL Jr, Becker RF. Injuries of the cervical spine. In: *The Radiology of Vertebral Trauma.* Vol 3. Philadelphia, PA: WB Saunders; 1980:89–256.

9. Hanson JA, Blackmore CC, Mann FA, et al. Cervical spine injury: a clinical decision rule to identify high-risk patients for helical CT screening. *Am J Roentgenol.* 2000;174:713–717.

10. Harris JH Jr, Burke JT, Ray RD, et al. Low (type III) odontoid fracture: a new radiographic sign. *Radiology.* 1984;153(2):353–356.

11. Harris JH Jr, Carson GC, Wagner LK. Radiologic diagnosis of traumatic occipitovertebral dissociation: 1. Normal occipitovertebral relationships on lateral radiographs of supine subjects. *AJR Am J Roentgenol.* 1994;162(4):881–886.

12. Harris JH Jr, Carson GC, Wagner LK, et al. Radiologic diagnosis of traumatic occipitovertebral dissociation: 2. Comparison of three methods of detecting occipitovertebral relationships on lateral radiographs of supine subjects. *AJR Am J Roentgenol.* 1994;162(4):887–892.

13. Harris JH Jr, Mirvis SE. *The Radiology of Acute Cervical Spine Trauma.* 3rd ed. Baltimore, MD: Williams & Wilkins; 1996.

14. Hoffman JR, Mower WR, Wolfson AB, et al. Validity of a set of clinical criteria to rule out injury to the cervical spine in patients with blunt trauma. National Emergency X-Radiography Utilization Study Group. *N Engl J Med.* 2000;343(2):94–99.

15. Hogan GJ, Mirvis SE, Shanmuganathan K, et al. Exclusion of unstable cervical spine injury in obtunded patients with blunt trauma: is MR imaging needed when multi-detector row CT findings are normal? *Radiology*. 2005;237(1):106–113.

16. Holmes JF, Akkinepalli R. Computed tomography versus plain radiography to screen for cervical spine injury: a meta-analysis. *J Trauma*. 2005;58(5):902–905.

17. Jefferson G. Fracture of the atlas vertebra: report of four cases and a review of those previously recorded. *Br J Surg*. 1919–1920;7(27):407–422.

18. Keats TE, Anderson MW. *Atlas of Normal Roentgen Variants that may Simulate Disease*. 8th ed. Philadelphia, PA: Mosby; 2007:155–372.

19. Kulkarni MV, Bondurant FJ, Rose SL, et al. 1.5 Tesla magnetic resonance imaging of acute cervical spine trauma. *Radiographics*. 1998;8(6):1059–1082.

20. Lee C, Woodring JH, Goldstein SJ, et al. Evaluation of traumatic atlantooccipital dislocations. *AJNR Am J Neuroradiol*. 1987;8(1):19–26.

21. Mirvis SE, Diaconis JN, Chirico PA, et al. Protocol-driven radiologic evaluation of suspected cervical spine injury: efficacy study. *Radiology*. 1989;170(3, pt. 1):831–834.

22. Powers B, Miller MD, Kramer RS, et al. Traumatic anterior atlanto-occipital dislocation. *Neurosurgery*. 1979;4(1):12–17.

23. Roaf R. A study of the mechanics of spinal injuries. *J Bone Joint Surg Br*. 1960;42-B(4):810–823.

24. Schoenfeld AJ, Bono CM, McGuire KJ, et al. Computed tomography alone versus computed tomography and magnetic resonance imaging in the identification of occult injuries to the cervical spine: a meta-analysis. *J Trauma*. 2010;68(1):109–113.

25. Smoker WR, Dolan KD. The "fat" C2: a sign of fracture. *AJR Am J Neuroradiol*. 1987;8:33–38.

26. Stiell IG, Clement CM, McKnight RD, et al. The Canadian C-spine rule versus the NEXUS low-risk criteria in patients with trauma. *N Engl J Med*. 2003;349(26):2510–2518.

27. Stiell IG, Wells GA, Vandemheen KL, et al. The Canadian C-spine rule for radiography in alert and stable trauma patients. *JAMA*. 2001;286(15):1841–1848.

28. Tomycz ND, Chew BG, Chang YF, et al. MRI is unnecessary to clear the cervical spine in obtunded/comatose trauma patients: the four-year experience of a level I trauma center. *J Trauma*. 2008;64(5):1258–1263.

29. Vaccaro AR, Kreidl KO, Pan W, et al. Usefulness of MRI in isolated upper cervical spine fractures in adults. *J Spinal Disord*. 1998;11(4):289–293.

30. Vandemark RM. Radiology of the cervical spine in trauma patients: practice pitfalls and recommendations for improving efficiency and communication. *AJR Am J Roentgenol*. 1990;155(3):465–472.

31. Young JW, Resnik CS, DeCandido P, et al. The laminar space in the diagnosis of rotational flexion injuries of the cervical spine. *AJR Am J Roentgenol*. 1989;152(1):103–107.

CHAPTER 6

The Pediatric Cervical Spine

Leonard E. Swischuk ■ John H. Harris, Jr.

This chapter deals with trauma of the cervical spine in infants and children and how things differ from adults. It will not deal with all cervical spine fractures for many of them are no different than seen in adults. In addition, in the growing child especially the infant and young child, because of natural ligament laxity, hypermobility of the cervical spine abounds. As a result, many findings in infants and young children that would be considered abnormal in adults are normal.[1,2] Furthermore, the skeleton still is growing in children, and to accommodate this in the extra-axial skeleton, epiphyseal plates are present. In the spine, synchondroses serve the same function. If one is not familiar with these synchondroses, one may erroneously misdiagnose them for fractures. The most problematic of these occur in the second cervical vertebra and will be addressed later. This chapter also deals with congenital anomalies, which can go on to present in adulthood but often first present in the pediatric age group.

PREVERTEBRAL SOFT TISSUE SWELLING

Prevertebral soft tissue swelling often is difficult to evaluate because of problems in obtaining good images. To properly evaluate the soft tissues of the neck, the airway needs to be fully distended on inspiration and the neck needs to be extended. However, this can be difficult to accomplish, especially with the patient on the emergency medical service (EMS) backboard, but on the lateral view of the well-positioned normal airway, the posterior pharyngeal wall is always more posterior than the posterior tracheal wall and this results in a step-off of the air column at this level (Fig. 6.1A). This latter finding is helpful because even if the airway is not fully distended, if a step-off is retained, the findings likely are normal (Fig. 6.1B). When the study is obtained in expiration, tracheal buckling with a pseudomass frequently results (Fig. 6.1C) and the study needs repeating with proper technique (Fig. 6.1D).

In the end however, with all of this considered, I have come to this conclusion about the prevertebral soft tissues. If they are not sending a definite message, then do not spend too much time on them. Go on to evaluate the radiographs for signs of vertebral column instability. These include (1) anterior displacement of vertebral bodies (rotation-flexion injuries), (2) posterior displacement of vertebral body (hyperextension injury), (3) narrow disk space (flexion, rotational injuries), (4) wide disk space (hyperextension injuries), (5) pedicles seen "en face" (rotary subluxation), and (6) increased predental distance (C1-C2 dislocation).

SYNCHONDROSES

Synchondroses occurring in the third through the seventh cervical vertebra are not usually a problem. The problem is with synchondroses in the first and second cervical vertebrae.[1,2] With the first cervical vertebra, the problem is not as difficult for the synchondroses often are very symmetric, and once one appreciates this, there is little chance of misdiagnosing them for a fracture (Fig. 6.2).

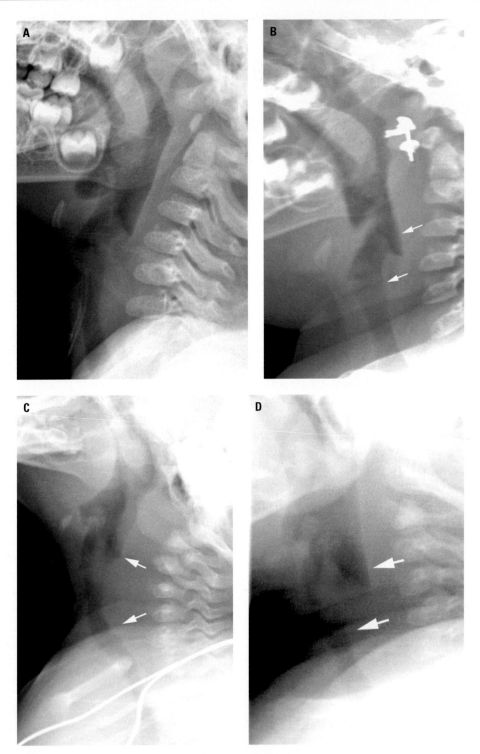

Figure 6.1. Airway: Normal and buckling. **A:** Normal fully distended airway in extension. Note that the posterior hypopharyngeal wall is posterior to the posterior tracheal wall. **B:** In this patient, thickening of the prevertebral soft tissues is suggested but because the step-off between the posterior pharyngeal wall and posterior tracheal wall is retained *(arrows)*, the study likely is normal. This was a normal patient. **C:** Pseudomass *(arrows)* caused by the study being obtained during expiration. The neck is extended, but the study was obtained in expiration. **D:** With full inspiration, the airway is normal and the pharyngeal/tracheal step-off is retained *(arrows)*. Even though the prevertebral soft tissues look a little prominent, the study is normal.

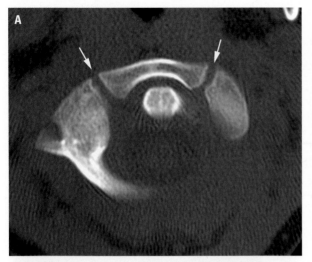

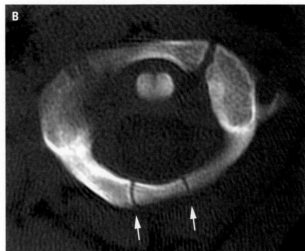

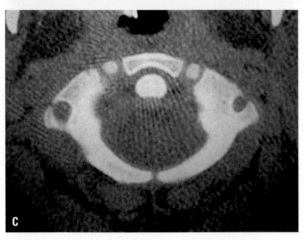

Figure 6.2. Synchondroses C1. **A:** Note symmetric anterior synchondroses *(arrows)*. **B:** Similar posterior synchondroses *(arrows)*. **C:** Numerous anterior and posterior synchondroses.

The synchondroses of C2 are a different matter (Figs. 6.3A, 6.3B). Until one learns their configurations, it is very easy to misinterpret them for fractures. In previous days, on oblique views of the cervical spine, these synchondroses produced a Y-shaped radiolucent line configuration (Fig. 6.3C). With the advent of computed tomography (CT) imaging, the same configuration is seen on extreme lateral sagittal reconstructed views of the cervical spine (Fig. 6.3D). Aberrant synchondroses may appear very bizarre but they generally have smooth edges (Fig. 6.4).

NEURAL ARCH DEFECTS

Neural arch defects can be fractures or congenital defects. Fractures in the upper cervical spine usually result from hyperextension injuries such as the

hangman's fracture or axial loading injuries such as sustained in the Jefferson fracture of C1. The resultant defects usually are relatively thin and/or sharp-edged. They do not show sclerosis whereas congenital defects, although variable in their configuration, generally have smooth and sclerotic edges (Fig. 6.5).

Neural arch defects in the lower cervical spine are not particularly common.[3–5] They are much more common at the C1 and C2 levels,[1,2,6–10] but even here, they are much more common at the C1 level. At the C2 level, they need to be differentiated from hangman's fractures, which do occur in infants and children.[11–14] In infants, these fractures maybe clinically silent and this is especially important because they can occur in the battered child syndrome.[13,14] C1 defects are very bizarre and extremely variable (Fig. 6.6). In spite of the bizarre and alarming appearance of all these defects, they are stable[9,15]

(text continues on page 247)

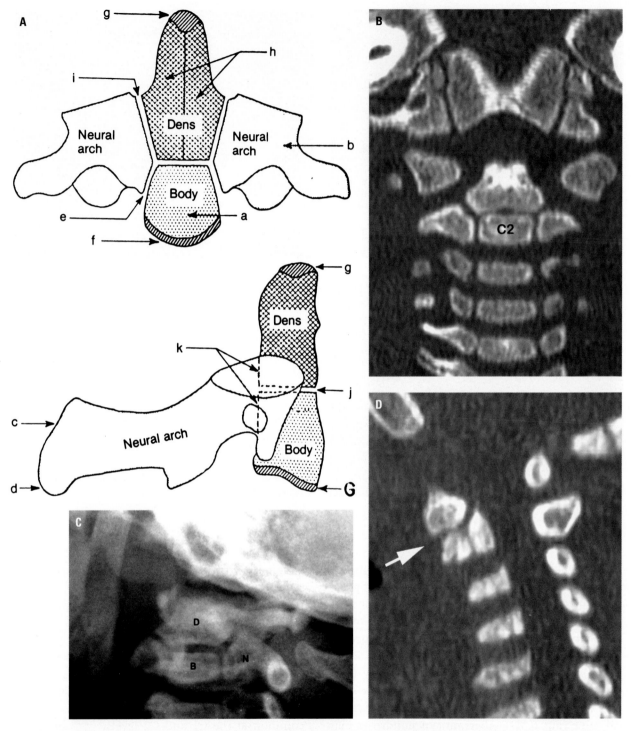

Figure 6.3. Synchondroses C2. **A:** Schematic representation of the ossification centers and synchondroses of the axis vertebra. The neurocentral synchondrosis is represented by *e*; the subdental (subchondral) synchondrosis, by *j*; and the synchondrosis between the dens and the neural arches, by *i*. (From Bailey DK. Normal cervical spine in infants and children. *Radiology.* 1952;59:713–714, with permission.) **B:** Coronal reconstruction of the C-spine demonstrates all of the synchondroses outlined in figure (**A**). Radiograph oblique view (**C**) demonstrates the triradiate synchondroses between the dens *(D)*, body *(B)*, and neural arch *(N)* of C2. Far lateral sagittal CT reconstruction (**D**) demonstrates the same findings *(arrow).*

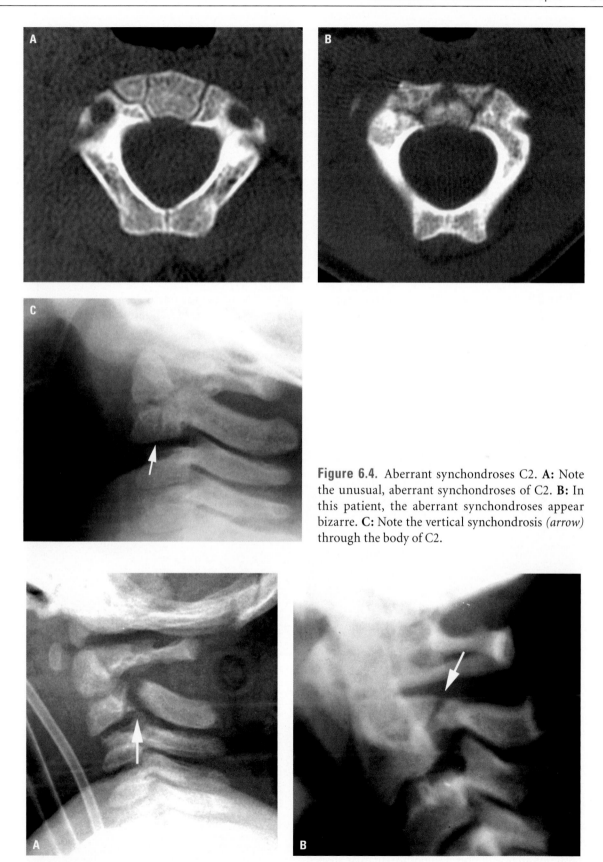

Figure 6.4. Aberrant synchondroses C2. **A:** Note the unusual, aberrant synchondroses of C2. **B:** In this patient, the aberrant synchondroses appear bizarre. **C:** Note the vertical synchondrosis *(arrow)* through the body of C2.

Figure 6.5. Posterior neural arch fracture verses defect. **A:** Hangman's fracture in an infant *(arrow)*. Note that the edges are sharp. **B:** Congenital defect *(arrow)* in a child. Note that the edges are smooth and slightly sclerotic. This spine was completely stable on flexion/extension. *(continued)*

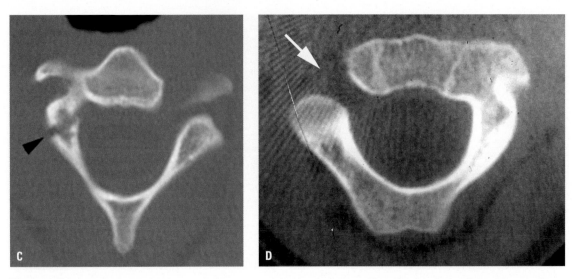

Figure 6.5. *(continued)* **C:** Hangman's fracture on CT *(arrow)*. Note that the fracture edges are very sharp and that there is no sclerosis. **D:** Congenital defect on CT *(arrow)* demonstrates smooth, sclerotic edges.

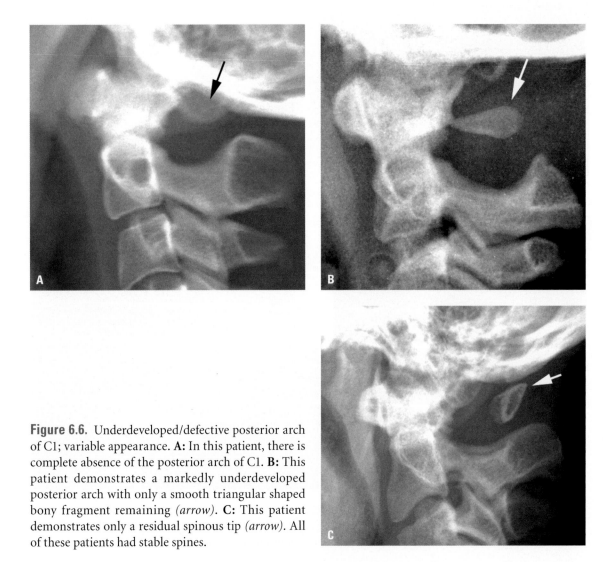

Figure 6.6. Underdeveloped/defective posterior arch of C1; variable appearance. **A:** In this patient, there is complete absence of the posterior arch of C1. **B:** This patient demonstrates a markedly underdeveloped posterior arch with only a smooth triangular shaped bony fragment remaining *(arrow)*. **C:** This patient demonstrates only a residual spinous tip *(arrow)*. All of these patients had stable spines.

and flexion/extension views can be confirmatory (Fig. 6.7).

Having considered all of the foregoing, there is one exception to the rule of stability with posterior neural arch defects of the upper cervical spine. This exception occurs when the dens is congenitally hypoplastic.[4] In such cases, the transverse ligaments that stabilizes the dens and the lateral masses of C1 are underdeveloped and weak. All of this leads to excessive motion at the C1-C2 level and an increase

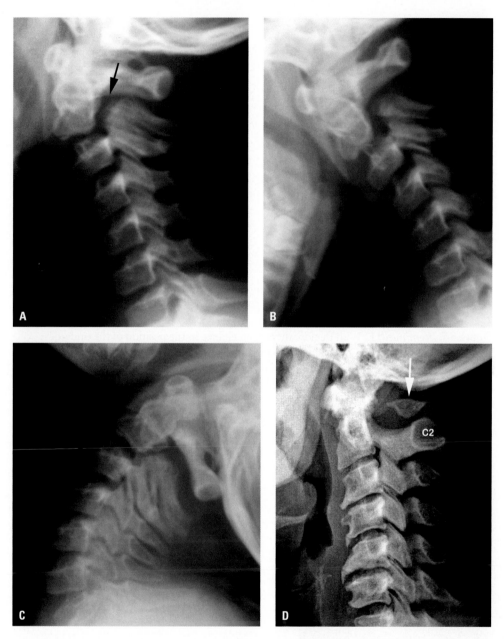

Figure 6.7. Congenital defect C1-C2; demonstration of stability. **A:** Note the smooth-edged defect *(arrow)* in the posterior arch of C2. C2 is slightly anterior-displaced and the disk space is wide anteriorly. **B:** With flexion, there is very little change in the width of the defect and C2-C3 alignments are basically unchanged. **C:** With extension, all of the vertebral bodies align up normally and there is very little evidence of excessive movement. This patient basically was stable but activity such as wrestling, football, gymnastics, and so forth might be discouraged. **D:** Note the underdeveloped posterior arch of C1 *(arrow)* and its relationship to the posterior arch of C2. This was a study in a 75-year-old male (note the degenerative changes in the mid-cervical spine region). *(continued)*

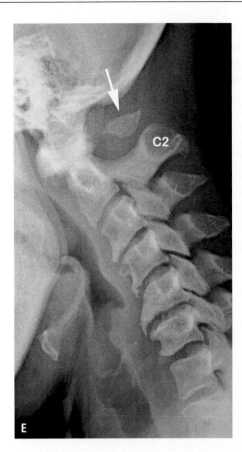
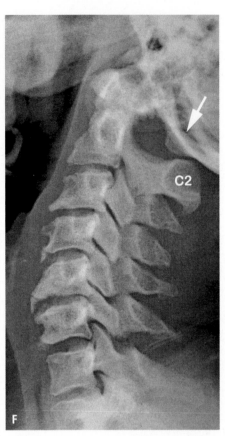

Figure 6.7. *(continued)* **E:** With flexion, there is no change in the position of the underdeveloped posterior arch of C1 *(arrow)* and the spinous tip of C2. **F:** With extension, both the posterior arch of C1 *(arrow)* and the spinous tip of C2 retained their original relationship. How many times do you think this 75-year-old male has flexed/extended his neck in his life?

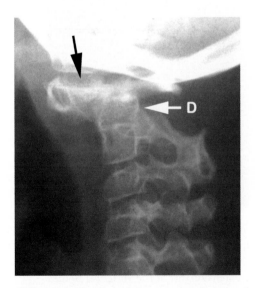

Figure 6.8. Underdeveloped C1 neural arch, hypoplastic dens, and instability. In this patient, the dens *(D)* is hypoplastic. The posterior arch of C1 is underdeveloped and there is marked anterior dislocation *(black arrow)* of C1 on C2. This is an unstable configuration.

in the predental distance—all discussed in the next section. In such cases, even though one might first note that the posterior arch of C1 is hypoplastic or deformed when the hypoplastic dens is also noted, the whole problem takes on a completely different and more serious complexion (Fig. 6.8). It usually requires surgical stabilization.

THE OS TERMINALE–OS ODONTOIDEUM COMPLEX

The normal os terminale is located at the top of the dens and fits into a V-shape groove (Figs. 6.9A–C). If the os terminale is not ossified, the groove for the dens may make the dens appear bifid (Fig. 6.9D). The os terminale is derived from an occipital sclerotome and not from a cervical sclerotome. The dens itself is actually the body of C1 and it is separated from the body of C2 by the dens/body

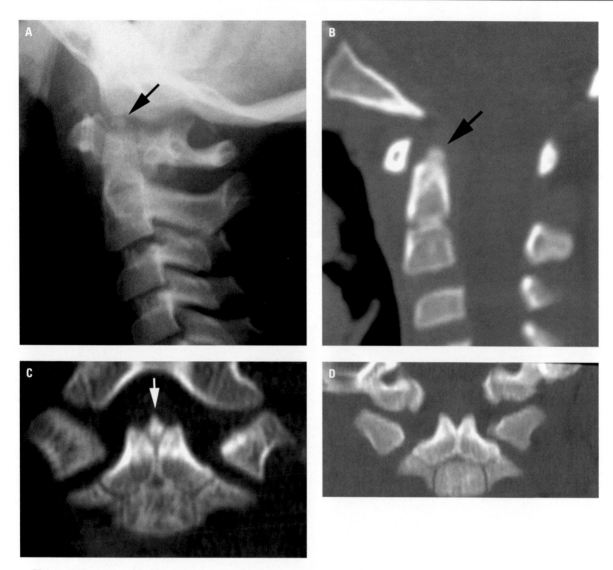

Figure 6.9. Os terminale: Normal. **A:** Note the small os terminale *(arrow)* at the tip of the dens. **B:** Similar findings of the os terminale *(arrow)* on a sagittal reconstructed CT study. **C:** Coronal reconstructed CT study demonstrates the os terminale *(arrow)* sitting in the V-shaped groove of the dens. **D:** In this patient, the os terminale is unossified and the tip of the dens appears bifid.

synchondrosis. In some cases, the os terminale can be somewhat more posteriorly located and a little enlarged (Fig. 6.10). In other cases, the os terminale can appear rather fragmented (Fig. 6.11). This should not be misinterpreted for a fracture because actually, it would be difficult to fracture the dens in such a fashion.

When the dens is hypoplastic, the os terminale overgrows to form the os odontoideum (Fig. 6.12).[16,17] At the same time, there often is overgrowth of the anterior arch of C1. At any rate, the cervical spine at the C1–C2 level becomes unstable because the transverse dens ligaments are underdeveloped and C1 on

C2 subluxation/dislocation is common (Fig. 6.12D). Overall, the os odontoideum configurations often are bizarre (Fig. 6.13). In still other cases, the dens can be entirely absent or fused to the lateral masses of C1 so as to become the body of C1 (Fig. 6.14). The latter problem/configuration usually is stable. The dens also may be come the body of C1 (Fig. 6.15). Rarely, the os odontoideum can be acquired. In these cases, when a fracture occurs through the dens, there is loss of blood supply followed by necrosis and then by resorption of the dens. The os terminale then overgrows and becomes an acquired os odontoideum.[18]

(text continues on page 254)

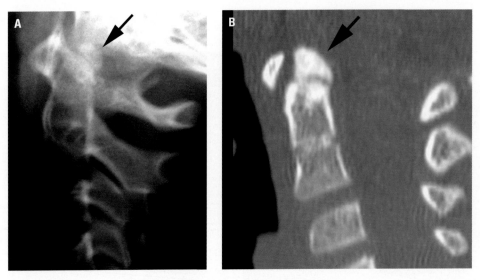

Figure 6.10. Os terminale: Normal, slightly posterior position. **A:** In this patient, the os terminale *(arrow)* is a little larger than usual. It is also somewhat posteriorly angulated. This is normal. **B:** CT study demonstrates the same findings. Os terminale *(arrow).*

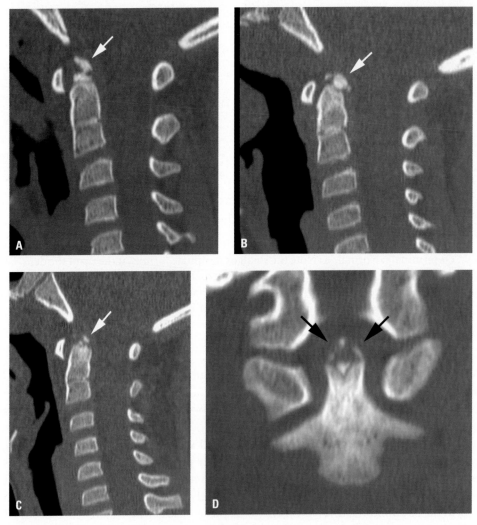

Figure 6.11. Os terminale: Irregular ossification. **A:** In this patient, the os terminale *(arrow)* appears very irregular and almost bipartite. **B:** In this patient, the os terminale *(arrow)* has a main ossification center but then two other ossified small fragments. **C:** This patient demonstrates a small fragmented os terminale *(arrow).* **D:** Coronal reconstructed CT study demonstrates the same findings *(arrows).* All patients were normal.

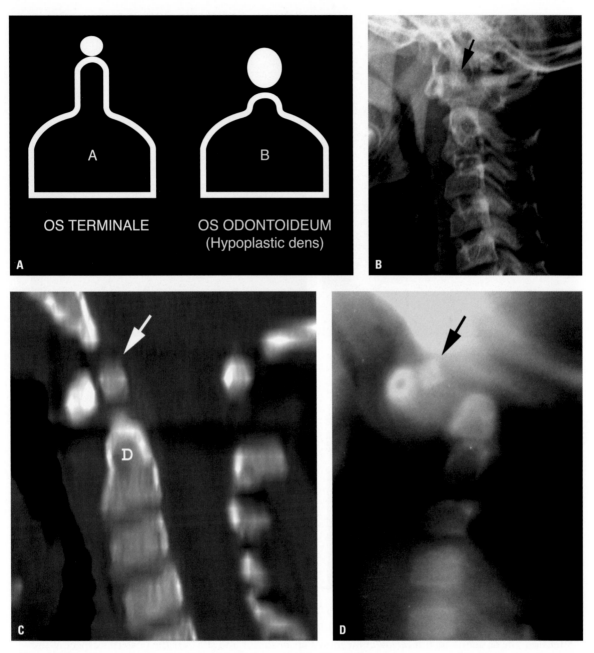

Figure 6.12. Os terminale–Os odontoideum complex. **A:** Diaphragmatic representation. The normal os terminale sits atop a well-developed dens *(A)*. The os odontoideum is larger than the os terminale and sits atop a hypoplastic dens *(B)*. **B:** In this patient, an os odontoideum *(arrow)* is seen atop a hypoplastic dens. The skeletal imaging details are difficult to discern. **C:** With a sagittal reconstructed CT study however, the os odontoideum *(arrow)* and the hypoplastic dens *(D)* are now clearly visualized. **D:** In this patient, the os odontoideum *(arrow)* is markedly anteriorly dislocated along with the anterior arch of C1, which is slightly overgrown. The dens is hypoplastic and the overall configuration is unstable.

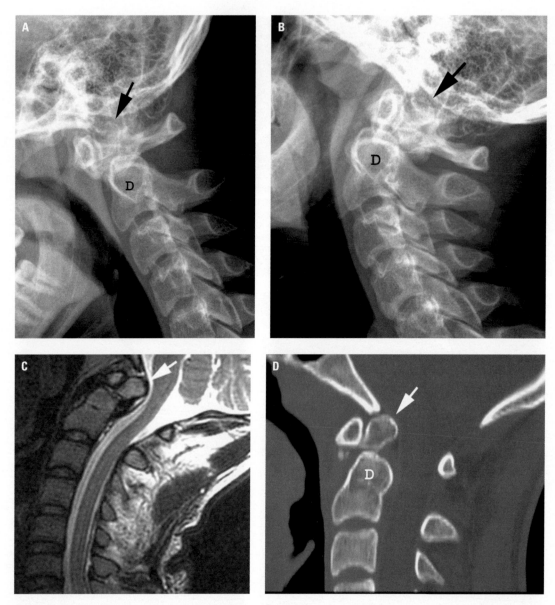

Figure 6.13. Os odontoideum hypermobility. **A:** Note the large malformed os odontoideum *(arrow)* sitting atop a hypoplastic dens *(D)*. The os odontoideum is slightly anteriorly subluxed. **B:** With extension, the os odontoideum *(arrow)* now moves far posterior and sits over the posterior aspect of the hypoplastic dens. Also note that the anterior arch of C1 is a little overgrown and now sits over the dens *(D)*. **C:** Sagittal T2-weighted magnetic resonance (MR) study. Note how the posteriorly displaced os odontoideum is causing slight pressure on the spinal cord *(arrow)*. **D:** CT study in the same patient clearly demonstrates the malformed os odontoideum *(arrow)* and the hypoplastic dens *(D)*.

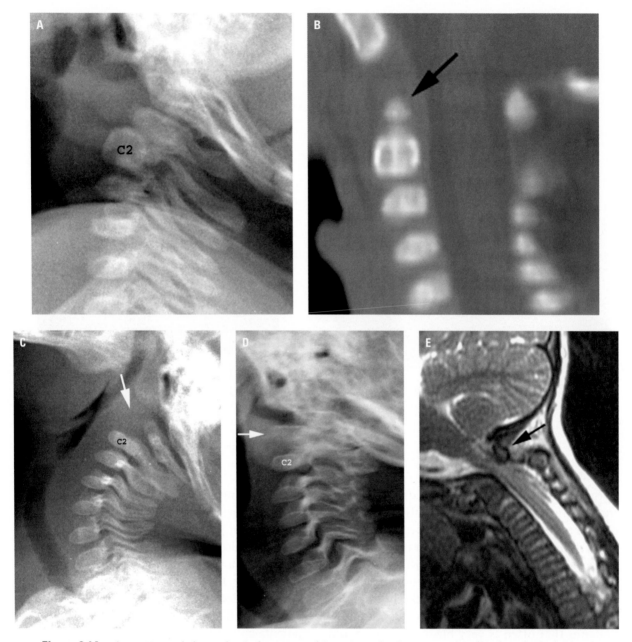

Figure 6.14. Absent/Severely hypoplastic dens. **A:** In this patient, the dens is not visualized. Only the body of C2 *(C2)* is seen. The lateral masses of C1 lie atop and somewhat posterior to the dens. **B:** Reconstructed CT study demonstrates the severely hypoplastic dens *(arrow)*. **C:** In this patient, the dens is absent *(arrow)* and only the body of C2 *(C2)* is seen. Note the position of the posterior arch of C1. **D:** With flexion, the lateral masses of C1 come into view *(arrow)* and sit atop the body of C2 *(C2)*. **E:** T2-weighted sagittal MR study demonstrates how the posterior arch of C1 *(arrow)* is pressing on the spinal cord.

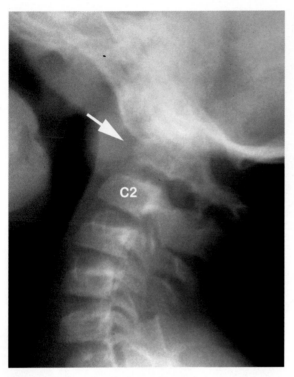

Figure 6.15. Dens as body of C1. Note the body of C2 *(C2)*. What appears to be the dens *(arrow)* is actually the body of C1.

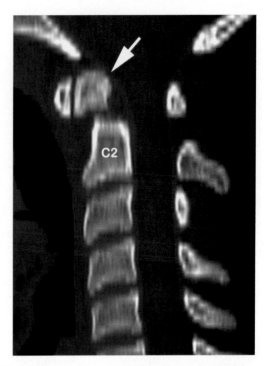

Figure 6.16. Ununited dens fracture. In this teenager, note the fractured and anteriorly displaced dens *(arrows)*. It is not malformed. Body of C2 *(C2)*. Compare with an os odontoideum in Figure 6.13D.

In adolescents and adults, an ununited dens fracture in the past often was confused with the os odontoideum. This should not occur very often because these cases are relatively rare in this day and age. However, in any case with an ununited dens fracture, the dens appears normal except that it is not firmly fused with the body of C2 (Fig. 6.16). This is different from the os odontoideum that often is very bizarre in shape and location.

DENS FRACTURES AND TILTING OF THE DENS

Fractures of the dens in infants and young children usually are a little different than fractures seen in older children, adolescents, and adults. In this regard, although typical type I, II, and III fractures of the dens occur in adolescents and older children, in the young child and infant (5 years and younger), fractures tend to occur through the synchondroses between the dens and body of C2 (Fig. 6.17A).[19] This is important because one may not have to endlessly

pursue getting a good open-mouth odontoid view in these young infants. The reason is that these fractures generally are visible on the lateral view. For this reason also, one may not need to go on to obtain a CT study, a very important consideration in this day and age. I have always basically depended on the lateral view of the cervical spine to assess dens fractures in these young patients. If it is normal in patients up to 5 years of age or so, then it is likely normal.[20]

Tilting of the dens can be normal or abnormal, and it can tilt anteriorly, posteriorly, or laterally. Anterior tilting most often is seen with flexion-induced fractures (Fig. 6.17A) but occasionally it can be seen as a normal variation (Fig. 6.17B). Normal posterior tilting of the dens, on the other hand, is very common.[21] This can be seen both on radiographs (Fig. 6.17C) and sagittal reconstructed CT studies. Of course, posterior tilting also can occur with hyperextension-induced fractures through the base of the dens, but in all age groups, normal posteriorly tilted is far more common.

Lateral tilting of the dens on anteroposterior (AP) views of the cervical spine in the past was relatively

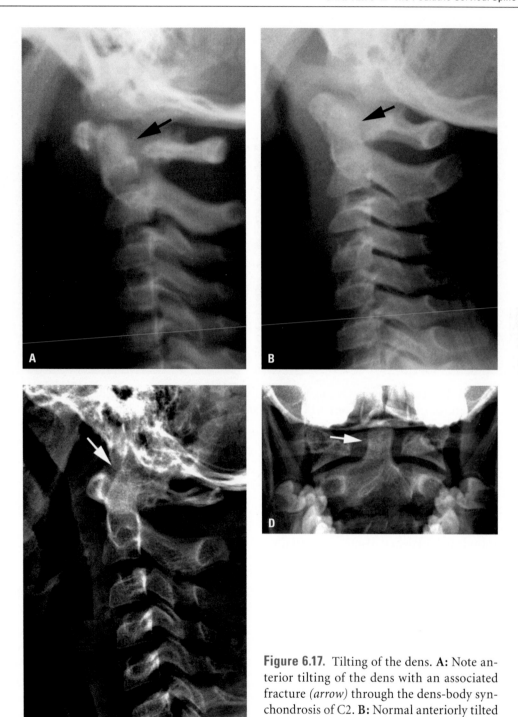

Figure 6.17. Tilting of the dens. **A:** Note anterior tilting of the dens with an associated fracture *(arrow)* through the dens-body synchondrosis of C2. **B:** Normal anteriorly tilted dens *(arrows)*. **C:** Normal posteriorly tilted dens *(arrow)*. **D:** Normal laterally tilted dens.

uncommon. In fact, if one saw a laterally tilted dens on the open-mouth odontoid view, one became suspicious that a fracture was present. This is not the case with CT studies where the spine frequently is rotated on the EMS backboard. This being the case, the normal dens now frequently appears laterally tilted (Fig. 6.17D).

THE PREDENTAL DISTANCE AND THE C1-C2 INTERSPINOUS DISTANCE

The predental distance in children often is wider than the accepted norm in adults. Indeed, 2 mm is common and 3 mm is nearly as common.[22,23] In addition, in a few cases, even 5 mm is normal and an

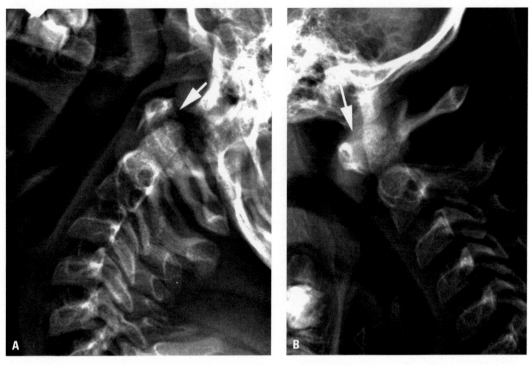

Figure 6.18. Predental distance: Normal movement. **A:** With the neck extended, the predental distance appears completely normal *(arrows)*. With flexion, the space increases but only by 2 mm *(arrow)*.

increase in the distance by up to 2 mm with flexion is usually normal (Fig. 6.18). However, all of this notwithstanding, one still needs to know how to deal with an abnormal predental distance, especially in infants and young children.

The predental distance, on a pathologic basis, becomes increased with traumatic anterior dislocation of C1 on C2, the previously referred to hypoplastic dens/os odontoideum complex, and in hypotonic individuals such as those with the trisomy 21 syndrome (Fig. 6.19). On the other hand, the interspinous distance in normal infants and young children on flexion (e.g., on the backboard for a CT study) can become alarmingly wide. One needs to appreciate that the range of normal is very wide and that most increases in the interspinous distance are normal. In this regard, in our experience and in an ongoing study, we have noted that this distance can increase with flexion by up to 11 to 12 mm in normal children. So how do we deal with this?

I have found that the best way to determine whether the interspinous distance is abnormally wide is to look at the predental distance. If the predental distance is wide then true dislocation is

likely present. However, if the predental distance is normal, it is most likely that the generous interspinous distance also is normal (Fig. 6.20).

C1 LATERAL MASS OFFSET AND DENS-LATERAL MASS C1 DISTANCE

Lateral mass offsetting, be it unilateral or bilateral, is characteristic of Jefferson fractures. In these cases, the space between the dens and the lateral mass is increased either unilaterally or bilaterally, depending on whether the fracture is unilateral or bilateral. However, in young infants, lateral mass offsetting maybe pronounced and yet normal, and in this regard, it has been demonstrated that lateral mass offsetting is normal up to 2 years of age.[24] In addition, infants and young children are so mobile that the lateral mass of C1, as it relates to the dens on rotation, can appear alarmingly displaced (Fig. 6.21A). Very often, one needs to proceed to fluoroscopy to determine whether true pathology is present (Fig. 6.21B).

Finally, when one is dealing with rotation, a specific configuration of the dens-lateral masses

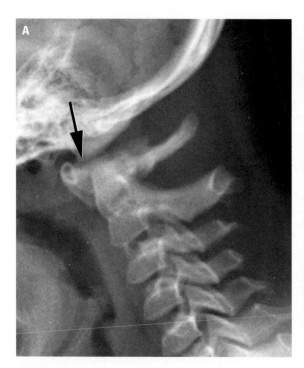 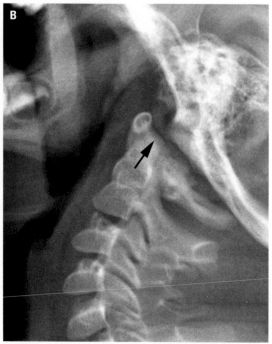

Figure 6.19. Predental distance: Abnormal. **A:** With flexion in this patient with trisomy 21, the predental distance *(arrow)* is increased. In addition, notice that the dens basically lines up with the clivus. **B:** With extension, the occipital condyles now lie posterior to the dens *(D)* and the predental distance has closed. This patient had instability at the C1-occiput and C1-C2 levels.

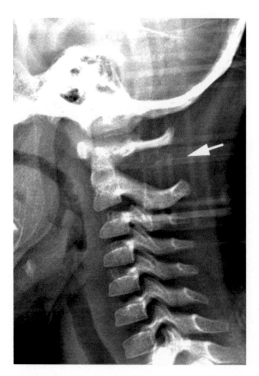

Figure 6.20. C1-C2 interspinous distance prominent: Normal. In this patient, the C1-C2 interspinous distance is quite prominent *(arrow)*. However it is normal. One can be sure of this by noting that the predental distance also is normal.

of C1 occurs. One will be presented with a lateral mass–dens distance that appears wider than normal on one side but narrower than normal on the other side. This indicates that the problem is rotation (Fig. 6.22) and, over the years, I have found this to be a good rule to follow.

ANTERIOR ANGULATION OF C2 AND WEDGING OF C3

Anterior angulation of C2 and wedging of C3 occur with hyperextension/compression fractures, but both are seen much more commonly on a normal basis.[25] Most anterior wedging/compression fractures occur in the midcervical spine and are more common in older children. In infants and young children, these injuries more often occur in the upper cervical spine and unfortunately, physiologic wedging also is common in this area.

Many times, normal anterior angulation of C2 and wedging of C3 are seen in the same patient (Fig. 6.23A). In other cases, the wedging is the predominant finding (Fig. 6.23B). In such cases, if

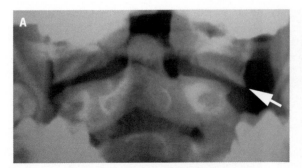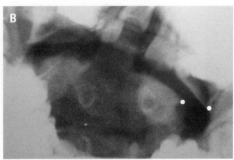

Figure 6.21. C1 lateral mass hypermobility. **A:** On this open-mouth odontoid view, note offsetting of the lateral mass *(arrow)* on the left. **B:** Under fluoroscopic control, the patient was asked to turn his head to the left. Offsetting *(dots)* became even more pronounced. This patient could do the same thing on the other side and was asymptomatic.

one needs to distinguish the findings from a true compression fracture, one can do so by noting that there is no associated disruption of the apophyseal joints at the C2-C3 level if the problem is physiologic (Fig. 6.23B). In this regard, as long as there is 50% coverage of the apophyseal joint, then the wedging deformity is likely normal. The wedging deformity results from chronic physiologic compression of the upper growth plate from repeated normal flexion of the neck. It eventually disappears and is not a finding seen in adolescents and adults. When there are multiple levels of wedging the problem is almost surely normal (Fig. 6.23C). In any case, if there is a question about where a fracture is present, one can perform a CT study that will show no fracture. When wedging is pathologic

and caused by a fracture, the fractures are apparent on CT studies.

PHYSIOLOGIC ANTERIOR SUBLUXATION OF C2-C3

Physiologic subluxation of C2 on C3 during flexion is a very common and normal phenomenon.[26–28] Once again, the problem is underlying ligament laxity and during flexion, C2 slides forward on C3. A similar phenomenon occasionally can be seen at the C3-C4 level but usually is not isolated. It will be seen together with subluxation of C2 on C3. When subluxation is limited to the C2-C3 level, it needs to be distinguished from the same configuration seen

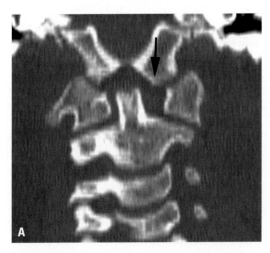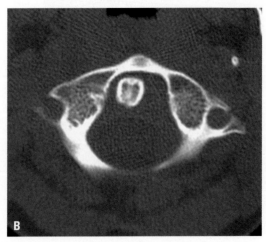

Figure 6.22. Rotation and pseudoabnormal dens-lateral mass distance. **A:** CT-reconstructed coronal study demonstrates a wide dens to lateral mass distance *(arrow)* on the left. However, note that the same distance on the right is narrower than normal. This is what is seen with rotation. **B:** Same findings on the axial CT study.

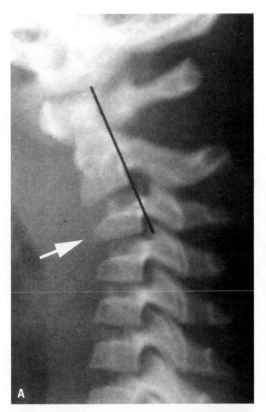

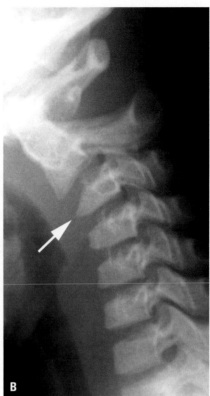

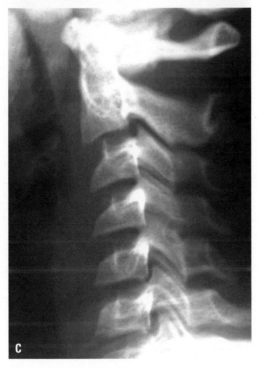

Figure 6.23 Anterior angulation C2 and wedging of C3. **A:** Note angulation of C2 on C3 *(line)*. There is no dislocation and the apophyseal joints are normal. Also note slight anterior wedging of C3 *(arrow)*. **B:** In this patient, more pronounced wedging of C3 *(arrow)* is seen. Note that the apophyseal joints are normal. Neither one of these patients had any fractures or neurologic findings. **C:** Note anterior wedging of C3 and C4 and to a slight extent of C5. When multiple wedging deformities are seen, the study is normal.

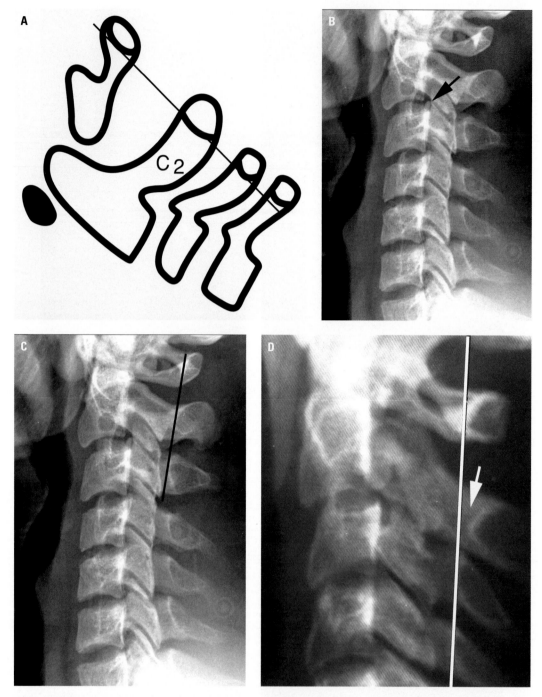

Figure 6.24. C2-C3 physiologic subluxation. **A:** Posterior cervical line. Note that the line drawn from the anterior cortex of the spinous tip of C1 to the same cortex of C3 passed through the anterior cortex of the spinous process of C2. It can just touch the anterior cortex or miss it by 1 mm and still be normal. **B:** In this patient, note offsetting of C2 on C3 *(arrow)*. Is it normal? **C:** Same patient. Anterior spinal line passes through the cortex of the spinous tip of C2 and thus the spine is normal. **D:** In this patient, the posterior line misses the anterior cortex of C2 by 2 mm *(arrow)*. There also is offsetting of C2 on C3 and a subtle hangman's fracture through the posterior arch of C2.

with an underlying hangman's fracture. Some time ago, I was confronted with the question, "How do you know that subluxation is truly physiologic?" I decided to look at this and after reviewing scores of cases, it became apparent to me that with hangman's fractures, all of C2 anterior to the fracture site, along with C1 moved forward as a unit with resultant anterior subluxation of C2 on C3. With physiologic subluxation, this did not occur. Rather, C2 in its entirety moved forward on C3. To aid in differentiating one configuration from the other, I devised the posterior cervical line.[26] This line is drawn from the anterior cortex of the spinous tip of C2 to the same anterior cortex of the tip of C3. If physiologic subluxation is present, the line will go through the anterior cortex of C2, touch the anterior cortex over its anterior surface, or miss it by only 1 mm (Figs. 6.24A–C). I have found this line to be very helpful, and it can be readily applied both on radiographs and sagittal-reconstructed CT studies. With the hangman's fracture, this line misses the anterior cortex of the spinous tip of C2

by 2 mm or more (Fig. 6.24D). The posterior cervical line has also been termed the spinolaminar line but involves the entire cervical spine. The posterior cervical line is designed only for determining pseudosubluxation of C2-C3 in the upper cervical spine. Finally, when one encounters multiple subluxations, the problem is invariably normal physiologic movement (Fig. 6.25).

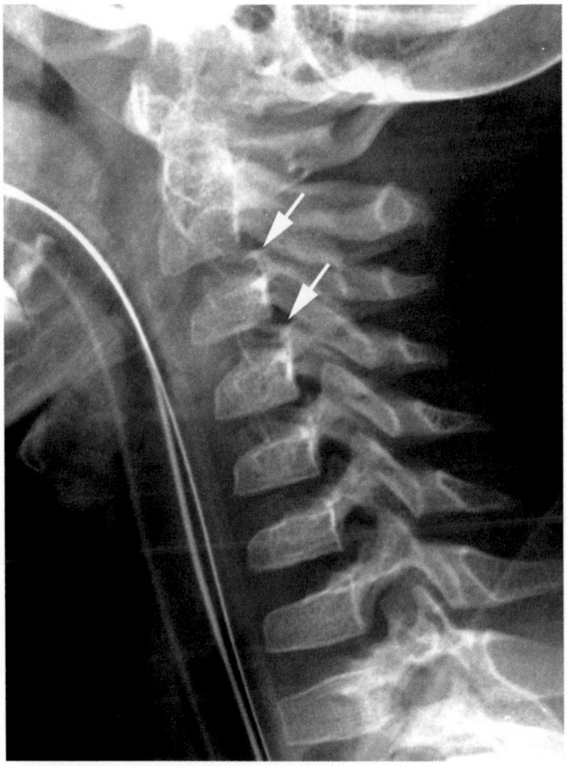

HIGH ANTERIOR ARCH OF C1

There is so much flexibility in the infants and young child's spine that with normal extension, C1 often looks as though it were going to slide over the top of the dens (Fig. 6.26). This is a normal finding and can be very pronounced. It would be very difficult to explain it on a traumatic basis.

APOPHYSIS OF THE VERTEBRA MIMICKING TEARDROP FRACTURES

The ring apophysis is a common and normal finding in the growing child. It usually is seen as a thin wedge-like structure along the lower anterior corner

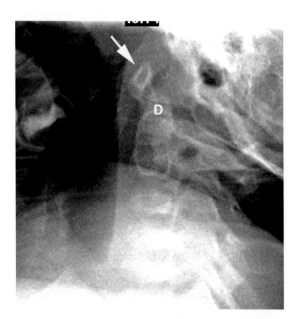

Figure 6.25. Physiologic subluxation: Multiple levels. Note subluxation of C2 on C3 and C3 on C4 *(arrows)*. When multiple subluxations are seen, the study basically will be normal.

Figure 6.26. High anterior arch of C1. Note the high position of the anterior arch *(arrow)* of C1. Note its relationship to the tip of the dens *(D)*. This cervical spine was seen on a lateral chest radiograph in this patient. The finding was entirely coincidental. This is very common in infants.

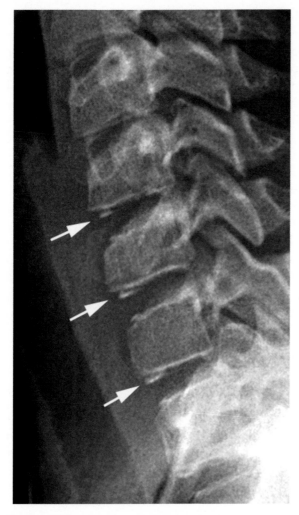

Figure 6.27. The ring apophysis. Note the numerous ring apophysis *(arrows)*.

of the vertebral body on lateral view (Fig. 6.27). The apophysis usually are seen at multiple levels and generally do not pose any problem. It is interesting, however, that the ring apophysis can be avulsed as part of a teardrop fracture.[29]

REFERENCES

1. Lustrin ES, Karakas SP, Ortiz AO, et al. Pediatric cervical spine: normal anatomy, variants and trauma. *Radiographics.* 2003;23(3):539–560.
2. Swischuk LE. Normal cervical spine variations mimicking injuries in children. *Emerg Radiol.* 1999;6(5):299–306.
3. Charlton OP, Gehweiller JA, Morgan CL, et al. Spondylolysis and spondylolisthesis of the cervical spine. *Skeletal Radiol.* 1978;3(2):79–84.
4. Forsberg DA, Martinez S, Vogler JB III, et al. Cervical spondylolysis: imaging findings in 12 patients. *AJR Am J Roentgenol.* 1990;154(4):751–755.
5. Prioleau GR, Wilson CB. Cervical spondylolysis with spondylolisthesis. Case report. *Journal Neurosurg.* 1975;43(6):750–753.
6. Riebel GD, Bayley JC. A congenital defect resembling the Hangman's fracture. *Spine (Phila Pa 1976).* 1991;16(10):1240–1241.
7. Smith JT, Skinner SR, Shonnard NH. Persistent synchondrosis of the second cervical vertebra simulating a hangman's fracture in a child. Report of a case. *J Bone Joint Surg Am.* 1993;75(8):1228–1230.
8. Williams JP III, Baker DH, Miller WA. CT appearance of congenital defect resembling the Hangman's fracture. *Pediatr Radiol.* 1999;29(7):549–550.
9. Currarino G. Primary spondylolysis of the axis vertebra (C2) in three children, including one with pyknodysostosis. *Pediatr Radiol.* 1989;19(8):535–538.
10. Parisi M, Lieberson R, Shatsky S. Hangman's fracture or primary spondylolysis: a patient and a brief review. *Pediatr; Radiol.* 1991;21(5):367–368.
11. Pizzutillo PD, Rocha EF, D'Astous J, et al. Bilateral fracture of the pedicle of the second cervical vertebra in the young child. *J Bone Joint Surg Am.* 1986;68(6):892–896.
12. Howard AW, Letts RM. Cervical spondylolysis in children: is it posttraumatic? *J Pediatr Orthop.* 2000;20(5):677–681.
13. Kleinman PK, Shelton YA. Hangman's fracture in an abused infant: imaging features. *Pediatr Radiol.* 1997;27(9):766–777.
14. McGrory BE, Fenichel GM. Hangman's fracture subsequent to shaking in an infant. *Ann Neurol.* 1977;2(1):82.
15. Kim HK, Laor T. Bilateral congenital cervical spondylolysis. *Pediatr Radiol.* 2010;40(1):132.
16. Torklus DV, Gehle W. *The Upper Cervical Spine.* London, United Kingdom: George Thieme Verlag; 1972.
17. Swischuk LE, John SD, Moorthy C. The os terminale-os dontoideum complex. *Emerg Radiol.* 1997;4(2):72–81.
18. Ricciardi JE, Kaufer H, Louis DS. Acquired os odontoideum following acute ligament injury. Report of case. *J Bone Joint Surg Am.* 1976;58(3):410–412.
19. Connolly B, Emery D, Armstrong D. The odontoid synchondrotic slip: an injury unique to young children. *Pediatr Radiol.* 1995;25(suppl 1):S129–S133.
20. Swischuk LE, John SD, Hendrick EP. Is the open-mouth odontoid view necessary in children under 5 years? *Pediatr Radiol.* 2000;30(3):186–189.
21. Swischuk LE, Hayden CK Jr, Sarwar M. The posteriorly tilted dens. A normal variation mimicking a fracture dens. *Pediatr Radiol.* 1979;8(1):27–28.

22. Locke GR, Gardner JI, Van Epps EF. Atlas-dens interval (ADI) in children: a survey based on 200 normal cervical mass spines. *Am J Roentgenol Radium Ther Nucl Med*. 1966;97(1):135–140.

23. Swischuk LE. *Emergency Imaging of the Acutely Ill or Injured Child*. 3rd ed. Philadelphia, PA: Williams & Wilkins; 1994.

24. Suss RA, Zimmerman RD, Leeds NE. Pseudo-spread of the atlas: false sign of Jefferson fracture in young children. *AJR Am J Roentgenol*. 1983;140(6):1079–1082.

25. Swischuk LE, Swischuk PN, John SD. Wedging of C-3 in infants and children: usually a normal finding and not a fracture. *Radiology*. 1993;188(2):523–526.

26. Swischuk LE. Anterior displacement of C2 in children: physiologic or pathologic. *Radiology*. 1977;122(3):759–763.

27. Harrison RB, Keats TE, Winn HR, et al. Pseudosub-luxation in the axis in young adults. *Can J Can Assoc Radiol*. 1980;31(3):176–177.

28. McIntosh A, Pollack AN. Pseudosubluxation. *PEC*. 2010;26(9):691–692.

29. Gooding CA, Hurwitz ME. Avulsed vertebral rim apophysis in a child. *Pediatr Radiol*. 1974;2(4):265–268.

CHAPTER 7

Imaging Thoracolumbar Spine Trauma

Mark P. Bernstein ■ Alexander B. Baxter ■ John H. Harris, Jr.

INTRODUCTION

Epidemiology

Motor vehicle crashes, falls, violence, and sports-related injuries contribute to 12,000 new spinal cord injuries each year in the United States. More than 80% of spinal cord injury victims are male, with an average age of 40 years. Forty-four percent of thoracolumbar spine fractures are associated with spinal cord injuries, and spinal cord injuries complicate 10% to 30% of all traumatic spinal fractures.

Four percent to 18% of blunt trauma victims suffer thoracolumbar spine fractures and these are often associated with major injuries in the head, chest, abdomen, pelvis, and extremities. Up to 25% of patients with spinal fractures and dislocations have multilevel injuries, as do 1.3% of spinal cord injury patients.

Half of all major spine injuries are unrecognized in the prehospital setting. Once in hospital, clinical diagnosis during the initial trauma resuscitation and evaluation may be challenged by altered consciousness, intoxication, and distracting injuries. Hasler et al., in a European cohort study of 24,000 spine fractures identified in more than 250,000 adult major trauma patients, determined predictors for spinal fracture.[1] These were age younger than 45 years, Glasgow Coma Scale (GCS) less than 9, falls greater than 2 m, sports injuries,

and vehicular accidents. Predictors of associated spinal cord injury were male sex, age younger than 45 years, GCS less than 15, falls greater than 2 m, sports injuries, vehicle accidents, shooting, and associated chest injury.

Fractures of the thoracolumbar spine may be difficult to diagnose, and missed diagnosis contributes to neurologic deficit in 10.5% of patients with delayed diagnosis compared with 1.4% whose fractures are diagnosed at presentation. In one study, 12.7% of lumbar spine fractures were missed on plain radiographs in multitrauma patients. When evaluated with nonreformatted abdominal computed tomography (CT) images, the same study showed an even higher missed rate of 23.2%, underscoring the importance of high-resolution CT images with multiplanar reformations (MPRs).

ANATOMY

The thoracolumbar spine is the principal load-bearing structure of the skeleton and is subject to axial compression, flexion and extension forces in different planes, and rotation. Flexion and extension forces act around a transverse fulcrum located in the posterior third of the vertebral body (Fig. 7.1). The direction and magnitude of these forces determine characteristic injury patterns.

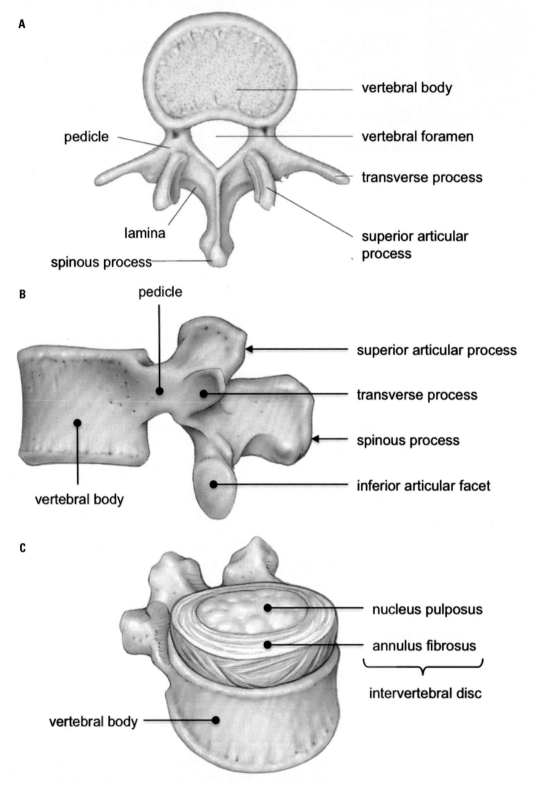

Figure 7.1. Spinal anatomy. **A:** Transaxial view of typical lumbar vertebra. **B:** Side view of typical lumbar vertebra. **C:** Oblique view of typical lumbar vertebra and disk. *(continued)*

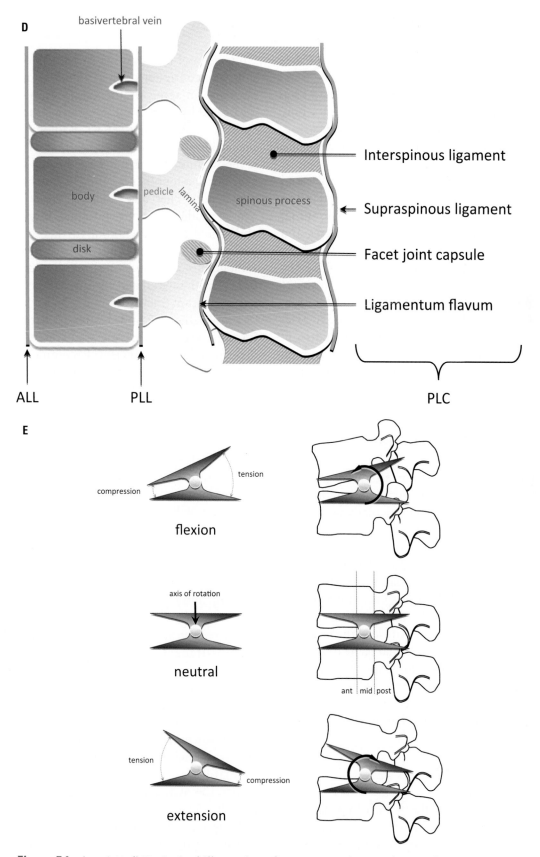

Figure 7.1. *(continued)* **D:** Sagittal illustration of 3 representative vertebrae and 2 intervertebral disks with associated ligaments. **E:** Schematic of flexion and extension forces compared with neutral acting upon 2 adjacent vertebrae.

Thoracic Segment T1-T10

The wedge shape of thoracic vertebrae establishes the normal kyphosis of the upper spine where the anterior vertebral body is generally 2 to 3 mm shorter than the posterior body. The anterior portion of the vertebral body supports load bearing, and the posterior arch resists tension/distraction. The T1-T10 facets are coronally oriented, protecting against anterior translation. The spinal canal is narrowest through the thoracic segment and in contrast to the lumbar spine, the thoracic spinal cord is easily injured in traumatic fractures and dislocations.

The intact rib cage and sternum stabilize the upper spine. The rib cage adds stiffness, restricts extension, and limits flexion and lateral rotation. This relationship allows a fourfold increase in axial loading capacity. Consequently, injuries that disrupt the upper thoracic spine typically result from high energy transfer mechanisms such as motor vehicle collisions and falls.

Thoracolumbar Segment T11-L2

Approximately two-thirds of all thoracolumbar spine injuries occur at the junction zone between T11 and L2. This segment is particularly susceptible to injury for several reasons. First, the stabilizing effects of the rib cage and sternal articulations are no longer present (T11 and T12 are floating ribs), resulting in a transition from a relatively rigid thoracic spine to a more mobile lumbar spine. Moreover, the conformation of the spine transitions from thoracic kyphosis to lumbar lordosis. And last, the facet orientation changes from the coronal plane to the sagittal plane distally. Because this segment of the spine is mobile and joins the relatively fixed thoracic cage and pelvis, compression fractures are most commonly seen at the thoracolumbar junction.

Lumbar Segment L3-L5

Lumbar lordosis balances the thoracic kyphosis such that axial loads are propagated through the posterior third of vertebral bodies. As a result, compressive loads produce burst fractures, which predominate in this region.

IMAGING

Up to 25% of multitrauma patients have concomitant, noncontiguous spinal injuries and in these patients, imaging of the entire spine has been advocated by several authors and by the American College of Radiology (ACR). Radiographs of the thoracolumbar spine are typically reserved for less severely injured patients who do not require CT examination for other reasons. In patients undergoing CT of the chest and abdomen, MPRs of the spine can be produced from the original thoracic and/or abdominal datasets without further scanning. In patients with abnormal, incomplete, or inadequate radiographs, a single acquisition thoracic and lumbar CT with sagittal and coronal MPRs can exclude any significant fracture.

In 2009, the ACR updated the spine trauma imaging appropriateness criteria after conducting an independent literature review.[2] Recommendations are not as definitive as those for the cervical spine, as there is less supporting data in the trauma literature. Current recommendations for imaging the thoracolumbar spine are any of the following: (1) back pain or midline tenderness, (2) local signs of thoracolumbar injury, (3) abnormal neurologic signs, (4) cervical spine fracture, (5) GCS <15, (6) major distracting injury, and (7) alcohol or drug intoxication. The ACR advocates the use of reconstructed spine imaging from thoracoabdominal CT, which are superior to radiographs (Table 7.1).

Radiography

Chest radiography for evaluation of the thoracic spine is fraught with difficulty. Fifty percent of such studies are nondiagnostic. Furthermore, there is significant overlap of radiographic findings of thoracic spine injury with those of traumatic aortic injury (Fig. 7.2). Dedicated overpenetrated coned down anteroposterior (AP) and breathing lateral thoracic spine radiographs are superior to standard chest radiograph. However, as outlined earlier, the ACR appropriateness criteria only support thoracic and lumbar spine radiographs for localizing signs. It is important to view radiographs as a screening study only with a low threshold for advanced imaging with multidetector computed tomography (MDCT).

TABLE 7.1	ACR Appropriateness Criteria for Suspected Spine Trauma as It Applies to the Thoracolumbar Spine

Clinical Condition: Suspected Spine Trauma
Variant 9: Blunt trauma meeting criteria for thoracic or lumbar imaging. With or without localizing signs.

Radiologic Procedure	Rating	Comments	RRL*
CT thoracic or lumbar spine without contrast	9	Dedicated images with sagittal and coronal reformat or derived from TAP (thorax-abdomen-pelvis) scan.	☢☢☢
MRI thoracic or lumbar spine without contrast	5	Depends on clinical findings and results of the CT. If suspected cord or soft-tissue injury.	O
Myelography and post myelography CT thoracic or lumbar spine	3	If MRI contraindicated.	☢☢☢☢
X-ray thoracic or lumbar spine	3	Useful for localizing signs.	☢☢☢

Rating Scale: 1, 2, 3 Usually not appropriate; 4, 5, 6 May be appropriate; 7, 8, 9 Usually appropriate   *Relative Radiation Level

Variant 10: Blunt trauma meeting criteria for thoracic or lumbar imaging. Neurologic abnormalities.

Radiologic Procedure	Rating	Comments	RRL*
CT thoracic or lumbar spine without contrast	9	Dedicated images with sagittal and coronal reformat or derived from TAP scan.	☢☢☢
MRI thoracic or lumbar spine without contrast	9	For cord abnormalities.	O
Myelography and post myelography CT thoracic or lumbar spine	7		☢☢☢☢

Rating Scale: 1, 2, 3 Usually not appropriate; 4, 5, 6 May be appropriate; 7 ,8, 9 Usually appropriate   *Relative Radiation Level

CT, computed tomography. From American College of Radiology. *ACR Appropriateness Criteria: suspected spine trauma.* 2009, with permission.

Thoracic Spine

The routine radiographic examination of the thoracic spine includes AP (Fig. 7.3A) and lateral (Fig. 7.3B) projections. CT is required for complete and sensitive assessment of osseous anatomy and alignment, whereas an MRI is superior in evaluating soft tissues including acute disc herniation, ligamentous, and spinal cord injuries.

On the AP radiograph of the thoracic spine (Fig. 7.3A), the lateral margin of the descending thoracic aorta extends to the diaphragm in an obliquely downward course. The left paraspinal stripe smoothly parallels the thoracic spine medial to the aorta and is visible from T5 to T10 in approximately 96% of patients. The left paraspinal stripe is not visible in patients who have little body fat. Changes in contour of the left paraspinous stripe may be secondary to infection, neoplasm, or traumatic hematoma. Focal or diffuse paraspinous hematoma may be the most obvious radiographic sign of a minor thoracic vertebral fracture, and bilateral paraspinous hematoma is commonly associated with major fractures and fracture dislocations.

Normally, in the frontal projection, the thoracic vertebral bodies are square or slightly rectangular. The end plates should appear as thin parallel densities separated by the lucency of the intervertebral disk spaces. The lateral margins of the thoracic vertebral bodies are usually smoothly and

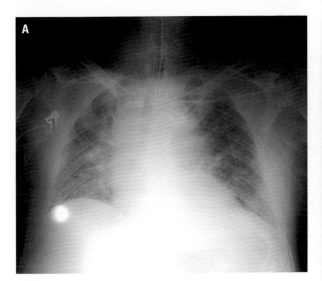

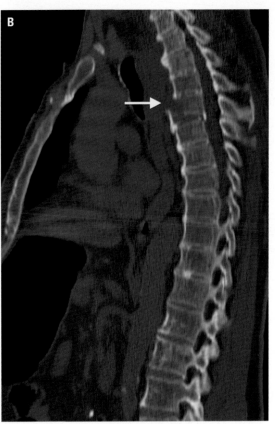

Figure 7.2. Hyperextension thoracic spine fracture. **A:** Abnormal AP admission chest radiograph in multi-trauma patient sustaining a thoracic spine fracture. Loss of the normal aortic contour, thickening of the right paratracheal stripe, and rightward deviation of the trachea are signs more commonly associated with traumatic aortic injury. Bilateral rib fractures are also present. **B:** Sagittal CT reformation reveals rigid spine hyperextension thoracic spine fracture. No aortic injury was present.

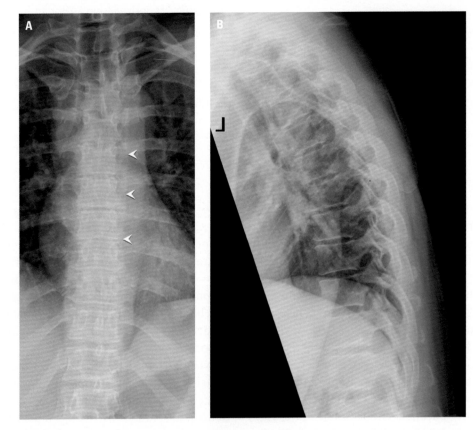

Figure 7.3. Normal thoracic spine radiographs. **A:** AP projection. Left paraspinal stripe outlined by *arrowheads*. **B:** Lateral projection with breathing technique to produce "autotomogram" with blurred out ribs.

gently concave. Spinous processes should be in the midline and roughly equidistant. Pedicles are normally round to slightly oval in shape, bilateral, and at each vertebra.

On the lateral projection, only the mid thoracic spine is evaluated. The upper segments are typically obscured by the superimposed shoulders, and the lower segments by subdiaphragmatic soft tissues. Superimposed ribs, lung tissue, the scapulae, and occasionally the descending thoracic aorta compromise evaluation of the spine on lateral radiographs, but it is possible to obtain clearer delineation by having the patient either inspire or expire slowly during a long radiographic exposure time. This maneuver, often referred to as an "autotomogram," is intended to blur superimposed structures (Fig. 7.3B). The costovertebral joints, laminae, and spinous processes are all seriously obscured by superimposed normal skeletal parts in the lateral projection.

Multiplanar CT is indicated in all patients in whom conventional radiography is abnormal,

equivocal, or inconsistent with the patient's clinical findings.

Lumbar Spine

The AP examination of the lumbar spine should include the lower thoracic vertebrae, the lower ribs, and portions of the pelvis (Fig. 7.4A).

In lateral projection (Fig. 7.4B), the lumbar vertebral bodies are slightly rectangular. Normally, both the anterior and posterior cortical margins are smoothly concave. Central interruptions of the posterior cortical margin of the lumbar vertebral bodies represent ostia for the basivertebral veins.

Because of the frequency of anomalies at the lumbosacral segments, particularly when the 12th ribs are absent, it may be difficult to enumerate the lumbar segments. However, the transverse processes of L4 are usually canted slightly cephalad, in distinction to the remainder of the lumbar vertebrae. When this characteristic is present, it serves as a useful landmark in identifying the lumbar segments.

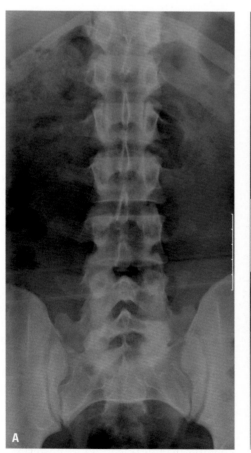 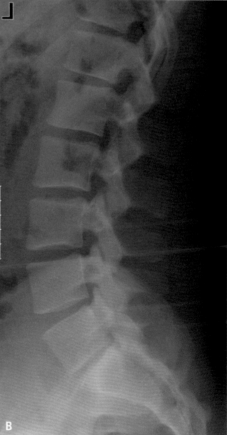

Figure 7.4. Normal lumbar spine radiographs. **A:** AP projection. **B:** Lateral projection.

Multidetector Computed Tomography

MDCT is more accurate than radiographs for assessment of bony injury and alignment and is ideal for characterization of fracture extent, morphology, and location of fracture fragments. High-quality MPRs are essential for interpretation.

MDCT is the imaging procedure of choice in the multitrauma setting where an evaluation of the chest and abdomen is also required. For these patients, reformatted images from thin, overlapping, trans-axial data from torso imaging provide high-quality sagittal and coronal reformations. There is no need with current technology to acquire dedicated spine CT when reformations come at no additional cost or radiation.

Magnetic Resonance Imaging

An MRI is indicated in patients with neurologic deficits and potentially unstable fracture patterns to assess injury to the spinal cord, nerve roots, intervertebral disks and ligaments, and to establish or exclude the diagnosis of epidural hematoma. Because an isolated unstable ligamentous injury in the absence of fracture or subluxation is rare, a screening MRI in the setting of a normal CT is not indicated.

INJURY PATTERNS

Classification

At present, there is no universally accepted thoracolumbar spine injury classification system. The ideal classification system would include a uniform methodology for injury description, a determination of stability, and facilitate clinical decision making.

Boehler published the first classification of thoracolumbar spine injuries in 1929.[3] Based on radiographic studies of World War I spine injury patients, together with mechanism of injury, five injury categories were described: compression fractures, flexion-distraction injuries, extension fractures, rotational injuries, and shear fractures. In 1938, Watson-Jones furthered Boehler's work by advocating that the integrity of the posterior ligamentous complex (PLC) was necessary to maintain spinal stability.[4]

In 1970, Holdsworth introduced the "column concept" of spinal stability, a biomechanical interpretation of injury mechanisms implied from radiographic studies.[5] In his conception, the vertebra is divided into an anterior and posterior column (Fig. 7.5). The anterior column consists of the vertebral body, intervertebral disk, anterior longitudinal ligament (ALL), and posterior longitudinal ligament (PLL). The posterior column comprises the facets, neural arch, and posterior ligament complex (interspinous and supraspinous ligaments, facet capsule, and ligamentum flavum). The integrity of the posterior column served as the major determinant of spinal stability. Holdsworth's classification categorized thoracolumbar spine fractures into anterior compression fractures, fracture dislocations, rotational fracture dislocations, extension injuries, shear injuries, and burst fractures. According to Holdsworth, burst fractures were structurally stable as they were confined to the anterior column. Subsequent experimental studies

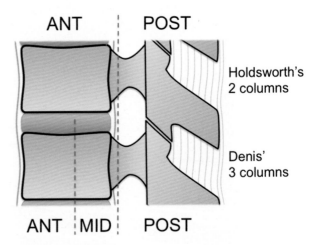

Figure 7.5. Column concept of the spine. Upper vertebral segment shows Holdsworth's two columns composed of anterior column (anterior longitudinal ligament, vertebral body, intervertebral disk, posterior longitudinal ligament) and posterior column (posterior bony arch and posterior ligament complex). Lower vertebral segment shows Denis' three columns comprised of anterior column (ALL, anterior vertebral body, and intervertebral disk), middle column (posterior vertebral body and intervertebral disk, PLL), and posterior column (unchanged from Holdsworth). ALL, anterior longitudinal ligament; PLL, posterior longitudinal ligament.

were unable to produce instability with only PLC disruption. Instability required, in addition to PLC disruption, rupture of the PLL and a portion of the annulus fibrosus.

Based on CT findings and newer experimental instability determinants, Denis modified the Holdsworth two-column model. In 1983, he published a review of 412 thoracolumbar spine injury patients and introduced the concept of the pivotal middle column defined as "the posterior longitudinal ligament, the posterior annulus fibrosus, and the posterior wall of the vertebral body" (Fig. 7.5).[6] Consequently, Denis' anterior column consists of "the anterior longitudinal ligament, the anterior annulus fibrosus, and the anterior part of the vertebral body." The posterior column, as in Holdsworth's model, is formed by the posterior bony arch and PLC.

Denis described four major types of spinal injuries along with their mechanisms: compression fractures, burst fractures, seat belt type (flexion distraction), and fracture-dislocations (Table 7.2). Instability, according to the Denis' three-column model, occurs with failure of two adjacent columns. The middle column represents the key to stability, as it fails either in association with the anterior column, the posterior column, or both. Denis also considered neurologic injury to be a marker of instability and used both mechanical and neurologic features to rate injury severity: first degree for isolated mechanical instability, second degree for isolated neurologic injury, and third degree for combined mechanical and neurologic instability.[6]

The classification proposed by Magerl et al. in 1994 groups all thoracic and lumbar spine fractures into three primary types that have a progressive relationship to one another based on increasing severity of the fracture pattern and degree of soft tissue involvement (Fig. 7.6).[7] This classification emphasizes the recognition and importance of ligamentous injury, particularly in the type B and C fractures.

Type A fractures are, in this schema, all the result of axial loading with or without an element of flexion. Type A fractures are limited to the vertebral body with loss of anterior vertebral body height but without posterior ligament complex injury or anterior translation. Type A fractures correspond to simple compression fractures due to hyperflexion.

Type B injuries involve both anterior and posterior columns and are associated with distraction of adjacent vertebrae due to ligamentous injury anteriorly (uncommon, hyperextension) or posteriorly (common, hyperflexion). In typical hyperflexion injuries, the posterior column injury is usually bony as in the Chance fracture or, less commonly, ligamentous as in the "soft tissue" Chance. Anterior translation is common in type B injuries.

Type C injuries include the characteristics of type B with the added element of rotation/shear and are by definition unstable. These injuries most closely correspond to the dislocations or fracture-dislocations of traditional classifications.

Each of these three main fracture types is divided into three groups, which are further divided into three subgroups, and finally into specifications

TABLE 7.2 Basic Modes of Failure of Denis' Three Columns in the Four Major Types of Spinal Injuries

Fracture Type	Column		
	Anterior	Middle	Posterior
Compression	Compression	None	None
Burst	Compression	Compression	None
Seat-belt type (flexion distraction)	None or compression	Distraction	Distraction
Fracture dislocation	Compression, rotation, shear	Distraction, rotation, shear	Distraction, rotation, shear

From Denis F. The three column spine and its significance in the classification of acute thoracolumbar spinal injuries. *Spine.* 1983;8(8):817–831, with permission.

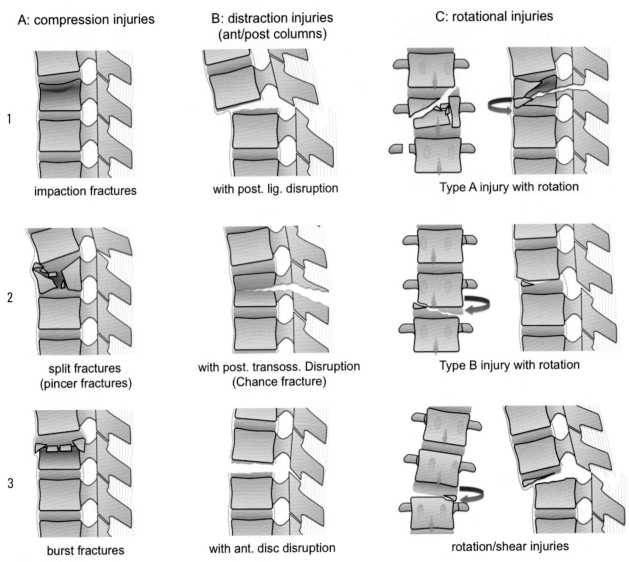

A: compression injuries

1 — impaction fractures

2 — split fractures (pincer fractures)

3 — burst fractures

B: distraction injuries (ant/post columns)

1 — with post. lig. disruption

2 — with post. transoss. Disruption (Chance fracture)

3 — with ant. disc disruption

C: rotational injuries

1 — Type A injury with rotation

2 — Type B injury with rotation

3 — rotation/shear injuries

Figure 7.6. Magerl spinal classification types and groups. (Modified from Magerl F, Aebi M, Gertzbein SD, et al. A comprehensive classification of thoracic and lumbar injuries. *Eur Spine J*. 1994;3(4):184–201.)

(Table 7.3). Together, the Magerl classification scheme is comprehensive, but also complex, as it catalogues 53 thoracolumbar injury patterns. Injuries are stratified from least severe A1 to most severe C3. No defined criteria for stability are inherent in the Magerl classification. In designing this classification, Denis' three-column concept is abandoned in favor of Holdsworth's two columns.

Stability

Predicting thoracolumbar spine fracture stability from an imaging study is difficult. Stability depends on the integrity of the vertebral bodies, including costal and sternal contributions in the thoracic segment, the ligaments, and joints of the spine. The practical definition of stability by White and Panjabi states that a stable spine is able to withstand physiologic loads without producing mechanical deformity or progressive neurologic injury or pain.[8] From both clinical and radiologic perspective, the three-column concept of Denis is most widely applied for determining thoracolumbar spine stability. According to Denis, failure of two or three columns yields instability, with disruption of the middle column representing the key contributing factor.

To simplify the imaging approach to stability, six radiologic signs of spinal instability have been described: (1) displacement, (2) wide interspinous space, (3) abnormal facet joints, (4) posterior vertebral body line disruption, (5) wide interpediculate distance, and (6) wide intervertebral disk space (Table 7.4). The presence of any one of these features indicates major injury to the supporting bone, ligaments, or joints and is felt to be sufficient to diagnose instability. Although originally described for radiographs, these features are applicable to, and in many cases, better seen with CT.

The common major fracture patterns described by Denis are compression, burst, flexion distraction (or Chance-type fractures), and fracture dislocations.

TABLE 7.3 Classification Scheme According to Magerl

Type A Injuries: Groups, Subgroups, and Specifications

Type A. Vertebral body compression

A1. Impaction fractures

A1.1. End plate impaction

A1.2. Wedge impaction fractures
  1 Superior wedge impaction fracture
  2 Lateral wedge impaction fracture
  3 Inferior wedge impaction fracture

A1.3. Vertebral body collapse

A2. Split fractures

A2.1. Sagittal split fracture

A2.2. Coronal split fracture

A2.3. Pincer fracture

A3. Burst fractures

A3.1. Incomplete burst fracture
  1 Superior incomplete burst fracture
  2 Lateral incomplete burst fracture
  3 Inferior incomplete burst fracture

A3.2. Burst-split fracture
  1 Superior burst-split fracture
  2 Lateral burst-split fracture
  3 Inferior burst-split fracture

A3.3. Complete burst fracture
  1 Pincer burst fracture
  2 Complete flexion burst fracture
  3 Complete axial burst fracture

Type B Injuries: Groups, Subgroups, and Specifications

Type B. Anterior and posterior element injury with distraction

B1. Posterior disruption predominantly ligamentous (flexion-distraction injury)

B1.1. With transverse disruption of the disc
  1 Flexion-subluxation
  2 Anterior dislocation
  3 Flexion-subluxation/anterior dislocation with fracture of the articular processes

B1.2. With Type A fracture of the vertebral body
  1 Flexion-subluxation + Type A fracture
  2 Anterior dislocation + Type A fracture
  3 Flexion-subluxation/anterior dislocation with fracture of the articular processes + Type A fracture

B2. Posterior disruption predominantly osseous (flexion-distraction injury)

B2.1. Transverse bicolumn fracture

B2.2. With transverse disruption of the disc
  1 Disruption through the pedicle and disc
  2 Disruption through the pars interarticularis and disc (flexion-spondylolysis)

B2.3. With Type A fracture of the vertebral body
  1 Fracture through the pedicle + Type A fracture
  2 Fracture through the pars interarticularis (flexion-spondylolysis) + Type A fracture

B3. Anterior disruption through the disc (hyperextension-shear injury)

B3.1. Hyperextension-subluxations
  1 Without injury of the posterior column
  2 With injury of the posterior column

B3.2. Hyperextension-spondylolysis

B3.3. Posterior dislocation

(continued)

| TABLE | 7.3 | **Classification Scheme According to Magerl (continued)** |

Type C Injuries: Groups, Subgroups, and Specifications

Type C. Anterior and posterior element injury with rotation

C1. Type A injuries with rotation (compression injuries with rotation)

C1.1. Rotational wedge fracture

C1.2. Rotational split fractures
1 Rotational sagittal split fracture
2 Rotational coronal split fracture
3 Rotational pincer fracture
4 Vertebral body separation

C1.3. Rotational burst fractures
1 Incomplete rotational burst fractures
2 Rotational burst-split fracture
3 Complete rotational burst fracture

C2. Type B injuries with rotation

C2.1. B1 injuries with rotation (flexion-distraction injuries with rotation)
1 Rotational flexion subluxation
2 Rotational flexion subluxation with unilateral articular process fracture
3 Unilateral dislocation
4 Rotational anterior dislocation without/with fracture of articular processes

5 Rotational flexion subluxation without/ with unilateral articular process + Type A fracture
6 Unilateral dislocation + Type A fracture
7 Rotational anterior dislocation without/ with fracture of articular processes + Type A fracture

C2.2. B2 injuries with rotation (flexion-distraction injuries with rotation)
1 Rotational transverse bicolumn fracture
2 Unilateral flexion spondylolysis with disruption of the disc
3 Unilateral flexion spondylolysis + Type A fracture

C2.3. B3 injuries with rotation (hyperextension-shear injuries with rotation)
1 Rotational hyperextension-subluxation without/with fracture of posterior vertebral elements
2 Unilateral hyperextension-spondylolysis
3 Posterior dislocation with rotation

C3. Rotational-shear injuries
C3.1. Slice fracture
C3.2. Oblique fracture

| TABLE | 7.4 | **Radiologic Signs of Instability** |

Sign	Column	Comment	Typical Injuries
Displacement	A/M/P	Dislocation or subluxation >2 mm	Fracture dislocation
Wide interspinous distance	M/P	Greater than 2 mm between adjacent levels	Flexion distraction (Chance-type fractures)
Abnormal facet joints	M/P	Widening or subluxation >2 mm or dislocation	Flexion distraction (Chance-type fractures)
Posterior vertebral body line disruption	A/M	Any defect including buckling, fracture, retropulsion, or rotation	Burst fractures
Wide interpediculate distance	A/M/P	Sagittal plane injury involving all columns	Burst fractures
Wide intervertebral disk space	A/M/P	Extension injuries; injury to ALL, PLL, and PLC	Hyperextension fracture dislocation

ALL, anterior longitudinal ligament; PLL, posterior longitudinal ligament; PLC, posterior ligamentous complex.

Compression Fractures

The compression fracture results from an axial loading force on a flexed spine with failure of the anterior column and loss of anterior vertebral height. The posterior vertebral body cortex and the posterior elements, including the PLC, are intact (Fig. 7.7). Because only one column is involved, compression fractures are stable injuries. No neurologic deficit results from this injury.

Imaging

Radiographically, the compression fracture appears as a wedge-shaped vertebra with features including disruption of the superior end plate, anterior vertebral body height loss with angulation, anterior cortical "step-off," or impaction (Fig. 7.8). Impacted trabeculae often cause a vague increase in density of the upper vertebral body (Fig. 7.8C). Associated paraspinous hematoma

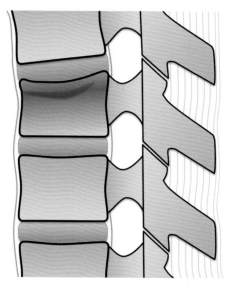

Figure 7.7. Compression fracture. Drawing illustrating failure of the anterior column only in flexion with anterior loss of vertebral body height. The posterior vertebral body cortex is uninvolved, and the facet joints remain intact. (Modified from Magerl F, Aebi M, Gertzbein SD, et al. A comprehensive classification of thoracic and lumbar injuries. *Eur Spine J.* 1994;3(4):184–201.)

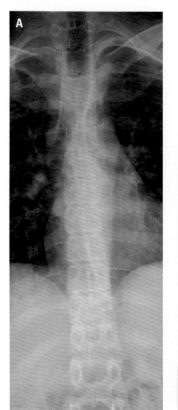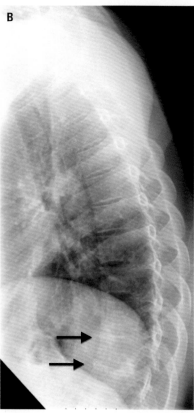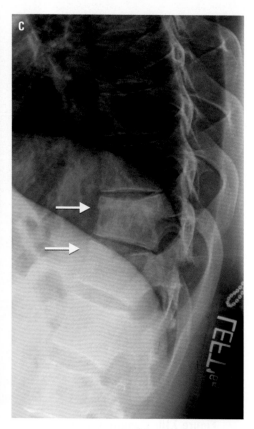

Figure 7.8. Compression fractures. **A:** AP views show subtle loss of height of T11 and T12. Lateral (**B**) and coned down lateral views (**C**) show loss of anterior vertebral body height with anterosuperior cortical buckling (*arrows*). Impacted trabeculae produce a vague linear density of the upper vertebral body.

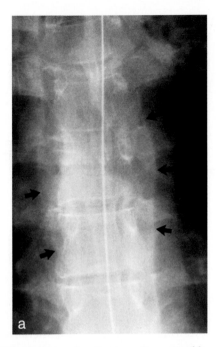

Figure 7.9. Compression fracture. Paraspinal hematoma.

causes focal displacement of the left paraspinal stripe (Fig. 7.9). These same findings are also seen at CT (Fig. 7.10). The stable anterior compression fracture can mimic more severe and unstable injuries such as pincer fractures, burst fractures, or flexion-distraction injuries, and once identified, or if plain radiographs are compromised by technique or patient body habitus, MDCT imaging should be pursued.

Posterior vertebral body cortical disruption or buckling are clues on lateral radiographs and sagittal CT reformations to middle column involvement and potentially unstable fractures. Interpedicular and interspinous widening are corresponding findings on AP radiographs and coronal CT.

Pincer fractures are unstable, coronal split vertebral body fractures (Magerl A2.3; Fig. 7.11) in which the fracture line extends from the superior end plate to the inferior end plate, and the

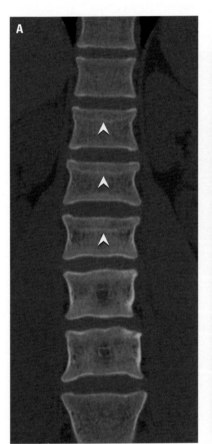
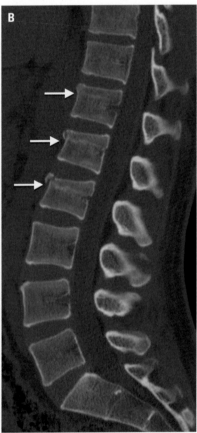
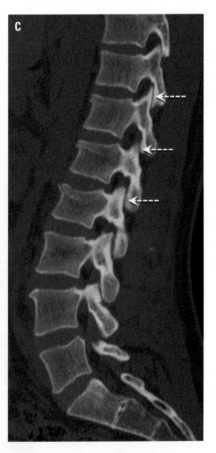

Figure 7.10. Compression fractures on CT. Coronal (**A**), midsagittal (**B**), and parasagittal (**C**) CT reformations show consecutive compression fractures from T12 to L2. Progressive buckling of the anterior cortex (*solid arrows* in **B**) and impacted trabeculae (*arrowheads* in **A**) are seen to better advantage than radiographs. Note the intact facet joints (*dashed arrows* in **C**) of the PLC. (*continued*)

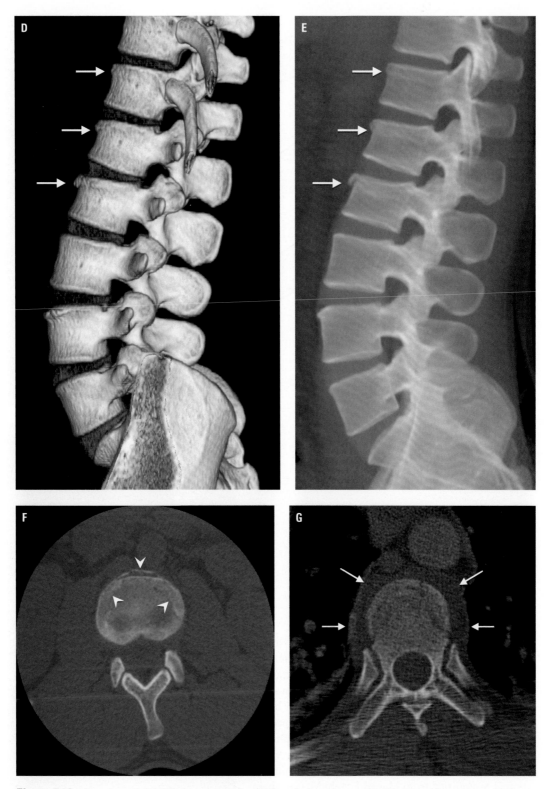

Figure 7.10. *(continued)* 3D CT reconstruction (**D**) and virtual x-ray (**E**, 3D image in transparent bone algorithm) show the same findings. Transaxial CT images show undisplaced anterosuperior vertebral peripheral fractures in the lumbar spine (**F**) and thoracic spine (**G**) with paraspinal hematoma *(arrows)*.

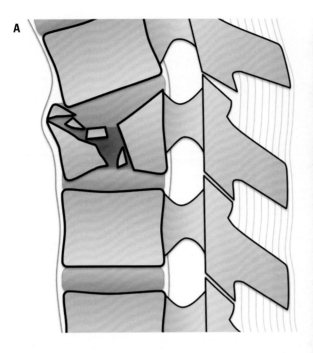

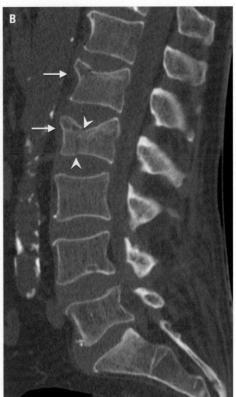

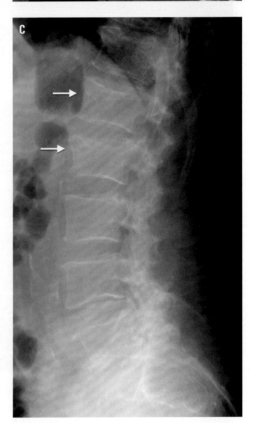

Figure 7.11. Pincer fracture. **A:** Illustration shows comminuted coronal vertebral body split fractures with herniation of disc material. **B:** Midsagittal CT reformation shows L2 coronal split fracture from superior to inferior cortices *(arrowheads)*. Anterior buckling of L1 and L2 vertebral bodies *(arrows)* appear as simple compression fractures on the radiograph (**C**), underscoring the need for CT evaluation with MPRs in all cases of acute thoracolumbar spine injuries. (Panel **A** modified from Magerl F, Aebi M, Gertzbein SD, et al. A comprehensive classification of thoracic and lumbar injuries. *Eur Spine J*. 1994;3(4):184–201.)

resulting gap is filled with disc material, further separating the fracture fragments. As a result, the vertebral body is not able to support axial loading and if untreated, these fractures may collapse further and result in focal kyphosis or pseudo-arthrosis (Fig. 7.12). Treatment for pincer fractures involves posterior fixation, and in some cases, additional anterior fixation is necessary if the anterior vertebral body fragment remains displaced.

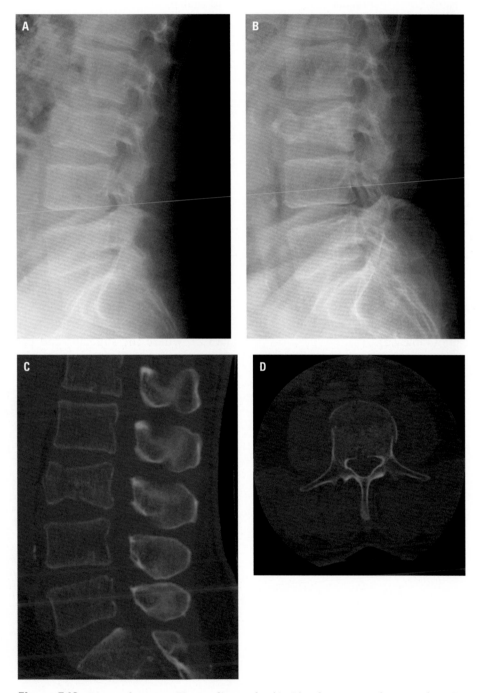

Figure 7.12. Pincer fracture. Two radiographs (**A**, **B**) taken 1 month apart show L3 coronal split vertebral body fracture with interval collapse and straightening of the lumbar lordosis. Midsagittal CT reformation (**C**) at the time of initial injury shows comminuted fracture of L3 with coronal fracture from superior to inferior cortices, separating this injury from a simple compression fracture. Transaxial CT image (**D**) shows the coronal fracture plane.

TABLE 7.5	Imaging Features Distinguishing Acute from Chronic Spine Fractures	
	Acute	**Chronic**
Margins	Sharp nonsclerotic	Smooth sclerotic
Paraspinal hematoma	Present	Absent
Gas	Absent	Present in disk or vertebral body
Bone scan	Uptake	Absent or minimal uptake
MRI	Low T1 signal	Fatty marrow on T1, no increased signal on T2, or IR

Distinguishing between acute and remote compression fractures is straightforward. Signs of a remote fracture include sclerotic margins of the fracture fragment and contiguous vertebral body, calcification of the anterior longitudinal ligament and bony bridging between the deformed vertebra and adjacent vertebrae, gas within the vertebral body or disk, and absence of a paraspinal hematoma on CT imaging. Additionally, chronic compression fractures will show minimal or no uptake of radiotracer on bone scan, whereas an MRI reveals fatty marrow on T1 and no increased signal on T2 or inversion recovery (Table 7.5).

Burst Fractures

Burst fractures result from an axial force on the nonflexed or neutral spine. Axial loading comminutes the vertebral body, fracturing the anterior and middle columns and disperses fracture fragments in a radial fashion. CT often reveals subtle posterior column failure in the form of a vertical fracture through the lamina or spinous process (Fig. 7.13). Variations include the incomplete burst (A3.1) in which only the superior or inferior end plate bursts; the burst-split (A3.2), where the superior end plate bursts and

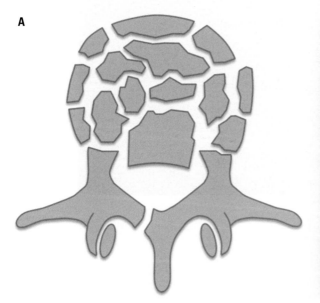
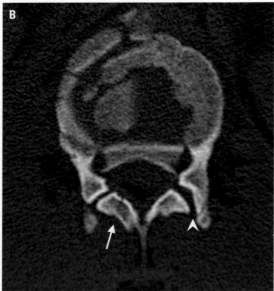

Figure 7.13. Burst fracture. Illustration (**A**) and transaxial CT image (**B**) show marked comminution of the vertebral body with radial dispersement of fracture fragments including retropulsion of the posterior vertebral body into the spinal canal. Commonly seen at CT is the associated vertical laminar fracture *(arrow)* and occasionally the widening of the facet joint *(arrowhead)*. (Panel **A** from Magerl F, Aebi M, Gertzbein SD, et al. A comprehensive classification of thoracic and lumbar injuries. *Eur Spine J.* 1994;3(4):184–201.)

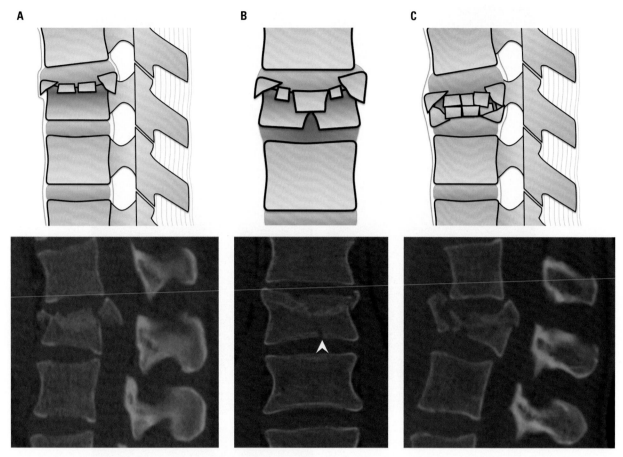

Figure 7.14. Burst fracture types. **A:** Incomplete burst fracture with superior body fragmentation and retropulsion. **B:** Burst-split fracture with superior body comminution and retropulsion with sagittal split of the inferior body *(arrowhead)*. **C:** Complete burst with fragmentation of the entire vertebral body. (From Magerl F, Aebi M, Gertzbein SD, et al. A comprehensive classification of thoracic and lumbar injuries. *Eur Spine J*. 1994;3(4):184–201.)

the lower vertebral body is split sagittally; and the complete burst (A3.3), where the entire body is burst (Fig. 7.14).

Disruption of the posterior vertebral body cortex is the hallmark of the burst fracture. The posterior body fragment is retropulsed into the spinal canal and is primarily responsible for acute neurologic compromise, which occurs in 48% to 77% of patients.

Imaging

AP radiographs may show loss of vertebral body height and widening of the vertebral body. Increased interpedicular distance indicates posterior column involvement (Fig. 7.15). The most obvious indirect radiographic sign on a frontal radiograph is focal paraspinous hematoma (Fig. 7.16). Lateral radiographs reveal compression of the vertebral body and poor definition or buckling of its posterior margin (Fig. 7.17). These findings are more clearly defined on a CT with MPRs. Because disruption of the posterior vertebral body cortex and retropulsed fragment may be subtle or obscured in 30% of radiographs, apparent anterior compression deformities in the setting of acute trauma should be evaluated with CTs and MPRs (Figs. 7.18 and 7.19).

MDCT is indicated to properly characterize the injury pattern. Transaxial images demonstrate vertebral body comminution, posterior body cortex fracture with buckling (Fig. 7.19B) or frank retropulsion (Fig. 7.13B), and often split vertical posterior neural arch fractures (signifying a three-column injury).

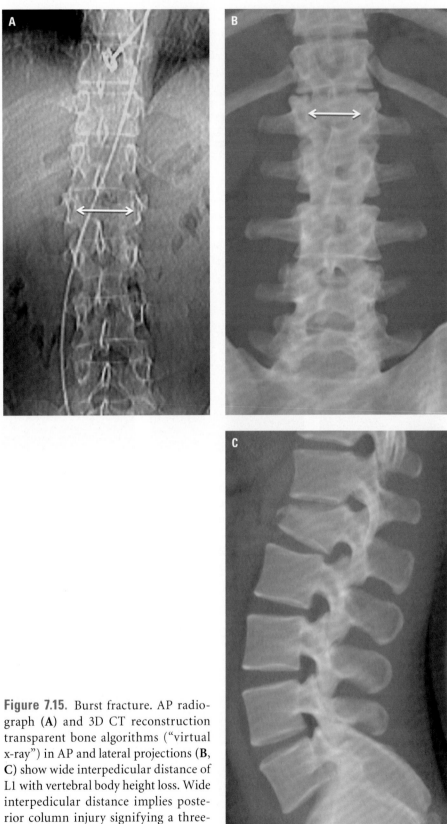

Figure 7.15. Burst fracture. AP radiograph (**A**) and 3D CT reconstruction transparent bone algorithms ("virtual x-ray") in AP and lateral projections (**B**, **C**) show wide interpedicular distance of L1 with vertebral body height loss. Wide interpedicular distance implies posterior column injury signifying a three-column, mechanically unstable injury.

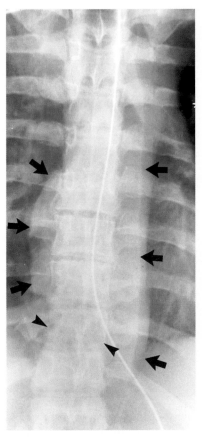

Figure 7.16. Burst fracture. Paraspinal hematoma.

Sagittal MPRs provide the best measure of canal compromise (Fig. 7.14 A,C). Posterior cortex buckling may be subtle. Figure 7.20 compares the difference between a compression fracture and a subtle burst fracture in the same patient.

An MRI is indicated for those patients with acute neurologic deficits. An MRI evaluates integrity of the posterior ligamentous complex, spinal cord injury, traumatic disc herniations, and epidural hematomas.

Burst Fracture Stability

Tremendous controversy exists over the concept of the "stable" burst fracture. Some consider all burst fractures unstable. Employing the six signs described earlier and in Table 7.4 would support this. Yet there are many surgeons who will treat certain burst fracture patterns nonoperatively and with success. For the remainder, determining stable from unstable burst fractures is fraught with difficulty. The question that arises is, "Can instability be predicted and can it be better predicted by imaging?" Willen et al. suggest that anterior compression greater than 50%, spinal canal narrowing greater than 50%, and

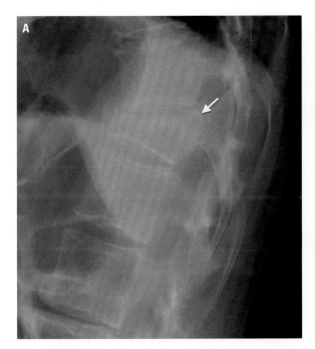

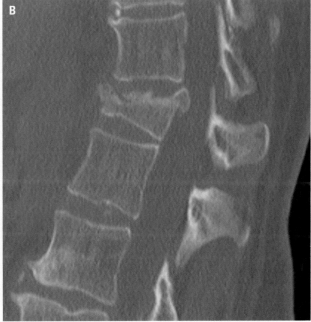

Figure 7.17. Burst fracture. Lateral radiograph (**A**) and midsagittal CT reformation (**B**) show anterior compression and posterior cortical buckling of T12, separating this injury from a simple compression fracture.

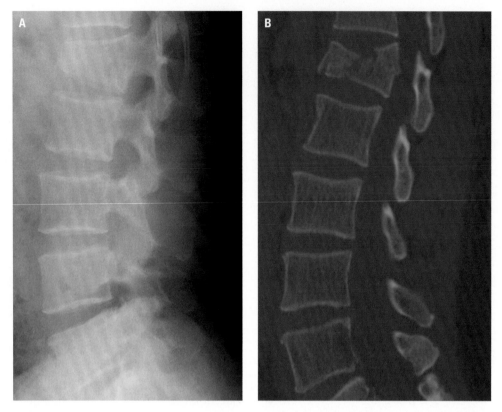

Figure 7.18. Burst fracture. Lateral radiograph (**A**) shows anterior compression deformity of L1 and was thought to represent a simple compression fracture. Midsagittal CT reformation (**B**) reveals failure of both the anterior and middle columns with posterior cortical fracture and buckling, thus representing a burst fracture.

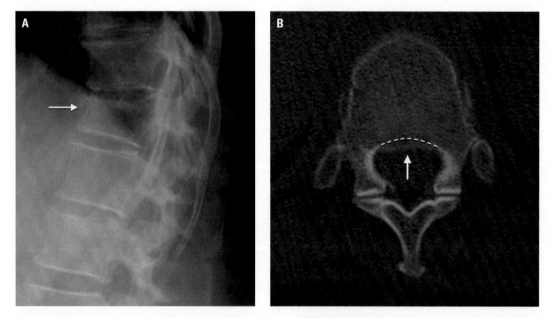

Figure 7.19. Burst fracture. Lateral radiograph (**A**) shows anterior compression deformity of T12. The posterior vertebral body cortex is obscured by overlapping ribs. Transaxial CT image (**B**) shows retropulsion of the posterior vertebral body cortex *(arrow)*. The expected posterior vertebral body contour is shown by the *dashed white lines*.

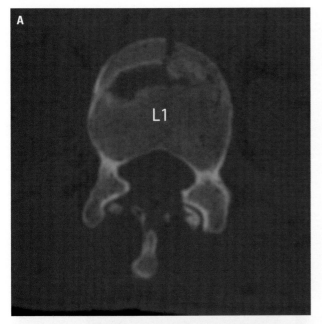

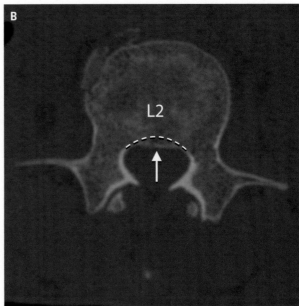

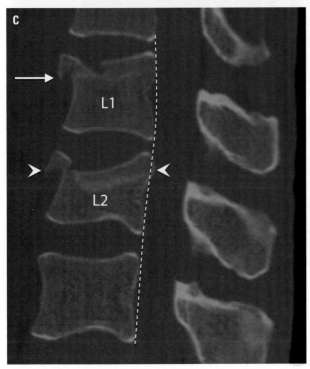

Figure 7.20. Compression fracture versus subtle burst fracture in the same patient. **A:** Transaxial CT image at L1 shows anterior vertebral cortex fracture. Posterior cortex is intact. **B:** Transaxial CT image at L2 in the same patient demonstrates posterior vertebral body cortical fracture with subtle retropulsion *(arrow)* in addition to anterior cortical fractures. **C:** Midsagittal CT reformation in this patient more readily confirms compression fracture of L1 *(arrow)* and burst fracture at L2 *(arrowhead)*. *Dashed white lines* in **B** and **C** show the expected contour of the posterior vertebral body cortex.

evidence of rotational malalignment are predictors of instability.[9] Many agree that posterior column injury including interpedicular widening, laminar fractures, and facet subluxation constitute instability as all three columns are injured. James et al. argue that the posterior ligaments, not the bones, represent the critical stabilizers.[10] Finally, the American Academy of Orthopaedic Surgeons has endorsed the determinants of instability reported by Vaccaro et al. as

progressive neurologic deficit, progressive kyphosis, substantial posterior column injury, and greater than 50% loss of vertebral height with substantial kyphosis.[11] Unfortunately, one cannot apply "progressive" to initial imaging alone, and it remains unclear what constitutes "substantial" injury or "substantial" kyphosis. Consequently, if nonoperative management is pursued, close radiologic follow-up is recommended to identify signs of failure (Fig. 7.21).

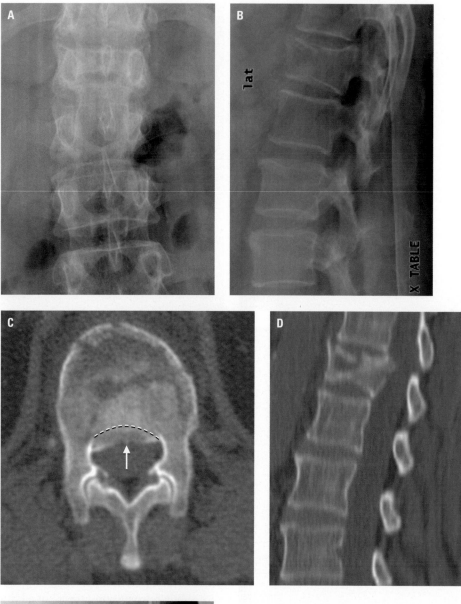

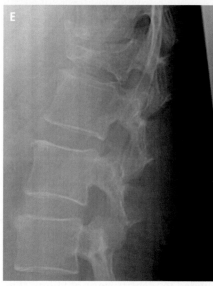

Figure 7.21. Missed burst fracture. AP (**A**) and cross-table lateral (**B**) radiographs at initial presentation reported as compression fracture of T12 with minimal loss of vertebral height anteriorly. Patient discharged. Patient returned 2 days later for dedicated spine CT (**C, D**). **C:** Transaxial CT image of T12 shows posterior cortical disruption with retropulsion. No posterior column injury is present. **D:** Midsagittal CT reformation better demonstrates the T12 burst fracture. **E:** Follow-up radiograph performed 9 days after initial presentation shows failure of nonoperative management. There is marked collapse of T12 with increased kyphosis consistent with an unstable burst fracture.

TABLE 7.6A	Thoracolumbar Injury Classification and Severity Score (TLISS)	
Injury Characteristic		**Points**
Mechanism	Compression	1
	Burst	2
	Translation/rotation	3
	Distraction	4
Neurologic status	Intact	0
	Complete cord injury	2
	Incomplete cord injury	3
PLC integrity	Intact	0
	Suspected/indeterminate	2
	Disrupted	3

PLC, posterior ligamentous complex.

In 2005, the Spine Trauma Study Group, an international group of spine surgeons, designed the thoracolumbar injury severity score (TLISS) as a tool to determine operative from nonoperative spine fractures, perhaps most importantly to address burst fractures.[12] Three areas are scored: mechanism of injury, PLC integrity, and neurologic status. Total score guides treatment (Table 7.6).

Scores <4 are managed nonoperatively, and scores >4 require stabilization with or without surgical decompression. A score of 4 is left for physician preference regarding management. When applied to burst fractures, the score begins at 2 for mechanism. If the patient is neurologically intact, and imaging

TABLE 7.6B	Thoracolumbar Injury Classification and Severity Score (TLISS)	
TLISS Score	**Management**	
<4	Nonoperative	
4	Physician preference	
>4	Require stabilization with or without surgical decompression	

TLISS, thoracolumbar injury severity score.

suggests an intact PLC, the score remains at 2 and is placed in the nonoperative group. With an indeterminate PLC, the score becomes 4 and the patient may or may not receive stabilization. Of note, the validity of the TLISS has never been studied outside of the Spine Trauma Study Group. Again, close radiologic follow-up should be considered in nonoperative cases of all but simple compression fractures.

Flexion Distraction

Flexion distraction, or Chance-type fractures, of the thoracolumbar spine are unstable injuries resulting from distraction of the posterior and middle columns and variable compression of the anterior column (Fig. 7.22). In flexion-distraction injuries, the fulcrum lies at the anterior abdominal wall. Forward flexion over a fixed object, such as a lap seat belt, subjects the entire spinal column to distractive forces. The lap seat belt injury is usually manifested by an anterior abdominal wall contusion or abrasion coinciding with the location of the seat belt. Typically, patients with flexion-distraction injuries are neurologically intact.

The Chance-type fracture is unique with respect to other flexion injuries of the spine because of the incidence of associated intraperitoneal and retroperitoneal injuries. Approximately 40% of patients with this fracture suffer intra-abdominal injuries, most commonly of the bowel and mesentery. Both the flexion-distraction fracture itself and associated visceral injuries may be subtle.

History

In 1948, Chance first identified a unique hyperflexion injury of the lumbar spine described as "horizontal splitting of the spine and neural arch" without ". . . any cord damage."[13]

In the 1960s, a spectrum of abdominal injuries distinct to vehicular crash occupants wearing lap seat belts was observed. Garrett and Braunstein first coined the term *seat belt syndrome* in 1961 where they identified pancreatic and duodenal ruptures in lap-belted automobile occupants.[14] Subsequently, Doersch and Dozier revealed a disproportionate number of victims with severe bowel and mesenteric injuries, although no specific connection with vertebral injuries was established.[15]

The following year, Smith and Kaufer published a series of 24 lumbar spine injuries related to lap belt use.[16] Twenty patients had unusual transverse

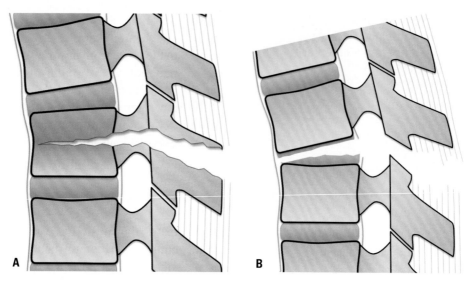

Figure 7.22. Flexion distraction or Chance-type fractures. **A:** Bony Chance-type fracture shows transverse fracture line through the spinous process extending anteriorly through the pedicles. Involvement of the vertebral body is variable. **B:** Flexion distraction "soft tissue Chance-type fracture" shows transverse ligamentous injuries from posterior to anterior through the supraspinous ligament, the interspinous ligament, the facet capsule, ligamentum flavum, and posterior longitudinal ligament and posterior annulus fibrosus. (Panels **A** and **B** from Magerl F, Aebi M, Gertzbein SD, et al. A comprehensive classification of thoracic and lumbar injuries. *Eur Spine J.* 1994;3(4):184–201.)

vertebral fractures with disruption and wide separation of the posterior elements. They termed this injury pattern the "Chance" fracture. Three patients in their series had reported intra-abdominal injuries.

By 1970, the connection between flexion-distraction injuries of the spine and intra-abdominal visceral injuries was made, and Ritchie et al. expanded the term "seat belt syndrome" to include the Chance fracture.[17] Upon review of the previously published 37 cases, Ritchie found a delay in diagnosis beyond 24 hours in more than half of patients, with small bowel and mesenteric lacerations most frequent but including injuries to all abdominopelvic organs. These findings led to the redesign of the seat belt to include the shoulder strap. Consequently, the Chance fracture is now more commonly seen as the result of a severe hyperflexion mechanism injury such as from a fall.

Radiography

Radiographic diagnosis of Chance-type fractures is challenging, but the key lies in careful evaluation of the posterior elements. The most common radiographic finding is the "empty body" sign on frontal view (Fig. 7.23). PLC injury causes

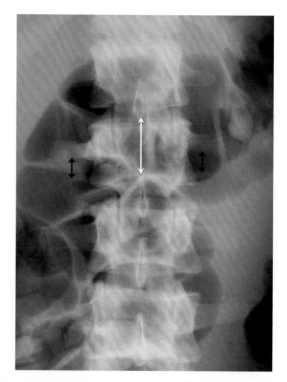

Figure 7.23. Chance-type fracture. AP radiograph shows vertical separation of spinous processes *(white double arrow)* leaving an L1 "empty body." Transverse fracture line also splits the transverse processes *(black double arrows).*

widening of the interspinous distance as a result of distraction and vertical separation of the posterior elements, producing a vertebral body without its superimposed spinous process. Horizontal fractures through the pedicles or transverse processes are also commonly seen. Widening of the interpedicular distance suggests a coexisting burst component.

The lateral view shows distraction of posterior elements to advantage. In Chance-type fractures, the fracture line extends from posterior to anterior through the spinous process with "fanning" of the spinous process fragments (Fig. 7.24). The fracture propagates into the pedicles, and variably, if at all, into the vertebral body. The ligamentous-only variant shows separation of intact bony spinous processes and facet joints. When present, increased vertical distance across the posterior intervertebral disk indicates disruption of the posterior annulus fibrosus (Fig. 7.25).

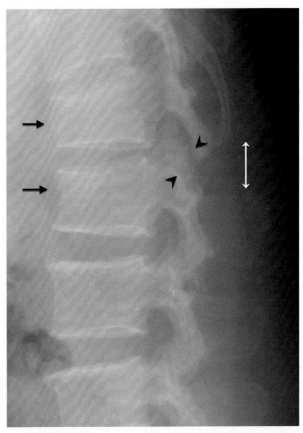

Figure 7.25. Flexion-distraction injury. Also referred to as a "soft tissue Chance," this injury at L1/L2 shows vertical separation of the spinous processes *(white double arrow)* and distraction of the facets *(black arrowheads)* from failure of the PLC in tension. Note accompanying compression of the L1 and L2 anterior vertebral bodies *(black arrows).*

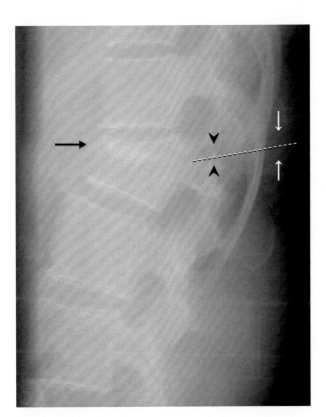

Figure 7.24. Chance-type fracture. Lateral radiograph shows transverse fracture line through the spinous process and pedicles of L1 *(dashed line)* with vertical separation of these structures *(white arrows, black arrowheads)*, respectively. Anterior vertebral body compression is present *(black arrow).*

Anterior subluxation (Fig. 7.26A), unilateral interfacetal dislocation (UID) (Fig. 7.26B), and bilateral interfacetal dislocation (BID) (Fig. 7.26C) thoracolumbar injuries are all flexion-distraction injuries and are commonly referred to as "soft tissue Chance" injuries. These injuries carry the same association with intra-abdominal soft tissue injury as the Chance fracture and require abdominal CT to evaluate abdominal viscera and better delineate fracture anatomy.

Computed Tomography

A CT is the optimal modality for depicting fractures of the thoracolumbar spine and should be obtained in all cases of radiographically detected Chance fractures. A combined CT of the chest,

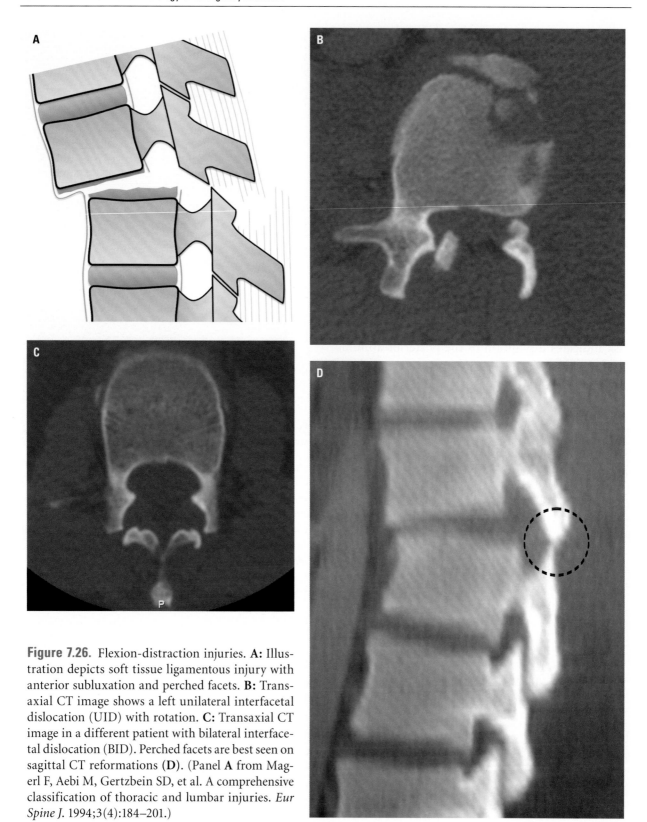

Figure 7.26. Flexion-distraction injuries. **A:** Illustration depicts soft tissue ligamentous injury with anterior subluxation and perched facets. **B:** Transaxial CT image shows a left unilateral interfacetal dislocation (UID) with rotation. **C:** Transaxial CT image in a different patient with bilateral interfacetal dislocation (BID). Perched facets are best seen on sagittal CT reformations (**D**). (Panel **A** from Magerl F, Aebi M, Gertzbein SD, et al. A comprehensive classification of thoracic and lumbar injuries. *Eur Spine J.* 1994;3(4):184–201.)

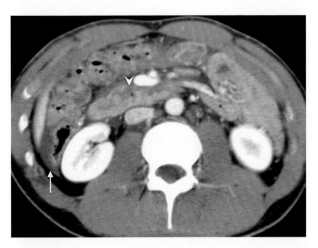

Figure 7.27. Intra-abdominal injuries in patient with Chance-type fracture. Transaxial contrast-enhanced CT image shows bowel contusion, seen as mural thickening, with free fluid *(arrow)* and a duodenal injury *(arrowhead)*.

abdomen, and pelvis with spinal reformations is the most efficient imaging strategy for patients at risk for flexion-distraction injuries. A CT defines the fracture pattern in detail, identifies any spinal canal compromise, and permits evaluation of the critical middle column to identify patients at risk of subsequent acute neurologic compromise. An abdominopelvic CT is necessary to exclude intraperitoneal and retroperitoneal organ injury (Fig. 7.27).

The "dissolving pedicle" sign, seen in 76% of bony Chance fractures on transaxial CT images, represents the gradual loss of definition of the pedicle on serial images as the image plane crosses the horizontal pedicle fracture (Fig. 7.28A–C). The comparable spinal ligamentous injury (soft tissue Chance) is the "naked facet" sign, seen in 40%, and reflects separation of the facet joint (Fig. 7.28D). These injuries may be asymmetric, with pedicle fracture on one side and facet disruption on the other. Both of these signs may therefore be present in the same patient, on the same transaxial image (Fig. 7.28E).

Sagittal CT reformations confirm the radiographic signs seen on the lateral projection and show the characteristically distracted posterior elements and pedicle fractures more accurately (Fig. 7.29). Any burst fracture component (i.e., the Chance-burst fracture) is clearly visible on sagittal images, which permit accurate assessment of canal

compromise (Fig. 7.30). Coronal CT reformations similarly improve on the AP radiograph by more clearly depicting transverse posterior element fractures (Fig. 7.31).

Magnetic Resonance Imaging
An MRI accurately evaluates the integrity of the posterior column ligaments, facet capsules, annulus fibrosus, and spinal cord in neurologically injured patients and reveals the presence of disc herniations and epidural hematoma. T2-weighted and inversion recovery (IR) images assess soft tissue edema, bone bruise, and spinal cord injury (Fig. 7.32). Ligamentous integrity is optimally demonstrated on proton density–weighted images.

The Chance-Burst Fracture

In 15% to 50% of patients with Chance-type fractures, buckling or frank retropulsion of the posterior vertebral body cortex indicates an associated burst component. Many of these patients suffered spinal cord injury, not unexpected in burst fractures, yet very unusual in typical Chance-type fractures.

Detection of a burst component has a significant impact on injury management. Application of an extension cast in a patient with a retropulsed burst fracture fragment may cause further retropulsion with consequent spinal cord injury. The degree of instability will dictate management, as patients with spinal canal compromise may benefit from anterior decompression (Gertzbein).[18]

Pathogenesis/Mechanism of Injury
In his original publication, Chance surmised that a flexion mechanism would be responsible for this horizontal fracture pattern, although he could not "think of any anatomical explanation of the peculiar site and direction of the fracture."[13] Smith and Kaufer explained that the lap seat belt at the anterior abdominal wall served as the fulcrum, thus subjecting all spinal elements to flexion and distraction forces.[16] This theory explains the high concurrence of intra-abdominal injuries but does not account for the compression or burst features. Rennie and Mitchell placed the axis or rotation in line with the posterior longitudinal ligament to account for anterior compression and posterior distraction.[19] Gertzbein postulated

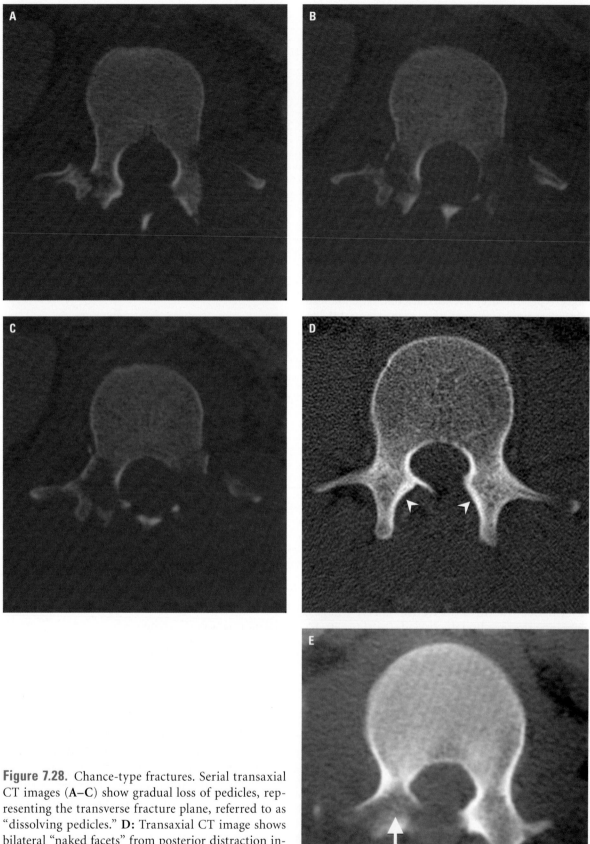

Figure 7.28. Chance-type fractures. Serial transaxial CT images (**A–C**) show gradual loss of pedicles, representing the transverse fracture plane, referred to as "dissolving pedicles." **D:** Transaxial CT image shows bilateral "naked facets" from posterior distraction injury or "soft tissue" Chance. Not uncommonly, these features may be present together from an asymmetric injury with both fracture and ligamentous injury, as seen in (**E**) with right-sided "dissolving pedicle" and left "naked facet" signs.

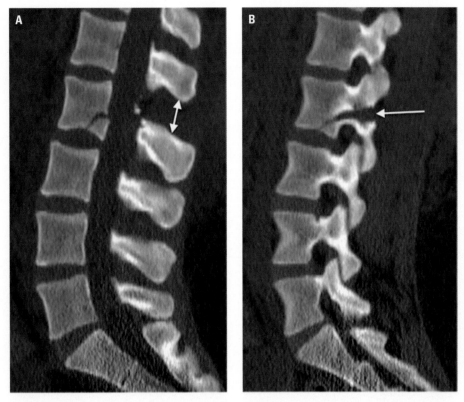

Figure 7.29. Chance-type fracture. Midsagittal **(A)** and parasagittal **(B)** CT reformations show interspinous widening *(double arrow)* and transverse fracture through the pedicle *(arrow)* extending into the vertebral body.

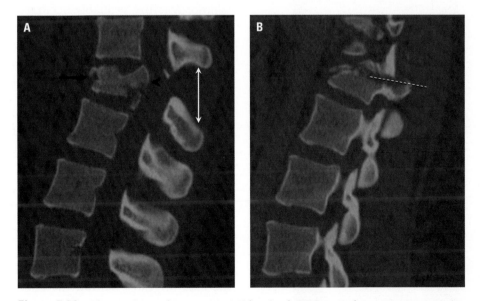

Figure 7.30. Chance-burst fracture. **A:** Midsagittal CT image demonstrates anterior compression *(black arrow)* and retropulsion of posterior body fracture fragment into the canal *(black arrowhead)*, seen in burst fractures. Unlike burst fractures, however, there is wide spacing between the spinous processes *(white double arrow)*. **B:** Parasagittal CT reformation shows transverse fracture through the pedicle, characteristic of Chance-type fractures.

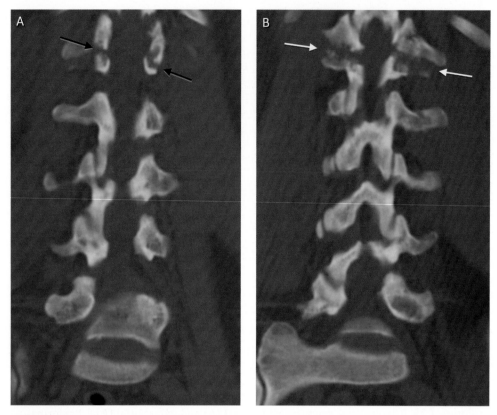

Figure 7.31. Chance-type fracture. Coronal CT reformations show transverse fractures through the pedicles (*black arrows*, **A**) and through the transverse processes (*white arrows*, **B**).

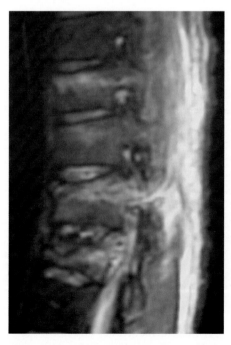

Figure 7.32. Chance-type fracture. Parasagittal inversion recovery MR image shows high signal in the posterior soft tissues and through the pedicle and into the vertebral body. Multilevel injury seen as high signal in the adjacent vertebral bodies including a burst fracture.

that the compression fracture component of the Chance fracture probably occurred at the initial axial load, but that the burst was the result of the final axial load, after the spine had already suffered the Chance fracture during the flexion phase of the injury.[18] Applying these ideas, Bernstein et al. hypothesized that the axis of rotation begins at the anterior abdominal wall at the time of impact and sudden deceleration.[20] As the spinal column begins to fail in tension, from posterior to anterior, the axis of rotation migrates from anterior to posterior. Once the interspinous ligaments tear or the spinous process fractures and flexion deformity results, the biomechanics begin to change. The initial flexion force is transformed into an axial load, driving the effective fulcrum posteriorly. With enough focal kyphosis, the axis migrates behind the anterior vertebral body cortex allowing for compression of the anterior column. With greater deceleration forces, the axial load further increases, and the axis of rotation migrates beyond the posterior longitudinal ligament allowing the vertebral body to burst (Fig. 7.33).

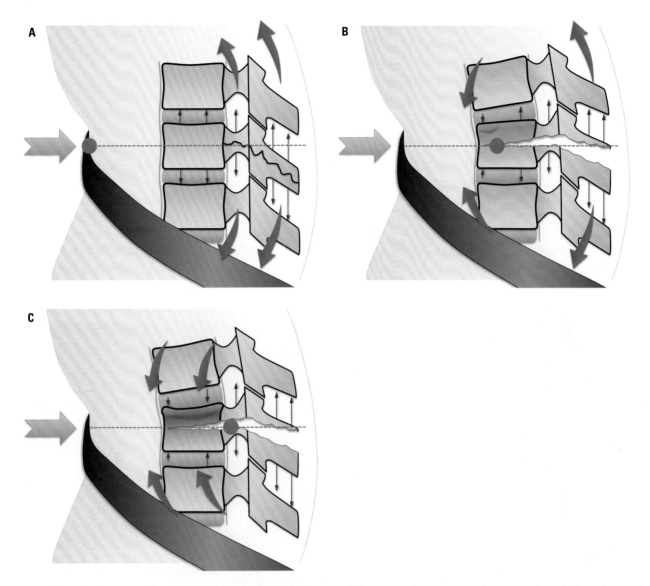

Figure 7.33. Chance-type fracture mechanism of injury. *Blue arrow* shows point of contact of seat belt and abdomen, and *straight brown arrows* depict forces. *Red circle* represents axis of rotation. **A:** Representative segment of lumbar spine is illustrated in abdomen restrained by seat belt. On sudden deceleration, point of contact of seat belt and abdomen serves as fulcrum, or axis of rotation, about which all structures posterior are subject to flexion and distractive (tensile) forces. With enough force, bone integrity is overcome and horizontal Chance fracture results. *Curved arrows* show rotational forces. **B:** With weakening of fractured spine, initial flexion-distraction force begins to involve an axial load component, driving axis of rotation *(red circle)* posteriorly. Once axis of rotation moves posterior to anterior vertebral body cortex, compression begins. **C:** With ongoing force in the further weakened spine, the axis of rotation *(red circle)* continues to migrate posteriorly. Once the axis is behind the posterior cortex, the load force ultimately causes the vertebral body to burst.

The Chance fracture requires special consideration because of its unique pathology as originally described, its unique occurrence in the thoracolumbar spine, but most importantly, its association with concomitant intra-abdominal soft tissue injury.

Fracture Dislocations

Fracture dislocations of the thoracolumbar spine result from complex, high-energy–transfer forces, with simultaneous hyperflexion, translation and/or rotation, and shear. These highly unstable injuries disrupt all three spinal columns, with most victims suffering spinal cord compression or disruption and consequent severe neurologic deficits.

Imaging

These injuries may be obvious (Fig. 7.34) or subtle (Fig. 7.35) on a properly exposed frontal radiograph. Radiographic signs of fracture dislocation include, in addition to gross skeletal abnormalities, focal scoliosis with bilateral paraspinous hematoma, pedicular and spinous process malalignment, abnormal interspinous distance(s), and loss of vertebral height secondary to vertebral body fracture. On a CT, the presence of any horizontal (Fig. 7.36) or rotational translation (Figs. 7.37 and 7.38), or two vertebral bodies on the same

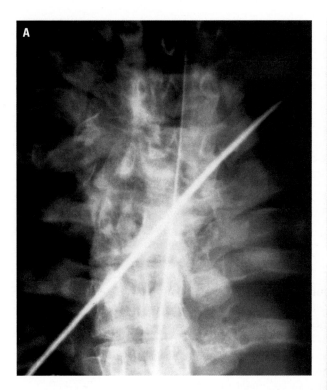

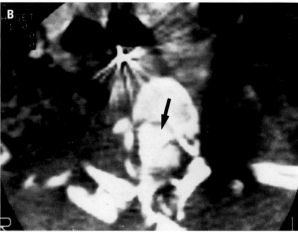

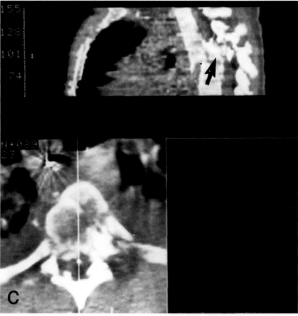

Figure 7.34. Fracture dislocation. Obvious injury on radiographs.

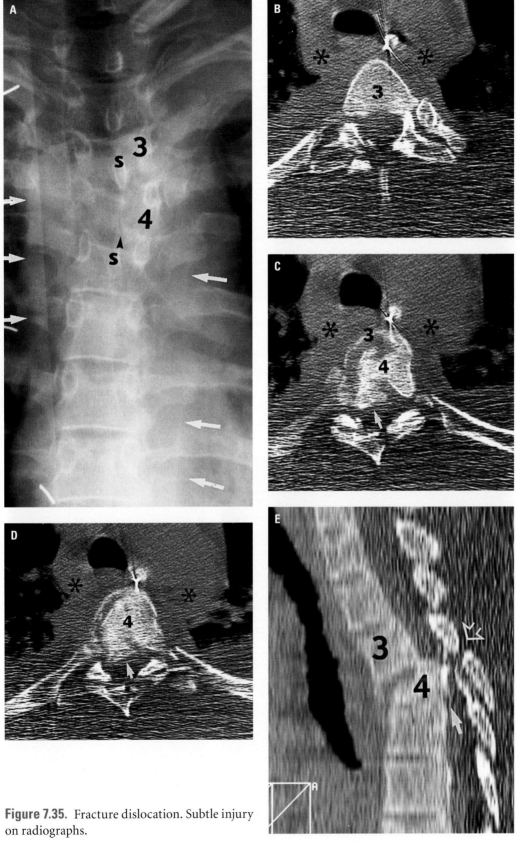

Figure 7.35. Fracture dislocation. Subtle injury on radiographs.

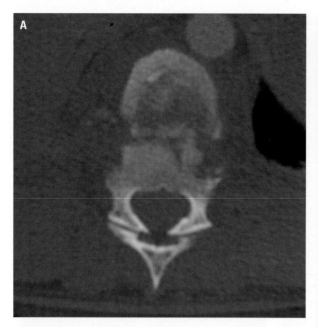

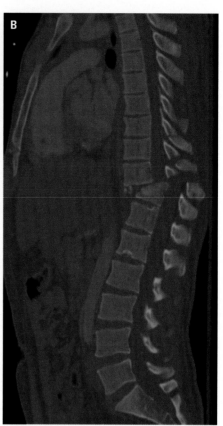

Figure 7.36. Fracture dislocation with translation. Transaxial CT image (**A**) shows comminuted and translated fracture fragments from two vertebral levels. Midsagittal CT reformation (**B**) better depicts the injury with the obliteration of the spinal canal at T10/T11. Findings are characteristic of a fracture dislocation injury.

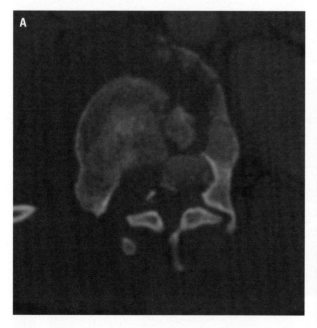

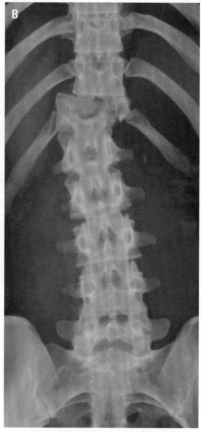

Figure 7.37. Fracture dislocation with rotation. Transaxial CT image (**A**) shows comminuted and rotated fracture fragments from two vertebral segments. 3D CT image (**B**) with transparent bone algorithm in AP projection shows T12 fracture with lateral translations and rotation.

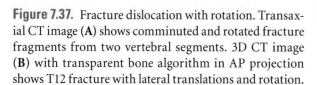

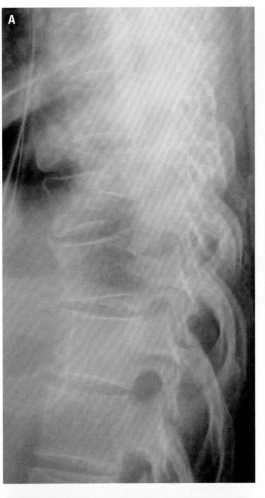

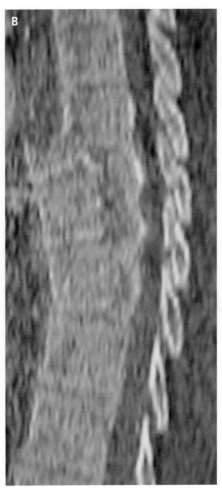

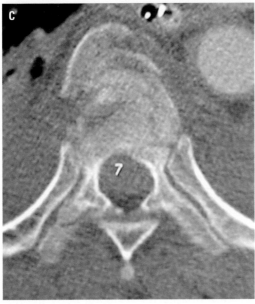

Figure 7.38. Shear fracture. Lateral radiograph (**A**) shows shearing fractures across three consecutive thoracic vertebral bodies with displacement. Sagittal CT reformation (**B**) shows the same findings. Transaxial CT image (**C**) of T7 shows the oblique shear fracture and displacement.

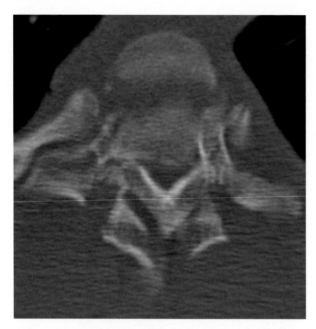

Figure 7.39. Fracture dislocation. Transaxial CT image shows comminuted vertebral fractures with fragments from two different segments, indicative of fracture dislocation.

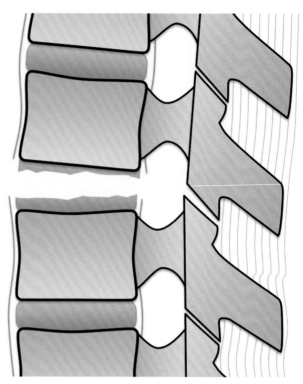

Figure 7.40. Hyperextension injury. Illustration shows soft tissue disruption from anterior to posterior (opposite of flexion distraction)—through the ALL, intervertebral disk, PLL, and facet joint capsule—characteristic of a hyperextension injury. (From Magerl F, Aebi M, Gertzbein SD, et al. A comprehensive classification of thoracic and lumbar injuries. *Eur Spine J.* 1994;3(4):184–201.)

transaxial image, defines a fracture dislocation (Figs. 7.36A, 7.37A, and 7.39).

Hyperextension Injuries

The hyperextension fracture is a unique subset of the fracture dislocation, representing less than 3% of all thoracolumbar spine fractures. Hyperextension injuries are usually the result of a fall on the back, with the patient landing across a narrow structure such as a fence or tree limb. With hyperextension forces, the entire spine fails under tension, beginning with the anterior column (Fig. 7.40).

Patients with a fused spine, as in ankylosing spondylitis or diffuse idiopathic skeletal hyperostosis (DISH), are particularly at risk (Fig. 7.41). These conditions produce a stiff, brittle, kyphotic, and osteoporotic spine where even minor trauma, such as a fall from standing, can result in devastating injury.

In the normal nonfused spine, hyperextension injuries are often produced by severe forces such as motor vehicle ejection (Fig. 7.42) and "lumberjack

paraplegia" where the individual is struck in the back by a falling tree.

The hyperextension fracture dislocation may be quite subtle, in contrast to typical fracture dislocation, and is often overlooked or misinterpreted. Osteoporosis and inadequately defined disc spaces in the ankylosed spine contribute to diagnostic difficulty. Moreover, the highly variable fracture plane may be seen crossing the spine at the disc, the end plate, or through the vertebral body (Fig. 7.41A,B). Injuries may cross vertebral segments. Lateral radiographs and sagittal reformations show anterior disc space widening or distraction of anterior vertebral body fracture fragments (Figs. 7.41A and 7.42). There may also be translation in the sagittal plane. As in all spine fractures, CT clearly demonstrates the fracture pattern, whereas an MRI best identifies the disrupted anterior longitudinal ligament and annulus fibrosus.

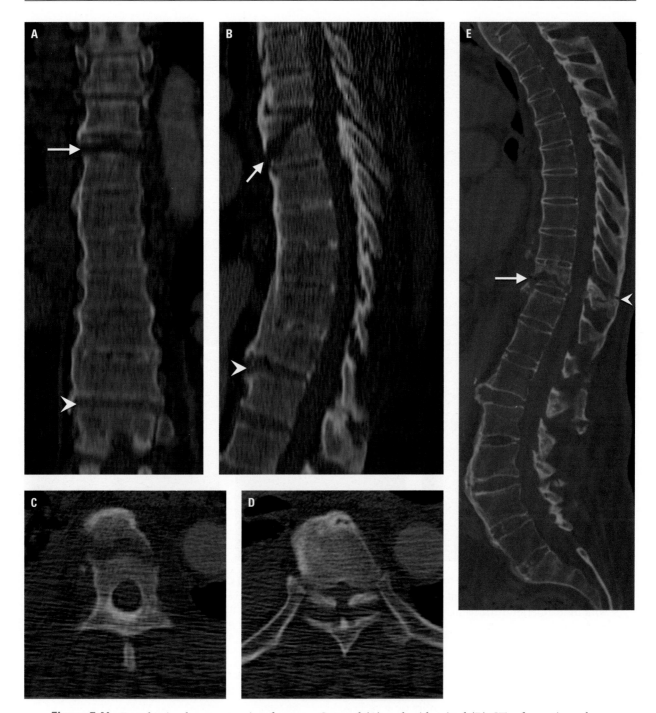

Figure 7.41. Fused spine hyperextension fracture. Coronal (**A**) and midsagittal (**B**) CT reformations show two separate hyperextension fractures in a patient with a fused spine. The transverse *(arrowheads)* and oblique *(arrows)* nature of these fractures are best seen on sagittal images. Anterior column distraction is present but subtle. Transaxial CT images of T4 (**C, D**) show the vertebral body fracture and wide facets. **E:** Midsagittal CT reformation in a different patient with a fused spine shows transverse fracture across the entire T10 vertebra with anterior distraction.

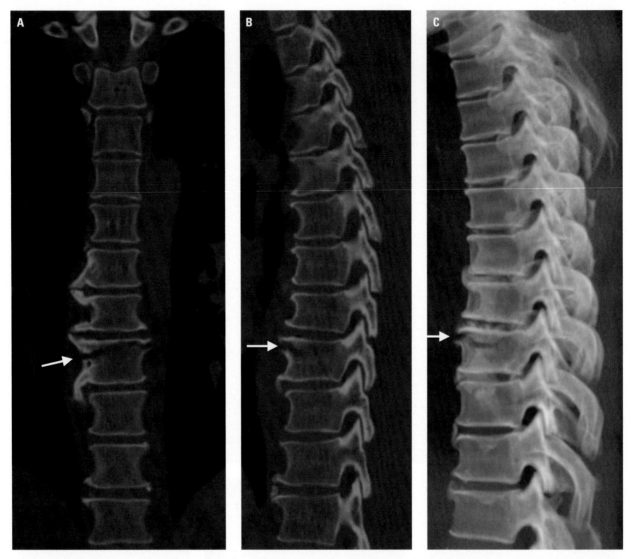

Figure 7.42. Hyperextension fracture. Coronal (**A**) and parasagittal (**B**) CT reformations and 3D CT reconstruction (**C**) with transparent bone algorithm in lateral projection reveal a transverse fracture across T8 with mild anterior distraction.

REFERENCES

1. Hasler RM, Exadaktylos AK, Bouamra O, et al. Epidemiology and predictors of spinal injury in adult major trauma patients: European cohort study. *Eur Spine J.* 2011;20(12):2174–2180.

2. American College of Radiology. ACR Appropriateness Criteria: suspected spine trauma. 2009. http://www.acr.org/SecondaryMainMenuCategories/quality_safety/app_criteria/pdf/ExpertPanelonPediatricImaging/Othertopics/SuspectedSpineTrauma.aspx. Accessed May 20, 2012.

3. Boehler L. *Die Techniek der Knochenbruchbehandlung im Grieden und im Kriege.* Vienna, Austria: Verlag von Wilheim Maudrich; 1930:9–11.

4. Watson-Jones R. The results of postural reduction of fractures of the spine. *J Bone Joint Surg Am.* 1938;20:567–86.

5. Holdsworth F. Fractures, dislocations, and fracture-dislocations of the spine. *J Bone Joint Surg Am.* 1970;52:1534–51.

6. Denis F. The three column spine and its significance in the classification of acute thoracolumbar spinal injuries. *Spine.* 1983;8(8):817–831.

7. Magerl F, Aebi M, Gertzbein SD, et al. A comprehensive classification of thoracic and lumbar injuries. *Eur Spine J.* 1994;3(4):184–201.

8. White AA, Panjabi MM. *Clinical Biomechanics of the Spine.* Philadelphia, PA: Lippincott; 1978.

9. Willen JA, Gaekwad UH, Kakulas BA. Burst fractures

in the thoracic and lumbar spine. A cliniconeuropathologic analysis. *Spine.* 1989;14(12): 1316–1323.

10. James KS, Wenger KH, Schlegel JD, Dunn HK. Biomechanical evaluation of the stability of thoracolumbar burst fractures. *Spine.* 1994;19:1731–1740.

11. Vaccaro AR, Kim DH, Brodke DS, et al. Diagnosis and management of thoracolumbar spine fractures. *J Bone Joint Surg Am.* 2003;85:2456–2470

12. Spine Trauma Group: Vaccaro AR, Zeiller SC, Hulbert RJ, et al. The thoracolumbar injury severity score: a proposed treatment algorithm. *J Spinal Disord Tech.* 2005;18:209–15.

13. Chance GQ. Note on a type of flexion fracture of the spine. *Br J Radiol.* 1948;21:452–453.

14. Garrett JW, Braunstein PW. The seat belt syndrome. *J Trauma.* 1962;2:220–238.

15. Doersch KB, Dozier WE. The seat belt syndrome: the seat belt sign, intestinal and mesenteric injuries. *Am J Surg.* 1968;116:831–833.

16. Smith WS, Kaufer H. Patterns and mechanisms of lumbar injuries associated with lap seat belts. *J Bone Joint Surg Am.* 1969;51A:239–253.

17. Ritchie WP Jr, Ersek RA, Bunch WL, et al. Combined visceral and vertebral injuries from lap type seat belts. *Surg Gynecol Obstet.* 1970;131(3):431–435.

18. Gertzbein SD, Court-Brown CM. Flexion-distraction injuries of the lumbar spine: mechanisms of injury and classification. *Clin Orthop Relat Res.* 1988;227:52–60

19. Rennie W, Mitchell N. Flexion distraction fractures of the thoracolumbar spine. *J Bone Joint Surg Am.* 1973;55A:386–390

20. Bernstein MP, Mirvis SE, Shanmuganathan K. Chance-type fractures of the thoracolumbar spine: imaging analysis in 53 patients. *AJR.* 2006;187(4):859–868.

SUGGESTED READINGS

1. el-Khoury GY, Whitten CG. Trauma to the upper thoracic spine: anatomy, biomechanics, and unique imaging features. *AJR.* 1993;160(1):95–102.

2. Daffner RH, Deeb ZL, Goldberg AL, et al. The radiologic assessment of post-traumatic vertebral stability. *Skeletal Radiol.* 1990;19(2):103–108.

3. Patel AA, Vaccaro AR. Thoracolumbar spine trauma classification. *J Am Acad Orthop Surg.* 2010;18(2): 63–71.

4. Denis F, Burkus JK. Shear fracture-dislocations of the thoracic and lumbar spine associated with forceful hyperextension (lumberjack paraplegia). *Spine.* 1992;17(2):156–161.

5. Bernstein M. Easily missed thoracolumbar spine fractures. *Eur J Radiol.* 2010;74(1):6–15.

CHAPTER 8

Shoulder, Including Clavicle and Scapula

John H. Harris, Jr.

For the purpose of this discussion, the shoulder shall be considered to consist of the clavicle, including the sternoclavicular joint, the scapula, the scapulohumeral joint, and the proximal third of the humerus. This concept is anatomically and radiographically imprecise but has practical clinical relevance. The anatomy of the shoulder includes only the distal clavicle, the glenohumeral joint, and the proximal humerus, which governs positioning for the radiographic examination of the shoulder.

Clinically, injuries to the shoulder may include the entire clavicle (sternoclavicular separation, scapulothoracic dislocation). For this reason, it seems appropriate to include the entire clavicle in the discussion of the shoulder. One must remember that this inclusion is for clinical purposes only and that, as described in the text that follows, positioning for radiographic examination of the shoulder is completely different than positioning to examine either the clavicle or the scapula. The clavicle and scapula are discussed separately later in the chapter.

Although the shoulder is a large, seemingly relatively simple joint, its "motions are more extensive than those of any other joint in the body," and therefore it must not be considered an uncomplicated structure radiographically.[1] The anatomy of the shoulder and its relation to the trunk are the basis of serious radiographic diagnostic pitfalls peculiar to this joint. For example, partial or complete acromioclavicular separation, fracture of the coracoid process, and direct posterior dislocation of the shoulder present special radiographic diagnostic problems. If disruption of the acromioclavicular fibers is complete while the coracoclavicular ligament remains intact, separation of the acromioclavicular space may not occur unless the acromioclavicular joint is stressed. Consequently, when an acromioclavicular separation is suspected, special views of the shoulder must be obtained. The radiographic examination of the uninjured shoulder serves as a normal baseline study for comparison with the similar examination obtained of the injured side. A minimally displaced fracture of the coracoid process of the scapula may be established only on the axillary projection of the shoulder. Direct posterior dislocation of the shoulder is extremely difficult to diagnose on routine anteroposterior (AP) radiographs of the shoulder. Superimposition of the humeral head on the glenoid fossa or widening of the space between the humeral head and the glenoid fossa has been described as a sign of posterior dislocation of the shoulder. However, neither is sufficiently consistent to be reliable, and special views are necessary to establish this diagnosis. Apophyses are common about the shoulder. These normal structures, as well as the proximal humeral epiphysis, may create radiographic enigmas. Sternoclavicular separation and scapulothoracic dissociation are major injuries that are commonly radiographically subtle.

RADIOGRAPHIC EXAMINATION AND ANATOMY

The routine radiographic examination of the shoulder is made with the patient in the AP position with the arm rotated both internally (Fig. 8.1A) and externally (Fig. 8.1B). When these projections are

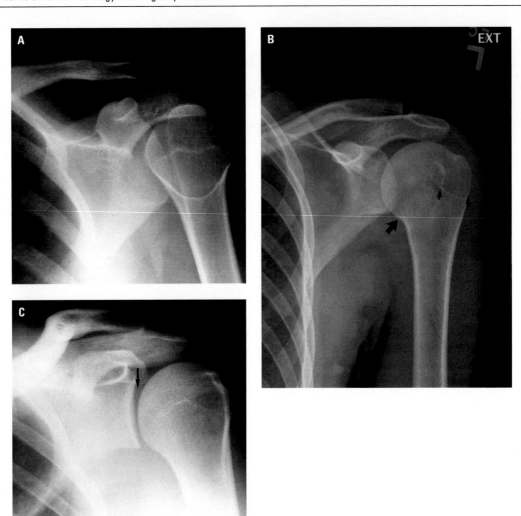

Figure 8.1. AP projections of the shoulder in internally (**A**) and externally (**B**) rotated projections; AP radiograph of the glenohumeral joint (**C**). In the internally rotated radiograph of the shoulder (**A**) obtained with the forearm flexed across the abdomen, the appearance of the humeral head has been likened to a light bulb or rifle barrel. The externally rotated view is taken with the humerus rotated outward so that the flexed forearm is perpendicular to the sagittal plane of the body. On this view, the inferior margin of the surgical neck *(arrow)*, between the humeral shaft and head, is clearly visible. The cortex of the lesser *(medial small arrow)* and greater *(lateral small arrow)* tuberosities and the intervening bicipital groove are visible to varying degrees. The AP view of the glenohumeral joint (**C**) is the true frontal projection of the shoulder designed to show the glenohumeral joint space *(arrow)* and its contiguous surfaces.

made in the usual position, neither provides a true frontal view of the glenohumeral joint space. The latter requires rotation of the body into the posterior oblique position of the injured shoulder so that the plane of the scapula parallels that of the cassette with the central x-ray beam directed just medial to the articulating surface of the humeral head. The resulting radiograph (Fig. 8.1C) is the true AP projection of the glenohumeral joint and provides a true assessment of the glenohumeral joint space.

These projections, which may be made with the patient either erect or supine, provide an adequate "survey" examination of the shoulder. However, as noted earlier, they frequently do not provide definitive data relative to some of the traumatic lesions involving the shoulder.

It is frequently necessary to obtain views of the shoulder made in planes other than the frontal projection. These may be either the axillary view (Fig. 8.2A) or "Y" projection (Fig. 8.2B).

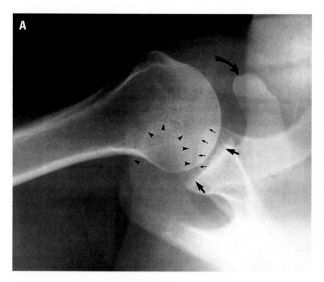

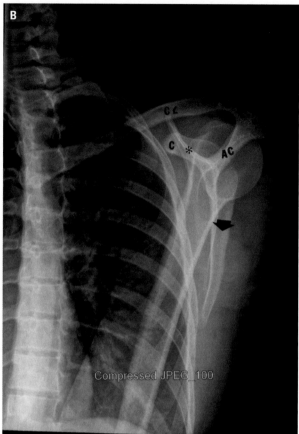

Figure 8.2. Axillary (**A**) and Y (**B**) radiograph of a normal adult shoulder. In the axillary projection (**A**), the relationship between the humeral head and glenoid fossa *(large straight arrows)* is obvious. The *curved arrow* indicates the anteriorly projecting coracoid process; *small straight arrows* indicate the distal clavicle; and *arrowheads* indicate the acromion. **B:** Y view of the left shoulder. In this slightly off-true axial projection, the supraspinous portion of the scapula (C) and the acromion process (AC) represent the arms of the Y. The infraspinous portion of the scapula *(arrowheads)* is the stem of the Y.

The axillary view (Fig. 8.2A) should be considered in the radiographic examination of the shoulder in all cases of trauma to the shoulder. Although it is frequently overlooked, the axillary view provides more information about the shoulder than any other single projection. It is the only view in which minimally displaced fractures of the coracoid process of the scapula, cortical fractures of the anterior or posterior surfaces of the humeral head, posterior dislocation of the humerus, and direction of angulation of proximal humeral fracture fragments can be conclusively demonstrated. Positioning for the axillary view is very simple, and the demonstration of the anatomy of the shoulder is clear. The axillary view is best obtained with the patient supine.

A few words of caution are necessary relative to the use of the axillary projection in the evaluation of acute skeletal injury involving the shoulder. First, the axillary projection should be obtained only if the routine frontal projections do not permit a definitive radiographic diagnosis. Stated differently, the axillary view should not be part of the "routine" shoulder series of a patient who has sustained shoulder trauma. The axillary view is intended primarily for evaluation of glenohumeral joint injuries and may be contraindicated in patients with fractures of the proximal humerus. Second, contrary to the positioning described for the axillary projection in standard textbooks of radiologic positioning, it is not necessary to abduct the arm 90 degrees from the body to obtain a satisfactory axillary projection. Diagnostic axillary views (see, for example, Figs. 8.24, 8.25, 8.27, and 8.28) can be obtained with only sufficient abduction of the arm (10 to 15 degrees) to permit placing the x-ray tube between the hand and the hip with the central beam directed to the apex of the axilla. The cassette is placed above the shoulder in a plane perpendicular to the central x-ray beam. Finally, the radiologist should personally abduct the arm in order to ensure maximum control and minimum movement during positioning. The purpose for this caveat is, obviously, to prevent any unnecessary motion of the injured shoulder during this diagnostic examination.

The radiographic appearance of a normal child's shoulder is seen in Figure 8.3.

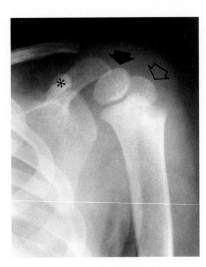

Figure 8.3. Frontal projection of the normal shoulder of a child. *Arrows* indicate the ununited humeral head epiphyses, and the *asterisk* marks the coracoid process of the scapula.

Figure 8.4A illustrates the radiographic appearance of the normal adolescent shoulder. The apophysis of the coracoid process is clearly seen. The radiographic characteristics of the proximal humeral physis, namely, its dense sclerotic margins, variable width, and anatomic location, are illustrated at the anatomic neck of the humerus. This figure also illustrates the effect of position on the appearance of the physis and indicates how an arc of the physis may be projected in such a way as to resemble a fracture line. The ability of the proximal humeral physis to simulate a metaphyseal fracture is due to this physis being an essentially circular plane.

Consequently, when the arm is displaced anteriorly or posteriorly from the coronal plane of the body during the radiographic exposure, the plane of the physis will be tangent to the x-ray beam and either the anterior or the posterior margin of the physis will project through the metaphysis, often resembling a metaphyseal fracture (Fig. 8.4B).

Routine radiographic examination of the noninjured contralateral part "for comparison purposes," although advocated by Swischuk, may not be necessary in all instances.[2] However, it is occasionally necessary to examine the contralateral shoulder radiographically because of the great variability of the proximal humeral physis and alterations in its radiographic appearance—usually secondary to positioning—that may simulate a fracture. For this reason, the shoulder is the part of the growing skeleton that is most frequently examined for comparison purposes.

The apophysis at the tip of the acromion (Fig. 8.5) and the apophyses at the base (Fig. 8.6) and tip (Fig. 8.4) of the coracoid process are normal structures that should not be misinterpreted as fractures. Again, the radiographic appearance of the apophyseal line surfaces and their characteristic locations should make this distinction relatively straightforward.

The scapula is difficult to visualize in AP projection because of its configuration, its orientation with respect to the posterolateral chest wall, its mobility, and superimposition of the clavicle, ribs, and humerus. The routine radiographic examinations of the shoulder described earlier do not

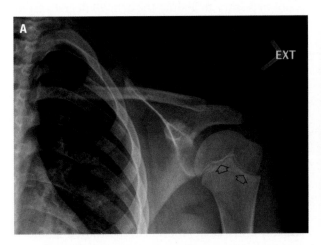
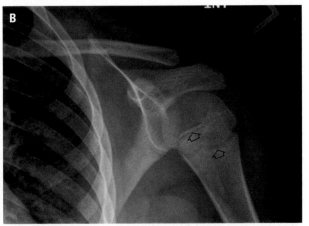

Figure 8.4. Straight AP radiograph of an adolescent left shoulder (**A**) showing the proximal humeral physis (*open arrows*) to be in the same plane. In the same patient, with the shoulder abducted (**B**), the physis is tangentially seen so that one margin could be misinterpreted as a metaphyseal fracture (*open arrows*).

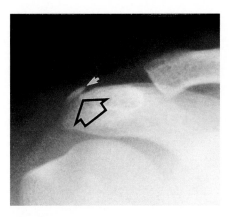

Figure 8.5. Physis at the tip *(open arrow)* of the acromial process. The location and radiographic appearance of this anatomic structure and the age of the patient should distinguish it from a fracture line. The lucent physis, in this instance, lies adjacent to the distal acromial apophysis *(white arrow)*.

provide an adequate radiologic study of the scapula. Therefore, when injury of the scapula is suspected, special scapular views must be obtained.[3] These consist of AP (Fig. 8.7A) and lateral (Fig. 8.7B) (transscapular, tangential, axial, "Y") projections. The AP radiograph of the scapula (Fig. 8.7A) is obtained with the patient either erect or supine and, optimally, rotated into approximately 45 degrees of ipsilateral posterior obliquity or sufficient obliquity so that the coronal plane of the scapula parallels that of the cassette. In the frontal projection, the medial border, varying amounts of the infraspinous portion, and the tip of the scapula are usually at least partially obscured by overlying ribs and lateral chest wall soft tissue. The coracoid process, which projects anteriorly, is seen essentially en face. This normal anatomy may render infraspinous and coracoid fractures invisible on frontal projections. In severely injured patients, the radiographic examination of the scapula may be limited to its appearance on the supine chest radiograph.

When the patient's condition will permit, the axial projection (Fig. 8.7B) of the scapula is obtained with the ipsilateral arm adducted anteriorly while the patient is rotated into ipsilateral anterior obliquity. In this position, the central x-ray beam is tangent to the coronal plane of the scapula, which, in turn, is perpendicular to the plane of the cassette. In this projection, the anteriorly projecting coracoid process represents the anterior arm of the Y; the scapular spine, its posterior arm; and the body, the vertical stem. The glenoid fossa, which forms the confluence of the Y, being en face to the central x-ray beam and covered by the humeral head, is usually not well seen on this projection.

The routine radiographic examination of the clavicle (Fig. 8.8) consists of a straight AP and a tangential AP projection with the central beam angled rostrally and tangent to the anterior chest wall to project the clavicle off the ribs as much as possible.

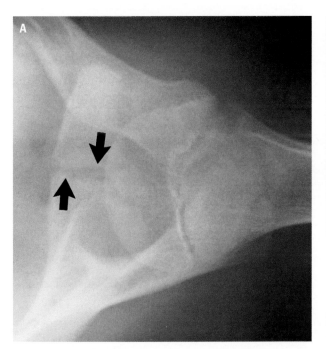

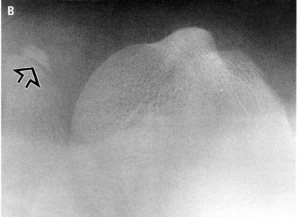

Figure 8.6. Normal physis at the base *(arrows,* **A**) and tip *(open arrow,* **B**) of the coracoid process.

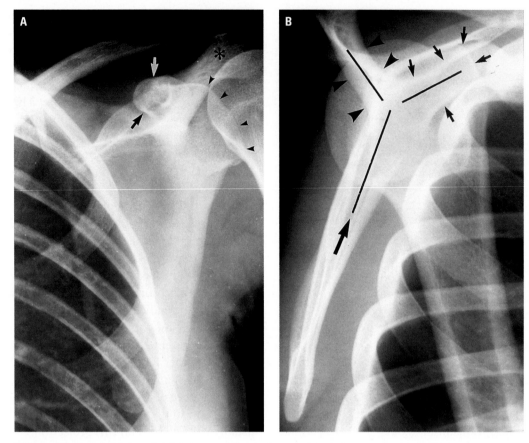

Figure 8.7. Frontal (**A**) and (*Y*) (**B**) projections of a normal adult scapula. In the frontal projection (**A**), *arrowheads* indicate the posterior margin of the glenoid fossa; the *asterisk* indicates the acromial process; and *arrows* indicate the anteriorly projecting coracoid process. On the Y projection of the scapula (**B**), the humeral head is superimposed on the glenoid fossa, which is at the junction of the coracoid process (*small arrows*), the spine (*arrowheads*), and the infraspinous portion of the scapula (*large arrow*).

The inner third of the clavicle is best visualized on conventional radiography by projections designed to demonstrate the sternoclavicular joints. Individualized projections with varying degrees of tube angulation and patient rotation are frequently required to demonstrate this area radiographically. Computed tomography (CT) is the most definitive modality for diagnosis of subtle fractures and dislocations of the sternoclavicular joint. Because routine views of the clavicle may not demonstrate inner third fractures

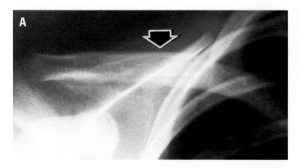
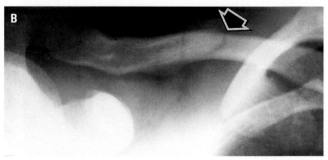

Figure 8.8. The complete fracture in the middle third of the right clavicle (*arrow*) can only be suspected in the straight AP projection (**A**). The presence of the fracture is clearly established, however, on the radiograph made with 15 degrees cephalad angulation of the x-ray tube (**B**).

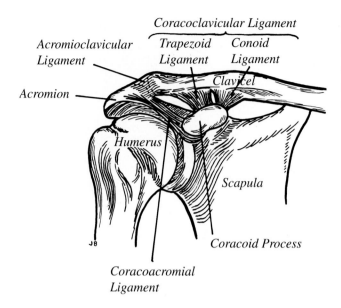

Acromioclavicular Ligament

Coracoclavicular Ligament
Trapezoid Ligament   Conoid Ligament

Acromion

Clavicel

Humerus

Scapula

Coracoid Process

Coracoacromial Ligament

JB

Figure 8.9. Schematic representation of the normal ligamentous attachments between the acromion and the coracoid process of the scapula and the clavicle. (Modified from Conwell HE, Reynolds FC. *Key and Conwell's Management of Fractures, Dislocations and Sprains.* 7th ed. St Louis, MO: Mosby; 1961.)

and because special projections may be necessary to establish the diagnosis, it is critical that the clinical impression be transmitted to the radiologist so that the appropriate views may be obtained.

RADIOGRAPHIC MANIFESTATIONS OF TRAUMA

Acromioclavicular Separation

The diagnosis "acromioclavicular separation" refers to abnormal widening of the acromioclavicular (AC) joint due to disruption of the AC ligament, usually as the result of a direct trauma to the point of the shoulder. This terminology completely ignores the importance of the coracoclavicular (CC) ligament in the support of the upper extremity. Furthermore, the term *AC separation* is misleading because there is no reference to CC separation, which is the most important soft tissue injury caused by this type of trauma. The normal ligamentous anatomy between the clavicle and the scapula is indicated in Figure 8.9. Radiographically, the location of the AC and CC ligaments is seen in Figure 8.10.

Normally, the AC joint space should not exceed 4 mm in width in adults, and the distal inferior cortical margin of the clavicle and of the acromion should be on the same plane or arc (Figs. 8.1B, 8.5B, and 8.10). However, developmental variations in this relationship have been reported to be as high as 19%.[4] Hypoplasia of the anterior tip of the

acromion (Fig. 8.11) can result in apparent abnormal widening of the AC space and simulate a grade I AC separation.[5]

Both the AC and the CC ligaments play a role in the radiographic appearance of the effects of a blow or fall on the point of the shoulder. The AC joint is enclosed by a thin capsule that is reinforced superiorly and inferiorly by AC ligaments. The principal ligament between the clavicle and the scapula, however, is the CC ligament, which is thick, dense, and strong and is the principal ligament of attachment of the upper extremity to the torso through the clavicle. The extent of the CC separation has a direct bearing on the degree of AC separation.

Injuries of the AC (and CC) ligaments are traditionally classified as either sprain (type I), subluxation (type II), or dislocation (type III).[6] More recently, types IV, V, and VI have been described.[7-9]

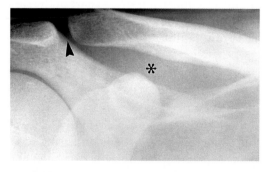

Figure 8.10. Normal adult shoulder. The location of the acromioclavicular and coracoclavicular ligaments is indicated by the *arrowhead* and *asterisk*, respectively.

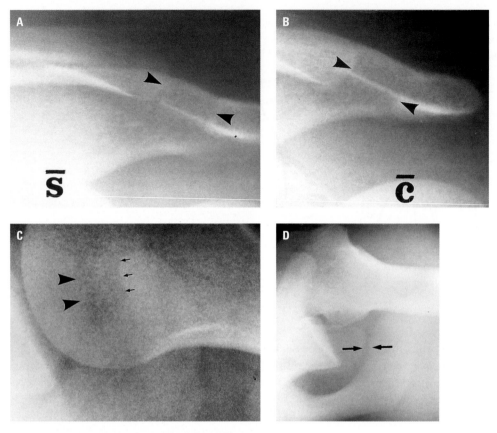

Figure 8.11. Anomalous acromial process simulating a grade I acromioclavicular separation. In the erect frontal radiographs of the shoulder without (**A**) and with (**B**) weights, the distance between the distal clavicle and acromion *(arrowheads)* is abnormally wide but does not change its contour with stress. On the axillary projection (**C**), the hypoplastic acromial process *(arrows)* is demonstrated to be the basis for the wide acromial *(arrows)*-clavicular *(arrowheads)* distance. The normal acromioclavicular relationship *(arrows)* is clearly depicted in the axillary view of a patient with an anterior shoulder dislocation (**D**).

Type I AC separation (sprain) consists of stretching or tearing of a few fibers of the AC ligament. The AC joint remains stable, and the CC ligament is intact. This injury can be confirmed radiographically only by comparing stress views of the injured and uninjured shoulders. The radiographic sign of AC sprain is minor widening of the AC space (Fig. 8.12).

Partial or complete rupture of the AC ligament may exist with only partial disruption of the CC ligament (type II, subluxation) (Fig. 8.13), and the separation of the AC joint may not be evident on routine radiographs of the shoulder. Therefore, when "shoulder separation" is clinically suspected but not apparent on the routine shoulder radiographs, stress radiographs are required. These examinations are made with the patient in the erect AP position both with and without 10- to 15-lb weights being attached to each wrist. The weight is intended to stress the AC and/or CC ligaments of the affected shoulder, resulting in widening of the AC space as well as minimal widening of the CC space.

Inferior displacement of the scapula causes disruption of the continuous arc formed by the inferior cortices of the acromion and distal clavicle (Fig. 8.14). These alterations of normal anatomy indicate complete tearing of the AC ligament and either attenuation or partial disruption of the CC ligament.

The distinction between type I and type II AC separation is of greater theoretical than clinical importance because the radiologic distinction is frequently subjective and the treatment is usually nonsurgical.[10]

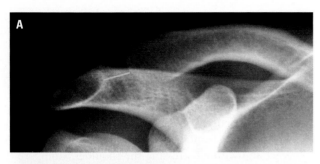

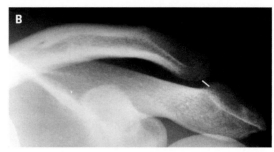

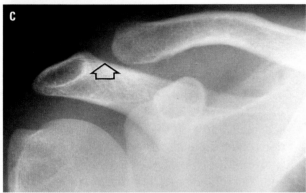

Figure 8.12. Type I acromioclavicular (AC) separation. This high school wrestler landed on the "point" of his right shoulder and experienced severe pain and point tenderness over the AC joint. The initial AP radiograph of his right shoulder (**A**) demonstrated only minor widening of the AC joint space *(long white line)* compared with a comparable projection of the left shoulder *(short white line,* **B**). Frontal views of the injured right shoulder (**C**) with weights confirm the widened AC space *(open arrow).*

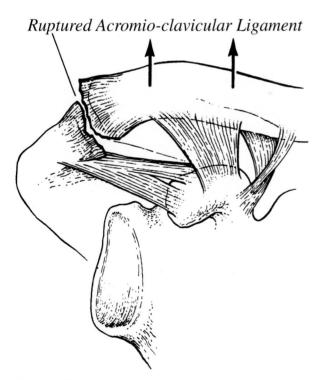

Ruptured Acromio-clavicular Ligament

Figure 8.13. Schematic representation of type II acromioclavicular (AC) separation. Note that only the AC ligament is ruptured and that there is a slight separation of the AC space. (From Schultz RJ. *The Language of Fractures.* Baltimore, MD: Lippincott Williams & Wilkins; 1972. Used with permission.)

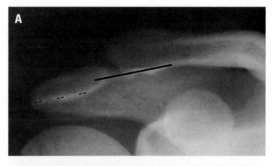

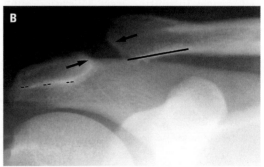

Figure 8.14. Type II acromioclavicular (AC) separation. In the non–weight-bearing frontal projection (**A**), the plane of the inferior cortex of the distal end of the clavicle *(solid line)* is superior to that of the inferior cortex of the acromial process *(broken line).* With weight (**B**), not only is the acromion more inferior to the clavicle, but the AC space *(arrows)* is abnormally widened, indicating disruption of the AC ligament. The coracoclavicular space is normal without and with weights, indicating that the coracoclavicular ligament is intact, although some of its fibers may be disrupted.

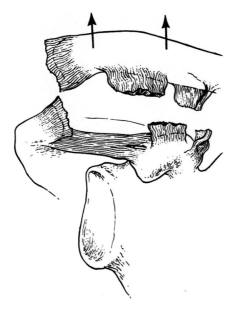

Figure 8.15. Type III acromioclavicular (AC) separation. This line drawing depicts complete disruption of the AC and the coracoclavicular ligaments. (From Schultz RJ. *The Language of Fractures.* Baltimore, MD: Williams & Wilkins; 1972. Used with permission.)

When the force applied to the point of the shoulder is sufficient to disrupt both the AC and the CC ligaments, the scapula and its acromion are displaced inferiorly by the effect of gravity in the erect position, resulting in both AC and CC separation, for example, type III AC separation (Fig. 8.15). Radiographically, complete ligamentous disruption is represented by obvious widening of the AC and CC spaces in routine erect AP radiographs of the shoulder (Fig. 8.16). Type III AC separation is

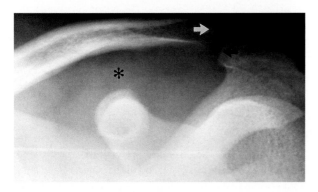

Figure 8.16. Erect AP radiograph of a type III acromioclavicular separation. The upper extremity, including the scapula, is displaced inferiorly by its own weight and the effect of gravity, resulting in inferior displacement of the acromion with respect to the distal clavicle *(arrows)* and widening of the coracoclavicular space *(asterisk)*.

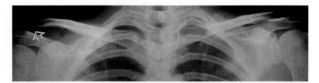

Figure 8.17. Type III right acromioclavicular *(open arrow)* and coracoclavicular separation *(asterisk)* is obvious on this frontal projection made with the patient erect and without stressing the shoulder. Compare the changes on the right with the appearance of the normal left shoulder.

usually clinically obvious, and the diagnosis will be confirmed with only an erect AP radiograph of the shoulder (Fig. 8.17). When a type III AC separation is demonstrated on the erect radiograph, examinations of the shoulder with weights are not indicated. Conversely, a type III AC separation may be present and not radiographically visible on the supine frontal shoulder radiograph (Fig. 8.18). The common AC separation injuries are summarized in Table 8.1.

The type IV (posterior) AC separation occurs when the AC and CC ligaments are disrupted while the coracoacromial ligament remains intact (Fig. 8.19A). Radiographically, in AP (Fig. 8.19B)

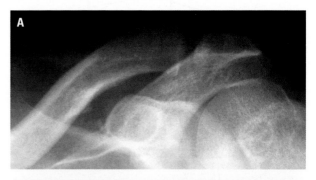

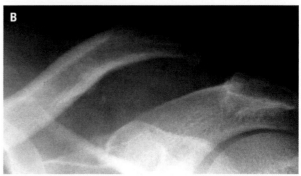

Figure 8.18. Type III acromioclavicular separation not visible in recumbency (**A**) but clearly evident in the erect frontal projection (**B**).

TABLE 8.1	Acromioclavicular Dislocation: Classification and Prognosis	
Classification	**X-ray**	**Prognosis**
Type I. Ligament sprain, a few ligament fibers torn	Normal	No instability; excellent
Type II. Rupture of the capsule and acromioclavicular ligaments	Joint wide; clavicle may be slightly elevated	May require arthroplasty if symptoms persist; 90% recovery, 10% may require surgery
Type III. Rupture of capsule, acromioclavicular ligaments, and coracoclavicular ligaments	Elevated clavicle; increased coracoclavicular distance	Internal fixation; 80% good, 20% reoperation

From Neer CS II, Rockwood CA Jr. Chapter 11. In: Rockwood CA Jr, Green DP, eds. *Fractures.* Philadelphia, PA: JB Lippincott Co; 1975:721–756.

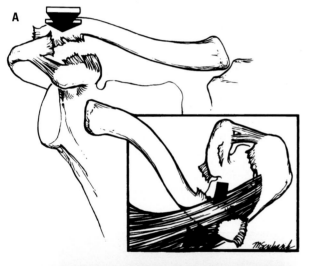

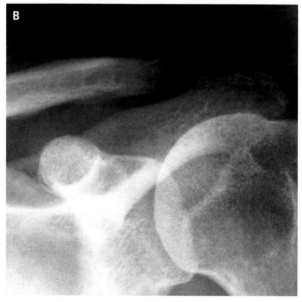

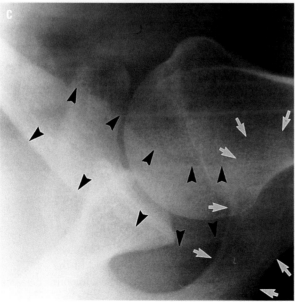

Figure 8.19. Type IV acromioclavicular (AC) separation. The schematic representation (**A**) shows disruption of the AC and coracoclavicular ligaments, the intact coracoacromial ligament and posterior displacement of the distal end of the clavicle. The inset (**A**) shows the posterior displacement of the distal end of the clavicle as seen in the axiliary projection. It is difficult to appreciate the posterior displacement of the distal end of the clavicle on the AP radiograph (**B**), although it is clear that the AC joint *(arrow)* is abnormal. The axillary projection (**C**) shows the posterior dislocation of the distal end of the clavicle *(arrowheads)* with respect to the acromial process *(arrows)*.

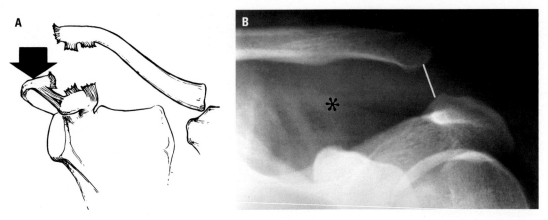

Figure 8.20. Type V acromioclavicular (AC) separation. The schematic (**A**) illustrates the mechanism of injury to be marked inferior displacement of the scapula by severe downward force delivered to the acromial process with only the coracoacromial ligament remaining intact. Subluxation (or dislocation) occurs at the sternoclavicular joint as well. On the AP radiograph (**B**), The AC *(line)* and coracoclavicular *(asterisk)* spaces are grossly wide and, because of the cephalad retraction of the proximal end of the clavicle by the sternocleidomastoid muscle, the clavicle assumes an almost horizontal attitude.

and axillary (Fig. 8.19C) projections, the distal end of the clavicle lies inferior and posterior to the acromion.

Type V (inferior) AC separation refers to the severe inferior displacement of the scapula and occurs when, in addition to disruption of the AC and CC ligaments, some degree of sternoclavicular separation occurs as well (Fig. 8.20A). The latter allows the proximal end of the clavicle to be rostrally distracted by the unopposed action of the sternocleidomastoid muscle. The result, radiographically, is that the entire clavicle appears more severely rostrally located with respect to the scapula (Fig. 8.20B) than with type III AC separation. Conceptually, the type V AC separation can be considered a severe type III separation.

In the type VI AC separation, the distal end of the clavicle is displaced anteroinferiorly and comes to rest deep to the conjoined tendon of the biceps and coracobrachialis muscles (Fig. 8.21A).

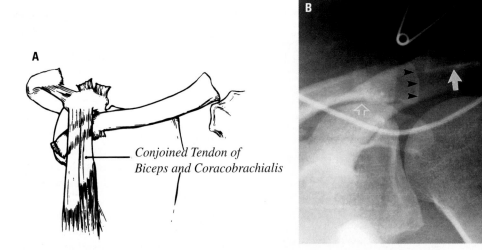

Conjoined Tendon of Biceps and Coracobrachialis

Figure 8.21. Type VI (anterior) acromioclavicular separation refers to the location of the distal end of the clavicle relative to the scapula. In the schematic (**A**), the distal end of the clavicle is depicted inferior to the coronoid process. The AP radiograph (**B**) shows the distal end of the clavicle *(arrowheads)* inferior to the acromion *(arrow)* but impinging on the top of the coracoid process *(open arrow)*. (The glenohumeral joint is also posteriorly dislocated.)

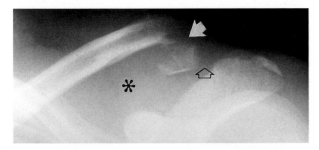

Figure 8.22. Fracture of the distal end of the clavicle *(arrow)* with disruption of the coracoclavicular ligament *(asterisk)* and an incomplete tear of the acromioclavicular ligament.

The ligamentous injuries and sternoclavicular disruption are the same as in the type V AC separation. On the AP radiograph (Fig. 8.21B), the distal end of the clavicle is located inferior to the coracoid process.

Fracture of the coracoid process associated with AC dislocation has been reported in approximately 20 cases.[11] Recognition of this rare association has patient management implications.

Fracture of the distal end of the clavicle is commonly associated with tearing of the CC ligament with (Fig. 8.22) or without separation (Fig. 8.23) of the AC ligament. As with AC separations, the distal end of the clavicle is not retracted upward; rather, the effect of gravity and the weight of the upper extremity pull the distal fragment and scapula downward. In these kinds of fractures, the important injury is that to the CC ligament.

Glenohumeral Dislocation

The shoulder is the most frequent site of dislocation of any joint in the body, with dislocation of the shoulder constituting approximately 50% of all dislocations.[12] The explanation for this incidence reflects the configuration of the humeral head and the glenoid fossa, the relative size of each, the weakness of the shoulder capsule, and the fact that this major joint is frequently subject to injury.

Dislocations of the shoulder, also referred to as glenohumeral instability and shoulder dislocation, are classified as "traumatic," "atraumatic," and "voluntary."[13,14] Traumatic dislocations of the shoulder are the result of direct or indirect trauma, constitute 96% of glenohumeral dislocations,[14] are usually

unilateral, are the etiology of the Hill-Sachs fracture and the Bankart "lesion",[13] and usually ultimately require surgical management.[13]

Atraumatic dislocations occur as the result of a sudden forceful normal motion of the arm, as might occur during a seizure. Voluntary dislocations are those in which the patient is able to dislocate the glenohumeral joint at will. The latter two categories constitute only approximately 4% of glenohumeral instabilities. Voluntary instability is usually of congenital or developmental etiology, is usually bilateral, and usually responds to a rehabilitation program.[13]

Dislocations of the glenohumeral joint are also classified on the basis of the final resting place of the humeral head with respect to the glenoid fossa and are designated, therefore, as anterior, inferior, posterior, and superior.[13,15–19] Of these, the anterior dislocation, occurring most often as a subcoracoid (infracoracoid) dislocation (Figs. 8.24 and 8.25), is the most common. The inferior (subglenoid) (infraglenoid) dislocation is next in

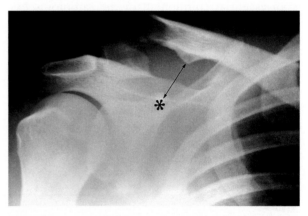

Figure 8.23. Fracture of the lateral third of the clavicle, resulting from severe force directed downward against the superolateral aspect of the shoulder. In this injury, the distal clavicular fragment retains its normal relationship to the acromial process indicating the acromioclavicular (AC) ligament is intact. The clinically significant injury associated with this type of clavicular fracture is disruption of the coracoclavicular ligament, indicated by the abnormally wide coracoclavicular distance *(double-headed arrow)*. The *asterisk* indicates the coracoid process. Contrary to a common misconception, the distal end of the proximal fracture is *not* displaced upward by the sternocleidomastoid muscle, which inserts at the medial end of the clavicle. Rather, the entire upper extremity is displaced inferiorly by its own weight and the effect of gravity.

frequency. Posterior and superior dislocations are rare, as is luxatio erecta, a unique form of anterior dislocation. Glenohumeral dislocations have also been classified, perhaps more simply, into *anterior* (98%), which includes infracoracoid (most common), infraglenoid, infraclavicular, luxatio erecta, and the rare intrathoracic; *posterior* (2%), which may be subacromial (most common), subglenoid, and subspinous.[19] Most posterior dislocations are subacromial and are fixed fracture-dislocations with the humeral head impacted on the posterior glenoid rim.

In each classification system, the anterior dislocation, occurring most often as subcoracoid (infracoracoid) dislocation, is the most common. The inferior (subglenoid) dislocation is next in frequency.

Dislocations of the shoulder are usually clinically obvious. The indications for radiographic evaluation before reduction include establishing the type of dislocation, the relationship of the humeral head to the glenoid fossa, and the possible presence of associated fractures, particularly the impacted Hill–Sachs fracture. The axillary view is an essential component of the radiologic examination of patients suspected of having glenohumeral dislocation to confirm the direction of dislocation, assess impaction of the humeral head on the glenoid fossa in anterior dislocation and posterior fracture-dislocation, and after reduction to assess for Hill–Sachs fractures, which may be ambiguously depicted on the postreduction radiograph.

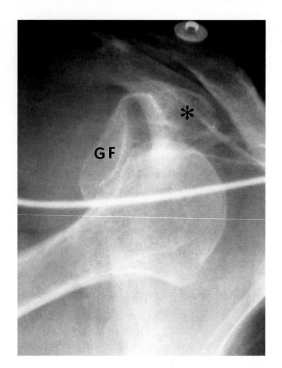

Figure 8.24. Anterior (infracoracoid) glenohumeral dislocation. The humeral head is displaced out of the glenoid fossa *(GF)* inferior to the coracoid process *(asterisk)* of the scapula. GF, glenoid fossa.

Anterior dislocation is characterized by the humeral head coming to rest anterior to the glenoid fossa, typically inferior to the coracoid process (Fig. 8.24), hence the term *infracoracoid dislocation*. When it is difficult to distinguish infracoracoid from infraglenoid dislocation, the axillary view provides the definitive diagnosis (Fig. 8.25).

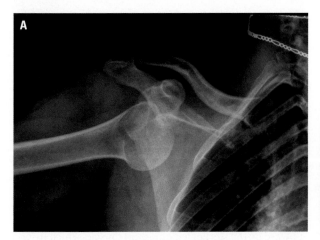

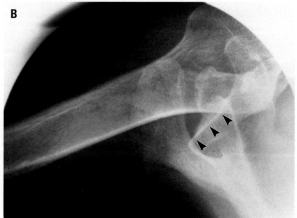

Figure 8.25. Infracoracoid dislocation in the axillary projection. (**A**) is the AP projection. Whether the glenohumeral dislocation is infracoracoid or infraglenoid is ascertained by the axillary projection (**B**), which indicates the infracoracoid position of the humeral head with respect to the glenoid fossa *(arrowheads)*.

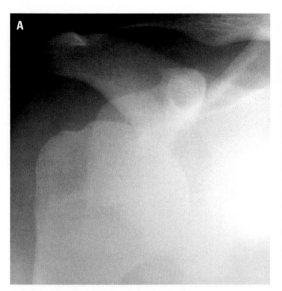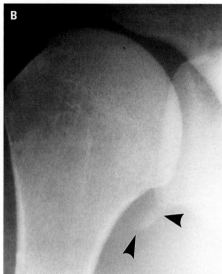

Figure 8.26. Anterior (infracoracoid) dislocation (**A**) with thin osteochondral fracture fragment (Bankart lesion) *(arrowheads)* of the anteroinferior glenoid labrum visible only in the postreduction radiograph (**B**).

Glenohumeral dislocations—particularly the infracoracoid type—are commonly associated with injury to either the anterior or anteroinferior rim of the glenoid labrum (Bankart lesion) or the Hill–Sachs fracture. Each of these features may occur with the initial dislocation. Therefore, the presence of either fracture does not necessarily imply a previous or recurrent dislocation.[20]

The Bankart lesion, pathologically, may consist of disruption of the fibrocartilaginous labrum, detachment of a cartilaginous fragment, or an osteocartilaginous fracture fragment.[21–23] The injury is caused by the humeral head impacting on the labrum during dislocation. Since most glenohumeral dislocations are infracoracoid, the anterior or anteroinferior arc of the glenoid rim is most commonly involved. Ribbans et al. found anterior labral "damage" in all patients younger than age 50 and in 75% of patients above age 50 years by computerized arthrotomography.[24] Arthroscopically, Hintermann and Gachter found 87% of patients examined had anterior labral "tear," and 68% sustained Hill–Sachs fractures following acute glenohumeral dislocation.[25] The Bankart lesion, being primarily cartilaginous, may be seen radiographically only when the separate fragment includes an osseous component (Fig. 8.26). Magnetic resonance imaging (MRI) is the imaging modality of choice for the detection of the labral type of injury.

The Hill–Sachs fracture was originally described as "a large defect or groove in the posterolateral aspect of the head of the humerus," as illustrated in Figure 8.27.[26] The authors further noted the defect was "not as a late result of dislocation of the shoulder, but as a true fracture."

Although sometimes referred to as the Hill–Sachs "lesion," the injury is, very simply, a fracture of the humeral head caused by whatever adjacent bony structure the humeral head impacts upon. This fact also determines the location of the fracture on the humeral head, with the posterolateral aspect being most commonly involved because of the most common infracoracoid dislocation. For the same reason, the fracture is most commonly seen on the AP internally rotated view of the shoulder. Contrary to a common misconception, the Hill–Sachs fracture is not a sign of prior glenohumeral dislocation. Because the Hill–Sachs fracture occurs in as many as 68% of initial glenohumeral dislocations,[25] it is reasonable to expect to find a Hill–Sachs fracture in the majority of patients with recurrent shoulder dislocation.

The radiographic appearance of the Hill–Sachs fracture defect may vary from that originally described and illustrated (Fig. 8.27), as seen in Figures 8.28 through 8.31. The direction of humeral head dislocation is also confirmed on the Y scapular

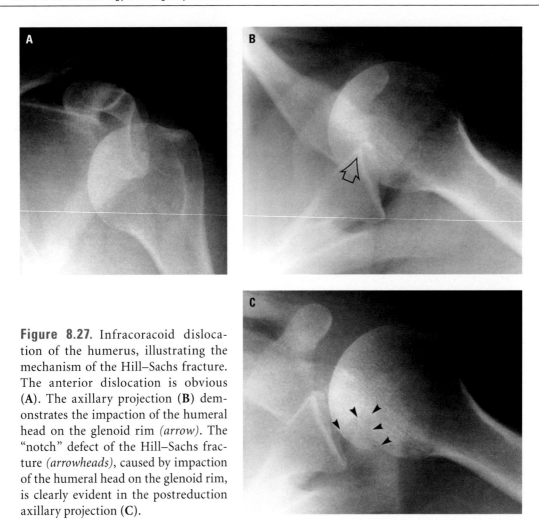

Figure 8.27. Infracoracoid dislocation of the humerus, illustrating the mechanism of the Hill–Sachs fracture. The anterior dislocation is obvious (**A**). The axillary projection (**B**) demonstrates the impaction of the humeral head on the glenoid rim *(arrow)*. The "notch" defect of the Hill–Sachs fracture *(arrowheads)*, caused by impaction of the humeral head on the glenoid rim, is clearly evident in the postreduction axillary projection (**C**).

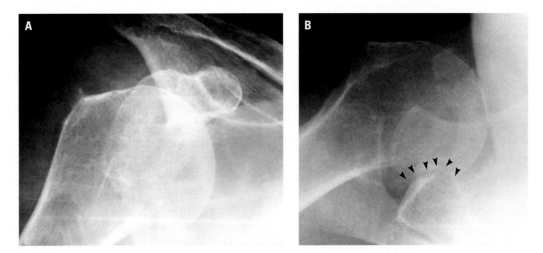

Figure 8.28. Direct infracoracoid dislocation (**A**) with Hill–Sachs groove fracture *(arrowheads)* of posterior aspect of humeral head (**B**).

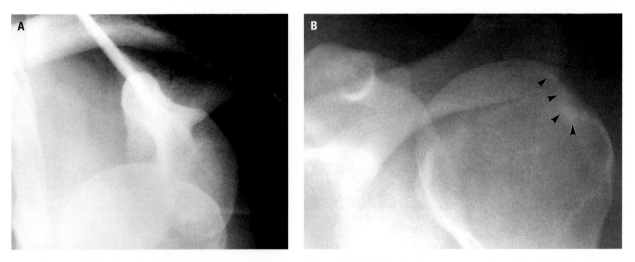

Figure 8.29. Anterior (infracoracoid) dislocation (**A**), with Hill–Sachs fracture manifested by ill-defined area of increased density *(arrowheads)* of the posterolateral aspect of the humeral head (**B**).

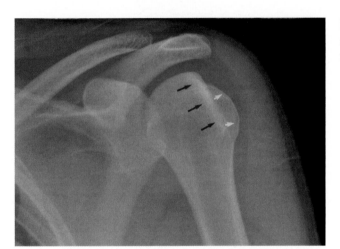

Figure 8.30. Frontal radiograph of the left shoulder showing what sclerotic margin of the healed Hill–Sachs fracture *(arrows)*.

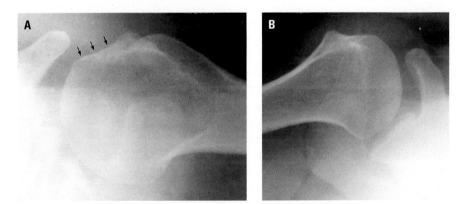

Figure 8.31. Impaction variety of Hill–Sachs fracture *(arrows)* of the humeral head in externally rotated AP projection (**A**). The normal right shoulder (**B**) is shown for comparison. Flattening of this arc of the humeral head with subchondral cortical sclerosis is abnormal and represents an impaction fracture differing from that described by Hill and Sachs.

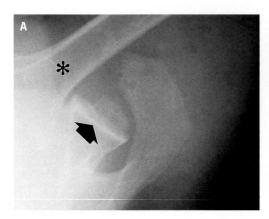

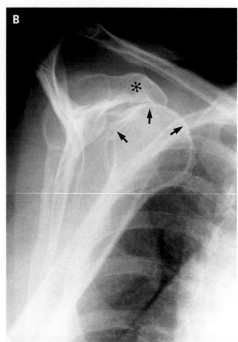

Figure 8.32. Infracoracoid dislocation on axillary (**A**) and scapular Y (**B**) views. On the axillary projection (**A**), the humeral head is not visible, but the humeral neck *(asterisk)* is anterior to the glenoid fossa *(arrow)*, implying an infracoracoid dislocation. The Y view conclusively demonstrates the humeral head *(arrows)* to lie beneath the coracoid process *(asterisk)*.

view (Fig. 8.32). Infracoracoid dislocation may be associated with other fractures in addition to the Hill–Sachs or Bankart, such as of the greater tuberosity of the humerus (Fig. 8.33) or the surgical neck of the humerus (Fig. 8.34).

Rare instances of irreducible anterior glenohumeral dislocation, without associated neck fractures, have been reported.[27,28] Irreducible anterior dislocations usually occur in middle-aged and elderly patients and are frequently associated with

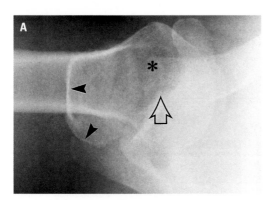

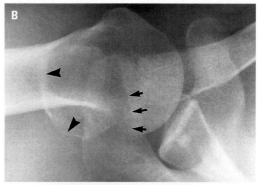

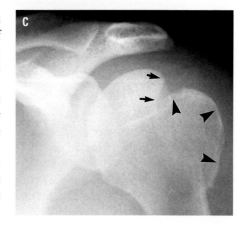

Figure 8.33. Infracoracoid dislocation with Hill–Sachs fracture and greater tuberosity fractures. Impaction of the humeral head *(asterisk)* on the anterior lip of the glenoid fossa *(open arrow)* is readily apparent on the initial axillary view (**A**). A separate fragment *(arrowheads)* superimposed on the humeral head should be considered a greater tuberosity fragment. The postreduction axillary projection (**B**) shows one edge of the notch defect of the Hill–Sachs fracture *(arrows)* and the persistent separate fragment *(arrowheads)*. The postreduction AP radiograph (**C**) confirms the greater tuberosity fragment *(arrowheads)*, as well as one margin of the Hill–Sachs fracture defect *(arrows)* of the humeral head.

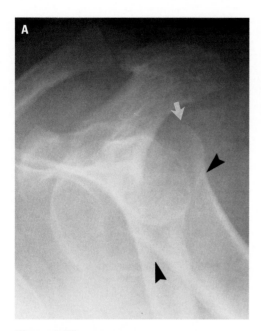 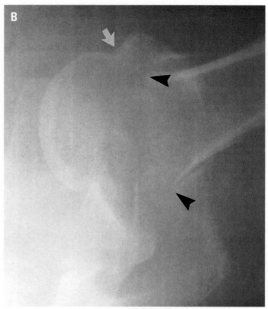

Figure 8.34. Infracoracoid dislocation with a comminuted displaced fracture of the surgical neck *(arrowheads)* and greater tuberosity *(arrow)* of the humerus in AP **(A)** and axillary **(B)** views.

greater tuberosity fractures. Seradge and Orme suggest that although the incidence of greater tuberosity fractures is greater (approximately 57%) and the fragment is larger than those associated with reducible anterior dislocations, the separate fragment is usually not the cause of the irreducibility.[28] Instead, the tuberosity fracture permits interposition of the biceps tendon between the glenoid fossa and the humeral head. A large greater tuberosity fragment and dislocation of the humeral head medial to the coracoid process on the AP radiograph are frequently seen with biceps interposition (Fig. 8.33).[29] Additionally, infracoracoid dislocation may occur with humeral surgical neck fractures with (Fig. 8.34) or without greater tuberosity fractures.

Inferior (infraglenoid or subglenoid) dislocation (Fig. 8.35) is characterized by the humeral head being dislocated below the inferior rim of the glenoid into the subglenoid space created by the neck of the scapula. Inferior dislocation may be associated with a Bankart fracture of the inferior labrum of the glenoid (Fig. 8.36).

Luxatio erecta (erect dislocation of the humerus) is a rare form of anterior dislocation in which, as a result of severe hyperabduction of the arm, the humeral head is levered out of the glenoid fossa by the acromium, and in the process, tears the joint

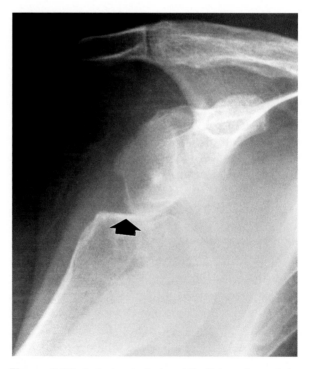

Figure 8.35. Inferior (subglenoid) dislocation of the humerus with Hill–Sachs fracture. The *arrow* indicates the flattened segment of the humeral head adjacent to the greater tuberosity of the humerus, caused by the impacted cortical fracture. This fracture, commonly associated with subglenoid dislocations, is the result of forceful impaction of the humeral head with the inferior rim of the glenoid fossa, that is, the Hill–Sachs fracture.

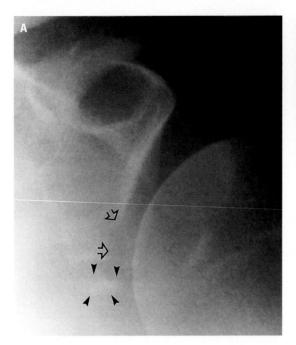
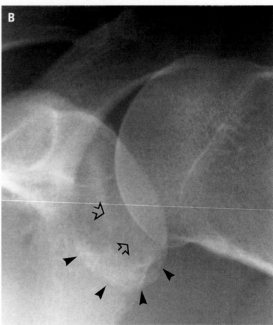

Figure 8.36 Inferior subluxation with Bankart fracture of the inferior labrum of the glenoid fossa. On the initial radiograph **(A)**, the labral defect *(open arrows)* is recognizable. The osteochondral fragment is difficult to see because of its thin bony component. On the postreduction radiograph **(B)**, the defect remains visible *(open arrows)*, and the Bankart fragment *(arrowheads)* is more obvious.

capsule.[30, 31] The entire capsule may be avulsed, or the humeral head and neck may be button-holed through the capsule. Usually the head comes to rest adjacent to either the corocoid process or, less commonly, into the subglenoid fossa. (The latter variety of luxatio erecta has been referred to as an "inferior" dislocation.)[32] In either location, the humerus is locked in position and cannot be voluntarily reduced. The usual mechanism of injury is a fall in which the arm is forced into hyperabduction, such as by a tree limb or the edge of a hole through which a construction worker falls. Clinically, the arm is in extreme abduction and superiorly elevated so that the arm is adjacent to the side of the head with a forearm flexed over the top of the head.

In the AP radiograph of the shoulder of luxation erecta, the humeral head is typically located in the subcoracoid fossa with the humeral shaft pointed upward so that its long axis is parallel to that of the spine of the scapula (Figs. 8.37 and 8.38.).

With infraglenoid luxatio erecta, the humeral head comes to rest in the infraglenoid fossa and, while directed superiorly, the long axis of the humeral shaft is described as being perpendicular to

the lateral chest wall (Figs.8.39 and 8.40). As with any glenohumeral dislocation, the association of Hill–Sachs (Figs. 8.37B, 8.39, and 8.41), as well as fractures of other components of the shoulder is common (Figs. 8.34, 8.40, and 8.41). Occlusion of the axillary artery secondary to intimal rupture and thrombosis associated with luxatio erecta has been reported.[33]

Posterior dislocation of the shoulder, with or without humeral head fracture, is rare, constituting 1.5%, 2.5%, and 4% of shoulder dislocations.[34–36] Pure posterior dislocation (without humeral head fracture) is even more uncommon. In addition to direct backward trauma, posterior dislocation is often the result of violent muscle contraction such as occurs in the convulsive seizures of epilepsy or electric shock, causing the humerus to rotate severely internally and to adduct.

Clinically, in posterior dislocation, the shoulder deformity is not great and is best appreciated by viewing the shoulder from above downward and noting a posterior protuberance caused by the humeral head. In obese or well-muscled individuals, even this is difficult to recognize. Abduction of the arm is usually limited in posterior dislocation but

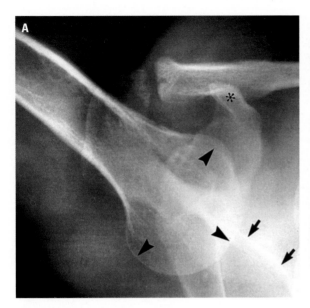
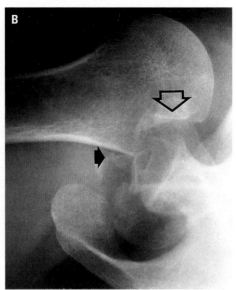

Figure 8.37. Luxatio erecta. On the AP radiograph (**A**), the humeral head *(arrowheads)* is situated inferior to the coracoid process *(asterisk)*. The long axis of the humerus coincides exactly with the long axis of the scapular spine *(arrows)*. The axillary projection (**B**) shows a Hill–Sachs fracture *(open arrow)* of the humeral head and a smaller separate fragment *(solid arrow)* of unknown origin.

may be sufficiently possible to be clinically misleading. In a series of 40 patients with 41 posterior fracture dislocations reported by Hawkins et al.,[37] the diagnosis was initially clinically missed "in the majority," and the average interval from injury to diagnosis was 1 year.

Radiologically, posterior dislocation is reported to be unrecognized in as many as 50% of cases.[26] This is due to several factors. The humeral head–glenoid relationship may appear normal on the frontal radiograph of the shoulder[38–41]; patient positioning in frontal projections may present a misleading

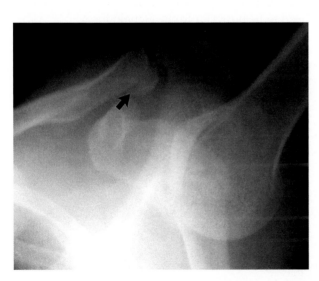

Figure 8.38. Typical appearance of luxatio erecta on frontal radiograph of the shoulder with the humeral shaft obviously rostrally oriented. The unusual finding in this patient is the concomitant distal clavicular fracture *(arrow)*.

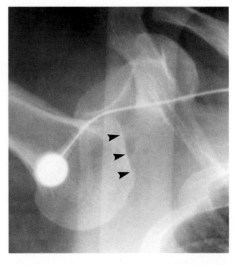

Figure 8.39. Inferior (infraglenoid) luxatio erecta with Hill–Sachs fracture. The humeral head lies in the infraglenoid fossa. While the orientation of the humeral shaft is directed superiorly, it is also referred to as being perpendicular to the rib cage. The flattened arc of the humeral head *(arrowheads)* is a Hill–Sachs fracture.

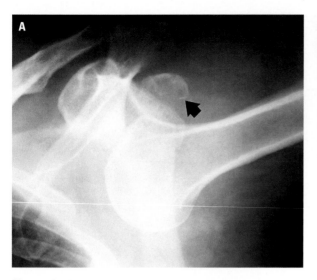

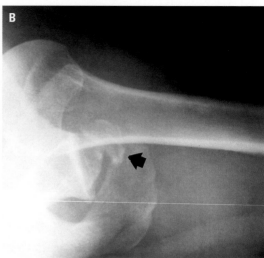

Figure 8.40. Luxatio erecta associated with fracture of the superior rim of the glenoid fossa *(arrows)* in AP (**A**) and axillary (**B**) projections.

appearance of the glenohumeral relationship; or mutually exclusive signs of the glenohumeral relationship have been ascribed to posterior dislocation of the shoulder (e.g., widened glenohumeral joint or "positive rim sign") and superimposition of the humeral head on the anterior glenoid rim (e.g., a "negative rim sign").

Radiographic recognition of the rare pure posterior dislocation of the shoulder on the frontal projection is dependent on two radiographic signs. The first is the appearance of the severely internally rotated humeral head resembling a rifle barrel or a light bulb and, second, a positive rim sign in which the distance between the articular cortex of the humeral head

and the anterior glenoid rim is wider than normal.[38] When these signs are present in concert and are as obvious as in Figure 8.42, the diagnosis of posterior humeral dislocation may be made with certainty.

However, should the patient purposefully or inadvertently be placed in the ipsilateral anterior oblique frontal position, the humeral head may be superimposed on the glenoid fossa, resulting in a negative distance between the head and anterior glenoid rim, for example, a false-negative rim sign. This potential ambiguity can be eliminated by either an axillary or Y projection, which will clearly reveal the humeral head to lie posterior to the glenoid fossa.

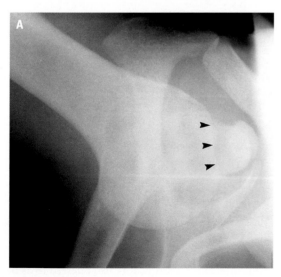

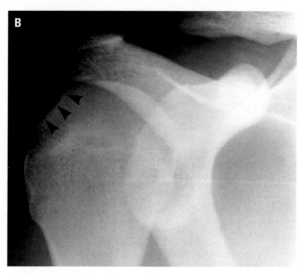

Figure 8.41. Luxatio erecta with Hill–Sachs fracture secondary to impaction of the humeral head on the coracoid process. The impaction fracture *(arrowheads)* is evident in both the initial axillary (**A**) and the post-reduction frontal (**B**) projection.

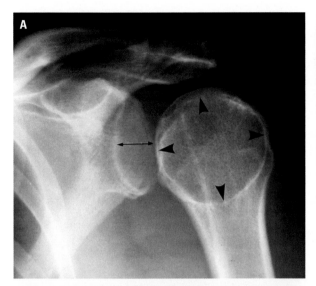

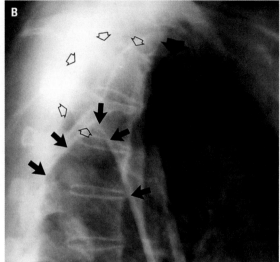

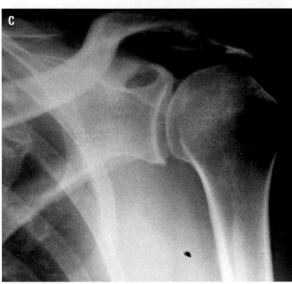

Figure 8.42. Pure posterior dislocation of the left shoulder in frontal projection (**A**). The through-the-chest lateral radiograph (**B**) shows the humeral head *(open arrows)* posterior to the glenoid fossa *(black arrowhead)*. The spine of the scapular and the posterior margin of the humeral shaft *(black arrows)* indicate narrow humero-scapular angle. The AP radiograph of the normal opposite shoulder (**C**) has been reversed for ease of comparison.

Posterior fracture-dislocation of the humeral head is the much more common manifestation of posterior displacement, and the radiologic signs of posterior fracture-dislocation are much more easily discernible and reliable. Posterior fracture-dislocation of the shoulder is actually only a partial posterior displacement of the humeral head with respect to the glenoid fossa. The anteromedial articulating surface of the humeral head, usually just posterior to the level of the lesser tuberosity, impacts on the posterior rim of the glenoid fossa (Fig. 8.43). By a mechanism identical with that causing the Hill–Sachs fracture of anterior shoulder dislocation, impaction of the humeral head on the posterior glenoid labrum typically results in a groove or "V" defect, which is usually large and comminuted and involves the contiguous arc of the humeral head. As seen in the axillary projection (Fig. 8.44B), the

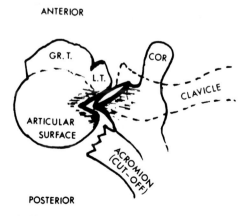

Figure 8.43. Diagrammatic representation of the pathologic basis of the "trough line" sign of posterior fracture dislocation of the shoulder. Gr. T., greater tuberosity; L. T., lesser tuberosity. From Wilson JC, McKeever FM. Traumatic posterior dislocation of humerus. *J Bone Joint Surg Am.* 1946;31A(1):160–172, with permission.

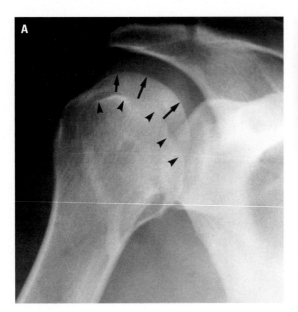
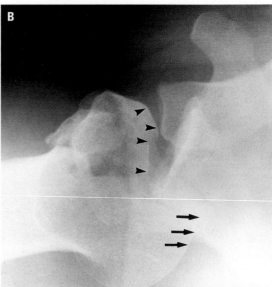

Figure 8.44. Classic appearance of the trough sign of posterior fracture-dislocation of the shoulder. In the frontal radiograph (**A**), the humerus is in severe internal rotation. The lateral edge of the trough line *(arrowheads)* is formed, in part, by the greater tuberosity cortex and the comminuted, depressed humeral head fracture. The medial edge of the trough is the humeral head cortex *(arrows)*. In this patient, the rim sign is equivocal but also unnecessary. The posterior fracture-dislocation is confirmed in the axillary projection (**B**), in which the impacted fracture fragments that contribute to the lateral edge of the trough *(arrowheads)* and the humeral head articular cortex *(arrows)* are clearly evident. (Compare **B** with Fig. 8.38)

lateral (anterior) margin of the wedge-shaped defect is the basis of the "trough line" popularized by Cisternino et al.[41] which is characteristic of posterior fracture-dislocation on the frontal projection (Fig. 8.44A).[38,39,42]

In posterior fracture-dislocations with severe comminution of the humeral head, the trough line, even though not well defined, can usually be recognized (Fig. 8.45A, B). The trough sign is usually not useful in the AP radiograph of eccentric posterior

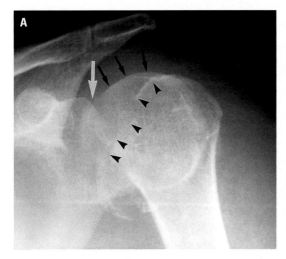
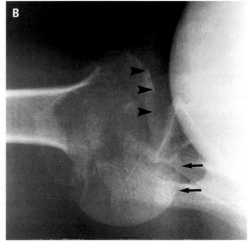

Figure 8.45. Comminuted posterior fracture-dislocation. On the AP radiograph (**A**), the humeral head cortex is very close to the anterior cortex of the glenoid *(white arrow)* (negative rim sign). Although comminuted, the lateral margin of the trough *(arrowheads)* is discernible, while the humeral head cortex *(black arrows)* constitutes the medial margin of the trough. The posterior fracture-dislocation is clearly evident on the axillary view (**B**), as are the margins of the trough.

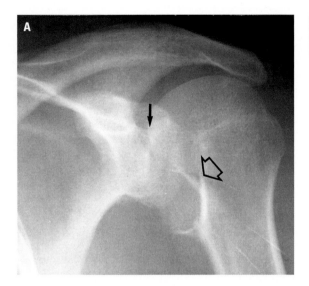
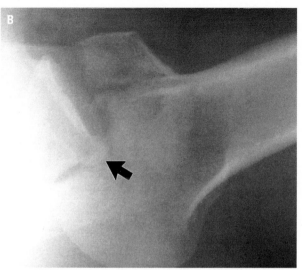

Figure 8.46. Eccentric posterior fracture-dislocation. The negative rim sign *(arrow)*, superior displacement of the humeral head, and fracture of the inferior cortex of the humeral neck *(open arrow)* on the AP radiograph **(A)** is consistent with posterior fracture-dislocation, which is confirmed on the axillary view **(B)** *(arrow)*.

fracture-dislocation, although the negative rim sign (Fig.8.46) should be. In any event, the axillary projection establishes the diagnosis of posterior fracture-dislocation.

As discussed earlier, although a positive rim sign is valuable in the recognition of pure posterior humeral dislocation (Fig. 8.42), a normal (Fig. 8.47A) or narrowed (Fig. 8.47C) glenohumeral joint space (e.g., normal or negative rim sign) is common in posterior fracture-dislocation.[38]

Figure 8.47 is an example of rare bilateral posterior fracture-dislocation of the shoulder

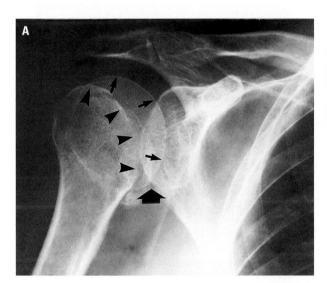
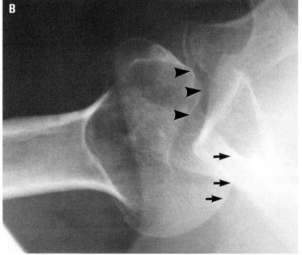

Figure 8.47. Bilateral shoulder posterior fracture-dislocation. In the frontal projection of the right shoulder **(A)**, the trough line *(arrowheads)* is the most obvious radiographic sign of the posterior fracture-dislocation and roughly parallels the humeral head articular cartilage *(smaller arrows)*. The *large arrow* indicates a normal glenohumeral relationship. The degree of internal humeral rotation is difficult to assess, and the rim sign is ambiguous. The diagnosis is confirmed on the axillary projection **(B)**, in which the groove fracture margin *(arrowheads)* that causes the trough line and the arc of the humeral head *(arrows)* that causes the humeral head cortex shadow in the frontal projection are clearly apparent. *(continued)*

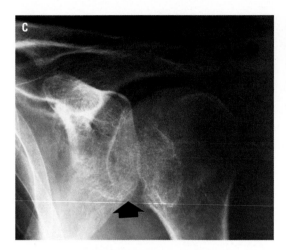

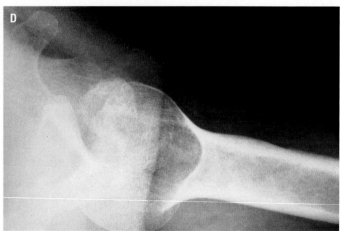

Figure 8.47. *(continued)* In the frontal projection of the left shoulder (**C**), the only sign suggestive of posterior fracture-dislocation is the severely narrowed glenohumeral joint space (negative rim sign) *(arrow)*. The degree of humeral head internal rotation is difficult to assess, and a trough line is not visible. Posterior fracture-dislocation is confirmed in the axillary projection (**D**).

that occurred during an epileptic seizure. In each frontal projection (Figs. 8.47A,C), the trough line is the most obvious sign of the posterior fracture-dislocation. The diagnosis is confirmed by the axillary projections (Figs. 8.47B,D).

Pseudosubluxation of the shoulder refers to inferior displacement of the humerus (head) with respect to the glenoid fossa that may or may not be related to the acute traumatic event. As the name implies, this entity is not a true dislocation of the glenohumeral joint, as discussed earlier, but is instead a "drooping" of the humeral head with respect to the glenoid fossa, secondary to distention of the joint capsule by hemarthrosis or lipohemarthrosis, as may occur in acute shoulder injuries or by disruption of the joint capsule associated with chronic or recurrent shoulder dislocations (Figs. 8.48, 8.49, and 8.50).[43] Pseudosubluxation is usually apparent only in erect examinations of the shoulder when the humerus can "droop" with respect to the glenoid fossa within the distended or lax joint capsule. Pseudosubluxation may be suspected on supine AP radiographs by the incongruity between the contiguous surfaces of the humeral head and glenoid fossa (Figs. 8.49A and 8.50A). However, glenohumeral incongruity is not a reliable finding, and clinical suspicion of pseudosubluxation should prompt an erect AP radiograph of the shoulder (Fig. 8.51).

Fractures of the Shoulder: Proximal Humeral Fractures

Primary fractures of the proximal humerus are traditionally identified by the Neer classification system (Fig. 8.51): type I—minimally or

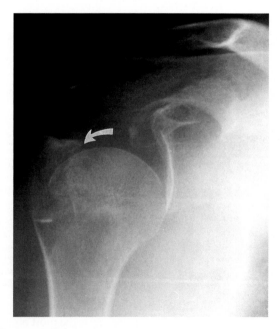

Figure 8.48. Pseudosubluxation of the humerus ("drooped" shoulder). The joint capsule is distended by a large hemarthrosis secondary to the tuberosity fracture *(curved arrow)*.

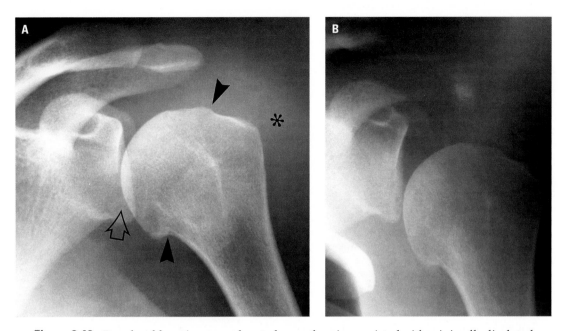

Figure 8.49. Pseudosubluxation secondary to hemarthrosis associated with minimally displaced surgical neck fracture *(arrowheads)*. On the supine radiograph (**A**), pseudosubluxation is reasonably suspected because of the glenohumeral incongruity *(open arrow)*. The large intracapsular density *(asterisk)* represents the hemarthrosis. The erect AP radiograph (**B**) clearly demonstrates the "drooped" humerus of pseudosubluxation.

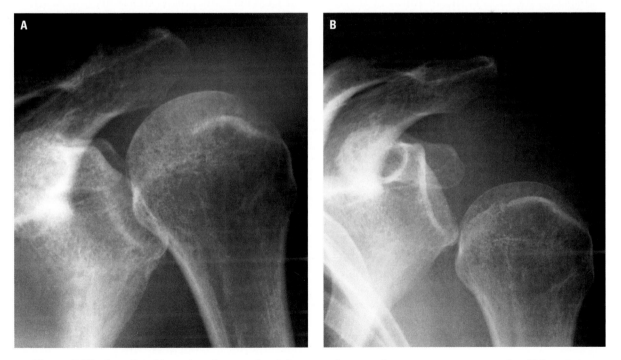

Figure 8.50. Pseudosubluxation due to a lax joint capsule secondary to recurrent posterior dislocation. (Note the marked internal rotation of the humeral head) (**A**). The pseudosubluxation is not apparent on the supine (**A**) radiograph but is clearly evident on the erect (**B**) projection.

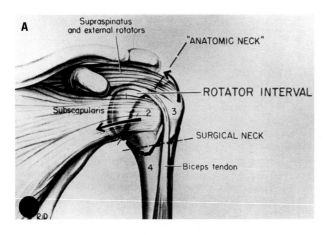

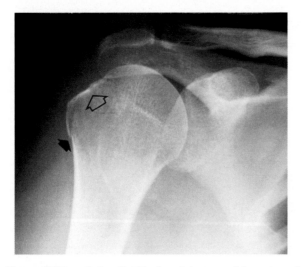

Figure 8.51. Neer classification system of displaced proximal humeral fractures. (From Neer CS. Displaced proximal humeral fractures. I. Classification and evaluation. *J Bone Joint Surg Am.* 1970;52(6):1077–1089, with permission.)

nondisplaced fractures of the anatomic or surgical neck or of either tuberosity (Fig. 8.52); type II—displaced two-part fractures involving the anatomic neck (Fig.8.53); type III—displaced surgical neck fracture (Fig. 8.54); type IV—fracture of the

Figure 8.52. Minimally displaced, impacted fracture of the greater tuberosity of the humerus (one of the variety of Neer type I fractures). *Open arrow* indicates the flattened segment of the greater tuberosity. *Closed arrow* indicates the cortical fracture site.

surgical neck and greater tuberosity (Fig. 8.55); and type V—fracture of the surgical neck and lesser or both tuberosities (Fig. 8.56).[44]

Recent literature has questioned the clinical application of the Neer classification only because of the difficulty of identifying the number of tuberosity fragments and their degree of displacement by routine radiographic examinations of the shoulder.[45–47]

Although CT is now routinely used in an attempt to better define the fragments of the Neer type IV through VI injuries, Bernstein et al. found that the addition of CT produced only a slight increase in intraobserver reliability and no increase in interobserver reproducibility relative to application of the Neer classification.[47]

The effect of position (patient or x-ray tube) on the proximal humeral physis to simulate a proximal metaphyseal fracture is described and illustrated (Fig. 8.4) earlier in this chapter. The distinction between the positional illusion (Fig. 8.4) and a proximal humeral metaphyseal fracture is shown in Figure 8.57. The Salter–Harris physeal injury most commonly seen at the proximal humerus, as elsewhere, is type II (Fig. 8.58).

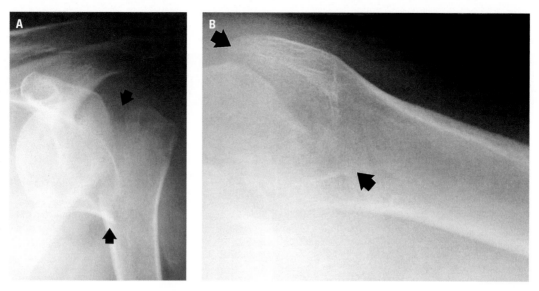

Figure 8.53. Neer type II oblique fracture *(arrows)* through the anatomic neck of the humerus in AP (**A**) and lateral (**B**) projections.

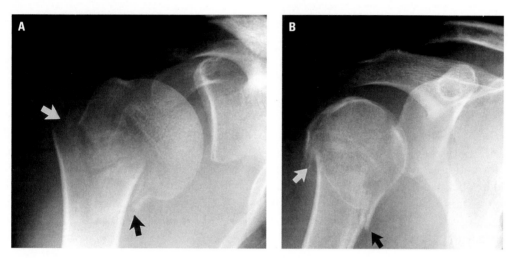

Figure 8.54. Neer type III comminuted, displaced fracture of the surgical neck *(arrows)* of the humerus in externally (**A**) and internally (**B**) rotated AP projections.

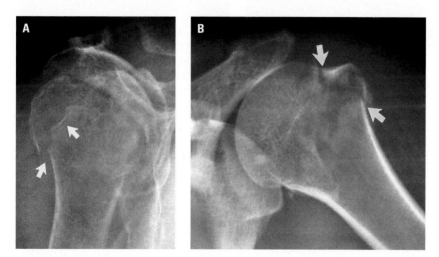

Figure 8.55. Neer type IV proximal humeral fracture of the greater tuberosity *(arrows)* may occur as an isolated fracture (Neer description, **A**) or in conjunction with a surgical neck fracture (**B**).

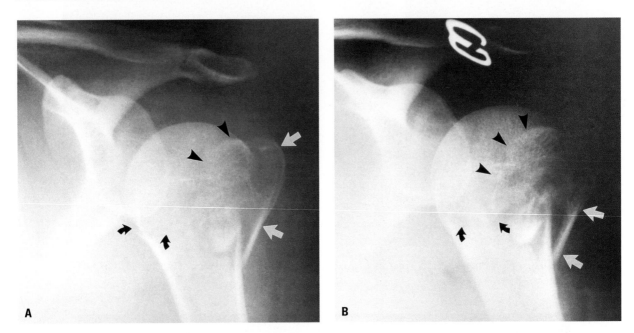

Figure 8.56. Neer type V fracture. The surgical neck fracture *(curved arrows)* is visible in both externally (**A**) and internally (**B**) rotated frontal projections. The greater tuberosity fragment is indicated by *straight arrows* and the lesser tuberosity fragment by *arrowheads*.

Fractures of the Clavicle

Detailed information relative to the mechanism of injury could be obtained from 81% of 150 consecutive patients sustaining clavicular fractures.[48] Of these, the fracture was caused by a fall or direct blow in 94%. Clavicular fractures occur most commonly in the middle third and are usually isolated injuries, although clavicular fractures occur commonly in patients who sustain major blunt thoracic or thoracoabdominal trauma.[49,50]

Nondisplaced or minimally displaced fractures of the mid-third of the clavicle, poorly demonstrated in the straight frontal projection, will

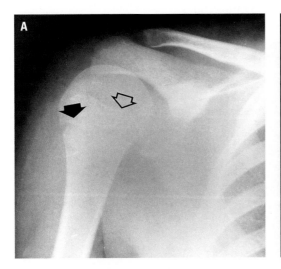
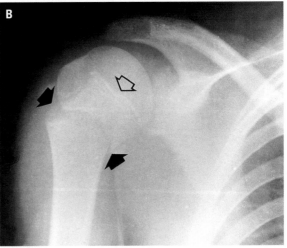

Figure 8.57. Fracture of the proximal humeral metaphysis. In the internally rotated projection (**A**), the fracture line *(closed arrow)* could be misinterpreted as the posterior arc of the physis *(open arrow)*. However, the externally rotated radiograph (**B**) clearly demonstrates the relationship between the physis and the fracture line. Note the difference in the radiographic characteristics of the fracture line and physis.

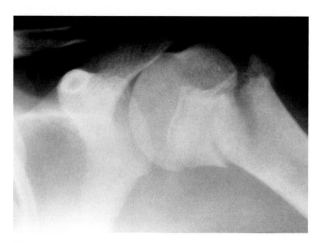

Figure 8.58. Salter II epiphyseal injury of the proximal humerus.

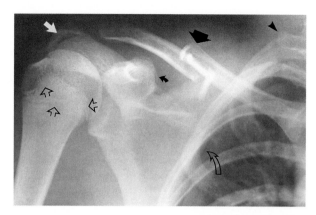

Figure 8.60. Comminuted, displaced middle-third clavicular fracture *(black arrow)* and concomitant right pneumothorax *(open curved arrow)*. The proximal humeral physis *(open arrows)* and the apophyses of the acromion *(white arrow)*, the coracoid *(curved arrow)*, and the right first thoracic transverse process *(arrowhead)* all have radiographic characteristics that should distinguish each from acute fractures. (Adapted from Harris RD, Harris JH Jr. The prevalence and significance of missed scapular fractures in blunt chest trauma. *AJR Am J Roentgenol.* 1988;151(4):747–750, with permission.)

usually be seen in the tangential frontal view (Fig. 8.8). Occasionally, however, such a fracture may be difficult to recognize in either projection (Fig. 8.59A, B). The presence of the fracture line on either examination or the physical findings confirm the fracture.

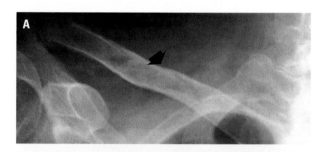

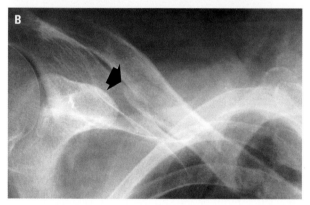

Figure 8.59. **A** and **B:** The subtle, minimally displaced fracture *(arrow)* in the middle third of the clavicle is not well seen in either projection. However, the fact that portions of the fracture line can be seen in each projection indicates that it is a real finding.

Figures 8.60 and 8.61 demonstrate the typical deformity associated with mid-third clavicular fractures. The distal fragment is retracted inferiorly by the force of the pectoralis minor muscle, which inserts on the coracoid process, and by the weight of the upper extremity.

Mid-third clavicular fractures may, obviously, be the result of major blunt chest trauma and in those patients they may be associated with, or even considered harbingers of, other injuries of greater clinical significance, such as pneumothorax, hemopneumothorax, or pulmonary contusion (Figs. 8.61 and 8.62). This association, as well as that of clavicular fractures as a non-predictor of acute traumatic aortic injury caused by major blunt chest trauma, is discussed in greater detail in Chapter 13. Mid-third clavicular fractures may infrequently occur with concomitant distal-third fractures, resulting in a separate segmental (Fig. 8.62).

Fractures of the distal (outer) third of the clavicle are usually caused by direct trauma to the shoulder top that is very similar to the mechanism of injury of AC injuries. Outer-third clavicular fractures are usually transverse and nondisplaced, with the distal fragment being fixed by the AC ligament and the proximal fragment being fixed by the CC ligament.

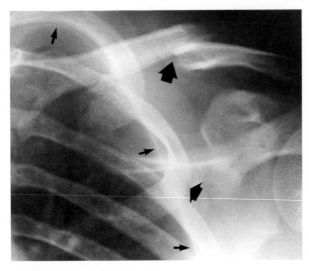

Figure 8.61. Complete, displaced mid-third clavicular fracture (*large arrow*) associated with minimally displaced fracture of the anterior end of the second left rib (*medium arrow*) and a tiny hemopneumothorax (*small arrows*).

If the distal end of the proximal fragment is superiorly displaced and distance between the clavicle and coracoid process is wide, it indicates the coracoclavicular ligament is disrupted. If the distal clavicular fragment remains normally aligned with the acromion process, it indicates that the AC ligament is intact (Fig. 8.23).

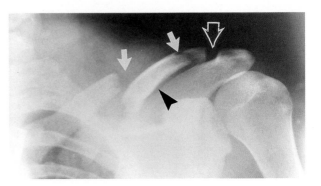

Figure 8.62. Segmental fracture of the clavicle. Fracture sites (*arrows*) in the midportions and distal portions of the clavicle create the separate (segmental) fragment (*arrowhead*). The acromioclavicular joint is disrupted as well (*open arrow*).

Fractures of the inner third of the clavicle (Fig. 8.63) are uncommon and are particularly difficult to recognize because of the many superimposed osseous shadows. Fractures close to the sternoclavicular joint may be demonstrable radiographically only by oblique views (Fig. 8.63) or CT.

Other injuries associated with fractures of the clavicle may be missed clinically because of the pain and deformity of the clavicular injury (Fig. 8.64). The responsible physician must have a high index of suspicion for associated injury and must be satisfied

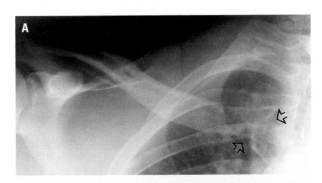

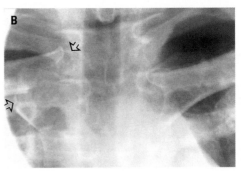

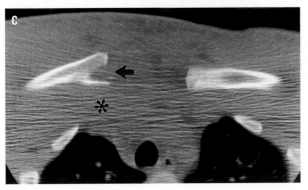

Figure 8.63. The fracture of the innner third of the clavicle (*open arrows*) is the subtle on the AP radiograph (**A**) because the minimal displacement of its fragments and the superimposed ribs and transverse process. A slight left anterior oblique projection (**B**) shows the fracture (*open arrows*) to better advantage. The fracture (*arrows*) is confirmed on axial CT (**C**). A hematoma (*asterisk*) of nonarterial origin (negative arteriogram) is present posterior to the proximal end of the clavicle.

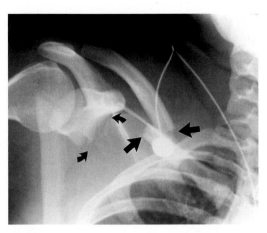

Figure 8.64. Displaced clavicular *(arrows)* and scapular neck *(curved arrows)* fracture. Although the clavicular fracture site is partially obscured by the electrocardiograph lead, it is visible, and its presence is confirmed by the displacement of the distal fragment. The scapular neck fracture could be overlooked because the glenohumeral relationship is normal. However, the position of the displaced shoulder joint with respect to the lateral cortex of the scapula and the position of the humeral head in relation to the acromion should clearly establish the presence of the fracture.

that associated injuries have not been overlooked because of an obvious clavicular fracture. Because sternoclavicular separation is usually the result of major blunt chest trauma, it is discussed and illustrated in Chapter 12.

Fractures of the Scapula (Scapular Fractures)

Because the scapula is an integral part of the shoulder, some of the traumatic lesions affecting it, or the related soft tissues, have been discussed earlier. In each of those instances, however, the scapula has not been the site of the primary injury. This section deals with trauma affecting the scapula primarily.

The scapular secondary growth centers, their locations, and the radiographic characteristics of their physeal lines must be considered when radiographs of the scapula of children and adolescents are being evaluated for fracture. The medial (vertebral) border of the scapula ossifies from two centers, one for the majority of the border and one at its inferior angle. The latter may not unite with the infraspinous portion of the scapula until age 25 years, and thus may simulate a fracture fragment. The typical radiographic appearance of this center is seen in Figure 8.65. The location and radiographic appearance of the acromial and coracoid apophyseal lines appear in Figures 8.5 and 8.6, respectively, and Figure 8.60.

Fractures of the scapula typically result from major, direct blunt trauma—such as a fall with the patient landing supine, a motor vehicle accident, or a direct blow to the shoulder—because most of the scapula is protected by rather large muscle masses.[51] Fractures of the scapula are commonly encountered

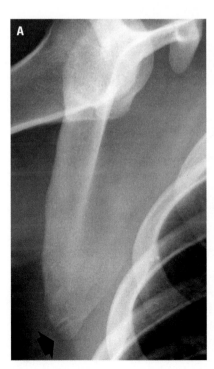
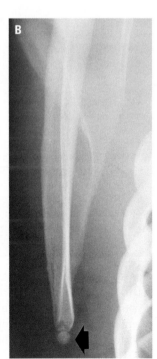

Figure 8.65. The ossification center at the inferior angle of the scapula *(arrow)* is a normal finding generally seen between the ages of 15 and 25 years. It should not be misinterpreted as a fracture fragment. The location of the center and its smooth, sclerotic margins are characteristics that should help distinguish it from an acute fracture.

in massive blunt chest trauma.[52] This association is discussed in Chapter 12. Treatment by open reduction and internal fixation of glenoid and scapular neck fractures has made the radiographic identification of these fractures on initial examinations of the shoulder (or chest) of major clinical relevance.[53] That the remainder, and majority, of fractures of the scapula continue to be treated nonoperatively is not rationalization for failure to identify scapular fractures, especially those involving the neck and/ or glenoid fossa.[54]

Fractures of the scapula are commonly radiologically subtle, may be obscured by superimposed clavicle and ribs and, particularly in patients with massive blunt trauma, are commonly obscured by subcutaneous emphysema, monitoring or life-support equipment, or patient radiograph identification markers or labels applied to the cassette. The observer's attention is frequently distracted from the scapula by other skeletal or soft tissue injuries. Consequently, the radiographic diagnosis of fractures of the scapula is dependent on knowledge of the mechanism of injury, a very high index of suspicion, and concentrated attention to the analysis of the radiographic image of the scapula. Failure to observe these guidelines will most assuredly result in failure to promptly diagnose fractures of the scapula and will possibly result in suboptimal patient care (Fig.8.66).[52]

For the reasons mentioned earlier, scapular fractures are missed on approximately 40% of initial chest radiographs following blunt chest.[52] This tenet is illustrated in Figure 8.67, in which various subtle signs of infraspinous fractures present on the AP radiograph of the scapula, are ambiguously dem-

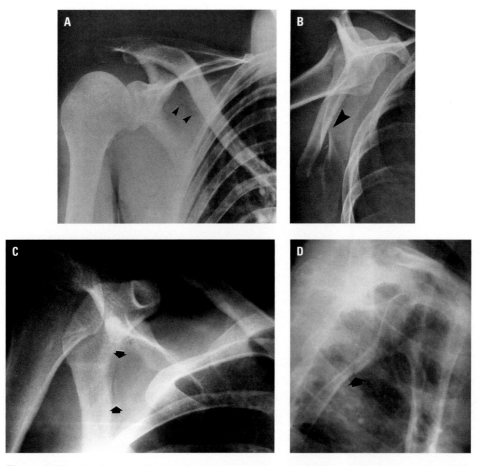

Figure 8.66. The fracture line in the infraspinous portion of the scapula *(arrowheads)* is not well seen in the frontal projection (**A**). However, the fracture line *(arrowhead)* is clearly evident on the Y view (**B**). In another patient, the fracture line in the infraspinous portion of the scapula *(arrows)* is barely perceptible in the frontal projection (**C**), being represented by a vague, radiolucent, slightly curvilinear defect paralleling the sweep of the lateral margin of the scapula. The lateral view (**D**), however, clearly defines a displaced fracture.

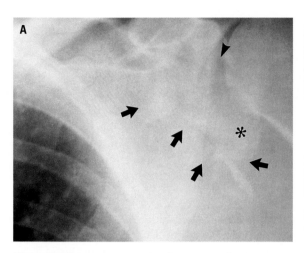
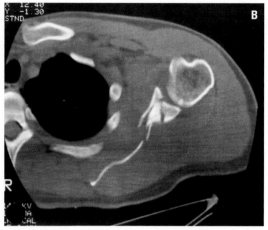

Figure 8.67. Comminuted infraspinous fracture *(arrows)* in AP projection (**A**). The neck component is suggested by inappropriate orientation of the glenoid fossa *(asterisk)*, and a superior glenoid fossa fracture is indicated by subtle disruption of its posterior labrum *(arrowhead)*. CT (**B**) of the shoulder clearly delineates the extent of the fracture into the scapular neck and glenoid fossa.

onstrated by CT (Fig. 8.67B). In Figure 8.67, the comminuted infraspinous fracture is obvious on the frontal projection, but the neck and glenoid components, confirmed by CT, are only suggested by the inappropriate orientation of the glenoid fossa and a subtle disruption of its superior labrum. Similarly, a supraspinous process fracture confirmed on the Y view is suggested by disruption and discontinuity of the medial border of the scapula on the frontal radiograph (Figs. 8.68 and 8.69). The reader

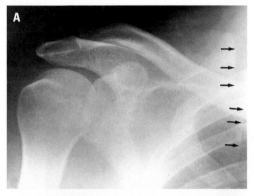
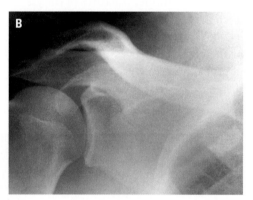
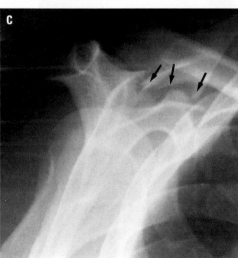

Figure 8.68. On the AP view of the shoulder (**A**), the only indication of the presence of a supraspinous fracture is disruption and discontinuity of the superior medial cortex of the scapula *(arrows)*. The fracture is not visible in the AP view of the glenohumeral joint (**B**) but is clearly evident *(arrows)* on the Y projection (**C**).

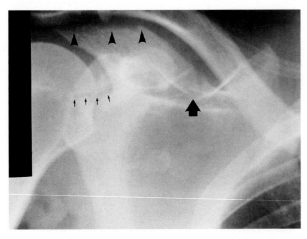

Figure 8.69. On the frontal projection of the shoulder, the comminuted fracture of the spinous process *(large arrow)* and the fracture of the acromial process *(arrowheads)* could easily divert attention from the subtle fracture of the glenoid fossa *(small arrows)*. (From Harris RD, Harris JH Jr. The prevalence and significance of missed scapular fractures in blunt chest trauma. *AJR Am J Roentgenol.* 1988;151(4):747–750, with permission.)

will find other examples of the common subtlety of scapular fractures in this section.

Minimally displaced (subtle) fractures of the glenoid fossa, which may be visible on conventional radiographs (Fig. 8.67), are best demonstrated by CT.

Fracture of the coracoid process or its base is a rare injury but probably occurs more frequently than has been reported.[51,55–59] In a review of 67 patients

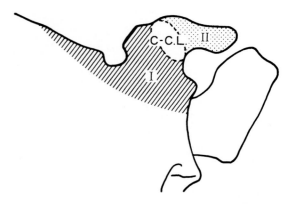

Figure 8.70. Classification of coracoid process fractures proposed by Ogawa et al. *C-CL* is the site of attachment of the coracoclavicular ligament. (From Ogawa K, Yoshida A, Takahishi M, et al. Fractures of the coracoid process. *J Bone Joint Surg Br.* 1997;79(1):17–19.)

with coracoid process fractures, Ogawa et al. classified these fractures into type I (most common), located posterior to the coracoclavicular (C-CL) ligament, and type II, those anterior to the CC ligament (Fig. 8.70).[60]

The type I fractures involve the base of the coracoid process, are usually associated with multiple shoulder injuries, and result in dissociation of the scapula and clavicle. These injuries are best demonstrated by CT. However, when they are ambiguous on the AP shoulder radiograph, the precise distribution and significance of type I fractures may be established with oblique views (Figs 8.71, 8.72, and 8.73).

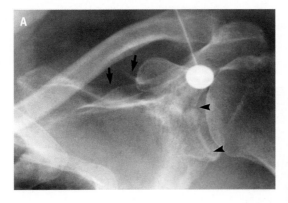
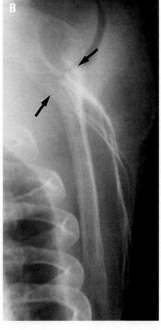

Figure 8.71. Subtle type I coracoid fracture with extension into the glenoid fossa confirmed by CT. On the AP radiograph (**A**), fractures involve the supraspinous portion of the scapula *(arrows)* and the anterior rim of the glenoid fossa is disrupted *(arrowheads)*. The Y view (**B**) suggests a fracture of the base of the coracoid process *(arrows)*. *(continued)*

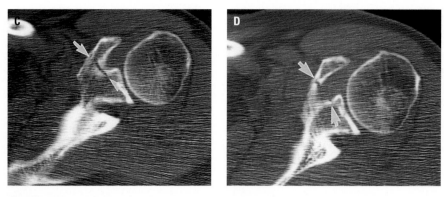

Figure 8.71. *(continued)* Axial CT images (**C, D**) confirm the type I coracoid fracture *(arrows)* extending into the glenoid fossa.

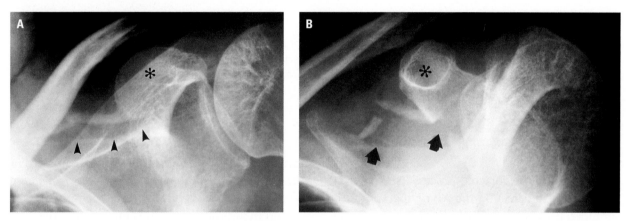

Figure 8.72. Comminuted type I coracoid fracture. On the frontal projection of the shoulder (**A**), the coracoid process *(asterisk)* appears in normal position. A horizontal lucent defect *(arrowheads)* suggests a fracture of the base of the coracoid process. The displacement of the coracoid process *(asterisk)* and the degree of comminution of its base fracture *(arrows)* is recorded in the oblique view (**B**).

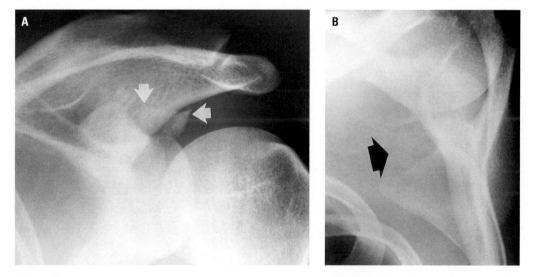

Figure 8.73. The location and significance of the fracture on the AP radiograph *(white arrows,* **A**) is not apparent from this perspective. The widened coracoclavicular space should suggest a type I coracoid fracture, which is clearly evident on the scapular Y view (**B**) *(arrow).*

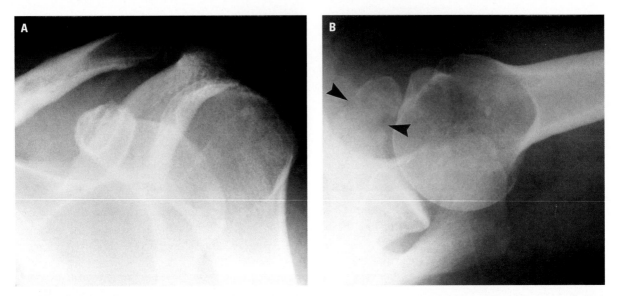

Figure 8.74. Type II fracture of the coracoid process of the scapula. On the internally rotated frontal projection (**A**), the fracture is not discernible. On the axillary projection (**B**), however, the transverse, slightly displaced, and distracted fracture is clearly evident *(arrowheads)*.

The treatment usually requires open reduction and internal fixation.

Fractures of the coracoid process itself (type II) are difficult to detect on the AP radiograph of the shoulder, because the coracoid process projects almost directly anteriorly on this projection. The long axis of the coracoid process is essentially parallel to the central x-ray beam, and unless the coracoid fragments are grossly displaced, they are usually not visible on frontal examinations of the shoulder. Fractures of the coracoid process are clearly delineated in the axillary projection (Figs. 8.74 and 8.75). These type II injuries are typically treated conservatively.

Acromial process fractures may involve the base (spinous process) (Fig. 8.76), the acromion itself (Fig. 8.77), or its tip (Fig. 8.78). Acromial process fractures do not usually occur at the site of the normal acromion apophysis (Fig. 8.6).

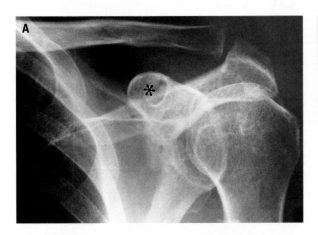

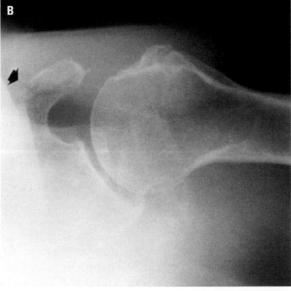

Figure 8.75. The coracoid process *(asterisk)* appears normal in the AP shoulder radiograph (**A**). The minimally displaced type II coracoid fracture, however, is clearly evident *(arrow)* on the axillary projection (**B**).

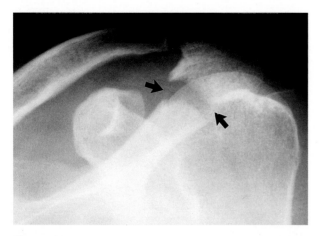

Figure 8.76. Distracted fracture of the acromial process (*arrows*).

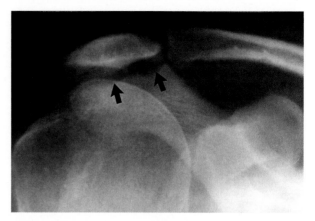

Figure 8.78. Fracture of tip of the acromial process (*arrows*).

The radiographic characteristics of the apophyseal physes are sufficiently different from those of a fracture line that the radiologic distinction should be readily apparent. These differences have been described and illustrated earlier.

Scapulothoracic Disassociation

Scapulothoracic dissociation is lateral displacement of the scapula with respect to the thorax, usually as a result of massive blunt chest trauma.[61–63]

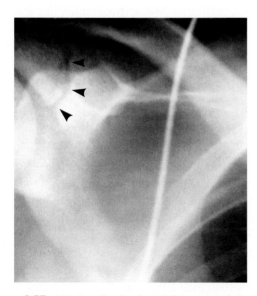

Figure 8.77. Minimally displaced fracture of the base of the acromion (*arrowheads*) in a mature adult. The fracture line, while at approximately the level of the apophyseal physis, is comminuted, curves dorsally, and has none of the characteristics of a physis.

Clinically, scapulothoracic disassociation is manifested by a large hematoma involving the axilla that extends into the adjacent anterolateral chest wall and arm and by some expression of brachial plexus injury.

Radiographically, the diagnosis is typically not readily apparent on the initial supine chest radiograph, because the scapulae are usually not sufficiently included for the lateral displacement to be recognized. Therefore, the radiographic diagnosis must depend on a high index of suspicion prompted by such findings as lateral sternoclavicular separation (Fig. 8.79), distracted clavicular fragments (Fig. 8.80), segmented clavicular fracture, and AC separation or fracture-separation (Fig. 8.81), particularly when the AC space is widened transversely. As a consequence of these injuries, the AP radiograph of the shoulder will demonstrate the scapula to be laterally displaced with respect to the lateral chest wall.

Soft Tissue Injuries of the Shoulder

Acute soft tissue injuries of the shoulder may prompt an emergency center visit because of pain, tenderness, and limitation of motion of the shoulder. The history and physical examination are usually sufficient to reasonably suspect the diagnosis. The indication for radiograph examination of the shoulder is to exclude other possible etiologies for the patient's complaints, since most soft tissue injuries of the shoulder are not visible on conventional radiographs. Traditional arthrography (without

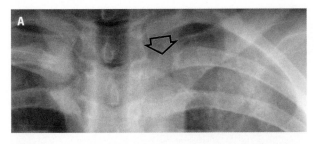

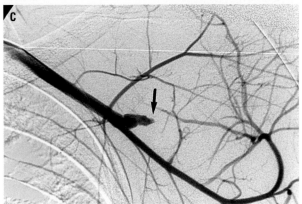

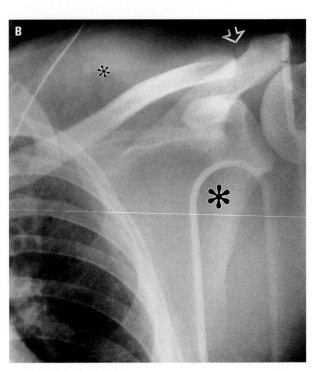

Figure 8.79. Scapulothoracic dissociation. On the AP radiograph of the sternoclavicular joints (**A**), the left sternoclavicular joint is widened *(open arrow)*. The AP radiograph of the shoulder (**B**) shows a large ill-defined soft tissue density filling the supraclavicular space *(small asterisk)* and the axilla and extending onto the chest wall and arm *(large asterisk)*. Additionally, the left acromioclavicular joint is wide *(open arrow)*. The left brachial artery (**C**) shows complete transection of one of its major branches *(arrow)* and compressive attenuation of the distal brachial artery and its branches by the hematoma.

CT or MRI) is rarely indicated today. CT and MRI are both useful in assessing for glenohumeral joint instability, glenoid labrum, and supraspinatus injury. MRI is currently the imaging modality of choice because of excellent soft tissue contrast, the ability to recognize fractures, and multiplanar capability.[64–66]

MRI, including MR arthrography, has a greater than 90% sensitivity in detection of full-thickness tears of the rotator cuff but is less sensitive in the detection of partial-thickness tears.[67–70]

NONTRAUMATIC CONDITIONS

Nontraumatic conditions affecting the shoulder may produce acute or severe symptoms. One of the most common of these is bursitis, which may be inflammation of either a periarticular bursa or a tendon. Periarticular soft tissue calcification, or "calcifying peritendinitis," associated with acute periarticular inflammation may resemble a thin cortical fracture fragment (Fig. 8.82). The radiographic characteristics of the calcific deposit and the absence of an acute traumatic history aid in establishing the true etiology of this soft tissue calcification. The presence of periarticular calcification

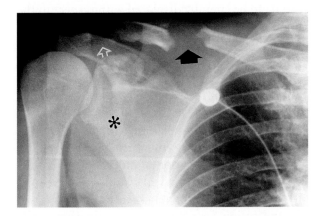

Figure 8.80. Scapulothoracic dissociation secondary to laterally distracted clavicular fragments *(arrow)* and acromioclavicular separation *(white open arrow)*. The large, ill-defined axillary soft tissue mass *(asterisk)* represents the hematoma.

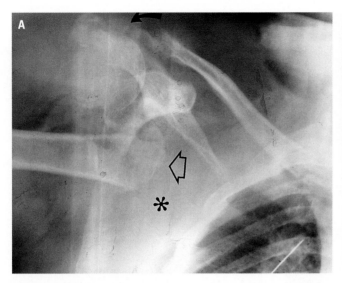

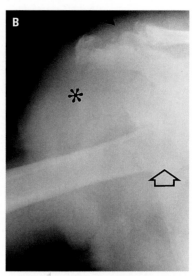

Figure 8.81. Scapulothoracic dissociation with acromioclavicular (AC) fracture-separation and displaced surgical neck humeral fracture. Both the AP (**A**) and axillary (**B**) radiographs show the horizontally distracted AC fracture-separation *(curved arrows)*. The fractures involve both the distal clavicle and the acromion. The scapula is laterally displaced and a large hematoma involves the axilla *(asterisk, **A**)* and shoulder *(asterisk, **B**)*. The humeral surgical neck fracture with infraglenoid displacement of the distal fragment *(open arrow)* is visible on each projection.

has no relevance to the presence or absence of clinical signs or symptoms.

Pathologic fractures occurring in benign (Fig. 8.83) or malignant (Fig. 8.84) bone lesions may occur spontaneously or as the result of minimal, commonly unrecognized trauma. These fractures may produce all of the clinical signs and symptoms of an acute fracture of normal bone. Osteomyelitis

of the humeral head (Fig. 8.85) and areas of avascular necrosis in the proximal third of the humerus secondary to hemophilia disease may cause acute symptoms relative to the shoulder (Fig. 8.86).

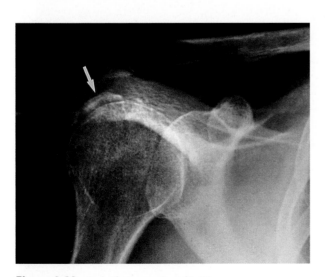

Figure 8.82. Calcifying peritendinitis.

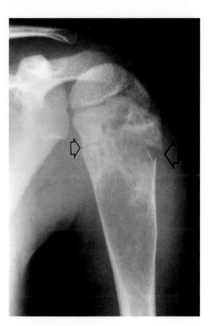

Figure 8.83. Pathologic fracture *(open arrows)* through an aneurysmal bone cyst.

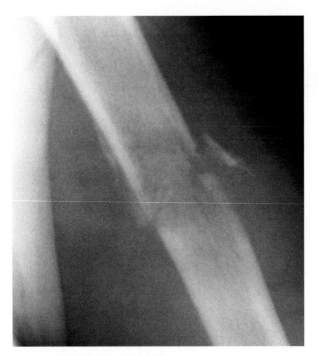

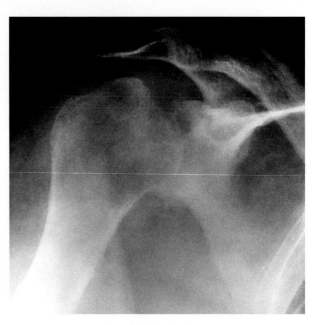

Figure 8.84. Pathologic fracture of lytic metastatic focus in the proximal third of the humerus. All the radiographic characteristics of this process, including the periosteal reaction, are those of an aggressive lesion.

Figure 8.85. Osteomyelitis of the humeral head. Note the irregular demineralization of the head and neck as well as destruction and erosion of the articulating surface of the head and glenoid fossa.

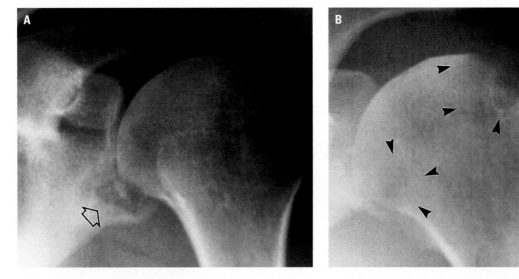

Figure 8.86. Avascular necrosis of the glenoid fossa (*open arrow*, **A**) and the humeral head (*arrowheads*, **B**) in a patient with hemophilia.

REFERENCES

1. Inman VT, Saunders JB, Abbott LC. Observations on function of the shoulder joint. 1944. *Clin Orthop Relat Res.* 1996;(330):3–12.
2. Swischuk LE. *Emergency Imaging of the Acutely Ill or Injured Child.* 3rd ed. Baltimore, MD: Lippincott Williams & Wilkins, 1994.
3. Pavlov H, Freiberger RH. Fractures and dislocations about the shoulder. *Semin Roentgenol.* 1978;13(2):85–96.
4. Keats TE, Pope TL Jr. The acromioclavicular joint: normal variation and the diagnosis of dislocation. *Skeletal Radiol.* 1988;17(3):159–162.
5. Kern JW, Harris JH Jr. Case report 752: normal variant of the acromion simulating grade I acromioclavicular separation. *Skeletal Radiol.* 1992;21(6):419–420.
6. Cave EF, Burke JF, Boyd RJ. *Trauma Management.* Chicago, IL: Year Book Medical Publishers; 1974.
7. Søndergård-Petersen P, Mikkelsen P. Posterior acromioclavicular dislocation. *J Bone Joint Surg Br.* 1982;64(1):52–53.
8. Schwarz N, Kuderna H. Inferior acromioclavicular separation. Report of unusual case. *Clin Orthop Relat Res.* 1988;(234):28–30.
9. Hastings DE, Horne JG. Anterior dislocation of the acromioclavicular joint. *Injury.* 1979;10(4):285–288.
10. Georgiadis GM, Wilson RF. Musculoskeletal trauma. In: Wilson RF, Walt AJ, eds. *Management and Trauma.* 2nd ed. Baltimore, MD: Lippincott Williams & Wilkins; 1996:648.
11. Carr AJ, Broughton NS. Acromioclavicular dislocation associated with fracture of the coracoid process. *J Trauma.* 1989;29(1):125–126.
12. Conwell HE, Reynolds FC. *Key and Conwell's Management of Fractures, Dislocations and Sprains.* 7th ed. St Louis, MO: Mosby; 1961.
13. Rockwood CA Jr, Green DP, Bucholz RW, eds. *Rockwood and Green's Fractures in Adults.* 3rd ed. Philadelphia, PA: JB Lippincott Co.; 1991.
14. Rowe CR. Instabilities of the glenohumeral joint. *Bull Hosp Joint Dis.* 1978;39(2):180–186.
15. Berquist TH, ed. *Imaging of Orthopaedic Trauma and Surgery.* Philadelphia, PA: WB Saunders; 1986.
16. Rockwood CA Jr, Green DP, Bucholz RW. *Rockwood and Green's Fractures in Adults.* 4th ed. Philadelphia, PA: JB Lippincott Co.; 1996:1213–1237.
17. Green A, Norris TR. Glenohumeral dislocations. In: Browner BD, Jupiter JB, Levine AM, Trafton PG, eds. *Skeletal Trauma: Fractures, Dislocations, Ligamentous Injuries.* 2nd ed. Philadelphia, PA: WB Saunders; 1998:1639–1640.
18. Weissman BNW, Sledge CB. *Orthopedic Radiology.* Philadelphia, PA: WB Saunders; 1986.
19. Green A, Norris TR, Glenohumeral dislocations. In: Browner BD, Jupiter JB, Levin AM. Trafton PG, eds. *Skeletal Trauma: Fractures, Dislocations, Ligamentous Injuries.* 2nd ed. Philadelphia, PA: WB Saunders; 1998:1649.
20. Hovelius L, Augustini BG, Fredin H, et al. Primary anterior dislocation of the shoulder in young patients. A ten-year prospective study. *J Bone Joint Surg Am.* 1996;78(11):1677–1684.
21. Bankart AS. Recurrent or habitual dislocation of the shoulder-joint. *Br Med J.* 1923;2(3285):1132–1133.
22. Helms CA. *Fundamentals of Skeletal Radiology.* Philadelphia, PA: WB Saunders; 1989.
23. Pavlov H, Freiberger RH. Shoulder. In: Felson B, ed. *Roentgenology of Fractures and Dislocations.* New York, NY: Grune & Stratton; 1978:79–90.
24. Ribbans WJ, Mitchell R, Taylor GJ. Computerized arthrotomography of primary anterior dislocations of the shoulder. *J Bone Joint Surg Br.* 1990;72(2):181–185.
25. Hintermann B, Gächter A. Arthroscopic findings after shoulder dislocation. *Am J Sports Med.* 1995;23(5):545–551.
26. Hill HA, Sachs MD. The grooved defect of the humeral head: a frequently unrecognized complication of dislocations of the shoulder joint. *Radiology.* 1940;35:690–700.
27. Kuhnen W, Groves RJ. Irreducible acute anterior dislocation of the shoulder: case report. *Clin Orthop Relat Res.* 1979;(139):167–168.
28. Seradge H, Orme G. Acute irreducible anterior dislocation of the shoulder. *J Trauma.* 1982;22(4):330–332.
29. McLaughlin HL. Dislocation of the shoulder with tuberosity fracture. *Surg Clin North Am.* 1963;43:1615–1620.
30. Freundlich BD. Luxatio erecta. *J Trauma.* 1983;23(5):434–436.
31. Downey EF Jr, Curtis DJ, Brower AC. Unusual dislocations of the shoulder. *AJR Am J Roentgenol.* 1983;140(6):1207–1210.
32. Rockwood CA, Wirth MA. Subluxation and dislocations about the G-H joint. In: Rockwood CA, Green DR, Burkolz RW, Heckman JD, eds. *Rockwood and Green's fractures in Adults.* 4th ed. Philadelphia, PA: Lippincott–Raven Publishers; 1996:1306–1309.
33. Lev-El A, Adar R, Rubinstein Z. Axillary injury in erect dislocation of the shoulder. *J Trauma.* 1981;21(4):323–325.
34. Wilson JC, McKeever FM. Traumatic posterior dislocation of humerus. *J Bone Joint Surg Am.* 1946;31A(1):160–172.
35. Wood JP. Posterior dislocation of head of humerus and diagnostic value of lateral and vertical view. *U.S. Navy Medical Bulletin.* 1941;39:532–535.

36. Nobel W. Posterior traumatic dislocation of the shoulder. *J Bone Joint Surg Am.* 1962;44A:523–538.

37. Hawkins RJ, Neer CS II, Pianta RM, et al. Locked posterior dislocation of the shoulder. *J Bone Joint Surg Am.* 1987;69(1):9–18.

38. Arndt JH, Sears AD. Posterior dislocation of the shoulder. *Am J Roentgenol Radium Ther Nucl Med.* 1965;94:639–645.

39. Detenbeck LC. Posterior dislocations of the shoulder. *J Trauma.* 1972;12(3):183–192.

40. Brown WH, Dennis JM, Davidson CN, et al. Posterior dislocation of the shoulder. *Radiology.* 1957;69(6):815–822.

41. Cisternino SJ, Rogers LF, Stufflebaum BC, et al. The trough line: a radiographic sign of posterior shoulder dislocation. *AJR Am J Roentgenol.* 1978;130(5):951–954.

42. Figiel SJ, Figiel LS, Bardenstein MB, et al. Posterior dislocation of the shoulder. *Radiology.* 1966;87(4):737–740.

43. Laskin RS, Schreiber S. Inferior subluxation of the humeral head: the drooping shoulder. *Radiology.* 1971;98(3):585–586.

44. Neer CS II. Displaced proximal humeral fractures. I. Classification and evaluation. *J Bone Joint Surg Am.* 1970;52(6):1077–1089.

45. Kristiansen B, Andersen UL, Olsen CA, et al. The Neer classification of fractures of the proximal humerus. An assessment of interobserver variation. *Skeletal Radiol.* 1988;17(6):420–422.

46. Brien H, Noftall F, MacMaster S, et al. Neer's classification system: a critical appraisal. *J Trauma.* 1995;38(2):257–260.

47. Bernstein J, Adler LM, Blank JE, et al. Evaluation of the Neer system of classification of proximal humeral fractures with computerized tomographic scans and plain radiographs. *J Bone Joint Surg Am.* 1996;78(9):1371–1375.

48. Stanley D, Trowbridge EA, Norris SH. The mechanism of clavicle fracture. A clinical and biomechanical analysis. *J Bone Joint Surg Br.* 1988;70(3): 461–464.

49. Allman FL Jr. Fractures and ligamentous injuries of the clavicle and its articulation. *J Bone Joint Surg Am.* 1967;49(4):774–784.

50. Lee J, Harris JH Jr, Duke JH Jr, et al. Noncorrelation between thoracic skeletal injuries and acute traumatic aortic tear. *J Trauma.* 1997;43(3):400–404.

51. Rowe CR. Fractures of the scapula. *Surg Clin North Am.* 1963;43:1565–1571.

52. Harris RD, Harris JH Jr. The prevalence and significance of missed scapular fractures in blunt chest trauma. *AJR Am J Roentgenol.* 1988;151(4):747–750.

53. Hardegger FH, Simpson LA, Weber BG. The operative treatment of scapular fractures. *J Bone Joint Surg Br.* 1984;66(5):725–731.

54. McGahan JP, Rab GT, Dublin A. Fractures of the scapula. *J Trauma.* 1980;20(10):880–883.

55. Imatani RJ. Fractures of the scapula: a review of 53 fractures. *J Trauma.* 1975;15(6):473–478.

56. Findlay RT. Fractures of the scapula and the ribs. *Am J Surg.* 1937;38:489–494.

57. Mariani PP. Isolated fracture of the coracoid process in an athlete. *Am J Sports Med.* 1980;8(2): 129–130.

58. Zilberman Z, Rejovitzky R. Fracture of the coracoid process of the scapula. *Injury.* 1981;13(3):203–206.

59. Martín-Herrero T, Rodriguez-Merchán C, Munuera-Martínez L. Fractures of the coracoid process: presentation of seven cases and review of the literature. *J Trauma.* 1990;30(12):1597–1599.

60. Ogawa K, Yoshida A, Takahishi M, et al. Fractures of the coracoid process. *J Bone Joint Surg Br.* 1997;79(1):17–19.

61. Oreck SL, Burgess A, Levine AM. Traumatic lateral displacement of the scapula: a radiologic sign of neurovascular disruption. *J Bone Joint Surg Am.* 1984;66(5):758–763.

62. Rubenstein JD, Ebraheim NA, Kellam JF. Traumatic scapulothoracic dissociation. *Radiology.* 1985;157(2):297–298.

63. Mirvis SE, Sheafor DH. Scapulothoracic dissociation: report of five cases and review of the literature. *Emerg Radiol.* 1995;2(5):279–284.

64. Hodler J. Imaging methods. *Ther Umsch.* 1998; 55(3):169–174.

65. Deutsch AL, Klein MA, Mink JH, et al. MR imaging of miscellaneous disorders of the shoulder. *Magn Reson Imaging Clin N Am.* 1997;5(4):881–895.

66. Tan RK. A review of the role of magnetic resonance imaging in the evaluation of shoulder impingement syndrome and rotator cuff tendon tears. *Ann Acad Med Singapore.* 1998;27(2):243–247.

67. Zlatkin MB, Dalinka MK, Kressel HY. Magnetic resonance imaging of the shoulder. *Magn Reson Q.* 1989;5(1):3–22.

68. Rafii M, Firooznia H, Sherman O, et al. Rotator cuff lesions: signal patterns at MR imaging. *Radiology.* 1990;177(3):817–823.

69. Uri DS. MR imaging of shoulder impingement and rotator cuff disease. *Radiol Clin North Am.* 1997;35(1):77–96.

70. Rafii M. Shoulder. In: Firooznia H, Golimbu CN, Rafii M, eds. *MRI and CT of the Musculoskeletal System.* St. Louis, MO: Mosby–Year Book; 1992:515.

SUGGESTED READINGS

1. Helms, CA. *Fundamentals of Skeletal Radiology.* 3rd ed. Philadelphia, PA: WB Saunders; 2005.
2. Taylor JAM, Resnick D. *Skeletal Imaging: Atlas of the Spine and Extremities.* Philadelphia, PA: WB Saunders; 2000: 808, 813, 863.
3. Greenspan A. *Orthopedic Imaging: A Practical Approach.* 4th ed. Philadelphia, PA: Lippincott Williams and Wilkins; 2004.
4. Chew FS. *Musculoskeletal Imaging.* Philadelphia, PA: Lippincott Williams and Wilkins; 2003: 58–60, 72–75.
5. Nordin M. Frankel VH, eds. *Basic Biomechanics of the Musculoskeletal System.* 3rd ed. Philadelphia, PA: Lippincott Williams and Wilkins; 2001: 318–339.
6. Jeffery RB, Manaster BJ, Gurney JW, et al. *Diagnostic Imaging: Emergency Radiology.* Salt Lake City, UT: Amirsys Inc.; 2007: I436–I455.
7. Manaster BJ, May DA, Disler DG. *Musculoskeletal Imaging.* 3rd ed. Philadelphia, PA: Mosby; 2007: 67–76.

CHAPTER 9

Elbow

Sarah Yanny ■ Eugene McNally ■ Thomas L. Pope Jr.

GENERAL CONSIDERATIONS

Radiographic Examination

Standard radiographic examination of the elbow includes anteroposterior (AP) and lateral views (Fig. 9.1). The AP view should be obtained with the elbow fully extended, the forearm fully supinated (if possible), and the fingers slightly flexed. The central beam is directed perpendicular to the elbow joint. There should be no rotation of the forearm. The lateral view should be obtained with the elbow at 90 degrees of flexion and the forearm in a neutral position with the thumb pointing upward. The vertical central beam is centered over the lateral epicondyle of the humerus. If the limb cannot be moved, two perpendicular projections can be taken by rotating the x-ray tube.

When a fracture of the radial head, coronoid process, or capitellum is suspected, a radial head-capitellar view, a variant of the lateral view, should be obtained (Fig. 9.2). The elbow is positioned at 90 degrees of flexion, the forearm resting on its ulnar side with the thumb pointing upward, and the central beam directed at the radial head with a 45 degrees angle to the forearm.

In children, oblique projections may be useful if the routine views do not demonstrate a fracture but a joint effusion is present. Internal oblique views are valuable when humeral lateral condylar fractures are suspected. Comparison views of the other elbow should not be part of routine radiographic practice and should only be performed in exceptional circumstances.

Computed tomography (CT) may be indicated in the context of severe or complex injuries, dislocations, and foreign bodies. Magnetic resonance imaging (MRI) is useful in the detection of soft tissue and ligamentous injury, radiographically occult fractures, osteochondral injuries, and is of particular use in children to detect injury of the nonossified epiphysis. Ultrasound (US) is widely used in the context of soft tissue injuries, whether acute or chronic, and can detect intra-articular injury following trauma by demonstration of a lipohemarthrosis.

Anatomy

The elbow is a complex pivotal-hinge synovial joint with three articulations (the humeroulnar, radiocapitellar, and proximal radioulnar joints). Flexion-extension occurs mostly at the humeroulnar articulation (uniaxial joint), whereas pronation-supination occurs at the radiocapitellar and radioulnar articulations. The joint is held together by a fibrous capsule, the deep surface of which is lined by synovium. Three fat pads rest in the radial, coronoid, and olecranon fossae. They are enveloped by fibers of the joint capsule separating the fat pads from the synovial lining, making them intracapsular and extrasynovial. The articulating surfaces of the head of the radius and ulna are held together by the annular ligament. The capsule is weak anteriorly and posteriorly, but joint stability is reinforced by the medial (ulnar)

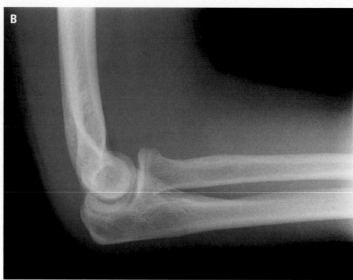

Figure 9.1. Routine radiographic examination of the elbow. Anteroposterior (**A**) and lateral view (**B**).

and lateral (radial) collateral ligament complexes. The flexor-pronator group of muscles originates from the medial epicondyle, whereas the extensor-supinator muscles attach to the lateral epicondyle. The ulnar nerve courses posterior to the medial epicondyle and is closely applied to the ulnar collateral ligament, passing between the heads of flexor carpi ulnaris.

Ossification of the elbow is complex. Careful and systematic assessment of the pediatric elbow is essential, particularly in the context of avulsion of the epicondylar apophyses. The distal humerus has four secondary ossification centers; those for the capitellum and trochlea, which comprise the articular surface, and those for the medial and lateral epicondyles (Fig. 9.3). The acronym "CRITOL" is often used to describe the usual order of the six ossification centers of the elbow (capitellum, radial head, internal [medial] epicondyle, trochlea, olecranon, lateral [external] epicondyle). The capitellar ossification center appears at 1 to 2 years of age, the radial head at 2 to 4 years, the internal epicondyle at 4 to 6 years, the trochlea at 8 to 11 years, the olecranon at 9 to 11 years, and the lateral epicondyle at 10 to 11 years. The age at which these centers are first seen varies considerably and usually proceeds earlier in girls than in boys. The main role of CRITOL is to highlight that the medial epicondyle center should be present before the trochlea. If following trauma a trochlear center is visible and the medial epicondyle is not, a displaced medial epicondyle should be suspected.

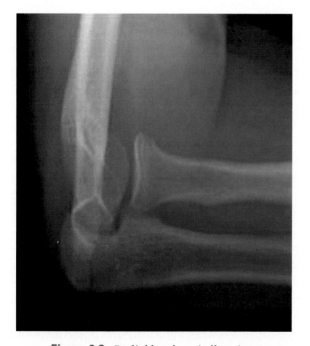

Figure 9.2. Radial head-capitellar view.

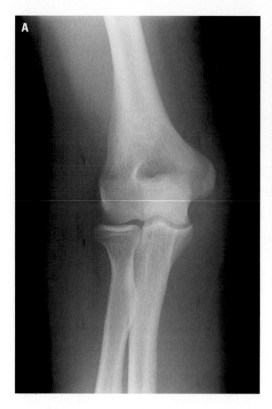

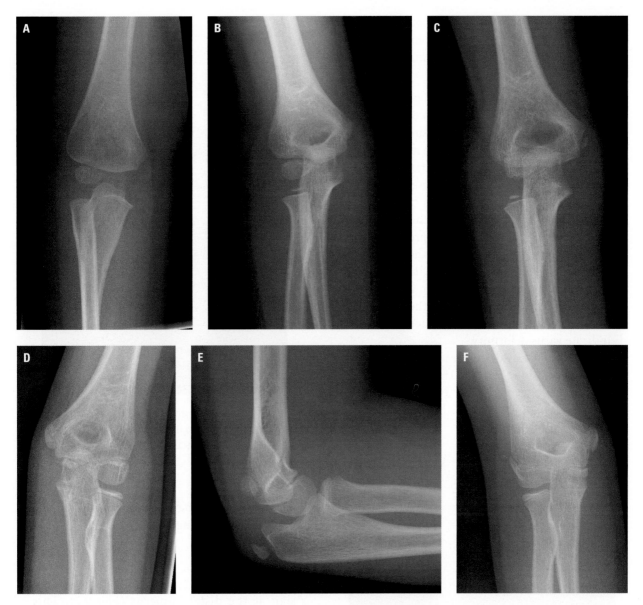

Figure 9.3. Serial radiographs showing the typical sequence of appearance of ossification centers of the elbow. "CRITOL": capitellum, radial head, internal (medial) epicondyle, trochlea, olecranon, lateral (external) epicondyle.

Ununited ossification centers may persist unfused into adulthood and may be confused with avulsion fractures. The trochlea has two or more ossification centers, which may result in a fragmented appearance. The olecranon may also be very irregular during its normal development. The medial epicondyle fuses directly with the humerus, whereas the lateral epicondyle fuses first with the capitellum, then both fuse with the humeral shaft. This often causes the lateral epicondyle to appear widely separated from the humerus due to the thicker cartilaginous plate associated with it.

Landmarks

Fracture lines can be difficult to visualize after acute elbow injury, particularly in children. Important landmarks should be reviewed to confirm the adequacy of the radiograph and aid in recognition of occult signs of injury.

Anteroposterior View

A common complication of supracondylar fracture is an abnormal carrying angle. In full extension and supination, the forearm lies at 165 degrees to the humerus (15 degrees of valgus) to clear the hips. The angle is greater in females. Various angles are measured on AP radiographs to determine the proper alignment of the distal humerus.

1. The humeroulnar angle is the angle formed between the long axis of the humerus and the long axis of the ulna, and normally measures 154 degrees to 178 degrees (Fig. 9.4). This angle most accurately depicts the true carrying angle of the elbow.
2. Baumann's angle or the shaft-physeal angle is the angle created between the longitudinal axis of the humerus and a line through the physis of the lateral condyle (Fig 9.5), and is predictive of an acceptable carrying angle. This should measure approximately 70 degrees and within 5 degrees that of the contralateral uninjured elbow. This angle is helpful in determining the adequacy of reduction of a supracondylar fracture and may indicate varus deformity.
3. The metaphyseal-diaphyseal angle is formed between the long axis of the humerus and a line connecting the lateral and medial epicondyles (Fig. 9.6). This ranges from 72 degrees to

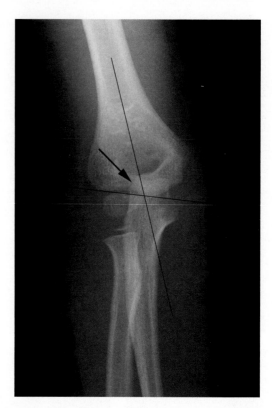

Figure 9.5. Baumann's angle *(arrow)* is the angle created between the longitudinal axis of the humerus and the coronal axis of the capitellar physis.

95 degrees but is the least reliable estimate of the clinical carrying angle.

Lateral View

1. The "hourglass," "teardrop," or "figure eight" sign at the distal humerus (Fig. 9.7). This is formed by the anterior margin of the olecranon fossa and the posterior margin of the coronoid fossa. The inferior portion of the teardrop should be the ossification center of the capitellum. The capitellum and trochlea should be superimposed. If not, the image is likely not a true lateral and interpretation of the remaining observations is less reliable.
2. The fat pad sign. Normally on a lateral radiograph, lucency that represents fat is present along the anterior aspect of the distal humerus, and no lucency is visualized along the posterior cortex. An elevated anterior lucency—the radiographic "sail sign"—and/or a visible posterior lucency is described as a positive fat pad sign (Fig. 9.8), although this is not as specific as a positive posterior fat pad.

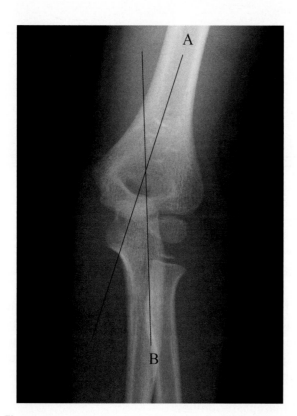

Figure 9.4. The humeroulnar angle formed between the long axis of the humerus (**A**) and long axis of the ulna (**B**). This angle most accurately depicts the true carrying angle of the elbow.

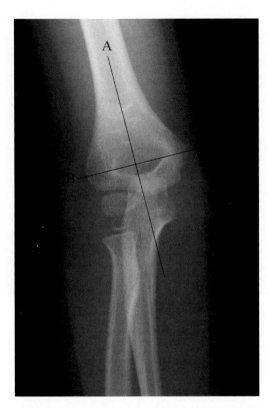

Figure 9.6. The metaphyseal-diaphyseal angle formed between the long axis of the humerus (A) and a line connecting the lateral and medial epicondyles (B).

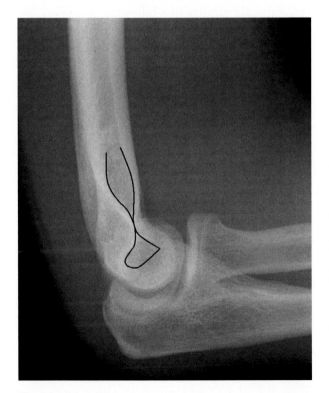

Figure 9.7. Teardrop or figure eight sign at the distal humerus. This is formed by the anterior margin of the olecranon fossa and the posterior margin of the coronoid fossa.

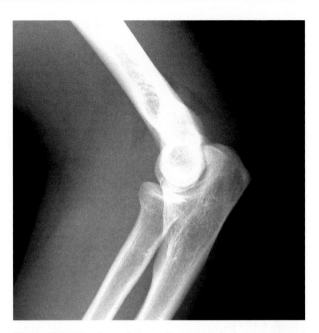

Figure 9.8. The fat pad sign. The elevated anterior fat pad and posterior fat pad are, following trauma, consistent with hemarthrosis.

3. The anterior humeral line (Fig. 9.9). A line drawn along the anterior cortex of the humerus should intersect the middle third of the capitellum on the lateral view. Supracondylar fractures usually result in displacement of the capitellum posteriorly with resultant displacement of the anterior humeral line anteriorly.
4. The radiocapitellar line (Fig. 9.10). A line drawn along the center of the proximal radius should

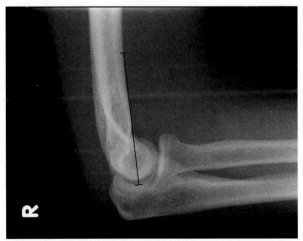

Figure 9.9. The anterior humeral line. A line along the anterior cortex of the humerus should intersect the middle third of the capitellum.

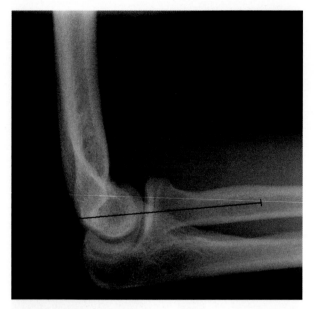

Figure 9.10. Radiocapitellar line. A line along the center of the radius should intersect the capitellum.

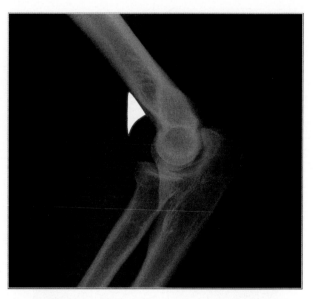

Figure 9.11. A visible anterior fat pad may be normal, but is displaced anteriorly and superiorly in the presence of joint distention to form a triangular shape, with a convex anterior margin similar to a billowing spinnaker sail.

normally bisect the capitellum on both the lateral and the AP elbow radiograph. Failure of alignment suggests dislocation of the radial head. This requires prompt reduction because neurovascular compromise may ensue.

RADIOGRAPHIC MANIFESTATIONS OF TRAUMA

Evaluation of the soft tissues is important in elbow trauma. Soft tissue swelling may often be the most obvious radiographic abnormality in the setting of subtle or undisplaced fractures. Extracapsular soft tissue swelling may be diffuse or localized, such as to the radial or ulnar borders of the elbow in fractures of the lateral condyle or medial epicondyle, respectively.

As previously mentioned, three intracapsular fat pads are present between the synovium of the elbow and the joint capsule. The anterior fat pad is a summation of the radial and coronoid fat pads, which are normally pressed into the shallow radial and coronoid fossae by the brachialis muscle during extension. The posterior fat pad is normally pressed into the deep olecranon fossa by the triceps brachii tendon and anconeus muscle during flexion and the third lies over the supinator as it wraps over the radius.

Hemarthrosis or effusion into a structurally intact joint capsule causes distention of the joint

and displacement of the fat pads. A visible anterior fat pad may be normal, but if displaced anteriorly and superiorly in the presence of joint distention, it will form a triangular shape, with a convex anterior margin similar to a billowing spinnaker sail (Fig. 9.11). An atraumatic sail sign implies intra-articular fluid of an inflammatory nature (Fig. 9.12),

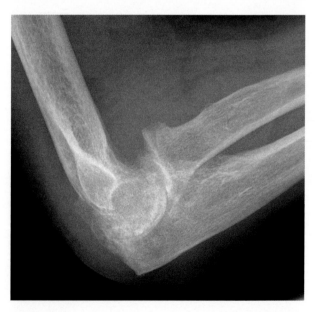

Figure 9.12. Advanced rheumatoid arthritis of the elbow with concentric joint space narrowing, subluxation of the radiocapitellar joint, and a moderate joint effusion.

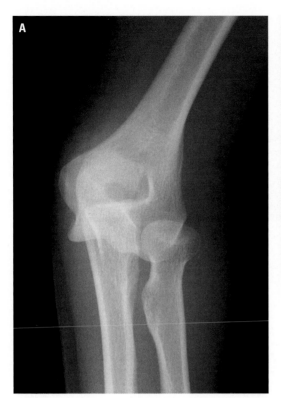
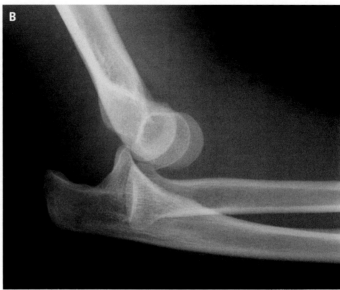

Figure 9.13. AP (**A**) and lateral (**B**) views of the elbow demonstrate simple posterior dislocation of the elbow.

although with chronicity, infiltration of the fat pad may obscure it. A visible posterior fat pad is always regarded as abnormal, signifying fluid in the intra-articular space. In the setting of acute trauma, an occult fracture should be sought, particularly of the radial head in adults or a supracondylar fracture in children. It must be remembered that an absent fat pad sign does not exclude a fracture. This may occur with poor positioning, capsular rupture (e.g., dislocations, displaced intra-articular fractures), or an extracapsular injury (e.g., medial and lateral epicondylar fractures).

Although one of the most stable joints in the body, dislocation and fracture-dislocation of the elbow are not uncommon. Elbow dislocations are second in frequency only to shoulder dislocations in adults, and the elbow is the most frequently dislocated joint in children. Elbow dislocations are classified as simple or complex. Simple dislocations are classified according to direction of displacement of the radius and/or ulna in relation to the distal humerus, namely posterior (Fig. 9.13), posterolateral, posteromedial, lateral, medial, or divergent. Fracture-dislocations are referred to as complex, the most common complex dislocation involving concomitant fracture of the radial head

(Fig. 9.14). Complications include vascular injury, particularly in the setting of open and/or anterior dislocations, where the brachial artery is disrupted by forcible hyperextension, and neuropraxia, most commonly involving the ulnar nerve or anterior interosseous branch of the median nerve. Long-term sequelae include valgus or posterolateral instability, which may result in recurrent elbow dislocation.

PEDIATRIC INJURIES

In children, the most common elbow fractures are supracondylar (60%), lateral condylar (15%), and medial epicondylar (10%).

Supracondylar Fractures

Supracondylar fractures are the most common pediatric fractures around the elbow and have a peak incidence in the first decade of life. They are extraarticular, lying beyond the proximal extensions of the joint capsule. They occur at a potential site

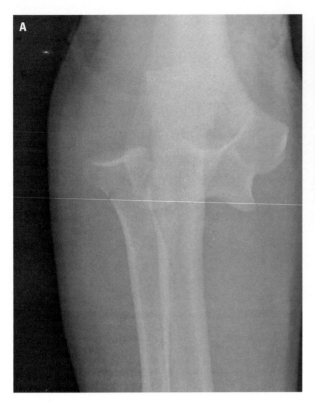

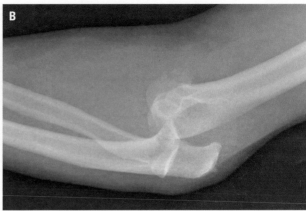

Figure 9.14. AP (**A**) and lateral (**B**) radiographs demonstrating a complex fracture-dislocation involving concomitant fracture of the radial head.

of weakness in the humeral metaphysis, which is relatively under-trabeculated in children. There are two types based on the mechanism of injury. The vast majority (96%) are extension injuries. Such fractures result from a fall on the outstretched hand with the elbow hyperextended. They result in posterior displacement or angulation of the distal fracture fragment. Conversely, the rarer flexion-type fractures are usually caused by a blow to the posterior aspect of the elbow resulting in anterior displacement of the distal fragment and are potentially very unstable. Supracondylar fractures may be complete or incomplete.

The anterior humeral line is useful in the diagnosis of supracondylar fractures, passing anterior to the middle third of the capitellum in most cases (Fig. 9.15). The most commonly used classification for extension fractures is the Gartland classification as modified by Wilkins, which divides them into three categories. Type I fractures are those with no or minimal displacement of the posterior fragment such that the anterior humeral line still intersects part of the capitellum (Fig. 9.16). Type II fractures are those with more posterior displacement or angulation but with an intact posterior cortical hinge (Fig. 9.17). Type III fractures are

displaced fractures with complete disruption of the cortex (Fig. 9.18).

Complications are common with a high incidence of malunion and nerve injury and a 0.5% to 5% incidence of vascular compromise. Vascular injury may be severe and results from injury to the brachial artery from posterior displacement of the distal fragment.

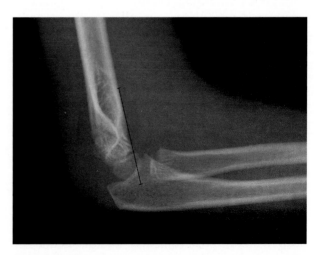

Figure 9.15. Supracondylar fracture. The anterior humeral line passes anterior to the middle third of the capitellum.

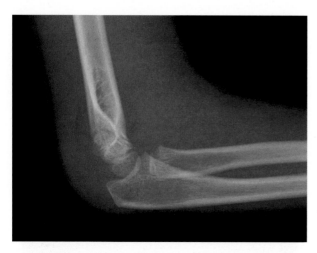

Figure 9.16. Gartland type I (undisplaced) supracondylar fracture. There is minimal displacement of the posterior fragment such that the anterior humeral line still intersects part of the capitellum.

This requires prompt reduction as delay may result in Volkmann's ischemic contracture, a permanent contracture of the forearm flexors resulting from ischemia/necrosis. Nerve injury occurs in approximately 5% of cases and most commonly involves the anterior interosseous branch of the median nerve.

Cubitus varus or valgus are late sequelae primarily resulting from inadequate fracture alignment rather than physeal injury. Varus deformity may

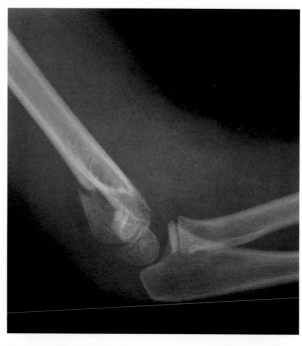

Figure 9.18. Gartland type III supracondylar fracture. This is a displaced fracture with complete disruption of the posterior cortex.

require treatment with an osteotomy at any age after stiffness has resolved.

Lateral Humeral Condyle Fractures

Fractures of the lateral condyle are the second most common elbow fracture in children and have a typical age range of 5 to 10 years. There are two primary mechanisms of injury. Most commonly, an acute varus stress is applied to an extended supinated forearm causing traction on extensor carpi radialis longus and brevis with avulsion of the lateral condyle. Alternatively, fall on an outstretched arm with an extended abducted forearm causes axial loading of the radius on the capitellum with consequent fracture of the lateral condyle.

Lateral condylar fractures are classified according to position of the fracture line.[1] A type I fracture is a Salter-Harris IV injury where the fracture line passes through the ossified capitellum (Fig. 9.19). These fractures enter the articular surface in the capitellar trochlear groove lateral to the lateral crista of the trochlea so that the ulnar articulation remains intact. The commoner Milch type II fractures are Salter-Harris II injuries where the fracture line

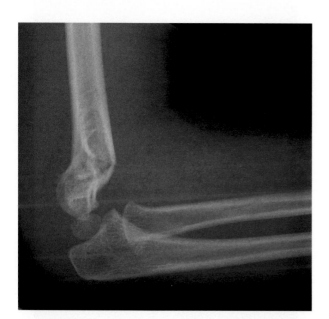

Figure 9.17. Gartland type II supracondylar fracture. Type II fractures are those with more posterior displacement or angulation, but with an intact posterior cortical hinge.

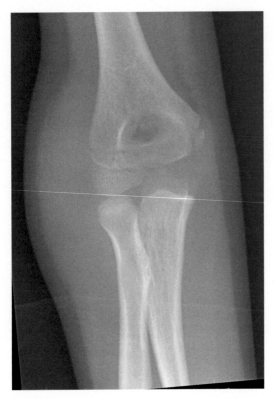

Figure 9.19. Type I Milch fracture. The fracture line passes through the ossified capitellum lateral to the lateral crista of the trochlea so that the ulna articulation remains intact.

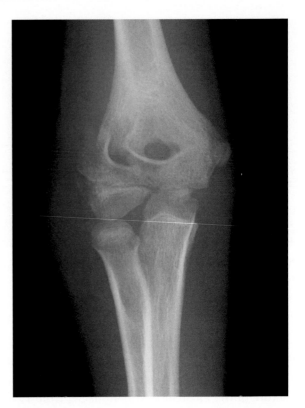

Figure 9.20. Milch type II fracture. The fracture line exits medial to the lateral crista, leading to humeroulnar joint instability.

passes medial to the lateral crista leading to joint instability (Fig. 9.20).

Radiographic diagnosis can be challenging and depends on the degree of capitellar ossification and the extent of displacement. Often, the only radiographic sign is a small sliver of displaced metaphyseal bone (Fig. 9.21). Depiction of undisplaced lateral condylar fractures may be subtle and may rely on lateral soft tissue swelling and the presence of a joint effusion.

Lateral humeral condylar fractures are unstable and are prone to displacement even when immobilized. Because these fractures are intra-articular, they are prone to non-union because the fracture is bathed in synovial fluid. Other complications include malunion and progressive cubitus valgus with lateral growth arrest and possible secondary ulnar nerve palsy.

Medial Epicondylar Fractures

Medial epicondylar fractures are the third most common fracture in the pediatric population, accounting for approximately 10% of fractures in

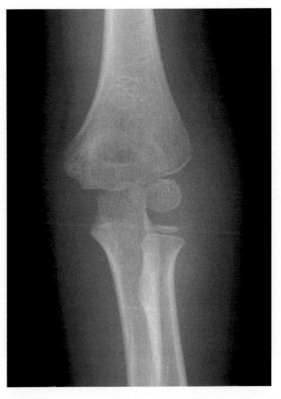

Figure 9.21. Lateral condylar fracture. Often the only radiographic sign is a small sliver of displaced metaphyseal bone.

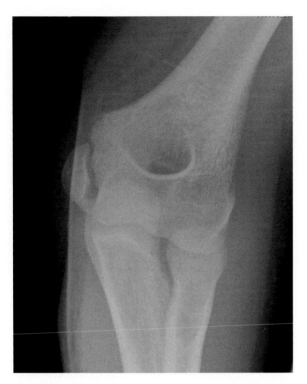

Figure 9.22. Rang type I medial epicondylar fracture.

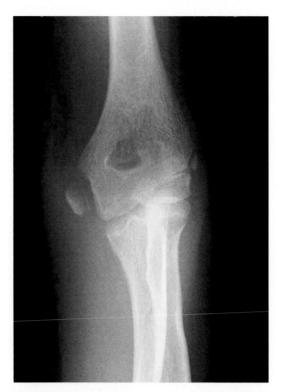

Figure 9.23. Moderately displaced Rang type II fracture of the medial epicondyle. There is localized soft tissue swelling medially.

children. They typically occur in boys (80%) in early adolescence between 9 and 14 years of age after the apophysis becomes a separate ossification nucleus and before it fuses with the distal humerus. Fractures of the medial epicondylar apophysis are avulsion injuries caused by traction from the ulnar collateral ligament or flexor forearm muscles and are almost always extraarticular.

The major mechanisms of injury include an acute valgus force on an outstretched elbow usually following a fall, frequently in association with elbow dislocation, and occasionally from acute or chronic traction from the flexor-pronator group of muscles such as that caused by throwing ("little leaguers elbow"). Occasionally, ulnar neuropraxia may occur due to intra-articular displacement and entrapment of the ulnar nerve.

Medial epicondylar apophyseal avulsions are classified based on the extent and pattern of displacement.[2] Rang Type I avulsions are minimally displaced (<2 mm) (Fig. 9.22); type II avulsions are moderately displaced (Fig. 9.23); type III avulsions are severely displaced with intra-articular interposition of the avulsed apophysis (Fig. 9.24); and type IV avulsions are displaced and associated with elbow dislocation (Fig. 9.25).

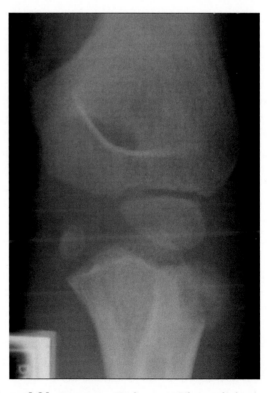

Figure 9.24. Rang type III fracture. The medial epicondyle is severely displaced with intra-articular interposition of the avulsed apophysis.

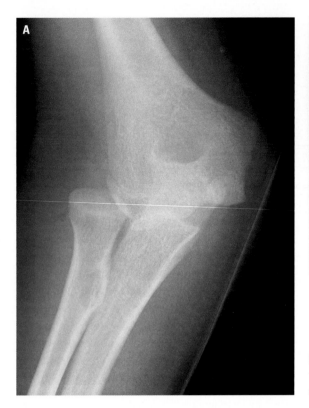

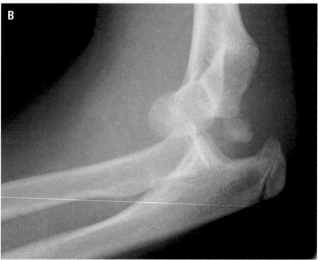

Figure 9.25. Rang type IV fracture, AP (**A**) and lateral (**B**) views. There is a displaced fracture of the medial epicondyle associated with elbow dislocation.

Radiographic diagnosis is based on AP and lateral views, where the normal alignment of the medial epicondyle is disrupted. With nondisplaced or minimally displaced fractures, the physis of the medial epicondyle may appear wider than normal. Correct identification of the normal sequence of ossification is necessary in the diagnosis of type III fractures. A displaced medial epicondyle lying within the elbow joint must not be confused with the expected position of the trochlear ossification center (Fig. 9.26) and may be best appreciated on the lateral view. The medial epicondyle is always ossified before the trochlea; thus, the trochlea should not be seen unless the medial epicondyle is also identified.

Avulsion fractures of the medial epicondyle may occur before ossification and may be suspected on plain radiographs due to the presence of localized tenderness, soft tissue swelling, and posterolateral dislocation. In such cases, US, MRI and/or CT arthrography may be useful in identification and depiction of the displaced cartilaginous fragment. MRI is also useful in the diagnosis of "little leaguers elbow" with demonstration of physeal widening and irregularity, periapophyseal edema, and signal changes in the common flexor origin.

Nursemaids Elbow

Subluxation of the radial head is the most common traumatic injury of the elbow in children and is known as "nursemaids elbow" or "pulled elbow." This is a relatively common injury seen in children between 1 and 5 years of age after longitudinal traction and forced pronation to the upper extremity. This usually occurs after a child is lifted up by the wrist, such as when an adult prevents a child from falling. The child refuses to use his or her arm and there is painful restricted supination. The mechanism of injury is either tear or slippage of the annular ligament over the radial head, allowing radial head subluxation. This occurs in young children because at this age the radial head is spherical and composed mainly of cartilage.

The diagnosis is largely clinical; however, imaging may be indicated if the history is unusual, reduction is unsuccessful, or to exclude more severe injuries such as radial head dislocation or fracture. Subluxation may be evident radiographically if the relative positions of the radius and capitellum are carefully assessed, with displacement of the radiocapitellar line. US and MRI can be used to demonstrate interposition of the annular ligament between the

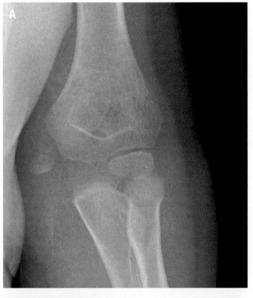

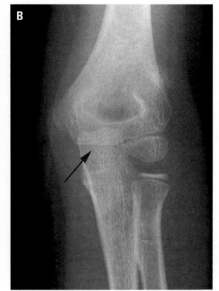

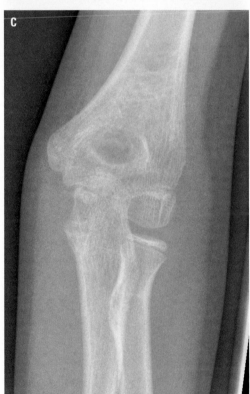

Figure 9.26. A displaced medial epicondyle lying within the elbow joint (**A**) must not be confused with the expected position of the trochlear ossification center (**B**, *arrow*). The trochlea should not be seen unless the medial epicondyle is also identified (**C**).

radial head and capitellum but are seldom needed to confirm the diagnosis.

ADULT INJURIES

In adults, 50% of fractures involve the radial head and neck, 20% involve the olecranon, and 10% are supracondylar.

Radial Head/Neck Fractures

Radial head fractures are the most common type of elbow fracture in adults, whereas fractures of the radial neck are more common in children. Radial head and neck fractures are usually the result of a fall on the outstretched hand with the force of the impact driving the radial head axially into the capitellum. The anterolateral aspect of the radial head

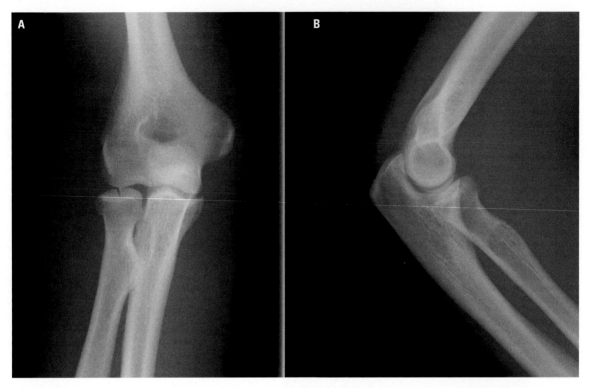

Figure 9.27. Mason type I (minimally displaced) radial head fracture. There is no mechanical block to rotation.

is particularly susceptible to injury due to its lack of strong subchondral bone. The most widely accepted classification of radial head and neck fractures was described.[3] Type I fractures are undisplaced (<2 mm, or marginal lip fracture) with no mechanical block to rotation (Fig. 9.27), type II are displaced (>2 mm) and may produce a mechanical block to motion (Fig. 9.28), and type III are comminuted and always cause a mechanical block (Fig. 9.29). The Johnston modification added a fourth type of radial fracture where there is concomitant dislocation of the elbow (Fig. 9.30).[4]

Associated injuries include posterior dislocation of the elbow, dislocation of the distal radioulnar joint (Essex Lopresti), fractures of the proximal ulna (Monteggia fracture), capitellum, coronoid process, or olecranon, and valgus instability due to medial collateral ligament rupture. The "terrible triad" is a term used to describe posterior dislocations of the elbow associated with both fractures of the radial head and coronoid process (Fig. 9.31) because of the difficult challenges involved in its management.

Diagnosis relies on standard AP and lateral views. The radiocapitellar view, a modified lateral view with the forearm in neutral rotation and the x-ray tube angled 45 degrees cephalad, can be useful

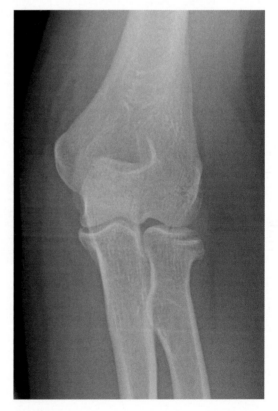

Figure 9.28. Mason type II radial head fractures are displaced (>2 mm) and may produce a mechanical block to rotation.

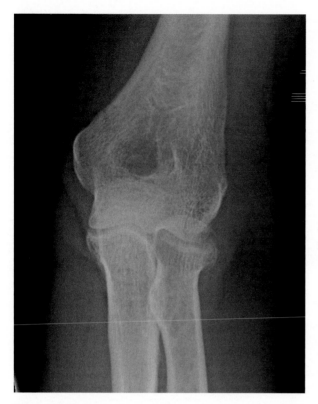

Figure 9.29. Comminuted Mason type III radial head fracture. This results in a mechanical block to rotation.

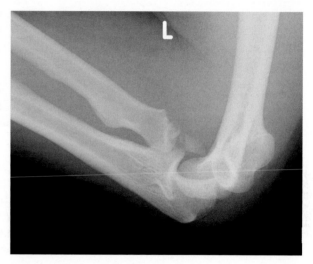

Figure 9.30. Comminuted radial head fracture with concomitant dislocation of the elbow.

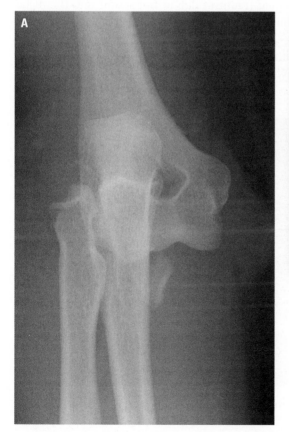

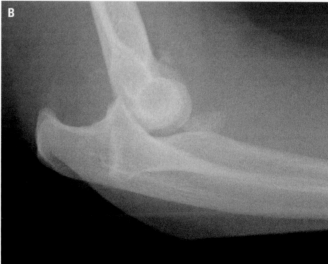

Figure 9.31. The "terrible triad." There is posterior dislocation of the elbow associated with fractures of the radial head and coronoid process.

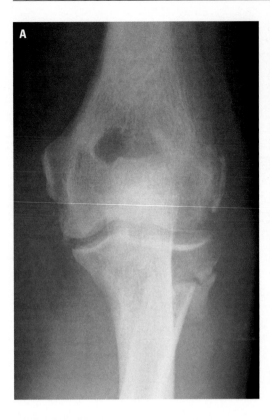

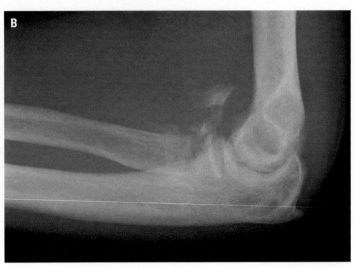

Figure 9.32. AP and lateral views of radial head nonunion with surrounding heterotopic ossification.

in identifying fractures of the posterior half of the radial head. Displacement of fat pads on the lateral radiograph indicates hemarthrosis and is the most frequent and obvious sign of an undisplaced intra-articular fracture. CT may better delineate fracture configuration in complex cases and can be of value in preoperative planning.

Complications of radial head fracture include contracture; posttraumatic osteoarthrosis (OA); instability; wrist pain due to interosseous, distal radioulnar, or triangular fibrocartilage injury; heterotopic ossification (Fig. 9.32); osteonecrosis; nonunion; and pain related to hardware.

Olecranon Fractures

Olecranon fractures may be direct or indirect. They are most common in the adult population because the pediatric olecranon is short, thick, and relatively strong in relation to the distal humerus. Indirect fractures occur as a result of forceful contraction of the triceps often during a fall to an outstretched arm and are most common in the elderly. The amount of fracture displacement is influenced by contraction of the triceps muscle as well as any disruption of the triceps aponeurosis or periosteum. Fractures in

younger patients are more often high-energy injuries, resulting from direct trauma, often producing comminuted fractures due to impaction into the distal humerus or concomitant fractures of the ulnar shaft.

Olecranon fractures are classified according to Colton based on displacement and fracture characteristics.[5] Type I fractures (Fig. 9.33) are undisplaced

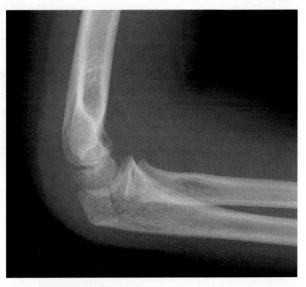

Figure 9.33. Colton type I olecranon fractures are undisplaced or minimally displaced (<2 mm) and are stable.

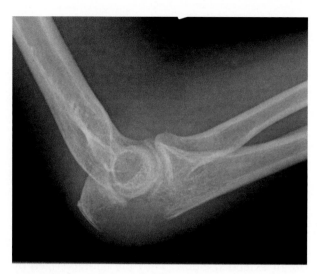

Figure 9.34. Colton type IIA avulsion fracture of the olecranon with moderate displacement.

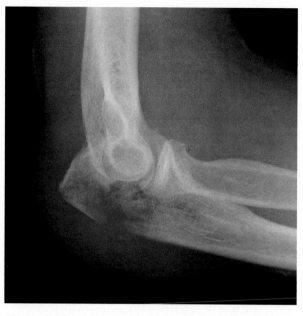

Figure 9.36. Colton type IIC comminuted fracture of the olecranon.

or minimally displaced (<2 mm) and are stable. Type II fractures are unstable and divided according to the fracture pattern: type IIA are avulsion fractures (Fig. 9.34), type IIB are oblique or transverse fractures (Fig. 9.35), type IIC are comminuted (Fig. 9.36), and type IID are fracture dislocations (Fig. 9.37).

Radiographic diagnosis is based on AP and lateral radiographs of the elbow. Because all fractures of the olecranon process are intra-articular, a hemarthrosis will invariably be present. Although fractures of the olecranon are usually isolated injuries, care

should be taken in the exclusion of fractures of the coronoid and radial head, as well as Monteggia fracture-dislocations, which have significant implications on elbow stability.

The main complication following internal fixation is pain and irritation caused by hardware,

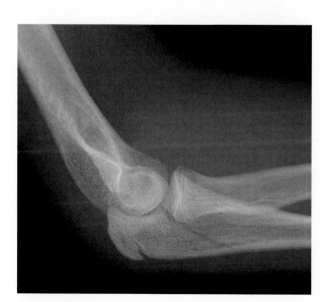

Figure 9.35. Colton type IIB oblique fracture of the olecranon.

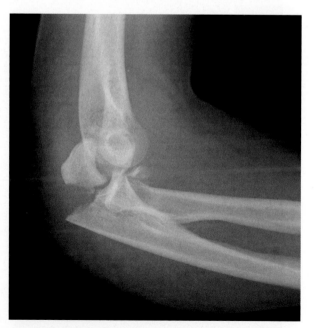

Figure 9.37. Colton type IID fracture-dislocation of the olecranon associated with a displaced fracture of the radial head.

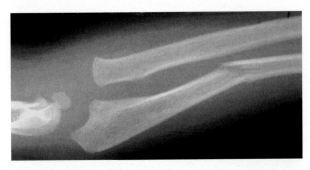

Figure 9.38. Bado type I (extension type) injury. They are characterized by fracture of the ulnar diaphysis at any level with anterior dislocation of the radial head and anterior angulation of the fracture fragments.

mostly related to tension-band wiring. Other complications include ulnar nerve paresthesia, nonunion (1%), and loss of extension typically by 10 degrees to 15 degrees.

Monteggia Fracture-Dislocation

Fractures of the proximal ulna with dislocation of the proximal radioulnar joint are known as Monteggia fractures. They were first described in 1814 and subclassified into four types by Bado in 1967 based on the direction of dislocation of the radial head.[6] Bado type I (extension type) injuries account for 60% of cases and are due to hyperpronation injury of the forearm. They are characterized by fracture of the ulnar diaphysis at any level with anterior dislocation of the radial head and anterior angulation of the fracture fragments (Fig. 9.38). Bado type II (flexion type) injuries account for 15% and are "reversed" Monteggia fracture-dislocation injuries with fracture of the ulnar diaphysis with posterior dislocation of the radial head and posterior angulation of the fracture fragments (Fig. 9.39). Bado type III injuries (20%) are due to varus stress on an extended elbow. They are characterized by fracture of the proximal ulnar metaphysis with lateral or anterolateral dislocation of the radial head (Fig. 9.40). Type IV fractures account for 5% and are characterized by fractures of the proximal thirds of the radius and ulna at the same level and anterior dislocation of the radial head (Fig. 9.41).

Radiographic diagnosis relies on standard AP and lateral views. The ulnar fracture is usually clinically and radiographically apparent. Findings associated with the concomitant radial head dislocation are often subtle; thus, review of the

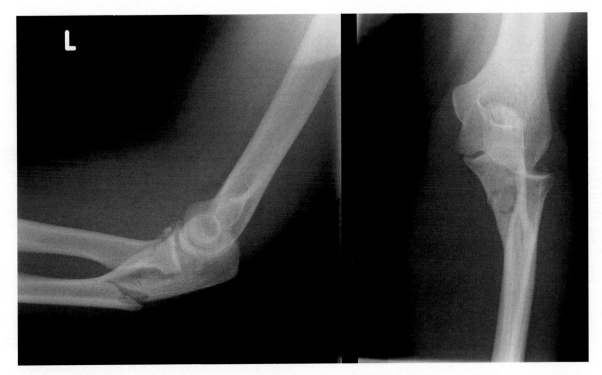

Figure 9.39. Bado type II (flexion type) Monteggia fracture-dislocation with fracture of the ulnar diaphysis with posterior dislocation of the radial head and posterior angulation of the fracture fragments.

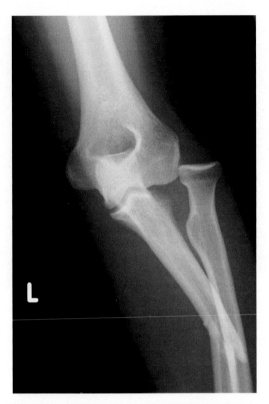

Figure 9.40. Bado type III injury with fracture of the proximal ulna and lateral dislocation of the radial head.

radiocapitellar line is mandatory to assess its position.

Nerve complications are rare and most commonly involve the posterior interosseous nerve with type III injuries. Other associations include ulnar nonunion, recurrent radial head dislocation, radiohumeral or radioulnar ankylosis, periarticular

ossification with chronic radial head dislocations, and myositis ossificans.

COMPUTED TOMOGRAPHY

CT is a valuable imaging modality in the setting of acute trauma and polytrauma. Multislice imaging provides rapid radiologic assessment and allows multiplanar and 3D reconstructions. CT is particularly useful in the context of severe or complex fractures and fracture-dislocations to determine the extent of injury, involvement and congruity of the articular surfaces and growth plates, size of fracture fragments, and the need for surgical intervention (Fig. 9.42). CT may also be performed when conventional radiography is insufficient or when no fracture is identified in the presence of a joint effusion. It is useful in the assessment of fracture healing and alignment to demonstrate pseudarthroses, intra-articular loose bodies, or myositis ossificans.

MAGNETIC RESONANCE IMAGING

MRI is helpful in the setting of acute and chronic trauma as a result of its multiplanar characteristics and superior soft tissue resolution. Its nonionizing nature renders it preferable to CT in the setting of pediatric trauma, although sedation may be required. Plain radiographs do not demonstrate trabecular microfracturing (bone bruising) or cartilaginous or soft tissue damage and may underestimate physeal

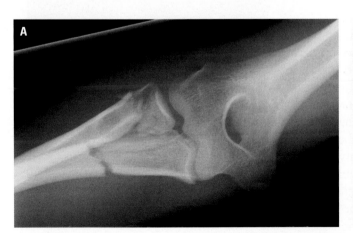
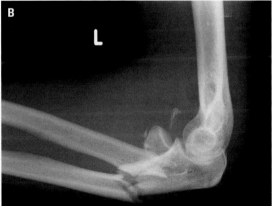

Figure 9.41. AP (**A**) and lateral (**B**) views demonstrating Bado type IV Monteggia fracture-dislocation. There are fractures of the proximal thirds of the radius and ulna and anterior dislocation of the radial head.

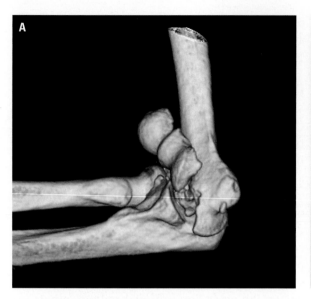
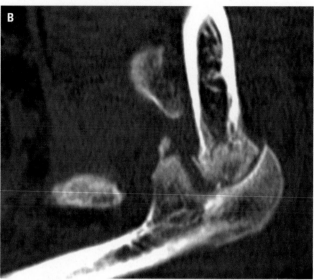

Figure 9.42. 3D VR image (**A**) demonstrates a complex fracture dislocation of the elbow with craniad displacement of a large fracture fragment involving the capitellar and trochlear articular surfaces. Parasagittal MPR image (**B**) reveals concomitant fracture of the coronoid process.

injury. MRI is particularly useful in the setting of radiographically occult fractures (Fig. 9.43), osteochondral injuries (Fig. 9.44), and muscle or ligamentous injury. MRI and/or US are valuable in imaging soft tissue structures about the elbow; common injuries include rupture of the biceps (Fig. 9.45) and/or triceps tendons, lateral or medial epicondylitis, and injury to the collateral ligament complexes (Fig. 9.46).

NONTRAUMATIC CONDITIONS

There are several bursal structures around the elbow. These include the superficial olecranon bursa, which occurs in the subcutaneous tissue over the olecranon; the subtendinous olecranon bursa between the triceps tendon and olecranon (inflamed with repetitive flexion and extension of the elbow); the radioulnar bursa between extensor digitorum, the radioulnar joint, and supinator muscle; and the cubital bursa between the distal biceps tendon and radial tuberosity.

The superficial olecranon bursa is particularly vulnerable to traumatic and inflammatory processes and is the most common superficial bursitis in the body. Clinically, it appears as a lump over the olecranon process due to fluid distention or synovial hypertrophy, with or without local erythema. Trauma can cause both septic and non-septic bursitis, although

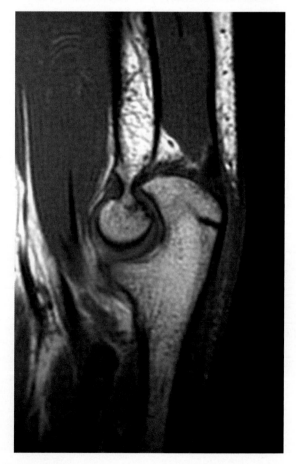

Figure 9.43. Sagittal T1W image demonstrating a stress fracture of the olecranon. This was not visible on radiograph.

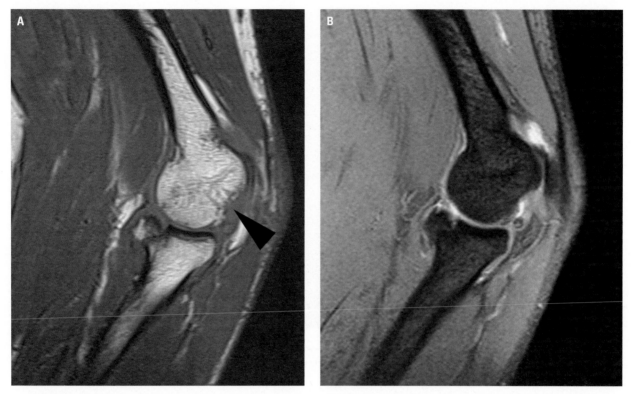

Figure 9.44. Sagittal T1 (**A**) and T2-weighted (T2W) image with fat suppression (**B**) demonstrating a minimally displaced radial head fracture and concomitant osteochondral lesion of the capitellum (**A**, *arrowhead*).

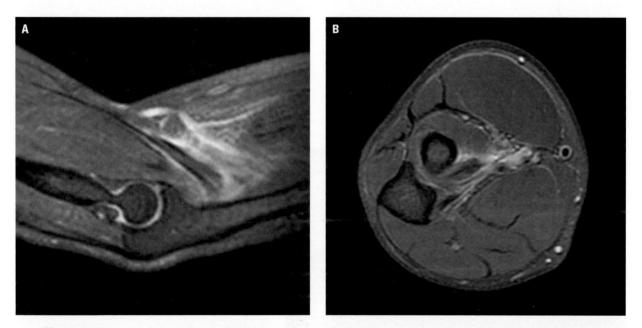

Figure 9.45. Sagittal (**A**) and axial (**B**) short tau inversion recovery (STIR) images demonstrating a partial tear of the long head of biceps tendon. There is intrasubstance high signal within the distal tendon and fluid surrounding its insertion into the radial tuberosity.

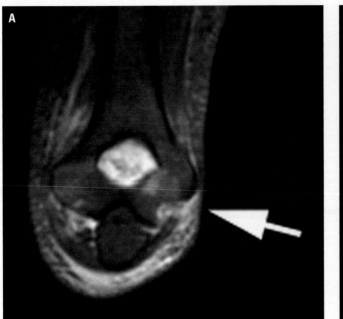 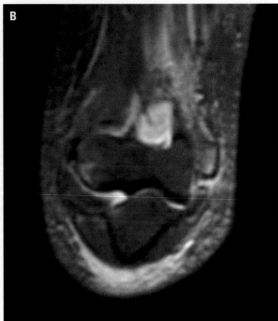

Figure 9.46. Coronal STIR images in a 17-year-old male with a history of previous elbow dislocation. There is disruption of the ulnar collateral ligament and common flexor origin (**A**, *arrow*) with posttraumatic edema in the medial epicondylar enthesis (**B**).

the most common cause is direct repetitive micro-trauma (student's elbow). Approximately one-third of cases of olecranon bursitis are septic, most commonly due to *Staphylococcus* infection and should be treated by aspiration and antimicrobial therapy. A variety of inflammatory and systemic disorders may also produce distention of the bursa including rheumatoid arthritis, crystal arthropathy, tuberculosis, autoimmune disorders, and chronic renal disease (due to uremia or long-term hemodialysis).

Plain radiographs are indicated if there is a history of significant trauma to exclude fracture of the olecranon. They may also demonstrate enthesopathy of the distal triceps insertion or features of inflammatory arthropathy. US is particularly helpful early in the course of the disease demonstrating effusions, synovial proliferation, calcifications, inflammatory nodules, hyperemia, and in guiding diagnostic or therapeutic intervention (Fig. 9.47). In crystal deposition diseases, US typically

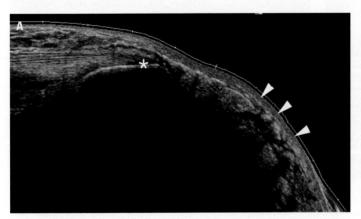 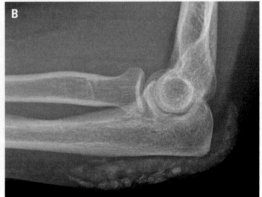

Figure 9.47. US image (**A**) demonstrating marked thickening of the olecranon bursa containing extensive echogenic calcifications *(arrowheads)* in keeping with calcific bursitis. Note a normal distal triceps enthesis *(asterisk)*. Findings were confirmed with a plain radiograph (**B**). There are no signs of underlying inflammatory arthropathy or systemic disease.

demonstrates hyperechoic fluid with thickened echogenic bursal walls. In septic bursitis, there may be a more complex appearance with extensive peribursal inflammatory change. Rarely, MRI may be indicated in the exclusion of concurrent osteomyelitis.

REFERENCES

1. Milch H. Fractures and fracture-dislocations of the humeral condyles. *J Trauma*. 1964;4:592–607.
2. Rang M. *Injuries of the epiphysis, growth plate, and the perichondral ring. Children's fractures*. Philadelphia: JB Lippincott; 1983.
3. Mason ML. Some observations on fractures of the head of the radius with a review of a hundred cases. *Br J Surg*. 1954;42:123–32.
4. Johnston GW. A follow-up of one hundred cases of fractures of the head of the radius with a review of the literature. *Ulster Med J*. 1962;31:51–56.
5. Colton CL. Fractures of the olecranon in adults: classification and management. *Injury*. 1973;5(2):121–129.
6. Bado JL. The Monteggia lesion. *Clin Orthop Relat Res*. 1967;50:71–86.

SUGGESTED READINGS

1. Johnson KJ, Bache E, Baert AL. *Imaging in Pediatric Skeletal Trauma*. Berlin, Germany: Springer–Verlag; 2008.
2. Bianchi S, Martinoli C. *Ultrasound of the Musculoskeletal System*. Heidelberg, Germany: Springer–Verlag; 2007.
3. Goswami GK. The fat pad sign. *Radiology*. 2002;222(2):419–420.
4. Beltran J, Rosenberg ZS, Kawelblum M, et al. Paediatric elbow fractures: MRI evaluation. *Skeletal Radiol*. 1994;23(4):277–281.
5. Ring D, Jupiter JB, Simpson, NS. Monteggia fractures in adults. *J Bone Joint Surg Am*. 1998;80(12):1733–1744.
6. Griffith JF, Roebuck DJ, Cheng JC, et al. Acute elbow trauma in children: spectrum of injury revealed by MR imaging not apparent on radiographs. *AJR Am J Roentgenol*. 2001;176(1):53–60.
7. Zuazo I, Bonnefoy O, Tauzin C, et al. Acute elbow trauma in children: role of ultrasonography. *Pediatr Radiol*. 2008;38(9):982–988.
8. Snyder HS. Radiographic changes with radial head subluxation in children. *J Emerg Med*. 1990;8(3):265–269.

CHAPTER 10

Wrist

Robert SD Campbell ■ John H. Harris Jr.

INTRODUCTION

Radiography remains the primary investigation for trauma of the wrist. The requirement for implementing secondary imaging modalities is dictated by clinical and x-ray findings. Computed tomography (CT) is commonly used for surgical planning of complex fractures, detecting occult fractures, and assessment of fracture union. Magnetic resonance imaging (MRI) is useful for detecting occult fractures and assessment of ligament injuries. Both CT and MRI may be combined with arthrography to improve diagnostic accuracy of ligament injury.

This chapter concentrates on interpretation of radiographic examinations of wrist trauma. The indications for CT and MRI are discussed, but a full description of the complex soft tissue anatomy and pathology is beyond the scope of this text.

RADIOLOGIC TECHNIQUE

Radiographs

The wrist includes the articulations of the distal radius and ulna, the carpus, and the carpometacarpal joints. Attending physicians should indicate precisely the anatomic area for radiologic evaluation based on the clinical history and physical examination. It is important to acquire radiographs with appropriate positioning and beam centering in order to adequately evaluate wrist trauma. Properly positioned radiographs are essential for assessing carpal relationships. The distal radioulnar joint (DRUJ) and the radiocarpal, midcarpal, and carpometacarpal (CMC) joints should be fully included on all images.

A minimum of two radiographic projections (posteroanterior [PA] and lateral) should be acquired to fully evaluate injuries of the distal radius and ulna (Fig. 10.1). It is important to remember that injuries may affect more than one anatomic area. However, it is not necessary to routinely image both the wrist and the elbow in the instance of a suspected distal radial fracture if the physical examination of the elbow is negative and when the patient is alert, responsive, and communicative. It is also not necessary to routinely obtain radiographs of the normal contralateral wrist in children simply "for comparison." Physicians interpreting skeletal radiographs of children and adolescents should be sufficiently familiar with the appearance of normal growing bones to be able to determine normality.

The routine radiographic study of the carpus should include at least a frontal, lateral, and a PA oblique projection (Fig. 10.2A–C).[1] The PA oblique is obtained by elevating the radial border of the wrist by 30 degrees. An additional PA in ulnar deviation, the scaphoid (navicular) view, should be obtained in all patients with pain in the anatomical snuffbox to optimally demonstrate the waist of scaphoid. The scaphoid view is obtained with the hand in pronation and in maximum possible ulnar deviation. The central x-ray beam is centered over

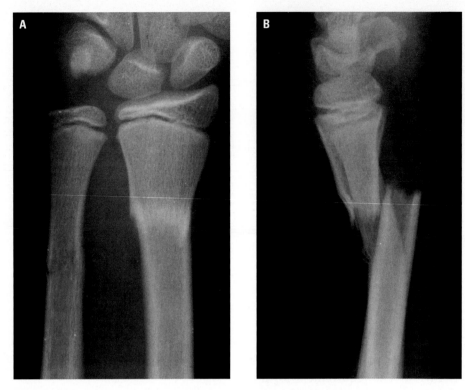

Figure 10.1. The distal radial and ulnar fractures are obvious in the frontal projection (**A**), but the marked displacement can only be appreciated in the lateral radiograph (**B**).

the anatomic "snuffbox" and angled approximately 10 degrees in both an ulnar and proximal direction (Fig. 10.3). The radial surface of the scaphoid is seen in greater detail and in different perspective than in the PA projection. The normal dorsal ridge appears as a localized irregularity of the radial aspect of its cortex and should not be confused

as a cortical buckling or incomplete fracture. The scaphoid view is not required in infants and very young children because scaphoid fractures are rare in this age group and the scaphoid does not ossify until 6 years of age.

Other radiographic projections have largely been abandoned in favor of CT imaging for acute trauma

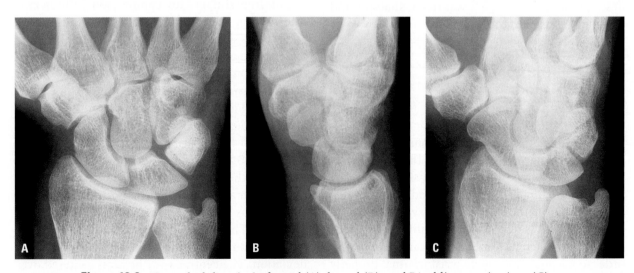

Figure 10.2. Normal adult wrist in frontal (**A**), lateral (**B**), and PA oblique projections (**C**).

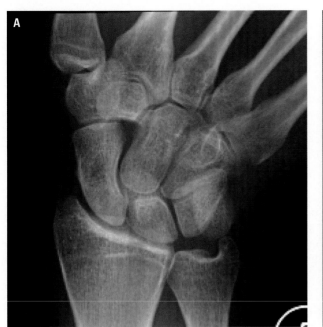
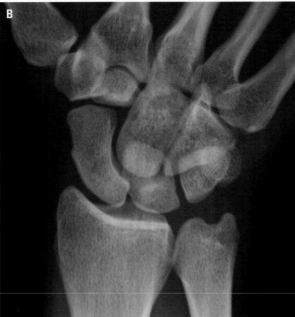

Figure 10.3. Additional radiographic projections for suspected scaphoid fracture include either a PA in ulnar deviation (**A**) or a PA with cranial and ulnar beam angulation (**B**). Both views show the long axis of the scaphoid in profile.

(Fig. 10.4). Multiple projections may be indicated for suspected carpal instability.

Computed Tomography

High-resolution multiplanar reconstructed (MPR) images are obtained with multidetector computed tomography (MDCT), which provide specific information about fracture morphology in complex wrist fractures that assist surgical planning.[2] Up to 30% of fractures are occult on plain radiographs, and MDCT has been shown to identify fractures with up to 100% sensitivity.[3] This includes not only occult scaphoid fractures but also fractures of the lunate, triquetrum,

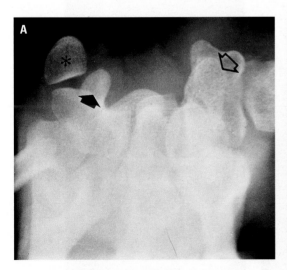
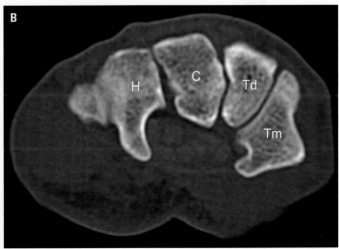

Figure 10.4. Carpal tunnel view demonstrating the pisiform *(asterisk)*, the hook of the hamate *(closed arrow)*, and the scaphoid bone *(open arrow)* (**A**). An axial CT image demonstrates more detail of the morphology and articulation of the carpal bones (**B**). *H*, hamate; *C*, capitate; *Td*, trapezoid; *Tm*, trapezium.

capitate, and hamate, which are often poorly visualized or easily missed on radiographs.[4] Caution is advised in interpreting radiographs of patients with marked osteopenia because fracture lines may be subtle.

CT of the wrist is performed with the patient prone and the arm outstretched above the head within the bore of the CT (the "superman" position). This may not be achievable in some trauma patients, in which case the patient is placed supine with the hand on the abdomen or by the patient's side. However, image quality is compromised by beam-hardening effects. Alternatively, it is possible to sit the patient on a chair on the opposite side of the CT gantry with the shoulder abducted and the wrist positioned within the bore (Fig. 10.5).

Thin section volumetric scanning of the wrist (≤1 mm) is performed with a small field of view using bone algorithms that enhance bony detail. MPR images are acquired in the coronal, sagittal, and axial plane. Non-orthogonal MPR imaging in the oblique sagittal plane provides optimal visualization of the scaphoid (Fig. 10.6), which improves diagnostic accuracy and delineation of fracture patterns. The benefits of 3D MPRs of the wrist for surgical planning have not been proven.

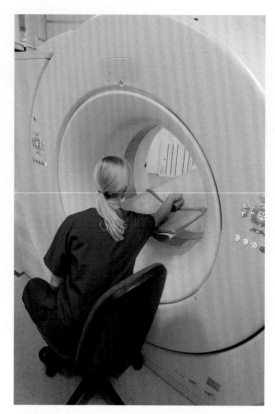

Figure 10.5. CT examinations of the wrist can be performed with the patient seated behind the gantry. This is a useful alternative to the supine position with the arm by the side to avoid beam-hardening artifact.

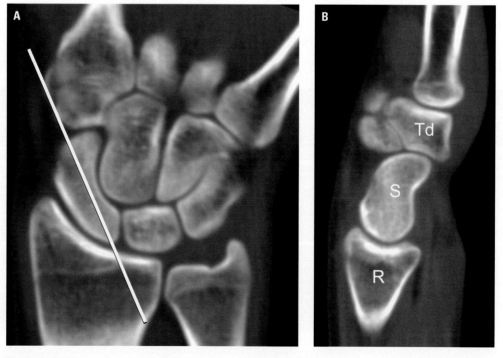

Figure 10.6. A coronal MPR CT image of the wrist (**A**) demonstrating the plane for obtaining an oblique sagittal long axis view of the scaphoid (**B**). *R*, radius; *S*, scaphoid; *Td*, trapezoid.

Magnetic Resonance Imaging

MRI is indicated for evaluation of ligamentous injury and carpal instability. It may be used as an alternative to CT for early detection of occult trauma, especially in the context of scaphoid fractures.[5,6] Patient positioning is important for wrist imaging because of several potential problems. Movement artifacts may occur if the patient experiences pain or discomfort when the arm is placed above the head. With the arm by the side, the wrist lies in the periphery of the magnetic field, and field inhomogeneities may degrade image quality. Placing the hand on the abdomen results in breathing movement artifact. Phased-array wrist coils or knee coils with a 6 to 8 cm field of view provide the best image quality (Fig. 10.7). MRI of the wrist can be performed in a plaster cast, but this will limit coil selection.

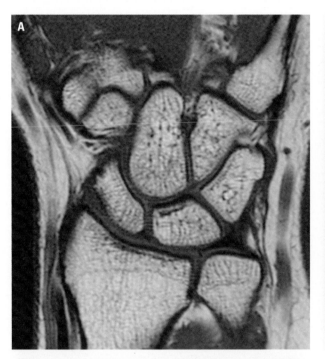

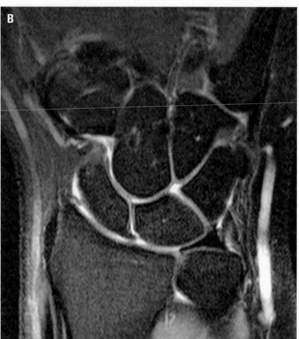

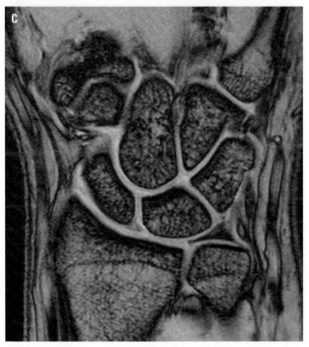

Figure 10.7. High-resolution MR images obtained on a 1.5T system with four channel wrist coil and an 8 × 8 cm field of view. The combination of a T1W sequence (**A**), a T2W fat saturation sequence (**B**) and T2* gradient echo sequence (**C**) provides excellent detail of bone, articular cartilage, fibrocartilage, and ligament anatomy.

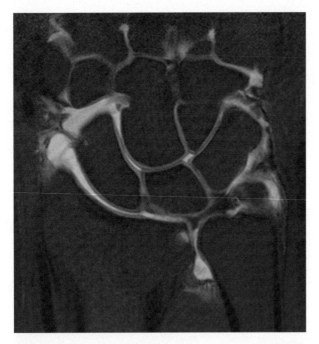

Figure 10.8. T1W fat saturation images are used to supplement other pulse sequences for MR arthrography. There is good delineation of articular cartilage in joints filled with dilute Gadolinium.

Standard protocols for the wrist include T1W and fluid sensitive sequences such as T2W fat saturation or STIR sequences for optimal visualization of marrow edema associated with fractures and soft tissue edema in acute ligamentous injuries. A variety of gradient echo sequences can be used for cartilage imaging and delineation of small, thin ligaments. Images are obtained in coronal, sagittal, and axial planes.

Magnetic resonance (MR) (or CT) arthrography may be preferred for demonstration of the carpal ligaments and triangular fibrocartilage (TFC) in nonacute cases. Arthrography is usually performed under fluoroscopic guidance. A dilute solution of gadolinium is mixed with iodinated contrast in order to obtain images during joint injection and to identify sites of abnormal communication between joint compartments.[7] T1W fat saturation sequences are used to supplement the other standard sequences in conventional MR wrist imaging (Fig. 10.8).

RADIOLOGIC ANATOMY

The radius and ulna articulate with the proximal carpal row through the radiocarpal and ulnocarpal joint. The ulnocarpal joint also contains the TFC complex. The distal radius is divided into radial and ulnar facets that articulate with the scaphoid and lunate, respectively. The articular surfaces of the ulna and radius should be approximate (Fig. 10.9), although the length of the ulna can vary in some individuals, being either longer (ulnar plus variance) or shorter (ulnar minus variance). In addition, there is an increase in ulnar plus variance in full pronation and on fist clenching, compared to

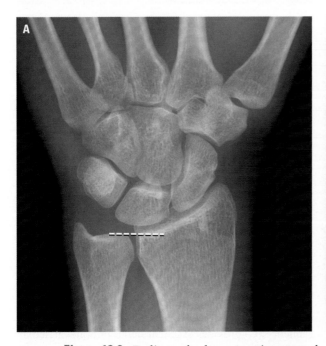
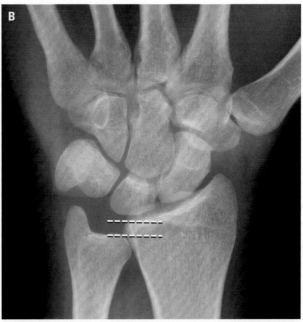

Figure 10.9. Radiographs demonstrating normal ulnar variance (**A**) and ulnar minus variance (**B**).

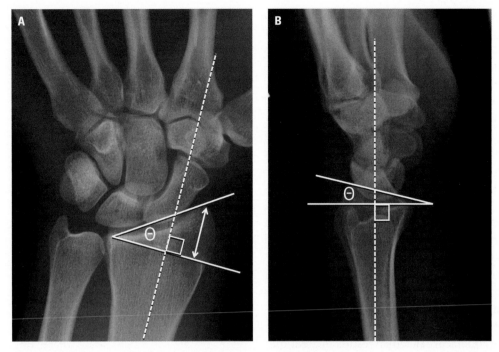

Figure 10.10. Normal wrist measurements. The radial inclination angle is subtended between a line drawn perpendicular to the long axis of the radius and a line drawn along the length of the articular surface of the radius (**A**). The normal radial inclination angle Θ is approximately 22 degrees. The radial height *(double arrow)* is approximately 11 degrees. The degree of normal volar radial tilt measured on a lateral radiograph is approximately 11 degrees (**B**).

forearm supination. Radiographic analysis should include an evaluation of the radial height, radial inclination, and volar tilt (Fig. 10.10). Other measurements may include the radiocarpal angle and the carpal height ratio.

The eight carpal bones are divided into two horizontal rows. The proximal row consists of the scaphoid, lunate, and triquetrum. The pisiform is a sesamoid bone formed within the tendon of the flexor carpi ulnaris and articulates with the volar aspect of the triquetrum. The proximal row of carpal bones forms the intercalated segment of the wrist. The main function of these bones is to coordinate the complex range of movements that occurs between the distal radius and the distal carpal row, thereby maintaining the stability of the wrist joint. The distal carpal row consists of the trapezium, trapezoid, capitate, and hamate. They have a more rigid configuration with less movement than the proximal row.

On a PA radiograph, the articular surfaces of the proximal and distal carpal row form continuous arcs (the arcs of Gilula) (Fig. 10.11).[8] There should be no

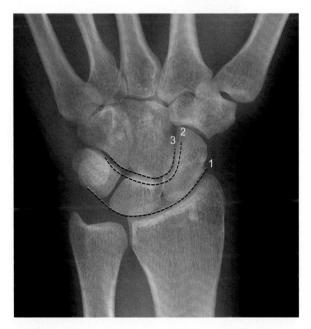

Figure 10.11. The three arcs of Gilula comprise the proximal and distal articular surfaces of the proximal carpal row and the proximal articular surfaces of the distal carpal row *(broken lines)*. These should be continuous smooth arcs with no steps between joints.

interruption of the congruity of the arcs. The width of the scapholunate space must be measured at, or distal to, its midpoint and should be equivalent to the other intercarpal joints and measure <3 mm.

On a well-positioned lateral radiograph of a normal adult wrist, the axis of the distal radius, lunate, and capitate should be linear, with congruence between the articular surfaces (Fig. 10.12). The long axis of the lunate and capitate should align with an angle of 0 degree ± 15 degrees. The scapholunate angle is important for assessment of carpal instability. This is the angle subtended between the long axis of the scaphoid bone and the lunate, and it should normally measure between 30 degrees and 60 degrees (Fig. 10.13).[9]

The carpometacarpal joints are arthrodial (gliding) diarthroses except for the fifth, which is a modified saddle joint. All metacarpal bones articulate with the distal row of carpal bones and with each adjacent metacarpal, which results in great mechanical stability. The third CMC articulation provides very little movement and is a prime stabilizing

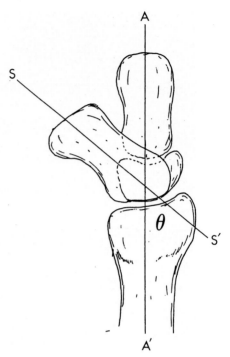

Figure 10.13. Schematic representation of the normal alignment of the distal radius, lunate, scaphoid, and capitate in lateral projection. The axis of the distal radius, lunate, and capitate should be linear. The long axis of the scaphoid bone (*S–S′*) should normally be at an angle of 30 to 60 degrees to the linear axis (*A–A′*). The scapholunate angle is indicated by *Θ*. (From Mirvis SE, Young JWR, eds. *Imaging in Trauma and Critical Care.* Baltimore, MD: Lippincott Williams & Wilkins, 1992:470. Used with permission.)

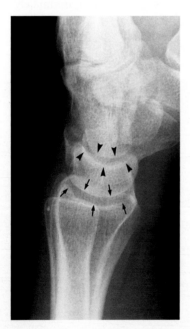

Figure 10.12. Lateral radiograph of the normal wrist. The contiguous concave surface of the distal radius and the proximal convex surface of the lunate *(arrows)* are normally congruous, as are the contiguous concave distal articulating surface of the lunate and the proximal convex surface of the capitate *(arrowheads)*. Normally, a line drawn to the midsagittal plane of the carpus should bisect both the lunate and capitate bones. In this case, the capitate is rotated slightly posterior to this line.

factor of the carpometacarpal joint. Greater flexibility and mobility are present at the fourth and fifth carpometacarpal joints.

The ligaments of the wrist are complex and are interconnected in their actions. They are divided into the intrinsic and extrinsic ligaments.[9] The intrinsic ligaments (scapholunate and lunotriquetral ligaments) stabilize the intercalated segments of the proximal carpal row. Each intrinsic ligament consists of three parts. There are relatively strong volar and dorsal components, with a thinner central membranous portion (Fig. 10.14). The extrinsic ligaments of the wrist are situated over both the volar and dorsal aspects of the wrist and help stabilize movement between rows (radiocarpal joint and midcarpal joint). They include the volar radioscaphocapitate and radiolunate-triquetral ligaments and the dorsal radioscaphoid, radiolunate, and radiotriquetral ligaments.[10]

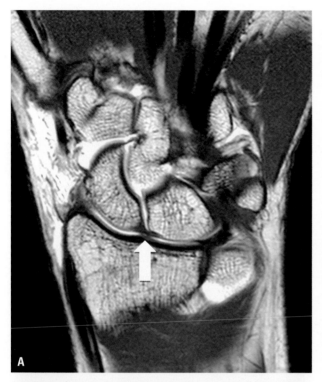

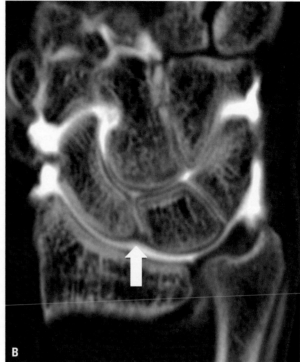

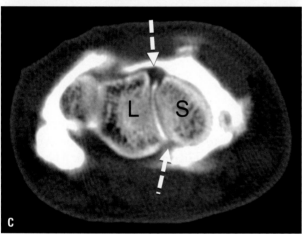

Figure 10.14. T1W image of an MR arthrogram demonstrating the normal scapholunate ligament *(arrow)*. A three joint compartment injection has been performed, and both aspects of the ligament are outlined by contrast **(A)**. A CT image from the same patient also clearly demonstrates the scapholunate ligament *(arrow)* **(B)**. The axial CT image **(C)** demonstrates the dorsal and volar components of the ligament *(broken arrows)*. L, lunate; S, scaphoid.

RADIOLOGIC MANIFESTATIONS OF TRAUMA

Distal Radius and Ulna Fractures

Distal radial fractures are the most common fractures around the wrist. The most common mechanism of injury is a fall on the outstretched hand with the hand and wrist in dorsiflexion, which results in a variety of injuries depending on the patient's age. This may be as a result of either a high-energy injury in young patients or low-energy injury in the older osteoporotic individual.

Localized soft tissue swelling about the wrist may be the most obvious radiographic finding in instances of subtle skeletal injury (Fig. 10.15). The pronator quadratus muscle is a quadrangular muscle that passes transversely from the distal radius to the distal ulna. Superficially, it is covered with a layer of loose fatty areolar tissue, which is visible as a linear area of low density on the lateral radiograph of the wrist (Fig. 10.16A). Hemorrhage beneath the pronator quadratus muscle causes muscle bulging, which either displaces or obliterates the pronator fat stripe (Fig. 10.16B).[11] This is a useful sign in the presence of subtle injuries of the distal third of the radius or ulna.

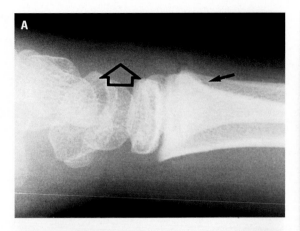

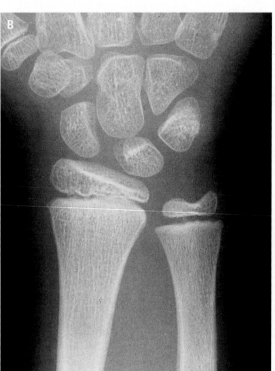

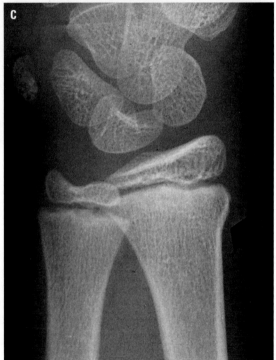

Figure 10.15. Soft tissue swelling over the dorsum of the wrist *(open arrow)* on the lateral projection (**A**) is the most prominent sign of the subtle cortical buckling fracture of the distal radius *(solid arrow)*, which was not visible on the PA radiograph (**B**) but was confirmed *(arrow)* on the oblique projection (**C**).

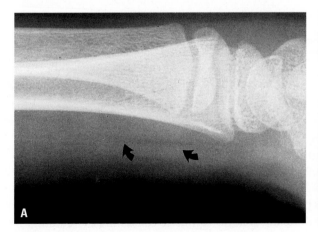

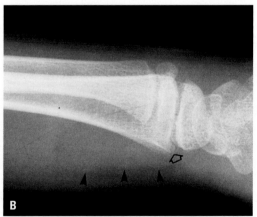

Figure 10.16. Normal pronator fat stripe *(black arrows)* (**A**). The abnormal pronator quadratus muscle sign *(arrowheads)* on the lateral radiograph (**B**) represents the hematoma associated with the minimally displaced distal radial metaphyseal fracture *(open arrow)*.

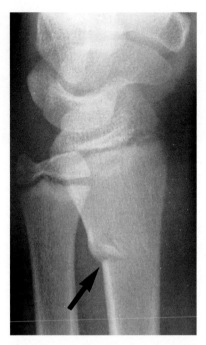

Figure 10.17. Cortical buckling or greenstick fracture *(arrow)* of the dorsal cortex of the distal radius.

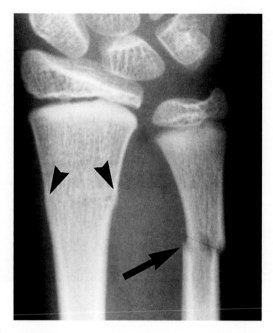

Figure 10.19. Torus fracture *(arrowheads)* of the distal radius with a minimally displaced complete fracture of the distal ulna *(arrow)*.

Distal Radial Fractures in Children

In the young child, a fall on the outstretched hand may produce a greenstick (cortical buckling) fracture of the distal radius (Fig. 10.17); a "torus" fracture, which is a circumferential impacted cortical buckling fracture (Fig. 10.18); a complete fracture

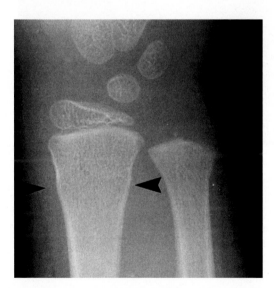

Figure 10.18. Torus fracture *(arrowheads)* of the distal radial metaphysis. The fracture is indicated by the very short, focal convexities of the distal cortex. No fracture line or trabecular impaction is visible.

of the distal third of one forearm bone with a cortical buckling fracture of the other (Fig. 10.19); or one of the Salter-Harris injuries, primarily of the distal radial physis. Colles fractures are uncommon in children (Fig. 10.20).

The Salter-Harris physeal injuries of the wrist are usually of the type I or type II variety caused by the shearing or twisting mechanism of injury associated with falls on the outstretched hand. The type I injury may be very subtle (Fig. 10.21) or obvious (Fig. 10.22) as may be the type II injury (Figs. 10.23 and 10.24).

The distal radial physis fuses in the mid-to-late teens. The physeal "scar" may simulate an incomplete or minimally displaced impacted fracture (Fig. 10.25). The absence of soft tissue swelling, the smooth sclerotic margins, and the typical location should aid differentiation from a genuine fracture.

Distal Radial Fractures in Adults

A variety of different fractures of the distal radius occur dependent on the mechanism of injury.[1] They may be extraarticular or intra-articular. Historically, many of these fractures have been given eponymous titles, some of which remain in common usage.

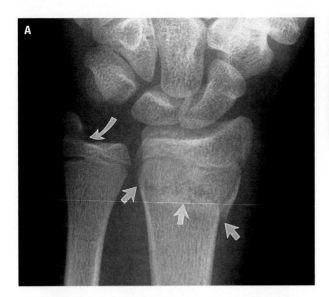

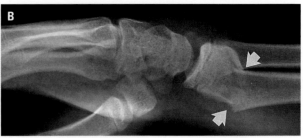

Figure 10.20. Extra-articular (Colles) distal radial fracture *(arrows)* in PA (**A**) and lateral (**B**) projections associated with a fracture of the base of the ulnar styloid *(curved arrow, **A**).*

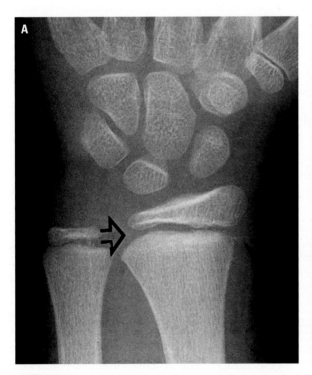

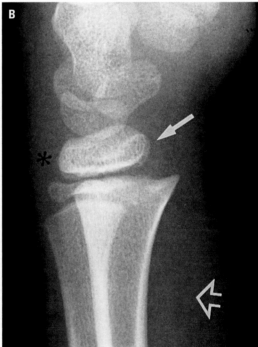

Figure 10.21. Subtle Salter-Harris I physeal injury. On the PA radiograph (**A**), the distal radial physis is minimally displaced *(open arrow)*, and a tiny metaphyseal fragment *(arrow)* is present along the radial aspect of the physis. The strict definition of the Salter-Harris I injury does not include a fracture. However, tiny fragments of this size in or adjacent to the physis (which may arise from either the epiphysis or metaphysis) do not fulfill the criteria of a Salter-Harris II injury. The lateral radiograph (**B**) shows soft tissue swelling of the dorsum of the wrist *(asterisk)*, an absent pronator quadratus muscle shadow *(open arrow)*, and dorsal displacement of the distal radial physis *(arrow)*.

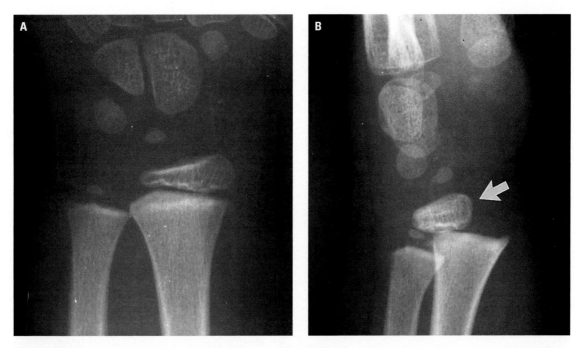

Figure 10.22. Displaced Salter-Harris type I distal radial physeal injury. On the PA projection (**A**), the relationship of the distal radial epiphysis to its metaphysis appears normal. On lateral projection (**B**), however, dorsal displacement of the distal radial epiphysis *(arrow)* is clearly evident.

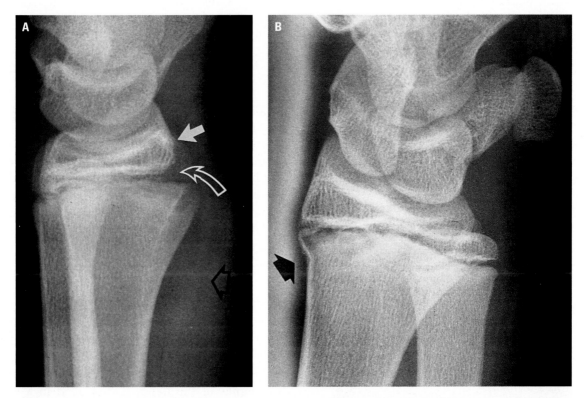

Figure 10.23. Volar bulging of the fascial plane *(open arrow)* covering the abnormally thickened pronator quadratus muscle shadow on the lateral projection (**A**) is the most prominent radiographic sign of the very subtle Salter-Harris II injury. The distal radial epiphysis *(arrow)* is slightly, but definitely, dorsally displaced and the volar aspect of the physis is wide *(curved arrow)* on the lateral (**A**) projection. The metaphyseal component of the type II injury *(arrow)* is evident on the oblique radiograph (**B**).

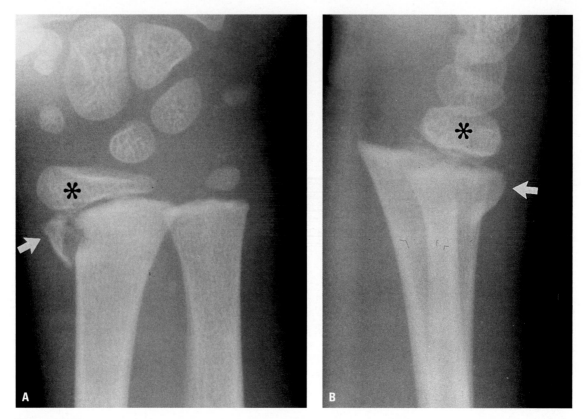

Figure 10.24. Salter-Harris type II distal radial physeal injury. The distal fragment of the Salter-Harris II consists of the distal radial epiphysis *(asterisk)* and a triangular metaphyseal fragment *(arrow)* adherent to the epiphysis through the intact physis. The distal fragment is radially displaced on the PA view **(A)** and dorsally displaced on the lateral **(B)** radiograph.

Colles Fracture

The Colles fracture is the most common distal radial fracture. It is a transverse fracture of the distal metaphysis with dorsal angulation and dorsal and proximal displacement of the distal

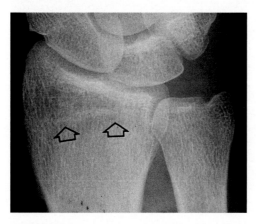

Figure 10.25. Normal appearance of the scar of the distal radial physis *(open arrows)*. It appears as a thin sclerotic line and should not be mistaken for a fracture.

fragment (Figs. 10.20 and 10.26). The classic "dinner fork" deformity is typically evident on lateral radiographs (Fig. 10.26B). A Colles fracture is frequently associated with an avulsion of the base of the ulnar styloid process caused by the intact ulnar collateral ligament (Fig. 10.27). Intra-articular fracture extension is a common occurrence (Fig. 10.28). Impacted or depressed articular fragments are sometimes referred to as "die-punch" fractures.

Smith Fracture

The Smith fracture is the reverse of the Colles fracture, but it occurs less commonly. It typically results from a fall on the flexed wrist. The distal radial fragment, together with the carpus and bones of the hand, is displaced in a volar direction and rotated proximally (Figs. 10.29 and 10.30). Smith fractures may also be intra-articular or extraarticular. They are uncommon in children.

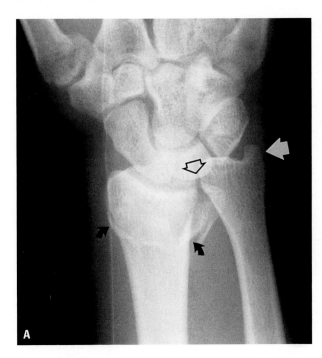

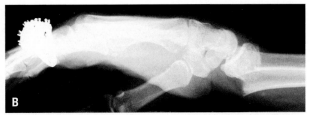

Figure 10.26. A typical Colles fracture as originally described. The PA view (**A**) shows the intact ulnar styloid process *(arrow)*, radiocarpal diastasis *(open arrow)*, and the transverse distal radial fracture *(curved arrows)* without intra-articular extension. In the lateral projection (**B**), dorsal and proximal displacement of the distal radial fragment, together with the bones of the wrist and hand, has resulted in the typical dinner fork deformity.

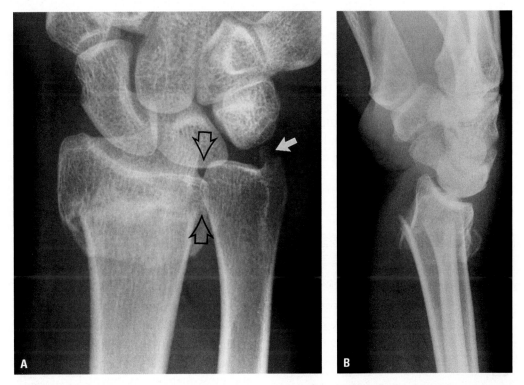

Figure 10.27. Colles fracture with characteristic distal radial fracture line and displacement of the distal radial fragment (**A** and **B**). Displacement of the ulnar styloid fragment *(arrow)* suggests avulsion by an intact triangular fibrocartilage. Dorsal displacement of the distal radial fragment causes disruption of the distal radioulnar joint *(open arrows)*.

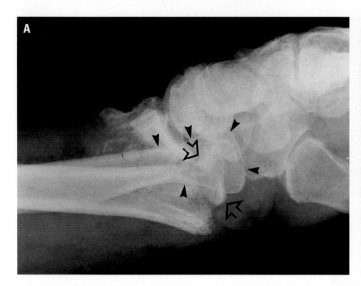

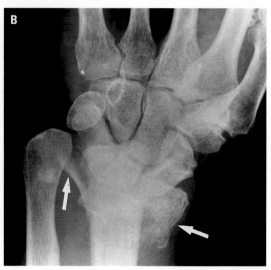

Figure 10.28. Severely comminuted intra-articular distal radial fracture. The widely separated, comminuted distal radial fragments *(arrows)* are more evident on the PA view **(B)** than on the lateral **(A)** projection. On the lateral view **(A)**, the distal ulna *(arrowheads)* largely obscures one of the distal radial fragments *(open arrows)*.

Barton Fracture

The Barton fracture differs from the Colles and the Smith fracture in that the distal radial fracture line is obliquely, rather than transversely, oriented and is intra-articular. The oblique fracture line runs primarily in the coronal plane and may involve the either the dorsal aspect of the distal radius (Fig. 10.31) or the volar aspect (Fig. 10.32). The volar pattern fracture is most common. The fragment size may vary. The radiocarpal separation may be minimal, or there may be a complete dislocation (Fig. 10.33).

Other Fracture Patterns

Fracture of the base of the radial styloid process (Fig. 10.34) (Chauffeur fracture) is also intra-articular. It is distinguished from the Barton fracture by the sagittal orientation of the fracture line and the absence of radio-carpal dislocation and carpal displacement.

The Galeazzi fracture-dislocation consists of a fracture of the distal third of the radius associated with dislocation of the DRUJ (Figs. 10.35 and 10.36). The DRUJ separation is the result of radial shortening caused by angulation or overriding of the fracture site. The degree of distal radioulnar diastasis may be subtle. A "reversed" Galeazzi fracture is a fracture of the distal third of the ulna with distal radioulnar dislocation. Both types may occur in children but are uncommon (Fig. 10.37).

Concomitant Injuries

Fractures of the distal radius are often associated with other injuries that should prompt careful radiologic evaluation of the entire wrist. These associated injuries may influence fracture classification and subsequent management. Cross-sectional imaging may be required in some cases.

Distal radius fractures have a high association with ulnar styloid fractures. Ulnar styloid nonunion is common. The fracture may involve any part of the styloid process. Fractures of the base of ulnar styloid are associated with TFC disruption and tears of the

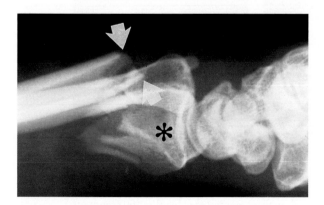

Figure 10.29. Smith fracture characterized by a transverse fracture *(arrows)* of the distal radius with volar and proximal displacement of the distal radial fragment *(asterisk).*

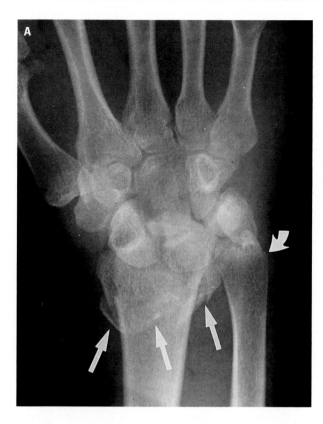

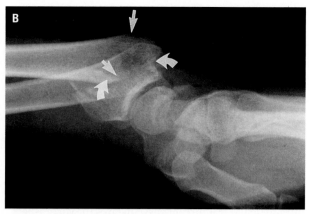

Figure 10.30. Smith fracture associated with distal ulnar shaft fracture. On the PA radiograph (**A**), the distal radial fragment *(arrows)*, together with the proximal row of carpal bones, is superimposed on the radius. A minimally displaced fracture *(curved arrow)* involves the distal ulnar shaft with slight radial displacement of the distal fragment. On the lateral radiograph (**B**), the radial fracture line is very distal and slightly oblique *(arrows)*. The ulnar fracture line *(curved arrows)* is also slightly oblique. The distal radial and ulnar fragments, together with the carpus and hand, are displaced in a volar direction and rotated clockwise.

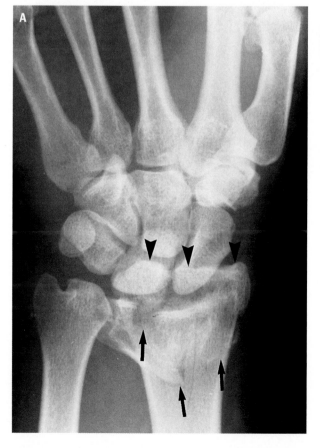

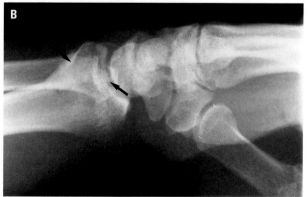

Figure 10.31. Dorsal Barton fracture of the distal radius. The PA radiograph (**A**) shows a comminuted fracture of the distal radius *(arrows)*. The proximal row of carpal bones is superimposed on a segment of the distal radial articulating surface *(arrowheads)*, implying an oblique fracture. The lateral radiograph (**B**) confirms the oblique, intra-articular fracture of the distal radius *(arrows)* with posterior displacement of the dorsal fragment together with the bones of the wrist and hand.

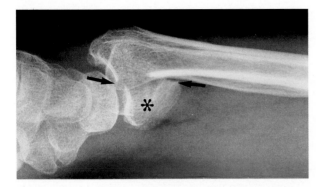

Figure 10.32. Classic volar Barton fracture. The oblique intra-articular fracture *(arrows)* involves the volar aspect of the distal radius. The separate fragment *(asterisk)* and the bones of the wrist and hand are displaced proximally and in a volar direction.

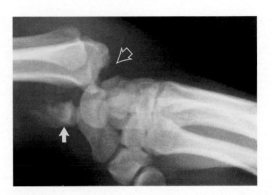

Figure 10.33. Volar Barton fracture-dislocation. The volar fragment *(arrow)* is relatively small and, together with the bones of the wrist and hand, is so severely displaced that the radiocarpal joint *(open arrow)* is dislocated.

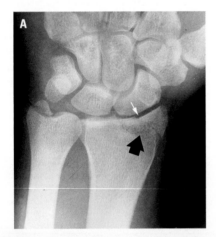

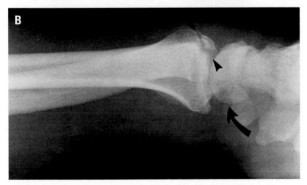

Figure 10.34. Radial styloid (Chauffeur) fracture with ulnar styloid fracture. On the PA radiograph (**A**), the distal radial fracture *(arrow)* extends obliquely across the base of the radial styloid process into the distal radial articulating surface *(small arrow)*. There is an ulnar styloid process fracture *(arrowhead)*. On the lateral radiograph (**B**), the radial styloid fragment *(arrowheads)* is minimally displaced and the proximal row of carpal bones *(curved arrow)* maintains the normal relationship to the radius.

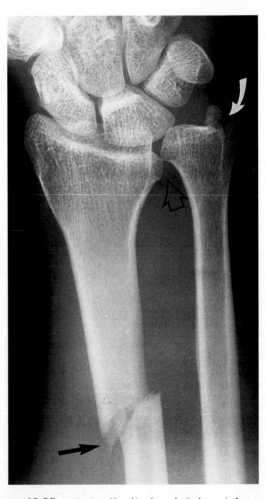

Figure 10.35. Minimally displaced Galeazzi fracture-dislocation. There is minor, but definite, shortening of the distal radial fracture site *(straight arrow)*, which has resulted in diastasis of the distal radioulnar joint *(open arrow)*. A fracture is present at the base of the ulnar styloid process *(curved arrow)*.

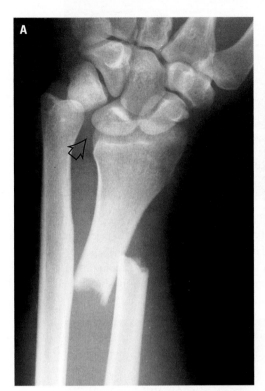
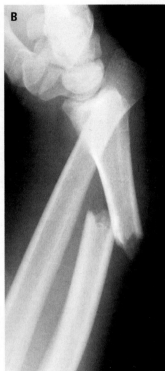

Figure 10.36. Severely displaced Galeazzi fracture-dislocation in PA (**A**) and lateral (**B**) projections. The distal radioulnar dislocation *(open arrow)* is secondary to the marked shortening of the radius caused by the severe ulnar displacement and dorsal angulation of the distal radial fragment.

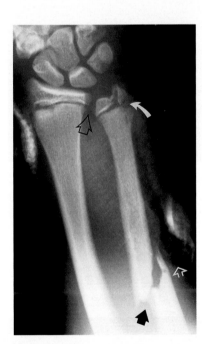

Figure 10.37. Reversed Galeazzi fracture-dislocation. In this instance, the fracture is at the junction of the middle and distal thirds of the ulna *(closed arrow)*. Shortening of the ulna has resulted in disruption of the distal radioulnar joint *(open arrow)*. A comminuted fracture involves the ulnar styloid process and the adjacent metaphysis *(curved arrow)*. The laceration and subcutaneous emphysema along the ulnar aspect of the distal forearm *(open white arrow)* indicate an open injury.

volar and dorsal radioulnar ligaments, which may lead to instability of the DRUJ.[12] Chronic DRUJ instability is usually a clinical diagnosis. MRI and MR arthrography can be used to demonstrate disruption of the TFC complex (Fig. 10.38).[13] However, traumatic tears that affect the peripheral attachments are more accurately diagnosed with MR arthrography.[14] CT or MRI performed in both supination and pronation can demonstrate dynamic DRUJ instability (Fig. 10.39).

Acute traumatic subluxation (Fig. 10.40) or dislocation of the DRUJ is usually the result of dorsal angulation of the distal fragment of either a distal radial or ulnar fracture (Fig. 10.41). A congenitally long ulna has the radiographic appearance of traumatic distal radioulnar dissociation, particularly on the lateral view (Fig. 10.42). However, the absence of an ulnar fracture and the anomalous location are distinguishing features.

It is important to stress the association of interosseous membrane (IOM) tears with longitudinal radioulnar dissociation injuries such as the Galeazzi fracture and other complex forearm (or elbow) injuries. The IOM maintains longitudinal stability of the forearm, and unrecognized injury can lead to poor outcome following fracture reduction and fixation. Signs of IOM tears have been described

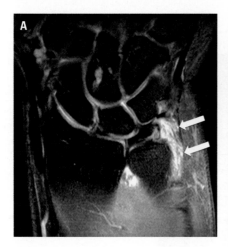
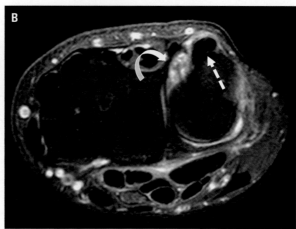

Figure 10.38. Triangular fibrocartilage (TFC) disruption. The coronal T2W fat saturated image (**A**) shows traumatic detachment of the peripheral attachments of the TFC on the ulna. There is high SI edema and hemorrhage around the distal ulna *(arrows)*. The axial T2W fat saturated image (**B**) shows the dorsal radioulnar ligament *(curved arrow)*, which is deficient laterally, and subluxation of the extensor carpi ulnaris tendon *(broken arrow)* secondary to a tear of the tendon subsheath.

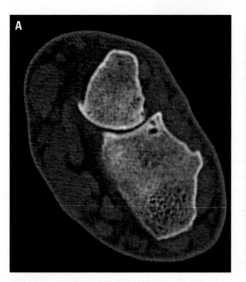
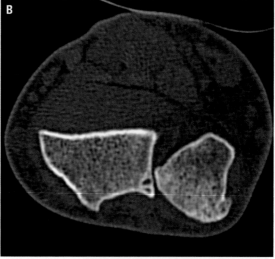

Figure 10.39. Dynamic CT of DRUJ instability in a patient with previous wrist fracture and secondary OA in the DRUJ. The lateral radiograph showed normal alignment of the DRUJ with normal variance. The axial CT image in pronation (**A**) shows the OA changes but normal alignment of the DRUJ. The instability becomes evident in supination (**B**), with dorsal subluxation of the joint.

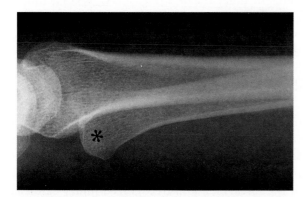
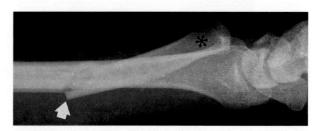

Figure 10.40. Subluxation of the distal radioulnar joint secondary to volar displacement of the distal ulna *(asterisk)*.

Figure 10.41. Distal radioulnar dislocation secondary to a distal ulnar fracture *(arrow)* with dorsal angulation of the distal ulnar fragment *(asterisk)*.

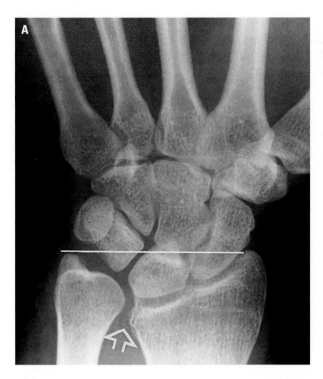

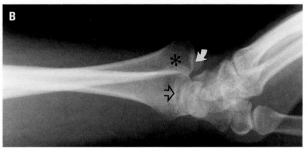

Figure 10.42. Congenitally long ulna simulating distal radioulnar dissociation. On both the PA (**A**) projections, the radial and ulnar styloid processes are on essentially the same plane *(line)*. The distal radioulnar space *(open arrow)* appears wide. On the lateral projection (**B**), the ulna *(asterisk)* is dorsal to the distal radius, and its articulating surface *(curved arrow)* is distal to that of the radius *(open arrow)*.

on both MRI and ultrasound (US), but current studies include only small patient numbers, and the accuracy of imaging for detection of IOM tears is unknown.[15]

There is also a common association of scapholunate ligament disruption and scapholunate dissociation with distal radial fractures (Fig. 10.43), occurring in up to half of all cases. Patients may subsequently develop carpal instability.[16] Other carpal dislocations or fractures occur less frequently.

Classification of Distal Radius Fractures

There is no absolute consensus on a single classification system for distal radial fractures.[17] However, the Fernandez classification is widely adopted by hand surgeons to help determine fracture management (Table 10.1). Following closed reduction, stable fractures may be maintained in a cast split or brace. Open reduction may be necessary for unstable fractures, and the fracture is fixated by any combination of pins, plating, or external fixation. A variety of biologics may be required to fill destabilizing defects.

Eight fracture characteristics help determine optimal treatment options:

- Location (intra-articular or extraarticular)
- Configuration (simple or comminuted)
- Displacement

- Ulnar styloid integrity
- Distal radioulnar joint integrity
- Stability
- Associated injuries
- Bone mineralization

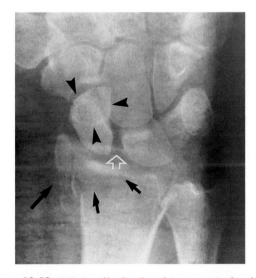

Figure 10.43. Minimally displaced intra-articular distal radial fracture *(arrows)* with the scaphoid "ring" sign *(arrowheads)* and abnormally wide scapholunate space *(open arrow)* consistent with scapholunate instability (rotary subluxation of the scaphoid) caused by disruption of the scapholunate ligament.

TABLE 10.1	The Fernandez Classification of Distal Radial Fractures	
Fernandez Classification		
1	Bending	One cortex of the metaphysis fails due to tensile stress and the opposite cortex undergoes some degree of comminution (Colles and Smith fractures)
2	Shearing	Fracture of the joint surface (Barton's fracture, reversed Barton's styloid process fracture, simple articular fracture)
3	Compression	Fracture of the surface of the joint with impaction of the subchondral and metaphyseal bone (die-punch); intra-articular comminuted fracture.
4	Avulsion	Fracture of the ligament attachments to ulnar and radial styloid process; radiologic fracture-dislocation.
5	Combinations	Combination of types; high-energy injuries

Characteristics that define fracture instability include >10 degree angulation, >5 mm axial shortening, >2 mm articular incongruity, comminution of the palmar and dorsal cortex, and an irreducible fracture.

There are no absolute indications for which fractures require evaluation with CT, but it is common practice to perform CT for comminuted intra-articular fractures to help define fracture configuration and displacement prior to surgical fixation (Fig. 10.44). MRI is not usually required in the immediate postinjury period, and the presence of hemorrhage may make interpretation of associated soft tissue injury difficult. However, MRI may be indicated at a later stage if there are symptoms of associated carpal instability or triangular fibrocartilage disruption.

Carpal Fractures

The scaphoid is the most frequently fractured of the carpal bones and is second only to fractures of the distal radius for all wrist fractures.[18] Fractures of the other carpal bones are less common but now more frequently recognized with increasing use of CT.[3] Carpal fractures may occur in isolation or in combination with other carpal bones.

Scaphoid

Scaphoid fractures are high-risk injuries. Up to 90% occur in male patients, with an average age of 26 years.[19] Complications include fracture nonunion, avascular necrosis (AVN) of the proximal fragment, and associated scapholunate ligament disruption and instability. This has significant implications for young manual workers or athletes whose livelihood may depend on the use of their hands.

Patients present with pain and tenderness in the region of the anatomic snuffbox. This finding is not specific for a scaphoid fracture and may be produced by injury to any of the bones along the radial aspect of the wrist. Scaphoid fractures are often subtle and easily missed. A scaphoid view should always be obtained, in addition to the routine projections, for any patient with blunt trauma to the wrist and clinical signs and symptoms referable to the anatomic snuffbox. It is common for the fracture to be visible on only one projection (Fig. 10.45).

The scaphoid fat stripe is a rhomboid lucency between the radial cortex of the scaphoid bone and the tendon of the extensor pollicis brevis muscle (Fig. 10.46). Blood from an occult scaphoid fracture obliterates the fat stripe.[20] This sign is not as reliable as other fat stripe signs because radial adduction of the wrist can obliterate the normal fat stripe and is not specific for scaphoid fractures (Fig. 10.47).

Scaphoid fractures are usually classified on the basis of the location of the fracture line. The waist of scaphoid is the most common site, with fractures occurring with lesser frequency in the proximal and distal poles. Distal tubercle fractures are rare (Fig. 10.48). Scaphoid fractures are uncommon in children (Fig. 10.49).

A scaphoid fracture may not be initially visible. If symptoms persist and there is strong clinical suspicion of a scaphoid fracture, then further investigations are imperative. It has been traditional practice to repeat the radiographic study after 10 to 14 days with immobilization. At this time, the fracture

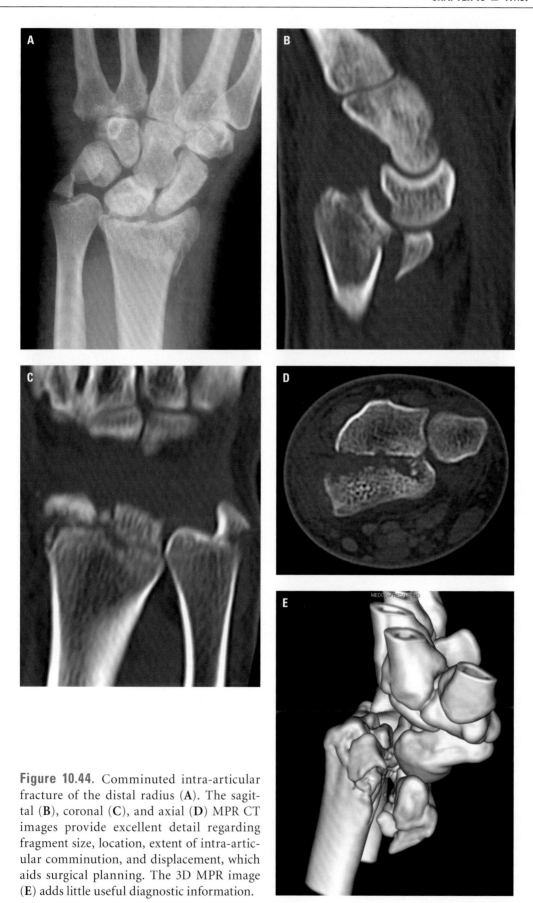

Figure 10.44. Comminuted intra-articular fracture of the distal radius (**A**). The sagittal (**B**), coronal (**C**), and axial (**D**) MPR CT images provide excellent detail regarding fragment size, location, extent of intra-articular comminution, and displacement, which aids surgical planning. The 3D MPR image (**E**) adds little useful diagnostic information.

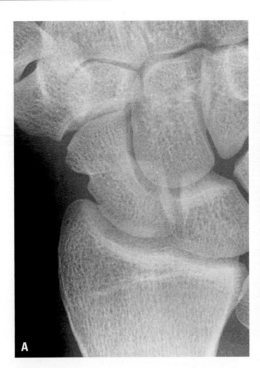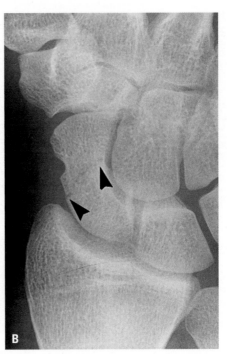

Figure 10.45. Scaphoid fracture. On the initial PA radiograph (**A**), the scaphoid bone appears normal. A minimally displaced fracture of the waist of the scaphoid *(arrowheads)* is visible on the scaphoid view (**B**).

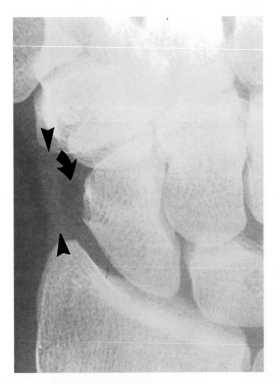

Figure 10.46. The vague, rhomboid lucency *(curved arrow)* between the radial aspect of the scaphoid and the density of the extensor pollicis brevis tendon *(arrowheads)* is the normal scaphoid fat pad.

line will be more visible because of bony resorption adjacent to the fracture line. If the subsequent radiographs remain negative and symptoms persist, imaging with MRI or CT is indicated. Three-phase nuclear medicine bone scans may be positive within 24 hours postfracture but are now rarely used.

MRI accurately demonstrates occult scaphoid fractures and is more sensitive and specific than isotope bone scans.[21] The signs of a fracture are a low-signal intensity fracture line on T1W images and intraosseous edema on T2W fat saturated or STIR images (Fig. 10.50).[22,23] MRI performed within 14 days of the initial injury will significantly influence clinical management.[24] It may be justified to perform MRI immediately following the first negative radiographic examination in order to exclude a fracture in patients with strong clinical findings. MDCT is also accurate for diagnosis of occult scaphoid fractures and may be appropriate when MRI is not readily available.[3,4] Although current evidence suggests that both MRI and MDCT are appropriate modalities to exclude an acute scaphoid fracture, caution is advised because fracture lines may be subtle within the first few days following injury (Fig. 10.51).

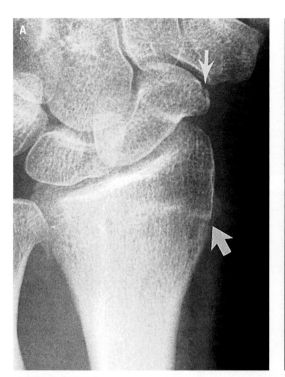

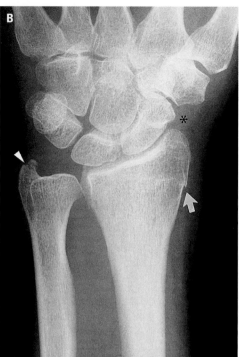

Figure 10.47. Minimally displaced distal radial fracture associated with a fracture of the scaphoid tubercle. The distal radial fracture *(large arrows)* is clearly visible on the externally rotated oblique projection (**A**) in which the minimally displaced scaphoid tubercle fracture *(small arrow)* is also evident. On the PA projection (**B**), the scaphoid fat stripe is obliterated *(asterisk)*, and a minimally displaced ulnar styloid fracture *(arrowhead)* is evident.

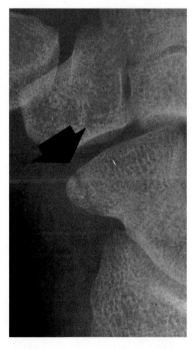

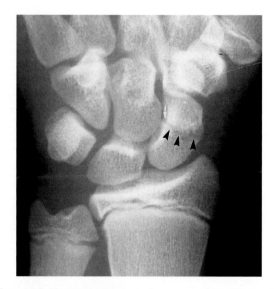

Figure 10.49. PA radiograph demonstrating a minimally displaced fracture of the waist of scaphoid *(arrowheads)* in a child. The fracture defect might be considered part of the normal cortex of the distal pole. However, disruption of the ulnar cortex *(arrow)* establishes the presence of the fracture.

Figure 10.48. Fracture of the scaphoid tubercle *(arrow)* evident on an oblique projection of the wrist.

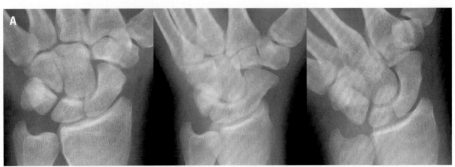

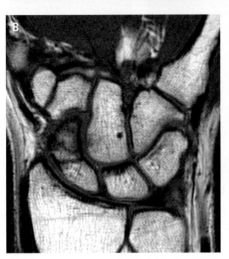

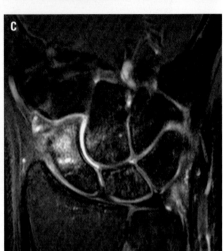

Figure 10.50. Occult scaphoid fracture. The radiographic series (**A**) are normal with no fracture line visible. However, MRI performed a few days later show a low-signal intensity fracture line on the T1W Image (**B**) and diffuse high-signal intensity marrow edema in the distal pole on the T2W fat saturation image (**C**), confirming an undisplaced scaphoid fracture.

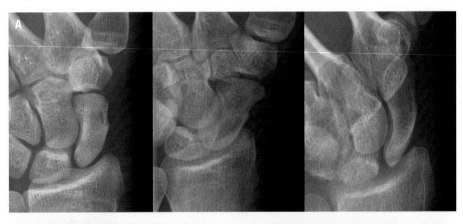

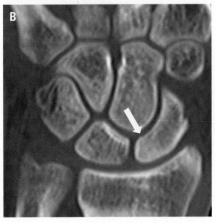

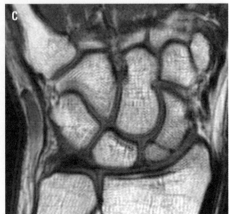

Figure 10.51. An initial radiographic series of a patient with suspected scaphoid fracture (**A**) shows a possible lucent line in the proximal pole on the PA view only. A CT performed the same day was interpreted as normal (**B**). No fracture line is visible, and the only abnormality is a very subtle step in the articular surface *(arrow)*. The patient had persistent pain, and an MRI scan acquired 2 weeks later clearly shows the scaphoid fracture (**C**).

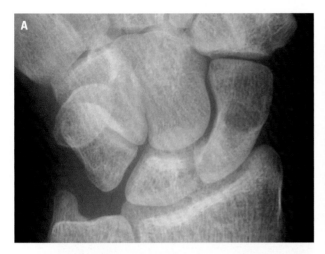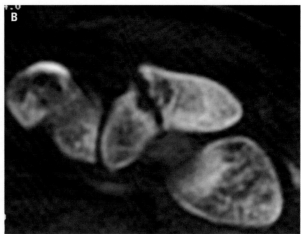

Figure 10.52. Scaphoid fracture nonunion. Follow-up radiographs acquired to monitor fracture healing apparently show a united fracture with an intramedullary cyst (**A**). However, the patient had residual pain, and CT clearly demonstrates fracture nonunion (**B**). (From Waldman SD, Campbell RSD. *Imaging of Pain.* 1st ed. Philadelphia, PA: Saunders Elsevier; 2011, with permission.)

Failure to diagnose a scaphoid fracture increases the incidence of fracture nonunion and AVN. Nonunion or delayed union occurs in 5% to 40% of patients dependent on displacement and fracture location.[25] Assessment of bony union is best achieved with CT when radiographs are indeterminate and may help determine the need for surgical fixation (Fig. 10.52). Fracture malunion and development of a "humpbacked deformity" may be associated with carpal instability.[1] This deformity is well demonstrated by CT and can help determine surgical management.

The blood supply to the scaphoid is variable, but 70% to 80% have a distal arterial supply that also provides a feeding vessel to the proximal pole. Fractures of the waist of the scaphoid have a very high probability of disrupting the artery to the middle and proximal pole of the scaphoid. AVN of the proximal pole occurs in as many as 30% of patients and in up to 100% of displaced fractures. The more proximal the fracture line, the greater the incidence of AVN.[26] AVN is indicated by increased density of that portion of the scaphoid devoid of blood supply (Fig. 10.53). Cystic change may be seen around the fracture line. Eventually, there may be subchondral collapse and fragmentation of the avascular segment. MRI is used to detect early AVN and predict viability of the proximal fragment. Low signal intensity (SI) of the marrow of the proximal scaphoid on T1W images is a reason-

able indicator for AVN.[27] Lack of enhancement on post-contrast images improves diagnostic accuracy (Fig. 10.54).[28]

Hamate

Fractures of the hamate may occur as isolated injuries (Fig. 10.55). However, they are commonly associated with dorsal dislocation of the base of the

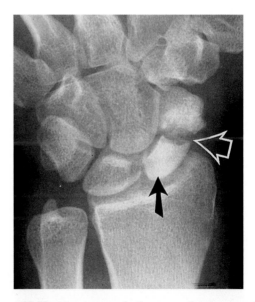

Figure 10.53. Nonunion of a fracture of the waist of the scaphoid *(open arrow)*. The proximal pole is sclerotic due to secondary AVN *(closed arrow)*.

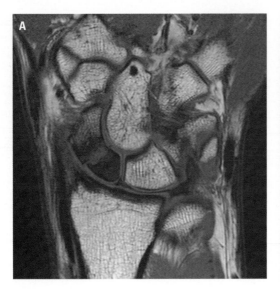

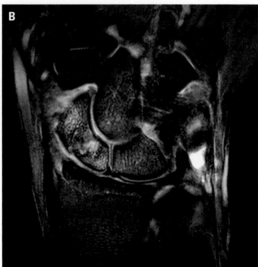

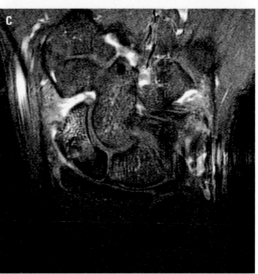

Figure 10.54. AVN of the proximal pole following a waist of scaphoid fracture. The proximal pole is low-signal intensity on the T1W image (**A**). The diffuse marrow edema on the T2W fat saturation image (**B**) suggests there may be residual vascularity, but there is no enhancement of the proximal pole on the post-contrast T1W fat saturation image (**C**) indicating nonviable (From Waldman SD, Campbell RSD. *Imaging of Pain.* 1st ed. Philadelphia, PA: Saunders Elsevier; 2011, with permission.)

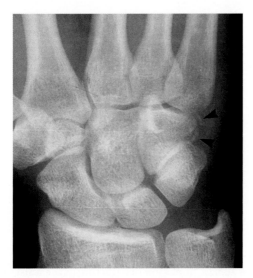

Figure 10.55. Minimally displaced, comminuted, isolated fracture of the ulnar aspect of the hamate *(arrowheads)*.

fourth and fifth metacarpals (Fig. 10.56). These fractures may be complex and CT may be required to aid surgical planning (Fig. 10.57). Fracture of the base of the hook of the hamate is a rare injury that is frequently missed (Fig. 10.58). Occult hook of hamate fractures may be a cause of prolonged pain and discomfort along the palmar aspect of the ulnar side of the wrist and are best demonstrated with MRI or CT (Fig. 10.59)

Triquetrum

The most common fracture of the triquetrum involves the dorsal surface and is only seen on a lateral radiograph (Fig. 10.60). The mechanism of injury is avulsion of the dorsal radiotriquetral ligament after forced hyperflexion or impaction of the dorsal triquetrum against the dorsal rim of the

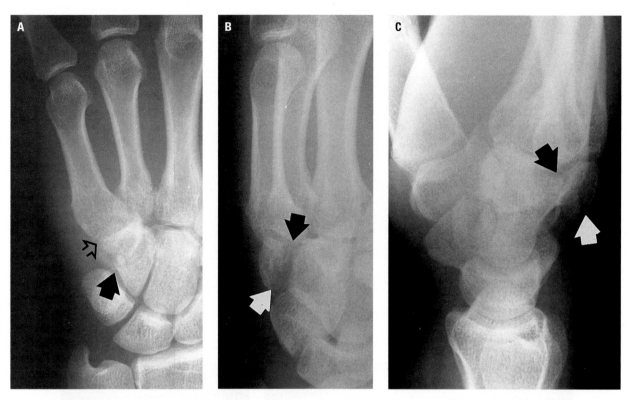

Figure 10.56. Comminuted, displaced fracture of the dorsum of the hamate *(arrows)*, associated with dorsal dislocation of the fifth metacarpal *(open arrow)* as seen on PA (**A**), oblique (**B**), and lateral (**C**) projections.

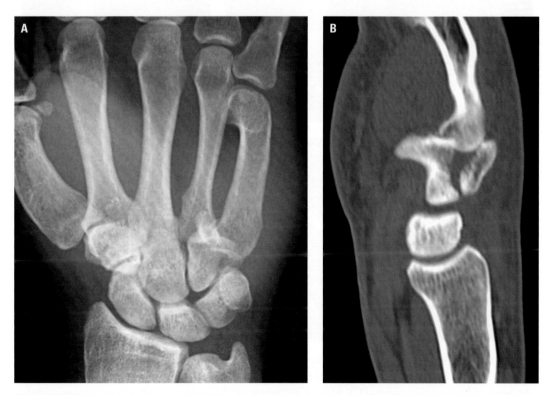

Figure 10.57. Fracture-dislocation of the fourth and fifth CMC joint. The radiograph shows disruption of the joint line and an associated hamate fracture (**A**). On the sagittal CT MPR image, there is a coronal hamate fracture, and the base of the fifth metacarpal is displaced into the fracture line (**B**). If the dislocation is not reduced, it will result in nonunion or malunion of the hamate.

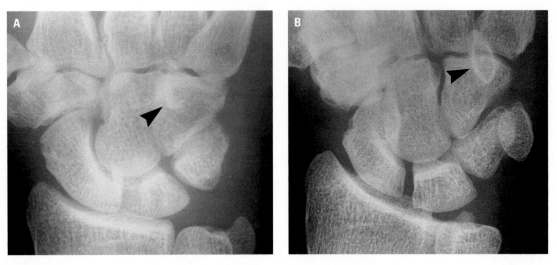

Figure 10.58. Fracture of the hook of the hamate *(arrowheads)* evident only by the abnormal location on the PA (**A**) and oblique (**B**) projections.

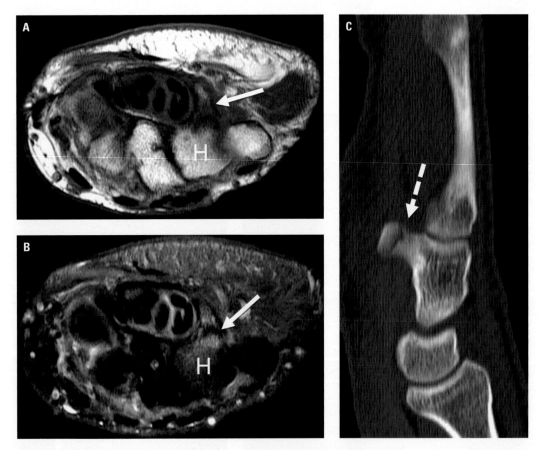

Figure 10.59. MRI of an occult hamate fracture in a golfer with chronic wrist pain. There is marrow edema *(arrows)* on both the axial T1W image (**A**) and the axial T2W fat saturation image (**B**) in the hook of hamate. The sagittal CT MPR (**C**) confirms the diagnosis of a fracture *(broken arrow)*. H, hamate. *Images courtesy of Dr. Phil O'Connor, Leeds Teaching Hospitals, UK.*

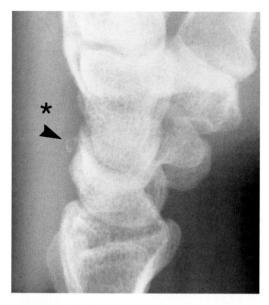

Figure 10.60. Isolated fracture of the dorsal aspect of the triquetrum *(arrowhead)*. Soft tissue swelling *(asterisk)* of the dorsum of the wrist is usually the most prominent sign of this fracture.

distal ulnar articulating surface. However, avulsion injuries involving the extrinsic dorsal wrist ligaments may affect other carpal bones. Triquetral body fractures may occur alone (Fig. 10.61) or in association with fractures of the pisiform or hamate (Fig. 10.62).

Other Carpal Fractures

Isolated fractures of other carpal bones occur infrequently and are easily overlooked (Fig. 10.63). Fracture of the pisiform is caused by a fall on the outstretched hand with the impact on the ulnar side of the wrist. Pisiform fractures may be simple, seen best on the lateral radiograph (Fig. 10.64), and may be associated with triquetral fractures. Dislocation of the pisiform may occur (Fig. 10.65). Lunate dislocations are discussed in the section on carpal instability. Comminuted or multiple fractures of the carpal bones are best documented on CT.

Carpal Instability

Stability of the wrist is maintained by the complex articulations between the individual carpal bones and the intrinsic and extrinsic wrist ligaments.[9] Any disturbance of the static or dynamic forces that act around the wrist can lead to instability. This can occur as a result of fracture, ligament disruption, or a combination of both. Failure to recognize the presence of instability may result in inadequate or inappropriate treatment with impairment of wrist function and progressive secondary arthrosis.[29]

Following acute injury, ligamentous disruption may be evident by easily recognizable radiographic

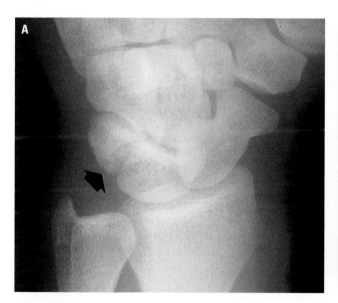
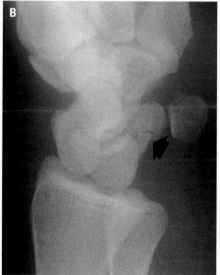

Figure 10.61. Isolated, comminuted, minimally displaced fracture of the triquetrum *(arrow)* seen on oblique (**A**) and lateral (**B**) projections.

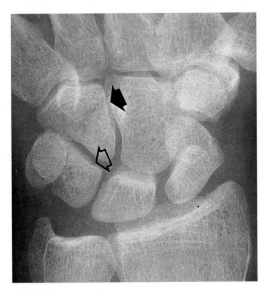

Figure 10.62. Concomitant fractures of the hamate *(closed arrow)* and triquetrum *(open arrow).*

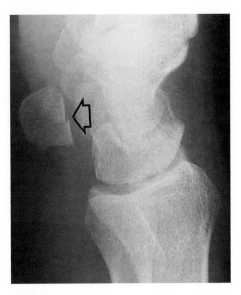

Figure 10.64. Isolated fracture of the pisiform *(open arrow).*

abnormalities. However, in some cases, these findings may be subtle or undetectable on conventional radiographic projections. A wide range of radiologic investigations may be undertaken to identify instability for patients with chronic wrist pain following trauma.[9]

Carpal malalignment may only be evident on an "instability or stress series" of radiographs acquired with the wrist in different positions. Instability radiographs may include PA views in radial and ulnar deviation and a clenched fist view. Lateral views may be taken in flexion and extension. Alternatively, dynamic fluoroscopy may be performed to detect dynamic alterations of the complex movements of the wrist. The radiographic signs of carpal instability involve disruption of the arcs of Gilula (Fig. 10.11), asymmetry of the intercarpal joint spaces, and alteration of the contour of individual carpal bones.

Arthrography identifies abnormal communication between different wrist compartments caused by ligament disruption. MRI is able to directly visualize many of the wrist ligaments. MR arthrography and CT arthrography provide the benefits of both cross-sectional imaging and the delineation of joint compartments with contrast media. Decisions regarding optimum imaging pathways are best achieved through dialogue between radiologists and hand surgeons and are dependent on clinical findings.

There are many classification systems for defining the patterns of wrist instability, and a complete discussion is beyond the scope of this text. The analysis of carpal instability is dependent on several factors, including chronicity, reducibility, etiology, location, and direction.[30] The four patterns of instability are described as

- dissociative,
- nondissociative,
- complex, and
- adaptive.

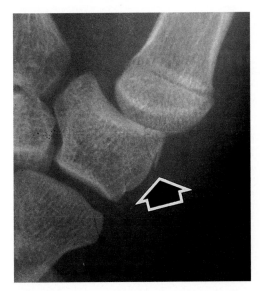

Figure 10.63. Minimally displaced fracture of the trapezium *(arrow).*

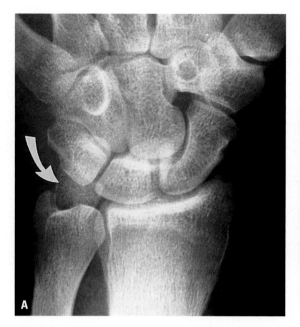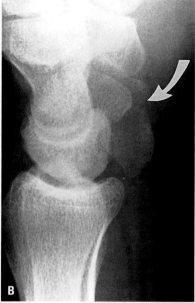

Figure 10.65. Fracture-dislocation of the pisiform *(curved arrows)* seen on PA (**A**) and lateral (**B**) projections. The dislocation of the pisiform is evident in the PA projection, whereas the fracture and dislocation are demonstrated on the lateral view.

Only the most common and most important patterns are described.

Carpal Instability Dissociative

Disruption of the intrinsic ligaments between the bones of the proximal carpal row (scapholunate and lunatotriquetral) leads to abnormal motion segments centered on the lunate, which is described as the keystone of the wrist.

Dorsal Intercalated Instability

When the scapholunate ligament is torn, it allows an increase in the palmar flexion of the scaphoid (also termed rotatory instability of the scaphoid) and dorsal tilt of the lunate. There is widening of the scapholunate articulation on the PA wrist view (diastasis >3 mm), which may be exaggerated on a clenched fist view. The scaphoid "ring" sign represents the cortex of the distal pole of the scaphoid seen end-on secondary to palmar rotation (Figs. 10.66 and 10.67A). On a true lateral projection, the scapholunate angle is increased (>60 degrees) (Fig. 10.67B). Diagnosis is dependent on the presence of one or more of these signs, and there are four stages of scapholunate instability.[9] Scapholunate ligament tears may be associated with scaphoid fractures (Fig. 10.68) and distal radial fractures (Fig. 10.43).

When the radiographic signs are equivocal, arthrography will demonstrate leak of contrast through a tear of the scapholunate joint (Fig. 10.69). MRI can directly visualize a torn ligament or may show partial tears and ligament laxity in cases of subtle instability (Fig. 10.70). Early diagnosis of scapholunate disruption enables ligament repair.

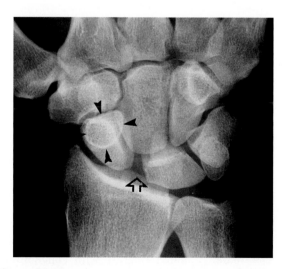

Figure 10.66. Classic appearance of scapholunate dissociation on the PA view including scapholunate diastasis *(open arrow)* and the scaphoid ring sign *(arrowheads)*.

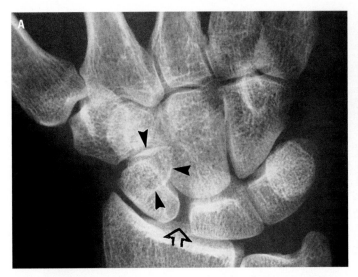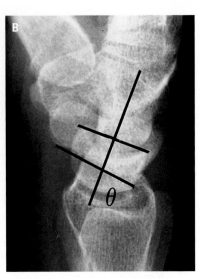

Figure 10.67. Scapholunate dissociation. On the PA radiograph (**A**), the diastasis *(open arrow)* is obvious, but the ring sign *(arrowheads)* is subtle. On the lateral projection (**B**), the dorsal tilt of the lunate is obvious and the scapholunate angle (θ) is greater than 60 degrees.

In the chronic situation, ligament reconstruction may be required. If left untreated, the patient may develop severe secondary arthrosis, termed *scapholunate advanced collapse* (SLAC). Scaphoid fracture with nonunion or malunion without ligament disruption is also a cause of instability. Arthrosis associated with scaphoid nonunion is termed *scaphoid nonunion advanced collapse* (SNAC) (Fig. 10.71).

Volar Intercalated Instability

Rupture of the lunatotriquetral ligament is less common. There is no widening of the lunatotriquetral interval, although there is often a step at the proximal lunotriquetral joint, which is often most evident on PA radiographs in ulnar deviation. On a lateral view, the lunate tilts in a volar direction, reducing the scapholunate angle (<30 degrees) (Fig. 10.72). On fluoroscopy, there may be opposite rotational movement of the scapho-lunate segment and the triquetrum.[9] The lunatotriquetral ligament is less reliably demonstrated on conventional MRI than the scapholunate ligament, and MR or CT arthography may be preferred. Contrast leak between the lunatotriquetral joint is seen on arthrography (Fig. 10.73).

Both the dorsal intercalated segment instability (DISI) and volar intercalated segment instability (VISI) types of instability may be associated with more complex patterns of instability. Some patterns of instability may be difficult to classify. The presence or absence of instability probably depends on an association of tears (partial or complete) of both intrinsic and extrinsic ligaments rather than intrinsic ligaments alone.[31]

Figure 10.68. Scaphoid fracture with concomitant scapho-lunate dissociation. There is scapholunate diastasis *(open arrow)* and the waist of scaphoid fracture is obvious *(arrow)*.

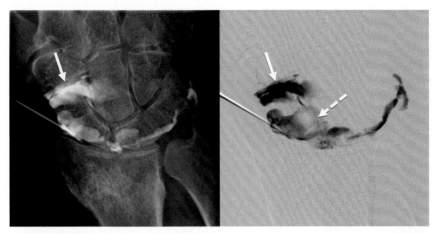

Figure 10.69. Arthrogram images of a scapholunate ligament tear. The spot films acquired during a radiocarpal joint injection demonstrate contrast not only within the radiocarpal joint but also the midcarpal joint *(arrows)*. The digital subtraction image more clearly demonstrates the track of contrast extending through the scapholunate joint line *(broken arrow)*.

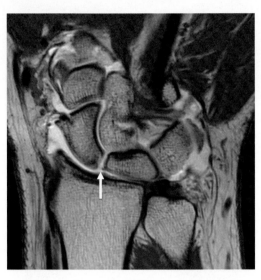

Figure 10.70. T1W coronal MR arthrogram image of a scapholunate ligament tear. No scapholunate ligament is visible *(arrow)*, and high-signal intensity contrast extends throughout the scapholunate joint space. There is no associated joint diastasis.

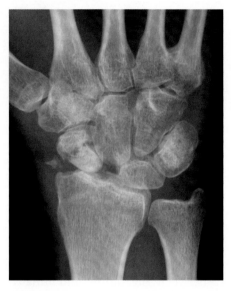

Figure 10.71. Scaphoid nonunion advanced collapse (SNAC). There is an un-united scaphoid fracture, and the proximal pole is sclerotic consistent with associated AVN. There is scapho-lunate diastasis and narrowing of the radioscaphoid joint, the scaphocapitate joint, and the lunatocapitate joint indicating secondary arthrosis.

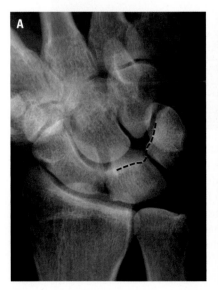
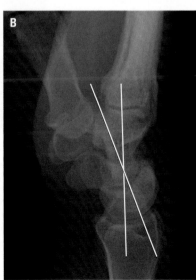

Figure 10.72. Lunatotriquetral ligament tear. The PA radiograph (**A**) in radial deviation shows a step at the margin of the lunatotriquetral articulation *(broken lines)* and widening of the midcarpal joint line. The lateral projection demonstrates volar tilt of the lunate and an increase of the capitolunate angle (**B**).

411

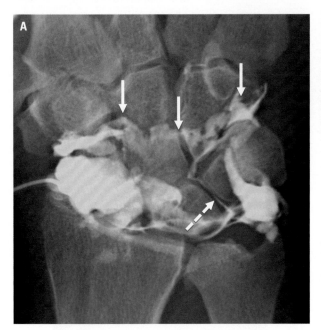

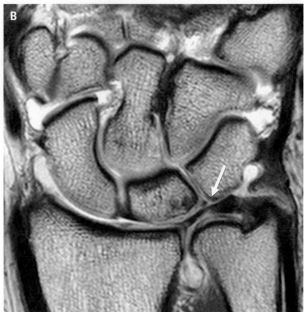

Figure 10.73. Lunatotriquetral ligament tear. Radiographs were normal. The arthrogram image acquired during radiocarpal joint injection shows contrast leak into the midcarpal joint *(arrows)*, and the track of contrast within the lunatotriquetral joint line *(broken arrow)* (**A**). The ligament is deficient on the corresponding coronal T1W MR arthrogram image *(arrow)* (**B**).

Carpal Instability Nondissociative

The extrinsic ligaments of the wrists provide stability between the radius and ulna and the proximal carpal row, and between the proximal and distal carpal row. Ligament disruption, or stretching, leads to instability between the carpal rows (radiocarpal or midcarpal instability) rather than instability between individual bones of a single row. The abnormal alignment may be seen on a lateral radiograph or may be evident on dynamic fluoroscopy.

Radiocarpal instability is most commonly associated with distal radial fractures (adaptive type). Pure ligamentous radiocarpal dislocations are rare. Ulnar translation is the most common pattern and occurs due to tears of the radioscaphoid, radioscaphocapitate, and radiolunate-triquetral ligaments. Radiocarpal instability may also occur in a dorsal or volar direction (Fig. 10.74).

Midcarpal instability (MCI) is more common. It is a complex group of conditions for which the etiology, terminology, and treatment remains controversial (Fig. 10.75).[32] Combined instability of the radiocarpal and midcarpal joints is common. There may be both VISI and DISI patterns, and the lunatocapitate angle is abnormal.

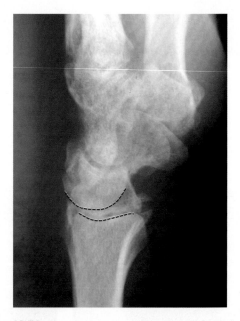

Figure 10.74. Acute rupture of the dorsal radiolunate-triquetral ligament with dorsal radiocarpal instability. There is subtle dorsal subluxation of the lunate with respect to the radius *(dotted lines)*. The lunate is also tilted in a volar direction with secondary increase in the lunatocapitate angle. The instability was successfully treated by reattachment of the torn ligament. *Image courtesy of Mr. Doug Campbell, Consultant Orthopedic Hand Surgeon, Leeds Teaching Hospitals, UK.*

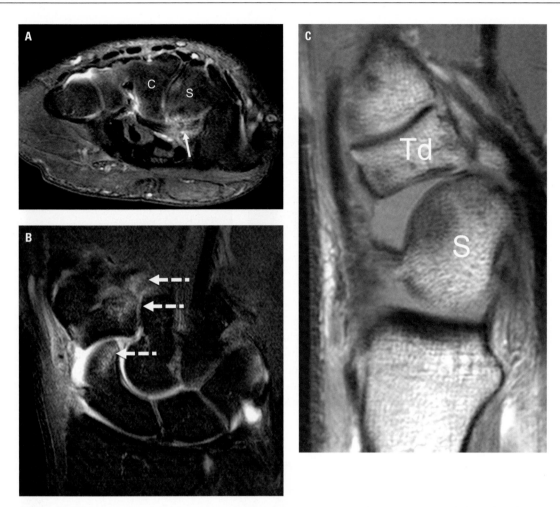

Figure 10.75. Acute tear of the volar scapho-trapezio-trapezoidal ligament with subtle midcarpal instability. The axial T2W fat saturation image demonstrates thickening and high-signal intensity edema within the ligament *(arrow)* (**A**). There is associated bone marrow edema within the distal pole of scaphoid, the trapezoid, and the base of the second metacarpal *(broken arrows)* on the coronal T2W fat saturation image (**B**). There is malalignment of the scapho-trapezoid articulation of the sagittal PD image (**C**). *S*, scaphoid; *C*, capitate; *Td*, trapezoid.

Carpal Instability Complex

These types of instability are rare. However, acute peri-lunate and lunate dislocations are severe injuries that are important to diagnose and treat early. They may be complicated by AVN of the lunate.

Perilunate Dislocation

A variety of instability patterns occur with progressive failure of scapholunate, capitolunate, and lunatotriquetral ligaments. In perilunate dislocation, the lunate retains its normal position with respect to the distal radius, whereas the scaphoid, triquetrum, and all other carpal bones are dislocated dorsally with respect to the lunate. On a frontal projection, there is loss of congruity of each of the three carpal arcs. The lunate assumes a triangular configuration, with

the apex being distal, caused by volar rotation. On the lateral projection, the lunate is normally related to the distal radius, whereas the capitate and other carpal bones are dislocated in a dorsal direction (Fig. 10.76). It is most commonly associated with a fracture of the waist of the scaphoid (transscaphoid perilunate dislocation) (Fig. 10.77).

Lunate Dislocation

Lunate dislocation is the most severe of the carpal instabilities, involving all of the intercarpal joints with disruption of the majority of the intercarpal ligaments. On the frontal projection, the lunate assumes a triangular configuration similar to that seen with perilunate dislocation (Fig. 10.69). On the lateral projection, the lunate is displaced and rotated in a volar

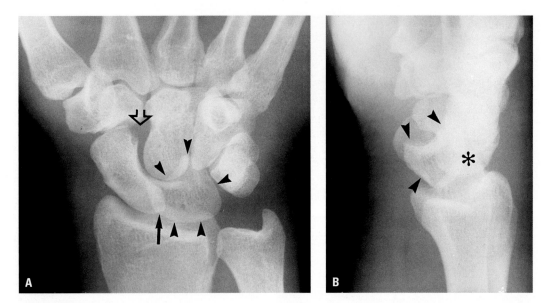

Figure 10.76. Pure posterior perilunate dislocation. The precise diagnosis cannot be made on the PA projection (**A**). Signs of carpal instability include scaphocapitate *(open arrow)* and scapholunate *(arrow)* separation and a minor triangular configuration of the lunate *(arrowheads)*. The lateral projection (**B**) confirms posterior dislocation of the capitate *(asterisk)* and all other carpal bones with respect to the lunate *(arrowheads)*. The minor volar rotation of the lunate accounts for the triangular configuration on the PA radiograph (**A**).

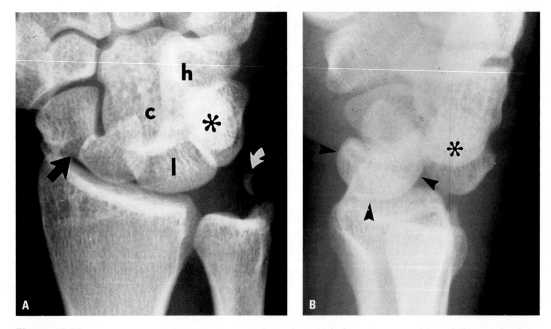

Figure 10.77. Transscaphoid fracture–posterior perilunate dislocation carpal instability with ulnar styloid process fracture. The signs of this complex injury on the PA radiograph (**A**) include the transscaphoid fracture *(arrow)*, ulnar subluxation and triangular shape of the lunate, and malalignment of the capitate, hamate, triquetrum, and pisiform *(asterisk)*, with superimposition of each on the lunate. There is an associated fracture of the tip of the ulnar styloid process *(curved arrow)*. The perilunate dislocation is seen on the lateral radiograph (**B**) by the position of the capitate *(asterisk)* and other carpal bones lying posterior to the lunate *(arrowheads)*, which remains the normal relationship to the distal radius. *L*, lunate; *C*, capitate; *H*, hamate.

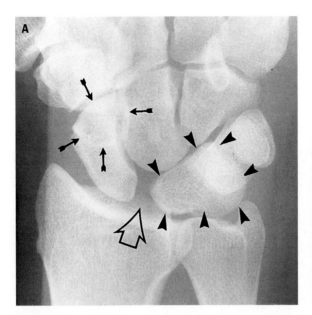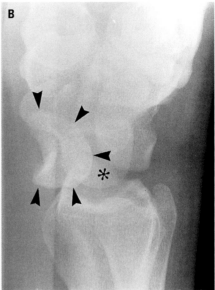

Figure 10.78. Lunate dislocation. On the PA projection (**A**), the lunate is dislocated with a characteristic triangular configuration *(arrowheads)*. Additionally, there is scapholunate diastasis *(open arrow)*, and a scaphoid ring sign *(arrows)* is present. In the lateral projection (**B**), the lunate *(arrowheads)* is completely dislocated and rotated in a volar direction. The capitate *(asterisk)* and the remainder of the carpal bones lie posterior to the lunate.

direction with loss of the normal relationship to the radius. The volar rotation is typically about 90 degrees. The capitate and the remaining carpal bones lie posterior to the lunate, with the capitate occupying the space vacated by the lunate but maintaining its

alignment with the radius (Fig. 10.78). An associated transscaphoid fracture is common (Fig. 10.79).

The key to differentiating the lunate and perilunate dislocation is the relationship between the lunate and radius on the lateral radiograph. These

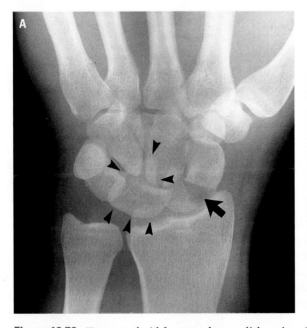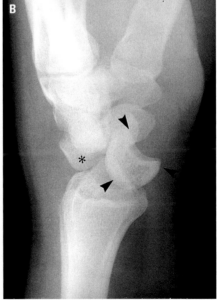

Figure 10.79. Transscaphoid fracture–lunate dislocation. On the PA radiograph (**A**), the scaphoid fracture *(arrow)* is readily apparent. The triangular configuration of the dislocated lunate *(arrowheads)* is less obvious. On the lateral radiograph (**B**), the volar dislocation of the lunate *(arrowheads)* is less marked than in Figure 10.78. The capitate *(asterisk)* and other carpal bones lie posterior to the dislocated lunate.

injuries may be complex, and associated injuries other than scaphoid fractures may occur. CT is helpful in defining the relationship between the carpal bones, the presence of associated fractures, and the degree of fracture displacement (Fig. 10.80).

Carpal Instability Adaptive

The adaptive instabilities are the result of acquired or congenital abnormalities around the wrist. The most common patterns are associated with malunion of distal radial or scaphoid fractures.

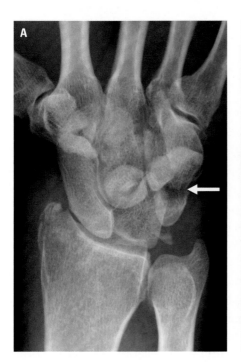
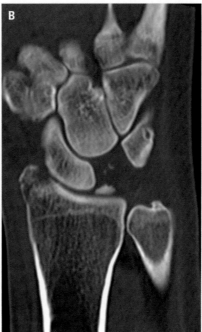
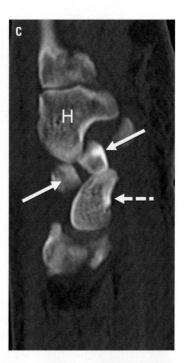
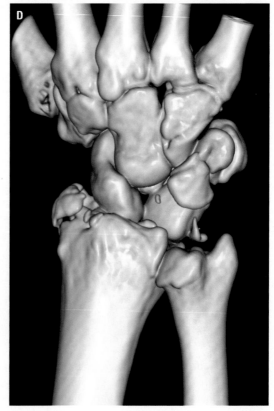

Figure 10.80. Transtriquetral fracture and lunate dislocation. The radiograph (**A**) shows the abnormal triangular configuration of the lunate and a fracture of the triquetrum *(arrow)* (**A**). There is also a fracture fragment in the ulnocarpal joint and a radial styloid fracture. The coronal CT MPR image shows preservation of the articulation with the scaphoid and absent lunate (**B**). The sagittal MPR demonstrates the fractured triquetral fragments *(arrows)*, and the rotated and displaced lunate *(broken arrow)* (**C**). The 3D MPR image shows the volar displacement of the lunate (**D**). *H,* hamate.

Adaptive instability may also be seen with different types of Madelung's deformity.

Carpometacarpal Fractures

The complex anatomy of the interlocking articulations and the network of short, dense CMC and intermetacarpal ligaments limit injuries to the second to fifth CMC joints. Fracture-dislocations require significant force, usually a major crushing or punching injury, and are most common at the fourth and fifth CMC joints, which are more mobile than the second and third CMC joints. They are frequently associated with a fracture of the hamate. These injuries may be subtle on the PA radiograph of the hand, which necessitates careful analysis of the CMC joint space (Fig. 10.81). A true lateral radiograph of the hand will demonstrate the dorsal dislocation of the metacarpal base (Fig. 10.56). On occasion, the metacarpal may dislocate into a coronal plane fracture of the hamate (Fig. 10.57). If this dislocation is not adequately reduced, it will prevent fracture union. Pure ligamentous dislocation

of the fifth metacarpal may occur without associated fracture (Fig. 10.82).

Isolated fractures of the base of the second and third metacarpal are less common (Fig. 10.83). Pure ligamentous volar dislocation of the second to fifth CMC joints is a rare injury (Fig. 10.84).

CONCLUSION

Wrist fractures may be subtle and require good quality radiographs and careful radiologic analysis in order to avoid missing a potentially serious injury that, left untreated, may be associated with a high incidence of comorbidity. Radiologists should be alert to the common occurrence of ligament injury that may or may not be accompanied by a fracture. Optimal imaging pathways for the diagnosis of ligament injury require a good dialogue between the radiologist and hand surgeon. The reader is encouraged to read some of the excellent cited references for a fuller description of the patterns of carpal instability and diagnosis of TFC disruption.

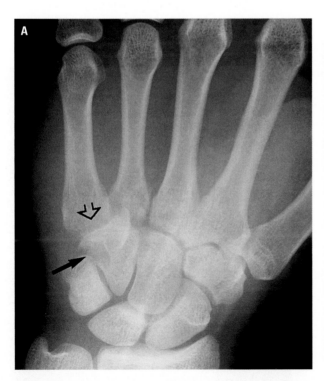
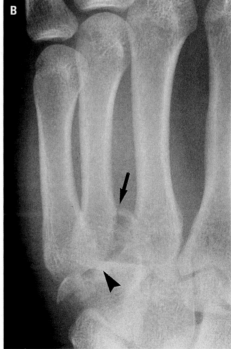

Figure 10.81. Complex fourth and fifth metacarpal fracture-dislocation. On the PA radiograph (**A**), it appears as though only the fifth metacarpal is dislocated *(open arrow)* and is associated with a hamate fracture *(arrow)*. The oblique projection (**B**) demonstrates a concomitant posterior subluxation of the fourth metacarpal *(arrowhead)* with an oblique fracture of the radial aspect of its base *(arrow)*.

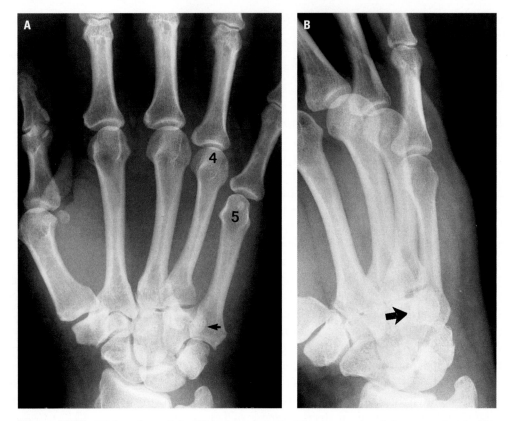

Figure 10.82. Dislocation of the fifth metacarpal without associated fracture. On the PA projection (**A**), dislocation of the fifth metacarpal is indicated by superimposition of the base over the hamate *(arrow)* and apparent shortening of the fifth metacarpal with respect to the fourth metacarpal. Posterior dislocation is confirmed *(arrow)* on the oblique projection (**B**).

Figure 10.83. Isolated fracture of the base of second metacarpal *(arrow)*.

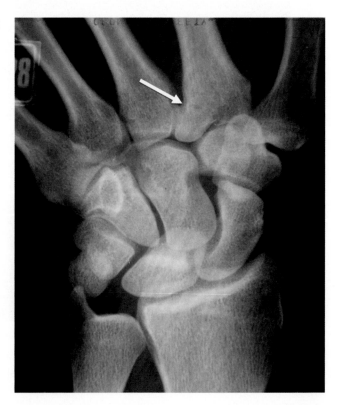

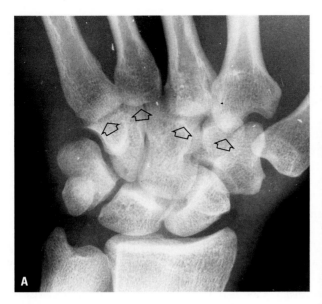
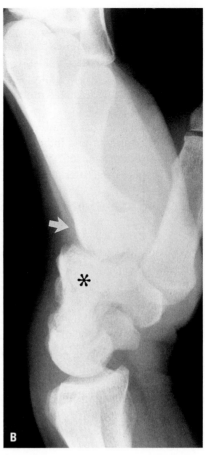

Figure 10.84. Pure ligamentous volar dislocation of the lateral four metacarpals. On the PA projection (**A**), the dislocation is indicated by the loss of the lateral four carpometacarpal joint spaces caused by superimposition of the metacarpal bases on the distal carpal row *(open arrows)*. The lateral radiograph (**B**) demonstrates the volar dislocation of the third metacarpal *(arrow)* with respect to the capitate *(asterisk)*.

REFERENCES

1. Goldfarb CA, Yin Y, Gilula LA, et al. Wrist fractures: what the clinician wants to know. *Radiology.* 2001;219(1):11–28.
2. Kiuru MJ, Haapamaki VV, Koivikko MP, et al. Wrist injuries; diagnosis with multidetector CT. *Emerg Radiol.* 2004;10(4):182–185.
3. Welling RD, Jacobson JA, Jamadar DA, et al. MDCT and radiography of wrist fractures: radiographic sensitivity and fracture patterns. *AJR Am J Roentgenol.* 2008;190(1):10–16.
4. Ilica AT, Ozyurek S, Kose O, et al. Diagnostic accuracy of multidetector computed tomography for patients with suspected scaphoid fractures and negative radiographic examinations. *Jpn J Radiol.* 2011;29(2):98–103.
5. Hunter JC, Escobedo EM, Wilson AJ, et al. MR imaging of clinically suspected scaphoid fractures. *AJR Am J Roentgenol.* 1997;168(5):1287–1293.
6. Pierre-Jerome C, Moncayo V, Albastaki U, et al. Multiple occult wrist bone injuries and joint effusions: prevalence and distribution on MRI. *Emerg Radiol.* 2010;17(3):179–184.
7. Grainger AJ, Elliot JM, Campbell, RS, et al. Direct MR arthrography: a review of current use. *Clin Radiol.* 2000;55(3):163–176.
8. Gilula LA. Carpal injuries: analytic approach and case exercises. *Am J Roentgenol.* 1979;133(3):503–517.
9. Schmitt R, Froehner S, Coblenz G, et al. Carpal instability. *Eur Radiol.* 2006;16(10):2161–2178.
10. Timins ME, Jahnke JP, Krah SF, et al. MR imaging of the major carpal stabilizing ligaments: normal anatomy and clinical examples. *Radiographics.* 1995;15(3):575–587.
11. MacEwan DW. Changes due to trauma in the fat plane overlying the pronator quadratus muscle: a radiologic sign. *Radiology.* 1964;82:879–886.
12. Mohanti RC, Kar N. Study of triangular fibrocartilage of the wrist joint in Colles' fracture. *Injury.* 1980;11(4):321–324.
13. Zlatkin MB, Rosner J. MR imaging of ligaments and triangular fibrocartilage complex of the wrist. *Radiol Clin North Am.* 2006;44(4):595–623, ix.
14. Rüegger C, Schmid MR, Pfirrmann CW, et al. Peripheral tear of the triangular fibrocartilage: depiction with MR arthrography of the distal radioulnar joint. *AJR Am J Roentgenol.* 2007;188(1):187–192.

15. Rodriguez-Martin J, Pretell-Mazzini J. The role of ultrasound and magnetic resonance imaging in the evaluation of the forearm interosseous membrane. A review. *Skeletal Radiol*. 2011;40(12):1515–1522.

16. Lee JS, Galla A, Shaw RL, et al. Signs of acute carpal instability associated with distal radial fracture. *Emerg Radiol*. 1995;2(2):77–83.

17. Ilyas AM, Jupiter JB. Distal radius fractures—classification of treatment and indications for surgery. *Orthop Clin North Am*. 2007;38(2):167–173, v.

18. Amadio PC. Scaphoid fractures. *Orthop Clin North Am*. 1992;23(1):7–17.

19. Filan SL, Herbert TJ. Herbert screw fixation of scaphoid fractures. *J Bone Joint Surg Br*. 1996; 78(4):519–529.

20. Terry DW Jr, Ramin JE. The navicular fat stripe: a useful roentgen feature for evaluating wrist trauma. *Am J Roentgenol Radium Ther Nucl Med*. 1975;124(1):25–28.

21. Fowler C, Sullivan B, Williams LA, et al. A comparison of bone scintigraphy and MRI in the early diagnosis of the occult scaphoid waist fracture. *Skeletal Radiol*. 1998;27(12):683–687.

22. Anderson MW, Kaplan PA, Dussault RG, et al. Magnetic resonance imaging of the wrist. *Curr Probl Diagn Radiol*. 1998;27(6):187–229.

23. van Gelderen W, Gale RS, Steward AH. Short tau inversion recovery magnetic resonance imaging in occult scaphoid injuries: effect on management. *Australas Radiol*. 1998;42(1):20–24.

24. Brydie A, Raby N. Early MRI in the management of clinical scaphoid fracture. *Br J Radiol*. 2003;76(905):296–300.

25. Neuhaus V, Jupiter JB. Current concepts review: carpal injuries—fractures, ligaments, dislocations. *Acta Chirurgiae Orthopaedicae et Traumatologiae Cechoslovaca*. 2011;78(5):395–403.

26. Kaye JJ. Fractures and dislocations of the hand and wrist. *Semin Roentgenol*. 1978;13(2):109–116.

27. Fox MG, Gaskin CM, Chhabra AB, et al. Assessment of scaphoid viability with MRI: a reassessment of findings on unenhanced MR images. *AJR Am J Roentgenol*. 2010;195(4):W281–W286.

28. Schmitt R, Christopoulos G, Wagner M, et al. Avascular necrosis (AVN) of the proximal fragment in scaphoid nonunion: is intravenous contrast agent necessary in MRI? *Eur J Radiol*. 2011;77(2):222–227.

29. Garcia-Elias M. The treatment of wrist instability. *J Bone Joint Surg Br*. 1997;79(4):684–690.

30. Larsen CF, Amadio PC, Gilula LA, et al. Analysis of carpal instability: I. Description of the scheme. *J Hand Surg Am*. 1995;20(5):757–764.

31. Theumann NH, Etechami G, Duvoisin B, et al. Association between extrinsic and intrinsic carpal ligament injuries at MR arthrography and carpal instability at radiography: initial observations. *Radiology*. 2006;238(3):950–957.

32. Toms AP, Chojnowski A, Cahir JG. Midcarpal instability: a radiological perspective. *Skeletal Radiol*. 2011;40(5):533–541.

CHAPTER 11 Hand

Emma L. Rowbotham ■ Dominic A. Barron ■ Thomas L. Pope Jr.

GENERAL CONSIDERATIONS

The hand and wrist are commonly considered together in the trauma setting by ED physicians, and although several systemic diseases and traumatic injuries involve both the hand and the wrist, it is important to emphasize that each is a separate anatomic region. The radiographic examination of the hand does not constitute an adequate study of the wrist, and the radiographic examination of the wrist does not constitute an adequate study of the hand. Furthermore, certain special views of the hand and wrist are particular to each and have no application to the other. Therefore, it is mandatory that the attending physician determine as precisely as possible which part is to be studied radiographically and transmit this information to the radiology department. As with all orthopedic radiology, two views of the injured region are mandatory and should be in two different planes—if this is not possible, then bony injury or dislocation cannot be excluded (Fig. 11.1A,B).

During childhood and adolescence, when the epiphyses are undergoing fusion, the extreme variability in the radiographic appearance of the physes may make interpretation of this region difficult. The mechanism, the location of the injury, the clinical findings, and the radiographic appearance of the soft tissues are all important in the radiographic evaluation of the injured part (Fig. 11.2).

The soft tissue shadows often show subtle changes, which provide valuable indirect signs related to subtle but significant bone abnormalities. The value of careful appraisal of these tissue shadows cannot be overemphasized.

IMAGING TECHNIQUES

Radiographic Examination

The optimum routine examination of the hand of patients of all ages should include PA (frontal), oblique, and lateral projections. The digits should be flexed to varying degrees in the oblique and lateral projections to eliminate superimposition (Fig. 11.3A,B). The lateral is the most difficult to interpret but is critical in the evaluation of carpometacarpal (CMC) fractures and fracture-dislocations (Fig. 11.3C).

When the clinical concern is for phalangeal injury, dedicated finger views should be taken with specific lateral views of the injured digits. These are readily obtained by having the patient flex the uninvolved digits.

The thumb requires special mention because none of the positions described affords a PA view of this digit. The frontal view of the thumb is generally obtained with the forearm placed midway between pronation and supination and with the thumb extended away from the volar surface of the hand (Fig. 11.4A–B).

Previously, special views of the hand, including carpal tunnel and reversed oblique views, were employed when the standard series of films could not answer the clinical question. These techniques are now rarely used and have largely been replaced by cross-sectional

421

Figure 11.1. A: AP view of the left little finger. An oblique fracture through the proximal phalanx is visible. The middle and distal phalanges appear normal. **B:** Lateral view of the left little finger in the same patient shows an intra-articular fracture through the base of the distal phalanx. This fracture is not visible on the AP view.

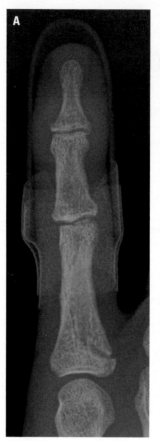

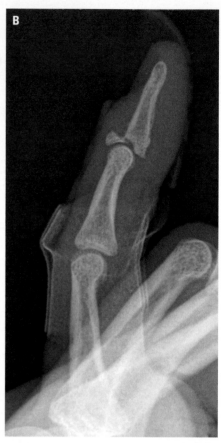

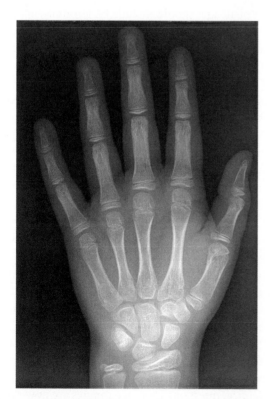

Figure 11.2. Normal AP view of the hand demonstrating the normal configuration of epiphyses in an 8-year-old boy.

imaging. When there is concern regarding, for example, CMC dislocation with equivocal radiography, then computed tomography (CT) is indicated.

Ultrasound

The advent of high-frequency ultrasound probes has revolutionized soft tissue imaging of the hand and wrist. Ultrasound is now increasing the imaging modality of choice in the assessment of ligaments, tendons, foreign body localization, and soft tissue pathology such as joint effusion or hematoma. This is because of the high resolution, accessibility, relatively low cost, and excellent temporal assessment that this modality provides.

Ultrasound of the hand and fingers can prove technically challenging because of the small surface area involved and relative inaccessibility of various areas. A small footprint probe is invaluable as well as a gel stand off or the use of a water bath (Fig. 11.5). These provide a good imaging window without the discomfort of direct pressure on the injured hand or fingers.

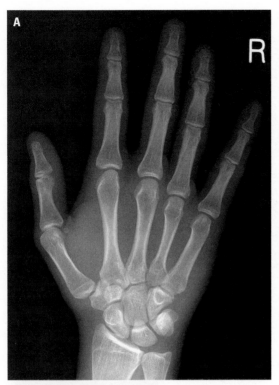

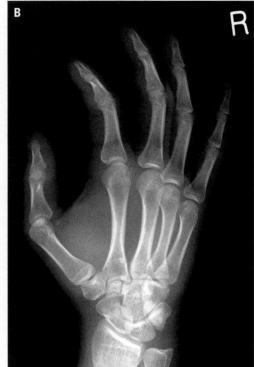

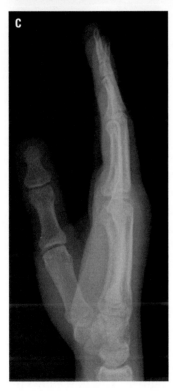

Figure 11.3. A: Normal AP view of the right hand in an adult patient. **B:** Normal oblique view of the right hand. **C:** Normal lateral view of the right hand showing normal alignment of the carpometacarpal joints and the metacarpophalangeal joints.

Figure 11.4. A: Normal AP view of the right thumb in an adult patient. **B:** Normal lateral view of the right thumb in an adult patient.

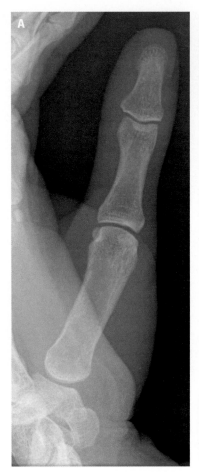 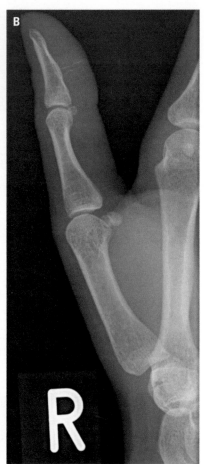

Ultrasound also has the benefit of allowing real time and dynamic evaluation of structures, which is particularly helpful in assessment of the tendons. A further immediate advantage for the operator is the ability to compare appearances with the contralateral side to help with interpretation of any

Figure 11.5. Ultrasound image of the left ring finger showing a linear echogenic foreign body. The *asterisk* denotes a water bath, hence high definition of the soft tissues.

abnormal findings. Studies have been published that have shown that ultrasound may be useful in detecting fractures with signs including a break in the hyperechoic line representing the bony cortex and local hematoma.[1] However, standard radiographs remain the mainstay of imaging all bony trauma, and the role of ultrasound remains an adjunct at present.

CT/MRI Uses in Trauma

The advent of multislice CT has transformed its use for hand imaging and has an important role in the management of trauma.[2] This now allows thin-slice, low-dose volumetric acquisitions of the affected areas in a short time period. The use of submillimeter acquisitions facilitates high-quality images with multiplanar and 3D reformations. These are particularly valuable across the CMC joints where they can accurately characterize the true extent of the injury or, in difficult cases, make the diagnosis.

Three-dimensional images can be particularly valuable when the angulation and rotation of the injured site is critical for surgical planning.

Magnetic resonance imaging (MRI) is rarely employed in the investigation and management of traumatic injuries to the hand, whereas ultrasound's superior resolution is preferred for soft tissue injuries.

RADIOGRAPHIC NORMAL ANATOMY

The locations of the epiphyses of the phalanges and metacarpals and the radiographic characteristics of the nutrient artery canals are key practical aspects of the radiographic anatomy of the hand. The phalangeal and metacarpal epiphyses are differently located, and even among the metacarpals, the location of the growth centers is not uniform (Fig. 11.2). The phalangeal epiphyses are proximally situated compared to the index, middle, ring, and little finger metacarpals that are located distally and constitute the metacarpal heads. The thumb metacarpal has its growth center at its base. Anomalous secondary ossification centers may involve the distal end of the thumb metacarpal or the base of any of the lateral metacarpals.

During childhood, when the physes are open, the epiphyseal plate should not be mistaken for a fracture line, and knowledge of the estimated age of fusion is essential when interpreting pediatric radiographs.

Nutrient artery canals (medullary foramen; Fig. 11.6) are located near the middle of the phalangeal and metacarpal shafts and enter the bone from each side, passing obliquely distally. The margins of these normal vascular grooves are uniformly smooth, sclerotic, parallel, and converge distally. Nutrient artery canals are not, however, constant features. When they are present, their location, course, and radiographic characteristics should distinguish them from incomplete fracture lines.

The sesamoids are small, rounded bones embedded in certain flexor tendons. Five sesamoid bones are commonly found in the hand. These include two lying volar to the thumb metacarpophalangeal (MCP) joint, one volar to the interphalangeal joint of the thumb, and one in the soft tissues anterior to the MCP joint of both the index and little fingers. Sesamoid bones are characterized by dense, smooth cortical margins and a normal trabecular pattern.

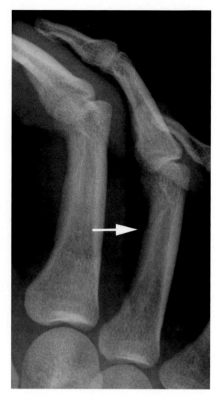

Figure 11.6. Lateral finger radiograph with the *arrow* pointing to a typical nutrient canal.

RADIOGRAPHIC MANIFESTATIONS OF TRAUMA

Knowledge of the common mechanisms of injury and their associated fracture patterns is essential when both examining a patient presenting with a hand injury and interpreting his or her radiographs. This will facilitate the appropriate imaging being performed for the suspected injury and aid diagnosis of subtle findings.

Mallet Finger

"Mallet" finger and "baseball" finger are terms given to the same flexion deformity at the distal interphalangeal joint, which results from a proximally retracted avulsion fracture of the dorsum of the base of the distal phalanx to which the extensor tendon is inserted. The flexion deformity is due, therefore, to the unopposed action of the flexor tendon inserted on the volar aspect of the phalanx. This injury most commonly involves the distal phalanx of the long finger (Figs. 11.7–11.8).

Figure 11.7. A: Mallet deformity of the index finger with a small subtle avulsion fracture at the base of the distal phalanx. **B:** A larger fracture fragment is seen at the base of the distal phalanx but with a less pronounced mallet deformity at the distal interphalangeal joint.

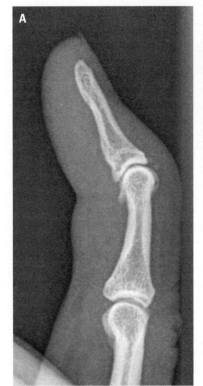
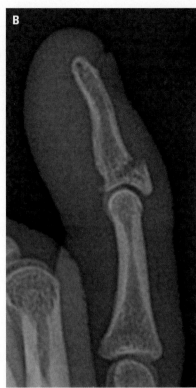

Figure 11.8. A: "Mallet" or "baseball" finger. The small triangular fragment *(arrows)* is proximally retracted by the common extensor tendon that inserts on this fragment. The flexion deformity results from the unopposed action of the flexor digitorum profundus tendon. **B:** Nondisplaced fracture of the dorsal aspect of the base of the distal phalanx. In this patient, the common extensor tendon inserts distal to the fracture fragment, and a mallet deformity did not result.

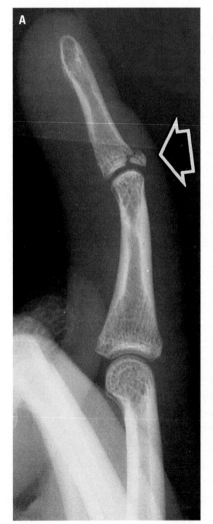
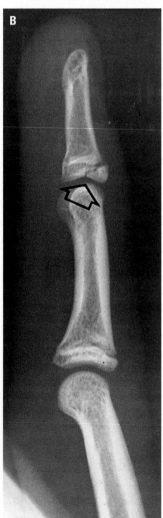

The "mallet" finger is the result of the tip of the finger being struck, such as in the act of catching a baseball, softball, or basketball, causing forceful hyperflexion of the distal interphalangeal joint when the extensor tendon is taut, or it is the result of forceful hyperextension of the distal interphalangeal joint. Proximal retraction of the dorsal fragment indicates that the common extensor tendon is attached to the separate fragment.

When the extensor tendon inserts distal to the fracture of the dorsum of the base of the distal phalanx, the separate fragment will neither be retracted nor will there be a flexion deformity at the distal interphalangeal joint (Fig. 11.8B).

Variations of the mallet finger deformity are dependent on the site of the fracture and the relation of the volar plate and of the extensor and flexor tendon insertions to the fragments. Figures 11.9 and 11.10 illustrate two such variants. It is important for the radiologist to have an understanding of the soft tissue anatomy of the interphalangeal joints so that the status of the ligaments and tendons can be incorporated into the interpretation of the radiographic examination.

Volar Plate Injury

The volar plate is a dense fibrous band that forms the palmar aspect of the capsule of the thumb MCP and finger proximal interphalangeal joints (Fig. 11.11). Distally, the volar plate is fibrocartilaginous at its insertion on the volar margin of the base of the adjacent phalanx. Volar plate injuries, although most commonly involving the proximal interphalangeal joints of the fingers, may also occur at the MCP joint of the thumb. These injuries, regardless of their anatomical location, are the result of hyperextension of the joint. In hyperextension, the volar plate itself may rupture, in which case routine radiographs of the digit will demonstrate only periarticular soft tissue swelling. When the hyperextension

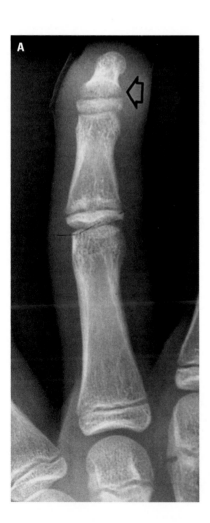
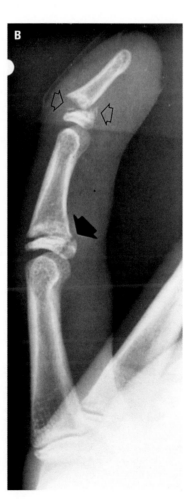

Figure 11.9. "Mallet" finger deformity in which the proximal fragment, by virtue of the transverse fracture line *(arrows)*, remains anatomically situated because of insertion of the extensor tendon dorsally and the volar plate volarly (**A** and **B**). The position of the distal fragment reflects the unopposed action of the flexor tendon, which is inserted distal to the fracture line (**B**).

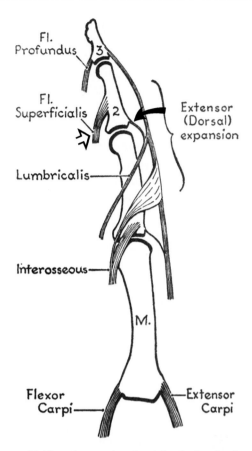

Figure 11.10. The pathophysiologic basis for the "mallet" deformity in this child is identical to that seen in Figure 11.9. The type II physeal injury *(open arrow)* of the child corresponds to the transverse fracture of the adult (Fig. 11.9). Additionally, this child sustained a volar plate fracture of the middle phalanx *(solid arrow)*.

force is sufficiently great and the volar plate remains intact, a characteristic thin fracture fragment may be avulsed from the volar aspect of the base of the phalanx (Fig. 11.12).

Volar plate fractures, unless recognized and appropriately treated, may lead to instability of the involved joint. These injuries are usually best appreciated on the lateral or oblique views but infrequently may be visible in the frontal projection. When associated with dorsal dislocation, the avulsion fragment attached to the volar plate will be retracted proximally. In this case, the separate fragment may not be recognized or, if recognized, its significance may not be appreciated. Following reduction of the proximal interphalangeal joint dislocation, the site of avulsion of the separate fragment and its significance should become apparent. Volar plate injuries of the thumb MCP joint may be indicated by dislocation or fracture of one or both sesamoids.

Thumb Fractures

Injuries to the thumb are common and often cause significant loss of function to the affected hand. The two main eponymous fractures involving this area are the Bennett and Rolando fractures—both of these are intra-articular fractures with extension into the CMC joint. If a fracture of the base of the thumb does not extend into this joint, then

Figure 11.11. Schematic representation of the ligamentous anatomy of an interphalangeal joint. (From Weeks PM. *Acute Bone and Joint Injuries of Hand and Wrist.* St. Louis, MO: Mosby; 1981:122. Used with permission.)

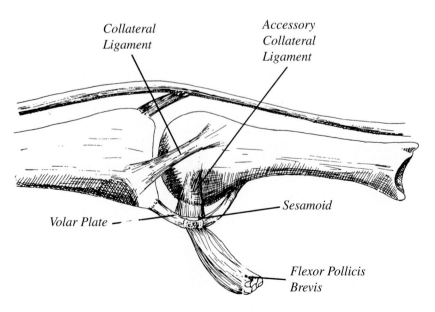

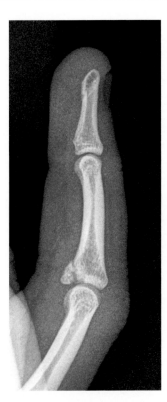

Figure 11.12. Volar plate fracture of the middle phalanx of the middle finger.

it is neither and should be described as either a transverse or oblique fracture of the thumb or first metacarpal. The Bennett and Rolando injuries have specific fracture characteristics and each fracture requires different management principles.

Bennett Fracture

This is an oblique intra-articular fracture of the base of the first metacarpal with a triangular fragment arising from the ulnar aspect of the base of the first metacarpal (Fig. 11.13A–B). This injury usually occurs as the result of an axial blow directed against the partially flexed metacarpal. The obliquity of the fracture line and its extension into the proximal articulating surface allow proximal retraction of the large distal fragment by the unopposed action of the abductor pollicis tendon that inserts on its dorsal surface. The smaller fragment retains its normal relationship to the concavity of the distal articulating surface of the trapezium via attachment of the intervening volar anterior oblique ligament (Fig. 11.14). The clinical importance of the Bennett fracture rests in its management, which usually requires

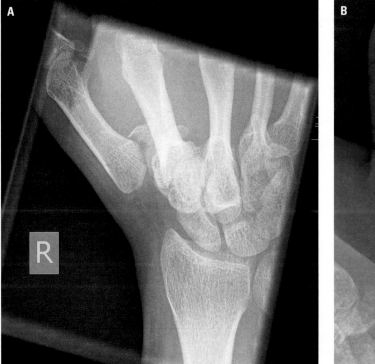
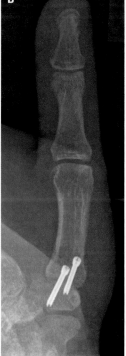

Figure 11.13. **A:** Bennett fracture of the right thumb showing intra-articular extension of the fracture and lateral displacement of the distal fracture fragment. **B:** Postoperative image of the same patient showing internal fixation at the first metacarpophalangeal (MCP) joint.

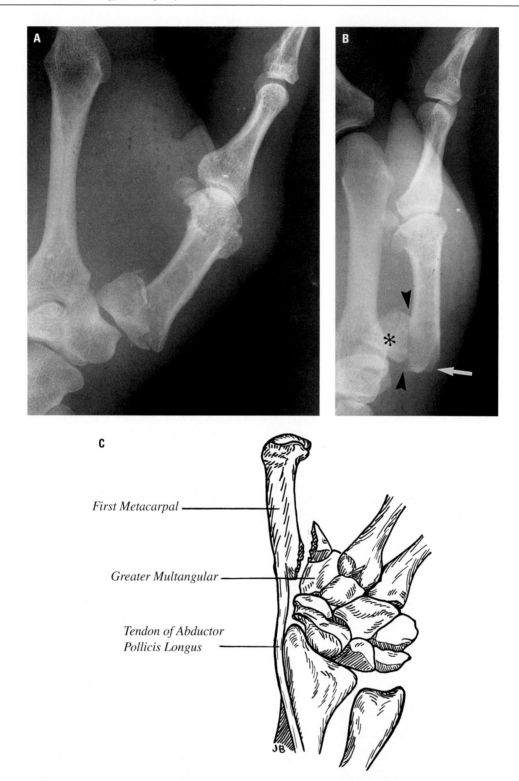

Figure 11.14. Bennett fracture-dislocation of the first metacarpal (**A**). The lateral radiograph (**B**) shows the oblique fracture of the base of the first metacarpal with extension into its proximal articulating surface *(arrowheads)*. The small proximal fragment *(asterisk)* remains in its anatomic position relative to the trapezium, whereas the long distal fragment is retracted proximally *(arrow)*. **C**: A schematic representation of the role of the abductor pollicis tendon in the Bennett fracture-dislocation.

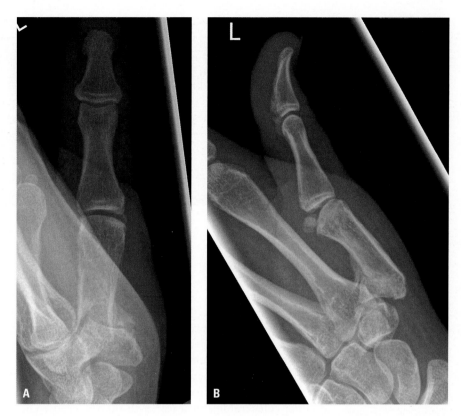

Figure 11.15. A: AP view of the thumb showing a Rolando fracture 6 weeks following initial injury. There is callous formation around the fracture site indicative of the subacute nature of the injury. **B:** Lateral view of the thumb in the same patient.

skeletal traction or open reduction and internal fixation to maintain the position of the distal fragment following reduction owing to the insertion of the adductors into the base of the thumb metacarpal.[3]

Rolando Fracture

This fracture also involves the proximal articulating surface of the thumb metacarpal. A Rolando fracture involves a three-part fracture at the base of the thumb metacarpal. In addition to a volar lip fracture (as seen with Bennett fracture), there is also large dorsal fragment resulting in Y- or T-shaped intra-articular fracture. This fracture is less common than the Bennett fracture but has a worse prognosis for the patient as would be expected with the more extensive fragmentation (Fig. 11.15A–B).

Thumb Ligamentous Injuries

Ligamentous injuries of the thumb are also common, but there will rarely be any radiographic manifestation of the injury unless associated with a fracture. Assessment of the ligaments is best performed by

clinical examination and, if necessary, ultrasound of the area.

Injury to the ulnar collateral ligament (UCL) of the thumb is a relatively common injury (Fig. 11.16). This ligament is situated on the ulnar

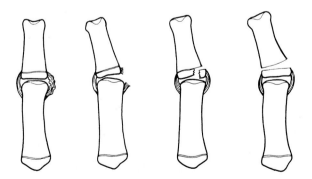

Figure 11.16. Schematic representation of the spectrum of injuries of the ulnar collateral ligament of the thumb metacarpophalangeal joint. (From O'Brien ET. Fractures of the hand and wrist region. In: Rockwood CA Jr, Wilkins KE, King RE, eds. *Fractures in Children*. 3rd ed. Philadelphia, PA: JB Lippincott & Co; 1991:364, with permission.)

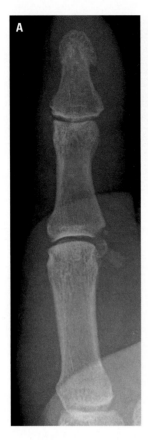

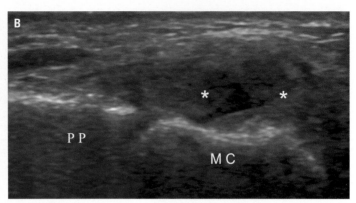

Figure 11.17. A: AP view of the thumb with an avulsion fracture adjacent to the ulnar aspect of the distal end of the thumb metacarpal. **B:** Longitudinal ultrasound image of the thumb at the level of the first MCP joint showing the thumb proximal phalanx (*PP*) and the thumb metacarpal (*MC*). *Asterisks* delineate the ends of an ulnar collateral ligament tear with fluid interposed between the ligament ends.

aspect of the thumb MCP joint, and injury to this structure usually occurs as a result of a valgus force on the thumb MCP joint. This injury is often referred to as a "skier's thumb" or a gamekeeper's thumb because of the high incidence of this injury in these activities. Avulsion injuries associated with the UCL may be appreciated on plain radiographs and are most common at the distal insertion of the ligament (Fig. 11.17A). Ultrasound examination should be performed both in a neutral position and during cautious valgus stress at the MCP joint (Fig. 11.17B).[4]

The adductor aponeurosis may become interposed between the two ends of a ruptured ligament, preventing healing of the rupture and negating conservative management of the lesion—this is termed a *Stener lesion*. Injuries to the radial collateral ligament (RCL) are approximately 10 times less frequent than UCL injuries and occur secondary to a varus force on the thumb MCP joint.

Most UCL and RCL injuries have no associated fracture and are best assessed by ultrasound. This will give high-definition information about their extent and stability and importantly can demonstrate the presence of adductor aponeurotic entrapment.

Physeal Injuries

Physeal injuries of the hand are common, usually affecting the phalanges, although the metacarpals may also be involved. As discussed previously, the approximate ages of physeal fusion are key to the interpretation of pediatric radiographs. The Salter-Harris classification system is widely used and is accepted by both radiologists and clinicians alike.[5] The most common are Salter-Harris Type I and II, with Type II injuries accounting for approximately 75% of all epiphyseal injuries.[6]

A Type I fracture is a transverse fracture through the hypertrophic zone of the physis. This leads to widening of the physis. Radiographic detection of this can be very difficult, and comparison with the contralateral digit may be helpful as well as a good clinical history.

The most common type of Salter-Harris fracture, a Type II fracture, occurs through the physis and metaphysis; the epiphysis is not involved in the

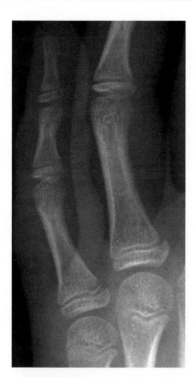

Figure 11.18. Salter-Harris Type II fracture of the base of the proximal phalanx of the little finger.

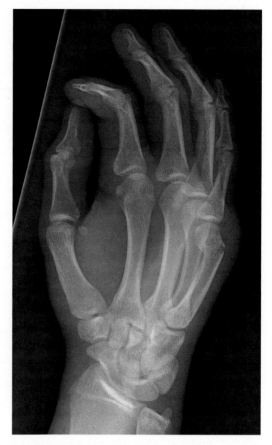

Figure 11.19. Oblique view of the hand showing a boxer's fracture of the fifth metacarpal with volar angulation of the distal fragment.

injury. These can be very subtle with often only a small fracture line at the corner of the physis being visible (Fig. 11.18).

A Type III fracture is a vertical fracture through the epiphysis and separation of the involved physis. This fracture passes through the hypertrophic layer of the physis and extends to split the epiphysis, inevitably damaging the reproductive layer of the physis.

A Type IV fracture involves the epiphysis, physis, and metaphysis and extends intra-articularly.

A Type V fracture is a compression or crush injury of the epiphyseal plate with no associated epiphyseal or metaphyseal fracture.

Metacarpal Fractures

Fractures of the metacarpal shaft are more commonly oblique or spiral than transverse. When minimally displaced, such fractures may be quite difficult to identify radiographically. As has been previously noted, radiographic examination of the acutely traumatized hand must include more than simply an AP projection. A common metacarpal fracture is the boxer's fracture (Fig. 11.19). This involves the metacarpal neck, commonly involving the little finger metacarpal, often as a result of a punch injury. Professional fighters more commonly injure their index or middle metacarpals because they are taught to punch directing the force through these stronger metacarpals rather than the roundhouse action favored by amateurs. There is often angulation of the distal fracture fragment in a palmar direction (Fig. 11.20A–B). Management of these fractures is largely determined by the degree of angulation, which if severe may need surgical intervention. The degree of rotation needs to be assessed both radiographically and clinically to determine the definitive management.[7]

Carpometacarpal Dislocation

Dislocation of the CMC joints, with the exception of the thumb, is a rare but commonly misdiagnosed injury. CMC dislocations without fractures

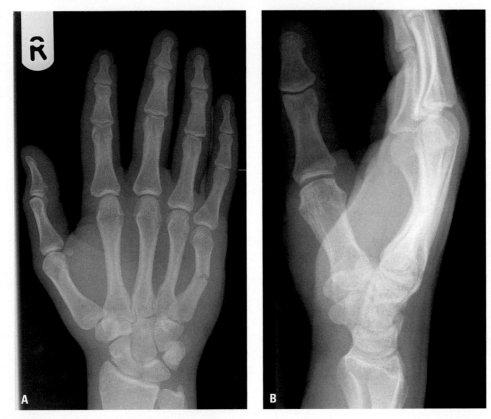

Figure 11.20. A: AP plain radiograph of the right hand showing a fracture through the midshaft of the fifth metacarpal. **B:** Lateral plain radiograph of the same patient that more readily shows the degree of volar angulation of the distal fragment.

are rare because these joints are supported by the strength and complexity of the CMC and intermetacarpal ligaments. The relatively mobile ring and little CMC joints are more susceptible to dislocation than the more immobile index and long finger joints.

The mechanism of injury is not clearly established but is most likely the result of a dorsally directed force applied to the palmar aspect of the hand with the wrist fixed in neutral position. This presumption is based on the fact that dorsal dislocation of the CMC joints is far more common than volar dislocation. The most common cause is a punch injury, usually when the assailant misses his or her intended victim and strikes a wall or lamp post instead. The standard teaching is that these are best appreciated on the lateral view. Unfortunately, this can be very difficult to interpret. On the frontal projections, it should be possible to clearly make out the CMC joints to all the fingers and the thumb. This gives a "wavy W" appearance. Overlap of the metacarpal bases on the carpal bones results in a

loss of the joint margins and therefore a disruption to the "W." This subtle sign should immediately alert the reader to the possibility of a major injury in this region (Fig. 11.21A).

The fifth metacarpal base fracture is usually easily recognized on the frontal projection and is associated with soft tissue swelling along the ulnar aspect of the hand. The subluxation or dislocation is best demonstrated in the AP (frontal), oblique, or lateral projections (Fig. 11.21B,C). Because the fracture-dislocation of the base of the fifth metacarpal is pathologically and radiographically similar to the Bennett fracture of the thumb metacarpal, it is sometimes referred to as a "reversed Bennett" or "ulnar Bennett" (Fig. 11.22). Like the Bennett fracture, the large distal fragment of the base of the fifth metacarpal is proximally retracted by the flexor and extensor carpi ulnaris muscles. Open reduction and internal fixation are recommended to reduce and stabilize the fracture fragments.

Dorsal dislocation of the thumb is caused by a hyperextension force applied to the MCP joint.

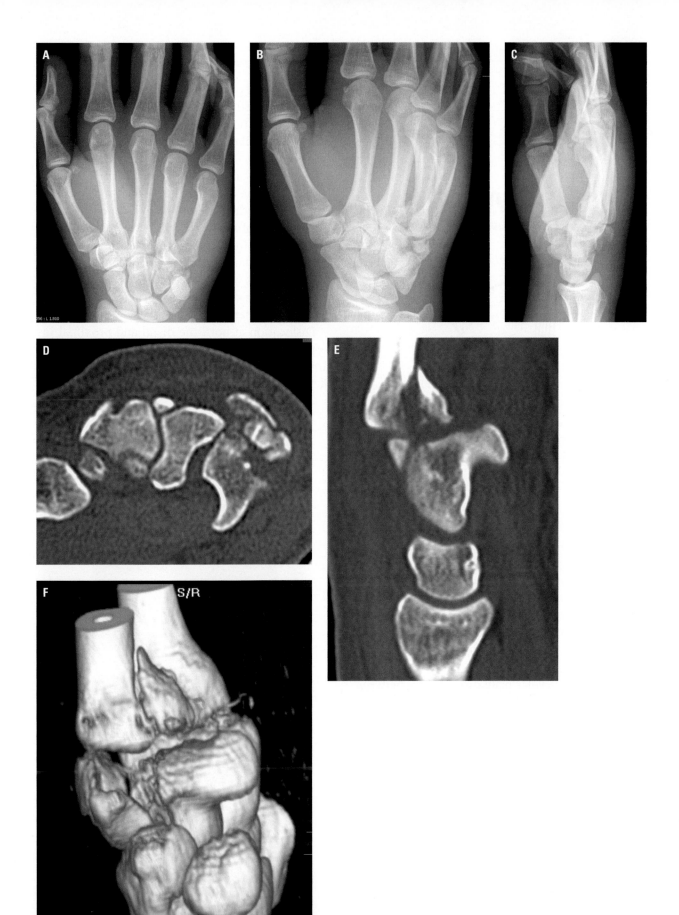

Figure 11.21. **A–F:** Series of radiographs and CT images showing a complex fracture-dislocation injury involving the proximal ends of the ring and little finger metacarpals and an intra-articular fracture of the hamate.

435

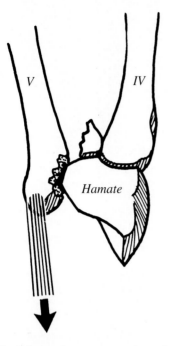

Figure 11.22. Schematic representation of the pathology of the "reversed" Bennett fracture of the base of the fifth metacarpal. (From Helal B, Kavanagh TG. Unstable dorsal fracture-dislocation of the fifth carpometacarpal joint. *Injury*. 1977;9:142, with permission.)

This may occur in both children and adults. This is associated with disruption of the volar plate and usually the volar aspect of the collateral ligaments. In adults, the relationship of the MCP sesamoid bones indicates the site of volar plate disruption. When the sesamoids accompany the dislocated proximal phalanx, the volar plate disruption is proximal to the sesamoids. If the sesamoids do not follow the proximal phalanx, the volar plate disruption is between the sesamoids and the base of the phalanx.

CT imaging is routinely used in the evaluation of CMC dislocation because it provides vital information regarding associated fractures, articular involvement, and the degree of fragmentation. Three-dimensional reconstructions will also allow the surgeon to visualize the injury pattern and degree of rotation deformity prior to surgical intervention (Fig. 11.21A–F).

Phalangeal Fractures

These fractures are very common and occur in children and adults alike. Fractures of the distal phalanx are the most common, accounting for more than 50% of all phalangeal fractures. Fractures of the phalanges are often multiple and may be classified as either intra-articular or extraarticular (Fig. 11.23). The distal phalanx is commonly injured during a perpendicular force and may be associated with soft tissue loss and nail bed injury. Intra-articular fractures of the distal phalanx usually result from either a mallet fracture or an avulsion of the flexor digitorum profundus tendon—the latter of these will present with the inability to flex the digit at the distal interphalangeal joint (Fig. 11.24A–B). Clinical examination is vital to the underlying pathology in both these cases, particularly when there is no bony avulsion fragment.

Dislocation at both the distal and proximal interphalangeal joints are commonly reduced at the time of injury (Fig. 11.25). Radiograph evaluation of the affected digit will often be normal by the

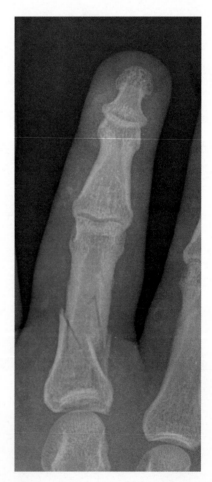

Figure 11.23. AP view of the ring finger showing an oblique fracture with intra-articular extension into the metacarpophalangeal joint.

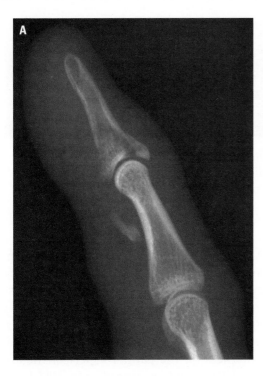

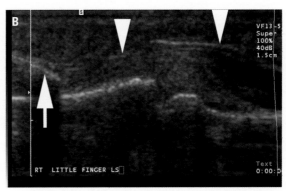

Figure 11.24. A: Lateral plain radiograph of the little finger that shows an intra-articular avulsion fracture of the base of the distal phalanx with proximal retraction of the avulsed tendon insertion. **B:** Longitudinal ultrasound image of the little finger in the same patient showing avulsion of the flexor digitorum profundus (FDP) tendon from the distal phalanx. A bony avulsion fragment is seen *(white arrow)* attached to the FDP tendon *(arrowheads)*.

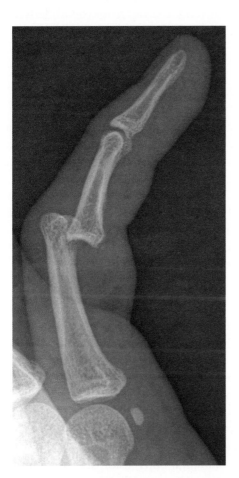

Figure 11.25. Lateral view of the little finger showing a dislocation of the proximal interphalangeal joint.

time the patient presents to the ED, but it is important to scrutinize the radiograph for small avulsion fragments.

Foreign Bodies

Retained foreign body following traumatic injury is a common cause of presentation to the ED. Patients will present with either ongoing pain at the site of injury or swelling around the affected area. As with bony injury, plain radiographs will often be the first line of imaging investigation but will only be beneficial if the foreign body is radiopaque. Using a high-frequency linear probe, typically 9 to 12 MHz, the soft tissues can be interrogated for the presence of foreign body (Fig. 11.26). These will usually manifest as a hyperechoic linear area within the subcutaneous tissues with no through transmission. The position, size, and depth of the foreign body can all be mapped out for the referring clinician to aid in removal.

Follow-up ultrasound may be of benefit when the initial scan is negative, but there is a strong clinical concern for a foreign body. This is because a foreign body reaction with hypervascularity will develop, making the foreign body more sonographically obvious (Fig. 11.27).

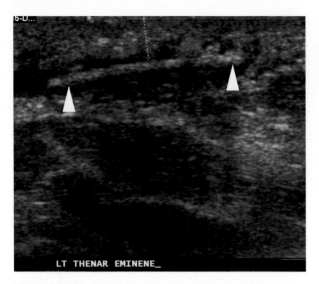

Figure 11.26. Ultrasound image of the thenar eminence of the right hand that shows a linear hyperechoic foreign body *(arrowheads)* lying in a longitudinal plane just deep to the skin surface.

Pulleys

Pulley Disruption

The five annular pulleys lie on the flexor aspect of the fingers and have a key role in stabilizing the flexor tendons of the fingers. The pulleys may be injured in the acute trauma setting, classically in rock climbers. There are five annular pulleys

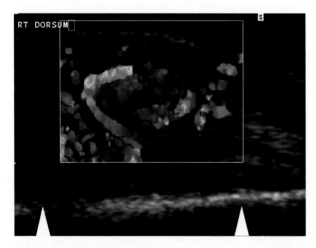

Figure 11.27. Ultrasound image of the dorsal aspect of the index finger middle phalanx 6 weeks after injury to this region with penetration of a foreign body. Hypoechoic soft tissue with markedly increased color Doppler flow in keeping with a foreign body reaction. *Arrowheads* indicate the underlying bony cortex.

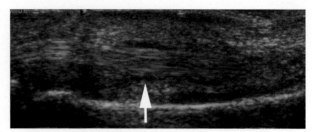

Figure 11.28. Longitudinal ultrasound image of the middle finger illustrating bowstringing of the flexor tendon following disruption of the A2 pulley.

(A1–A5) and three cruciform ligaments in each finger, which are situated on the palmar aspect of the flexor tendons and prevent the tendons bowstringing away from the bone during flexion of the fingers.[8] Rupture of the pulleys will usually manifest as sudden tearing pain with focal swelling and tenderness on the palmar aspect of the affected digit. Ultrasound imaging of a ruptured pulley will reveal thickening of the pulley itself with bowing of the flexor tendon away from the underlying phalanx (Fig. 11.28).

Trigger Finger

A trigger finger is a diagnostic challenge that may be solved by ultrasonography. Stenosing tenosynovitis is the most common cause when the tendon is caught underneath the A1 flexor pulley. "Triggering" occurs when the finger is moved from the fully flexed position to the extended position. This condition may often be progressive and, in severe cases, may result in a fixed flexion deformity of the involved finger.[9]

Nontraumatic Conditions

The radiographic appearances of normal variants and nontraumatic lesions may pose potential problems for the trauma radiologist. Benign incidental lesions will also be encountered, and it is important to recognize these lesions, thereby avoiding unnecessary investigation (Fig. 11.29). The most common benign bony lesion seen within the hand is an enchondroma. This is a cartilage-derived tumor most commonly seen in the short tubular

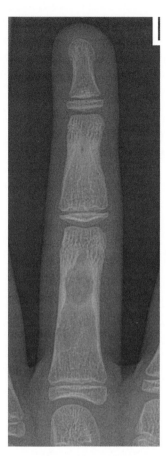

Figure 11.29. AP view of the middle finger in a pediatric patient that shows a simple bone cyst within the proximal phalanx.

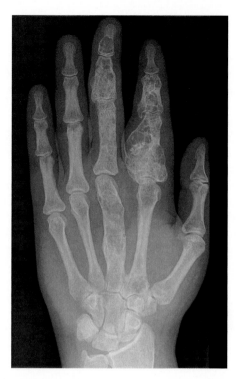

Figure 11.30. AP view of the left hand that shows multiple enchondromas throughout the phalanges and metacarpals. This is characteristic of Ollier disease.

bones of the hands and feet and usually seen in the diaphysis. These lesions are usually lytic, oval in shape, have well-defined margins, and contain small punctuate areas of calcification (Fig. 11.30). Occasionally, pathologic fractures through an enchondroma may occur and should be recognized as such.

Infection is commonly encountered and must not be missed. This may be associated with an earlier injury or may be hematologically transmitted. The appearances of osteomyelitis on plain radiographs can be very aggressive, and the history and clinical examination are key to radiograph interpretation (Fig. 11.31).

The arthritides are common conditions that will often be present in patients who have traumatic injury to their hands. A full description of these is outside the scope of this text, but there is no doubt that their presence can make interpretation of the acute radiographs very difficult.

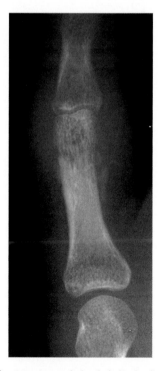

Figure 11.31. AP view of the left little finger shows a permeative appearance to the distal end of the proximal phalanx with florid periosteal reaction and marked surrounding soft tissue swelling in a patient with proven tuberculosis.

REFERENCES

1. Hauger O, Bonnefoy O, Moinard M, et al. Occult fractures of the waist of the scaphoid: early diagnosis by high-spatial-resolution sonography. *Am J Roentgenol.* 2002;178(5):1239–1245.
2. Davis A. *Making Best Use of Clinical Radiology Services.* 6th ed. London, United Kingdom: The Royal College of Radiologists; 2007.
3. Helms CA. Trauma. In: Helms CA, *Fundamentals of Skeletal Radiology.* 3rd ed. Philadelphia, PA: Elsevier Saunders; 2005:78.
4. McNally EG. Hand and wrist. In: McNally EG, *Practical Musculoskeletal Ultrasound.* Elsevier; 2005.
5. Rogers LF. The radiography of epiphyseal injuries. *Radiology.* 1970;96(2):289–299.
6. Salter RB. *Textbook of Disorders and Injuries of the Musculoskeletal System.* Baltimore, MD: Lippincott Williams & Wilkins; 1970.
7. Green DP, Rowland SA. Fracture and dislocations in the hand. In: Rockwood CA, Green DP, eds. *Fractures and Dislocations.* 2nd ed. Philadelphia, PA: JB Lippincott & Co; 1975:265–327.
8. Doyle JR. Anatomy of the flexor tendon sheath and pulley system: a current review. *J Hand Surg Am.* 1989;14(2, pt 2):349–351.
9. O'Connor PJ. Hands and wrist injuries. In: Robinson P, ed. *Essential Radiology for Sports Medicine.* New York, NY: Springer; 2010:168.

CHAPTER 12

Chest: Nontrauma

Bruce E. Lehnert ■ Eric J. Stern

GENERAL CONSIDERATIONS

Imaging plays a critical role in evaluating nontraumatic pathology in the chest because physical exam findings may not be reliable and the patient's symptoms are often not specific to a particular disease state. The chest radiograph remains the first-line imaging modality for evaluating the chest and often allows for rapid clarification or confirmation of clinically suspected pathology such as pneumonia, edema, and pleural gas or fluid or may suggest the need for cross-sectional imaging such as in the setting of an abnormal mediastinum in a patient with chest pain.

The clinical presentation of acute vascular pathology in the chest is often nonspecific, and an accurate evaluation of emergent vascular disease in the chest is typically not possible with clinical exam and chest radiography. The recent widespread availability of multidetector computed tomography (MDCT), which allows rapid, detailed imaging of the chest, has revolutionized the imaging workup of acute chest pathology, particularly in the setting of suspected acute aortic syndrome (AAS), pulmonary embolus, and most recently in suspected acute coronary syndrome (ACS). Magnetic resonance imaging (MRI) technology has also advanced significantly; however, the use of this modality in evaluating chest pathology in the emergency room is generally limited to a problem-solving role, particularly in the evaluation of AAS.

The current chapter reviews both the radiographic and cross-sectional imaging features of

thoracic pathology germane to the evaluation of patients presenting with signs and symptoms of nontraumatic disease of the chest. The radiographic and MDCT features of acute lung pathology including aspiration, infection, exacerbation of chronic obstructive airway disease, edema, and alveolar damage, as well as pleural pathology and mediastinitis, are reviewed. MDCT applications to vascular imaging in the setting of AAS, pulmonary embolus, and ACS are reviewed as well as potential emergent complications of aortic stent grafting.

Lungs

A comprehensive review of diseases affecting the lungs is beyond the scope of the current discussion; however, acute pathology relevant to the emergency department (ED) setting is addressed. Recognizing and accurately diagnosing acute nontraumatic pathology in the chest can be instrumental in directing appropriate therapy. The imaging features associated with aspiration, pulmonary infection in immunocompetent and immunocompromised patients, tuberculosis (TB), pulmonary abscess, atelectasis, foreign body aspiration, edema, and alveolar damage are reviewed.

Aspiration
Aspiration pneumonitis refers to the pulmonary reaction to a foreign substance aspirated into the tracheobronchial tree and is a common problem in patients presenting to the ED. Gastric contents

and oral secretions are the most commonly aspirated substances and risk factors include neurologic deficit, decreased level of consciousness, alcoholism, seizure, esophageal disease, and nasogastric or endotracheal intubation. Aspiration pneumonitis may present clinically with fevers, shortness of breath, and hypoxemia, which can be clinically difficult to differentiate from infectious pneumonia.

The distribution of imaging abnormalities resulting from aspiration are typically gravitationally dependent. In a supine position, this includes the right upper lobe apical and posterior segments, the left upper lobe apical posterior segment, and the superior segments on the lower lobes (Fig. 12.1).

The radiographic appearance of aspiration is also dependent on the type of aspirated material, volume of the aspirate, and on the time interval since the aspiration event. Aspiration of nonirritating substances such as neutralized gastric contents, secretions, blood, and water does not incite an inflammatory response. This so-called bland aspiration results in a gravitationally dependent segmental or subsegmental distribution of patchy opacities that clear rapidly with coughing or ventilation. Aspiration of acids, caustic material, vegetable matter, fatty acid, or hyperosmolar material may result in an inflammatory response manifesting as gravitationally dependent hazy nodules or confluent consolidation in a bronchovascular distribution (Fig. 12.2).

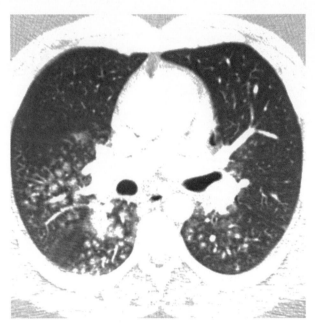

Figure 12.2. Aspiration pneumonitis. Rounded, hazy nodules in a bronchovascular distribution in lower lobes and dependent segments of the right upper lobe are typical of aspiration pneumonitis.

Another form of aspiration is seen in patients who suffer near-drowning events, which results in water filling alveoli. The clinical significance of water aspiration is more closely related to volume than to whether the aspirate is freshwater or saltwater. The radiographic features of mild near drowning are similar to those of aspiration, such as patchy, irregular perihilar opacities with relative sparing of the periphery. More severe radiographic manifestations of near drowning include diffuse, confluent fluffy opacities similar in appearance to pulmonary edema (Fig. 12.3). Computed tomography (CT) findings in near-drowning patients include bilateral patchy or diffuse areas of ground-glass attenuation as well as ill-defined centrilobular nodularity.

Smoke inhalation is the primary cause of death in victims of indoor fires, with approximately 50% to 80% of fire deaths demonstrating burns to the upper respiratory system. Inhalation injury also contributes significantly to the morbidity of burn survivors because it can result in acute lung injury and the development of acute respiratory distress syndrome (ARDS).

The golden standard for diagnosing acute smoke inhalation injury remains bronchoscopy. Acute smoke inhalation typically produces no recognizable changes on the initial chest x-ray (CXR), even with blood carboxyhemoglobin levels as high as 50%. CT may

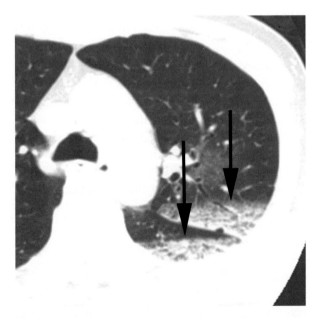

Figure 12.1. Aspiration. Axial CT image illustrates the dependent "settling" of aspirated material into the left upper lobe and the left lower lobe (arrows).

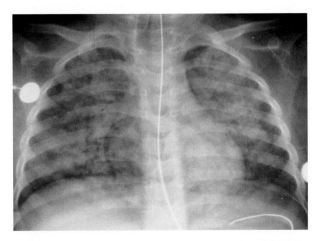

Figure 12.3. Near drowning. Extensive bilateral fluffy opacities resulting from a near-drowning episode are similar in appearance to those seen in alveolar pulmonary edema.

show ground-glass opacities in a peribronchial distribution and/or patchy peribronchial consolidations as early as a few hours after the inhalation injury.

Obstructive Lung Disease

The most common obstructive lung diseases include asthma, emphysema, and chronic bronchitis. These conditions are among the leading causes of mortality and morbidity in the United States and are frequently treated in the emergency setting.

Asthma affects up to 5% of the US population. The disease is characterized by increased airway reactivity to a variety of stimuli, airway inflammation with associated increased mucus exudate, and episodes of at least partially reversible smooth muscle-mediated bronchospasm resulting in small airway obstruction. The radiographic appearance of asthma predominantly includes increased lung volumes with the various manifestations of air trapping such as horizontal positioning of the posterior portions of the upper ribs and visible, bulging intercostal spaces; flattening and depression of the diaphragms; and an increase in the anteroposterior (AP) diameter of the chest. In infants and young children, a radiograph that appears to have been taken during deep inspiration is tantamount to air trapping (Fig. 12.4). Alternatively, asthma may present radiographically with a mix of air trapping and multifocal atelectasis or, less commonly, may mimic foreign body aspiration with unilateral hyperinflation (Figs. 12.5 and 12.6). At CT, manifestations of asthma may include bronchial wall thickening, luminal narrowing, regions of decreased lung parenchyma

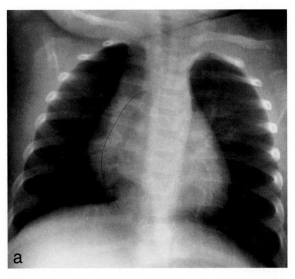

Figure 12.4. Asthma with air trapping in a pediatric patient. The frontal radiograph appears to have been taken during deep inspiration; however, the patient is too young to follow breathing instruction for a chest radiograph. There are large lung volumes, increased intercostal spaces, and relatively horizontal positioning of the upper ribs consistent with air trapping.

attenuation, and decreased vascularity during inspiration. Areas of air trapping may be present if the examination is taken during expiration (Fig. 12.7).

The National Heart, Lung, and Blood Institute defines emphysema as "abnormal permanent

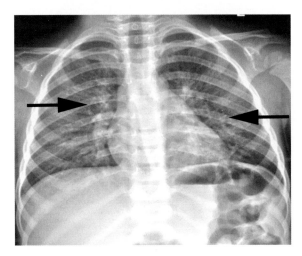

Figure 12.5. Reactive airway disease exacerbation may present with relative pulmonary hyperinflation, atelectasis, or a variable combination of these features. In this case, there are linear opacities in the central lungs bilaterally representing perihilar atelectasis (*arrows*); however, the overall lung volumes are greater than expected for age in this 3-year-old patient.

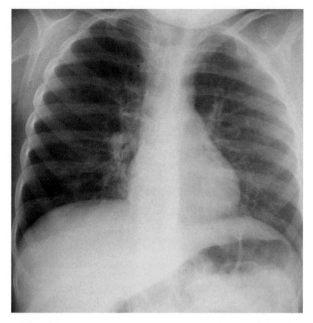

Figure 12.6. Reactive airway disease exacerbation may occasionally mimic foreign body aspiration in pediatric patients. Illustrated here is hyperinflation of the right lung with horizontal orientation of the ribs, widening of the right intercostal rib space, and leftward shift of the heart and mediastinum in this patient presenting with asthma exacerbation and ball-valve mucus plugging of the right mainstem bronchus. Short interval follow-up imaging after bronchodilator treatment and clinical improvement demonstrated normalization of lung volumes.

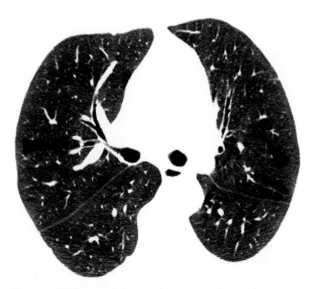

Figure 12.7. Multiple axial images of the chest in a patient presenting with respiratory distress demonstrate multiple small geographic regions of decreased attenuation throughout both lungs *(arrowheads)*, likely representing air trapping in the setting of reactive airway disease exacerbation. The patient's clinical status improved with bronchodilators.

enlargement of the airspaces distal to the terminal bronchioles, accompanied by destruction of the alveolar walls, and without obvious fibrosis." Centrilobular, panlobular, and paraseptal subtypes exist; however, centrilobular emphysema, typically seen in long-term cigarette smokers, is the most common form encountered in clinical practice. Chest radiographs are insensitive for detecting and grading emphysema; however, depression and flattening of the diaphragms, irregular radiolucency within the lungs caused by a heterogeneous distribution of parenchymal destruction, and increased retrosternal lucency on the lateral view may assist in making the diagnosis radiographically (Fig. 12.8). At CT, centrilobular emphysema typically manifests as numerous small foci of decreased attenuation without definable walls scattered in a background of relatively normal, homogeneous lung parenchyma. The lobular arteries may be visible in the center of the lucent regions, assisting in differentiating centrilobular emphysema from panlobular emphysema and cystic lung disease (Fig. 12.9). Exacerbation of chronic obstructive lung disease symptoms typically does not have a radiographic or CT correlate; however, patients may present with other complications including pneumothorax, pneumonia, and bulla infection (Figs. 12.10, 12.11, and 12.12).

Pneumonia

In the United States, pneumonia is among the leading causes of death and is very commonly evaluated and treated in the ED. Along with careful clinical and laboratory evaluation, radiography plays an important role in diagnosing, localizing, and characterizing pulmonary infections. Multiple pathogens can result in pulmonary infection, including bacteria, viruses, parasites, and fungi. The wide differential diagnosis for causative organisms can be narrowed by classifying pulmonary infections into clinical subsets such as community acquired, nosocomial, immunocompromised, pediatric, and so forth.

The most common pathogens found in community-acquired pneumonia are *Streptococcus pneumoniae* (40% of patients admitted to the hospital with pneumonia), *Mycoplasma pneumoniae*, *Chlamydia pneumoniae*, and *Legionella pneumophila*. Gram-negative organisms, especially *Klebsiella pneumoniae*, are also common causative organisms in persons at risk for aspiration, such as elderly patients and alcoholics.

Numerous viruses are implicated in lower respiratory tract infections of both immunocompetent

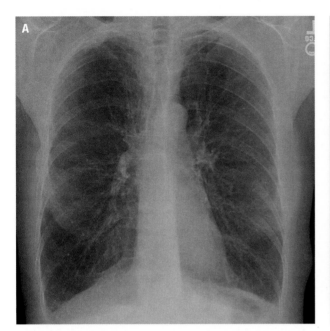
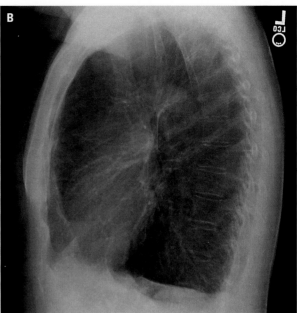

Figure 12.8. Severe pulmonary emphysema. **A:** The lungs are hyperinflated and there is a vertical orientation of the heart. **B:** Flattening of the diaphragms, increased AP diameter of the chest, and increased retrosternal lucency are evidence on the lateral view.

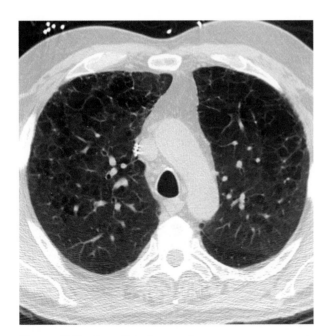
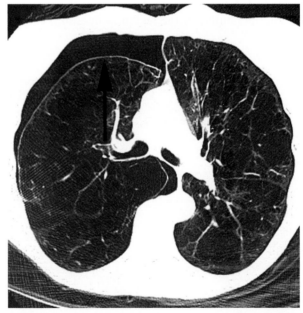

Figure 12.9. Centrilobular emphysema appears as apical predominant parenchymal lucencies with imperceptible walls, often with punctuate central densities representing the centrilobular arteries. In this case, extensive parenchymal destruction is evident representing moderate centrilobular emphysema.

Figure 12.10. Emphysema may be complicated by respiratory distress, a propensity for developing pneumonia, or, as in this case, pneumothorax in the setting of severe centrilobular emphysema with extensive and confluent regions of parenchymal destruction. The pneumothorax is clearly evident on the right with associated partial collapse of the right lung *(arrow).*

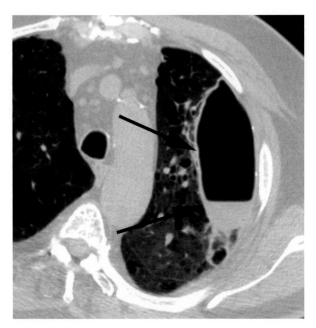

Figure 12.11. There is an air–fluid level in the left upper lobe with a smooth but thick wall superimposed on a background of moderate-to-severe centrilobular and bullous emphysema consistent with an infected bulla *(arrows)*. Differentiation from a loculated pleural fluid collection may be difficult and comparison with prior imaging, which may demonstrate the presence of multiple bullae in the region in question, can be helpful.

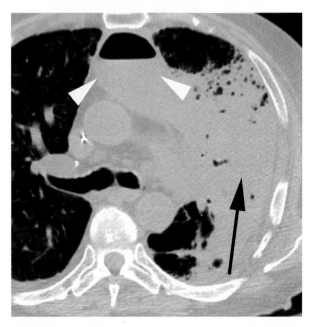

Figure 12.12. There is an air–fluid level centered in the anterior midchest *(white arrowhead)*, representing an infected lingular bulla in a patient with bullous emphysema and left upper lobar pneumonia *(black arrow)*.

and immunocompromised hosts and are commonly evaluated in the ED. Pulmonary viral infections can be classified into those occurring in immunocompromised patients and those occurring in patients with normal immune systems; however, there is considerable overlap in their radiographic appearance, and a specific imaging diagnosis is usually not possible. Most viral pneumonias in immunocompetent adults are the result of influenza types A and B infection, whereas immunocompromised patients are susceptible to a multitude of viruses such as parainfluenza, cytomegalovirus (CMV), herpes viruses, measles virus, and adenovirus.

The chest radiograph is typically the first line of imaging in the workup of a suspected lower respiratory infection. CT can be used for further characterization in the setting of complex pneumonia, suspected complication (such as pulmonary abscess or empyema), or to evaluate for an underlying disease process in the lung or mediastinum predisposing to pulmonary infection, such as an obstructing mass or lymphadenopathy (Fig. 12.13).

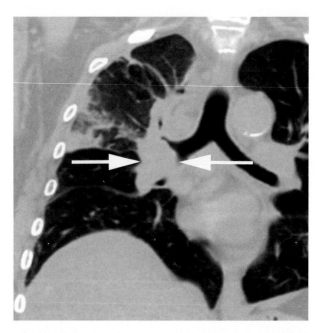

Figure 12.13. Postobstructive pneumonia may develop secondary to a hilar neoplasm centered in or invading the central airways. In this example, there is a soft tissue mass near the origin of the right upper lobe bronchus with near complete obstruction of the upper lobe bronchus and the bronchus intermedius *(arrows)*. There is patchy airspace consolidation and interstitial thickening in the right upper lobe and to a lesser degree in the right middle lobe consistent with postobstructive pneumonia.

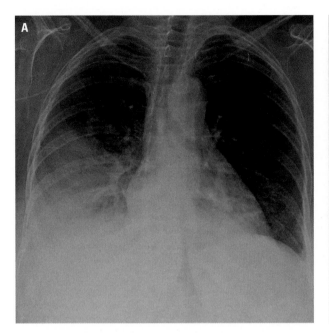
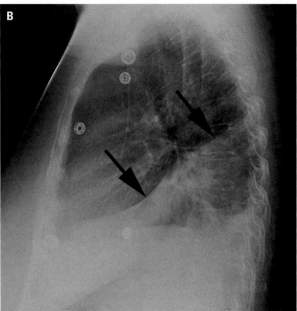

Figure 12.14. Right lower lobe pneumonia. Lobar pneumonia presenting with diffuse opacification of the right lower lobe and small right pleural effusion on the frontal (**A**) and lateral (**B**) radiographs *(arrows)*.

Pulmonary infection can be roughly classified into several radiologic patterns: lobar pneumonia, bronchopneumonia, and interstitial pneumonia. These patterns of infection tend to be associated with different organisms; however, significant overlap exists.

Lobar pneumonia typically appears as homogeneous consolidation involving predominantly a single lobe (Figs. 12.14, 12.15, 12.16, and 12.17). Multiple lobes may be involved; however, this is less common (Fig. 12.18). The lobar and segmental airways often remain patent within the region of

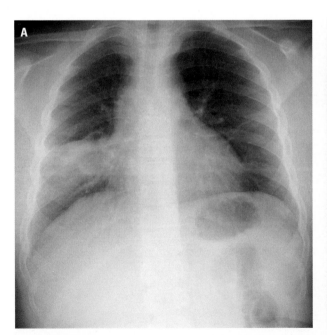
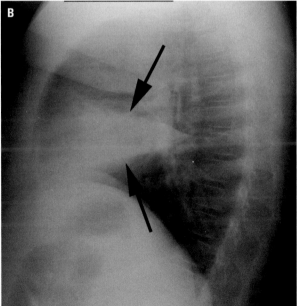

Figure 12.15. Right middle lobe pneumonia. Lobar pneumonia presenting with complete opacification of the right middle lobe on the frontal (**A**) and lateral (**B**) radiographs *(arrows)*.

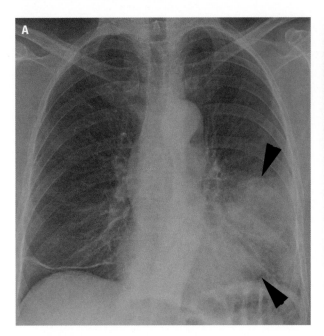
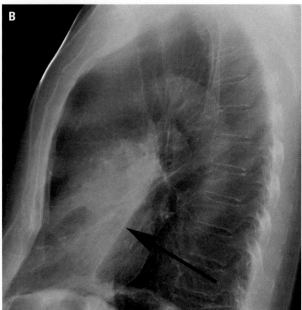

Figure 12.16. Lingular pneumonia. On the PA projection (**A**), there is increased density in the left midlung *(arrowheads)* resulting in desilhouetting of the left heart border. On the lateral view (**B**), there is a dense opacification anterior to the left major fissure in the lingula of the left upper lobe *(arrow)*.

consolidation, resulting in air bronchograms at chest radiography and CT.

Bronchopneumonia is often the result of infection with *Staphylococcus aureus* or gram-negative bacteria. Patchy parenchymal consolidation, usually surrounding a segmental or subsegmental airway, is a common radiographic appearance (Fig. 12.19). The spectrum of radiologic severity of bacterial bronchopneumonia ranges from peribronchial thickening and poorly defined bronchovascular

Figure 12.17. Lobar pneumonia with bulging fissure. There is dense consolidation of the right upper lobe resulting from *Staphylococcus* infection with posterior bulging of the right major figure *(white arrow)* and cavitation anteriorly *(black arrowhead)*.

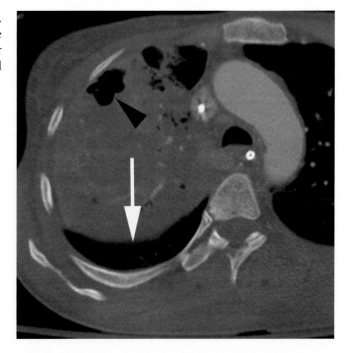

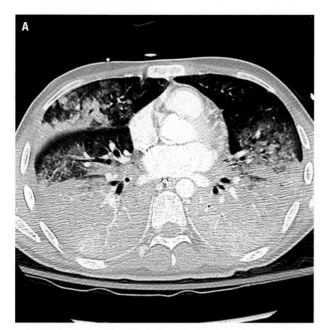
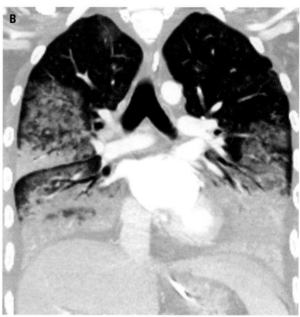

Figure 12.18. Multilobar bacterial pneumonia. Bacterial infection of the lungs may manifest with a variety of abnormalities on a chest radiograph or chest CT ranging from mild, focal involvement of terminal airways and acini to extensive multilobar infection with dense consolidation of multiple segments or lobes of the lungs. On the axial image (**A**) and the coronal reformat (**B**), there is dense, near-complete opacification of the lower lobes as well as patchy and confluent regions of airspace consolidation in the right middle lobe and in the upper lobes.

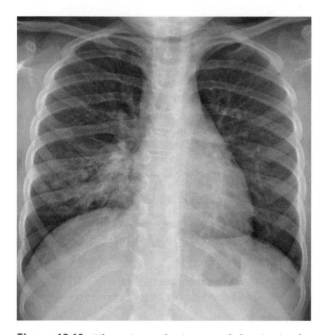

Figure 12.19. There is patchy increased density in the medial right lung with desilhouetting of the right heart border on the frontal radiograph, representing bronchopneumonia in the right middle lobe.

nodules (Figs. 12.20 and 12.21) to multifocal irregular regions of consolidation involving multiple lobes (Figs. 12.22, 12.23, and 12.24).

Infectious pneumonias involving predominantly the interstitium of the lung are commonly caused by viruses, *M. pneumoniae*, and *Pneumocystis jiroveci*. These organisms incite an interstitial cellular inflammatory infiltrate, resulting in the typical radiographic appearance of bilateral linear and reticular opacities (Figs. 12.25 and 12.26).

At CT, viral pulmonary infections typically manifest as multiple poorly defined nodules measuring up to 10 mm, patchy peribronchial ground-glass opacities, and airspace consolidation. Bronchiolar inflammation is also a common feature of viral pneumonia, resulting in air trapping and hyperinflation. Air trapping is most pronounced in pediatric patients, who also commonly demonstrate peribronchial infiltrates radiating from the hila.

Pulmonary Abscess

Pulmonary abscess occurs when a region of parenchymal infection undergoes tissue necrosis. The inciting organisms are most commonly mixed

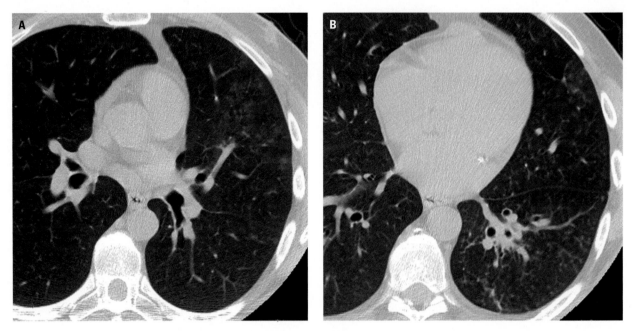

Figure 12.20. Multiple ill-defined ground-glass nodules in a bronchovascular distribution in the left upper (**A**) and left lower (**B**) lobes represent small airway infection in a patient with relatively mild bronchopneumonia.

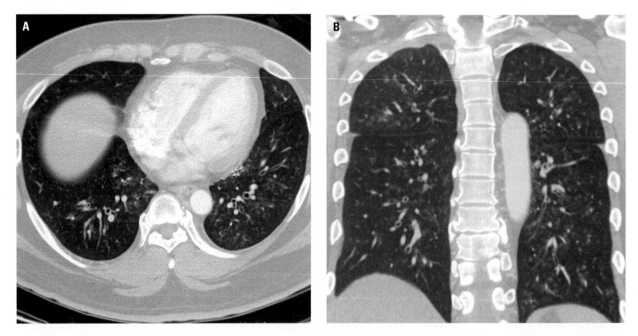

Figure 12.21. Axial (**A**) and coronal (**B**) CT images of the chest demonstrate tiny branching and nodular opacities in a "tree in bud" configuration in the bilateral upper and lower lobes, representing diffuse small airway infection in a patient with multifocal bronchopneumonia.

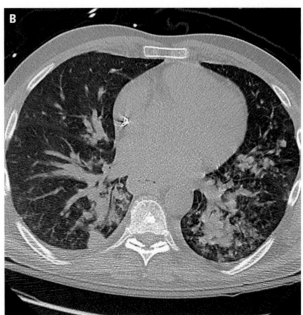

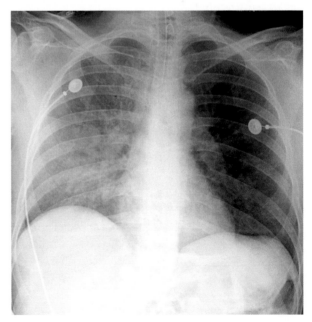

Figure 12.22. Severe bronchopneumonia. Axial CT images demonstrate patchy, irregular dense nodular opacities in the upper lobes (**A**) and in the lower lobes (**B**) along a bronchovascular distribution. The size and density of these nodules is greater than the fine "tree in bud" nodules seen in mild to moderate cases of bronchopneumonia (see Figs. 12.20 and 12.21). In the left upper lobe and in the medial lower lobes, the bronchovascular nodules are becoming confluent airspace consolidations in roughly segmental distributions.

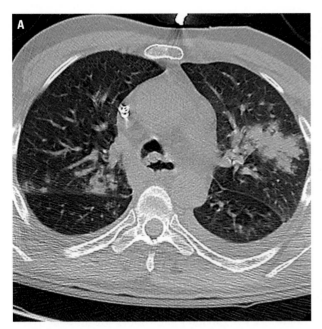

Figure 12.23. A spectrum of bronchopneumonia is seen in this CT examination. Severe infection is present in the left upper lobe with geographic confluent airspace opacities and interstitial thickening *(black arrow).* A mild focus of bronchopneumonia is present in the right upper lobe manifesting as multiple small "tree in bud" nodular opacities *(white arrowheads).*

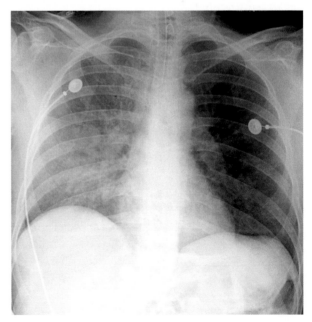

Figure 12.24. Pneumococcal pneumonia. Patchy opacities are present throughout the right lung, most prominently in the right lower lobe in a patient with pneumococcal pneumonia. Mild consolidation is also present around the lobar and segmental airways in the left lower lobe.

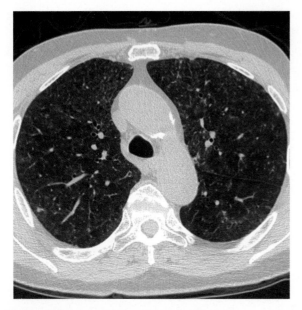

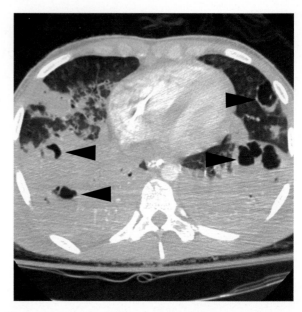

Figure 12.25. Varicella pneumonia. Ill-defined scattered small pulmonary nodules and mild peripheral interlobular septal thickening suggest a viral infection.

Figure 12.27. Cavitary multilobar pneumonia. Axial CT of the chest demonstrates dense consolidation in the lower lobes, patchy opacities in the right middle, and multifocal cavitation *(arrowheads)* resulting from *S. aureus* infection.

anaerobes, particularly in the setting of aspiration. Other causative organisms include *S. aureus* and *Pseudomonas aeruginosa* (Fig. 12.27). Multiple bilateral pulmonary abscesses may be seen secondary to septic emboli.

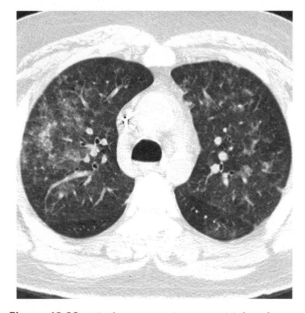

Figure 12.26. Viral pneumonia. Interstitial and scattered nodular airspace opacities suggesting an atypical (particularly viral) infection. In this case, the patient is immunocompromised due to stem cell transplant and has developed coronavirus pneumonia.

Differentiating an intrapulmonary abscess from an empyema can be difficult; however, the distinction is important for clinical management. The shape of a pulmonary abscess on radiographs and CT examinations tend to be round, whereas empyemas tend to appear ovoid or lenticular (Fig. 12.28). Pulmonary vessels may be observed to terminate abruptly at the margin of a pulmonary abscess while they tend to appear compressed or distorted along the margin of an empyema. The walls of a parenchymal abscess are typically, although not exclusively, more irregular and shaggy than those of an empyema (Fig. 12.29).

If a pulmonary abscess does not communicate with the bronchial tree, its radiographic appearance is that of a homogeneous density. Communication with the bronchus permits expulsion of necrotic material into the airways, resulting in cavitation and an air–fluid level.

The radiographic appearance of a cavitating pulmonary lesion typically does not allow for reliable differentiation between cavities caused by common bacterial pathogens, TB, vasculitis, or cavitating neoplasm. Although in many instances, the clinical findings, the location of the lesion, and the imaging appearance may suggest the etiologic agent, the correct diagnosis can be established only

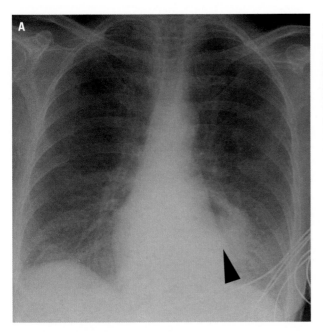
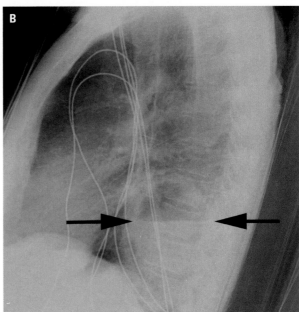

Figure 12.28. Pulmonary abscess. The PA radiograph (**A**) demonstrates a rounded retrocardiac opacity with an air–fluid level *(black arrowhead)*. On the lateral view (**B**), a round opacity with an air–fluid level *(black arrows)* is clearly visible in the left lower lobe.

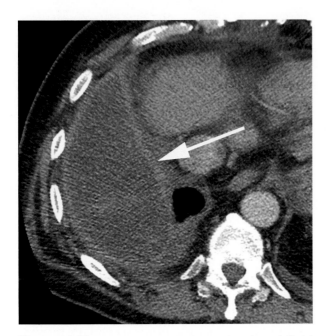

Figure 12.29. There is a complex right pleural fluid collection with abnormal pleural thickening and enhancement (split pleura sign) *(arrow)*. The normal pleura on contrast-enhanced chest CT is barely perceptible and does not appreciably enhance. Any thickening or enhancement of the pleura on contrast-enhanced CT is concerning for a complex pleural fluid collection, including empyema in the appropriate clinical setting.

by appropriate clinical evaluation and laboratory studies (Fig. 12.30).

Immunocompromised Patients

Immune compromise has multiple etiologies including HIV infection, solid organ transplantation, bone marrow transplantation, bone marrow suppression or replacement, and nonspecific reductions in immunity such as poorly controlled diabetes, alcoholism, and underlying malignancy. The various forms of iatrogenic and infectious immunosuppression are associated with unique time courses of susceptibility and unique opportunistic infections, and a comprehensive discussion of this complex topic is beyond the scope of this text.

The radiologic appearance of pulmonary infection in an immunocompromised patient is often nonspecific; however, there are three main radiologic patterns of pulmonary infection seen in immunocompromised patients: focal consolidation (patchy, segmental, or lobar), nodules (with or without cavitation), and diffuse or interstitial opacities.

A focal wedge-shaped opacity in an immunocompromised patient most likely represents a bacterial infection with a community-acquired pathogen. Infection with *Mycobacterium tuberculosis* (see later

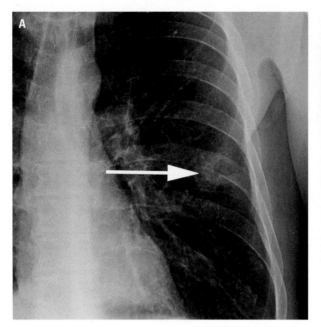

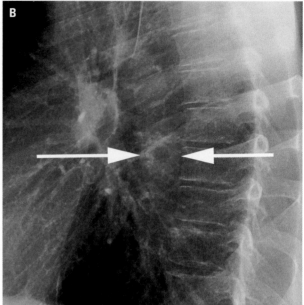

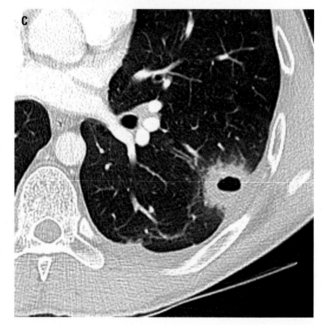

Figure 12.30. Pulmonary abscess. This small round cavitary nodule *(arrows)* on the PA **(A)** and lateral **(B)** radiographs represents a pyogenic pulmonary abscess. The abscess on chest CT **(C)** appears as a thick-walled cavitary nodule with spiculated margins and surrounding ground-glass attenuation. The appearance of this lesion is not specific for bacterial infection, and fungal infection should also be considered, particularly in an immunocompromised host. Vasculitis and neoplasm are also diagnostic considerations and such a lesion should be followed to complete resolution.

discussion) should be considered in the setting of severely compromised immunity, particularly in advanced HIV infection.

Pulmonary nodules (single or multiple) are commonly due to septic emboli, fungal infection (particularly *Cryptococcus neoforman* and *Aspergillus fumigates*), *Nocardia*, or mycobacteria (Fig. 12.31). Cavitation of nodules or associated parenchymal consolidation is concerning for angioinvasive aspergillosis or septic emboli. Cavitary lesions secondary to invasive *Aspergillus* may demonstrate a crescent of air between the infarcted, necrotic lung

centrally and the rim of surrounding viable lung tissue (Fig. 12.32).

Diffuse pulmonary opacities in an immunocompromised host are often secondary to viral infection such as CMV and varicella zoster or to the fungus *P. jiroveci* (particularly in advanced HIV infection). CMV pneumonia often manifests on chest radiograph as diffuse, bilateral reticular, and ground-glass opacities; however, the CXR may be normal despite significant clinical symptoms. CT may demonstrate multifocal ground-glass opacities, centrilobular nodules, and regions

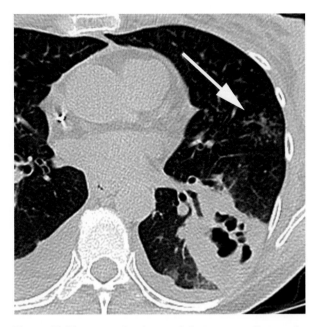

Figure 12.31. Dense focal consolidation extending to the pleura with central cavitation in the left lower lobe as well as "tree in bud" nodular opacities in a left upper lobe *(arrow)* are seen in this patient with cavitary *Nocardia* pneumonia and endobronchial spread of infection. Tuberculosis may have an identical appearance and is an important diagnostic consideration for cavitary lesions, particularly with evidence of endobronchial spread of disease.

of focal consolidation (Fig. 12.33). *P. jiroveci* infection manifests as bilateral perihilar ground-glass opacities and interstitial prominence during the early course of the disease (Fig. 12.34). CT demonstrates multifocal ground-glass opacities in a mid and upper lung distribution, often with mild interlobular septal thickening (Fig. 12.35). The infection may progress to more focal parenchymal consolidation (Fig. 12.36). Multiple small pneumatoceles may develop, predisposing the patient to develop a pneumothorax (Fig. 12.37).

Tuberculosis

The emergency radiologist can play a crucial role in diagnosing a patient with active TB. It is therefore important for the radiologist to have a high level of awareness of the various imaging features of this disease and alert the emergency physician to the possibility of active TB so that proper public health precautions can be instituted until the diagnosis is excluded or established. The radiologic presentation of TB depends on patient factors including age, immune status, and prior exposure.

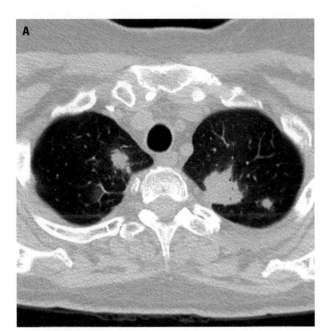

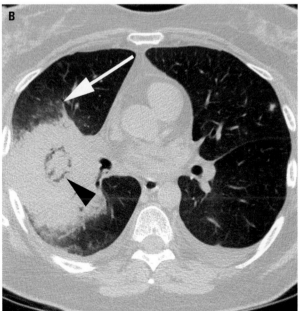

Figure 12.32. Invasive *Aspergillus*. Immunocompromised patients are at increased risk for opportunistic pulmonary infections. A relatively common pathogen is the fungus *A. fumigatus*, which may present as an aggressive, angioinvasive infection. Solitary or multiple irregular/spiculated pulmonary opacities are typical **(A)**. The lesions may cavitate *(black arrowhead)* and are characteristically surrounded by a halo of ground-glass attenuation *(white arrow)* **(B)**.

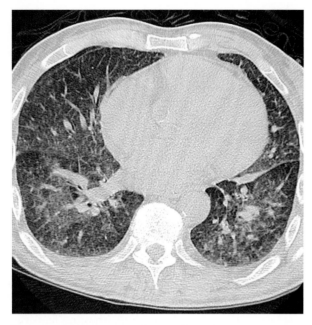

Figure 12.33. Cytomegalovirus (CMV) pneumonia. CT demonstrates multifocal and confluent ground-glass opacities, interlobular septal thickening, and regions of developing focal consolidation.

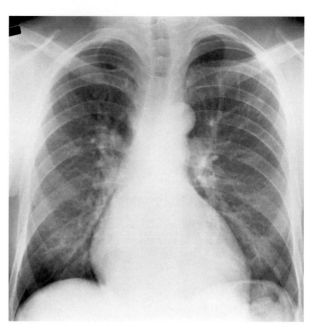

Figure 12.34. Diffuse ground-glass and fine reticular opacities represent *P. jiroveci* infection in a patient with AIDS.

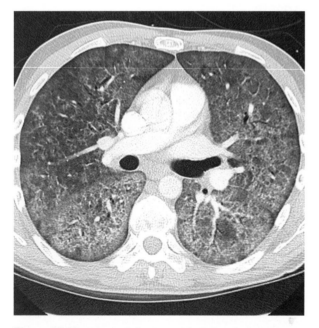

Figure 12.35. Severe infection with *P. jiroveci* in a patient with advanced HIV disease. There are extensive ground-glass opacities and interlobular septal thickening.

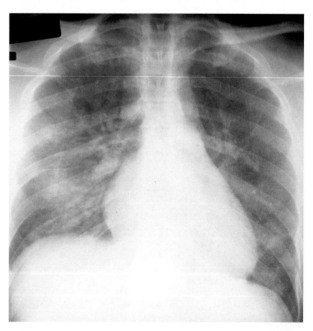

Figure 12.36. This example of *P. jiroveci* pneumonia is more advanced. There are fairly diffuse coarse reticular opacities and developing focal consolidations in the right upper and middle lobes.

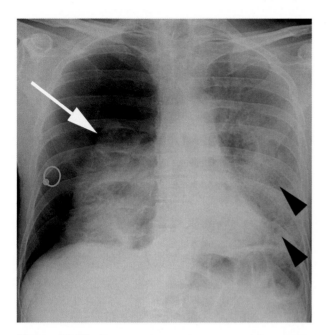

Figure 12.37. Pneumothorax is a potential complication of cystic *P. jiroveci* pneumonia, as in this case where diffuse opacities with multiple small rounded lucencies represent multiple cysts *(black arrowheads)* complicated by a large right pneumothorax *(white arrow)*.

In immunocompetent pediatric patients, intrathoracic lymphadenopathy (particularly in right paratracheal and hilar locations) is the most common manifestation of primary TB. The prevalence of lymphadenopathy decreases with patient age from nearly 100% in infants and toddlers to less that 10% by the sixth decade. Tuberculous lymphadenitis frequently demonstrates central low attenuation and peripheral rim enhancement on CT (Fig. 12.38). This feature, although suggestive of TB, is not pathognomonic and may be found in the setting of lymphoma, metastases, and infection by other mycobacteria species. Pulmonary parenchymal opacities frequently occur along with mediastinal lymphadenopathy in primary TB infection; however, unlike lymphadenopathy, this feature is more common in older patients than in the pediatric population. The airspace consolidation in primary TB is typically homogeneous and in a segmental or lobar distribution ipsilateral to mediastinal lymphadenopathy (Fig. 12.39).

Pleural effusion is an uncommon manifestation of primary TB infection in children <2 years of age; however, it may be seen in up to one-third

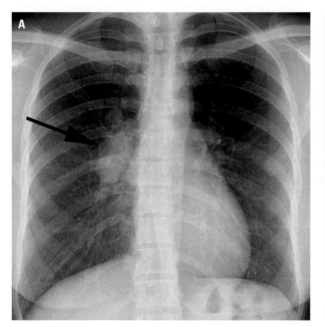
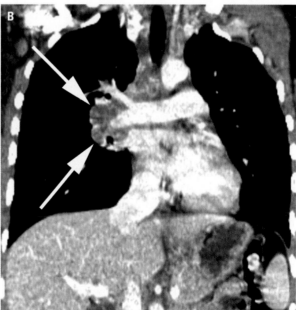

Figure 12.38. Primary tuberculosis infection, particularly in younger patients, may present with mediastinal and/or hilar lymphadenopathy. The abnormal soft tissue in the right hilum on the chest radiograph **(A)** *(arrow)* represents enlarged lymph nodes caused by primary tuberculosis infection. On CT **(B)**, the lymphadenitis in primary tuberculosis infection tends to be low in attenuation with thin peripheral rim enhancement *(arrows)*.

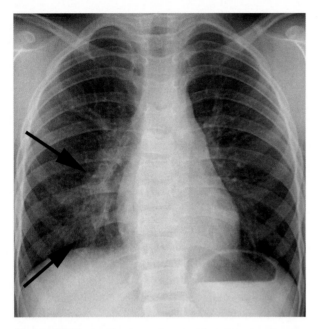

Figure 12.39. Pediatric patients with primary tuberculosis infection often present with isolated mediastinal lymphadenopathy; however, pulmonary involvement may coexist, as in this case with somewhat ill-defined right perihilar consolidation *(arrows)*.

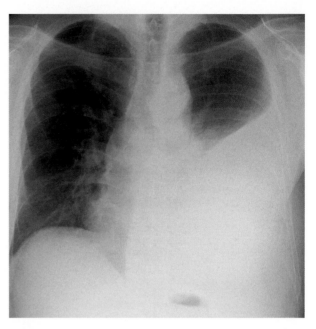

Figure 12.40. Primary tuberculosis infection may involve primarily the pleura and present with a (typically unilateral) pleural effusion.

of adults. Pleural effusion may be the only radiographic manifestation of infection in approximately 5% of adult cases (Fig. 12.40). The effusion typically develops 3 to 6 months after exposure, is most commonly unilateral, and occurs on the side of the initial TB infection. Effusions in primary TB infection are thought to be caused by a pleural hypersensitivity response rather than direct pleural infection. As a result, aspirated pleural fluid often does not yield positive cultures. Pleural effusions occur less commonly in postprimary than in primary TB infection. In contrast to the effusions in primary TB, those associated with reactivation disease tend to be complex, loculated, and may contain an air fluid level suggesting bronchopleural fistula.

Identifying active postprimary TB in the ED can be challenging because comparison examinations are frequently not immediately available, and a reliable differentiation between active and inactive disease can often only be made based on temporal radiographic evolution (Fig. 12.41). Mediastinal lymphadenopathy is an uncommon (5%) feature in postprimary TB. The most common manifestations of reactivated TB infection are heterogeneous parenchymal opacities in the apical and posterior upper

lobe segments and in the superior segments of the lower lobes. The opacities may appear to radiate from the hilum with distortion of adjacent pulmonary and mediastinal structures. These regions of consolidation often coalesce, and cavitation is seen in up to 45% of cases.

Endobronchial spread of TB is a very important entity to diagnose because it carries the most significant public health risk of all the forms of TB. This form of tuberculosis infection may be seen on chest radiograph in up to 20% of postprimary TB cases and occurs when a necrotic cavity develops communication with the bronchial tree, resulting in release of contents into the airways. Ill-defined bronchovascular nodules in a segmental or lobar distribution, remote from the cavitary lesions, are typical (Fig. 12.42). CT is very sensitive for detecting endobronchial spread, with up to 95% of cases of active postprimary TB infection demonstrating segmental or lobar centrilobular nodules remote from the necrotic cavity (Fig. 12.43).

Miliary TB typically presents with innumerable, randomly distributed 1 to 3 mm nodules throughout the lungs; however, these findings may not present radiographically until 3 to 6 weeks after the initial hematogenous dissemination

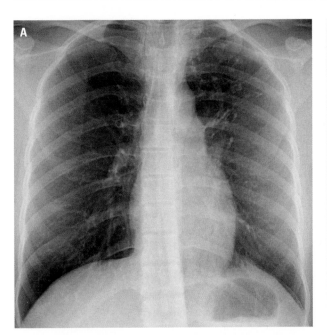
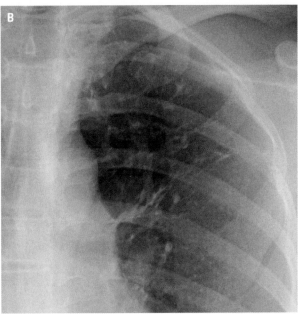

Figure 12.41. Fibrocalcific tuberculosis. The chest radiograph (**A**) and the coned, magnified view of the left apex (**B**) demonstrate fine branching linear opacities with small irregular apical nodules representing sequelae of prior active tuberculosis infection. Comparison with prior imaging is necessary to demonstrate stability of these fibrocalcific changes and to exclude reactivation of the tuberculosis infection.

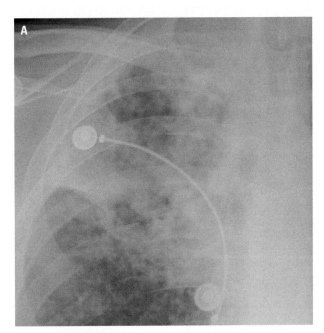
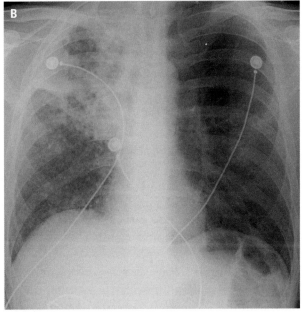

Figure 12.42. Active tuberculosis with endobronchial spread of disease. On the coned view of the left apex (**A**), there is heterogeneous consolidation in the right upper lobe with multiple small lucencies representing active cavitary tuberculosis. On the PA chest radiograph (**B**), multiple irregular and somewhat ill-defined nodules are present bilaterally, most prominently in the right lower lobe, which represent endobronchial dissemination of tuberculous bacilli and resultant multifocal tuberculous bronchopneumonia. Patients with this condition are contagious and should be placed in respiratory isolation as soon as possible.

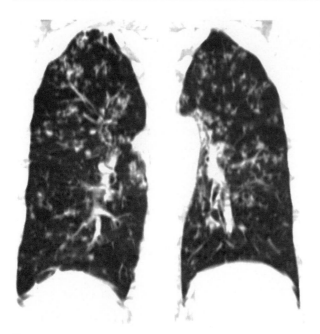

Figure 12.43. Tuberculosis with endobronchial spread of disease. Innumerable irregular small nodules in a bronchovascular distribution throughout both lungs in a patient with known active pulmonary tuberculosis represent endobronchial dissemination of tuberculous bacilli and tuberculous pneumonia.

(Fig. 12.44, 12.45). Histoplasmosis and cryptococcosis are also diagnostic consideration for a miliary nodular pattern in an immunocompromised patient.

Atelectasis

Atelectasis has been defined as "any pulmonary loss of volume without significant fluid filling of alveolar spaces" and can be classified in two principal groups: central and peripheral. Radiographic signs of atelectasis follow a theme of volume loss with associated positional changes in adjacent structures.

Central or lobar atelectasis is usually the result of bronchial obstruction. In pediatric patients, this is most commonly caused by aspirated foreign body or obstructive airway disease; however, neoplasm should be considered as an underlying etiology for an adult presenting with lobar collapse (Figs. 12.46, 12.47, 12.48, and 12.49). Peripheral (segmental or subsegmental) atelectasis has multiple etiologies, including small airway obstruction, mass effect from pleural gas or fluid, adjacent neoplasm or infection, and scarring.

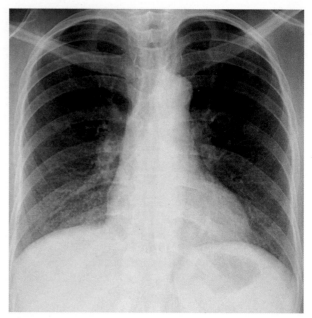

Figure 12.44. Miliary tuberculosis. The PA chest radiograph demonstrates diffuse 1 to 2 mm nodular densities resulting from hematogenous dissemination of tuberculosis.

Foreign Body

Foreign body aspiration is uncommon in adults but is the most common cause of airway obstruction in pediatrics. Frequently aspirated objects include food fragments, teeth, and small toys. Patients often

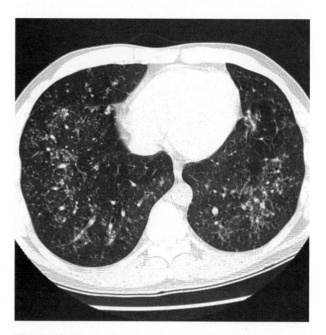

Figure 12.45. CT demonstrates innumerable 1 to 2 mm nodular densities in a random distribution resulting from hematogenous dissemination of tuberculosis.

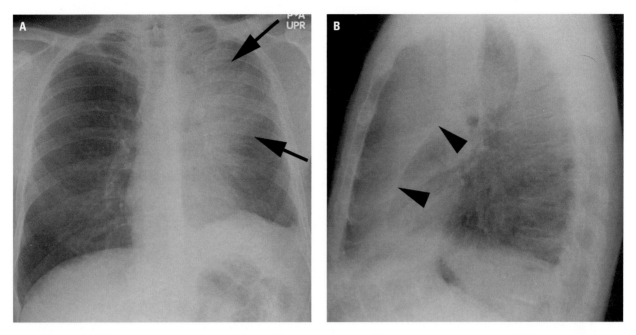

Figure 12.46. Left upper lobe collapse. On the frontal radiograph (**A**), there is a diffuse opacity obscuring the aortic arch, left hilum, and left heart border *(arrows)*. The left hemidiaphragm is elevated and there is leftward shift of the mediastinum. The right lung is relatively hyperinflated. On the lateral projection (**B**), there is a homogenous anterior opacity terminating abruptly at the left major fissure *(arrowheads)*.

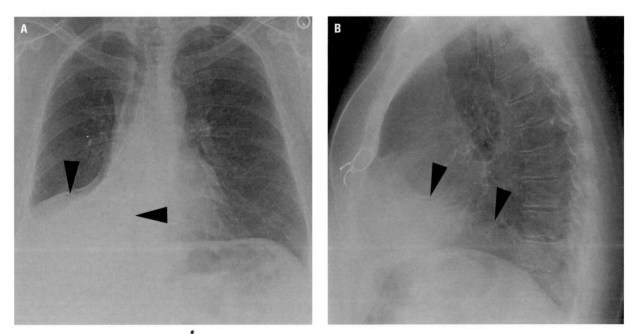

Figure 12.47. RML, RLL collapse. On the frontal radiograph (**A**), there is complete collapse of the right middle and lower lobes *(arrowheads)* with associated hyperinflation of the right upper lobe and rightward shift of the heart and mediastinum. On the lateral view (**B**), a homogeneous opacity is present in the inferior right lung with desilhouetting of the right hemidiaphragm *(arrowheads)*.

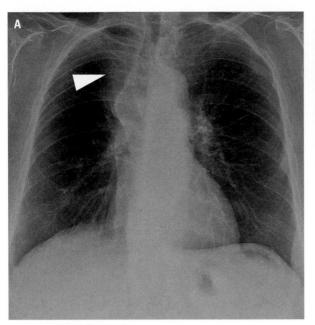 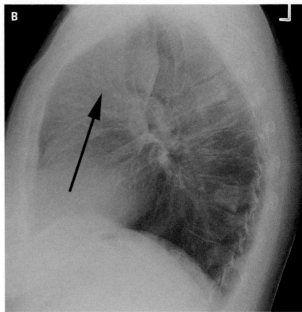

Figure 12.48. Right upper lobe collapse. On the frontal radiograph (**A**), hazy opacity in the medial right upper hemithorax abutting the mediastinum *(arrowhead)* with associated rightward deviation of the trachea, elevation of the right hilum, and relative hyperlucency of the right lung are consistent with right upper lobe collapse. On the lateral view (**B**), there is subtle increased density superiorly *(arrow)*. Multiple sclerotic bone metastases are present.

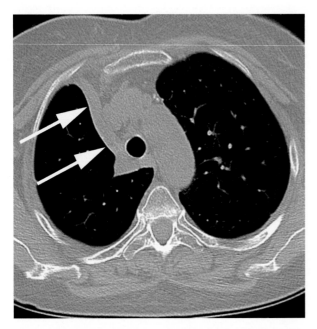

Figure 12.49. Right upper lobe collapse. The smooth, thin, roughly linear soft tissue density abutting the right mediastinum represents complete collapse of the right upper lobe *(arrows)*. There is relative mild compensatory hyperinflation of the right middle and right lower lobes.

present with a history of witnessed or suspected aspiration and cough. The aspirated foreign body is often radiolucent and may not be directly detected on a chest radiograph; however, secondary signs including obstructive lobar or segmental overinflation or atelectasis may be seen. Alternatively, the standard inspiratory chest radiograph may be entirely normal. In this setting, a radiograph obtained in expiration can be employed to demonstrating persistent asymmetric lung inflation due to air trapping from ball-valve motion by the aspirated foreign body. Decubitus radiographs are an alternative approach to demonstrate foreign body-induced air trapping. The dependent lung on decubitus radiographs is normally relatively poorly inflated due to extrinsic compression from the dependent chest wall. In the presence of a ball-valve endobronchial obstruction resulting in air trapping, the obstructed lung remains hyperlucent even when it is in the dependent position on the decubitus radiograph (Fig. 12.50).

CT is much more sensitive than chest radiography for demonstrating relatively radiolucent foreign bodies, such as subtle low-attenuation intraluminal

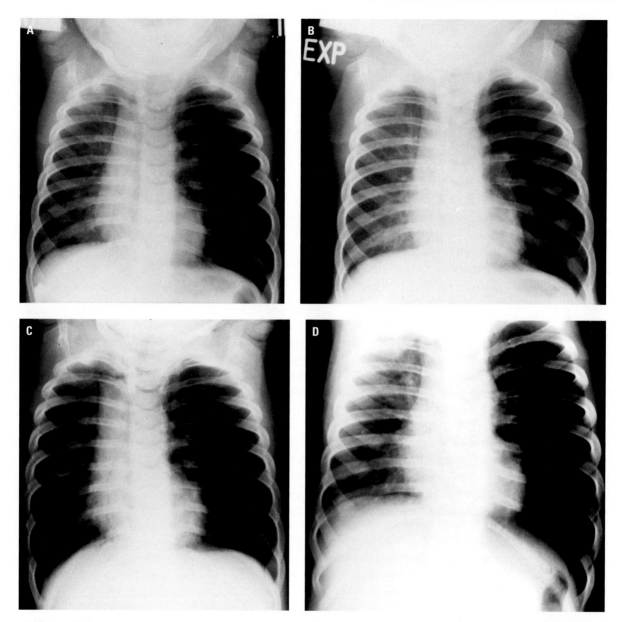

Figure 12.50. Nonradiopaque foreign body aspiration with resultant ball-valve effect in the left mainstem bronchus. There is severe left lung hyperinflation on the inspiratory radiograph (**A**) with rightward shift of the mediastinum. There is persistent hyperinflation of the left lung on the expiratory radiograph (**B**) with the expected expiratory decrease in volume of the right lung. This phenomenon can also be demonstrated with lateral decubitus chest radiographs. In the left lateral decubitus radiograph (**C**), the dependent left lung, which should normally decrease in volume, remains hyperinflated. In the right lateral decubitus radiograph (**D**), the left lung remains hyperinflated while the right lung demonstrates the expected decrease in volume.

vegetable material; however, this technique is infrequently performed on pediatric patients.

Pulmonary Edema

Pulmonary edema is defined as an abnormal accumulation of fluid in the extravascular compartments of the lungs. The relative amount of intravascular and extravascular fluid in the lung is primarily influenced by capillary permeability and intravascular oncotic pressure.

Pulmonary edema can be categorized on the basis of the underlying pathophysiology: increased hydrostatic pressure, increased capillary permeability secondary to alveolar damage, and increased capillary permeability without associated alveolar damage. Multiple etiologies for, and types of, pulmonary edema have been described. Those germane to the practice of emergency radiology including cardiogenic edema, ARDS, neurogenic edema, opiate overdose, and negative pressure edema are discussed.

Increased hydrostatic pressure in the pulmonary vasculature is most commonly the result of left heart failure, fluid overload, or both. Typically, no radiographic abnormalities are seen with pulmonary capillary wedge pressure less than 12 mm Hg. Above 12 mm Hg, cephalization of pulmonary vessels may be observed, particularly in the setting of chronic pulmonary venous hypertension (Fig. 12.51). Interstitial edema begins to manifest above 15 mm Hg as Kerley lines and loss of vascular definition, which may progress centrally to involve the perihilar vessels (Fig. 12.52). As pulmonary capillary wedge pressure rises above 25 mm Hg, fluid begins to accumulate in the alveoli resulting in small nodular opacities (representing fluid-filled acini), which coalesce into areas of confluent consolidation (Fig. 12.53).

Pulmonary edema may present asymmetrically at imaging due to underlying lung disease such as emphysema and fibrosis with alveolar filling occurring in regions of more normal lung parenchyma. The radiographic abnormalities also tend to distribute gravitationally within the lung, resulting in an asymmetric distribution of edema into the

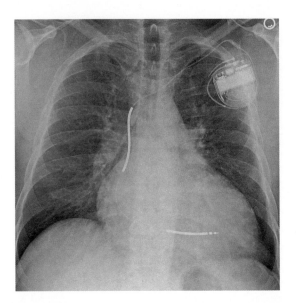

Figure 12.51. Vascular cephalization. The pulmonary vasculature is prominent in the upper lungs in this patient with cardiomegaly and a pacer/defibrillator, suggesting elevated central pulmonary venous pressures. No interstitial thickening or alveolar opacities are present to suggest pulmonary edema.

dependent portions of the lungs. Right upper lobe predominant edema may be caused by underlying mitral regurgitation resulting in the preferential jetting of refluxed blood into the right upper lobe pulmonary vein.

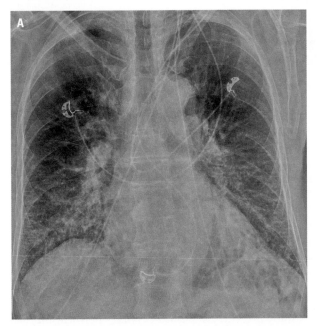

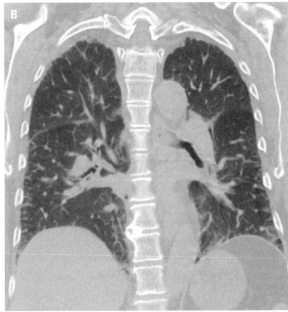

Figure 12.52. Interstitial thickening in the peripheral mid and lower lungs (Kerley B lines) on the PA chest radiograph (**A**) and on the coronal CT reformat of the chest (**B**) represent interstitial pulmonary edema.

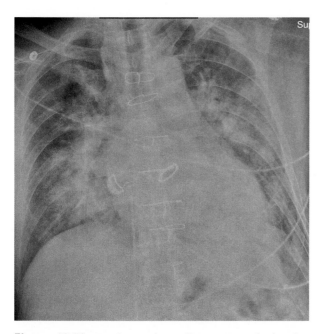

Figure 12.53. Patchy and confluent central alveolar opacities with relative sparing of the periphery are caused by rapidly developing alveolar edema. A leaflet from the prosthetic aortic valve malfunctioned, resulting in acute severe aortic regurgitation.

Occasionally, cardiogenic pulmonary edema may present with perihilar alveolar opacities that spare the lung periphery, resulting in a "bat wing" configuration on the chest radiograph (Figs. 12.54 and 12.55). This appearance is typically seen in the setting of acute heart failure, such as massive myocardial infarct, acute mitral regurgitation due to papillary muscle rupture or endocarditis, and renal failure.

Pulmonary edema occurs in up to 15% of patients presenting with opiate overdose. This type of pulmonary edema is likely the result of increased pulmonary capillary permeability related to hypoxia and acidosis. The radiographic manifestation consists of indistinct pulmonary vasculature and patchy airspace opacities, indistinguishable from other etiologies of pulmonary edema. Of note, there is often a marked gravitationally dependent radiographic asymmetry in the distribution of lung abnormalities because overdose patients are often immobile for long periods of time prior to receiving medical attention. Aspiration commonly coexists in these patients and can be difficult to distinguish from superimposed pulmonary edema.

Neurogenic pulmonary edema is uncommon sequelae of severe neurologic insult such as brain or spinal cord trauma, central nervous system (CNS)

infection, or cerebral vascular accident and likely results from a combination of increased hydrostatic pressure and increased capillary permeability without frank alveolar damage. Radiographic differentiation from the other etiologies for pulmonary edema cannot be reliably made by imaging, and neurogenic pulmonary edema is a diagnosis of exclusion. This form of pulmonary edema tends to resolve in 24 to 48 hours, allowing it to be distinguished from edema due to alveolar damage.

Negative pressure pulmonary edema can result from vigorous inspiration in the presence of an upper airway obstruction such as severe epiglottitis, laryngospasm, or foreign body impaction. The relatively extreme negative intrathoracic pressure generated by forced inspiration increases venous return to the heart, which transiently elevates pressure in the pulmonary vasculature, resulting in hydrostatic pulmonary edema. Imaging findings are similar to those found in the setting of cardiogenic pulmonary edema, including interlobular septal thickening, loss of vascular definition, and alveolar filling. This form of edema generally develops very rapidly and resolves spontaneously over the course of 24 to 48 hours after resolution of the upper airway obstruction.

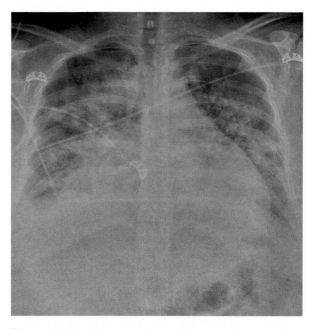

Figure 12.54. Patchy and confluent alveolar opacities, most prominently the perihilar region, represent alveolar pulmonary edema. The diagnosis is further supported by a small right pleural effusion and an enlarged cardiac silhouette.

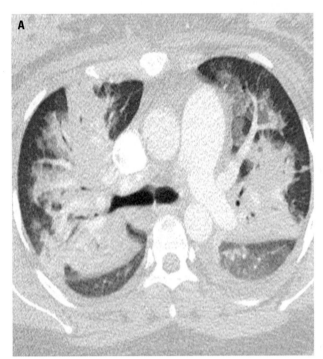
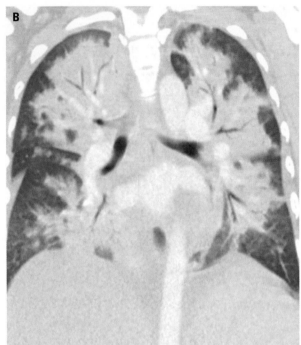

Figure 12.55. Perihilar edema. Axial (**A**) and coronal reformat (**B**) CT images demonstrate dense perihilar airspace opacities with relative sparing of the peripheral lungs and central air bronchograms in a patient with alveolar and interstitial pulmonary edema.

Acute Respiratory Distress Syndrome

In 1994, the American-European Consensus Conference developed a consensus definition for ARDS consisting of an acute onset of symptoms, bilateral pulmonary infiltrates with relative sparing of the costophrenic angles, a pulmonary artery wedge pressure <18 mm Hg, and a Pao_2:Fio_2 ratio of <200 mm Hg (200 to 300 mm Hg is defined as acute lung injury). Numerous risk factors for developing ARDS are recognized, including infection, inhalation injury, and trauma.

The radiographic presentation of ARDS is quite variable and reflects a diffuse alveolar epithelial injury (pathologically characterized by diffuse alveolar damage [DAD]) with resultant leak of proteinaceous fluid into the alveoli. Early manifestations on a chest radiograph or CT are primarily peripheral patchy alveolar opacities. These opacities often progress in size to become confluent and diffuse (Figs. 12.56 and 12.57). Notably, pleural effusions are typically not associated with this condition. The early alveolar opacities of ARDS may be difficult to distinguish from developing infection, edema, or hemorrhage; however, the radiographic abnormalities typically stabilize after several days,

whereas infection or untreated edema will continue to progress.

Pleura

The pleura represents a potential space in the chest that normally contains a trace amount of fluid (approximately 5 mL) and is maintained at a negative pressure relative to the atmosphere. A disruption of the equilibrium maintained by capillaries in the parietal pleura and lymphatics in the visceral pleura or of the negative pressure created by the chest wall, lungs, and diaphragm may manifest radiographically as abnormal pleural fluid or gas, respectively.

Pleural Effusion

Pleural effusions are typically classified as transudative or exudative. Transudative fluid is low in protein and has multiple etiologies, including congestive heart failure and associated pulmonary venous hypertension, decreased intravascular oncotic pressure in the setting of hypoalbuminemia, and transdiaphragmatic migration of peritoneal ascites. Exudative effusion has multiple etiologies

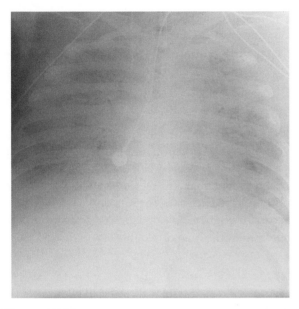

Figure 12.56. Acute respiratory distress syndrome (ARDS). This patient presented with H1N1 influenza infection and subsequently developed extensive, diffuse bilateral opacities with central air bronchograms, consistent with severe ARDS.

that typically result in increased pleural permeability, leading to accumulation of protein and cells, infection, inflammation, trauma, and malignancy. A chylous effusion may result from disruption of the thoracic duct.

Approximately 50 mL of fluid must be present to detect posterior costophrenic angle blunting on an upright lateral view radiograph. Pleural thickening may blunt the costophrenic angles and may be indistinguishable from a small free-flowing effusion on upright radiographs. The distinction may be established with lateral decubitus radiographs because thickened pleura will not change in configuration in the decubitus position. Conversely, a small loculated pleural effusion may be indistinguishable from thickened pleura by chest radiograph.

Subpulmonic pleural fluid that collects between the convexity of the diaphragm and the undersurface of the lower lobes can be difficult to detect with a chest radiograph. The effusion is often sharply margined and may be mistaken for an elevated hemidiaphragm (Fig. 12.58). An interlobar pleural fluid collection may simulate a pulmonary mass on the frontal radiograph (Fig. 12.59). The lateral projection may better demonstrate the interlobular location of the pleural fluid.

CT is a very sensitive technique for assessing pleural fluid, allowing for as little as 10 mL to be detected; however, this technique does not allow for reliable differentiation between transudative and exudative fluid. Intravenous contrast administration may demonstrate enhancing, thickened pleura that is suggestive of an exudative effusion; however,

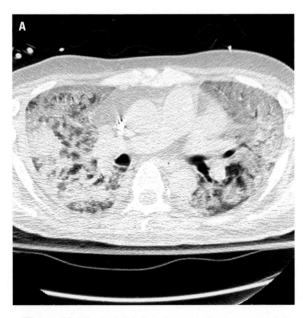
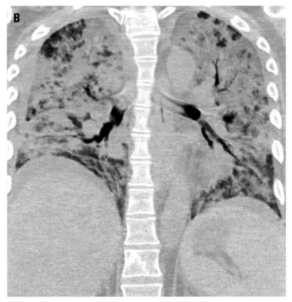

Figure 12.57. Axial (**A**) and coronal reformat (**B**) images from a CT scan of the chest demonstrated diffuse and confluent regions of consolidation throughout both lungs with scattered air bronchograms, consistent with ARDS. Pleural effusions are not typically seen in ARDS.

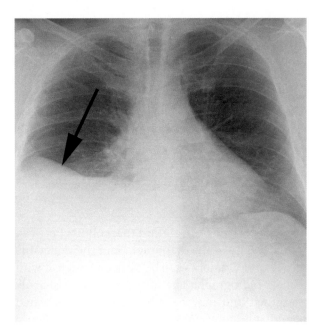

Figure 12.58. Subpulmonic pleural effusion *(arrow)* can be difficult to detect and may be mistaken for an elevated hemidiaphragm.

the absence of this finding does not exclude an exudate.

Ultrasound (US) is also a valuable modality for identifying and characterizing pleural fluid. Echogenic fluid and/or septations have been

demonstrated to reliably predict an exudative effusion; however, anechoic fluid on US does not allow reliable differentiation between transudate and exudates.

Hemothorax

Blood in the pleural space (hemothorax) is relatively high in attenuation and may contain layering or irregular high-density clot on CT. Hemothorax is most commonly caused by trauma; however, it can be atraumatic, such as in the setting of coagulopathy, aneurysm rupture, thoracic aorta dissection, and neoplasm of the lung or pleura (Fig. 12.60).

Empyema

An empyema is due to infection of pleural fluid resulting in the formation of an abscess in the pleural space. Bacterial seeding of the pleural space and resultant empyema most commonly occurs secondary to anaerobic, mixed anaerobic/aerobic, and tuberculous pneumonia. Therefore, empyema should be suspected in a patient who develops a pleural effusion in the setting of a bacterial pneumonia, particularly if the effusion appears loculated.

Radiographically, an empyema is typically well-defined and lenticular in shape. At CT, typical features of an empyema include thickened,

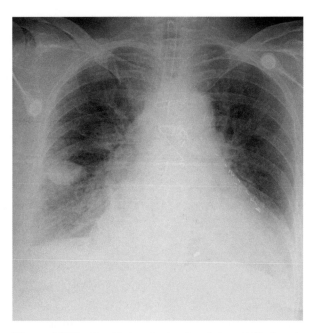

Figure 12.59. Ovoid density in the right middle hemithorax represents loculated fluid in the minor fissure.

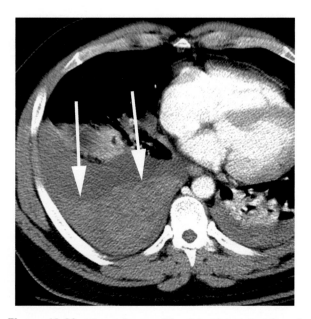

Figure 12.60. Hemothorax. Blood in the right pleural space presents as high attenuation material on this CT of the chest *(arrows).*

enhancing visceral and parietal pleura with well-defined margins. Gas within a suspected empyema may be caused by bronchopleural fistula (particularly in the setting of an adjacent necrotizing pneumonia or pulmonary abscess), recent thoracentesis, or less commonly caused by the presence of gas-forming organisms (Fig. 12.61).

Pneumothorax

The presence of gas within the pleural space is most commonly assessed with chest radiograph. This technique is most sensitive with the patient in the upright position, which allows the pleural gas to rise to the lung apices, where an air-pleural interface can be detected. Supine radiographs are not sensitive for detecting a small to moderate amount of pleural gas because the gas rises to the anterior hemithorax and pleural separation at the apex or laterally may not be present. A deep, lucent costophrenic angle (the deep sulcus sign) on a supine chest radiograph may suggest the presence of a large pneumothorax (Figs. 12.62 and 12.63).

Nontraumatic (spontaneous) pneumothorax may be classified as primary or secondary. Primary

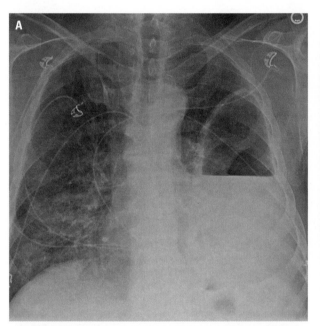

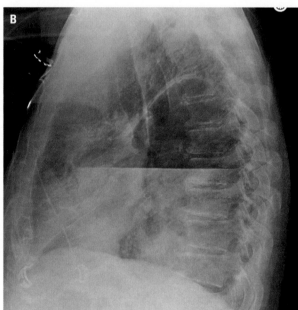

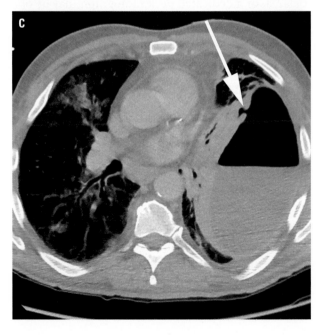

Figure 12.61. The PA (**A**) and lateral (**B**) chest radiographs demonstrate a large air–fluid level in the lateral left chest that is lenticular in shape and appears to be bordered by relatively normal lung along the superior margins, suggesting a pleural location. Gas within a pleural fluid collection is most commonly due to recent instrumentation or a bronchopleural fistula. On CT (**C**), a focal communication with the bronchial tree is evident at the anterior margin of the gas and fluid collection *(arrow)*. There is abnormal thickening and enhancement of the pleura, and the surrounding lung parenchyma appears displaced rather than disrupted, consistent with an empyema.

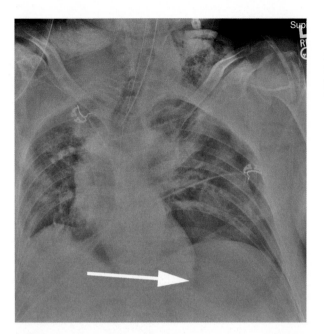

Figure 12.62. A large pneumothorax is present on the left with rightward shift of the mediastinum. The left costophrenic angle is deep and there is abnormal lucency over the left hemidiaphragm *(white arrow)*, illustrating the "deep sulcus" sign associated with a large pneumothorax on supine chest radiographs.

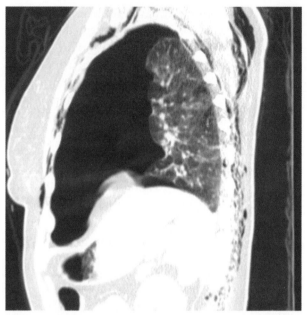

Figure 12.63. CT correlate of the deep sulcus sign in the setting of a large pneumothorax. Preferential, antidependent accumulation of gas within anterior pleural space extending to the anterior costophrenic margin results in the relative lucency of the left hemidiaphragm and prominence of the left costophrenic angle on a supine chest radiograph in the setting of a large pneumothorax.

spontaneous pneumothorax occurs in otherwise healthy individuals, most frequently in 20- to 40-year-old male smokers with tall, thin body habitus, and is thought to be caused by the rupture of an apical bleb. Same-side recurrence of a spontaneous pneumothorax is common and may prompt further evaluation of the lung parenchyma with CT to detect a bleb or bulla.

Secondary spontaneous pneumothorax occurs in patients with an underlying lung parenchyma abnormality, such as emphysema, asthma, cavitary infection, malignancy, cystic lung disease, and honeycombing caused by end-stage fibrosis.

Trachea/Airways

Acute abnormalities of the trachea are usually caused by trauma, inhalational injury, inflammation, and infection. Clinical presentation may include stridor, fever, cough, or acute respiratory decompensation. Tracheal infection and inflammation, as well as tracheal foreign body, are most commonly seen in the pediatric population. Viral laryngotracheobronchitis (LTB) *(croup)* and bacterial

LTB (pseudomembranous croup) are responsible for more than 90% of infectious tracheitis cases.

Radiographs can be helpful in establishing the diagnosis of LTB; however, they are relatively insensitive and may be normal in up to 50% of cases. The AP view of the chest may include the subglottic area, or a dedicated neck radiograph may be obtained to demonstrate soft tissue narrowing in this area ("steeple sign").

Pericardium

The pericardium is a sac surrounding the heart and roots of the great vessels, which consist of tough outer fibrous layer as well as visceral and parietal serous layers. This potential space normally contains approximately 15 to 50 mL of lubricating fluid. The most common cause of pericardial effusion is left heart failure; however, there are numerous other etiologies including trauma, renal failure, cardiac failure, infection (pericarditis), neoplasm, medication, radiation, and idiopathic.

Approximately 250 mL of fluid must accumulate to be detected on a chest radiograph. Signs of a

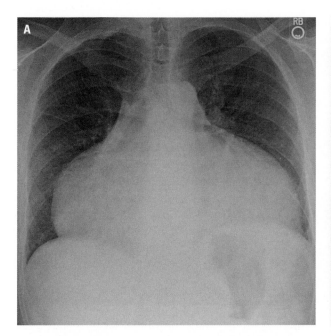

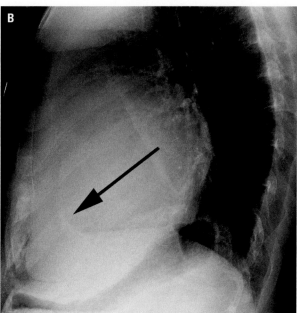

Figure 12.64. Large pericardial effusion. On the PA view of the chest (**A**), there is market globular enlargement of the cardiac silhouette. On the lateral view (**B**), the large pericardial effusion is visible as a rim of relatively high attenuation about the anterior and inferior margins of the heart *(arrow)*.

pericardial effusion include an enlarged cardiac silhouette on the posteroanterior (PA) or AP view and >2 mm separation of the retrosternal and epicardial fat stripes on the lateral view (the "Oreo cookie sign") (Fig. 12.64). CT and MRI are more sensitive for detecting small volumes of pericardial fluid; however, the modality of choice for rapidly evaluating and quantitating pericardial fluid remains echocardiography (Fig. 12.65).

Cardiac tamponade can develop in the setting of a rapidly accumulating pericardial effusion resulting in extrinsic pressure on the heart and poor ventricular filling. This is a critical condition that can result in rapid clinical deterioration and death if not treated. Tamponade physiology is typically clinically diagnosed; however, echocardiography can be employed to demonstrate pericardial fluid and mass effect on the ventricles. CT is less predictive of tamponade physiology.

Gas in the pericardial space may be the result of penetrating trauma, recent instrumentation, infectious pericarditis involving a gas-producing organism, as well as communication with the esophagus or stomach in the setting of visceral perforation (e.g., Boerhaave syndrome), inflammation, or malignancy.

Chest radiography may demonstrate air density on both sides of the pericardium, resulting in sharp definition of this structure. The heart may

also be partially or completely surrounded by air density (Figs. 12.66 and 12.67). This entity can be distinguished from the more commonly seen pneumomediastinum by the anatomic restriction of pericardial gas distribution to the pericardial reflection at the base of the great vessels.

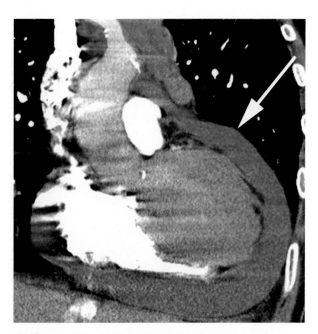

Figure 12.65. Coronal CT reformat demonstrating a moderate pericardial effusion *(arrow)*.

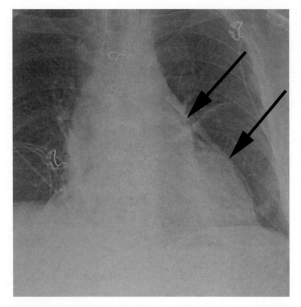

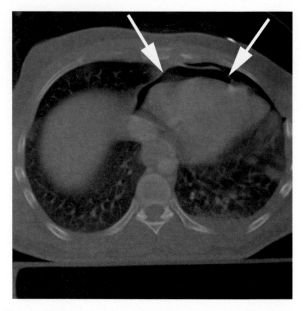

Figure 12.66. Pneumopericardium. Linear lucency along the left heart border represents gas within the pericardium *(arrows)*. Thin, linear soft tissue attenuation just lateral to this represents the dense, fibrous pericardium.

Figure 12.67. Pneumopericardium. Air surrounding the anterior heart is contained by the fibrous pericardium *(arrows)*.

Mediastinum

The mediastinum extends from the thoracic inlet to the diaphragms and between the medial boundaries of the right and left pleura and contains the heart, great vessels, central airways, the esophagus, lymphatics, and nerves. Most acute mediastinal ab-

normalities evaluated in the emergency room setting are secondary to trauma; however, familiarity with the radiographic appearance of acute nontraumatic mediastinal abnormalities is essential.

Acute mediastinitis is most commonly secondary to esophageal perforation (90%) or recent instrumentation/surgery (Fig. 12.68). Chronic or

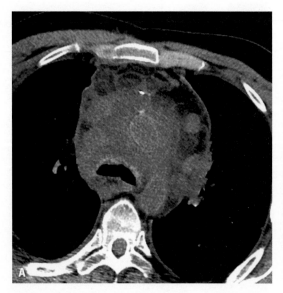

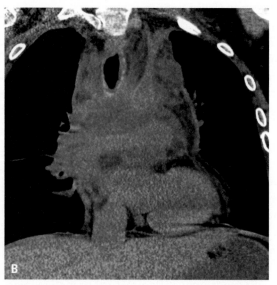

Figure 12.68. Mediastinitis. Axial (**A**) and coronal reformat (**B**) noncontrast CT images of the heart and mediastinum demonstrate irregular fat stranding throughout the mediastinal fat and multiple fluid collections, consistent with mediastinitis and multiple abscesses.

slowly progressing mediastinitis is usually caused by TB or fungal (particularly histoplasmosis) infection.

Esophageal perforation is generally caused by forceful vomiting (Boerhaave syndrome), ingestion of sharp objects, complication of endoscopy or surgery, or neoplasm. The diagnosis of esophageal perforation can typically be made with fluoroscopic esophagram; however, this is usually not the first line of imaging in the emergency room setting (Fig. 12.69). Early recognition is nonetheless critical because this condition is life threatening and prompt intervention greatly improves prognosis. Radiographic findings in acute mediastinitis caused by esophageal perforation

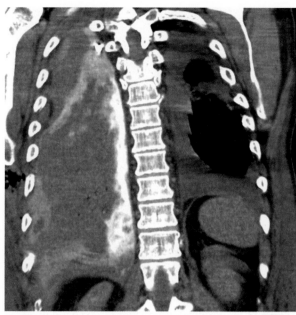

Figure 12.70. Boerhaave syndrome. High attenuation enteric contrast is present in the right pleural space as a result of esophageal perforation.

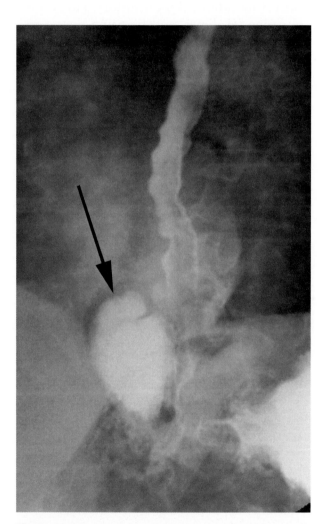

Figure 12.69. Boerhaave syndrome. Contrast extravasation can be seen from the distal esophagus on this single contrast esophagram in a patient with a history of vigorous emesis *(arrow)*.

or recent instrumentation may include widening of the mediastinum, pleural gas and fluid, pneumomediastinum, and mediastinal air-fluid levels. CT findings in esophageal perforation consist of esophageal wall thickening, extraluminal fluid collections, pneumomediastinum, pleural fluid, and possibly extraluminal enteric contrast in the mediastinum, pericardium, or pleural space (Figs. 12.70 and 12.71). Pneumomediastinum is the most sensitive sign and may be the only finding indicating underlying esophageal pathology.

Postoperative mediastinitis is not well evaluated by conventional chest radiograph as findings are often nonspecific, typically consisting of mediastinal widening, which can be commonly found in the expected evolution of noninfected postsurgical changes. Comparison of the position of midline sternotomy wires with prior examinations for interval change in position, suggesting sternal dehiscence, is critical (Fig. 12.72). CT can be helpful for characterizing the infection and the degree of involvement of adjacent structures as well as for directing image-guided treatment such as abscess drainage. Findings may include focal fluid collection, pleural or pericardial fluid, lymphadenopathy, and sternal abnormalities suggesting osteomyelitis such as osteolysis and sternotomy dehiscence (Fig. 12.73).

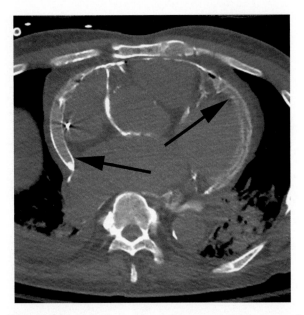

Figure 12.71. Esophageal perforation. Axial CT image of the chest after ingesting water-soluble enteric contrast demonstrates extension of the enteric contrast into the pericardium *(arrows)*. There is pneumopericardium as well.

Vasculature

Acute Pulmonary Embolism

Acute pulmonary embolism (PE) is the third leading cause of cardiovascular mortality in the United States. Rapid, adequate treatment

significantly reduces the mortality rate, thus making the timely, accurate diagnosis of acute PE critical. The clinical presentation is variable and nonspecific including, but not limited to, hypoxia, pleuritic chest pain, hemoptysis, cardiac arrhythmias, and syncope.

CT pulmonary angiography (CTPA) has become the standard first-line imaging modality for suspected PE due to the wide availability and speed of MDCT scanners, the high accuracy of CTPA for detecting acute emboli, and the ability of MDCT to demonstrate other chest pathology. The wealth of diagnostic information provided by CTPA and the speed at which this information can be obtained must be responsibly weighed against the relatively high radiation dose associated with the procedure. Appropriate use of CTPA can be directed by careful clinical history, physical examination, D-dimer, and by using pretest risk stratification tools.

The Prospective Investigation of Pulmonary Embolism Diagnosis II (PIOPED II) trial demonstrated CTPA negative predictive values (NPVs) of 96% and 89% for PE in patients with a low and moderate pretest probability, respectively. The NPV of CTPA in the setting of high pretest probability was only 60% in this trial. CT venography (CTV) to evaluate the deep veins in the proximal lower extremities and pelvis is possible with MDCT without requiring

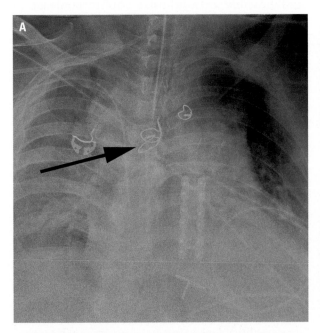 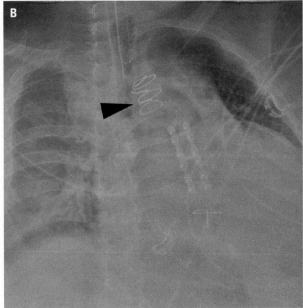

Figure 12.72. There has been interval displacement of sternal wires *(arrow)* **(A)** when compared with prior imaging *(black arrowhead)* **(B)**, indicating sternal dehiscence.

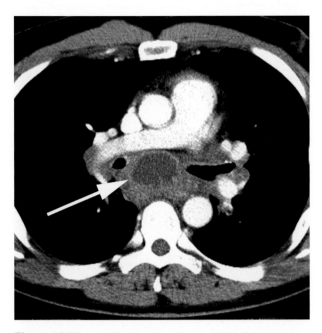

Figure 12.73. Axial contrast-enhanced CT demonstrates and peripherally enhancing fluid collection *(arrow)* and fat stranding, consistent with a mediastinal abscess and mediastinitis.

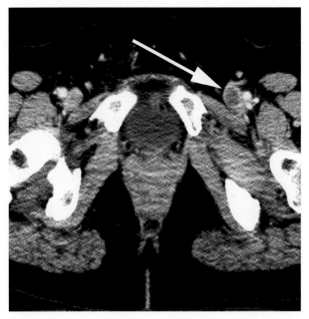

Figure 12.74. CT evaluation of the deep veins in the proximal lower extremities and pelvis in a patient with suspected pulmonary embolus demonstrates a filling defect in the left common femoral vein *(arrow)*, representing a deep vein thrombus. A negative CT venogram in a patient with a high pretest probability for pulmonary embolus significantly improves the negative predictive value of imaging.

additional contrast injection (Fig. 12.74). Employing this technique in patients with a high pretest probability increases the NPV of imaging from 60% to 82% (PIOPED II). Minimal improvement in NPV is observed in low- and moderate-risk patients by adding CTV to the imaging workup. The chest radiograph is not sensitive for detecting pulmonary embolus and is often normal despite significant clot burden at CTPA. Findings that may suggest acute pulmonary embolus on chest radiograph include enlarged pulmonary arteries or wedge-shaped peripheral opacities; however, these findings are not specific.

The appearance of an acute PE at CTPA is a low attenuation filling defect that may partially or completely occlude an otherwise well-opacified pulmonary artery (Fig. 12.75). Embolized thrombi are typically long, thin objects and accordingly are most commonly found draped across branch points in the pulmonary artery tree (Fig. 12.76).

The ability to visualize subsegmental pulmonary arteries with MDCT pulmonary angiogram has resulted in detection of isolated subsegmental pulmonary emboli (ISSPE) in up to one-third of pulmonary angiograms; however, management of these emboli remains controversial. Autopsy stud-

ies have demonstrated ISSPE in up to 90% of cases, suggesting that these are usually asymptomatic and may resolve without treatment in otherwise healthy individuals. Patients with severe cardiopulmonary comorbidities, such as cardiovascular disease or chronic pulmonary arterial hypertension, may benefit from anticoagulation for ISSPE.

Secondary CT findings of acute pulmonary embolus include wedge-shaped peripheral regions of consolidation and decreased enhancement, representing possible pulmonary infarcts, atelectasis, or hemorrhage (Fig. 12.77). A pleural effusion may also be found.

More ominous secondary findings of acute pulmonary embolus include enlargement of the right ventricle, straightening of the interventricular septum, compression of the left ventricle, and acute enlargement of the central pulmonary arteries, which suggest right heart strain (Fig. 12.78). These findings are concerning for impending circulatory collapse and should be communicated emergently to the referring physician. Reflux of contrast into

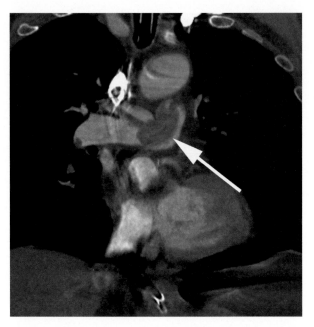

Figure 12.75. There is a large pulmonary embolus saddling the main pulmonary arteries *(arrow)*.

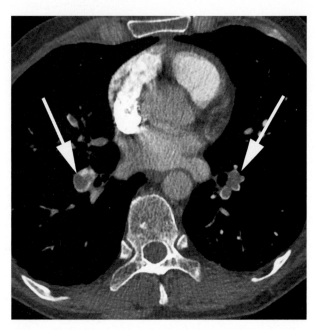

Figure 12.76. Multiple bilateral pulmonary emboli saddle the segmental pulmonary arteries *(arrows)*. The rims of contrast around the filling defects suggest that these are acute.

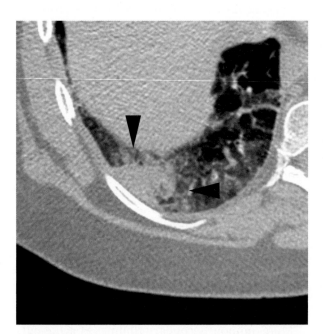

Figure 12.77. Somewhat indistinct wedge-shaped consolidation in the peripheral base of the right lower lobe *(arrowheads)* in a patient with multiple pulmonary emboli is consistent with an evolving pulmonary infarct. Infarcted parenchyma may demonstrate relatively decreased enhancement when compared with adjacent perfused lung.

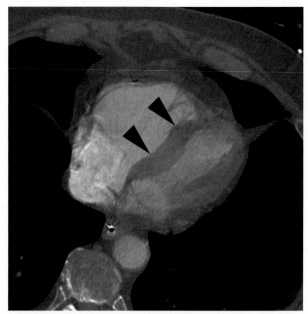

Figure 12.78. Massive pulmonary embolus resulting in right heart strain as evidenced on the axial CT by enlargement of the right ventricle and straightening of the interventricular septum *(arrowheads)*. Reflux of contrast into the hepatic veins is commonly seen with injection rates above 3 mL/sec and therefore is not a reliable indicator of right heart strain.

the hepatic veins is specific for right heart dysfunction at low injections rates (<3 mL/sec); however, it does not accurately predict right heart strain at the higher injection rates employed for MDCT pulmonary angiograms.

Septic Pulmonary Emboli

Emboli to the lungs containing microorganisms may develop into foci of infection in the lung parenchyma. Relatively common source of septic pulmonary emboli are tricuspid valve endocarditis and infected indwelling central venous catheter. Other predisposing conditions are recognized including alcoholism, immunodeficiency, and the complex of retropharyngeal abscess and jugular vein septic thrombophlebitis (Lemierre syndrome).

Multiple poorly defined nodular opacities, often with cavitation, may be seen on the chest radiograph (Fig. 12.79). At CT, multiple fairly well-defined nodules may be seen (Fig. 12.80). The nodules tend to predominate in the lower lungs, corresponding to the relatively larger blood flow to these regions. Cavitation is a common feature of septic emboli; however, the nodules may demonstrate variability in degree of cavitation and size, likely caused by multiple embolic showers (Fig. 12.81).

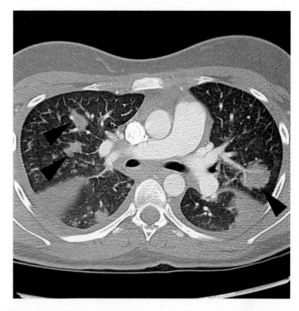

Figure 12.80. Lemierre syndrome. Multiple irregular nodules in a patient with jugular vein thrombophlebitis are concerning for septic emboli *(arrowheads)*. Peripheral interlobular septal prominence suggests interstitial edema.

Acute Aortic Syndrome

AAS is composed of penetrating atherosclerotic ulcers (PAUs), intramural hematomas (IMHs), and aortic dissections (ADs), which are generally considered to represent a spectrum of the same

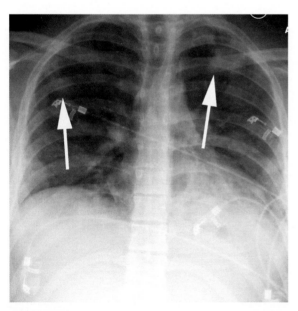

Figure 12.79. Lemierre syndrome. A patient with retropharyngeal abscess and jugular vein thrombophlebitis demonstrates multiple nodular opacities in the lungs *(arrows)*, consistent with septic emboli from the infected jugular vein thrombus.

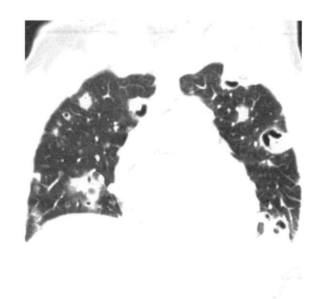

Figure 12.81. Multiple pulmonary nodules are present, which vary in size and degree of cavitation due to septic emboli. The variability in size of the pulmonary nodules and the degree of nodule cavitation is likely related to multiple episodes of embolization to the lungs.

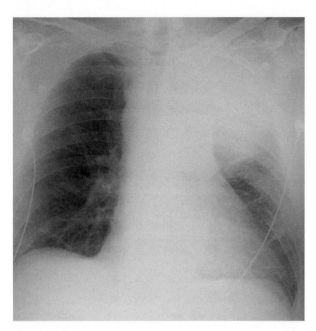

Figure 12.82. Ruptured aortic dissection. The frontal chest radiograph demonstrates a loss of the normal aortic contour and an ill-defined opacity occupying the superior left hemithorax, consistent with hemorrhage.

disease process with the primary risk factor of hypertension.

AAS, particularly AD, has a high mortality rate in the first 48 hours after the onset of symptoms; therefore, timely diagnosis and treatment is essential.

A chest radiograph is typically the first imaging study obtained for the evaluation of acute chest pain; however, this modality does not provide adequate sensitivity or specificity for acute pathology of the aorta. Radiograph findings that can suggest underlying acute aortic pathology include abnormal aortic contour and intimal aortic calcification displacement (>6 mm) (Fig. 12.82). MDCT is the current gold standard for imaging of aortic pathology with a sensitivity and specificity approaching 100%.

AD results from an intimal tear that allows blood to enter and longitudinally split the media along the course of the vessel, forming a false lumen, which may rejoin the true vessel lumen at a more distally located intimal tear. The proximal intimal tear tends to be located at points of maximal aortic pressure, such as along the lateral margin of the ascending aorta or the proximal descending aorta. The second, distal intimal tear tends to be located at a calcified atherosclerotic lesion, usually in the abdominal aorta or iliac arteries.

AD is most often categorized with the Stanford classification. Dissection involving the ascending aorta is classified as Stanford type A and is generally managed with emergent surgical intervention (Fig. 12.83). Descending aorta dissection (beginning after the origin of the left subclavian artery) is classified as Stanford type B and can typically be managed medically or with endovascular stent graft placement (Fig. 12.84).

An intimal flap separating the true and false lumens is frequently visible in ADs at MDCT. The site of intimal tear may be visible, allowing accurate differentiation of the true and false lumens (Fig. 12.85). The false lumen tends to have a larger diameter than the true lumen and tends to track along the outer border of the aorta. Other features of the false lumen include an acute angle with the outer vessel wall (the "beak" sign) (Fig. 12.86) and subtle fine linear low attenuation structures within the false lumen representing untorn fibers of the aortic media (the "cobweb" sign) (Fig. 12.87). Occasionally, the dissection may extend circumferentially around the aorta, resulting in a central true lumen completely surrounded by the false lumen (the "windsock" sign).

Complications associated with AD include cerebral infarction, limb ischemia, visceral organ ischemia, as well as proximal extension of the dissection

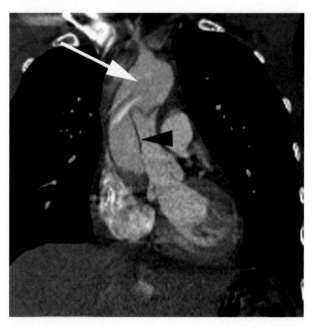

Figure 12.83. Stanford type A dissection. The intimal flap *(black arrowhead)* and false lumen *(white arrow)* in the ascending aorta are visible on this coronal reformat.

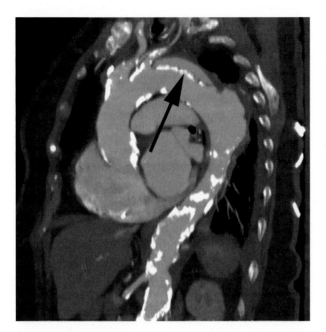

Figure 12.84. Sagittal maximum intensity projection (MIP) CT angiogram image of a heavily calcified thoracic aorta demonstrates displacement of calcified intima in the proximal descending thoracic aorta *(arrow)*, arising just distal to the origin of the subclavian artery, consistent with a Stanford type B dissection.

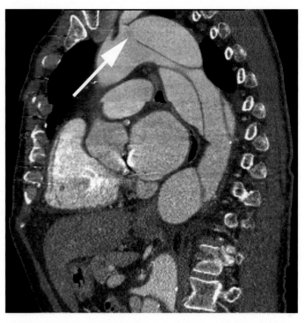

Figure 12.85. An intimal tear is visible *(arrow)* just distal to the origin of the left subclavian artery in this sagittal reformat of a Stanford type B aortic dissection.

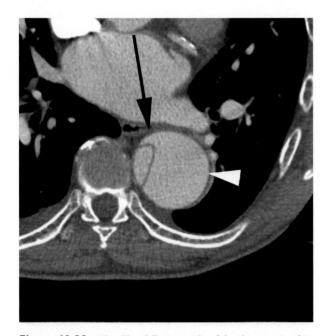

Figure 12.86. The "beak" sign. The false lumen in this aortic dissection *(white arrowhead)* forms an acute angle with the wall of the vessel *(black arrow)*.

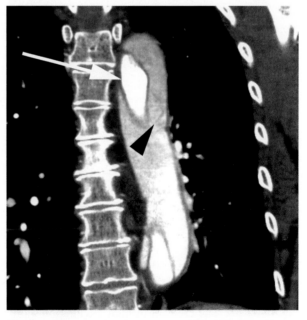

Figure 12.87. The "cobweb" sign. There is a type B thoracic aortic dissection with dense contrast opacification of the true (smaller) lumen *(arrow)*. The less densely classified false lumen nearly completely surrounds the true lumen. Close examination of the false lumen demonstrates thin, curvilinear low attenuation structures *(arrowhead)* representing residual, untorn vessel media fibers (cobweb sign).

to involve the coronary arteries resulting in myocardial infarction or into the pericardium, resulting in cardiac tamponade. Electrocardiogram (ECG) gating can improve evaluation of Stanford type A dissections, in particular to evaluate the coronary arteries and aortic valve and to reduce motion artifact in this region, which may otherwise result in a false-positive CT interpretation.

IMH may arise from rupture of the aortic vasa vasorum or a radiographically occult intimal disruption. The Stanford classification system for AD is used to classify IMH as type A or type B, based on location. As with AD, type A IMH is usually managed surgically, whereas type B IMH is frequently managed medically. The 5-year survival of untreated IMH is estimated to be less than 50% because this condition frequently progresses to frank AD.

The protocol for MDCT evaluation of suspected AAS should include a noncontrast series to evaluate for IMH because the crescentic high attenuation IMH may not be appreciated on the contrast phase of the examination (Fig. 12.88). No enhancement or free flow of contrast into the lesion should be present for the diagnosis of IMH. The high attenuation

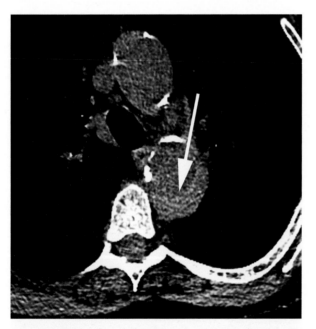

Figure 12.88. The crescent of high attenuation along the posterior descending thoracic aorta *(arrow)* on this noncontrast phase of an acute aortic syndrome CT scan represents a Stanford type B intramural hematoma. The relative high attenuation of the intramural blood is masked by intravenous contrast during the angiographic phase; therefore, noncontrast examination of the aorta in suspected acute aortic syndrome is critical.

of the IMH typically persists from 7 to 10 days, allowing for rough aging of the abnormality.

A PAU is an atheromatous plaque ulceration that has penetrated into the vessel media. Patients present with PAU are generally older than those with AD and IMH and have more advanced atherosclerotic disease. Most PAUs are found in the aortic arch and in the descending aorta. The ascending aorta is infrequently involved due to the relative absence of significant atheromatous plaques in this segment of the vessel. Uncomplicated cases are generally managed medically with periodic imaging surveillance; however, progression of the ulcer through the media resulting in pseudoaneurysm or through the adventitia, resulting in frank aortic rupture and hemorrhage into the mediastinum and/or pleural spaces, may necessitate urgent surgical or endovascular intervention.

The clinical presentation of this entity is not reliably distinguished from that of IMH and AD, and the MDCT workup is similar, consisting of a noncontrast series, followed by an arterial phase contrast-enhanced series. The noncontrast series may occasionally demonstrate an IMH at the site of ulceration. The contrast-enhanced series will demonstrate extension of contrast-enhanced arterial blood beyond the intima and focally into the media (Fig. 12.89). Focal vessel wall thickening and surrounding mild mediastinal fat stranding may be noted. Occasionally, the ulceration may be very superficial and confined to the intima, making detection of PAU more difficult.

Aortic Stent Grafts

Numerous complications associated with thoracic aorta stent graft treatment of AAS have been described including graft leak, stent graft migration, pseudoaneurysm, aortic perforation, stent kinking, thrombosis, fistula, and infection. Many complications are potentially life threatening, and familiarity with the appearance of common endovascular stent graft complications is essential.

Endoleak is a relatively common complication of stent grafting and is characterized by persistent blood flow outside the lumen of endovascular graft but within the aneurysm sac or vessel segment excluded by the stent graft. MDCT protocol for stent graft evaluation typically consists of a noncontrast series followed by arterial and delayed phases. The

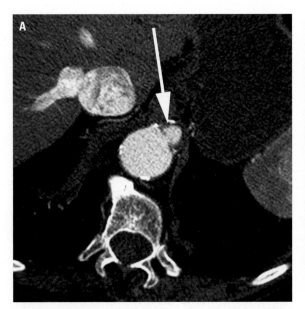 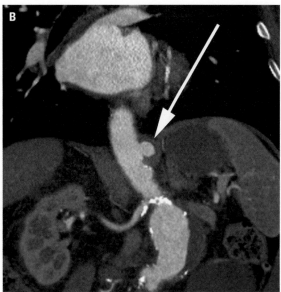

Figure 12.89. The focal outpouching containing arterial phase contrast-enhanced blood from the thoracic aorta at the diaphragmatic hiatus on axial (**A**) and coronal reformat (**B**) CTA represents a penetrating ulcer *(arrows)*. The aorta is atherosclerotic and there is focal vessel wall thickening at the site of penetration.

combination of these different phases results in a near 100% sensitivity for endoleak.

Five types of endoleak have been described based on imaging findings. Type 1A (proximal) and 1B (distal) leaks occur at the ends of the stent graft at the vessel attachment sites (Fig. 12.90 and 12.91).

Type 2 leak results from collateral vessel formation or retrograde venous flow, which drains into the excluded portion of the aneurysm or vessel wall (Fig. 12.92). Type 3 leak is caused by a structural defect in the graft itself or a junctional separation of overlapping grafts (Fig. 12.93). Type 4 leaks are

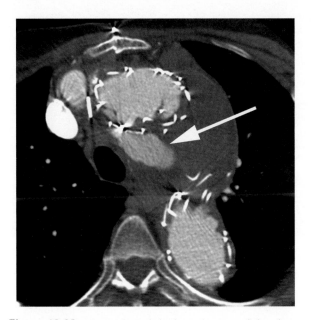 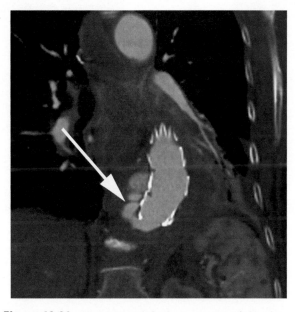

Figure 12.90. Type 1A endoleak. A stent graft has been placed across the proximal segment of a Stanford type A aortic dissection. Arterial phase contrast enters the excluded segment of the aorta from the proximal margin of the stent graft *(arrow)*.

Figure 12.91. Type 1B endoleak. A stent graft has been placed to treat a thoracic aorta dissection. Arterial phase contrast enters the excluded false lumen at the distal margin of the stent *(arrow)*.

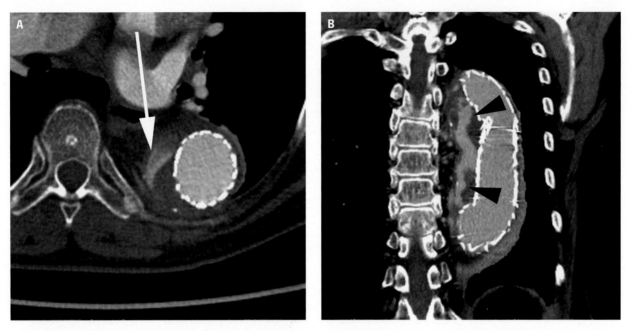

Figure 12.92. Type 2 endoleak. Axial (**A**) and coronal reformat (**B**) images status post endovascular stenting of a Stanford type B aortic dissection. Contrast can be seen entering the excluded, false lumen *(black arrowheads)* (**B**) of the dissection from adjacent thoracic intercostal veins *(white arrow)* (**A**).

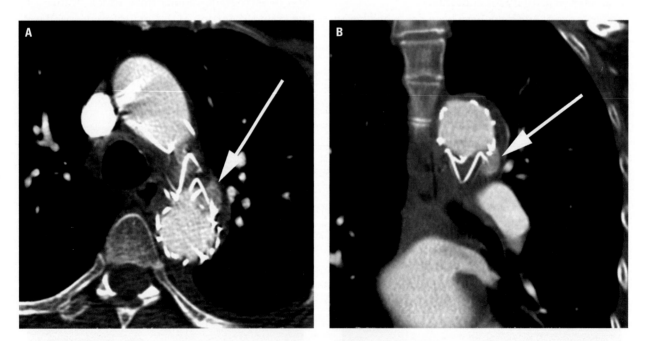

Figure 12.93. Type 3 endoleak. Axial (**A**) and coronal reformat (**B**) CTA images demonstrate contrast beyond the margins of the stent graft near the middle of a multicomponent graft construct, consistent with a type 3 endoleak *(arrows)*. This type of endoleak results in the exposure of the excluded segment of vessel to systemic arterial pressures and generally requires re-stenting.

seen transiently at the time of graft deployment, are thought to be caused by normal graft porosity, and are not seen at follow-up imaging. Type 5 endoleaks are described as interval aneurysm sac enlargement without imaging evidence of a leak. Type 1 and 3 endoleaks usually require reintervention because the excluded segment of vessel is being exposed to arterial blood pressures whereas type 2 leaks can typically be observed or the feeding collateral vessel can be embolized.

Acute Coronary Syndrome

Coronary artery disease is the leading cause of death in the United States. The high prevalence of this disease and its associated morbidity and mortality has resulted in a low clinical threshold to evaluate patients for ACS. Despite this low threshold to thoroughly evaluate patients with chest pain, up to 6% of acute myocardial infarctions are missed at the initial presentation.

The majority of patients presenting with chest pain to the ED fall into a low-risk category for ACS based on the Thrombolysis in Myocardial Infarction (TIMI) Risk Score (a widely accepted system for predicting the risk of death and cardiac ischemic events in patients presenting with unstable angina/Non–ST-Elevation Myocardial Infarction [NSTEMI]) and have an approximately 5% prevalence of ACS. ECG, serial cardiac enzymes, and myocardial perfusion analysis constitute the typical evaluation for low and moderate risk patients for ACS in the ED setting, which is time consuming and costly.

Although endovascular coronary angiography remains the gold standard for evaluating the coronary arteries and provides the additional benefit of real-time treatment with coronary artery stent placement, up to two-thirds of endovascular angiography does not result in intervention. The invasive nature of this examination and the high rate of negative examinations has driven the evolution of noninvasive coronary artery imaging, particularly coronary CT angiography (CCTA), to exclude significant coronary arteries stenosis. The development of 64-channel MDCT and the ability to gate examinations to the patient's ECG allows for imaging of the coronary arteries with high spatial resolution and near-complete elimination of cardiac and respiratory motion artifacts. CCTA has been demonstrated to have a high (>97%) NPV for significant (≥50%) coronary artery stenosis; however, the role

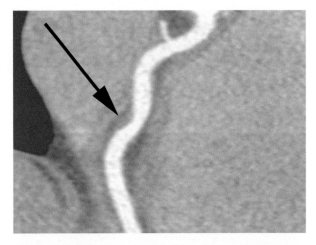

Figure 12.94. RCA vulnerable plaque: There is a smooth-walled, centrally low attenuation noncalcified plaque in the right coronary artery resulting in approximately 50% luminal narrowing *(arrow)* on this reformatted image from a coronary artery CTA. Coronary plaques at risk for rupture tend to have lipid-rich, necrotic (low attenuation) central regions with a thin fibrous covering.

for this examination in the setting of acute chest pain continues to evolve. The examination has been shown to safely rule out significant coronary artery stenosis in low-risk patients presenting with acute chest pain to the ED and may allow for a decreased length of stay in the ED and reduced medical costs in this select group when compared to standard evaluation with serial cardiac enzymes and myocardial perfusion analysis.

Plaque within the coronary arteries places a patient at increased risk for ACS; however, the composition and size of the plaque play an important role in risk stratification. In particular, lesions with a thin cap and central low attenuation (representing lipid and necrosis) (Fig. 12.94) as well as those resulting in severe (>90%) stenosis (Figs. 12.95 and 12.96) at CCTA are considered major risk factors for ACS.

Tubes and Lines

The use of various types of tubes and catheters is an integral part of the practice of emergency medicine. It is a routine practice to obtain chest radiographs following tube or line placement to ensure appropriate positioning and to evaluate for potential complications. Recognition of inap-

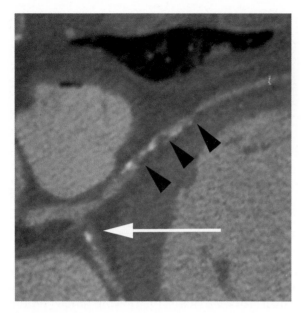

Figure 12.95. There is a complex, partially calcified plaque in the proximal LAD, resulting in severe vessel stenosis on this reformatted image of a coronary artery CTA *(black arrowheads)*. There is a more focal, partially calcified plaque at the origin of the circumflex artery as well *(white arrow)*.

propriate tube and line placement and associate complications is therefore an important part of emergency radiology.

Endotracheal tubes (ETTs) are often placed in the prehospital setting or during acute clini-

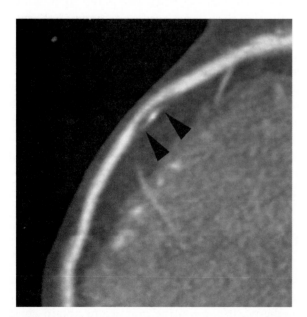

Figure 12.96. There is a focal, partially calcified fibrofatty plaque resulting in approximately 50% stenosis of the mid LAD *(arrowheads)* on this reformatted image of a coronary artery CTA.

cal decompensation in the ED. The rapidity with which endotracheal intubation must take place in emergent situations can frequently lead to tube malpositioning. Modern ETTs are equipped with CO_2 monitors, which decrease the frequency of esophageal intubations detected at chest radiography because this malpositioning is usually detected clinically very quickly and the tube is repositioned prior to obtaining the post intubation chest radiograph (Fig. 12.97). Clinically unrecognized intubation of the esophagus may also be difficult to recognize on the chest radiograph. The ETT may appear slightly to the left of the trachea and the ETT balloon may appear to extend beyond the normal margins of the air-filled trachea. Gaseous distention of the stomach may be present; however, this is nonspecific as patients are often ventilated with bag valve mask prior to intubation,

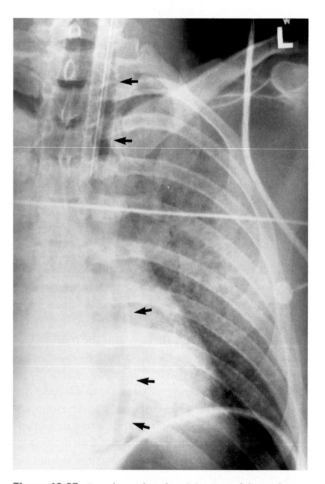

Figure 12.97. Esophageal malpositioning of the endotracheal tube. The endotracheal tube is positioned to the left of the trachea and there is air in the esophagus *(small arrows)* as well as in the stomach.

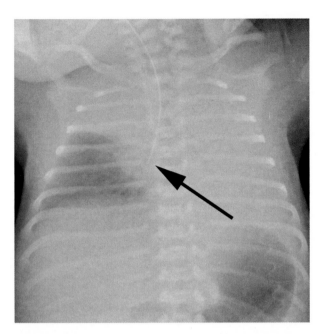

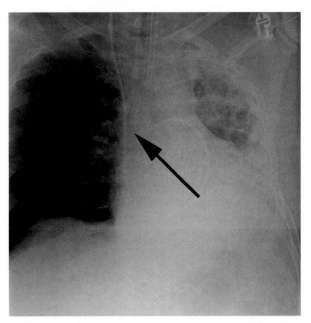

Figure 12.98. Malpositioned endotracheal tube. The endotracheal tube tip is in the bronchus intermedius *(arrow)*. There is resultant collapse of the right upper lobe and of the entire left lung with associated leftward shift of the heart and mediastinum. The right lower lobe is hyperinflated.

Figure 12.99. Right main stem intubation. The endotracheal tube tip is in the right main stem bronchus *(arrow)*. There is hyperinflation of the right lung, partial collapse of the left lung, and leftward shift of the heart and mediastinum.

which can introduce a significant amount of air into the stomach.

Mainstem bronchial intubation is the most frequent form of ETT malpositioning. The right mainstem bronchus is more frequently intubated than the left due to the relatively sharp angle of the left mainstem bronchus to the trachea. Secondary findings associated with mainstem bronchial intubation include ipsilateral lung hyperinflation and atelectasis of the contralateral lung with mediastinal shift (Figs. 12.98 and 12.99). Intubation of the tracheobronchial tree by an enteric tube is not uncommon and is usually readily apparent radiographically (Fig. 12.100).

Central catheters in the subclavian or jugular veins are also commonly placed in the ED, often under suboptimal conditions during rapid clinical decline. Optimal positioning for a standard central venous catheter tip is in the mid to distal superior vena cava (SVC); however, malpositioning is not uncommon (Fig. 12.101). Complications associated with central venous catheter placement are often detected on the postprocedure chest radiograph. Pneumothorax is the most commonly encountered complication and accordingly, postline placement

radiographs should be obtained in the upright position whenever possible to increase sensitivity. Inadvertent arterial placement, extraluminal placement, and mediastinal hematoma are less common but

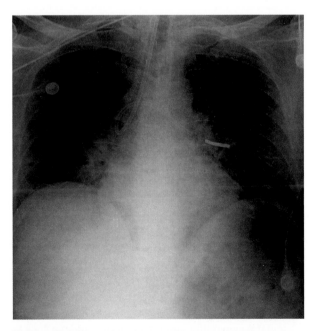

Figure 12.100. Malpositioned feeding tube. The malpositioned feeding tube loops in the right mainstem bronchus before terminating in a left lower lobe segmental bronchus.

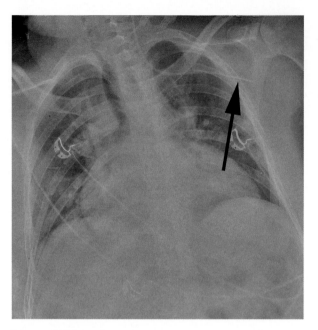

Figure 12.101. The left internal jugular central venous catheter is malpositioned in the left axillary vein *(arrow)*.

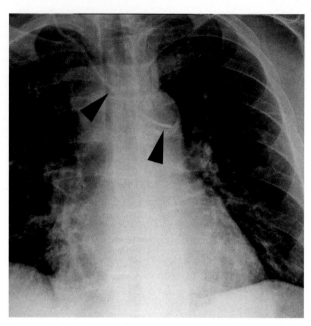

Figure 12.102. Arterial malpositioning of a central venous catheter. The central venous catheter does not follow the expected course of the right brachiocephalic vein or superior vena cava and terminates in the aortic arch *(arrowheads)*.

potentially very serious complications of central venous catheter placement that can be identified on the chest radiograph (Fig. 12.102).

SUGGESTED READINGS

1. Silva CI, Colby TV, Müller NL. Asthma and associated conditions: high-resolution CT and pathologic findings. *AJR Am J Roentgenol.* 2004;183(3):817–824.

2. Taylor AJ, Cerqueira M, Hodgson JM, et al. ACCF/SCCT/ACR/AHA/ASE/ASNC/NASCI/SCAI/SCMR 2010 Appropriate use criteria for cardiac computed tomography. A report of the American College of Cardiology Foundation Appropriate Use Criteria Task Force, the Society of Cardiovascular Computed Tomography, the American College of Radiology, the American Heart Association, the American Society of Echocardiography, the American Society of Nuclear Cardiology, the North American Society for Cardiovascular Imaging, the Society for Cardiovascular Angiography and Interventions, and the Society for Cardiovascular Magnetic Resonance. *J Cardiovasc Comput Tomogr.* 2010;4(6):407.e1–407.e33.

3. Stark DD, Federle MP, Goodman PC, et al. Differentiating lung abscess and empyema: radiography and computed tomography. *AJR Am J Roentgenol.* 1983;141(1):163–167.

4. LePage MA, Quint LE, Sonnad SS, et al. Aortic dissection: CT features that distinguish true lumen from false lumen. *AJR Am J Roentgenol.* 2001;177(1):207–211.

5. Akman C, Kantarci F, Cetinkaya S. Imaging in mediastinitis: a systematic review based on aetiology. *Clin Radiol.* 2004;59(7):573–585.

6. Tarver RD, Teague SD, Heitkamp DE, et al. Radiology of community-acquired pneumonia. *Radiol Clin North Am.* 2005;43(3):497–512, viii.

7. McMahon MA, Squirrell CA. Multidetector CT of aortic dissection: a pictorial review. *Radiographics.* 2010;30(2):445–460.

8. Franquet T, Giménez A, Rosón N, et al. Aspiration diseases: findings, pitfalls, and differential diagnosis. *Radiographics.* 2000;20(3):673–685.

9. Gluecker T, Capasso P, Schnyder P, et al. Clinical and radiologic features of pulmonary edema. *Radiographics.* 1999;19(6):1507–1531.

10. Bean MJ, Johnson PT, Roseborough GS, et al. Thoracic aortic stent-grafts: utility of multidetector CT for pre- and postprocedure evaluation. *Radio-*

graphics. 2008;28(7):1835–1851.

11. Kim EA, Lee KS, Primack SL, et al. Viral pneumonias in adults: radiologic and pathologic findings. *Radiographics.* 2002;(22 spec no):S137–S149.

12. Stein PD, Woodard PK, Weg JG, et al. Diagnostic pathways in acute pulmonary embolism: recommendations of the PIOPED II Investigators. *Radiology.* 2007;242(1):15–21.

13. Oh YW, Effmann EL, Godwin JD. Pulmonary infections in immunocompromised hosts: the importance of correlating the conventional radiologic appearance with the clinical setting. *Radiology.* 2000;217(3):647–656.

14. Leung AN. Pulmonary tuberculosis: the essentials. *Radiology.* 1999;210(2):307–322.

15. Webb WR, Higgins CB. *Thoracic Imaging: Pulmonary and Cardiovascular Radiology.* Philadelphia, PA: Lippincott Williams & Wilkins; 2005.

16. Collins J, Stern EJ. *Chest Radiology: The Essentials.* 2nd ed. Philadelphia, PA: Lippincott Williams & Wilkins; 2008.

John H. Harris Jr ■ Stuart E. Mirvis

GENERAL CONSIDERATIONS

For the purposes of this discussion, the chest shall include the thoracic cage and its soft tissues, portions of the shoulder girdles, the intrathoracic contents, and the diaphragm.

Whenever possible, the radiographic examination of the chest should be made with the patient erect because physiologic alterations of intrathoracic structures inherent in recumbency may simulate organic disease on the supine radiograph. However, in the practice of emergency radiology, it is required and expected that the physician interpreting emergency chest radiographs (CXRs) be solidly experienced in the evaluation of anteroposterior (AP) CXRs obtained in supine, semierect, and erect positions.

The technical factors employed in the production of a CXR are probably more critical than in the radiographic examination of any other body part. Pulmonary interstitial disease may be simulated by normal vascular and normal parenchymal markings made more prominent because of an underexposed CXR. Conversely, gross pulmonary or cardiovascular pathology may be obscured or obliterated by radiographic overexposure, poor radiograph-screen or patient-radiograph contact, or patient motion.

The radiographic examination of the chest may provide valuable information regarding the etiology or extent of acute intra-abdominal disease or trauma. Furthermore, intrathoracic abnormalities may produce symptoms referable to the upper abdomen. For these reasons, radiographic examination of the chest should always be considered in the evaluation of patients with acute symptoms that appear to arise within the abdomen.

The radiographic examinations of the chest of newborns, infants, and young children are inherently difficult to interpret. In these patients, strict adherence to established principles of positioning and radiographic technical factors is essential to accuracy of radiographic diagnosis.

The supine CXR can be expected to reflect the mediastinal hemorrhage and, when present, the left hemothorax, of exsanguinating acute traumatic aortic rupture (ATAR) in patients who survive this injury to reach the emergency center. On the contrary, conventional chest radiography does not display any direct signs of acute traumatic aortic tear (ATAT). However, the supine CXR, which is an essential component of the imaging assessment of the patient with blunt thoracic or thoracoabdominal trauma, coupled with a "coned-down" AP radiograph of the mediastinum using thoracic spine technique ("mediastinal" view, mediastinal radiograph [MXR]), very accurately demonstrates either a normal mediastinum (the absence of a mediastinal hematoma) in patients who therefore require no further consideration of acute traumatic aortic injury (ATAI) or signs consistent with a mediastinal hematoma in patients who therefore require additional imaging investigation for ATAT. In most institutions, multidetector computed tomographic aortography (MDCTA) is the initial examination for the detection of ATAT in the polytraumatized patient.

In some institutions, computed tomographic aortography (CTA) showing direct signs of ATAT is confirmed by catheter aortography. In most cases, CTA is the definitive study.

RADIOGRAPHIC EXAMINATION

The routine radiographic study of the adult chest consists of erect (standing) posteroanterior (PA) and lateral projections made in maximum inspiration (Fig. 13.1). Clinical situations occur in which it is impossible to obtain a standing erect PA radiograph of the chest. In these instances, and when possible, an erect sitting AP projection is preferable to a supine examination. However, in seriously ill or injured patients, the supine examination may be the only examination possible. One must therefore understand the physiologic changes that occur within the chest during recumbency and not interpret them as being abnormal.

Radiographs obtained in expiration may be misinterpreted as showing cardiomegaly and parenchymal densities at each base, suggesting atelectasis or developing pneumonitis (Fig. 13.2). As a general rule, if the posterior portion of the right ninth rib is visible above the diaphragmatic surface in the PA

CXR in an adult, an adequate degree of inspiration may be assumed.

Deep inspiration is particularly important in CXRs of infants and children (Fig. 13.3). This is because the poorly aerated lung produces a radiographic appearance that closely resembles pneumonia (Fig. 13.4).

In infants and children, it is preferable to attempt frontal (AP) and lateral radiographs in the erect position with the arms extended upward over the head and, when possible, the exposure timed to maximum inspiration. In these patients, maximum inspiration occurs in the quiet interval between crying—not when the patient is crying, which obviously represents expiration. If, for whatever reason, it is impossible to obtain erect frontal and lateral examinations of the chest of patients in this age group, perfectly adequate examinations can be obtained with the patient recumbent. However, again, it is essential that the arms be extended upward over the head and that the exposure be timed to maximum inspiration.

In the presence of major trauma, the radiographic examination of the chest is initially obtained in the supine position. Physiologically, the mediastinum is wider in this examination than in the erect chest examination, and the cardiac silhouette increases

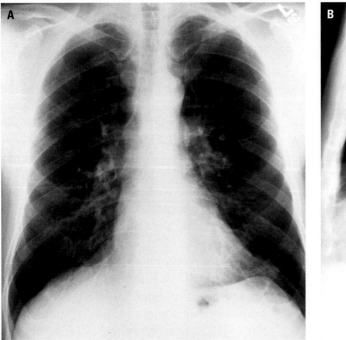
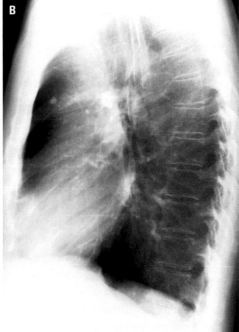

Figure 13.1. PA (**A**) and lateral (**B**) radiographs of a normal adult chest.

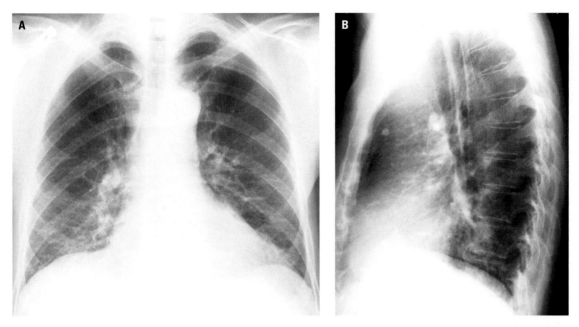

Figure 13.2. Effect of expiration on the chest radiograph of a normal adult subject. On the PA radiograph (**A**), expiration is characterized by increase in the transverse diameter of the cardiac silhouette and the superior medium, crowding of the interstitial markings and the basilar segmental arteries, and elevation of the diaphragm, all secondary to hypoventilation. Similar, although less obvious, changes occur on the lateral projection (**B**).

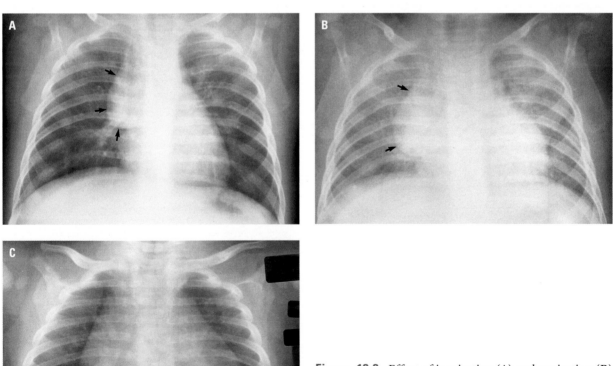

Figure. 13.3. Effect of inspiration (**A**) and expiration (**B**) on the appearance of the frontal radiograph of a normal child's chest. The sharply defined homogeneous soft tissue density in the right mediastinum *(arrows)* is the thymus. The normal frontal examination of a different child's chest is seen in (**C**).

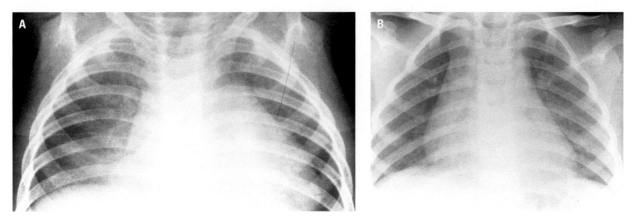

Figure 13.4. Crowding of parenchymal and vascular markings at the right base due to poor inspiration could be misinterpreted as pneumonia (**A**). These apparent parenchymal abnormalities have disappeared on the repeat CXR obtained with better inspiration (**B**).

in its transverse diameter. Although the superior mediastinum is wider, its margins remain distinct, and normal anatomic landmarks are identifiable (Fig. 13.5). Therefore, mediastinal widening alone in the supine examination of the chest does not constitute a radiographic sign of mediastinal hematoma, as is discussed subsequently.

The supine CXR has serious diagnostic limitations that must be borne in mind when that examination is interpreted. Small or even moderate pleural effusions that layer out in the posterior pleural space

in recumbency may not be easily discernible. Pneumothoraces may be impossible to detect in a supine radiograph because of air migration into the anterior pleural space. The pneumothorax suspected but not actually visible on a supine CXR may be confirmed by a lateral decubitus examination of the chest with the side of suspected pneumothorax up, by a horizontal beam supine lateral CXR, by computed tomography (CT), by an erect frontal CXR obtained during forced expiration (Fig. 13.6), or even by obtaining a frontal semierect CXR (Fig. 13.7). Some

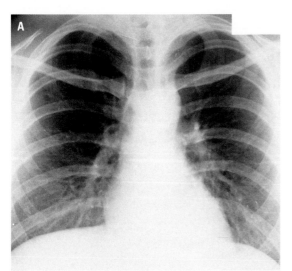
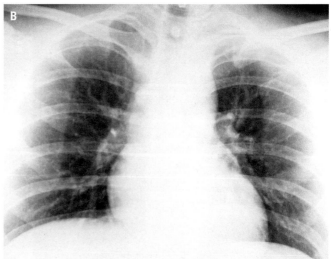

Figure 13.5. The effect of recumbency on the cardiovascular silhouette. Erect (**A**) and supine (**B**) radiographs of the chest of the same healthy subject. In recumbency (**B**), the superior mediastinal shadow and the transverse diameter of the heart increase in transverse dimension and the upperlobe pulmonary vessels increase in caliber. These changes are secondary to the physiologic redistribution of blood that occurs with recumbency.

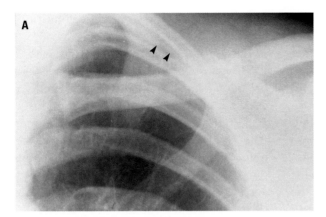

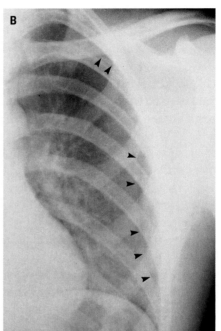

Figure 13.6. Effect of expiration on the detection of subtle pneumothorax. In the erect frontal examination of the chest made in deep inspiration (**A**), a very small, subtle apical pneumothorax *(arrowheads)* is barely perceptible. In the frontal examination of the chest made in forced expiration minutes later (**B**), the pneumothorax *(arrowheads)* is readily apparent.

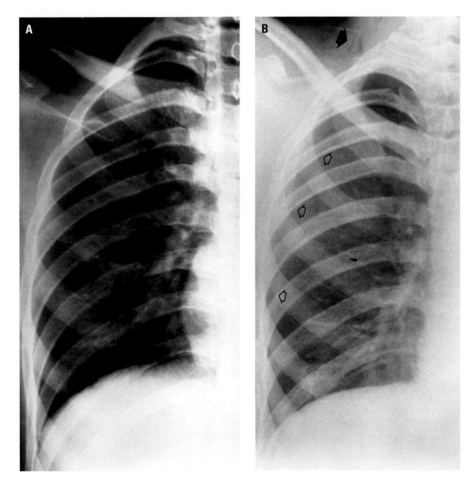

Figure 13.7. A: Supine chest radiograph of a patient stabbed in the right chest posteriorly. This examination is negative. **B:** Semierect chest radiograph taken shortly after **A** demonstrates both a pneumothorax *(open arrows)* and subcutaneous emphysema in the right side of the neck *(closed arrow).*

of the views mentioned to assist in the diagnosis of pneumothorax obviously depend on the patient's clinical condition and ability to assume, or be placed in, these positions. The frontal examination of the chest made in forced expiration is also very useful in the evaluation of possible nonopaque, endobronchial foreign bodies, as is subsequently illustrated in this chapter.

The apical lordotic view (Fig. 13.8) provides maximum visualization of the apices of the lungs. This examination is, as its name implies, made with the patient in the lordotic position and is designed to project the anterior ends of the upper ribs and the clavicle away from the underlying apical pulmonary parenchyma.

Oblique views are useful to assess cardiac configuration, the hila, and the lateral costophrenic angles and to help localize subtle pulmonary abnormalities (Fig. 13.9).

As mentioned earlier, an erect PA radiograph of the chest should be an integral part of every "abdominal series" to establish that an intrathoracic process is not the etiology of upper quadrant abdominal symptoms and to ensure detection of pneumoperitoneum (Fig. 13.10). If the patient cannot assume the erect position, the left lateral decubitus radiograph of the abdomen should be obtained to evaluate for pneumoperitoneum.

With experience gained from the increasing use of CT since publication of the third edition of *The Radiology of Emergency Medicine* in 1993, and particularly with the advent of multidetector CT (MDCT), CT has become the major—and frequently the definitive—imaging modality relative to traumatic and nontraumatic conditions of the chest.[1–9]

In spite of the extensive experience with CTA and its 90% sensitivity, 98% specificity, and 90% positive predictive value,[10] "thoracic aortography remains the standard of reference for the demonstration of acute traumatic aortic injury" (ATAI) according to Patel et al.[11] However, MDCT is now accepted in many institutions as the definitive imaging procedure for patients suspected of having acute thoracic aortic dissection. CTA is readily available, examination time is short (measured in seconds), and the sensitivity and specificity of CTA for detecting aortic dissection is nearly 100%.[12]

Magnetic resonance imaging (MRI) and magnetic resonance angiography (MRA), because of the exquisite soft tissue detail and imaging in all planes, are particularly valuable in assessing the thoracic aorta for acute tear in young children and demonstration of acute traumatic diaphragmatic rupture. Limitations of the use of magnetic resonance (MR) in these acute conditions are the generic limitations of MR units(e.g., limited availability, length of scan time, and the intrinsic physical difficulty)to accommodate the extensive life-support systems required by severely traumatized patients.

With the exception of transesophageal echocardiography (TEE) in the detection of ATAT,[13,14] ultrasound has little application in the imaging evaluation of traumatic or nontraumatic emergent conditions of the chest. The principal disadvantage of TEE in the assessment of ATAT is its limited accessibility on a round-the-clock basis.

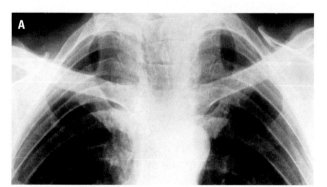
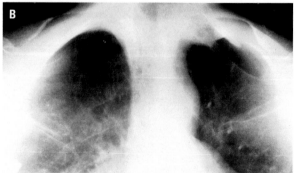

Figure 13.8. Apical lordotic view. In the erect frontal projection (**A**), the apex of each lung is largely obscured by superimposed densities of ribs, transverse processes, clavicles, calcified first costal cartilages, and the density of the sternocleidomastoid muscles. In the apical lordotic projection (**B**), the anterior chest wall structures have been projected free of the apices that are now clearly visible.

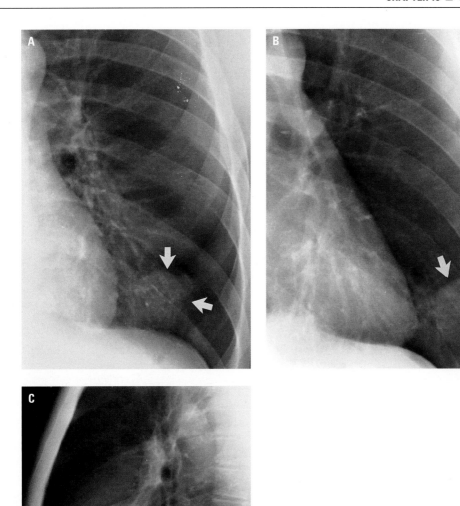

Figure 13.9. The location of the round pneumonia at the left base *(arrows)* on the PA CXR (**A**) is confirmed to be in the lingular segment of the left upper lobe by its position *(arrows)* on the left posterior oblique (**B**) and lateral (**C**) projections.

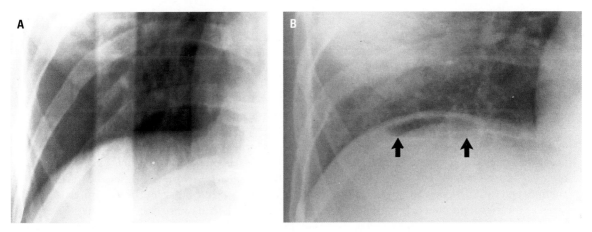

Figure 13.10. Supine examination of the abdomen (**A**) did not demonstrate the small pneumoperitoneum *(arrows)* seen beneath the right hemidiaphragm in the erect chest radiograph (**B**).

RADIOGRAPHIC ANATOMY

The erect PA and lateral radiograph of the normal chest is seen in Figure 13.11. The intrathoracic portion of the trachea and carina are usually visible through the density of the mediastinal structures and the spine in the PA projection (Fig. 13.11A). The aortic arch and the descending thoracic aorta lie to the left of the midline. The descending aorta passes obliquely from above downward toward the diaphragm. The shadow of the descending aorta, with its black Mach edge, must not be confused with the mediastinal stripe (left paraspinal line), which has a white Mach edge, is parallel to the thoracic vertebral bodies, and represents the interface of paraspinal fat with the mediastinal pleura of the left lung. This anatomy is described and illustrated in greater detail later in this chapter in the discussion of traumatic injuries of the aorta.

The hilar shadows are composed principally of the pulmonary arteries and veins, the walls of

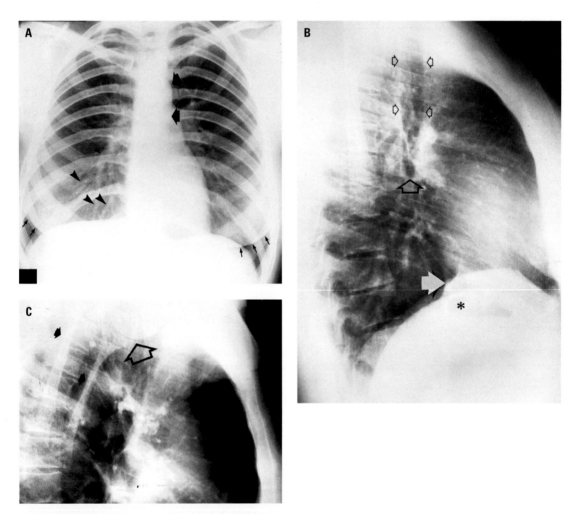

Figure 13.11. Normal adult chest radiograph. In the erect frontal projection (**A**), the aortic arch and descending thoracic aorta are indicated by the *closed (solid) arrows*. The curvilinear, tapering, branching soft tissue densities extending obliquely downward from the inferior portion of the right hilum represent right lower lobe segmental arteries *(arrowheads)*. The curved, sharply defined soft tissue densities superimposed on each base and extending across the middle third of each hemidiaphragm *(small stemmed arrows)* represent breast shadows. In the full lateral projection (**B**), the *small open arrows* indicate the tracheal air column, and the *large open arrow* indicates the carina. The *white arrow* indicates the inferior vena cava, whereas the gastric air bubble is indicated by the *asterisk*. In the lateral radiograph of the chest (**C**), it is important to realize that the infraspinous portions of the scapulae *(closed arrows)* and the humeral head *(open arrow)* may be superimposed on the middle and posterior mediastinum and should be recognized as being normal structures.

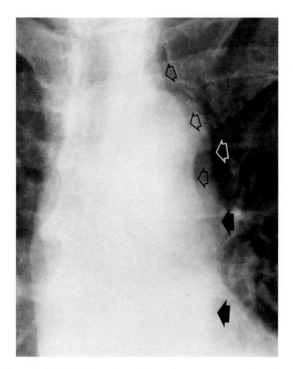

Figure 13.12. The "aorticopulmonary mediastinal stripe," which represents the mediastinal pleural reflection of the left upper lobe as it crosses the aortic arch and extends to the left hilum, is indicated by the *open arrows*. The lateral margin of the descending thoracic aorta with its black Mach margin is indicated by the *closed arrows*.

the stem bronchi and their segmental divisions, lymph nodes, and areolar tissue. Calcification of hilar nodes is a frequent finding and is usually of no clinical significance. The "aortic-pulmonary mediastinal stripe" (Fig. 13.12) represents the

mediastinal pleural reflection of the left upper lobe as it crosses the aortic arch and extends to the left hilum.[15]

The cardiophrenic angles are normally acute. A pericardial fat pad frequently occupies the right cardiophrenic angle. This normal structure may obscure the angle, but the cardiac and diaphragmatic margins are usually visible through it. The density of the fat pad is not as great and its margins are not as sharply defined as those of a pericardial cyst (Fig. 13.13).

The medial segment of the right middle lobe and the lingular segment of the left upper lobe wrap around the lateral heart borders. Consolidation of the entire middle lobe (Fig. 13.14) or its medial segment (Fig. 13.15) or of the lingular segment (Fig. 13.16) of the left upper lobe will obscure the contiguous arc of the heart border on the frontal radiograph. This phenomenon is referred to as the "silhouette" sign by Felson and Felson.[16] A corollary of the silhouette sign is that a basilar consolidation that obscures or obliterates the diaphragmatic surface and through which the appropriate heart border is clearly visible represents lower lobe pneumonia (Fig. 13.17). The heart border remains visible because of the normal aerated lung–cardiac margin interface.

An important radiographic anatomic observation is that the apices of the upper lobes extend well above the level of the clavicles (Fig. 13.11).

The thin, sharply defined homogeneous soft tissue density located above and parallel to the superior cortex of the clavicles is called the

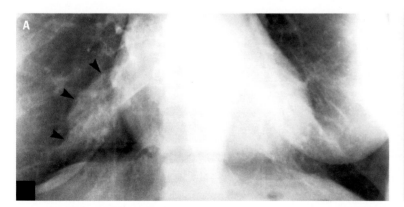

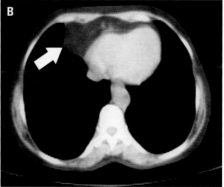

Figure 13.13. Cardiophrenic (pericardiac) fat pad. In the frontal radiograph of the chest (**A**), the rather sharply defined, irregularly rounded density through which pulmonary vascular structures are visible and which is located in the right cardiophrenic angle *(arrowheads)* has the characteristic radiographic findings of a pericardial fat pad. Axial CT (**B**) through the right cardiophrenic mass *(arrow)* demonstrates the low attenuation characteristic of fat, which is identical with that of the subcutaneous fat of the chest wall.

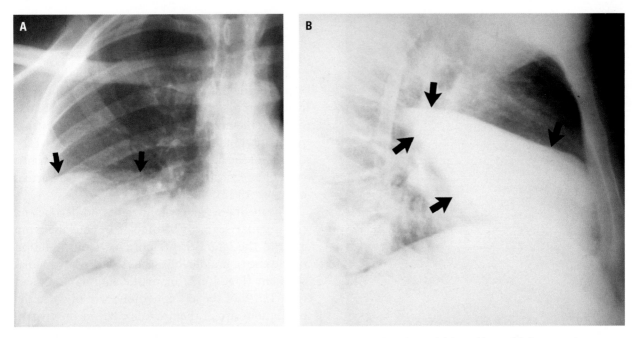

Figure 13.14. Consolidation of the entire right middle lobe *(arrows)* in frontal **(A)** and lateral **(B)** projections. In the frontal projection **(A)**, the right heart border is completely obscured by the consolidation of the medial segment of the right middle lobe. The lateral arc of the right hemidiaphragm remains visible because the lateral segment of the middle lobe does not extend into the costophrenic angle.

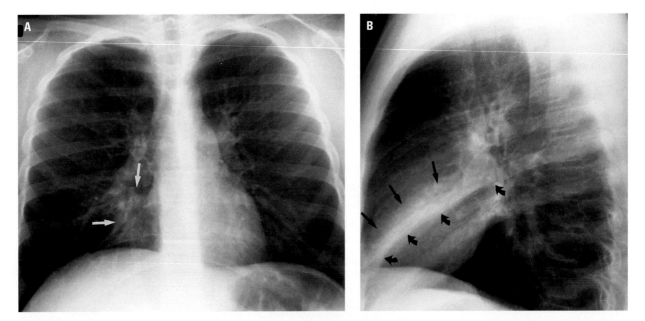

Figure 13.15. Inflammatory consolidation of the medial segment of the right middle lobe in frontal **(A)** and lateral **(B)** projections. In the frontal projection **(A)**, the ill-defined area of increased density *(arrows)* obscures the right heart border. In the lateral projection **(B)**, the area of consolidation is sharply defined inferiorly by the anterior portion of the major fissure *(curved arrows)*.

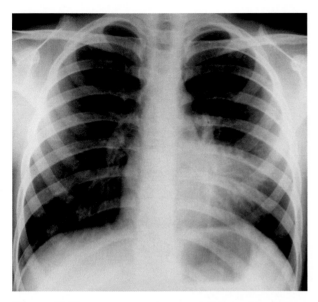

Figure 13.16. Obscuration of the left heart border by lingular segment pneumonia. Lingular segmental consolidation is an example of the "silhouette" sign.

"companion shadow" (Fig. 13.11). This density represents the skin and subcutaneous fat covering the clavicle made visible by the air that fills the concavity of the supraclavicular fossa when the shoulders are rotated anteriorly for the PA CXR.

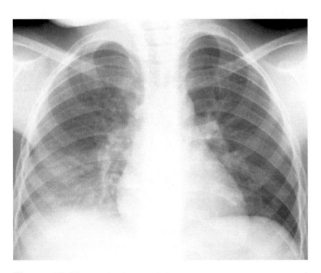

Figure 13.17. Right lower lobe pneumonia represented by the ill-defined area of increased density that involves all the basilar segments with obliteration of the right hemidiaphragmatic surface. That the right heart border remains visible through this density reflects the normal right middle lobe–right heart border interface and confirms that the right basilar density is in the right lower lobe.

Medially, the companion shadow is continuous with the lateral margin of the inferior portion of the sternocleidomastoid muscle. The companion shadow is effaced or obliterated when the supraclavicular fossa is filled with enlarged lymph nodes, which may not be clinically palpable.

The sternum is not well seen in the PA radiograph of the chest because it is almost completely obscured by the superimposed density of the mediastinal structures and the spine.

The lateral radiograph of the chest (Fig. 13.11B) dramatically illustrates the depth of the posterior costophrenic sulcus and the volume of the lower lobe that lies posterior to the dome of the diaphragm.

The posterior margin of the cardiac shadow is composed of the left atrium superiorly and the left ventricle inferiorly. The inferior vena cava (IVC) is commonly seen on the lateral radiograph of the chest as a posteriorly, sharply defined, homogeneous density extending upward through the diaphragm anterior to the posterior margin of the left ventricle (Fig. 13.18). Normally, at a distance 2.5 cm above the diaphragm, the posterior margin of the left ventricle should be less than 2.5 cm from the IVC.[17] Conversely, an IVC–left ventricle distance greater than 2.5 cm indicates cardiomegaly with left ventricular preponderance. This assessment of cardiac size is thought to be more accurate than the cardiothoracic ratio.[17]

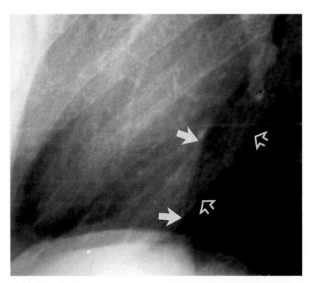

Figure 13.18. Normal relationship between the inferior vena cava (*solid arrows*) and the left ventricle (*open arrows*).

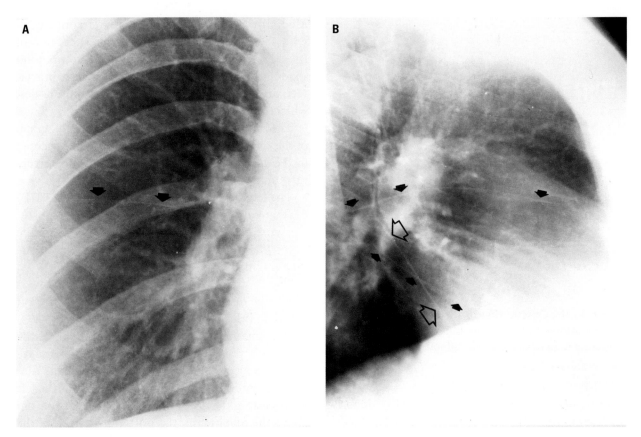

Figure 13.19. Interlobar fissures as seen in frontal (**A**) and lateral (**B**) projections. The right minor fissure *(closed arrows)* is seen in both projections. The inferior portion of the right major fissure *(closed arrows)* is obliquely vertically oriented in the lateral projection (**B**). In this projection, also, the inferior portion of the left interlobar fissure *(open arrows)* is visible. The inferior portions of the major fissures can be correctly identified by the fact that the right minor fissure crosses and extends posterior to the inferior portion of the left interlobar fissure *(open arrows)*.

The trachea is normally visible to the level of the carina (Fig. 13.11B).

The diaphragmatic surfaces can usually be lateralized on the lateral CXR by virtue of the air in the gastric fundus being related to the left hemidiaphragm (Fig. 13.11B).

When the patient's arms are elevated for the lateral CXR (Fig. 13.11C), the scapulae rotate anterolaterally and their lateral margins become superimposed on the posterior third of the chest. Frequently, the glenoid fossa and the humeral head are projected on the superior mediastinum. These normal structures should not be considered as representing abnormal radiographic densities.

Interlobar fissures are frequently normally visible as thin linear or curvilinear densities (Fig. 13.19). The minor fissure of the right lung may be visible in frontal, lateral, or both projections. The major interlobar fissures are usually seen only in the lateral projection. Occasionally, the diaphragmatic portion of the major fissure may be oriented so as to be visible in the frontal CXR (Fig. 13.20).

The azygos fissure (Fig. 13.21), which defines the azygos lobe, is the result of invagination of both the visceral and parietal pleura by an anomalous course of the azygos vein over the apex of the right upper

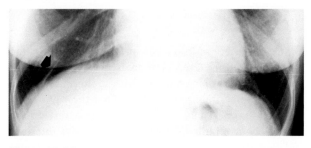

Figure 13.20. Inferior portion of the right major fissure *(arrow)* seen in frontal projection.

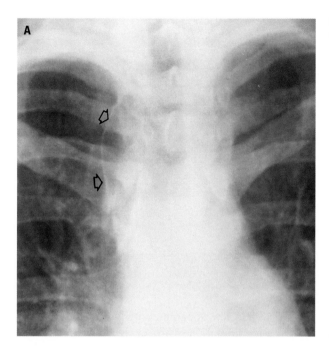

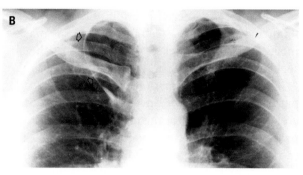

Figure 13.21. Configuration of the azygos lobe *(open arrows)* in two different patients (**A** and **B**).

lobe to its normal location at the junction of the trachea and the takeoff of the right stem bronchus. Because the azygos fissure results from the enfolding of both the visceral and the parietal pleura, it contains four layers of pleura. The location of the azygos fissure is variable in the medial aspect of the

right upper lobe. The azygos fissure and lobe have no clinical significance but could conceivably be mistaken for the wall of a bleb or bulla.

The breast shadow itself may produce an ill-defined haziness at either base simulating an inflammatory process (Fig. 13.22). The difference

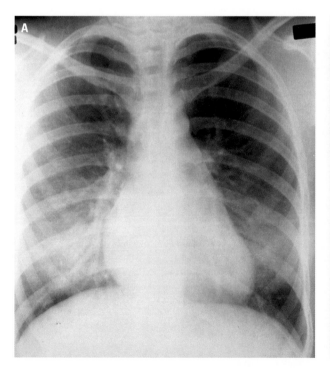

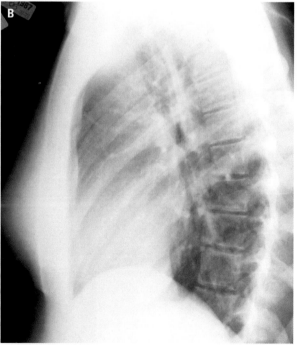

Figure 13.22. Vague, ill-defined, and poorly marginated densities at each base in the frontal projection (**A**) are caused by compression of the breast tissue. The lateral radiograph of the chest (**B**) is entirely normal. Specifically, there is no evidence of lower lobe pneumonia. The breast tissue accounted for the hazy densities at each base.

in density of the inferior portion of the lung fields following a radical mastectomy (Fig. 13.23) may be misleading if the observer is not aware of the absence of the breast shadow on the operated side.

The routine examination of the ribs, when the patient's condition will permit, must include an erect PA radiograph of the chest and each oblique projection of the affected side (Fig. 13.24). The indications for the erect frontal examination of the chest include, primarily, the detection of possible pneumothorax, pulmonary contusion, or pleural effusion and, secondarily, the recognition of preexisting or coexisting disease(i.e., left heart failure).

The purpose of examination of the affected hemithorax in each oblique projection is to visualize all segments of the ribs. Incomplete or minimally displaced rib fractures may be difficult or impossible to identify on the PA CXR alone and may frequently be recognized only in one of the oblique projections.

Portions of the lower ribs are obscured by the density of the upper abdominal contents and will not be visible using routine rib technique. When the clinical findings suggest an abnormality of the ribs below the diaphragm, an AP radiograph of

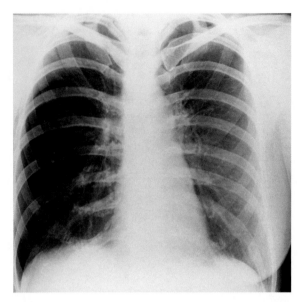

Figure 13.23. The apparent hyperlucency of the right lung is a manifestation of absent right anterior soft tissues subsequent to a right radical mastectomy.

the lower portion of the chest and upper abdomen using either abdominal or lumbar spine radiographic technique is required to evaluate the lower ribs as well as the lower thoracic and upper lumbar vertebrae.

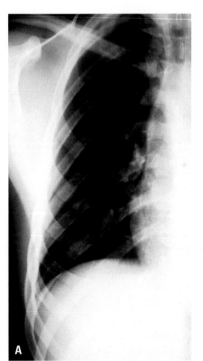
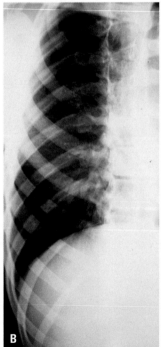
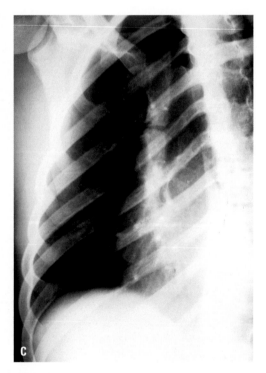

Figure 13.24. Routine radiographic examination for the ribs. This study must include erect CXR (**A**) and anterior (**B**) and posterior (**C**) oblique projections to demonstrate the full extent of each rib. The purpose of the erect frontal examination, in addition to visualizing the ribs, is to evaluate for pleural effusion, pneumothorax, or pulmonary contusion.

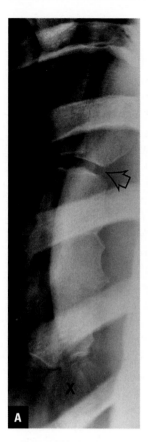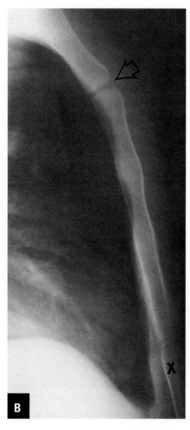

Figure 13.25. Routine radiographic examination of the sternum in frontal (**A**) and lateral (**B**) projections. The angle of Louis *(open arrow)* is clearly demonstrated in each projection. In this patient, the xiphoid *(X)* has not yet united.

Standard texts on radiographic positioning describe the routine radiographic examination of the sternum to consist of frontal views made with the patient prone and rotated slightly off the midline in each direction and a lateral projection (Fig. 13.25). The frontal sternal views require positioning difficult for a patient with a suspected sternal injury and are extremely difficult to interpret. A properly positioned lateral radiograph of the sternum provides the best opportunity for detecting sternal fracture or dislocation. Prior to their fusion, the location and smoothly sclerotic margins of the sternal segments (Fig. 13.26) should distinguish these normal defects from fracture lines.

RADIOGRAPHIC MANIFESTATIONS OF TRAUMA

Trauma to the chest usually involves multiple organ systems and different anatomic regions (e.g., the chest wall including the thoracic cage, the pleural space, and lungs; the extrapleural space and mediastinum; the heart and great vessels; and the spine and shoulders). To facilitate the discussion of the effects of trauma to the chest, an arbitrary decision has

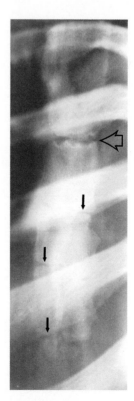

Figure 13.26. Normal appearance of the sternum in an adolescent. The angle of Louis is indicated by the *open arrow.* The body segments *(closed arrows)* are physiologically incompletely fused.

been made to discuss the effects of trauma on each of the components of the chest separately. Although it is certainly possible that individual components of the chest may be injured separately (e.g., isolated rib fracture[s] or pulmonary contusion without rib fractures), far more commonly multiple organ systems or anatomic regions are involved simultaneously. Despite the arbitrary organization of this chapter, the reader is reminded that, particularly in the severely or multiply traumatized patient, radiographic signs of multiple organ involvement will be the rule rather than the exception. That intellectual approach to the CXR of the massively injured patient should prompt an orderly and systematic approach to its interpretation.

Radiography is usually not needed to establish the presence of soft tissue trauma of the chest wall. Subcutaneous emphysema, which may be the most obvious sign of a subtle pneumothorax, can be detected only on the AP CXR (Fig. 13.27).

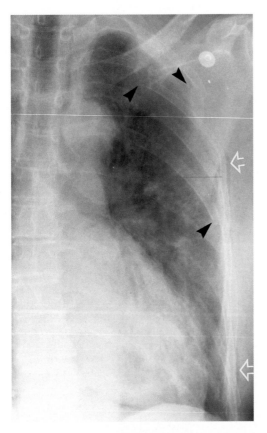

Figure 13.27. The small amount of subcutaneous emphysema along the left lateral chest wall *(open arrows)* in this patient with multiple minimally displaced rib fractures *(arrowheads)*, but with no left chest laceration, should alert the observer that a pneumothorax must be present.

Skeletal Injuries

The manubrium and body of the sternum are united by cartilage at the sternal synchondrosis (the angle of Louis). Blunt trauma to the anterior chest wall can result in dislocation at this site (Fig. 13.28).

Fracture of the sternum usually occurs in its body (Fig. 13.29) but may also involve the manubrium (Fig. 13.30). Clinically, the significance of sternal fracture lies in the mortality rate of 25% to 45%,[18] which results not from the fracture per se but from associated injuries within the chest, such as cardiac injury, ATAI, or tracheobronchial injury. Gibson and colleagues[19] reported a 75% incidence of head trauma associated with sternal fractures caused by motor vehicle accidents. Therefore, the clinician must maintain a high index of suspicion regarding the high association of sternal fractures and head trauma so that a sternal fracture, when present, may serve to alert the clinician to possible associated serious intrathoracic injury. The essential radiograph required to establish the diagnosis of sternal injury is the lateral projection, which may easily be obtained with the horizontal beam with the patient recumbent.

The anterior chest wall hematoma associated with sternal dislocation or fracture may produce the appearance of an ill-defined widening of the mediastinum (Fig. 13.29A) on the supine CXR similar to the appearance of the mediastinal hematoma associated with, but not caused by, ATAT. Some very salient observations regarding the relationship between mediastinal width and ATAT must be stated at this point, although these are amplified in greater depth subsequently in this chapter during the discussion of ATAI. In the first place, and contrary to much surgical and radiologic literature, a mediastinal width greater than 8.0 cm, with or without irregular margins, may be simply the normal appearance of the mediastinum due to recumbency. Second, although it has been established that an indirect relationship does exist between the presence of a mediastinal hematoma and acute aortic tear,[20–23] the hematoma is evidenced on the plain CXR by specific signs rather than simply "superior mediastinal widening." The radiographic signs of mediastinal hematoma are described and illustrated in considerable detail later in this chapter in the discussion of ATAI. The CXR illustrated in Figure 13.39A is insufficiently penetrated for

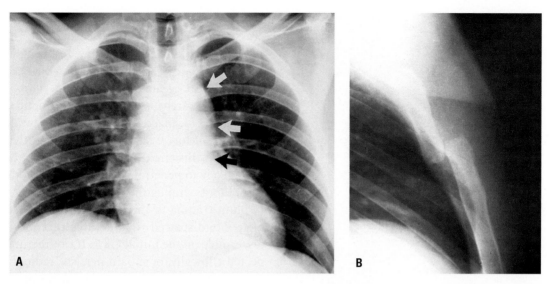

Figure 13.28. In the erect frontal examination of the chest (**A**) of this patient who received blunt trauma to the anterior chest wall in a motor vehicle accident, the superior mediastinum appears widened. However, the aortic arch and the descending thoracic aorta *(arrows)* remain visible. These structures are usually obscured or obliterated by a mediastinal hematoma. The lateral radiograph of the chest (**B**) demonstrates a complete posterior dislocation of the manubrium with respect to the body of the sternum. The superior mediastinal widening seen in the frontal projection (**A**) is caused by the anterior chest wall soft tissue swelling associated with the dislocation.

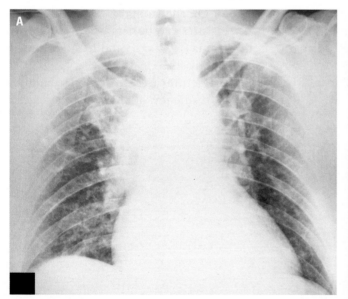
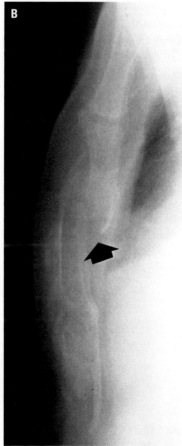

Figure 13.29. The frontal examination of the chest (**A**) of this patient involved in a motor vehicle accident demonstrates ill-defined mediastinal widening. In this instance, however, the apparent superior mediastinal widening was caused by anterior chest wall soft tissue hematoma secondary to the sternal body fracture *(arrow,* **B**). The frontal examination of the chest (**B**) is not sufficiently radiographically penetrated to evaluate the mediastinal structures for the presence of a mediastinal hematoma.

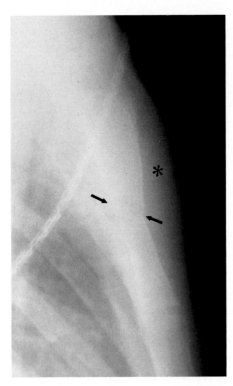

Figure 13.30. Fracture of the manubrium *(arrows)* with accompanying presternal hematoma *(asterisk).*

adequate evaluation of the presence of a mediastinal hematoma. It would be a major diagnostic error, if not an actual injustice, to suggest aortography based on the CXR illustrated in Figure 13.29A. Finally, there is no established relationship between sternal injury and aortic injury.

Rib fractures are usually the result of either compression of the chest or a direct blow to the chest wall. The former type of injury, resulting in a decrease in the arc of the ribs, causes an outward break at the site of greatest compression. This "spring fracture" is rarely associated with puncture of the lung. Direct localized trauma to the chest wall, when of sufficient force, results in fracture at the site of impact. In this circumstance, the fracture ends are more likely to penetrate the chest wall, producing a hemothorax or pneumothorax.

Blunt trauma to the chest may produce incomplete, nondisplaced rib fractures that may not be discernible on the initial CXR. If rib fracture is suspected clinically, or if pain persists, radiographs of the ribs obtained in 10 to 14 days will usually demonstrate callus formation at the fracture site, thereby establishing the diagnosis. Except for a densely calcified first costal cartilage (Fig. 13.31), costal cartilage fractures and costochondral separation are not radiographically visible.

Minimally displaced rib fractures or fractures occurring in the arc of the ribs between the anterior and posterior axillary lines are commonly demonstrated only in oblique projections (Figs. 13.32 and 13.33). On the frontal CXR, minimally displaced rib fractures may be heralded by a focal extrapleural hematoma (Figs. 13.33 and 13.34) or small pneumothorax (Fig. 13.35).

Rib fractures are uncommon in children because of the resiliency of the thoracic cage. However,

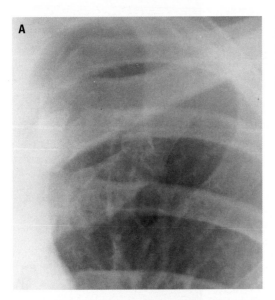
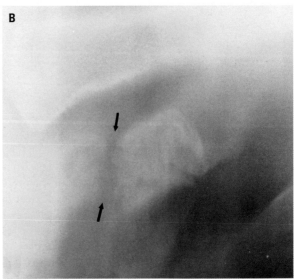

Figure 13.31 The fracture of the calcified left first costal cartilage that is not visible in the frontal projection (**A**) is clearly evident on the frontal tomogram (**B**, *arrows*).

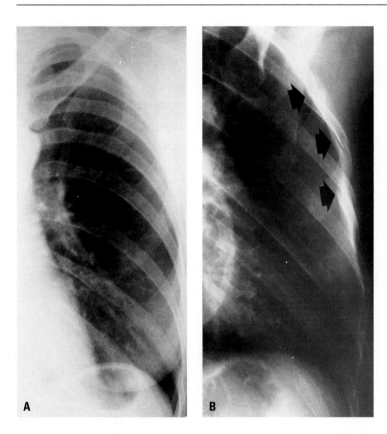

Figure 13.32. Minimally displaced, acute, complete fractures in the anterior axillary line of the left upper ribs are not visible in the frontal chest radiograph (**A**) but are clearly evident in the left posterior oblique projection (**B**, *arrows*).

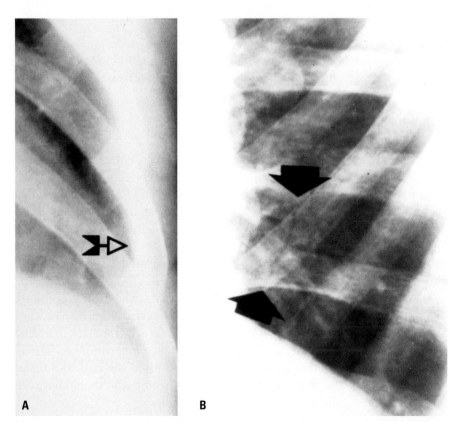

Figure 13.33. In the frontal projection (**A**), the localized extrapleural hematoma *(stemmed arrow)* marks the site of a rib fracture that is only radiographically visible in the left anterior oblique projection (**B**, *arrows*).

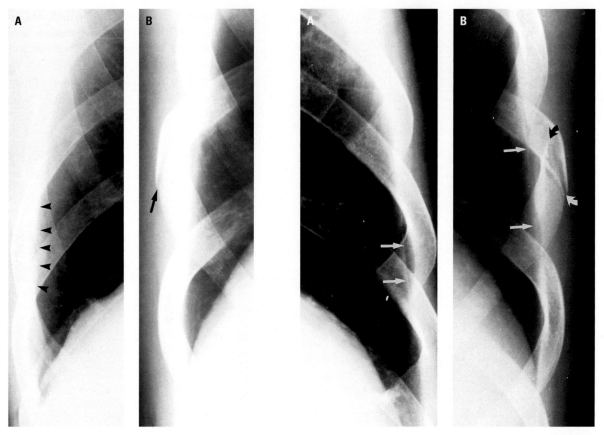

Figure 13.34. The small extrapleural hematoma *(arrowheads)* along the right lateral chest wall is the only sign in the frontal chest radiograph (**A**) suggestive of the rib fracture *(arrow)* demonstrated in the right anterior oblique projection (**B**).

Figure 13.35. The small, focal pneumothorax *(arrows)* is the only radiographic sign in the frontal chest radiograph (**A**) of the complete fracture *(curved arrows)* demonstrated in the left anterior oblique projection (**B**).

with a history of appropriate trauma, the possibility of a rib fracture in a child or any of its possible complications (e.g., pulmonary contusion, pneumothorax, or pleural effusion) must be actively considered during assessment of the radiograph (Fig. 13.36). Similarly, blunt thoracoabdominal trauma to a child may cause pulmonary and/or intraperitoneal injury without causing a rib fracture (Fig. 13.37).

Fractures of the upper ribs are uncommon because the upper ribs are protected by the clavicle, scapula, and large muscle masses of the anterior and posterior chest walls. When present, either alone or in conjunction with fracture of the bones of the shoulder girdle, these fractures indicate simply an injury of considerable force. Contrary to an opinion frequently cited in surgical and radiographic literature, upper (thoracic inlet) rib fractures are *not* associated with an increased incidence of aortic

injury. In fact, Fisher and colleagues,[24] in a study of approximately 200 patients, clearly demonstrated that there is no statistically significant difference in the frequency of acute aortic brachiocephalic arterial injury between patients with or without thoracic inlet rib fractures. Lee and colleagues,[25] in a comparative analysis of 62 patients with ATAT and 486 without ATAT, found that although fracture of the rib(s) was the most common thoracic skeletal injury associated with ATAT, "the positive predictive value of rib fractures in evaluating ATAT was only 14.7%, a rate similar to the incidence of ATAT at most trauma centers," and therefore of no value in determining who should have CTA or traditional aortography.

However, because of the magnitude of the causative force, upper rib fractures are commonly associated with pneumothorax or hemothorax, subcutaneous emphysema, pulmonary contusion, and

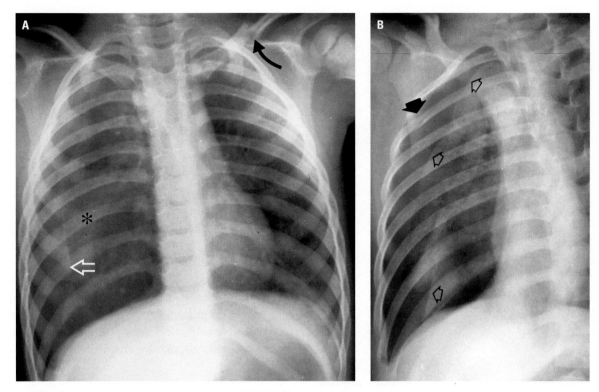

Figure 13.36. This 4-year-old child sustained blunt trauma to the chest. In addition to the displaced fracture in the middle third of the left clavicle *(curved arrow)*, the erect PA radiograph of the chest (**A**) revealed right pulmonary contusion *(asterisk)* and a right pneumothorax *(open arrow)*. The pneumothorax *(open arrows)* is seen to best advantage in the oblique radiograph (**B**). The only thoracic cage abnormality was a complete, minimally displaced fracture of the midaxillary line of the right third rib *(closed arrow)*.

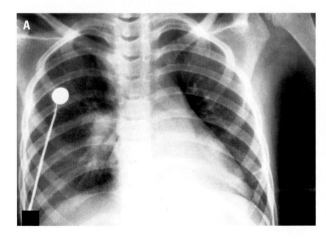

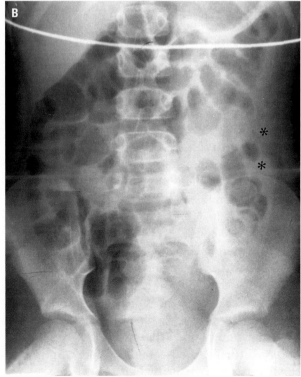

Figure 13.37. Blunt left thoracoabdominal trauma in a child without rib fracture. The AP chest radiograph (**A**) reveals atelectasis of the left lower lobe. In the supine radiograph of the abdomen (**B**), the soft tissue density *(asterisks)* displacing the descending colon from the left flank stripe represents blood in the left paracolic gutter from a ruptured spleen. The signs of hemoperitoneum require more definitive examination by orally and intravenously enhanced abdominal CT.

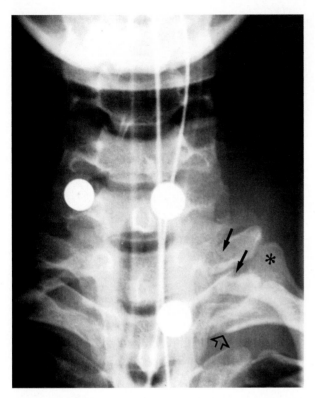

Figure 13.38. Fractures of the left first and second transverse processes *(stemmed arrows)*, dislocation of the left first rib *(asterisk)*, and fracture of the neck of the left second rib *(open arrow)* are all difficult to detect because of the superimposition of the skeletal parts at the thoracic inlet.

scapular fractures. All these associated injuries, in addition to the complex normal skeletal anatomy of the thoracic inlet, make the recognition of inlet rib fractures radiographically difficult (Fig. 13.38).

The lower ribs, being less securely attached anteriorly, are more mobile and less susceptible to fracture by blunt trauma. However, these ribs may be fractured by a forceful direct blow and, when such a fracture occurs on the left, splenic and/or renal injury should be automatically considered, and lower rib fractures on the right should prompt an automatic consideration of hepatic and/or renal injury.

Flail chest is defined as segmental fractures of three or more consecutive ribs. Segmental fracture refers to two fracture sites in the same rib, resulting in a separate fragment that is free floating. It is taught that flail chest is clinically diagnosed by recognition of paradoxical movement of the flail segment during respiration due to chest pain. The clinical difficulty with this concept is that the paradoxical movement is very difficult to observe even under optimum conditions and particularly in patients with shallow

respirations, in heavily muscled or obese patients, or in women with large breasts. Consequently, the primary responsibility for identification of a flail chest rests with the radiologist. That responsibility is not easily discharged because the diagnosis must almost invariably be made from a single supine CXR. Usually, the patient's condition precludes obtaining oblique radiographs of the ribs. Additionally, because of the chest trauma, the examination will have been obtained in relative hypoventilation. Pulmonary contusion, pneumothorax, pleural effusion, and subcutaneous emphysema, commonly present, further obscure rib delineation. Therefore, in patients with major blunt thoracic or thoracoabdominal trauma, the presence of multiple rib fractures must prompt a diligent search for segmental rib fractures. Recognition of flail chest is of clinical significance because of its effect on pulmonary physiology, which is usually also adversely affected by pulmonary contusion or hemopneumothorax. Figures 13.39 through 13.41

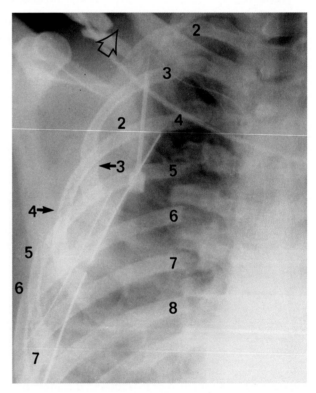

Figure 13.39. Right flail chest involving ribs 2 through 7. The posterior fracture sites are fairly readily apparent; those in the middle and anterior axillary lines are difficult to discern because they are only minimally displaced and are obscured by the density of the pleural effusion, pulmonary contusion, and the chest wall soft tissues. A comminuted, displaced fracture is present in the middle third of the right clavicle *(open arrow)*.

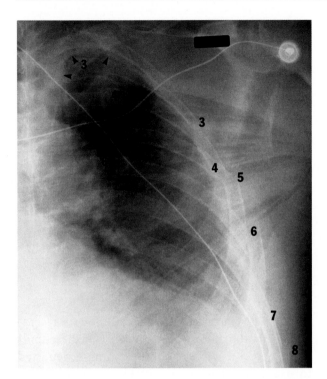

Figure 13.40. Left flail chest in which the lateral chest wall fracture sites are much more apparent than the posterior fracture sites in ribs 3 through 6. An apical pneumothorax *(arrowheads)* is barely perceptible. The oblique linear lucencies represent subcutaneous emphysema within the pectoral muscles.

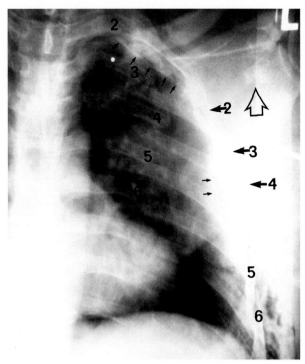

Figure 13.41. Subtle left flail chest involving ribs 2 through 6. A marginal pneumothorax *(small stemmed arrows)* is difficult to visualize but is imperative to identify. A fracture of the neck of the scapula is indicated by the *open arrow*, and subcutaneous emphysema is present along the left lateral chest wall and in the left supraclavicular fossa.

illustrate the difficulty in identifying the segmental fractures of flail chest as well as the evidence of the magnitude and diffusion of the force required to produce flail chest, such as the number of ribs fractured, pulmonary contusion, and the frequently associated clavicular and scapular fractures.

Harris and Harris[26] reported that scapular fractures were missed on the initial emergency center CXR in 43% of 100 patients with major blunt thoracic trauma. In 72% of the missed scapular fractures, the scapular fracture was visible on the initial supine CXR but may have been obscured by rib or clavicular fractures, pulmonary contusion, pleural effusion, subcutaneous emphysema, radiograph identification labels, or monitoring leads. Before 1984, when Hardegger and colleagues[27] advocated open reduction and internal fixation of fractures of the glenoid fossa or scapular neck as the preferred treatment for these injuries, the failure to diagnose a scapular fracture did not significantly adversely affect patient care. Because it is customary to treat all the orthopedic injuries requiring surgical

management at the same time and because open reduction and internal fixation is now the treatment of choice for displaced glenoid fossa and neck fractures, it is very important that scapular fractures be identified on the initial emergency center CXR. Consequently, instead of clavicular and upper rib fractures, pulmonary contusion, and subcutaneous emphysema being offered as excuses for not recognizing scapular fractures, these same injuries should be considered as indicators for a diligent search for scapular fractures.

Lee and colleagues[28] reported that although three or more rib fractures in patients 14 years or older carried an increased risk of splenic or hepatic injury, there was no association between the number of rib fractures and aortic injury.

Sternoclavicular dislocation is a rare injury, accounting for less than 1% of all types of dislocations.[29] The dislocation is usually posterior and may be caused by indirect trauma applied to the posterolateral aspect of the shoulder by a force that drives the lateral end of the clavicle anteriorly. The

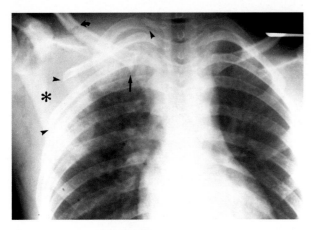

Figure 13.42. Massive direct right upper anterior chest wall trauma resulted in dislocation of the right sternoclavicular joint *(straight arrow)*; fractures of the right first, second, and third ribs *(arrowheads)*; a fracture in the middle third of the clavicle *(curved arrow)*; and a large right axillary hematoma *(asterisk)*.

taut costoclavicular ligament, acting as a fulcrum, causes the medial end of the clavicle to be levered posteriorly.[30] In our experience, however, the more common mechanism of injury is massive direct trauma to the anterior chest wall, driving the medial end of the clavicle posteriorly or posterolaterally (Fig. 13.42). Posterior dislocation at the left sternoclavicular joint is particularly clinically important because of the proximity of the left subclavian vein. Clinically, patients with sternoclavicular dislocation have a large hematoma and ecchymosis of the upper anterior chest wall and asymmetry of the

clavicles to palpation. Radiographically, the dislocation is difficult to diagnose on the AP CXR because displacement is usually minimal (Figs. 13.43 and 13.44), because the normal sternoclavicular anatomy may appear altered simply by rotation of the chest (Fig. 13.43A), and because of superimposed skeletal structures (Fig. 13.44). The dislocation is usually recognizable in a straight supine CXR by lateral displacement of the proximal end of the clavicle (Fig. 13.45) or by asymmetry of the proximal ends of the clavicle (Fig. 13.43A). The quickest and most accurate method to examine the sternoclavicular joint is by CT (Figs. 13.43B and 13.45B).

Pulmonary Contusion

Blunt chest trauma may cause pulmonary laceration, hematoma, and/or contusion. Of these, pulmonary contusion is the most common, reported to occur in 30% to 75% of blunt chest trauma patients.[31] In a review of 144 consecutive patients with pulmonary contusion and/or flail chest, isolated flail chest and pulmonary contusion each had a mortality rate of 16%. In combination, the mortality rate increased to 42%.[32] Pulmonary contusion may occur without rib fractures,[31,33,34] particularly in children in whom the chest wall is more compliant than in adults.[35]

Pulmonary contusion is the result of compressive force to the lung parenchyma at the time of impact and of a negative force applied to the lung during recoil after the causative force is dissipated.

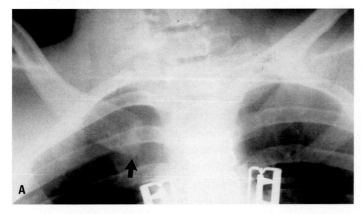
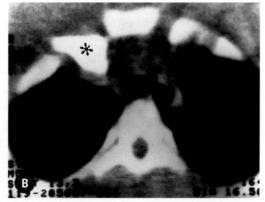

Figure 13.43. Right sternoclavicular dislocation. In the frontal projection of the thoracic inlet (**A**), the distal end of the right clavicle *(arrow)* is inferiorly displaced with respect to the left. The axial CT image (**B**) demonstrates the proximal end of the right clavicle *(asterisk)* to be posteriorly dislocated with respect to the manubrium.

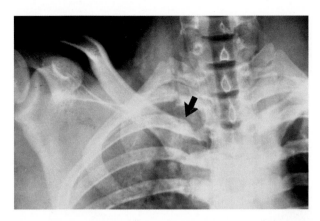

Figure 13.44. Minimally displaced right sternoclavicular dislocation. The medial end of the right clavicle *(arrow)* is both laterally and slightly caudally dislocated. The position of the clavicle is obscured by multiple rib fractures, hydropneumothorax, and pulmonary contusion, all indicating massive direct chest trauma.

Both of these forces result in alveolar and interstitial hemorrhage and edema.[35-37] The contusion may be focal and mild (Fig. 13.46) or extensive and severe (Fig. 13.47). Pulmonary contusion is usually mild, usually clears without producing significant

respiratory disturbance, and may be clinically masked by other conditions such as flail chest, pneumothorax, or hemothorax. Even when severe, the extent and significance of the lesion, which may not initially be appreciated either clinically or radiographically, is recognized only by arterial PO_2 levels reflecting hypoxia. Therefore, early in the post blunt chest trauma state, alteration of arterial blood gas values is the most sensitive indicator of the presence of pulmonary contusion.

Pathophysiologically, the blast effect of blunt chest trauma, which compresses the lung tissue, results in parenchymal hemorrhage and edema. When the initiating force is released, the lung rebounds, producing an abrupt negative pressure on the already damaged lung tissue. The hemorrhage occurs at the alveolar–capillary level, resulting in both intra-alveolar and interstitial extravasation of blood and edema. The ensuing cellular response to tissue damage combines with the hemorrhage and edema to produce a progressive O_2 diffusion barrier and hypoxemia, which may initially be paradoxical with respect to the clinical and radiographic appearance of the patient and which may become progressively more severe.

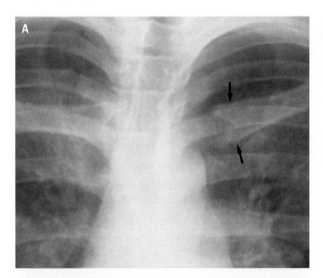

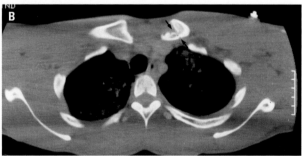

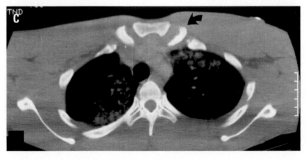

Figure 13.45. Left sternoclavicular fracture-dislocation. In the frontal projection of the chest (**A**), the medial end of the left clavicle *(arrows)* is laterally and slightly caudally displaced, and its inferomedial corner is not well delineated. The axial CT images (**B** and **C**) demonstrate posterior dislocation *(curved arrow)* and fracture *(arrows)* of the medial end of the left clavicle.

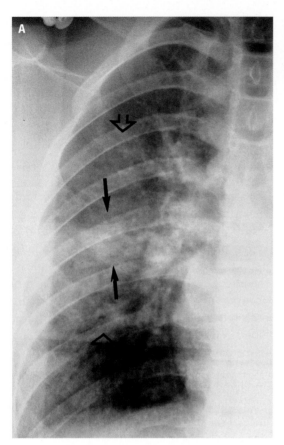

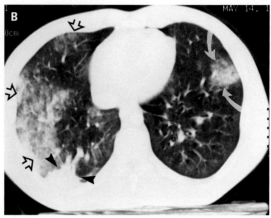

Figure 13.46. Mild pulmonary contusion limited to the right midlung zone (*open arrows*, **A**). Only in the center of the contusion is a smaller discrete area of focal consolidation *(arrows)*, which could represent an area of more severe contusion or a hematoma. The peripheral location of the pulmonary contusion is shown by CT (*open arrows*, **B**). CT also shows that the area of increased density thought to be a focal hematoma on the PA CXR is actually a focal area of atelectasis *(arrowheads)* posterior to the contusion. CT also shows a focal contusion of the left lung *(curved arrows)* not recorded on the CXR.

The natural history of uncomplicated pulmonary contusion is a dynamic process, with the area of contusion becoming progressively more extensive during the initial 24 hours, followed by a gradual clearing during the 48 to 72 hours after

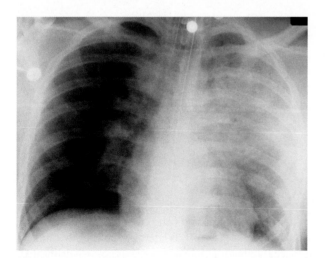

Figure 13.47. Extensive, severe pulmonary contusion involving the area of the majority of the left upper lobe and the atypical segment of the left lower lobe.

injury. This sequence is reflected radiographically in Figures 13.48 and 13.49. Consequently, the radiographic appearance of pulmonary contusion will vary not only with the magnitude of the causative force but also with the length of time between injury and the initial CXR. Because today's efficient patient transport systems frequently deliver the traumatized patient to the emergency center within an hour of the time of injury, the initial CXR may be negative for signs of pulmonary contusion. Conversely, the CXR of a patient seen initially several hours following blunt chest trauma will demonstrate well-established changes of pulmonary contusion (Fig. 13.50).

The radiographic signs of pulmonary contusion may not be present immediately but are visible in 70% of cases within 1 or 2 hours after injury.[31] In the remaining 30%, radiographic evidence of pulmonary contusion may not appear until 6 to 24 hours after injury.[31,34] For this reason, serial radiographs of the chest are indicated in patients whose initial chest examinations do not demonstrate changes of pulmonary contusion following significant blunt chest trauma.

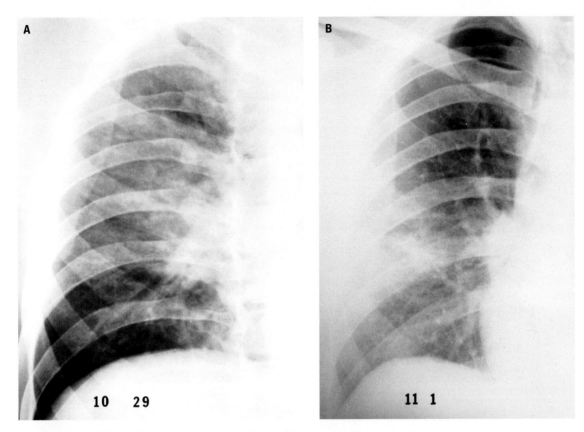

Figure 13.48. Pulmonary contusion. The initial chest radiograph (**A**) obtained approximately 3 hours postinjury demonstrates an extensive, ill-defined patchy parenchymal density that represents contusion of the right upper and middle lobes. The contusion had almost completely cleared on the frontal examination obtained approximately 72 hours postinjury (**B**).

In patients with massive blunt chest trauma, the radiographic signs of pulmonary contusion will be positive on the initial supine chest radiograph (Fig. 13.39). The characteristic radiographic appearance of pulmonary contusion consists of patchy, ill-defined areas of parenchymal density that may be either solitary and localized (Fig. 13.49), multiple, or diffuse (Fig. 13.51). Multiple foci of contusion in adjacent portions of the lung may coalesce. The area of contusion does not respect anatomic divisions of the lung, and therefore, the changes of pulmonary contusion on CXRs do not coincide with any of the anatomic divisions of the lung.

MDCT accurately reflects the pathophysiology of pulmonary contusion (Fig. 13.46B). On CT, the pulmonary contusion is peripheral and commonly contiguous with the adjacent pleura, involves adjacent segments and/or lobes of the lung without regard for segmental or lobar anatomic divisions, is variable in its degree of involvement, and shows signs of both airway and parenchymal involvement.

Complications of pulmonary contusion include pneumonia, pulmonary hemorrhage (hematoma), and traumatic pulmonary pseudocyst formation. Pneumonia is usually a relatively late complication and is associated with the usual clinical signs of pulmonary infection. Radiographically, postcontusion pneumonia resembles any other bacterial pneumonia except that in this instance, there is a direct radiographic continuum from the initial contusion to the subsequent area of inflammatory consolidation.

Pulmonary hematoma is a collection of blood in an area of pulmonary laceration. The hematoma is probably not a complication of the contusion per se but more likely was present at the time of initial chest trauma but was marked by the more extensive contusion and only became radiographically visible as the contusion cleared (Fig. 13.49). Pulmonary hematoma is usually described as a flame-shaped area (Figs. 13.49 and 13.52) of increased density that persists after the surrounding

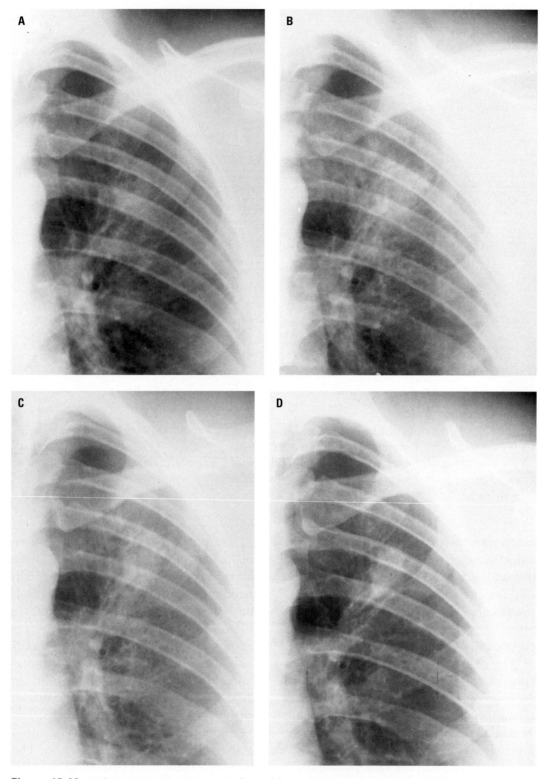

Figure 13.49. Pulmonary contusion complicated by pulmonary laceration and hemorrhage. The ill-defined patchy density in the left upper lobe on the initial chest radiograph (**A**) obtained shortly after the patient sustained blunt left upper chest trauma represents a pulmonary contusion. Twelve hours later (**B**), the area of contusion had increased in size radiographically. By 36 hours postinjury (**C**), the contusion had partially resolved, but within the area of contusion, a smaller, more discrete density is visible that represents the pulmonary hemorrhage, which persisted after the radiographic signs of contusion had completely cleared (**D**) 5 days postinjury.

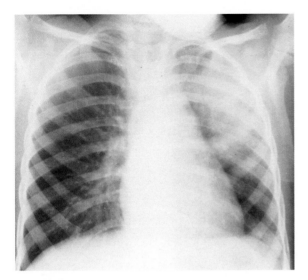

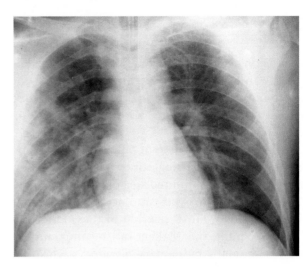

Figure 13.50. Well-established pulmonary contusion involving the majority of the left upper lobe and the apical segment of the left lower lobe subsequent to direct blunt trauma to the left hemithorax.

Figure 13.51. The mottled areas of increased density that are irregularly distributed throughout the entire right lung, that are more dense peripherally than centrally, and that show areas of consolidation are typical of the radiographic appearance of pulmonary contusion.

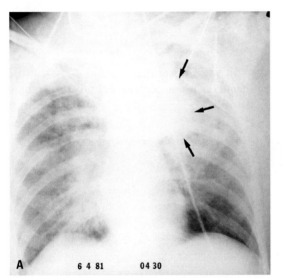

A   6 4 81   04 30

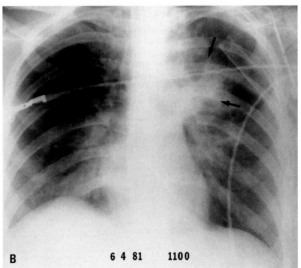

B   6 4 81   1100

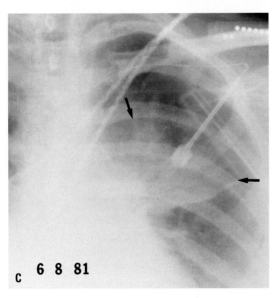

c   6 8 81

Figure 13.52. Concomitant left upper lobe pulmonary contusion and pulmonary hematoma in a patient who sustained massive blunt chest trauma. The initial chest radiograph (**A**) demonstrates changes of fluid overload. In addition, the extensive area of increased density in the left upper and middle lung fields, with a central homogeneous consolidation *(arrows)*, was thought to represent pulmonary contusion with probable pulmonary hematoma. Within 7 hours (**B**), the signs of fluid overload had cleared, and the left pulmonary contusion had significantly improved, leaving the central flame-shaped area of consolidation *(arrows)* consistent with pulmonary hematoma. Four days posttrauma (**C**), the contusion had cleared, but the pulmonary hematoma *(arrows)* persisted.

517

contusion clears. The hematoma may be visible on the initial CXR and distinguished from the surrounding contusion as a sharply defined area of homogeneous density within the contusion (Fig. 13.53).

The final complication of pulmonary contusion is the development of single or multiple thin-walled, air-filled spaces within the area of pulmonary contusion referred to as posttraumatic pneumatocele (Fig. 13.54).[38,39] Ellis[40] referred to these lesions as "cysts." Santos and Mahendra[41] recommend the term "traumatic pulmonary pseudocyst" because the pathologic definition of a cyst requires an epithelial lining, which these evanescent lesions do not have, and because the term *pneumatocele* has historically been associated with pneumonia. The important aspects of traumatic pseudocysts are that although they usually occur 4 to 5 days after closed chest trauma,[42] they may rarely be present on the initial CXR. They resolve spontaneously, do not require extensive workup, and do not require surgical intervention.[41]

As a reminder that the chest and abdomen must be considered as a single entity in the presence of blunt thoracic or thoracoabdominal trauma, basilar

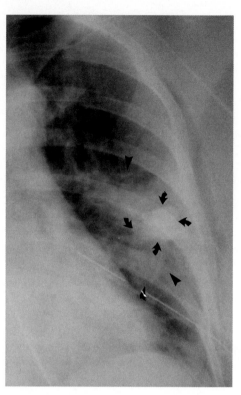

Figure 13.53. Concomitant pulmonary contusion *(arrowheads)* with a central pulmonary hematoma *(curved arrows)*.

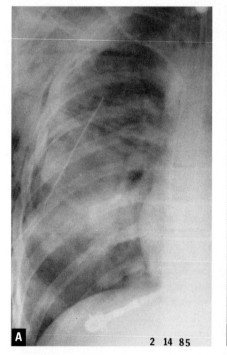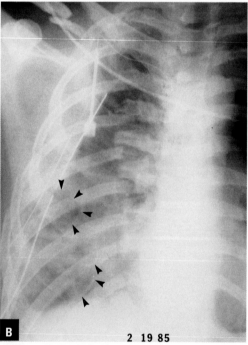

Figure 13.54. Posttraumatic pseudocysts. The initial chest radiograph (**A**) demonstrates multiple right rib fractures, pneumothorax, extensive pulmonary contusion and subcutaneous emphysema, and various tubes and catheters. On the frontal examination obtained 5 days post-trauma (**B**), sharply defined, rounded lucent areas with thin walls *(arrowheads)* are present at the right base. The lucencies represent posttraumatic pseudocysts.

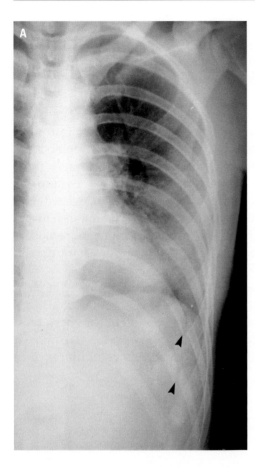
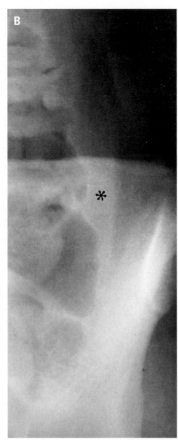

Figure 13.55. The frontal examination of the left hemithorax (**A**) demonstrates pulmonary contusion at the left base and complete, displaced fractures of the left ninth and tenth ribs *(arrowheads)* in the posterior axillary line. The left pulmonary contusion should force the observer to a diligent search for rib fracture. The presence of the left lower rib fractures should create a high index of suspicion for intra-abdominal (splenic or left renal) trauma. The frontal examination of the left flank (**B**) demonstrates medial displacement of the descending colon from the flank stripe by a soft tissue density *(asterisk)* within the left paracolic gutter. Laparotomy revealed a ruptured spleen and hemoperitoneum.

pulmonary contusion may be the most obvious radiographic finding in patients with lower rib fractures and intra-abdominal injury (Fig. 13.55). It must be apparent that pulmonary contusion may occur without rib fractures in both children (Fig. 13.50) and adults (Fig. 13.56). Finally, pulmonary contusion may resemble aspiration pneumonia in its radiographic appearance. However, the distinction may reasonably be made on the basis that aspiration pneumonia is usually more central, is of greater density medially than peripherally, and is limited to bronchial distribution(e.g., subsegmental or segmental). Pulmonary contusion, on the other hand, is usually more peripheral within the lung, is more dense laterally than medially, and does not respect the segmental or lobar anatomy of the lung (Figs. 13.46, 13.56, and 13.57).

Abnormal Intrathoracic Air

This section is devoted to the pathology and radiographic appearance of air in abnormal spaces within the chest (e.g., pneumothorax,

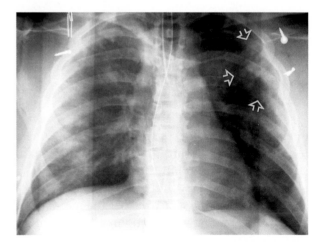

Figure 13.56. Bilateral pulmonary contusion more extensive on the right. The mottled, peripheral parenchymal densities are variable from the right apex to the diaphragm through the density of the transportation board. The distribution of these parenchymal abnormalities indicates that the injury does not respect the anatomic divisions of the lung, which, together with the very peripheral location, is entirely consistent with pulmonary contusion instead of aspiration. Similar but less extensive findings are present in the superolateral aspect of the left upper lobe *(open arrows)*.

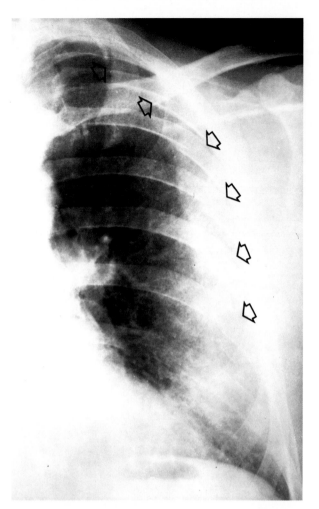

Figure 13.57. The diffuse haziness in the peripheral portion of the left lung represents pulmonary contusion associated with multiple rib fractures *(open arrows)*.

pneumomediastinum, paramediastinal pneumatocele, pneumopericardium). The radiographic appearance of air within these different spaces is peculiar to each, but within each space, the appearance of the air is the same whether the mechanism of injury is traumatic or nontraumatic. Therefore, the radiographic signs of abnormal air collections caused by both traumatic and nontraumatic etiologies are discussed together.

Pneumothorax

Air in the pleural space is usually the result of blunt or penetrating trauma that causes a tear in the visceral pleura, allowing air to collect within the pleural space. Pneumothorax secondary to blunt trauma most commonly results from a rib fracture that pierces the visceral pleura, but it may result from an abrupt increase in intra-alveolar pressure against a closed glottis with consequent rupture of a bleb or peripheral bulla. "Spontaneous" (nontraumatic) pneumothorax most commonly results from a rupture of alveolar blebs immediately beneath the visceral pleura. In more than 50% of patients, the etiology of the rupture is unknown. Many diseases may be associated with spontaneous pneumothorax, including such disparate conditions as spasmodic asthma, staphylococcal pneumonia, and pulmonary metastatic disease (Fig. 13.58).

A "closed" pneumothorax occurs when the chest wall is intact. An "open" pneumothorax, also referred to as a "sucking" wound of the chest, indicates direct communication between the ambient air and the pleural space. Pneumothorax may

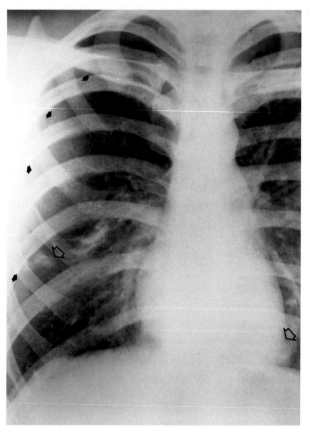

Figure 13.58. Spontaneous pneumothorax *(closed arrows)* associated with pulmonary metastasis *(open arrows)* from osteogenic sarcoma in a 17-year-old man.

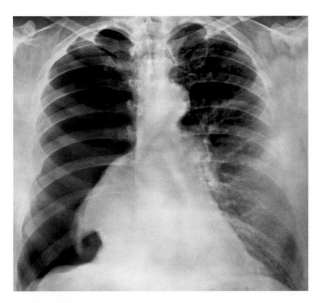

Figure 13.59. Massive right pneumothorax without mediastinal shift.

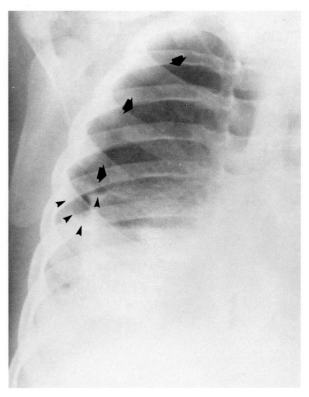

Figure 13.60. Right hydropneumothorax *(arrows)*. The pleural effusion is indicated by the meniscus sign and air–fluid level *(arrowheads)*.

also be classified based on magnitude of collapse as marginal (Fig. 13.35), moderate, or massive (Fig. 13.59).[43]

Conventional chest radiography—preferably erect PA and lateral projections, but even supine AP CXR—demonstrates most pneumothoraces and is the initial imaging modality of choice for this purpose. "Occult" pneumothorax is discussed subsequently in this section.

The radiographic diagnosis of pneumothorax depends on demonstration of the very thin, curved linear density of the visceral pleura with the lucency of air in the pleural space interposed between the visceral pleura medially and the parietal pleura and chest wall laterally. Obviously, there will be neither parenchymal nor vascular markings beyond the visceral pleura. When the magnitude of collapse is moderate or massive or when an associated hemopneumothorax or hydropneumothorax produces an air–fluid level within the pleural space (Fig. 13.60), the diagnosis is readily apparent.

The diagnosis of marginal pneumothorax may be exceedingly difficult because of superimposed skeletal shadows or the inherent difficulty in perceiving the faint density of the visceral pleural surface. The pneumothorax may be enhanced in a PA radiograph obtained during forced expiration (Figs. 13.6 and 13.61). The basis of this

phenomenon is that the collapsed lung decreases in volume during expiration while the air in the pleural space stays constant. Consequently, the lung "falls away" from the chest wall, rendering the pneumothorax more obvious. Other maneuvers to demonstrate pneumothoraces include placing the supine patient in the semierect (Fig. 13.7), erect (Fig. 13.62), or lateral decubitus position with the suspected side up in which event the pleural air will migrate to the uppermost portion of the pleural space. If the patient cannot be moved from the supine position, a horizontal beam lateral CXR may, and CT will, demonstrate air in the anterior pleural space.

The "deep sulcus" sign (Fig. 13.63) refers to an increase in the depth and width of the costophrenic angle associated with air in the pleural space and is an extremely valuable sign of a pneumothorax that is not visible on a poor quality radiograph. The deep sulcus sign may be the only indicator of pneumothorax on a supine CXR (Fig. 13.64).

Figure 13.61. Effect of inspiration (**A**) and expiration (**B**) on the volume of pneumothorax *(arrows)*.

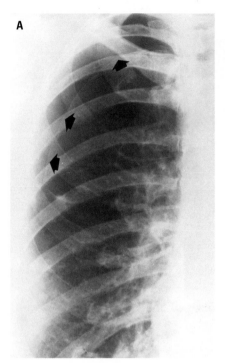
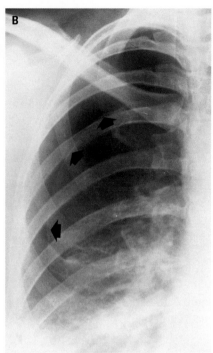

Figure 13.62. Supine examination of the chest (**A**) of a patient who was stabbed in the posterior right flank is negative. However, the semierect examination of the chest (**B**) demonstrates a pneumothorax *(open arrows)*, subcutaneous emphysema in the right side of the neck *(closed arrow)*, and subsegmental atelectasis at the right base.

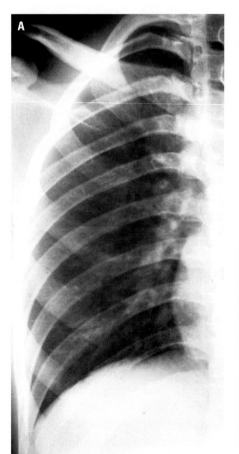
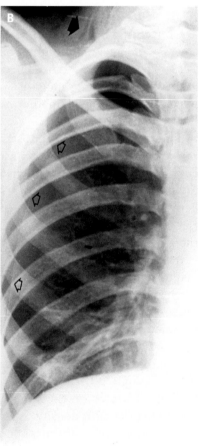

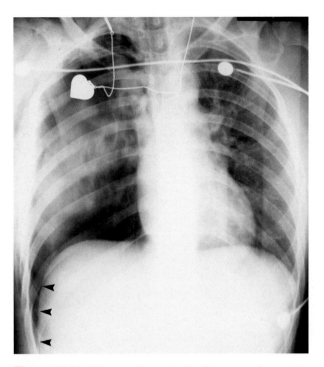

Figure 13.63. "Deep sulcus sign" of pneumothorax. In this supine frontal examination of the chest, the most obvious radiographic sign of the right pneumothorax is the abnormal depth and width of the right costophrenic angle *(arrowheads)* caused by air in the costophrenic pleural space.

Tension pneumothorax (Fig. 13.65) occurs when the communication that permits air to enter the pleural space acts as a flap valve so that air enters the pleural space during inspiration and cannot escape during expiration. The mediastinal structures are forced to the contralateral side, producing compression of the contralateral lung and impairment of venous circulation. If allowed to persist, a tension pneumothorax is rapidly fatal because of impaired venous return to the heart secondary to the mediastinal shift. Tension pneumothorax is usually traumatic but may also be spontaneous. As stated earlier, tension pneumothorax is a life-threatening emergency, and it is incumbent on the radiologist to be available for prompt interpretation of the CXR of a patient clinically suspected of having a pneumothorax and to promptly report the findings of tension pneumothorax to the attending physician.

Radiographically, tension pneumothorax, whether traumatic or spontaneous, is characterized by collapse of the lung on the affected side, air in the pleural space, and shifting of the mediastinal structures to the opposite side. Traumatic tension pneumothorax will, obviously, be identified by the patient history, physical findings, and radiographic signs of trauma (e.g., rib fractures) (Fig. 13.66).

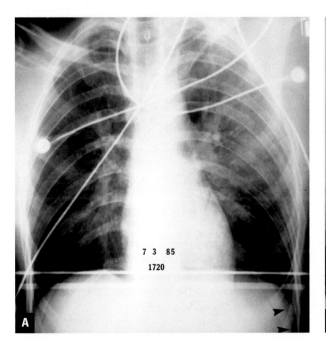

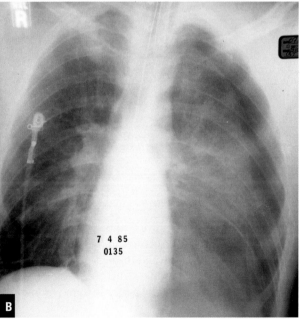

Figure 13.64. Missed left pneumothorax. On the initial supine examination (**A**), the ill-defined haziness in the left midlung field, representative of pulmonary contusion and the left fifth rib fracture, were recognized. However, the left deep sulcus sign *(arrowheads)* was not. The supine radiograph obtained approximately 8 hours later (**B**) demonstrated an obvious left tension pneumothorax.

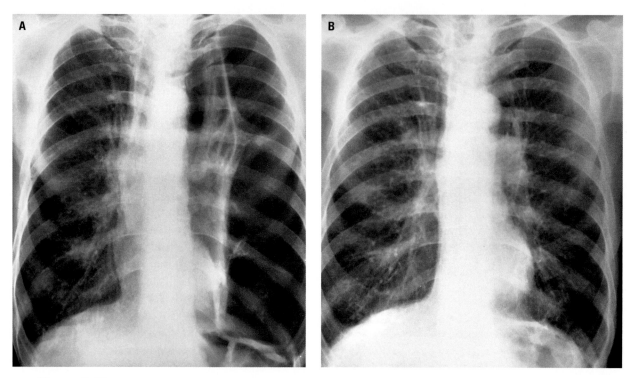

Figure 13.65. Spontaneous left tension pneumothorax with displacement of the mediastinal structures to the right (**A**) in a patient with severe chronic obstructive pulmonary disease. Following reexpansion of the left lung (**B**), the mediastinal structures returned to the midline.

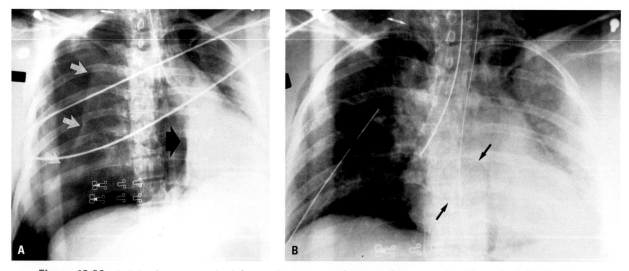

Figure 13.66. **A:** Massive traumatic right tension pneumothorax *(white arrows)* with marked displacement of the mediastinal structures to the left *(black arrow).* **B:** After insertion of a chest tube, the right lung has partially reexpanded, and the tension within the right pleural space has been diminished, as evidenced by return of the mediastinal structures to an almost normal position in spite of the endotracheal tube in the right stem bronchus. The perfectly round lucency overlying the spine *(arrows)* is an artifact.

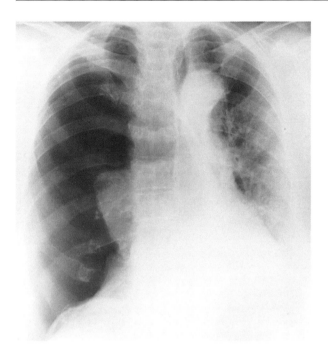

Figure 13.67. Massive spontaneous right tension pneumothorax.

There is no relationship between the magnitude of lung collapse and either the presence of a tension pneumothorax (Figs. 13.59 and 13.67) or the degree of mediastinal shift (Figs. 13.68 and 13.69). Occasionally, the mediastinal shift may be so subtle

that it is not fully appreciated until the mediastinum has returned to its normal position on the CXR obtained following insertion of the chest tube (Fig. 13.70). Therefore, the conservative radiologic attitude is to "overread" the CXR showing pneumothorax with only a suggestion of mediastinal shift as being a tension pneumothorax.

As noted in Figures 13.66 through 13.70, the side of the tension pneumothorax is usually lucent, and the contralateral hemithorax is relatively opaque because of the displaced mediastinal structures and compression atelectasis of the contralateral lung. Penetrating or blunt chest trauma may produce a tension hemopneumothorax in which the side of the tension is opaque on the supine CXR (Fig. 13.71) because of blood within the pleural space. On the supine CXR, instead of there being a lucent visceral pleura–air interface, the tension hemopneumothorax is characterized by a dense (blood) visceral pleural interface (visceral pleural line [VPL] sign) that demarcates the visceral pleural surface of the collapsed lung. The pathologic basis for the VPL sign is schematically illustrated in Figure 13.72.[44] The mediastinal shift is due to the air under tension within the pleural space rather than the accumulation of blood in the pleural space. With tension hemopneumothorax, the mediastinum is shifted to the lucent contralateral hemithorax. The proof of

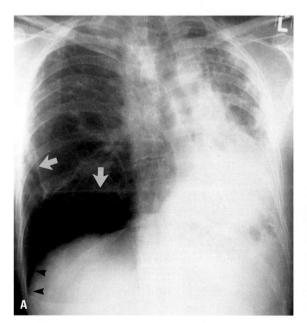

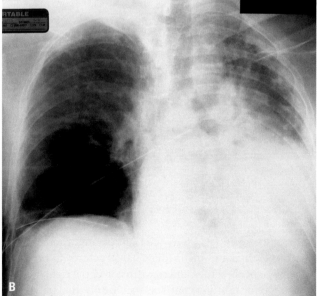

Figure 13.68. A: Massive spontaneous right tension pneumothorax *(white arrows)* in a patient with severe bullous emphysema. Pleural adhesions have restricted the collapse to primarily the middle and lower lobes. A deep sulcus sign *(arrowheads)* is present on the right. **B:** After insertion of two chest tubes, the right lung has reexpanded, and the mediastinal structures have returned to a more normal location.

Figure 13.69. Spontaneous left tension pneumothorax with deep sulcus sign *(arrowheads)*.

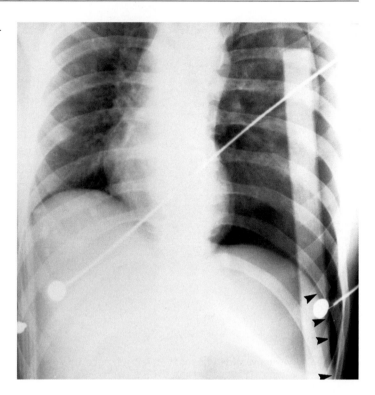

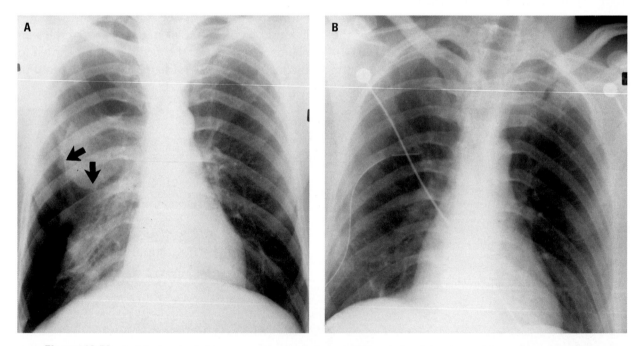

Figure 13.70. **A:** Moderate right pneumothorax *(arrows)* with minimal tension evidenced by very slight displacement of the mediastinal structures to the left in the initial chest radiograph. **B:** After insertion of the right chest tube and reexpansion of the right lung, return of the heart and mediastinal structures to their anatomic position confirms that the original pneumothorax was under tension.

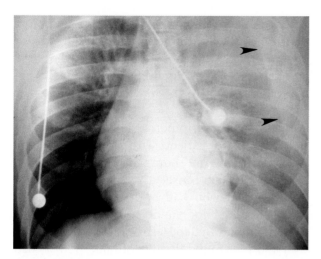

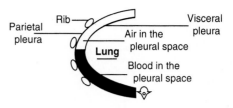

Figure 13.72. Schematic representation of hemopneumothorax and the "visceral pleural line" sign. (Adapted from Visweswaran A, Harris JH Jr. Identification of tension hemopneumothorax on supine chest radiograph: value of the visceral pleural line sign. *Emerg Radiol.* 1996;3:158–165, with permission.)

Figure 13.71. Tension hemopneumothorax on the left, secondary to blunt chest trauma. The sharply defined curvilinear density *(arrowheads)* roughly paralleling the left lateral chest wall is the visceral pleural surface of the partially collapsed left lung made visible by blood and air in the left pleural space.

this observation lies in the erect CXR that demonstrates an air–fluid level within the pleural space on the side of the tension (Fig. 13.73). All of the signs of tension hemopneumothorax due to blunt trauma that are visible on a supine radiograph are illustrated

in Figure 13.74. Obviously, tension hemopneumothorax may result from penetrating chest trauma such as stabbing or gunshot wound (Fig. 13.75). The essential importance of recognizing a blood-pleural interface associated with mediastinal shift is to be aware that these signs indicate an air leak under tension that requires immediate aspiration rather than a possibly slowly accumulating hydro(hemo)thorax, which carries a considerably lesser degree of urgency.

"Occult" pneumothorax is defined as a pneumothorax not visible on the initial supine CXR but identified by CT within 2 hours of

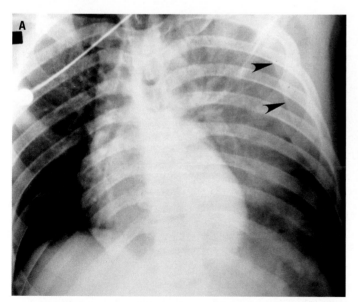

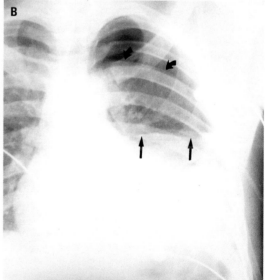

Figure 13.73. Left tension hemopneumothorax in supine (**A**) and erect (**B**) projections. On the supine projection (**A**), the partially collapsed left lung is indicated by the blood visceral pleural interface (VPL sign) *(arrowheads)*. On the erect projection (**B**), both the pneumothorax *(curved arrows)* and the blood–air level *(straight arrows)* verify the etiology of the changes seen in the supine projection (**A**).

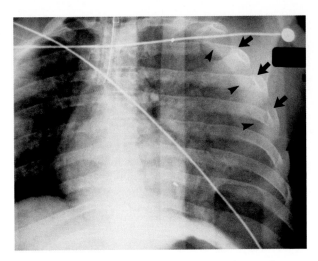

Figure 13.74. Left tension hemopneumothorax *(arrowheads)* resulting from massive left blunt chest trauma as evidenced by multiple rib fractures *(arrows)*.

hospital admission.[45] Pneumothoraces detected by CT have been classified as "miniscule,""anterior," and "anterolateral" by Wolfman and colleagues,[3] depending on size and location. Minuscule pneumothorax is defined as being less than 1 cm in thickness and seen on four or fewer images,

anterior pneumothorax is defined as being more than 1.0 cm in greatest thickness without extending posterior to the midcoronal plane of the chest, and anterolateral pneumothorax is defined as extending posterior to the midcoronal plane of the chest (Fig. 13.76).

Pneumothorax is reported to occur in between 10% and 22% of patients with blunt chest trauma and occult pneumothorax in 1.7% to 6%.[46–48] A review of 1,000 consecutive patients with blunt chest trauma who had both supine CXRs and unenhanced CT for the detection of mediastinal hematoma admitted to Hermann Hospital between 1991 and 1998 found that 128 of 1,000 (12.8%) had pneumothorax. Of these 128, 20 (15.6%) had occult pneumothorax. Of the 1,000 patients studied, 20 (2%) had occult pneumothorax. Once recognized by CT, the pneumothorax was treated as surgically indicated for any pneumothorax detected on the supine CXR. The principal indication for tube thoracostomy in the 20 patients with occult pneumothorax was pending patient mechanically assisted respiration.[49]

Penetrating wounds may cause simultaneous pneumothorax and pneumomediastinum with

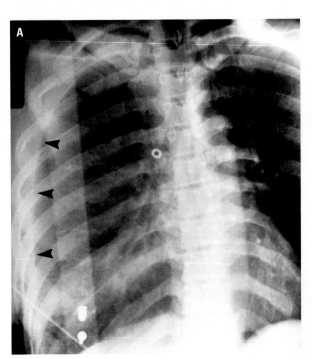

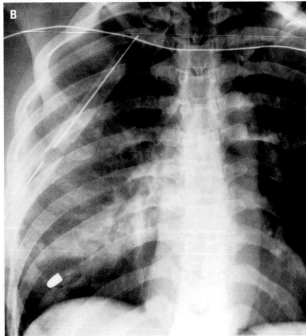

Figure 13.75. Right tension hemopneumothorax secondary to a gunshot wound to the chest. The initial supine CXR (**A**) shows a right visceral pleural line sign *(arrowheads)* with mediastinal shift to the left. The *metallic ring* marks the wounds of entrance. The bullet is above the right hemidiaphragm. **B:** After insertion of a right chest tube, the signs of hemopneumothorax disappeared and the mediastinal structures returned to the midline.

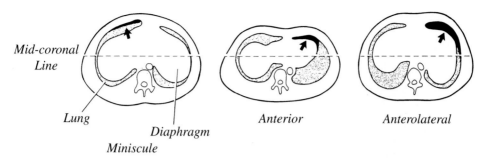

Figure 13.76. Schematic representation of occult pneumothorax on CT. (From Wolfman NT, Gilpin JW, Bechtold RE, et al. Occult pneumothorax in patients with abdominal trauma: CT studies. *J Comput Assist Tomogr.* 1993;17(1):56–59, with permission.)

mediastinal air tracking into the retropharyngeal fascial space (Fig. 13.77).

Pneumothorax may be simulated by the medial border of the scapula (Fig. 13.78) and various configurations of chest wall soft tissues in both adults (Figs. 13.79–13.82) and children (Fig. 13.83).

Because rupture of the tracheobronchial tree from blunt trauma more commonly involves the major bronchi than the trachea and because the site of bronchial rupture is usually intrapleural, resulting in pneumothorax,[50] rupture of the tracheobronchial tree is discussed here rather than under the heading "Extrapleural Air." The reader is referred to the comprehensive review article regarding acute tracheobronchial injury prepared by Mason and colleagues.[51]

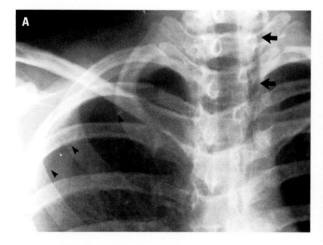

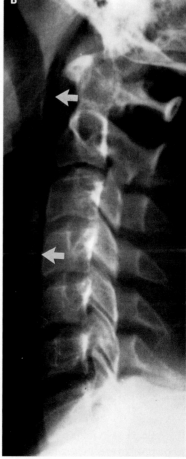

Figure 13.77. Simultaneous pneumothorax and pneumomediastinum secondary to a gunshot wound. In the supine frontal projection (**A**), both the right pneumothorax *(arrowheads)* and pneumomediastinum *(arrows)* are subtle but clearly present. In the lateral radiograph of the cervical spine (**B**), air is present in the retropharyngeal fascial space *(arrows)*, which is continuous with the mediastinum.

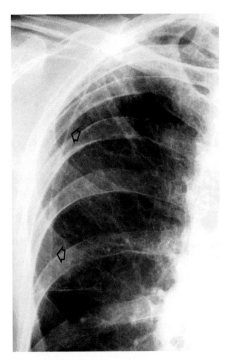

Figure 13.78. Pneumothorax simulated by the medial border of the scapula *(open arrows)*.

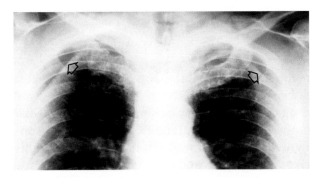

Figure 13.79. Skin folds *(open arrows)* simulating bilateral pneumothoraces in a supine chest radiograph.

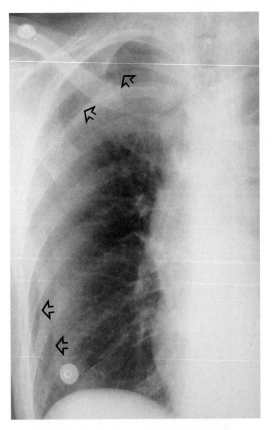

Figure 13.80. Multiple skin folds *(open arrows)* simulating pneumothorax in an erect chest radiograph.

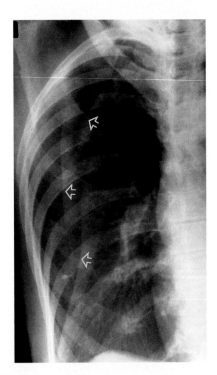

Figure 13.81. Skin folds *(open arrows)* simulating pneumothorax in a supine chest radiograph. The number of skin folds, their configuration and distribution, and, inferiorly, the presence of parenchymal and vascular markings lateral to the simulated visceral pleura should all help establish the true nature of these densities.

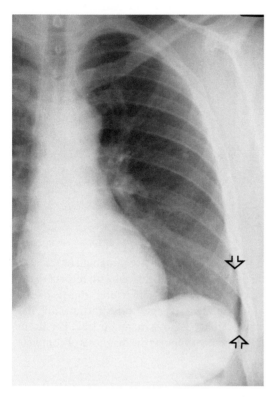

Figure 13.82. Left lower pneumothorax *(open arrows)* simulated by air trapped between the lateral aspect of the breast and the skin of the medial aspect of the arm.

Eighty percent of blunt injuries to the tracheobronchial tree occur within 2 to 3 cm of the carina.[50,51] The mechanism of injury is a combination of AP compression of the chest, abrupt increase in intraluminal pressure against the closed glottis, and lateral shearing forces caused by compression of the thoracic trachea and bronchi against the thoracic vertebral bodies, all the result of a high-velocity, abrupt deceleration injury.

Rupture of the cervical or thoracic trachea is usually fatal. Patients in whom the tracheal rent extends through the entire thickness of the trachea, but is not a major tear, have clinical and radiographic signs of massive cervical subcutaneous emphysema or pneumomediastinum, respectively, with the latter eventually resulting in rupture of the mediastinal pleura and the development of unilateral or bilateral pneumothorax.

Blunt injuries of the stem bronchi are most commonly incomplete tears that produce no immediate radiographic sign but that, with healing, result in cicatricial narrowing of the involved bronchial lumen with retention of endobronchial secretions and recurrent pneumonia. This diagnosis is usually established by endoscopic demonstration of the bronchial stenosis some time after the acute injury.

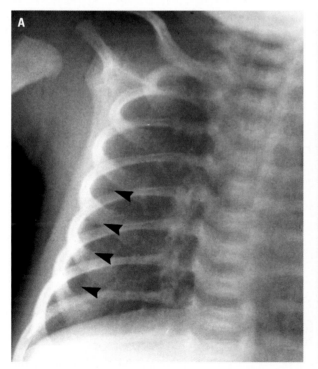
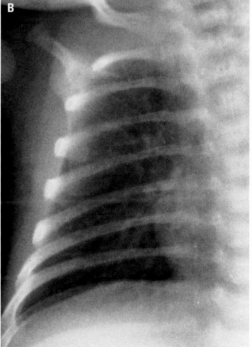

Figure 13.83. **A:** Skin fold *(arrowheads)* simulating a right pneumothorax in a child. **B:** In a subsequent radiograph obtained minutes later, the lung is hyperventilated, and the artifact simulating a pneumothorax has disappeared.

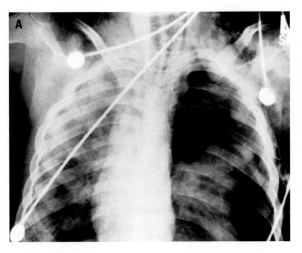
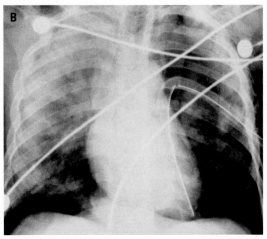

Figure 13.84. Traumatic rupture of the left stem bronchus. In the initial supine chest radiograph (**A**), a large left tension pneumothorax exists with a severely collapsed lung that is inferiorly displaced with respect to the normal location of the hilum. This positioning of the left lung, referred to as the "fallen lung" sign, is highly suggestive of a complete tear of the stem bronchus. **B:** After insertion of a left chest tube, the left lung has only partially reexpanded and the tension pneumothorax persists, indicative of a major air leak. Persistent tension pneumothorax in the presence of a functioning chest tube further supports the diagnosis of complete rupture of the left stem bronchus.

The radiologic diagnosis of rupture of the bronchial wall is usually difficult and begins with a high index of suspicion. The rare instance in which the bronchus is completely transected is typically radiographically manifested by a tension pneumothorax; a pneumothorax that persists in spite of one, or even two, functioning chest tubes because of the major air leak; and the "fallen"[52] or "dropped" lung sign (Fig. 13.84). The latter results when the root of the lung is sufficiently disrupted that the collapsed lung falls away from the hilum either inferiorly (Fig. 13.84) or laterally (Fig. 13.85). A persistent collapsed lung and a mediastinal pneumothorax, particularly in the presence of adequate and functioning chest tube drainage, either with (Fig. 13.86) or without

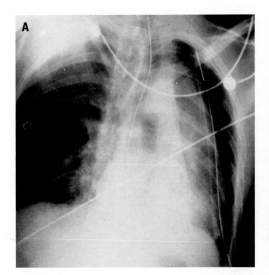
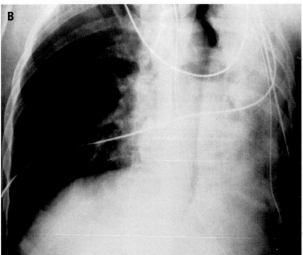

Figure 13.85. Large persistent left pneumothorax in the presence of a functioning chest tube in the supine radiograph (**A**) is consistent with a large air leak, and a bronchial injury must be a primary diagnostic consideration. The patient was placed in the left lateral decubitus position in which the collapsed left lung fell to the dependent left lateral chest wall (**B**), a variety of the fallen lung sign.

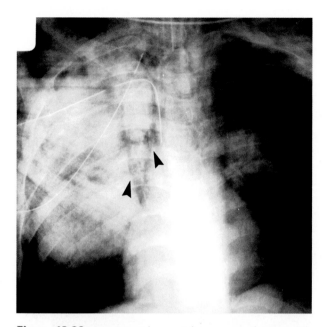

Figure 13.86. Persistent large right pneumothorax with a major collection of air in the medial pleural space *(arrowheads)* in the presence of two functioning chest tubes is extremely suggestive of a bronchial tear.

(Fig. 13.87) pneumomediastinum, are strongly suggestive of a bronchial tear. A small but persistent bronchial tear may not be radiographically recognizable initially. The gradual development of pneumothorax with the air collection principally located in the mediastinal pleural space, collapse of the lung, and pneumomediastinum should make traumatic bronchial tear the first diagnostic consideration (Fig. 13.88).

Paramediastinal pneumatocele is a collection of air either in the medial pleural space or the posterior mediastinum.[53] This collection, previously thought to be within the inferior pulmonary ligament, is seen most commonly in children and young adults following blunt chest trauma. The paramediastinal pneumatocele is almost always found on the left adjacent to or superimposed on the heart border and contains an air–fluid level in the erect CXR (Fig. 13.89). The paramediastinal pneumatocele, like other posttraumatic pneumatoceles, is of no clinical significance unless infected. Usually, it clears spontaneously. According to Heitzman,[54] paramediastinal pneumatoceles are usually present on the initial posttrauma CXR.

Extrapleural Air

Pneumomediastinum

Air may enter the mediastinum as a result of tracheal or esophageal rupture; from the deep fascial planes of the neck following penetrating injury or

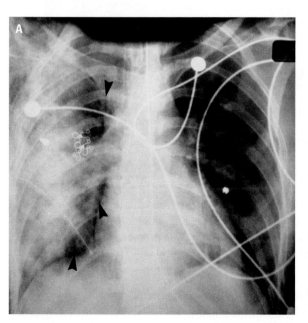
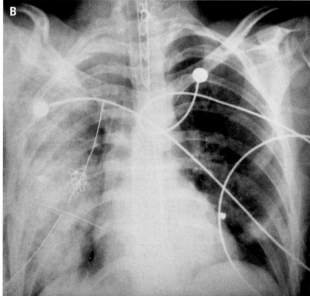

Figure 13.87. **A:** Large, persistent, primarily medial right pneumothorax *(arrowheads)* in the presence of a functioning chest tube and associated with pneumomediastinum is very suggestive of a bronchial tear. **B:** The diagnosis of a bronchial tear is made even more likely with persistence of the right pneumothorax with two functioning chest tubes in place.

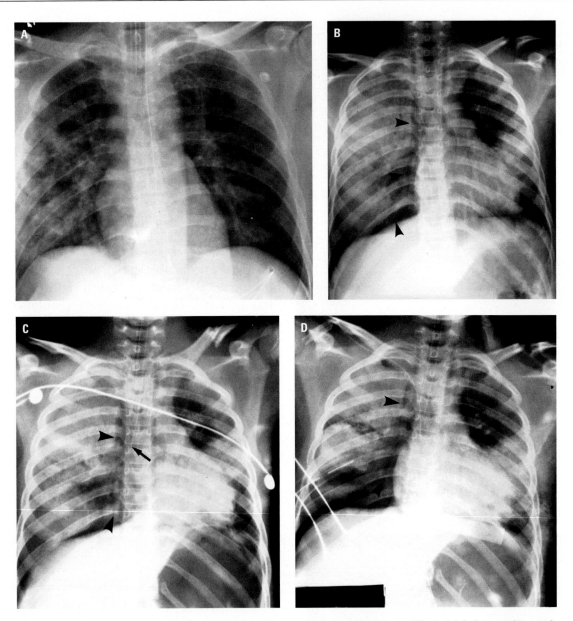

Figure 13.88. This child sustained major blunt thoracoabdominal trauma. The initial chest radiograph (**A**) demonstrates diffuse right pulmonary contusion without evidence of a pneumothorax. The second chest radiograph (**B**) demonstrates a right tension pneumothorax with pleural air at the base and medially *(arrowheads)*, pneumomediastinum, and left midlung contusion. The third radiograph (**C**) shows the endotracheal tube in the right stem bronchus *(arrow)* and an increase in the right tension pneumothorax with further collapse of the right lung and a greater accumulation of air in the medial pleural space *(arrowheads)* and pneumomediastinum. The left pulmonary contusion also increased. After the insertion of a right chest tube (**D**), the right lung was even further collapsed, and the medial pneumothorax had also increased further *(arrowheads)*. At autopsy, a full-thickness tear of the right stem bronchus was found.

rupture of the cervical trachea; rarely from the peritoneal or retroperitoneal space; or from an abrupt increase in intra-alveolar pressure, causing alveolar rupture and "interstitial emphysema" with air tracking proximally along the bronchovascular sheaths to the root of the lung and from there into the mediastinum.[31,54] The latter, which is probably the most common etiology, may be due to blunt chest trauma causing abrupt compression of pulmonary parenchyma or traumatically induced involuntary or voluntary abrupt increase in intraluminal pressure against the closed glottis. The voluntary increase in the intra-alveolar pressure may occur in any activity that results in straining, such as during

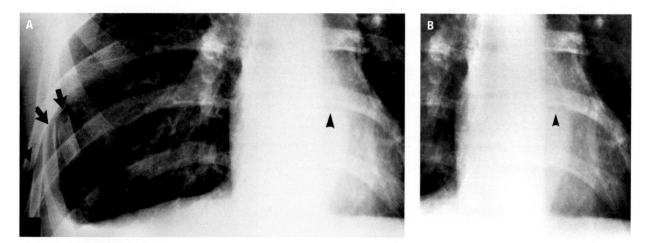

Figure 13.89. Paramediastinal pneumatocele containing an air–fluid level *(arrowhead)* in a patient who sustained acute chest trauma with multiple right lower rib fractures *(arrows,* **A**). The air–fluid level in the paramediastinal pneumatocele *(arrowhead)* is best seen in the "close-up" projection (**B**).

heavy lifting (e.g., in weight lifters, manual laborers, people lifting heavy furniture around the home, or musicians who play brass instruments). This type of nontraumatic pneumomediastinum is referred to as "spontaneous pneumomediastinum."

On the frontal CXR, the classic radiographic signs of pneumomediastinum include air between the heart and the mediastinal pleural surfaces (seen more commonly on the left than the right), air ex-

tending above the level of the pericardial reflection at the base of the heart, and air producing irregular radiolucent streaks in the paratracheal area that may extend into the neck. On the lateral projection, streaky, ill-defined lucencies are present throughout the mediastinum but particularly in the retrosternal space (Fig. 13.90). In the frontal CXR, in addition to the abnormal air collections already described, the mediastinal air may break through the fascial planes

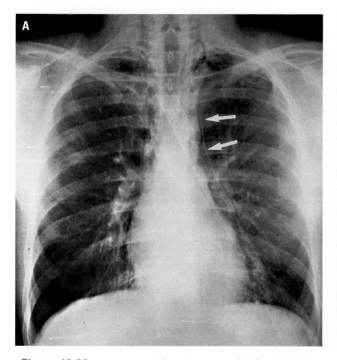
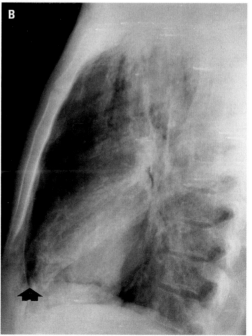

Figure 13.90. Pneumomediastinum. In the frontal projection (**A**), the mediastinal pleural reflection of the left upper lobe *(arrows)* has been laterally displaced and outlined by air in the mediastinum. In the lateral projection (**B**), an extrapulmonary collection of air is present in the retrosternal space *(arrow)*.

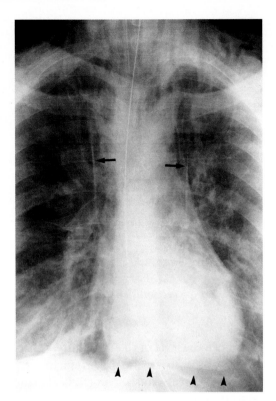

Figure 13.91. Pneumomediastinum. Air within the mediastinum outlines the mediastinal pleural surfaces of each lung *(arrows)*, and streaky, irregular radiolucencies present throughout the mediastinum extend upward into the neck. Further evidence of extrapleural air is the continuous diaphragm sign *(arrowheads)* and bilateral cervical subcutaneous emphysema caused by mediastinal air that has broken through the fascial planes at the thoracic inlet.

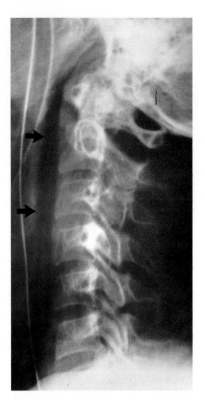

Figure 13.92. Air in the retropharyngeal fascial space *(arrows)* is the upward extension of pneumomediastinum.

of the thoracic inlet, resulting in irregular streaky lucencies of cervical subcutaneous emphysema (Fig. 13.91). On the lateral radiograph of the neck, in addition to the subcutaneous emphysema, mediastinal air usually extends into the retropharyngeal fascial space (Fig. 13.92).

Extrapleural air secondary to blunt chest trauma may accumulate in the space between the parietal pleura and the diaphragm as well as in the mediastinum itself. The intersection of these two extrapleural air collections results in a V-shaped lucency, usually on the left, referred to as the V sign of Naclerio (Fig. 13.93).[55] Figure 13.94 illustrates the V sign of extrapleural air, which also outlines the esophagus. Another sign of extrapleural (mediastinal) air is the "continuous diaphragm" sign described by Levin.[56] In this instance, the extrapleural air accumulates between the pericardium and the diaphragm (Figs. 13.91 and 13.95).

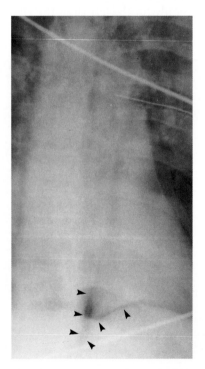

Figure 13.93. The V sign of Naclerio caused by the intersection of mediastinal air and extrapleural air between the pericardium and the diaphragm *(arrowheads)*.

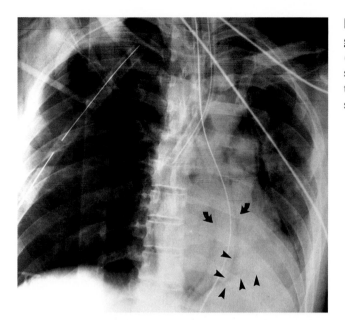

Figure 13.94. Extrapleural air outlines the esophagus *(curved arrows)* and forms the V sign of Naclerio *(arrowheads)*. The endotracheal tube is in the right stem bronchus, and the resultant hyperventilation of the right lung has resulted in shift of the mediastinal structures to the left.

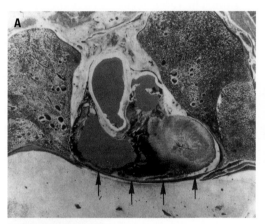

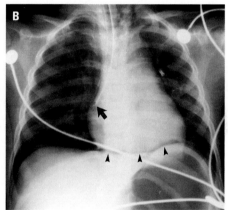

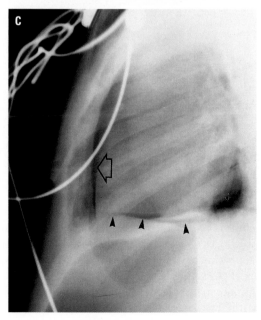

Figure 13.95. Anatomic basis and radiographic appearance of the continuous diaphragm sign of extrapleural air. The cadaver specimen **(A)** indicates the extrapleural space *(arrows)* between the pericardium and the diaphragm. The continuous diaphragm sign *(arrowheads)* is very clearly illustrated in the frontal **(B)** and lateral **(C)** radiographs of this child's chest. The *open arrow* **(C)** indicates the large pneumothorax. The endotracheal tube is in the right stem bronchus *(arrow,* **B**). (**A** is from Creasy JD, Chiles C, Routh WD, et al. Overview of traumatic injury of the thoracic aorta. *Radiographics.* 1997;17(1):27–45, with permission.)

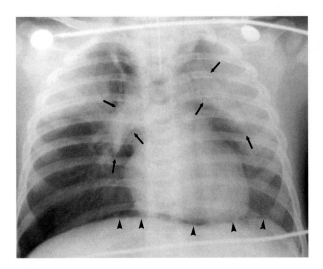

Figure 13.96. Extrapleural air (pneumomediastinum) evidenced by the continuous diaphragm sign *(arrowheads)* and the thymic spinnaker sail sign *(arrows)*.

In children, pneumomediastinum may be manifested by air delineating the thymus, the "spinnaker sail" sign,[57] as well as by the continuous diaphragm sign (Fig. 13.96).

Air in the mediastinum may rupture the mediastinal parietal pleura, resulting in pneumothorax. The reverse does not occur, according to Heitzman,[54] who states,"pneumothorax is a common complication of pneumomediastinum, but pneumothorax never causes pneumomediastinum." The radiographic signs of pneumomediastinum progressing to pneumothorax consist of the signs of both extrapleural air as well as air in the pleural space, especially the continuous diaphragm sign of pneumomediastinum and the deep sulcus sign and mediastinal shift of tension pneumothorax (Fig. 13.97).

Spontaneous pneumomediastinum, as described earlier, results from nontrauma-related excessive increase in intra-alveolar pressure causing alveolar rupture with air traversing along the bronchovascular sheaths ("interstitial emphysema") toward the hila, from which the air spills into the mediastinum. At the hila, the air becomes extrapleural. Because the mechanism of injury of spontaneous pneumothorax usually does not cause a major or persistent air leak, the pneumomediastinum is usually small and therefore is often difficult to identify radiographically on the frontal projection. The retrosternal area is the most sensitive for detecting small air collections within the mediastinum. Paratracheal streaky, ill-defined lucencies may be visible at the thoracic inlet, and air is usually present in the retropharyngeal fascial space (Fig. 13.98). Slightly larger air collections in the mediastinum cause bilateral displacement of the mediastinal pleural surface adjacent to the heart

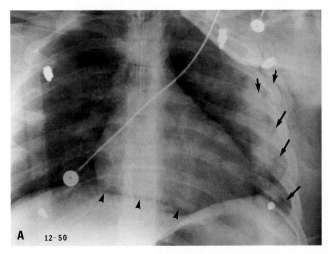

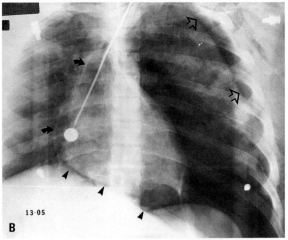

Figure 13.97. Pneumomediastinum leading to a left tension pneumothorax. **A:** In the initial supine chest radiograph, extrapleural air (pneumomediastinum) is evidenced by the continuous diaphragm sign *(arrowheads)*. Although fractures involve several of the left ribs *(arrows)*, there is no visible left pneumothorax. **B:** The examination of the same patient obtained approximately 15 minutes later demonstrated a tension pneumothorax on the left *(open arrows)* with a deep sulcus sign and shift of the heart and mediastinal structures to the right. The pneumomediastinum continues to be evidenced by the continuous diaphragm sign *(arrowheads)* and visualization of the right mediastinal pleural surface *(curved arrows)*.

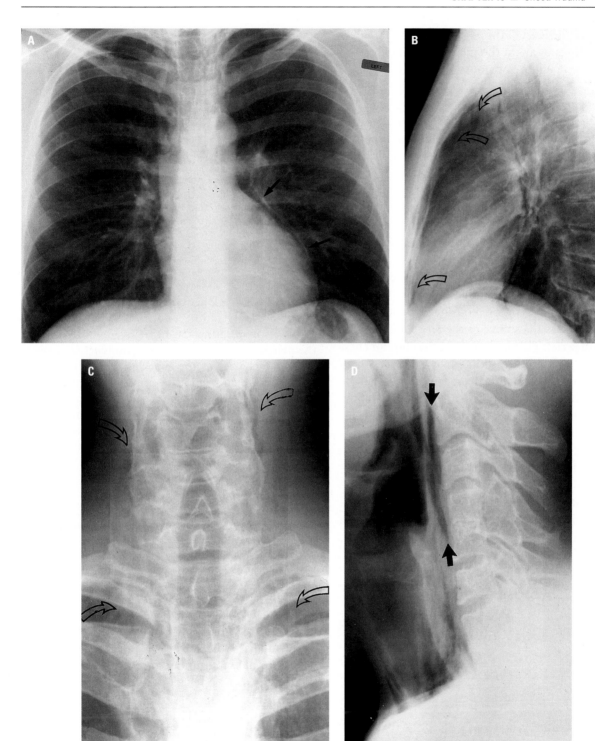

Figure 13.98. Spontaneous pneumomediastinum that occurred in a trumpet player. In the frontal radiograph of the chest (**A**), the left mediastinal pleural surface *(arrows)* is visible, and streaky, ill-defined lucencies are present in the mediastinum at the thoracic inlet. **B:** This subtle pneumomediastinum is clearly recognizable by streaky, ill-defined lucencies of air *(curved open arrows)* in the retrosternal space on the lateral projection. The frontal examination of the cervical spine and thoracic inlet (**C**) demonstrates streaky air lucencies *(curved open arrows)* in the superior mediastinum extending into the neck. The lateral radiograph of the neck (**D**) demonstrates both subcutaneous emphysema and air in the retropharyngeal space *(arrows)*.

and above the level of the aorta, and the characteristic findings of air in the mediastinum described earlier become more obvious.

Pneumopericardium

Air may gain access to the pericardial space through a tear in the pericardium due to blunt or penetrating chest trauma; alternatively, air in the pericardial space may be iatrogenic (diagnostic pneumopericardium) or secondary to infection with a gas-forming organism.[54] Traumatic pneumopericardium is rare, with only 142 patients found in a literature search including the years 1939 through 1983.[34] Pneumopericardium does not result from spontaneous pneumomediastinum[54] but requires the same massive anterior chest wall trauma that causes pneumomediastinum (which is the prerequisite for pneumopericardium and is the source of the air that enters the pericardial sac). That same force to the anterior chest wall may cause a shearing motion of the heart, which in turn causes a pericardial tear. The latter is usually found along the left heart border in the vicinity of the course of the left phrenic nerve. The pericardial tear may be very short or of sufficient length to accommodate extrapericardial herniation of the heart.[50]

The radiographic signs of pneumopericardium are frequently masked by the signs of the coexistent pneumomediastinum, and pneumomediastinum and pneumopericardium may be indistinguishable radiographically (Fig. 13.99).

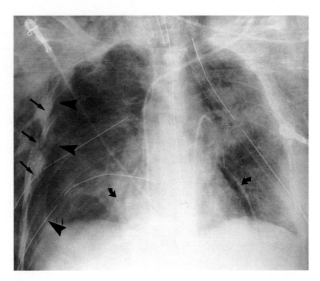

Figure 13.100. Concomitant pneumopericardium, pneumomediastinum, and right pneumothorax. The air surrounding the heart is contained within the distribution of the pericardium *(curved arrows)*. Streaky lucencies in the superior mediastinum and neck indicate pneumomediastinum. The right pneumothorax *(arrowheads)* resulted from fractures of multiple right ribs *(arrows)*. The patchy areas of increased density in the left perihilar area and at the right base represent either pulmonary contusion or aspiration pneumonitis.

Conversely, even in the presence of obvious pneumomediastinum, if the air surrounding the heart is limited to the distribution of the pericardial sac by a relatively thick, somewhat shaggy or unsharp curvilinear density representing the fibrous pericardium, which is outlined by air on either side and if there is no visible extension of that pericardial air to the streaky thoracic inlet lucencies characteristic of pneumomediastinum (Fig. 13.100), the diagnosis of pneumopericardium may be offered with considerable certainty. As an attempt to distinguish pneumomediastinum from pneumopericardium, some authors advocate obtaining CXRs in positions other than supine, particularly the lateral decubitus position, on the premise that the air within the pericardial sac will migrate away from the dependent position.[51] However, our experience has been that the magnitude of the chest trauma alone sustained by these patients usually precludes that option. Air within the pericardial sac usually does not completely outline the heart in the frontal (Fig. 13.101) or lateral (Fig. 13.102) projections. Anatomically, the pericardium is

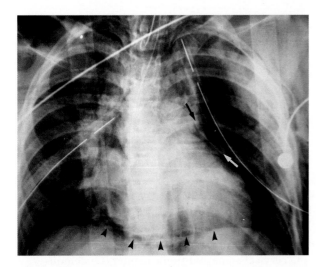

Figure 13.99. Concomitant pneumomediastinum and pneumopericardium. The extrapleural air is evidenced by the continuous diaphragm sign *(arrowheads)*. The *arrows* indicate the pericardium outlined by air in the pericardial sac.

considerably thicker (Fig. 13.103) than the mediastinal pleura. This fact helps distinguish the radiographic appearance of the pericardium as seen in Figures 13.100 through 13.102 from that of the mediastinal pleura seen in pneumomediastinum (Figs. 13.91, 13.94, and 13.98). This difference in the radiographic characteristics of the pericardium and the mediastinal pleura is a key element in the distinction between pneumomediastinum and pneumopericardium.

Cardiovascular Trauma

Cardiac injury is common in patients who sustain major blunt chest trauma. Rapid deceleration injuries, such as steering wheel accidents or falls from a height, constitute the most common cause of blunt cardiac injury. Pathologically, cardiac contusion is the most frequently encountered lesion. Myocardial rupture is the most rapidly fatal cardiac injury. Damage to the valve leaflets and damage to the chordae tendineae are not common and usually occur simultaneously. Blunt cardiac injury is rarely evident radiographically.

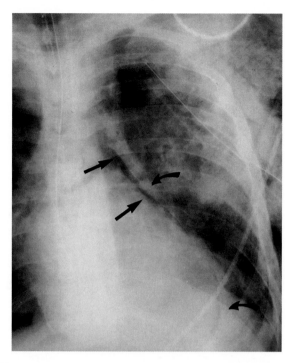

Figure 13.101. Pneumopericardium. Air surrounding the left heart border and extending only to the level of the pericardial reflection *(straight arrows)* is contained by the density of the thick fibrous pericardium *(curved arrows)*.

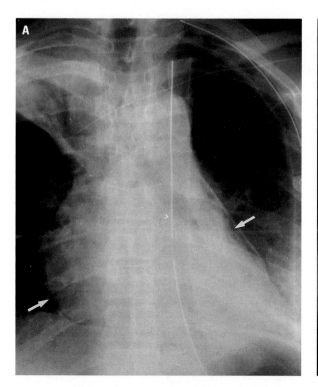 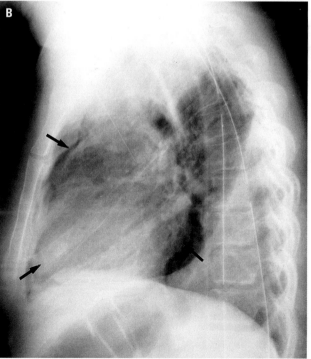

Figure 13.102. Pneumopericardium in frontal **(A)** and lateral **(B)** projections. The pericardial air *(arrows)* defines both the right and left heart borders in the frontal projection **(A)** and the anterior and posterior cardiac margins in the lateral projection **(B)**.

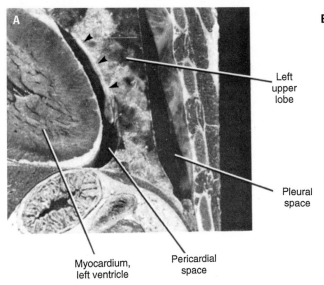

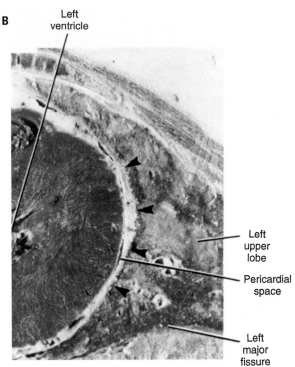

Figure 13.103. The irregular thickness of the fibrous pericardium *(arrowheads)* is illustrated in cadaver specimens (**A** and **B**). (From Wagner M, Lawson TL. *Segmental Anatomy: Applications to Clinical Medicine.* New York, NY: Macmillan; 1982, with permission.)

Radiology plays only a minor role in the diagnosis of penetrating injuries to the heart, other than simply to record the presence and location of the penetrating object, such as an impaling stake or knife blade. Gunshot wounds to the chest may penetrate the lung, mediastinum, and pericardium, resulting in pneumopericardium (Fig. 13.104).

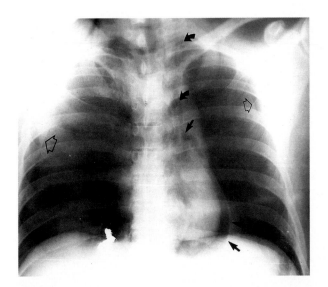

Figure 13.104. Concomitant bilateral pneumothoraces *(open arrows)*, pneumomediastinum *(curved arrows)*, and pneumopericardium *(straight arrows)* secondary to a gunshot wound to the chest. All these radiographic findings were confirmed at autopsy.

Acute Traumatic Aortic Injury

Terminology

Throughout the medical literature, the terms commonly used in reference to ATAI are pathologically incorrect and thus clinically diagnostically misleading. Correct pathologic terminology is essential to proper clinical management of patients suspected of having ATAI. Therefore, the following are the terms that should be used in describing blunt trauma to the thoracic aorta:

1. *Acute traumatic aortic injury (ATAI)* is a generic term that includes all pathologic varieties of blunt aortic injury.[11,58]
2. *Acute traumatic aortic rupture (ATAR)* is a through-and-through, full-thickness disruption of all layers of the aortic wall.[11,20,59]
3. *Acute traumatic aortic tear (ATAT)* is a partial disruption of the aortic wall limited to the intima and muscularis. The adventitia is intact (traumatic medial laceration).[11,20,60,61]
4. *Acute traumatic aortic intimal tear (ATAIT)* is disruption limited to the intima. The muscularis and adventitia are intact.[11,59–61]

The term traditionally used to refer to acute thoracic injury from blunt trauma or a high-velocity abrupt deceleration or "T-bone" injury—"rupture of the aorta," "acute aortic rupture," or "traumatic rupture of the aorta,"—is erroneous. Actually, most patients who sustain an acute aortic injury from high-speed decelerating trauma do indeed tear the full thickness of the aorta and exsanguinate at or shortly following injury. Consequently, patients with full-thickness tears rarely constitute a clinical or radiologic emergency. Patients who suffer *aortic injury* and survive the initial traumatic event do not have a "rupture" but an incompletely torn aortic wall, with at least the adventitia remaining intact. The integrity and flow of the aortic lumen is maintained by the intact adventitia that provides most (60%) of the tensile strength of the aorta (Fig. 13.105).[62]

Thus, the term acute traumatic aortic tear is the appropriate terminology to describe the *incomplete* aortic injury typically found in patients who survive to reach the hospital and which is demonstrated by CTA or, less commonly today, catheter aortography. Rarely, given the rapid transport potential of current medical evacuation systems, a patient with a complete tear who is usually actively bleeding into the mediastinum will also survive to reach medical treatment. This grave injury may be demonstrated by emergent chest CTA, but such patients have, in the author's experience, nearly 100% inhospital mortality even if they survive to have emergency thoracotomy. The terminology

described earlier is based on pathologic findings in the mediastinum and, most typically, the proximal descending thoracic aorta as found at autopsy or surgery.[58,63–75]

Injury Mechanism

Wilson and colleagues[75] believe, as do many others, that ATAI must be suspected in all patients who are involved in motor vehicle accidents in which speeds exceed 30 mph. Therefore, ATAI must be considered in the differential diagnosis of any patient sustaining major blunt chest trauma. The most widely accepted mechanism of aortic injury is high-velocity abrupt deceleration, as might occur in a motor vehicle accident or a fall from a height with the victim landing prone or secondary to a massive blow that strikes and compresses the anterior chest wall.[76–80]

The abrupt deceleration mechanism of injury is postulated to result from unequal rates of horizontal deceleration, with the more tensile or mobile portions of the aorta decelerating over a longer horizontal distance than the more fixed portions (Fig. 13.106), a shearing force. With a direct blow to the chest as the mechanism of injury, posterior displacement of the sternum causes marked posterior left lateral displacement of the heart, which in turn causes vertical elongation of the aorta and great vessels at their points of maximum fixation. This movement is thought to result in transverse aortic tears.[81] Others believe that the "water hammer" effect of abrupt increase in intraluminal aortic pressure plays a role in ATAI (Fig. 13.106).[82] It is probable that all of these mechanisms of injury play some role in ATAI. Although all the mechanisms described earlier are predicated on a force striking the chest in an AP direction, recent research found that 48 of 97 (49.5%) patients sustained ATAR as a result of lateral impact motor vehicle collisions. Although lateral impact crashes involved the drivers and passengers nearly equally, ATAR occurred more commonly in victims riding on the side of impact (ipsilateral, 38 of 81, or 47%) than on the contralateral side (10 of 81, or 12%).[83]

Regardless of the precise mechanism of injury, the natural history of ATAI as reported by Parmley and colleagues[59] Soyer and colleagues,[74] and Rizoli and colleagues[84] is that 80% to 85% of the patients exsanguinate through a full-thickness tear of the aorta at the time of initial injury or shortly thereafter and that only 15% to 20% survive to

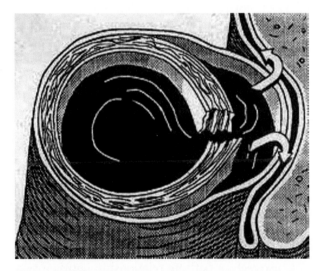

Figure 13.105. Schematic representation of the pathology of the pseudoaneurysm of acute traumatic aortic injury in patients who survive the initial injury according to Naclerio. (From Naclerio EA. *Chest Injuries: Physiologic Principles and Emergency Management.* New York, NY: Grune & Stratton; 1971, with permission.)

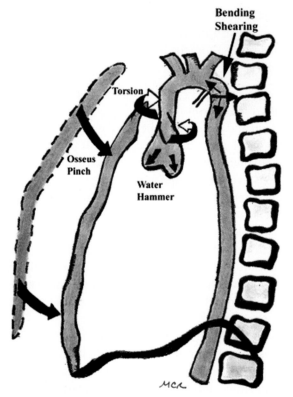

Figure 13.106. Schematic depicts various mechanisms of injury resulting in ATAI. The osseous pinch is shown by posterior translation of the sternum (*large arrows*), which traps the aorta at the narrowest point of the thorax. Torsion is depicted in the ascending aorta (*curved arrows*), resulting in twisting above the fixed aortic valve. Compression of lumen forces blood inferiorly toward the aortic valve resulting in the water hammer effect (*arrows in aortic root*). At ligamentum arteriosum, the aorta is affected by both bending and shearing stresses (*small arrows*) augmented by the anatomic changes from the osseous pinch against the thoracic spine and pressure changes from the water hammer effect. The combination of forces is concentrated at the fixed point of the descending thoracic aorta—the ligamentum arteriosum (parallel lines inferior to transverse aortic arch). (From Steenburg SD, Ravenel JG, Ikonomidis JS, et al. Acute traumatic aortic injury: imaging evaluation and management. *Radiology*. 2008;248(3):748–762, Fig. 1, with permission.)

reach the hospital. If untreated, approximately 49% of initial survivors exsanguinate within the first 24 hours after injury,[59] 80% by the end of the first week,[74] and approximately 95% by 4 months after injury. The remaining 2% to 5%[59,74] are long-term survivors whose life span is unaffected by a stable false aneurysm.[85–86] However, patients with minor aortic injuries such as intimal flaps, focal intramural hematomas, or shallow pseudoaneurysms that

are more often diagnosed by current high detector number CT scanners than before their common availability have a much better prognosis and may successfully be managed with follow-up CTA to verify healing on injury stability (M. Forman, SE Mirvis, unpublished data, March 2011).

Injury Location

The most common site of ATAI is the proximal descending thoracic aorta distal to the left subclavian artery in the region of the ligamentum arteriosum (50% to 71%).[50,78] The second most common site, in the author's experience, is the aortic arch (Fig. 13.107), and the third most frequent site is the ascending aorta (Fig. 13.108). In autopsy series, the ascending aorta is the second most common site because it has a higher mortality as a percent of injuries compared to other sites.[61] The distal thoracic aorta is the fourth most common site. Injuries at the root of the aorta, including those of the aortic valve, are usually acutely fatal,[61] with only approximately 7% surviving to reach the hospital.[87]

Clinical Considerations

The diagnosis of ATAI in patients who survive the initial traumatic event cannot be made clinically. Up to one-third of patients have only minimal clinical evidence of chest trauma.[75] Additionally, most of these patients have more clinically overt concomitant injuries that may detract from consideration of ATAI. For these reasons, Blair and colleagues[88] state that "the consistently most dramatic and lethal missed diagnosis in blunt chest trauma is transection [injury] of the aorta." Among commonly listed clinical signs and symptoms of acute traumatic rupture of the aorta (Tables 13.1–13.3),[89–91] there are none that are either sensitive or specific for ATAI. The same may be said for the predictive value of most of the associated injuries found in multiply traumatized patients who also sustain ATAI. Fisher and Hadlock[60] in particular have demonstrated an absence of correlation between thoracic inlet rib fractures and ATAI, and Lee and colleagues[25] have shown an absence of correlation between thoracic fractures and ATAI.

Conversely, a definite relationship between two remote skeletal injuries and ATAI has been documented as Ochsner and colleagues[92] reported that patients with pelvic ring disruption have a risk for an associated aortic injury two to five times greater than the overall blunt trauma population.

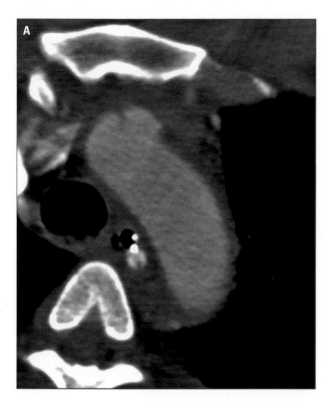

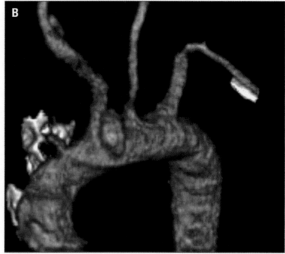

Figure 13.107. Pseudoaneurysm of aortic arch. **A:** Axial CT at level of arch shows pseudoaneurysm arising from anterior arch with surrounding mediastinal hematoma. The trachea is displaced to the right. **B:** Surface contour rendering demonstrates pseudoaneurysm *(white arrow)* arising from anterior proximal aortic arch just distal to right innominate artery.

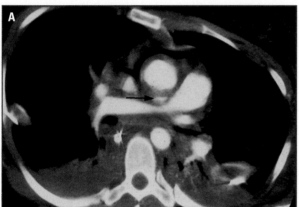

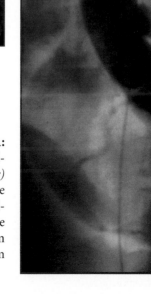

Figure 13.108. Ascending aortic pseudoaneurysm. **A:** Axial contrast-enhanced CT across proximal ascending aorta shows a small pseudoaneurysm *(black arrow)* arising from the posterior aspect of the aorta. Note the surrounding hematoma and compression of the proximal right pulmonary artery. There is bilateral lower lobe atelectasis. **B:** Image from digital subtraction aortogram shows pseudoaneurysm arising posteriorly from proximal ascending aorta.

TABLE 13.1	Clinical Signs of Great Vessel Injury

External evidence of major chest trauma (i.e., steering wheel imprint on chest)

Palpable fracture of sternum

Expanding hematoma at thoracic outlet

Intrascapular murmur

Upper extremity hypertension

Diminished or absent pulses (upper extremity from innominate or subclavian injury or lower extremity from pseudocoarctation syndrome)

Palpable fracture of thoracic spine

Left flail chest

Elevated central venous pressure

Hypotension

From Hood RM, Boyd AD, Culliford AT, eds. *Thoracic Trauma.* Philadelphia, PA: WB Saunders; 1989, with permission.

TABLE 13.3	Clinical Signs and Symptoms of Aortic Rupture

Acute hypertension

Upper extremity hypertension pseudocoarctation

Pulse pressure difference in upper extremities

New murmur and/or changing murmur

Precardial ecchymosis

Unexplained hypotension

Paraplegia

Interscapular pain

Dysphagia

Dyspnea

From Lee J, Harris JH Jr, Duke JH Jr, et al. Noncorrelation between thoracic skeletal injuries and acute traumatic aortic tear. *J Trauma.* 1997;43(3):400–404, with permission.

TABLE 13.2	Symptoms and Signs of Aortic Rupture

Symptoms
  Retrosternal pain
  Interscapular pain
  Hoarseness
  Dyspnea
  Dysphagia
  Paraplegia
  Distal ischemia
Signs
  Sternal fracture
  Fracture of upper ribs
  Fracture or dislocation of thoracic spine
  Fullness or hematoma at base of neck
  Tracheal deviation
  Hypertension in arms
  Hypotension in legs
  Bruits in chest and neck
  Hemothorax
  Stridor

From Townsend RN, Colella JJ, Diamond DL. Traumatic rupture of the aorta: critical decisions for trauma surgeons. *J Trauma.* 1990;30(9):1169–1174, with permission.

Marymont and colleagues[93] reported a 10% incidence of ATAI in patients with posterior dislocation or fracture-dislocation of the hip.

Pathology of Acute Traumatic Aortic Injury
Mediastinal Hematoma

The surgical literature describes a mediastinal hematoma as "massive" and "completely surrounding the proximal descending aorta,"[74] extending around the injury site,[73] and "often covering" most of the descending aorta and extending over the pericardium and the transverse aortic arch.[72,74,94–97] The only place this hematoma can accumulate is within the mediastinum within the confines of the parietal pleura.

The mediastinal hematoma has been identified as arising from tears of mediastinal vessels other than the aorta (i.e., the azygos and hemiazygos systems and the spinal, intercostal, and internal mammary arteries and veins).[11,72,96] The pathologic facts of (1) the intact aortic adventitia and (2) the mediastinal hematoma completely surrounding the injured aorta are key in understanding chest radiographic and thoracic CT findings of ATAI. The intact aortic adventitia indicates that the mediastinal hematoma is not of aortic origin, although some bleeding from the vasa vasorum of the aortic wall may also contribute.[97] Typically, the mediastinal hematoma "completely" surrounds and covers the aorta and

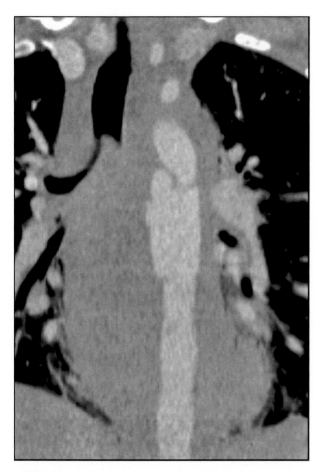

Figure 13.109. Descending aortic pseudoaneurysm with large surrounding hematoma. A large hematoma surrounds the aorta. There is an extensive aortic aneurysm shown on coronal CT reformation. The hematoma is limited by the parietal pleura. Note displacement of the airway to the right mainly from mass effect of hematoma.

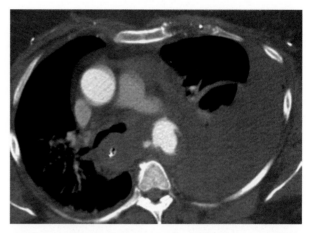

Figure 13.110. Mass effects of mediastinal hematoma. Axial IV contrast-enhanced CT shows proximal descending aortic pseudoaneurysm with a large amount of surrounding mediastinal hematoma. Note the displacement of the trachea and nasogastric tube to the right. There is also a large hemothorax on the left contributing to the mass effects.

It is reasonable to state that there are no specific clinical signs or symptoms of ATAI. Hemorrhagic shock is not associated with acute aortic trauma unless the aortic wall is completely transected in which event the patient typically exsanguinates. The

the pseudoaneurysm is between the aorta and the parietal pleura (Figs. 13.105 and 13.109).[72,96]

Although most of the mass effect on periaortic structures, mainly the trachea, esophagus, and left lower lobe bronchus, is attributed to the mediastinal hematoma, a large pseudoaneurysm may also contribute to these displacements or may even be the principal cause of displacement (Fig. 13.110). The mediastinal hematoma may extend along the entire aorta distal to the injury site to the level of the diaphragmatic crura, as described by Wong and colleagues.[98] The amount of mediastinal hemorrhage associated with ATAI is quite variable and, in fact, little or even no mediastinal blood may be found, particularly with minimal aortic injuries as more frequently diagnosed on state-of-the art MDCT (Figs. 13.111 and 13.112).

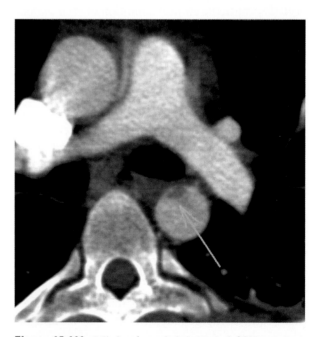

Figure 13.111. Minimal aortic injury. Axial IV contrast-enhanced CT image shows probable clot in proximal descending aorta *(white arrow)*. There is no other evidence of aortic injury or mediastinal hematoma.

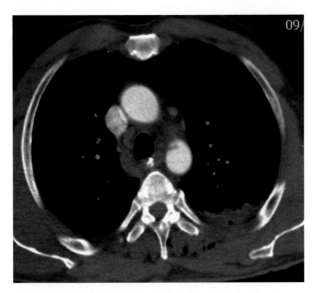

Figure 13.112. Minimal aortic injury. Axial IV contrast-enhanced CT image through level of proximal descending aorta shows intimal flap in anterior lumen *(arrow)*. There is no evidence of mediastinal blood. There are several periaortic lymph nodes.

important aspect of the clinical presentation of patients who sustain and survive ATAI (i.e., the lesion is clinically "silent")[59] is further emphasized by the report by Blair and colleagues[88] of three patients with ATAT in whom the diagnosis was originally unsuspected because the clinical condition of each patient was described as "good" when first seen by the emergency department, and by Plume and DeWeese,[76] who also observed that concomitant severe multiple trauma may result in delay in the diagnosis of ATAT.

Radiography

CXRs are still typically performed in patients with any history or clinical signs of significant chest trauma. Therefore, an understanding of the radiographic appearances of patients with ATAI is still vital. However, increasingly, screening CT angiography is being used to screen such patients for injuries from the head through the pelvis,[99] making knowledge of radiologic findings perhaps less relevant today. However, it is likely that chest radiography will continue to play a role in the rapid initial assessment of the chest for signs of many other injuries that require emergent treatment such as tension pneumothorax, large hemothorax, or tension pneumomediastinum. Radiologic signs of mediastinal hematoma must prompt the priority performance of CT angiography.

TABLE 13.4	Radiologic Findings Associated with Transection of the Descending Thoracic Aorta
Widening of superior mediastinum of more than 8 cm	
Depression of left mainstem bronchus of more than 140 degrees	
Obliteration of aortic knob	
Deviation of nasogastric tube, or trachea, to the right	
Fracture of first or second rib, scapula, or sternum	
Left apical hematoma	
Obliteration of aortopulmonary window on lateral chest radiograph	
Anterior displacement of trachea on lateral chest radiograph	
Fracture-dislocation of thoracic spine	
Calcium layering in aortic knob area	
Obvious double contour of aorta	
Multiple left rib fractures	
Massive hemothorax	

From Mattox KL. Injury to the thoracic great vessels. In: Moore EE, Mattox KL, Feliciano DV, eds. *Trauma.* 2nd ed. Norwalk, CT: Appleton & Lange, 1991;26:393–408, with permission.

Many plain chest radiographic findings have been described as being "associated with traumatic rupture of the aorta"[90,91,100] (Tables 13.4–13.6) or as being "signs of acute traumatic rupture of the aorta"[101–104] (Figs. 13.113–13.117). None of these

TABLE 13.5	Radiographic Changes of Aortic Rupture
Mediastinal widening	
Prominent aortic knob	
Obliteration of aortic outline	
Obliteration of aortic window	
Tracheal deviation	
Depression of left bronchus	
Widening of paravertebral stripe	
Deviation of esophagus	
Hemothorax	

From Hood RM, Boyd AD, Culliford AT. *Thoracic Trauma.* Philadelphia, PA: WB Saunders; 1989, with permission.

TABLE 13.6	X-ray Findings Associated with Traumatic Rupture of the Aorta Widened Mediastinum

Aortic knob obliteration
Aortopulmonary window opacification
Left pleural cap
Tracheal deviation
Depression of left mainstem bronchus
Nasogastric tube displacement
Paraspinous "stripe"
Fluid in pleural space

From Townsend RN, Colella JJ, Diamond DL. Traumatic rupture of the aorta: critical decisions for trauma surgeons. *J Trauma.* 1990;30(9):1169–1174, with permission.

signs is sensitive or specific enough to diagnose or completely exclude ATAI, but some are both sensitive and specific for the presence of a "mediastinal hematoma."

Of 1,000 patients admitted to Hermann Hospital emergency center and examined by unenhanced mediastinal CT (UMCT) because of equivocal CXR or MXR, 792 of 1,000 (79%) had no mediastinal hematoma and required no further imaging. These patients were discharged between 1 and 60 days (mean, 10 days) without subsequent evidence of cardiovascular trauma. Of the same 1,000 patients, 208 (21%) had a mediastinal hematoma diagnosed by UMCT and of these 208, in 176 (86%), the aorta was normal by CTA or catheter aortography. In 28 of the 208 (14%), ATAT was demonstrated by CTA or catheter aortography and confirmed surgically.

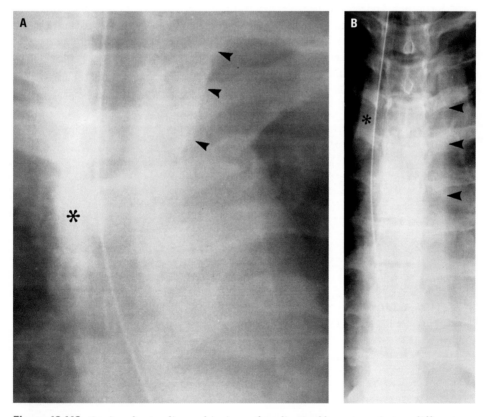

Figure 13.113. Supine chest radiographic signs of mediastinal hematoma in two different patients. In each, the superior mediastinum is abnormal. **A:** In the first patient, the left mediastinal stripe extends upward to form an apical cap *(arrowheads)*. The right paratracheal stripe *(asterisk)* is abnormally wide; its margin is indistinct; and the azygos arch is obscured. **B:** In the second patient, the left mediastinal stripe *(arrowheads)* extends above the level of the aortic arch. (The left apex was not included on the examination.) The right paratracheal stripe *(asterisk)* is abnormally wide, even though its lateral border is sharply delineated, and it has obliterated the azygos arch. In each of these patients, the nasogastric tube is displaced to the right.

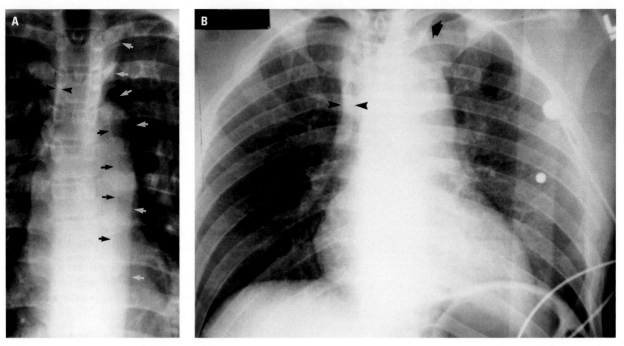

Figure 13.114. Radiologic signs of mediastinal hemorrhage. **A:** Properly exposed supine radiograph of the normal mediastinal soft tissue anatomy to display the right paratracheal stripe *(arrowheads)*; the left mediastinal stripe *(black arrows)* as it tapers medially and disappears at the level of the aortic arch; and the descending thoracic aorta, aortic arch, and left subclavian artery *(white arrows)*, which disappear beneath the medial end of the left clavicle. **B:** The relative underexposure of the supine chest radiograph of a patient with a mediastinal hematoma demonstrates the abnormally wide right paratracheal stripe *(arrowheads)* and the apical pleural cap *(arrow)* but is inadequate to demonstrate the left mediastinal stripe or the aorta. However, the abnormal configuration of the superior mediastinum, abnormal paratracheal stripe, and apical pleural cap are sufficient for the diagnosis of a mediastinal hematoma. This patient had acute traumatic aortic tear diagnosed by aortography.

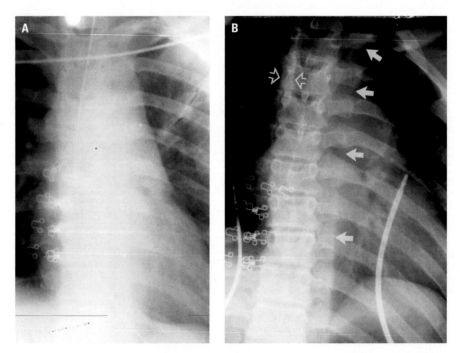

Figure 13.115. **A:** The routine supine chest radiograph of a patient involved in a high-speed motor vehicle accident. This examination demonstrates only an abnormal superior mediastinum that measured less than 8.0 cm. **B:** The overpenetrated supine radiograph demonstrates the left mediastinal stripe *(arrows)* extending above the level of the aortic arch to form an apical cap and an abnormally wide right paratracheal stripe *(open arrows)*.

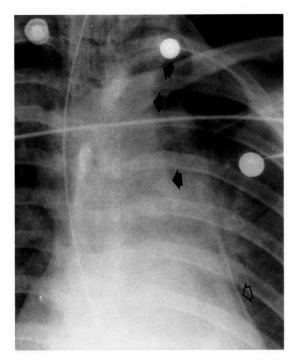

Figure 13.116. Mediastinal hematoma evidenced in the supine chest radiograph of a patient with pneumomediastinum *(open arrow)* by an ill-defined, abnormally wide superior mediastinum, complete obscuration of the right paratracheal stripe, and the left mediastinal stripe extending above the level of the aortic arch to form an apical pleural cap *(closed arrows)*. The value of naso-gastric tube displacement to the right is diminished by patient rotation to the right.

Therefore, the absence of mediastinal hematoma has a very high negative predictive value in excluding ATAT. Therefore, radiographic or noncontrast chest CT signs of a mediastinal hematoma in patients with a history of a major blunt chest trauma or a high-speed, abrupt deceleration injury require CTA or catheter aortography to exclude or establish ATAT. Patients with a similar history in whom there are no plain chest radiographic or CT signs of mediastinal hematoma do not require CTA or thoracic aortography (JH Harris Jr, A Trahan, D Kay, unpublished data, February 2012).

As noted earlier, some patients with minor aortic injury may have little or no mediastinal hemorrhage and thus could have a normal appearing CXR regarding the mediastinum.[105,106] Cleverley[105] found 3 of 34 patients with traumatic aortic injury (TAI) had no mediastinal hematoma on MDCTA; 2 having a pseudoaneurysm and 1 an intimal flap. Usually, these patients will be able to be successfully managed

without surgery or stent graft placement, although further research on this matter is required. Unfortunately, given the frequent limited technical quality of CXRs obtained in the acute trauma setting, patient motion, an expiratory respiratory phase, and occasionally large body habitus, the mediastinum cannot be declared normal.

Multidetector Computed Tomographic-Angiography

Some authors advocate thoracic aortography solely based on a high-velocity, abrupt deceleration mechanism of injury.[60,62,94,107] The inherent

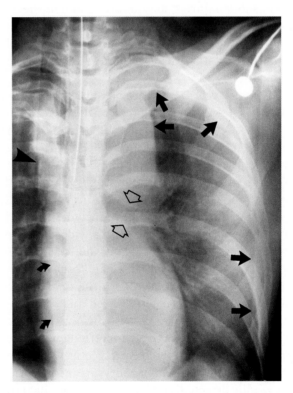

Figure 13.117. This young woman was involved in a high-speed, abrupt deceleration motor vehicle accident. She was intubated at the scene and brought by helicopter to the hospital with cardiopulmonary resuscitation in progress. This supine chest radiograph, obtained shortly after arrival in the trauma center and as she was being pronounced dead on arrival, demonstrates a massive mediastinal hematoma that has broken through the left pleura to form a left hemothorax *(closed arrows)*. The right paratracheal stripe *(arrowhead)* is grossly wide, and the presence of a right mediastinal stripe *(curved arrows)* indicates the magnitude of the mediastinal hematoma that was secondary to a full-thickness tear of the aorta. The mediastinal hematoma has also produced circumferential narrowing of the left stem bronchus *(open arrows)*. The highest *closed arrow* indicates the left apical cap.

disadvantage of this approach is the large number of negative aortic arteriograms that would be needed. Aortography is expensive, time consuming, invasive, and may delay the patient from receiving other indicated diagnostic or therapeutic procedures. There is the added risk of intravenous (IV) contrast-induced nephropathy (CIN), especially given additional IV contrast the patient may require for other studies as CT. Although catheter angiography has long been regarded as the gold standard study for aortic injury, there are in fact many studies that receive an uncertain interpretation due to atherosclerotic disease; aortic ulcers; anatomic variants, particularly in the ductus region; subtle injuries; and failure to obtain the appropriate projection to unequivocally reveal the injury. Currently, MDCT is accepted as the sole diagnostic method to determine the presence or absence of TAI.[108]

In recent years, with the introduction of very fast MDCT scanners and greater general availability in close proximity to the emergency admitting area, many centers are opting to perform whole-body CT from the head through the pelvis for patients with evidence of blunt polytrauma, with or without even obtaining an admission CXR. The logic behind this approach includes the ability to diagnose and characterize a wide variety of injuries in various body regions and to have high confidence in both identifying and excluding injury. The study is quick to perform, and the raw data can be quickly reconstructed and reformatted into other imaging planes with maximum or minimum intensity and volumetric depiction of anatomy from innumerable perspectives. Vascular injuries, including pseudoaneurysms and bleeding, are readily detected, and both images and diagnostic interpretation are often rapidly available. The use of both IV contrast, usually 100 mL of 300 or 350 mg% with a saline bolus push, is adequate for enhancement.

Unfortunately, the ease of performing "screening" whole-body CTA and its accuracy for a wide variety of injuries has led to a very low threshold for ordering the study even with a clear history of a low energy mechanism of injury and no significant injuries present. This approach increases the rate of fully normal CTA studies and suggests criteria are too liberal for obtaining this examination. More careful attention to details of history and careful physical examination to limit

use of this examination to more appropriate patients will hopefully evolve. The use and potential overuse of radiation in this manner is of great concern. Although there is steady progress in reducing radiation exposure using new techniques involving CT hardware and software, appropriate patient selection is most valuable in limiting unnecessary radiation.[109]

CTA is regarded to be at least as accurate as thoracic angiography for aortic injury and has numerous other advantages enumerated earlier.[108] A negative whole-body CTA also allows for more rapid discharge of patients with completely negative studies and can diagnose most clinically significant injuries, leading to earlier treatment and fewer or no additional diagnostic studies.

Computed Tomography Technique and Appearances of Aortic Injury

Many investigators, following the lead of Raptopoulos,[20,110–116] have demonstrated the value of CTA in the identification of ATAI, principally ATAT. It is vital to assess the appearance of the mediastinum in the arterial phase when the major arterial vascular structures are maximally opacified. Again, the assessment of the chest is frequently performed as a part of a whole-body survey from above the circle of Willis through the pelvis. In the authors' practice at the Maryland Shock Trauma Center, this study is generally performed on a 64-detector CT. The current technique for the whole-body blunt trauma MDCT-64 scanner at the University of Maryland Medical Center is described in Table 13.7. The scan is continued through the abdomen and pelvis and is followed by a portal venous phase study of the abdomen using lower exposure and increased slice thickness. Images of the chest, abdomen, and pelvis are routinely reformatted in the coronal plane.

In any study demonstrating a thoracic aortic injury, further postprocessing is usually performed including maximal intensity, volumetric, and endoluminal projections (Figs. 13.118–13.120). The report discussing the aorta should include the type of injury (minor, as described earlier, or major), the location and length of the injury, its diameter just above and below the injured segment, and its length from the nearest major branch (usually the left subclavian artery). The injury length should be measured along the longitudinal axis of the

TABLE 13.7	Total Body Survey for Blunt Polytrauma: 64-MDCT: 64 MDC

Arms at sides: Noncontrast head CT at 5 mm

Place arms over head for whole-body scan

Contrast dose—100 mL of 350 mg% at 50 mL at 6 mL/s, then 4 mm/s for 50 mL followed by 50 mL saline flush at 4 mL/s

No oral contrast for routine study

Dose reduction (z-DOM) throughout study

Arterial Phase

  Younger than 50 y—18 s delay from start of injection

  Older than 50 y—bolus timing (trigger 90 HU in proximal aorta)

  Total body scan in one sweep from vertex of skull through pubic femoral heads

Portal Venous Phase

  Includes abdomen only at 60 s delay postinitial injection at 250 m as tube current

  Renal collecting system scan (abdomen and pelvis) at 3–5 min postinjection as needed

Reconstruction and Display

  Chest, abdomen, pelvis: 3 mm at 3 mm axial display and routine MPR in coronal plane at 3 mm

  Cervical spine: Use 1 mm at 0.5 mm increment. Display at 2 mm

  Face: Use 1 mm at 0.5 mm. Display at 2 mm

  Thoracic and lumbar spine: Use 1.5 mm at 0.75 mm. Display at 2 mm

  For chest, abdomen, pelvis coronal reformation use 2 mm at 1 mm increments. Display coronal images 4 mm at 3 mm

  For cervical spine use 1 mm at 0.5 mm. Display coronal and sagittal MPR 2 mm at 2 mm

  Thoracic and lumbar spine use 1.5 mm at 0.75 mm. Display 2 mm at 2 mm for coronal and sagittal MPR.

  Dedicated thoracic and lumbar spine is an added (nonroutine) part of study

CT, computed tomography; *MPR,* multiplanar reconstruction.

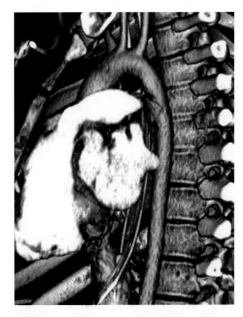

Figure 13.118. Postprocessed volume render view shows typical pseudoaneurysm arising from typical location in anterior proximal descending aorta.

erroneously referred to as an "indirect"[11,115] sign of ATAI—include an inhomogeneous or homogeneous density, depending on the amount of mediastinal blood admixed with the mediastinal fat. Mediastinal hemorrhage may be limited to the area around the injury, circumferentially around the aorta, or usually more extensively, pro-

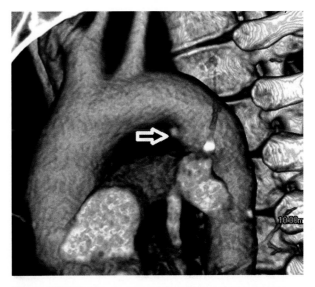

Figure 13.119. Postprocessed volume CT image shows relatively small pseudoaneurysm *(arrow)* arising from anterior proximal descending aorta.

aorta. Any aberrant artery branching should be described.

Major aortic injuries are almost always accompanied by adjacent hematoma. The MDCTA signs of a mediastinal hematoma—sometimes

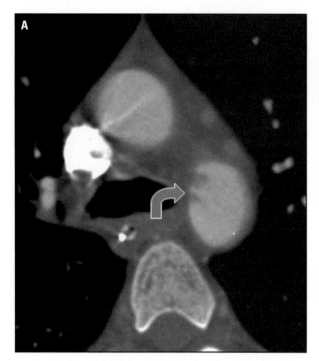
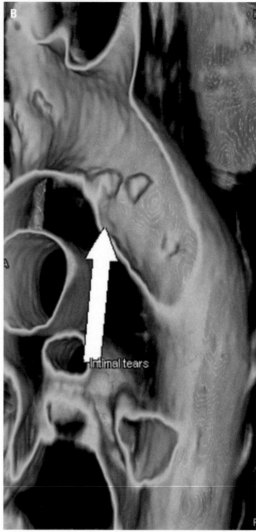

Figure 13.120. Postprocessed aortic pseudoaneurysm. **A:** Axial IV contrast-enhanced image shows intimal irregularity *(curved arrow)* in proximal descending aorta without adjacent hematoma. **B:** Postprocessed cut away view verifies intimal tears in aortic wall *(arrow)*.

ducing mass effects on adjacent structures as the esophagus, trachea, and left main stem bronchus (Figs. 13.109, 13.110, 13.121–13.124). Blood surrounds the descending aorta for a variable distance caudally (Figs. 13.123 and 13.124). Blood limited to the anterior mediastinum without blood in other compartments is very unlikely, if ever, a finding related to aortic injury.[116] In this circumstance, other lesions as injury to the sternum and/or internal mammary artery should be sought. Mediastinal hemorrhage can certainly occur without major arterial injury and could arise from a spinal or sternal injury, for instance (Fig. 13.125). MDCTA is regarded now as more sensitive than arteriography for diagnosing aortic injury.[117] If the aorta appears normal on a reasonably high-quality CTA study in all views, it should be declared intact despite the presence of mediastinal blood. If the MDCTA cannot be comfortably considered normal due to technical factors or difficulty distinguishing injury from anatomic variants, then catheter angiography can serve as an appropriate adjunct to help clarify the situation.

Typically, thoracic aortic injuries from blunt trauma occur at the level of the proximal descending aorta at the level of the right mainstem bronchus and left pulmonary artery. Generally, a pseudoaneurysm arises from the anterior aspect of the aorta (Figs. 13.121 and 13.123), although laterally oriented pseudoaneurysms are also seen (Fig. 13.124). Flaps arising from partial tears of the aortic wall, usually composed of intima and media, are seen at the base of the pseudoaneurysm (Figs. 13.107, 13.110, 13.121, 13.123, and

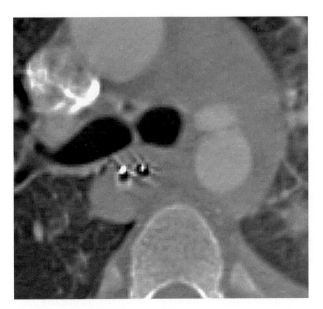

Figure 13.121. CT mediastinal hemorrhage. Axial IV contrast-enhanced CT shows pseudoaneurysm arising from anterior proximal descending aorta. There is large surrounding hematoma producing rightward displacement of the trachea and esophagus marked by nasogastric tubes. The pseudoaneurysm contributes to the mass effect.

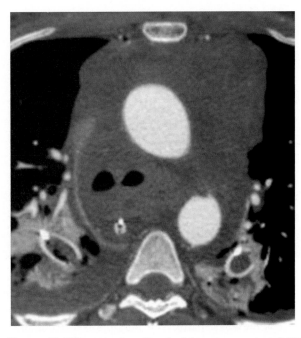

Figure 13.122. CT of mediastinal hematoma. Axial IV contrast-enhanced CT image demonstrates large hematoma (aortic injury not shown) displacing esophagus and trachea to the right and marked bowing azygous vein due to mass effect.

13.124). Classically, the contour of the pseudoaneurysm is hemispheric with its base adjacent to the aortic lumen (Figs. 13.110, 13.121, 13.123, and 13.124). The interior of the pseudoaneurysm may be smooth (Figs. 13.122–13.124) or irregular

(Figs. 13.109 and 13.126), and the edges are mainly attached to the aorta proper at acute (Figs. 13.126 and 13.127) or right angles (Figs. 13.110, 13.121, 13.123, and 13.124). The pseudoaneurysm may extend partially or near completely around the

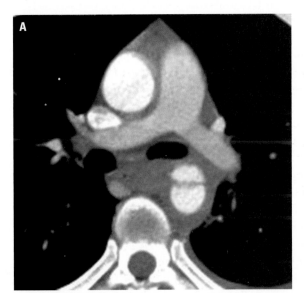

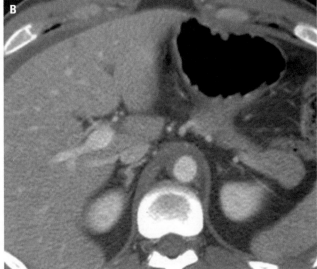

Figure 13.123. Pericrural mediastinal hematoma with aortic injury. **A:** Axial CT contrast-enhanced image shows anterior pseudoaneurysm arising from aorta at the level of the tracheal bifurcation. Hemorrhage surrounds the aorta, displacing the carina anteriorly and the esophagus to the right. **B:** A collar of blood tracts down along the aorta to the level of the diaphragmatic crura.

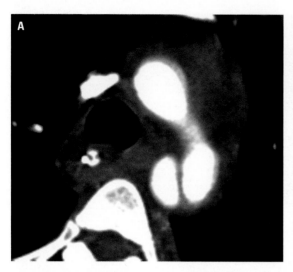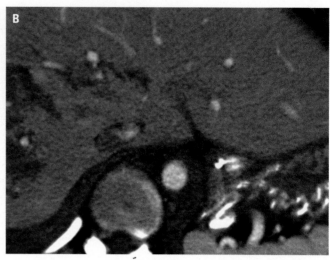

Figure 13.124. Pericrural mediastinal hematoma with aortic injury. **A:** Axial contrast-enhanced CT image shows pseudoaneurysm directed laterally to the right with surrounding mediastinal hematoma displacing esophagus mainly to the right. Blood also tracts along the left paraspinal space. **B:** Blood surrounds the aorta at the aortic hiatus. Note multiple liver lacerations.

aortic circumference (Figs. 13.121, 13.123, 13.124, 13.126, and 13.127). Direct findings of aortic injury had an 88% positive predictive value in a study by Ng and colleagues.[118] In this series, an intimal flap was the most sensitive and specific

sign of aortic injury.[119] Cleverley[105] found a pseudoaneurysm in 97%, a diffusely enlarged aorta in 32%, and an intimal flap in 91% of 34 patients with TAI.

Large pseudoaneurysms are under arterial pressure and may compress the intact portion of the aorta and diminish distal flow pressure. This compression results in a diminution in size of the distal aorta that can be appreciated in its lower thoracic portion but is often best appreciated in the upper abdomen (Figs. 13.123, 13.124, and 13.128). The aortic branches will also be narrowed in diameter. A similar appearance can also occur from extreme hypovolemia that should also be considered. Detection of the "small aorta sign" in the abdominal CT should draw attention to the thorax for proximal aortic injury. Periaortic hemorrhage extending to the diaphragmatic crura is also seen some patients with aortic injury (Figs. 13.123 and 13.124).[98] Wong and Gotway[98] reported that this finding had 70% sensitivity, 98% specificity, 74% positive predictive value, and negative predictive value of 92% for aortic injury. This finding had a likelihood ratio of 10.8 for the presence of TAI.[98] A study by Curry and colleagues[119] showed a sensitivity of 88% and positive predictive value of 97% for the association of periaortic hemorrhage and TAI. The major importance of this sign is to draw attention to the chest for potential TAI if the abdomen pelvis is scanned without including the thorax.

Figure 13.125. Axial contrast-enhanced CT image shows large periaortic mediastinal hemorrhage due to vertebral body fracture (arrow). Mediastinal structures are primarily displaced anteriorly in the case.

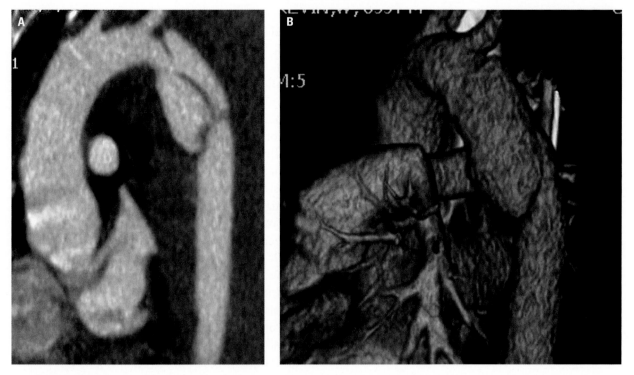

Figure 13.126. Irregular pseudoaneurysms with acute angles with aortic lumen. **A:** Reformatted image along axis of aorta shows complex pseudoaneurysm of proximal descending aorta with underlying intimal flaps connecting to aortic lumen at acute angles **B:** Volume rendering shows length of pseudoaneurysm, acute angle with aortic lumen, and proximity to left subclavian artery origin.

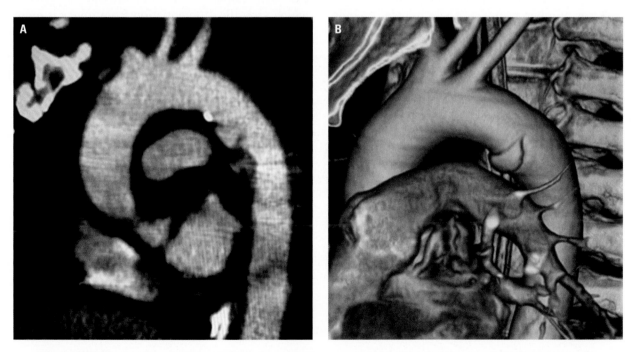

Figure 13.127. Small typical pseudoaneurysm forming acute angle with aortic lumen. **A:** Reformatted contrast-enhanced CT image along major axis of aorta demonstrates a small pseudoaneurysm with intimal flaps forming acute angles with aortic lumen. Small adjacent calcification is probably a remnant of the ductus arteriosus. **B:** Volume-rendered image shows shape of aneurysm and acute angles of its base with aortic lumen.

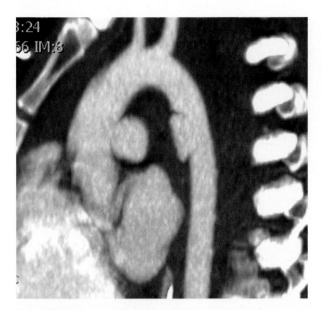

Figure 13.128. Coarctation of aorta by pseudoaneurysm. Volume-rendered image shows typical pseudoaneurysm in medial proximal descending aorta with decrease in aortic diameter below injury site.

As mentioned earlier, in the current generation of high-number multidetector scanners, it is more common to diagnose less overt injuries that were probably often not seen using conventional or low-detector number scanners. These injuries include

partial wall tears resulting in luminal flaps, intramural hemorrhage, abrupt contour changes in the aortic circumference, and shallow pseudoaneurysms. The precise definition of what constitutes a shallow pseudoaneurysmhas been suggested by Gavant and colleagues[120] but still is a subject for further research. Rarely, there is a full-thickness tear of the aortic wall allowing active bleeding, usually with a large surrounding hematoma. This is a highly unstable circumstance with only adjacent structures and the parietal pleural containing the high-pressure leak, naturally resulting in very high mortality.

There are variants of normal anatomy that can mimic aortic injuries. The most common is the ductus bump arising from the anterior aspect of the proximal descending aorta (Figs. 13.129 and 13.130). This structure usually occurs as a smooth outpouching from the aorta with obtuse margins with the aortic wall and smooth internal walls. A calcified ductus remnant may be present originating from the ductus approaching the left pulmonary artery or even rarely, a patent ductus can be occasionally found (Figs. 13.131 and 13.132). Unfortunately, sometimes the ductus does not conform to this classic appearance, manifesting acute or right angle contours with the aortic lumen or irregular internal margins in which case, the differentiation from injury is more

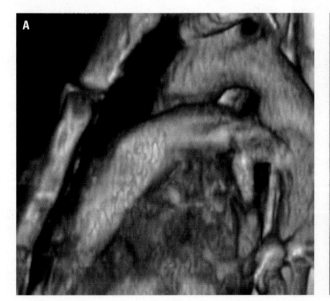
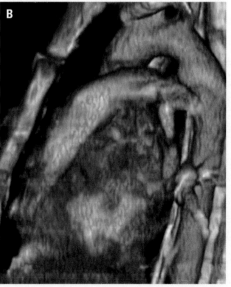

Figure 13.129. Ductus diverticulum. **A:** Axial contrast-enhanced CT image shows a contrast collection between ascending and descending aorta and mediastinal hematoma displacing carina and esophagus to the right. **B:** A reformatted image through the long axis of aorta shows a smooth outpouching without intimal flaps and 90-degree and obtuse interface margin with aorta. This was diagnosed as a ductus diverticulum without further evaluation.

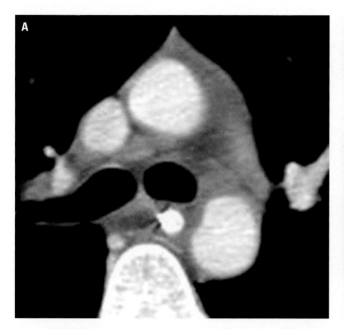

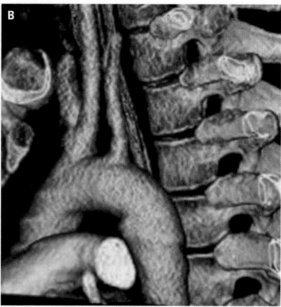

Figure 13.130. Ductus diverticulum. **A:** Axial contrast-enhanced CT image shows smooth outpouching of aorta at level of carina. Note lack of intimal flaps, lack of mediastinal blood, and obtuse angles of diverticulum makes with aortic lumen. **B:** 3D volumetric rendering of ductus in closer proximity to left pulmonary artery than case above.

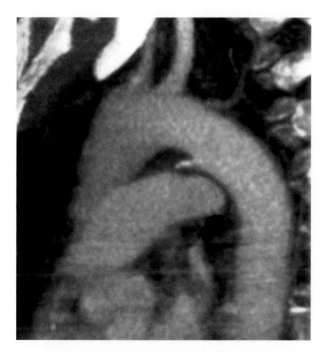

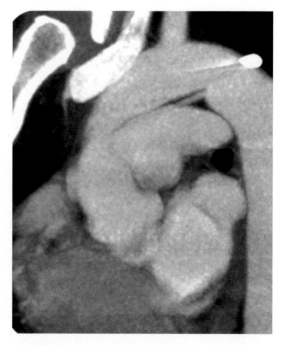

Figure 13.131. Ductus arteriosus remnant. An off-sagittal reformatted image through major axis of contrast-enhanced aorta shows partially calcified remnant of the ductus arteriosus pointing to left pulmonary artery.

Figure 13.132. Patent ductus arteriosus. An off-sagittal reformatted image through major axis of contrast-enhanced aorta shows small patent ductus between ductus diverticulum and left pulmonary artery. Again, typical ductus has a smooth contour, no intimal flaps, and obtuse margins with aortic lumen.

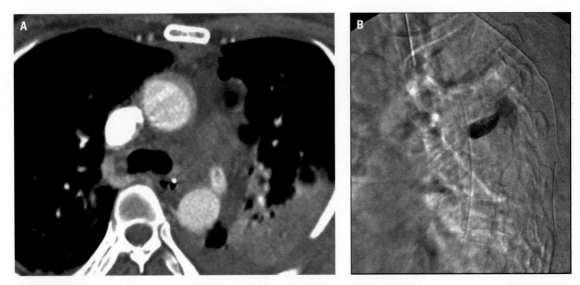

Figure 13.133. Atypical ductus. Contrast-enhanced axial CT image (**A**) from blunt trauma patient shows rectangular outpouching from anterior proximal descending aorta with surrounding hematoma but no mass effect on trachea or nasogastric tube. **B:** Catheter angiogram shows a smooth, rectangular outpouching from aorta. Although atypical in appearance, this finding was believed to be a ductus diverticulum rather than pseudoaneurysm of aorta. (From Steenburg SD, Ravenel JG, Ikonomidis JS, et al. Acute traumatic aortic injury: imaging evaluation and management. *Radiology.* 2008;248(3):748–762, with permission.)

challenging (Fig. 13.133). The lack of any surrounding periaortic hemorrhage is an extremely useful indicator that the finding is *not* an injury. The lack of intimal flaps at the base of the outpouching is additional strong evidence against a traumatic origin of the finding. Other entities that can mimic aortic injury include a diverticular origin of a bronchial artery, an aortic ulcer, and an irregular luminal contour from atherosclerosis (Fig. 13.134). Rarely, the author has found that performing an endoluminal

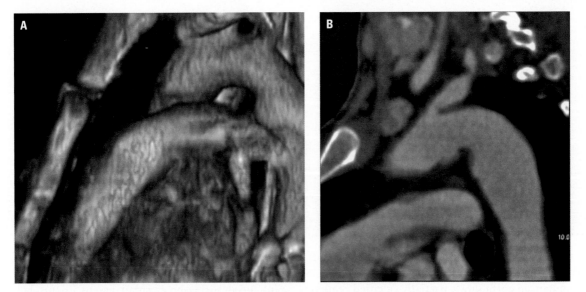

Figure 13.134. Probable atherosclerotic ulcer. **A:** Contrast-enhanced CT image shows outpouching arising from ascending aorta *(arrow)*. There is no mediastinal hematoma. **B:** Reformatted image through long axis of aorta shows a slightly irregular outpouching *(arrow)* opposite the left subclavian origin. Other irregularities of the aortic wall, location, and lack of mediastinal blood suggested this finding was more like the result of atherosclerosis.

view of the aorta and verifying an intact wall offers convincing evidence that the questionable finding is not due to trauma.

Less common sites of aortic injury include the aortic arch, ascending aorta (usually at the aortic root) (Fig. 13.135), and just above the diaphragm—all locations where there is an adjacent change in the degree of fixation of the aorta predisposing to greater shearing forces. Arch injuries typically involve one or more origins of great vessel branches (Fig. 13.136). Vascular injuries in the major branches can exist independently or concurrently with an aortic injury. Major branch vessels injuries usually are surrounded by predominantly superior mediastinal hematoma. Although quite rare, two injuries at different locations in the aorta should always be excluded.

Aortic Injury Treatment

The CT angiographic appearance of the aortic injury, considered in conjunction with the patient's overall clinical status, is vital to select optimal

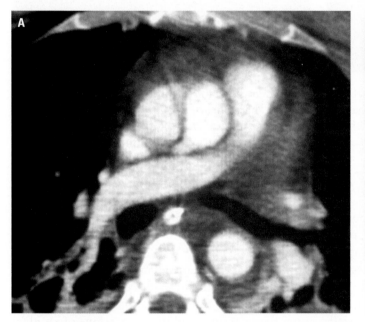

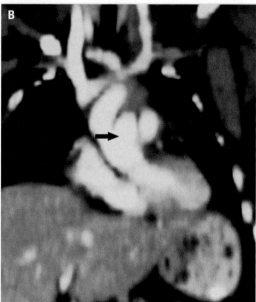

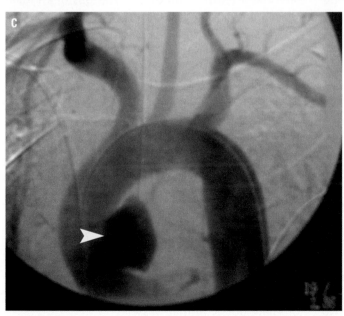

Figure 13.135. Ascending traumatic aortic pseudoaneurysm. **A:** Axial contrast-enhanced CT image of blunt trauma patient was initially interpreted as negative for aortic injury. The apparently wide ascending aorta is actually a pseudoaneurysm between the proximal ascending aorta and main pulmonary artery *(arrow)*. **B:** The pseudoaneurysm is better appreciated on a coronal reformation *(arrow)*. **C:** Catheter aortogram confirms ascending aortic pseudoaneurysm *(arrowhead)*.

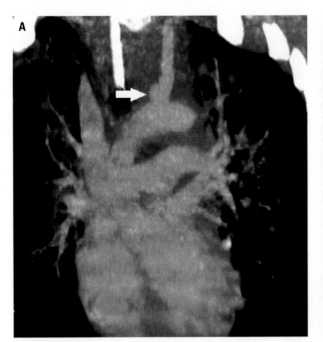
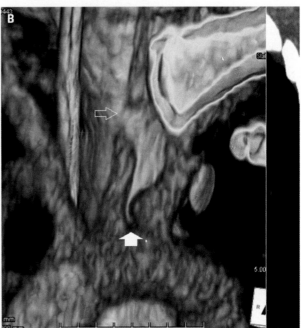

Figure 13.136. Pseudoaneurysm at great vessel root. **A:** Axial contrast-enhanced coronal reformatted image of blunt trauma patient shows pseudoaneurysm at root of left subclavian artery *(arrow)* with surrounding hemorrhage. **B:** Volume-rendered CT image shows pseudoaneurysm *(arrow)* extending to the aortic arch. Note second injury producing near occlusion of the left common carotid artery *(open arrow).*

treatment. In cases where the aortic injury appears minor and noninvasive treatment is initiated, early follow-up CT angiogram at 24 to 48 hours and again at 3 to 4 weeks to document stability, progression, or resolution of the injury is recommended. The clinical option of modulating blood pressure to diminish wall tension during this follow-up period may be prudent. Alternatively, minor injuries may be stented depending on management preference. Treatment with stent graft coverage has become the treatment of choice for ATAI over the past 5 years when technically feasible.[121] When necessary to achieve adequate injury coverage in an emergency setting, the left subclavian artery origin may need to be partially or completely covered by the stent graft, with a low, but not insignificant, incidence of complications including stroke, paraplegia, paralysis, and endoleak.[122] Some stents are fenestrated to allow placement into the left subclavian artery to maintain direct perfusion.[123] Mediastinotomy or left thoracotomy is performed if the injury cannot be stented for anatomic reasons or there are concurrent major vascular injuries, such as an ascending aorta or cerebrovascular artery, that require surgical repair. Stent grafts have been shown to decrease operative mortality, paraplegia, injury to the recurrent laryngeal nerve, and blood product usage compared to open surgical repair.[124–126]

Certain measurements are required to assist in stent graft placement as described earlier. If the midportion of the stent is placed at the injury site, the proximal and distal locations of an ideal placement can be determined. Diameters should be measured at right angles to the lumen walls perpendicular to the long axis of the aorta. The long axis distance from the proximal left subclavian or the nearest aortic branch (e.g., aberrant right subclavian artery) to the proximal injury site is required. The long axis aortic length of the injury is also obtained. Any abnormal aortic anatomy must be described (Fig. 13.137). Also, two-dimensional images through the long axis of the aorta and volumetric views of the injury from several perspectives are helpful to optimize the anatomy and, in some cases, decide if stent graft placement is a feasible option. A repeat CT-angiogram is necessary to confirm appropriate stent position with adequate coverage of the injury site without endoleak or unintended coverage of major aortic branch vessels.

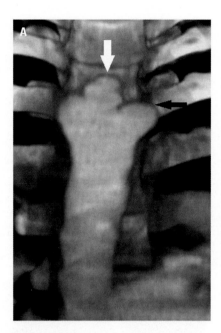 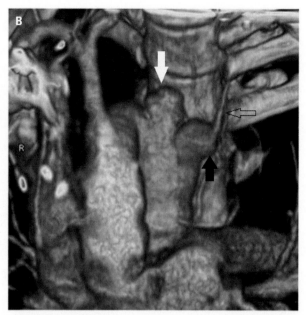

Figure 13.137. Aortic injury to congenitally variant thoracic aortic. **A:** Anterior view maximum intensity projection of contrast-enhanced CT shows pseudoaneurysm *(white arrow)* arising between right aortic arch and diverticulum of Kommerell *(black arrow)*. **B:** Volume-rendered image from anterior perspective shows superiorly directed pseudoaneurysm *(solid white arrow)*, diverticulum of Kommerell *(solid black arrow)*, and atretic left subclavian artery *(open arrow)* arising from diverticulum.

Complications of stent placement include migration, complete occlusion of uninjured aortic branches, oversizing the stent, suboptimal placement with proximal stent extending tangentially to the aortic wall and protruding into the aortic lumen promoting stent-collapse (Figs. 13.138 and 13.139),[127] inadequate injury coverage, endoleak, and procedural errors not directly related to stent positioning (Fig. 13.140). Some complications can be managed by additional stent placement within or adjacent to

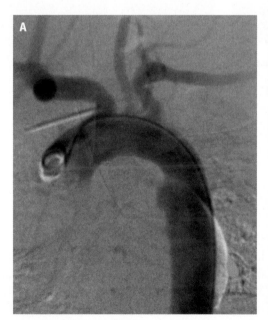 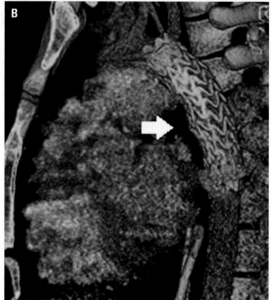

Figure 13.138. Proper stent graft positioning. **A:** Catheter aortogram shows typical proximal descending aortic pseudoaneurysm. **B:** Stent graft is centered over pseudoaneurysm with slight bulge at site of injury *(arrow)*.

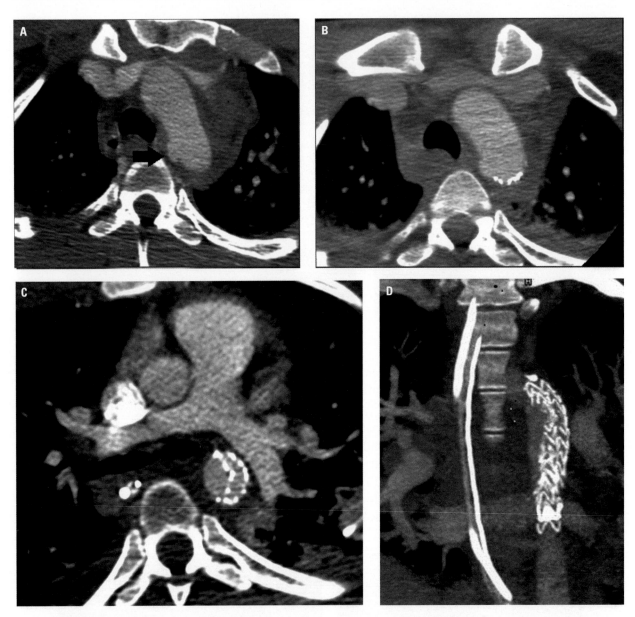

Figure 13.139 Inappropriate stent graft placement. **A:** Axial contrast-enhanced CT image shows small pseudoaneurysm arising from proximal descending aorta *(arrow)* surrounded by mediastinal blood. **B:** Proximal part of stent does not cover pseudoaneurysm. **C** and **D:** Exposed to high luminal pressure in the pseudoaneurysm portion that is not covered, the stent is compressed in its proximal portion, and the patient required surgical intervention.

(partially overlapping) the first stent (Fig. 13.141), but they may require surgical intervention.

Pediatric Aortic Injury

ATAI is rare in children younger than the age of 16 years. Trachiotis and colleagues[128] reported six patients, with the youngest being 8 years of age; Lowe and colleagues[129] also report ATAI in six children,

the youngest being 5 years of age; and Erb and colleagues[130] report three patients with ATAI ranging in age from 10 to 12 years. In all instances, the diagnosis was suspected based on the mechanism of injury and abnormal CXR. The diagnosis of ATAT was established by CXR, catheter aortography, and/or TEE and was confirmed surgically, except for one patient described by Lowe and colleagues

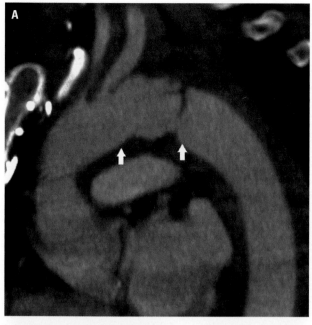

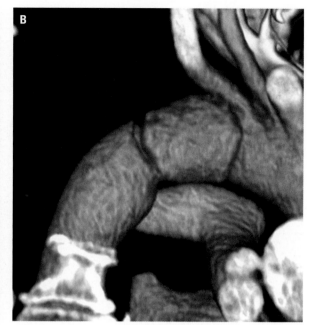

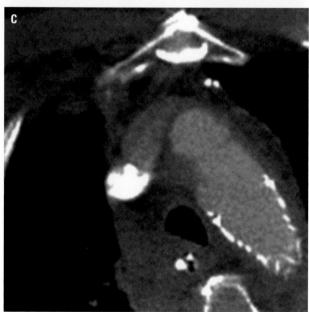

Figure 13.140 Inappropriate stent-graft placement. **A:** Reformatted CT image along axis of aorta shows extent of injury *(arrows)* extending proximally to origin of left subclavian artery. **B:** Volume-rendered image from posterior view clearly shows length of injury and proximity to left subclavian origin. **C:** Axial CT image after stent graft placement shows that proximal portion of injury is not covered by graft. The patient ultimately had surgical repair of the injury.

in whom the aortic "transection" was found at autopsy; the patient having died from closed head injury. In all reported patients, the mechanism of injury was motor vehicle collision.

CONCLUSION

The following factors should be considered in the imaging evaluation of patients sustaining major blunt trauma at risk for ATAI.

1. The only chest radiographic signs of ATAR (rupture) are those of exsanguination (e.g., massive or progressive hemomediastinum, left hemothorax).
2. Because of the pathology of ATAT (tear) and the etiology of the coexistent mediastinal hematoma, there are no plain chest radiographic signs of ATAT.
3. With the appropriate mechanism of injury, plain chest radiographic signs of (1) abnormal superior mediastinum contour, (2) a widened left mediastinal stripe extending above the aortic arch to

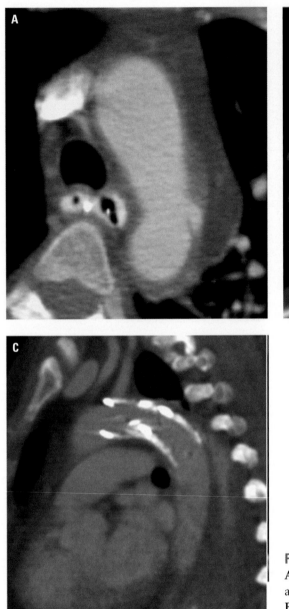

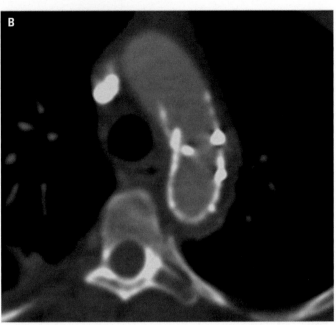

Figure 13.141. Two stent grafts to cover pseudoaneurysm. **A:** Contrast-enhanced axial CT image shows pseudoaneurysm arising from proximal descending aorta in atypical location. **B** and **C:** The initially placed stent graft did not entirely cover injury site, and a second tandem stent was required.

form an apical–pleural cap, (3) an abnormally wide right paratracheal stripe, and (4) displacement of the trachea and/or esophagus to the right of midline are relatively specific but not sensitive for mediastinal hematoma. An abnormal superior mediastinal contour is sensitive but not specific for mediastinal hemorrhage.

4. All patients with chest radiographic signs of mediastinal hematoma and an appropriate mechanism of injury require emergent MDCTA or catheter angiography (Generally, CTA is used as the initial study).

5. Patients who have technically high-quality CXRs without any signs of mediastinal hematoma, even with an appropriate mechanism of injury, do not typically require CTA or catheter aortography to exclude ATAI. However, rare cases of ATAI, usually with minimal injuries and without associated mediastinal hemorrhage, have been observed, and thus, this approach requires further validation.

6. There is an increasing reliance on CTA of the chest as part of a whole-body CT screening process for patients sustaining major blunt polytrauma.

7. A normal appearance of the aorta and proximal arterial branches on a technically satisfactory CTA study excludes major vascular injury, despite the presence of periaortic or generalized mediastinal hemorrhage.

8. Aortic stent graft placement is the most frequent technique for treating ATAI. Thus, accurate measurements of the injury length, proximity of aortic branch vessels, alterations of normal aortic anatomy, and aortic luminal diameter above and below the injury location are required.

Acute Traumatic Rupture of the Diaphragm

Acute traumatic rupture of the diaphragm (ATRD) can result from penetrating (34%) or blunt (66%) trauma. A literature review by Mueller and Pendarvis[131] of 1,345 cases of diaphragmatic rupture revealed that of all cases, 853 (67.2%) involved the left hemidiaphragm, 359 (28.3%) involved the right, and 58 (4.5%) were bilateral and involved the central tendons. Of the 887 ruptures secondary to blunt trauma, 606 (73.1%) involved the left and 195 (23.5%) the right hemidiaphragm, with 28 (3.4%) being bilateral. These statistics refute the traditional 90/10 left-to-right incidence of diaphragmatic rupture, particularly with reference to blunt trauma etiology. This observation should heighten our awareness of the radiographic subtlety of rupture of the right hemidiaphragm. The same study found that 94% of patients with ATRD had associated injuries. The study also found that the diagnosis of ATRD was suggested on the initial CXR in 70% of cases and correctly diagnosed in 50% of cases. Surgical literature reports the diagnosis of ATRD being made in approximately 45% of cases on the initial CXR examinations.[132] The study by Mueller and Pendarvis[131] found no fatalities directly related to ATRD. Surgical literature supports this observation as well.

With the statistics cited earlier relative to the accuracy of diagnosis of ATRD during patient assessment in the emergency center, it is obvious that none of the imaging modalities currently available is "best" for the diagnosis of ATRD in everyday practice. Most commonly recommended is the supine CXR, either before or after insertion of a nasogastric (NGT) tube. Shapero and colleagues[133] and Gelman and colleagues[134] report accuracy of 42% and 14%, respectively, in the diagnosis of

ATRD by CT. However, a recently described helical CT protocol has been shown to be accurate in a swine model.[135] Hoy and Shortsleeve[136] have demonstrated helical CT sagittal and coronal reformations to accurately show the site and extent of diaphragmatic tear. MR, because of all its intrinsic imaging advantages, optimally demonstrates the diaphragmatic "collar" and the herniated abdominal contents.[137] However, the intrinsic disadvantages of MR cited earlier relative to imaging the acutely injured patient make MR best suited for confirming a suspected diaphragmatic rupture in a clinically stable patient.

For all the reasons stated earlier, and because CXR is part of the initial blunt trauma patient evaluation, CXR remains the imaging modality with which the diagnosis of ATRD should be made. The traditional, and most common, CXR findings include, on the left, elevation of the hemidiaphragm; the presence of stomach, splenic flexure, and/or small bowel within the chest; compression atelectasis at the left base; and, usually, a left hemothorax and displacement of the heart and mediastinum to the right. Passage of an nasogastric tube (NGT) is commonly advocated in emergency medicine and surgical literature to establish the diagnosis by confirming the abnormal position of the stomach. The position of the NGT, by itself, cannot distinguish ATRD from a hiatal hernia or congenital eventration of the left hemidiaphragm [134] .

Acute traumatic rupture of the right hemidiaphragm is frequently difficult to diagnose on the initial CXR because the diaphragmatic rent is filled by the dome of the liver, leaving apparent elevation of the right hemidiaphragm as the only finding. Right hemothorax and basilar subsegmental atelectasis may be present.

REFERENCES

1. Haramati LB, Hochsztein JG, Marciano N, et al. Evaluation of the role of chest CT in the management of trauma patients. *Emerg Radiol.* 1996;3:1–6.
2. Hunink MG, Bos JJ. Triage of patients to angiography for detection of aortic rupture after blunt chest trauma: cost-effectiveness analysis of using CT. *Am J Roentgenol.* 1995;165(1):27–36.
3. Wolfman NT, Gilpin JW, Bechtold RE, et al. Occult pneumothorax in patients with abdominal trauma: CT studies. *J Comput Assist Tomogr.* 1993;17(1):56–59.

4. Karabulut N, Goodman LR. The role of helical CT in the diagnostic work-up for pulmonary embolism. *Emerg Radiol.* 1999;6(1):10–16.

5. Webb WR, Müller NL, Naidich DP. Diseases characterized primarily by nodular or reticulo-nodular opacities. In: *High-resolution CT of the Lung.* 2nd ed. Philadelphia, PA: Lippincott-Raven; 1996:149–191.

6. Kopecky KK, Buckwalter KA, Sokiranski R. Multi-slice CTspirals past single-slice CT in diagnostic efficacy. *Diagn Imaging.* 1999;21(4):36–42.

7. Fishman EK. Multislice technology raises the bar for spiral CT. *Diagn Imaging.* 1999;21:7.

8. Remy-Jardin M, Remy J, Artaud D, et al. Spiral CT of pulmonary embolism: technical considerations and interpretive pitfalls. *J Thorac Imaging.* 1997;12(2):103–117.

9. Goodman LR, Lipchik RJ, Kuzo RS. Acute pulmonary embolism: the role of computed tomographic imaging. *J Thorac Imaging.* 1997;12(2):83–86.

10. Mirvis SE, Shanmuganathan K, Miller BH, et al. Traumatic aortic injury: diagnosis with contrast-enhanced thoracic CT—five-year experience at a major trauma center. *Radiology.* 1996;200(2):413–422.

11. Patel NH, Stephens KE Jr, Mirvis SE, et al. Imaging of acute thoracic aortic injury due to blunt trauma: a review. *Radiology.* 1998;209(2):335–348.

12. Sebastià C, Pallisa E, Quiroga S, et al. Aortic dissection: diagnosis and follow-up with helical CT. *Radiographics.* 1999;19(1):45–60.

13. Cohn SM, Burns GA, Jaffe C, et al. Exclusion of aortic tear in the unstable trauma patient: the utility of transesophageal echocardiography. *J Trauma.* 1995;39(6):1087–1090.

14. Smith MD, Cassidy JM, Souther S, et al. Transesophageal echocardiography in the diagnosis of traumatic rupture of the aorta. *N Engl J Med.* 1995;332(6):356–362.

15. Keats TE. The aortic-pulmonary mediastinal stripe. *Am J Roentgenol Radium Ther Nucl Med.* 1972;116(1):107–109.

16. Felson B, Felson H. Localization of intrathoracic lesions by means of the postero-anterior roentgenogram;the silhouette sign. *Radiology.* 1950;55(3):363–374.

17. Hoffman RB, Rigler LG. Evaluation of left ventricular enlargement in the lateral projection of the chest. *Radiology.* 1965;85:93–100.

18. Ballinger WP, Rutherford RB, Zuidema GD, eds. *The Management of Trauma.* Philadelphia, PA: WB Saunders; 1968.

19. Gibson LD, Carter R, Hinshaw DB. Surgical significance of sternal fracture. *Surg Gynecol Obstet.* 1962;114:443–448.

20. Raptopoulos V, Sheiman RG, Phillips DA, et al. Traumatic aortic tear: screening with chest CT. *Radiology.* 1982;182(3):667–673.

21. Morgan PW, Goodman LR, Aprahamian C, et al. Evaluation of traumatic aortic injury: does dynamic contrast-enhanced CT play a role? *Radiology.* 1992;182(3):661–666.

22. Mirvis SE, Kostrubiak I, Whitley NO, et al. Role of CT in excluding major arterial injury after blunt thoracic trauma. *Am J Roentgenol.* 1987;149(3):601–605.

23. Harris JH Jr, Horowitz DR, Zelitt DL. Unenhanced dynamic mediastinal computed tomography in the selection of patients requiring thoracic aortography for the detection of acute traumatic aortic injury. *Emerg Radiol.* 1995;2(2):67–76.

24. Fisher RG, Ward RE, Ben-Menachem Y, et al. Arteriography and the fractured first rib: too much for too little? *Am J Roentgenol.* 1982;138(6):1059–1062.

25. Lee J, Harris JH Jr, Duke JH Jr, et al. Noncorrelation between thoracic skeletal injuries and acute traumatic aortic tear. *J Trauma.* 1997;43(3):400–404.

26. Harris RD, Harris JH Jr. The prevalence and significance of missed scapular fractures in blunt chest trauma. *Am J Roentgenol.* 1988;151(4):747–750.

27. Hardegger FH, Simpson LA, Weber BG. The operative treatment of scapular fractures. *J Bone Joint Surg Br.* 1984;66(5):725–731.

28. Lee RB, Bass SM, Morris JA Jr, et al. Three or more rib fractures as an indicator for transfer to a Level I trauma center: a population-based study. *J Trauma.* 1990;30(6):689–694.

29. Nettles JL, Linscheid RL. Sternoclavicular dislocations. *J Trauma.* 1968;8(2):158–164.

30. Cope R, Riddervold HO. Posterior dislocation of the sternoclavicular joint: report of two cases, with emphasis on radiologic management and early diagnosis. *Skeletal Radiol.* 1988;17(4):247–250.

31. Kirsh MM, Sloan H. *Blunt Chest Trauma.* Boston, MA: Little, Brown and Company; 1977.

32. Clark GC, Schecter WP, Trunkey DD. Variables affecting outcome in blunt chest trauma: flail chest vs. pulmonary contusion. *J Trauma.* 1988;28(3):298–304.

33. Fulton RL, Peter ET, Wilson JN. The pathophysiology and treatment of pulmonary contusions. *J Trauma.* 1970;10:719.

34. Alfano GS, Hale HW Jr. Pulmonary contusion. *J Trauma.* 1965;5(5):647–658.

35. Vyas PK, Sivit C. Imaging of blunt pediatric thoracic trauma. *Emerg Radiol.* 1997;4:16–25.

36. Williams JR, StembridgeVA. Pulmonary contusion secondary to nonpenetrating chest trauma. *Am J Roentgenol.* 1964;91:284.

37. Eddy AC, Carrico CJ, Rusch VW. Injury to the lung and pleura. In: Moore EE, Mattox KL, Feliciano DV, eds. *Trauma*. 2nd ed. Norwalk, CT: Appleton & Lange; 1991:358–359.

38. Greening R, Kynette A, Hodes PJ. Unusual pulmonary changes secondary to chest trauma. *Am J Roentgenol Radium Ther Nucl Med*. 1957;77(6):1059–1065.

39. Fagan CJ, Swischuk LE. Traumatic lung and paramediastinal pneumatoceles. *Radiology*. 1976;120(1):11–18.

40. Ellis R. Traumatic lung cysts. *JAMA*. 1976;236(17):1976–1977.

41. Santos GH, Mahendra T. Traumatic pulmonary pseudocysts. *Ann Thorac Surg*. 1979;27(4):359–362.

42. Reed JC. *Chest Radiology: Plain Film Patterns and Differential Diagnosis*. 2nd ed. Chicago, IL: Year Book; 1987.

43. Naclerio EA. *Chest Injuries: Physiologic Principles and Emergency Management*. New York, NY: Grune & Stratton; 1971.

44. Visweswaran A, Harris JH Jr. Identification of tension hemopneumothorax on supine chest radiograph: value of the visceral pleural line sign. *Emerg Radiol*. 1996;3:158–165.

45. Bridges KG, Welch G, Silver M, et al. CT detection of occult pneumothorax in multiple trauma patients. *J Emerg Med*. 1993;11(2):179–186.

46. Blaisdell FW. Pneumothorax and hemothorax. In: Blaisdell FW, Trunkey DD, eds. *Cervicothoracic trauma*. New York, NY: Thieme; 1994:215–253.

47. Enderson BL, Abdalla R, Frame SB, et al. Tube thoracostomy for occult pneumothorax: a prospective randomized study of its use. *J Trauma*. 1993;35(5):726–729.

48. Rhea JT, Novelline RA, Lawrason J, et al. The frequency and significance of thoracic injuries detected on abdominal CT scans of multiple trauma patients. *J Trauma*. 1989;29(4):502–505.

49. Yip D, Tsung S, Harris JH Jr. Occult pneumothorax: incidence and clinical significance. Manuscript in preparation.

50. Symbas PN. *Cardiothoracic Trauma*. Philadelphia, PA: WB Saunders; 1989.

51. Mason AC, Mirvis SE, Templeton PA. Imaging of acute tracheobronchial injury: review of the literature. *Emerg Radiol*. 1994;1:250–260.

52. Unger JM, Schuchmann GG, Grossman JE, et al. Tears of the trachea and main bronchi caused by blunt trauma: radiologic findings. *Am J Roentgenol*. 1989;153(6):1175–1180.

53. Godwin JD, Merten DF, Baker ME. Paramediastinal pneumatocele: alternative explanations to gas in the pulmonary ligament. *Am J Roentgenol*. 1985;145(3):525–530.

54. Heitzman ER. *The Mediastinum: Radiologic Correlations with Anatomy and Pathology*. 2nd ed. Berlin, Germany: Springer-Verlag; 1988.

55. Naclerio EA. The V sign in the diagnosis of spontaneous rupture of the esophagus (an early roentgen clue). *Am J Surg*. 1957;93(2):291–298.

56. Levin B. The continuous diaphragm sign. A newly-recognized sign of pneumomediastinum. *Clin Radiol*. 1973;24(3):337–338.

57. Moseley JE. Loculated pneumomediastinum in the newborn. A thymic "spinnaker sail" sign. *Radiology*. 1960;75:788–790.

58. Wilson D, Voystock JF, Sariego J, et al. Role of computed tomography scan in evaluating the widened mediastinum. *Am Surg*. 1994;60(6):421–423.

59. Parmley LF, Mattingly TW, Manion WC, et al. Nonpenetrating traumatic injury of the aorta. *Circulation*. 1958;17(6):1086–1101.

60. Fisher RG, Hadlock F. Laceration of the thoracic aorta and brachiocephalic arteries by blunt trauma. Report of 54 cases and review of the literature. *Radiol Clin North Am*. 1981;19(1):91–110.

61. Creasy JD, Chiles C, Routh WD, et al. Overview of traumatic injury of the thoracic aorta. *Radiographics*. 1997;17(1):27–45.

62. Verdant A, Mercier C, Pagé A, et al. Major mediastinal vascular injuries. *Can J Surg*. 1983;26(1):38–42.

63. Garland LH. The postero-medial pleural line. *Radiology*. 1943;41:29–33.

64. Brailsford JF. The radiologic postero-medial border of the lung, or the linear thoracic paraspinal shadow. *Radiology*. 1943;41:34–37.

65. Lachman E. A comparison of the posterior boundaries of the lungs and pleura as demonstrated on the cadaver and on the roentgenogram of the living. *Anat Rec*. 1942;83:521–542.

66. Woodring JH, Daniel TL. Mediastinal analysis emphasizing plain radiographs and computed tomograms. *Med Radiogr Photogr*. 1986;62(1):1–48.

67. Han MC, Kim CW. *Sectional Human Anatomy*. Tokyo, Japan: Igaku-Shoin; 1985.

68. Wagner M, Lawson TL. *Segmental Anatomy: Applications to Clinical Medicine*. New York, NY: Macmillan; 1982.

69. Sevitt S. Traumatic ruptures of the aorta: a clinicopathological study. *Injury*. 1977;8(3):159–173.

70. Strassmann G. Traumatic rupture of the aorta. *Am Heart J*. 1947;33(4):508–515.

71. Turney SZ, Attar S, Ayella R, et al. Traumatic rupture of the aorta. A five-year experience. *J Thorac Cardiovasc Surg*. 1976;72(5):727–734.

72. Turney SZ, Rodriguez A. Injuries to the great thoracic vessels. In: Turney SZ, Rodriguez A, Cowley RA, eds. *Management of Cardiothoracic Trauma*. Baltimore, MD: Lippincott Williams & Wilkins; 1990:229–260.

73. Saylam A, Melo JQ, Ahmad A, et al. Early surgical repair in traumatic rupture of the thoracic aorta (report of 9 cases and review of the current concepts). *J Cardiovasc Surg (Torino)*. 1980;21(3):295–302.

74. Soyer R, Brunet A, Piwnica A, et al. Traumatic rupture of the thoracic aorta with reference to 34 operated cases. *J Cardiovasc Surg (Torino)*. 1981;22(2):103–108.

75. Wilson RF, Arbulu A, Bassett JS, et al. Acute mediastinal widening following blunt chest trauma: critical decisions. *Arch Surg*. 1972;104(4):551–558.

76. Plume S, DeWeese JA. Traumatic rupture of the thoracic aorta. *Arch Surg*. 1979;114(3):240–243.

77. Lipchik EO, Robinson KE. Acute traumatic rupture of the thoracic aortic. *Am J Roentgenol Radium Ther Nucl Med*. 1968;104(2):408–412.

78. Griffith GL, Mattingly WT Jr, Tood EP. Current diagnosis and management of blunt thoracic aortic trauma. *J Ky Med Assoc*. 1981;79(9):588–593.

79. Newman RJ, Jones IS. A prospective study of 413 consecutive car occupants with chest injuries. *J Trauma*. 1984;24(2):129–135.

80. Jackson FR, Berkas EM, Roberts VL. Traumatic aortic rupture after blunt trauma. *Dis Chest*. 1968;53(5):577–583.

81. Crass JR, Cohen AM, Motta AO, et al. A proposed new mechanism of traumatic aortic rupture: the osseous pinch. *Radiology*. 1990;176(3):645–649.

82. Cohen AM, Crass JR, Thomas HA, et al. CT evidence for the "osseous pinch" mechanism of traumatic aortic injury. *Am J Roentgenol*. 1992;159(2):271–274.

83. Katyal D, McLellan BA, Brenneman FD, et al. Lateral impact motor vehicle collisions: significant cause of blunt traumatic rupture of the thoracic aorta. *J Trauma*. 1997;42(5):769–772.

84. Rizoli SB, Brenneman FD, Boulanger BR, et al. Blunt diaphragmatic and thoracic aortic rupture: an emerging injury complex. *Ann Thorac Surg*. 1994;58(5):1404–1408.

85. McCollum CH, Graham JM, Noon GP, et al. Chronic traumatic aneurysms of the thoracic aorta: an analysis of 50 patients. *J Trauma*. 1979;19(4):248–252.

86. Petty SM, Parker LA, Mauro MA, et al. Chronic posttraumatic aortic pseudoaneurysm. Recognition before rupture. *Postgrad Med*. 1991;89(6):173–174.

87. Lundervall J. The mechanism of traumatic rupture of the aorta. *Acta Pathol Microbiol Scand*. 1964;62:34–46.

88. Blair E, Topuzlu C, Davis JH. Delayed or missed diagnosis in blunt chest trauma. *J Trauma*. 1971;11(2):129–145.

89. Mattox KL. Injury to the thoracic great vessels. In: Moore EE, Mattox KL, Feliciano DV, eds. *Trauma*. 2nd ed. Norwalk, CT: Appleton & Lange; 1991:394.

90. Hood RM, Boyd AD, Culliford AT, eds. Thoracic *Trauma*.Philadelphia, PA: WB Saunders; 1989.

91. Townsend RN, Colella JJ, Diamond DL. Traumatic rupture of the aorta: critical decisions for trauma surgeons. *J Trauma*. 1990;30(9):1169–1174.

92. Ochsner MG Jr, Champion HR, Chambers RJ, et al. Pelvic fracture as an indicator of increased risk of thoracic aortic rupture. *J Trauma*. 1989;29(10):1376–1379.

93. Marymont JV, Cotler HB, Harris JH Jr, et al. Posterior hip dislocation associated with acute traumatic injury of the thoracic aorta: a previously unrecognized injury complex. *J Orthop Trauma*. 1990;4(4):383–387.

94. Beall AC Jr, Arbegast NR, Ripepi AC, et al. Aortic laceration due to rapid deceleration. *Arch Surg*. 1969;98(5):595–601.

95. DiSumma M, Ottino GM, Trucano G, et al. Traumatic rupture of the thoracic aorta. *J Cardiovasc Surg (Torino)*. 1981;22(2):181–1863–387.

96. Ayella RJ, Hankins JR, Turney SZ, et al. Ruptured thoracic aorta due to blunt trauma. *J Trauma*. 1977;17(3):199–205.

97. Mirvis SE, Shanmuganathan K. Diagnosis of blunt traumatic aortic injury 2007: still a nemesis. *Eur J Radiol*. 2007;64(1):27–40.

98. Wong H, Gotway MB, Sasson AD, et al. Periaortic hematoma at diaphragmatic crura at helical CT: sign of blunt aortic injury in patients with mediastinal hematoma. *Radiology*. 2004;231(1):185–189.

99. Mirvis SE, Kostrubiak I, Whitley NO, et al. Role of CT in excluding major arterial injury after blunt thoracic trauma. *Radiology*. 1987;163:487–493.

100. Mattox KL. Injury to the thoracic great vessels. In: Moore EE, Mattox KL, Feliciano DV, eds. *Trauma*. 2nd ed. Norwalk, CT: Appleton & Lange; 1991;26:393–408.

101. Tisnado J, Tsai FY, Als A, et al. A new radiographic sign of acute traumatic rupture of the thoracic aorta: displacement of the nasogastric tube to the right. *Radiology*. 1977;125(3):603–608.

102. Sefczek DM, Sefczek RJ, Deeb ZL. Radiographic signs of acute traumatic rupture of the thoracic aorta. *Am J Roentgenol*. 1983;141(6):1259–1262.

103. Seltzer SE, D'Orsi C, Kirshner R, et al. Traumatic aortic rupture: plain radiographic findings. *Am J Roentgenol*. 1981;137(5):1011–1014.

104. Peters DR, Gamsu G. Displacement of the right paraspinous interface: a radiographic sign of acute traumatic rupture of the thoracic aorta. *Radiology*. 1980;134(3):599–603.

105. Cleverley JR, Barrie JR, Raymond GS, et al. Direct findings of aortic injury on contrast-enhanced CT in surgically proven traumatic aortic injury: a multicentre review. *Clin Radiol*. 2002;57(4):281–286.

106. Exadaktylos AK, Sclabas G, Schmid SW, et al. Do we really need routine computed tomographic scanning in the primary evaluation of blunt chest trauma in patients with "normal" chest radiograph? *J Trauma.* 2001;51(6):1173–1176.

107. Kearney PA, Smith DW, Johnson SB, et al. Use of transesophageal echocardiography in the evaluation of traumatic aortic injury. *J Trauma.* 1993;34(5):696–701; discussion 701–703.

108. Downing SW, Sperling JS, Mirvis SE, et al. Experience with spiral computed tomography as the sole diagnostic method for traumatic aortic rupture. *Ann Thorac Surg.* 2001;72(2):495–501.

109. Haaga JR. Radiation dose management: weighing risk versus benefit. *Am J Roentgenol.* 2001;177(2):289–291.

110. Mirvis SE. Imaging of thoracic trauma. In: Turney SZ, Rodriguez A, Cowley RA, eds. *Management of Cardiothoracic Trauma.* Baltimore, MD: Lippincott Williams & Wilkins; 1990.

111. Agee CK, Metzler MH, Churchill RJ, et al. Computed tomographic evaluation to exclude traumatic aortic disruption. *J Trauma.* 1992;33(6):876–881.

112. Raptopoulos V. Chest CT for aortic injury: maybe not for everyone. *Am J Roentgenol.* 1994;162(5):1053–1055.

113. Gavant ML, Menke PG, Fabian T, et al. Blunt traumatic aortic rupture: detection with helical CT of the chest. *Radiology.* 1995;197(1):125–133.

114. Gavant ML, Flick P, Menke PG, et al. CT aortography of thoracic aortic rupture. *Am J Roentgenol.* 1996;166:955–961.

115. Dyer DS, Moore EE, Mestek MF, et al. Can chest CT be used to exclude aortic injury? *Radiology.* 1999;213(1):195–202.

116. Parker MS, Matheson TL, Rao AV, et al. Making the transition: the role of helical CT in the evaluation of potentially acute thoracic aortic injuries. *Am J Roentgenol.* 2001;176(5):1267–1272.

117. Pate JW, Gavant ML, Weiman DS, et al. Traumatic rupture of the aortic isthmus: program of selective management. *World J Surg.* 1999;23(1):59–63.

118. Ng CJ, Chen JC, Wang LJ, et al. Diagnostic value of the helical CT scan for traumatic aortic injury: correlation with mortality and early rupture. *J Emerg Med.* 2006;30(3):277–282.

119. Curry JD, Recine CA, Snavely E, et al. Periaortic hematoma on abdominal computed tomographic scanning as an indicator of thoracic aortic rupture in blunt trauma. *J Trauma.* 2002;52(4):699–702.

120. Gavant ML. Helical CT grading of traumatic aortic injuries. Impact on clinical guidelines for medical and surgical management. *Radiol Clin North Am.* 1999;37(3):553–574.

121. Morgan TA, Steenburg SD, Siegel EL, et al. Acute traumatic aortic injuries: posttherapy multidetector CT findings. *Radiographics.* 2010;30(4):851–867.

122. Dunning J, Martin JE, Shennib H, et al. Is it safe to cover the left subclavian artery when placing an endovascular stent in the descending thoracic aorta? *Interact Cardiovasc Thorac Surg.* 2008;7(4):690–697.

123. Kurimoto Y, Asai Y, Nara S, et al. Fenestrated stent-graft facilitates emergency endovascular therapy for blunt aortic injury. *J Trauma.* 2009;66(4):974–978; discussion 978–979.

124. Demetriades D, Velmahos GC, Scalea TM, et al. Diagnosis and treatment of blunt thoracic aortic injuries: changing perspectives. *J Trauma.* 2008;64(6):1415–1418.

125. Jonker FH, Giacovelli JK, Muhs BE, et al. Trends and outcomes of endovascular and open treatment for traumatic thoracic aortic injury. *J Vasc Surg.* 2010;51(3):565–571.

126. Broux C, Thony F, Chavanon O, et al. Emergency endovascular stent graft repair for acute blunt thoracic aortic injury: a retrospective case control study. *Intensive Care Med.* 2006;32(5):770–774.

127. Bandorski D, Brück M, Günther HU, et al. Endograft collapse after endovascular treatment for thoracic aortic disease. *Cardiovasc Intervent Radiol.* 2010;33(3):492–497.

128. Trachiotis GD, Sell JE, Pearson GD, et al. Traumatic thoracic aortic rupture in the pediatric patient. *Ann Thorac Surg.* 1996;62(3):724–731.

129. Lowe LH, Bulas DI, Eichelberger MD, et al. Traumatic aortic injuries in children: radiologic evaluation. *Am J Roentgenol.* 1998;170(1):39–42.

130. Erb RE, Stein SM, Mazer MJ, et al. Blunt thoracic aortic injury in children. *Emerg Radiol.* 1994;1:215–220.

131. Mueller CF, Pendarvis RW. Traumatic injury of the diaphragm: report of seven cases and extensive literature review. *Emerg Radiol.* 1994;1(3):118–132.

132. Morgan AS, Flancbaum L, Esposito T, et al. Blunt injury to the diaphragm: an analysis of 44 patients. *J Trauma.* 1986;26(6):565–568.

133. Shapero MJ, Heiberg E, Durham RM, et al. The unreliability of CT scans and initial chest radiographs in evaluating blunt trauma induced diaphragmatic rupture. *Clin Radiol.* 1996;51(1):27–30.

134. Gelman R, Mirvis SE, Gens D. Diaphragmatic rupture due to blunt trauma: sensitivity of plain chest radiographs. *Am J Roentgenol.* 1991;156(1):51–57.

135. Israel RS, McDaniel PA, Primack SL, et al. Diagnosis of diaphragmatic trauma with helical CT in a swine model. *Am J Roentgenol.* 1996;167(3):637–641.

136. Hoy JF, Shortsleeve MJ. Diagnosis of diaphragmatic rupture utilizing spiral computed tomographic reconstruction. *Emerg Radiol.* 1997;4(3):127–128.

137. Lawrason JN, Novelline RA, Rhea JT, et al. The magnetic resonance diagnosis of diaphragmatic rupture: a report of two cases. *Emerg Radiol.* 1996;3(3):137–141.

CHAPTER 14

Abdomen: Nontraumatic Emergencies

Amanda M. Jarolimek ■ John H. Harris Jr.

In this chapter, the abdomen is considered to include the solid organs and hollow viscera located between the diaphragm and the pelvic peritoneal reflections. This includes the pancreas, adrenal glands, kidneys, and ureters. This chapter discusses disease entities that are frequently encountered in patients seeking care for abdominal pain or related symptoms in the emergency center. Only disease entities for which diagnostic imaging plays an important role are included. Since the 1980s and 1990s, the role of diagnostic imaging has continued to change. Abdominal radiographs have limited use in the care of the emergency patient with abdominal signs and symptoms. Computed tomography (CT) and ultrasound (US) are the principal tools for imaging emergency patients and provide sensitive and specific means of diagnosing abdominal pathology. Selection of the appropriate diagnostic examination should be based on the clinical presentation of the patient.

GENERAL CONSIDERATIONS

The American College of Radiology (ACR) Appropriate Criteria for Imaging and Treatment Decisions provides guidelines for the symptom-based triage of patients to the appropriate diagnostic imaging study (Table 14.1). The ACR criteria outline the best uses for each modality. Radiography is the primary imaging study for screening patients with suspected small bowel obstruction or bowel perforation. It is also used to follow patients with urolithiasis. US is the primary diagnostic tool in evaluating patients with jaundice and acute right upper quadrant pain. It is highly sensitive in detecting biliary obstruction, cholelithiasis, choledocholithiasis, or acute cholelithiasis. In many institutions, in thin and average size children, US with graded compression is the preferred modality for evaluation of suspected appendicitis. US and computed tomography angiography (CTA) are the modalities used for evaluation of pulsatile abdominal masses when abdominal aneurysm is suspected. Computed tomography (CT) examinations with oral, intravenous (IV), and rectal contrast are preferred in the evaluation for abdominal abscess and appendicitis. Unenhanced multidetector CT (MDCT) of the urinary tract is used for patients with acute flank pain and hematuria with suspected urinary stones. Hepatobiliary scintigraphy (cholescintigraphy) is an additional modality used in the evaluation of right upper quadrant pain and is used to diagnose cholecystitis, particularly when an US of the right upper quadrant is normal. Barium studies are used less frequently than other modalities emergently. However, barium swallows are used for the evaluation of esophageal perforation as well as for identifying the presence of a foreign body, and upper gastrointestinal (GI) studies may be done for the evaluation of duodenal hematoma.

It is of utmost importance to correlate the patient's clinical presentation and physical exam

TABLE 14.1	Summary of American College of Radiology Appropriateness Criteria for Selected Gastrointestinal, Genitourinary, and Cardiovascular Conditions	
Clinical Presentation	**Imaging Procedure of Choice**	**Recommended Alternatives**
Suspected small bowel obstruction	CT	Supine and upright abdominal radiographs
Jaundice	US	CT MRI abdomen without contrast with MRCP ERCP
Acute right upper quadrant pain (suspect cholecystitis)	US	CT Cholescintigraphy
Acute right lower quadrant pain (suspect appendicitis)	US-graded compression (children, young women, or pregnant patients) CT (all other patients)	CT if US is equivocal
Suspected abdominal abscess	CT US	MRI Nuclear medicine white blood cell scan (postoperative)
Acute left lower quadrant pain (suspect diverticulitis)	CT	MRI (pregnant patient)
Acute pyelonephritis	No imaging in uncomplicated patient CT	Renal US CT with contrast
Acute onset flank pain (suspect stone disease)	CT low-dose renal stone protocol	Renal US with abdominal radiograph
Hematuria	CT urography IVU	US kidney and bladder
Pulsatile abdominal mass	US	CT without contrast CT with contrast CTA abdomen MRI with angiography (MRA)

CT, computed tomography; US, ultrasound; MRI, magnetic resonance imaging; IVU, intravenous urography; MRCP, magnetic resonance cholangiopancreatography; ERCP, endoscopic cholangiopancreatography; CTA, computed tomography angiography; MRA, magnetic resonance angiography.

with the imaging findings. False-positive and false-negative results are encountered in the evaluation of the acute abdomen. An imaging finding not commensurate with clinical presentation, physical exam, or laboratory studies must be viewed with some suspicion. Knowledge of detailed patient medical data facilitates the radiologist selecting the appropriate imaging modality and improves interpretation and detection of subtle diagnostic findings.

DIAGNOSTIC IMAGING MODALITIES

Conventional Abdominal Radiography

The single supine frontal view of the abdomen is also referred to as the anteroposterior (AP) or supine radiograph, or as kidney-ureter-bladder (KUB). Additional erect and decubitus views of the abdomen as well as erect view of the chest are included to supplement the evaluation of pneumoperitoneum.

This series of radiographs comprise the standard abdominal series.

The AP radiograph of the abdomen should include from above the diaphragm to the anus. The erect view of the abdomen is preferred as the second view of the abdomen if the patient is capable of standing. This allows the evaluation of air–fluid levels in the intestinal tract, whereas a semierect view fails to depict air–fluid levels. Detection of free intraperitoneal air is possible in erect and decubitus views of the abdomen. However, a semierect view may not allow free intraperitoneal air to migrate upward into an easily detected subdiaphragmatic region. Patients who are unable to stand must have a left lateral decubitus view of the abdomen.

Ultrasound

US examination of the abdomen in the acutely ill or injured patient must be tailored to the clinical indication. The three most common emergency center abdominal US examinations are (1) right upper quadrant examination for suspected gallbladder or biliary tract abnormalities, (2) right lower quadrant examination with graded compression for suspected appendicitis, and (3) examination of the aorta for patients with a pulsatile mass.

US examination of the gallbladder and the biliary tree begins with longitudinal and transverse views of the gallbladder. The gallbladder is imaged in at least one of the following positions: supine, right decubitus, erect, or prone. With a change in position, detection of mobile gallstones is facilitated. The gallbladder is also assessed for the presence of stones or sludge in the lumen, for increased thickness of the gallbladder wall, and for the presence of pericholecystic fluid. If pain is elicited upon compression of the right upper quadrant, a sonographic Murphy sign is present. Examination of the intrahepatic ducts includes transhepatic views of the right and left ducts, which lie adjacent to the portal veins. The extrahepatic bile ducts should be followed through the porta hepatis as distally as possible. The distal common bile duct should be visualized through its course to the pancreatic head.

In cases of suspected appendicitis in thin patients, graded compression often allows visualization of a dilated inflamed appendix, establishing the diagnosis of acute appendicitis. This technique, originally described by Puylaert, involves using a 7.5 MHz or 5.0 MHz linear array transducer to compress overlying bowel loops and bring the inflamed appendix into view. Although adequate compression must be applied to displace colon and intraluminal contents from the area of interest, compression should be gently released to ensure the patient remains as comfortable as possible. The technique requires tracing the ascending colon downward to the cecum and identifying the base of the appendix. The appendix is imaged in transverse and longitudinal planes. Sonographic criteria for the diagnosis of appendicitis include an outer diameter of the appendix greater than 7 mm, the lack of compressibility of the appendix mesenteric stranding, and the presence of periappendiceal fluid collection or free intraperitoneal fluid.

Abdominal US is used for rapid diagnosis of abdominal aortic aneurysm. Obesity and overlying bowel gas may render the examination inconclusive or nondiagnostic. The proper technique uses an acoustic window through overlying bowel gas loops to permit transverse and longitudinal views of the aorta. The diameter of the abdominal aorta should be measured perpendicular to the axis of insonation to avoid overestimation of the size of the aorta, which does occur if the image plane is oblique to the axis of the aorta. CTA of the chest, abdomen, and pelvis is commonly used in the emergent evaluation for aortic aneurysms or aortic dissection.

Computed Tomography

Multiplanar CT is the most valuable imaging modality in evaluating abdominal emergencies. Oral, IV, and rectal contrast improves diagnostic capabilities and allows differentiation of contrast differences between adjacent structures. When the clinical setting permits, oral contrast should be administered 30 to 45 minutes prior to a CT examination of the abdomen or pelvis. Additional oral contrast should be administered immediately before imaging, so the stomach and proximal small bowel are well opacified. A dilute barium sulfate solution or iodinated contrast medium are taken orally or given via a gastric tube. Examination of the colon and the appendix is performed best with the administration of iodinated rectal contrast or air.

Oral contrast is extremely helpful in evaluation of thin patients in whom the lack of intra-abdominal fat limits distinguishing adjacent separate structures. In larger patients or in urgent situations, oral contrast may be omitted, particularly if pathology in the GI tract is not the principal concern.

IV contrast material is administered to delineate the boundaries or solid organs and bowel from surrounding tissues and to increase relative attenuation values between normal and abnormal tissues. The intensity of contrast enhancement is a function of the dose and injection rate, the timing of the imaging examination, the patient's weight, and cardiac output. During the *vascular* phase, contrast material initially injected causes maximum vascular enhancement within the first 30 seconds after initial injection. During the *redistribution* phase, contrast rapidly redistributes to the extravascular space/tissues in the first 2 minutes after injection. At the end of redistribution, contrast enhancement of solid organs reaches its maximum. Over the next several minutes, in the *equilibrium* phase, contrast material within solid organs and vessels declines. Contrast material is excreted by the kidneys and excretion occurs over the next several hours. The proper CT scanning protocol should ensure the timing of the scan and contrast administration to allow accurate depiction of the area of interest. For most emergency

CT studies, imaging toward the end of the redistribution phase and in the early equilibrium phase maximizes the contrast between parenchymal structures and eliminates diagnostic confusion of evaluating the liver and spleen, which are affected by mixing in the early vascular phase.

Our standard examination technique consists of administration of 150 mL of low-osmolar IV contrast through an 18 gauge or larger antecubital IV catheter at 3.5 mL per second with helical scan acquisition beginning 60 to 70 seconds after the initiation of the bolus of contrast material. Delayed helical axial imaging is performed at 10 mm following a 5-minute delay following initial imaging. Children are imaged using a low radiation dose protocol. If children weigh less than 100 lb, a low-osmolar or iso-osmolar contrast is administered by hand injection if a 22 gauge or larger IV cannula can be placed in an antecubital fossa vein. The dose administered is 1.5 mL per kilogram and should not exceed 125 mL. In a child weighing greater than 100 lb, a power injection can be used via a central venous catheter or through a 24 gauge catheter if the rate of contrast injection is slow at 1 mL per second. Imaging begins at the end of contrast administration.

Technical parameters for common CT examinations of the abdomen and pelvis are detailed in Table 14.2. For the initial contrast-enhanced images, helical scanning with 5 mm collimation

TABLE 14.2   Recommended CT Techniques for Routine Abdomen and Pelvis Imaging

—	Initial scan, adults and children >100 lb	Delayed scan, >100 lb	Children–, <100 lb	Infants
IV contrast material	GFR ≥ 60: Low osmolar, 300 mg/mL; GFR 30–40: Iso-osmolar, 320 mg/mL	—	Low osmolar, 300 mg/mL	—
Volume	150 mL	—	1.5 mL/kg	—
Rate	3 mL/s	—	Hand injection	Hand injection
Scan delay	60–80 s	5 min	End of bolus	End of bolus
Collimation	5 mm (helical)	10 mm (helical)	5 mm (helical)	5 mm (helical)
Top slice	Base of heart	Top of kidneys	Base of heart	Base of heart
Bottom slice	Symphysis pubis	Bladder	Symphysis pubis	Symphysis pubis

IV, intravenous; GFR, glomerular filtration rate.

and a pitch of 1.0 to 1.5 is commonly used. Delayed scanning of the kidneys is performed for evaluation of renal excretion with helical axial imaging at 10 mm collimation.

CTA is the standard examination for the evaluation of the abdominal aorta and branches. CTA is an excellent preoperative assessment of aortic aneurysm, aortic dissection, arterial stenosis, and arterial occlusion. The 1.0 mm helical images in the axial, sagittal, and coronal planes as well as maximum intensity projection (MIP) images are used.

Gastrointestinal Contrast Examinations

In the emergency center patient requiring evaluation of the upper GI tract, endoscopy has nearly replaced the fluoroscopic upper GI series. Examinations involving enema administration of contrast have a role in the following circumstances: (1) to diagnose and reduce intussusceptions in children (enema of air, barium, or water-soluble iodinated contrast material) and (2) to distinguish distal small bowel obstruction from colonic obstruction in adults (enema of barium or water-soluble contrast).

High-quality single or double contrast examination of a properly prepared colon is not feasible in an emergency situation. Instead, a water-soluble contrast enema is performed on the unprepared colon. In colonic obstruction, barium is not used because it may convert a partial obstruction to a functional complete obstruction. If the colon perforates, extravasated water-soluble contrast material causes a less severe peritonitis than barium. Enema examinations are contraindicated in patients with known colonic perforation to prevent spillage of contrast and fecal material into the peritoneal cavity. Either barium or air may be used for the infant or child with suspected intussusceptions. In young children, high-osmolar water-soluble contrast material may cause problematic shifts in fluid balance.

Contrast enema examinations must be performed under the supervision of the radiologist. A digital rectal examination should be performed prior to placement of the enema tube tip to ensure safe placement. The tip should be placed by a physician or properly trained personnel. An inflatable cuff is useful, but it should be inflated carefully with a physician immediately available.

For examinations using water-soluble contrast material, a sufficient volume of commercially available preparation is administered per rectum via gravity to adequately distend the colon. Colonic distension is monitored fluoroscopically. The colon is manually compressed, and spot radiographs of suspicious areas are obtained. Spot radiographs are followed by a series of standard radiographs to evaluate the entire colon.

Nuclear Medicine

Nuclear medicine techniques are used infrequently in the care of emergency center patients. Hepatobiliary imaging using ^{99m}Tc iminodiacetic acid (IDA) analogues provides excellent quality accurate evaluation for acute and chronic biliary disease. Hepatobiliary scintigraphy (cholescintigraphy) is used in patients suspected of having acute cholecystitis but in whom US does not provide definitive diagnosis. Common indications are acute (calculous or acalculous) cholecystitis, biliary patency, and to identify biliary leaks.

GI bleeding studies are performed emergently to localize the site of bleeding. ^{99m}Tc-labeled red blood cells and ^{99m}Tc colloid are the most common radiopharmaceuticals used. The technique involves administering the ^{99m}Tc-labeled red blood cells and imaging the patient using a large field of view scintillation camera during the injection and for several minutes after the injection. If a site of bleeding is not initially detected, delayed images may be obtained within 24 to 36 hours. The detection of lower GI bleed by both ^{99m}Tc-labeled red blood cells and colloid has higher sensitivity than angiography and is noninvasive. Due to high background activity in the upper digestive tract and the diagnostic efficacy of endoscopy, nuclear imaging is used more commonly for evaluation of the lower GI tract. However, in evaluations of the GI tract, active, brisk bleeding in the duodenum and distal stomach are commonly detected in spite of background activity. Angiography may be negative with intermittent bleeding or in cases of bleeding rates lower than 1 mL per minute. With nuclear imaging, bleeding rates of .02 mL per minute are accurately detected. Although the accuracy of endoscopic diagnosis of upper GI bleeding is greater than 90%, tagged red blood cells are the agent of choice for diagnosis in slow or intermittent bleeding, with sensitivity of greater than 90%.

RADIOGRAPHIC ANATOMY

Boundaries of the Abdomen

The abdomen includes all of the structures contained within the transversalis fascia and extends from the diaphragm to the pelvis. It is divided by the peritoneum into a peritoneal cavity and several extraperitoneal spaces.

The rectus abdominis muscle comprises the anterior portion of the abdominal wall. This muscle extends from the xiphoid process and costal cartilages of the fifth through seventh ribs to attach inferiorly on the pubic symphysis. From superficial to deep the external oblique, internal oblique and transversus abdominis muscles form the lateral abdominal wall from its anterolateral to its posterolateral extent. The transversalis fascia arises from the transverse abdominis muscles and surrounds the entire abdomen. The posterior abdominal wall is made up of the latissimus dorsi muscles located laterally and the erector spinae muscles located medially (Fig. 14.1). A variably thick fat layer external

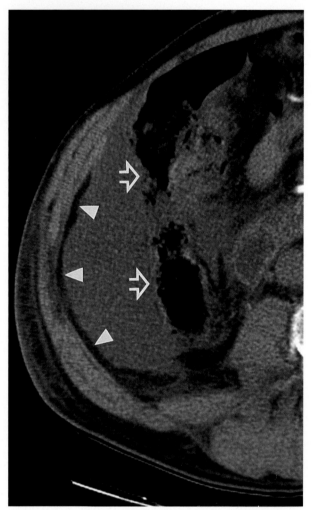

Figure 14.2. Fluid in the paracolic gutter. CT shows a collection of fluid in the right paracolic gutter displacing the ascending colon and hepatic flexure medially. The displacement is accentuated by the absence of the right kidney in this individual. The increased distance between the flank stripe *(white arrowheads)* and the lateral wall of the colon *(open arrows)* was evident on a conventional radiograph.

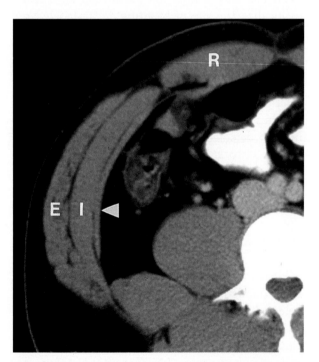

Figure 14.1. CT of the abdominal wall. CT image at the level of the upper portion of the umbilicus shows the muscles of the abdominal wall: external oblique *(E)*, internal oblique *(I)*, and transversus abdominis *(arrowhead)*. The rectus abdominis muscle *(R)* is seen anteriorly closer to the midline.

to the peritoneum surrounds the peritoneal cavity anteriorly, laterally, and posteriorly (Fig. 14.2). On conventional AP radiographs, the extraperitoneal fat between the transversalis fascia and the peritoneum is visible as the "flank stripe" described by Frimann-Dahl (Figs. 14.3 and 14.4). Normally, the ascending and descending colon are adjacent to the flank stripe. Processes that thicken the colonic wall or fill the peritoneal space between the colon and the parietal peritoneum (the paracolic gutter) displace the colon away from the flank stripe. The flank stripe is not visible in infants with a normal

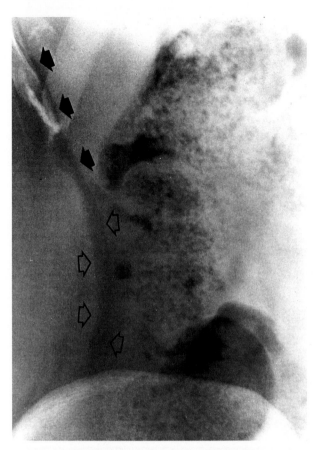

Figure 14.3. Radiographic appearance of the soft tissues of the right flank. The extraperitoneal fat ("flank stripe") produces the sharply defined, gently curved lucent band *(open arrows)* extending from below the iliac crest to above the lateral margin of the liver *(solid arrows)*. Gas and feces identify the ascending colon and the hepatic flexure and outline the inferior margin of the liver.

protuberant abdomen, debilitated patients, or patients with little body fat.

Superiorly, the abdomen is bounded by the diaphragm. The central tendon, the highest and thinnest part of the diaphragm, is located anterior to the inferior vena cava (IVC) and forms the margins of the esophageal hiatus. The radiographic appearance of the diaphragm depends on the patient's body habitus. Typically, the right hemidiaphragm is higher than the left, but the reverse situation is normal. Posteriorly, the diaphragm attaches to the lumbar spine via the right and left diaphragmatic crura. Posterior to the crura is the retrocrural space, bounded posteriorly by the lumbar vertebrae, through which pass the aorta and the azygos and hemiazygos veins (Fig. 14.5A).

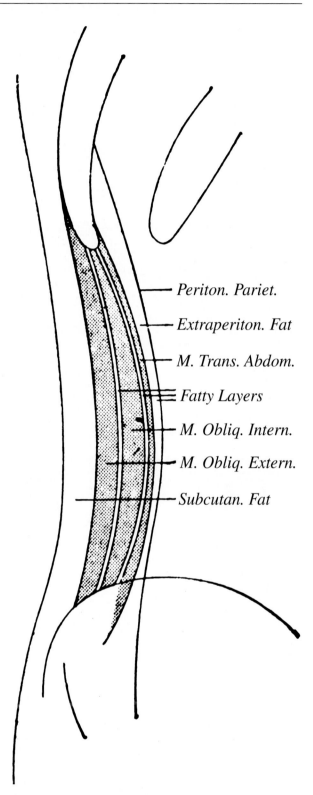

Periton. Pariet.

Extraperiton. Fat

M. Trans. Abdom.

Fatty Layers

M. Obliq. Intern.

M. Obliq. Extern.

Subcutan. Fat

Figure 14.4. Schematic drawing of the soft tissues of the flank. The extraperitoneal (preperitoneal, properitoneal, and retroperitoneal) fat produces the lucent shadow of the flank stripe. (From Soyer P. Segmental anatomy of the liver: utility of a nomenclature accepted worldwide. *Am J Roentgenol.* 1993;161(3):572–573, with permission.)

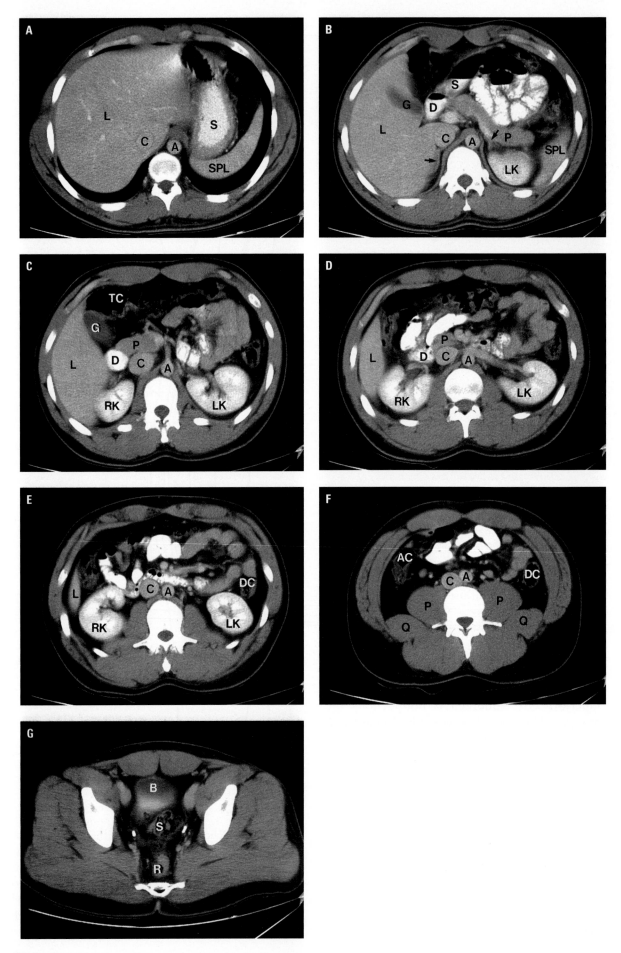

Inferiorly, the peritoneal cavity is bounded by the pelvic peritoneal reflection, which contains the pelvic loops of ileum (Fig. 14.5G).

The Peritoneal Spaces

The peritoneal cavity is divided into recesses, based on the proximity of adjacent structures and the complex embryology of each region (Fig. 14.6). The right peritoneal space includes the right perihepatic space and the lesser sac. The right perihepatic space surrounds the right lobe of the liver from the falciform ligament anteriorly to the coronary ligament, which surrounds the large, nonperitonealized, bare area of the liver. More caudally, the right perihepatic space surrounds the right lobe of the liver and forms a posterior recess (Morrison pouch) between the liver and the upper pole of the right kidney. The lesser sac is bounded by the stomach anteriorly, the porta hepatis on the right, the spleen on the left, and the pancreas posteriorly.

The left peritoneal space surrounds the left lobe of the liver from the falciform ligament to the left abdominal wall. Anteriorly, the space is termed the anterior left perihepatic space and posteriorly, the posterior left perihepatic space. The lateral extension of the left peritoneal space between the stomach and the diaphragm is called the left anterior subphrenic space. Further, posteriorly and laterally is the posterior subphrenic space, also termed the perisplenic space, which surrounds the spleen.

Caudal to Morrison pouch and the spleen, the peritoneal cavity does not have separate compartments, except for the paracolic gutters (Fig. 14.5F). In the pelvis, the peritoneum continues as an inferior recess (Fig. 14.5G). In men, this recess is termed the rectovesical pouch. In women, the recess is called the rectouterine pouch (pouch of Douglas) and the shallower, more anterior vesicouterine space.

The peritoneal spaces are easily defined on CT scans, and many of the compartments of the peritoneal cavity are visible by US. Although the peritoneal space is not directly visible on radiographs, the fat of the flank stripes and the perivesical fat between the peritoneum and the bladder serve mark the parietal peritoneum.

The Extraperitoneal Spaces

The extraperitoneal spaces are contained within the transversalis fascia but are outside the peritoneum. Although a large proportion of the retroperitoneum

Figure 14.5. Normal CT anatomy. **A:** Diaphragmatic hiatus. Note the collapsed esophagus immediately anterior to the aorta. *L*, liver; *C*, inferior vena cava; *A*, aorta; *S*, stomach; *SPL*, spleen. **B:** The pancreatic body and tail are located immediately anterior to the splenic vein. Note the superior end of the gallbladder fossa, which is located immediately caudal to the interlobar fissure. An air–oral contrast material level is present in the second portion of the duodenum. Both adrenal glands are visible in this section *(arrows)*. *L*, liver; *G*, gallbladder; *D*, duodenum; *C*, inferior vena cava; *S*, stomach; *A*, aorta; *P*, pancreatic tail; *LK*, left kidney; *SPL*, spleen. **C:** Pancreatic head. At the level of the superior mesenteric artery origin, an elongated but homogeneous pancreatic head has no contour abnormalities. The duodenum is filled with contrast material on this image. Note the close relationship between the hepatic flexure, the gallbladder, and the liver. *L*, liver; *G*, gallbladder; *TC*, transverse colon; *D*, duodenum; *RK*, right kidney; *P*, pancreatic head; *C*, inferior vena cava; *S*, stomach; *A*, aorta; *LK*, left kidney. **D:** The third portion of the duodenum. Note the contrast-filled duodenum crossing anterior to the inferior vena cava and the aorta immediately posterior to the superior mesenteric artery and vein at the upper end of the root of the small bowel mesentery. *L*, liver; *RK*, right kidney; *D*, duodenum; *P*, pancreatic head; *C*, inferior vena cava; *A*, aorta; *LK*, left kidney. **E:** Kidneys. Image at the level of the left splenic vein shows the inferior portion of the right lobe of the liver. The superior mesenteric vein and artery are visible in the root of the small bowel mesentery. *L*, liver; *RK*, right kidney; *C*, inferior vena cava; *A*, aorta; *DC*, descending colon; *LK*, left kidney. **F:** Paracolic gutters. In the normal individual, the paracolic gutter is a potential space between the parietal peritoneum of the body wall and the visceral peritoneum surrounding the ascending and descending colon. Note the multiple small arteries and veins coursing through the mesentery. *AC*, ascending colon; *P*, psoas muscle; *Q*, quadratus lumborum muscle; *C*, inferior vena cava; *A*, aorta; *DC*, descending colon. **G:** Peritoneal reflection. This image is below the anterior surface of the peritoneal reflection where the parietal peritoneum covers the dome of the bladder. *B*, bladder; *S*, sigmoid colon; *R*, rectum.

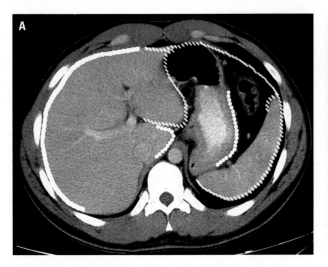

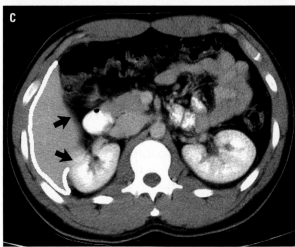

Figure 14.6. Peritoneal spaces. **A:** The *heavy white line* outlines the right perihepatic space. The *hash marks* outline the left peritoneal space, which is made up of the anterior left perihepatic space, the posterior left perihepatic space, and the perisplenic space. The series of *dots* outlines portions of the lesser sac around the caudate lobe and posterior to the stomach. **B:** At a lower level, the right perihepatic space, outlined by the *heavy white line*, is limited posteriorly by the coronary ligament, which defines the bare area of the liver. The left posterior hepatic space has ended below the liver. A small portion of the lesser sac is visible between the stomach and the pancreas. **C:** Caudally, the right perihepatic space continues as the hepatorenal recess (Morrison pouch) *(arrows)* between the liver and the right kidney.

is fat between other structures, the retroperitoneum also contains the great vessels, pancreas, portions of the duodenum and colon, the adrenal glands, kidneys, ureters, and bladder. The extraperitoneal spaces extend from the diaphragm to the floor of the pelvis and wrap around the entire peritoneal cavity. They are divided into the abdominal retroperitoneum, which is the subject of this section, and the pelvic perivesical space, which is described in conjunction with normal anatomy of the pelvis in Chapters 15 and 17.

Detailed description of the retroperitoneum is beyond the scope of this chapter; however, a basic understanding of the compartments within the retroperitoneum is essential in understanding the possible distribution of blood, pus, or fluid through the retroperitoneum. The aorta and IVC and their segmental and distal branches course through the retroperitoneum anterior to the vertebral bodies. Hemorrhage from these central vessels may extend throughout the retroperitoneum via the retroperitoneal fasciae.

At the level of the kidneys and pancreas, the retroperitoneum is divided into several compartments. The thin anterior and thicker posterior renal (Gerota) fasciae surround the kidneys. The anterior and posterior renal fasciae fuse laterally to form the lateroconal fascia, which extends anteriorly to fuse with the parietal peritoneum lateral to the ascending and descending colon (Fig. 14.7). Inside the renal fascia, the perirenal space contains the kidney, the adrenal gland, and perirenal fat. Below the kidneys, the perirenal space tapers in the shape of a cone (Fig. 14.8).

The posterior pararenal space is lateral to the lateroconal fascia and posterior to the posterior

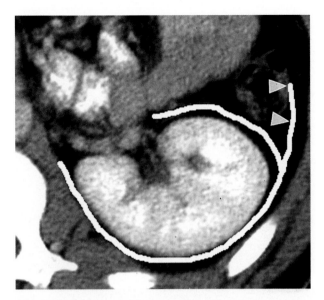

Figure 14.7. Perirenal space. The *heavy white line* outlines the renal fascia, which merges with the lateroconal fascia extending anteriorly to the descending colon *(arrowheads)*.

renal fascia and contains only fat. This space becomes important when inflammatory processes track into it.

The anterior pararenal space, lying between the anterior renal fascia and the posterior peritoneum, is continuous across the midline and contains most

of the duodenum, the ascending and descending colon, and the pancreas (Fig. 14.5B–E). The anterior pararenal space communicates readily with several peritoneal ligaments: the small bowel mesentery; the transverse mesocolon; the phrenicocolic, duodenocolic, and splenorenal ligaments; and the lesser omentum.

The psoas muscle and the quadratus lumborum muscles (Fig. 14.5F) communicate with the extraperitoneal spaces, allowing hematomas and fluid collections to track along these muscles.

Major Vessels

The abdominal aorta descends through the diaphragmatic hiatus in the retrocrural space to the left of midline at the ventral aspect of the lumbar vertebrae. At the L4 level, it bifurcates into the common iliac arteries. The normal aortic diameter does not exceed 3 cm and tapers progressively below the renal arteries. The common iliac arteries bifurcate at the pelvic brim into external and internal iliac arteries. The external iliac arteries extend anteriorly to the inguinal triangle, and the internal iliac arteries supply the pelvis.

The celiac axis originates at the level of the diaphragmatic hiatus (Figs. 14.9A and 14.9B). One centimeter inferiorly, the superior mesenteric

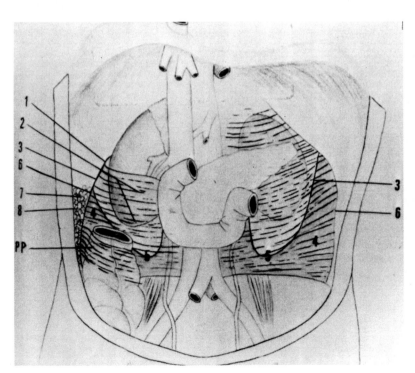

Figure 14.8. Schematic representation of the retroperitoneal compartments. This drawing clearly illustrates the conical configuration of the inferior portion of the perirenal space *(5)*. Other extraperitoneal structures represented include the posterior renal fascia *(1)*, anterior renal fascia *(2)*, line of fusion of anterior and posterior renal fasciae *(3)*, lateroconal fascia *(4)*, line of fusion of lateroconal fascia with posterior parietal peritoneum *(6)*, posterior pararenal fat extending into the flank stripe *(7)*, transverse fascia *(8)*, and parietal peritoneum *(PP)*. (From Meyers MA, Whalen JP, Peelle K, et al. Radiologic features of extraperitoneal effusions. An anatomic approach. *Radiology.* 1972;104(2):249–257, with permission.)

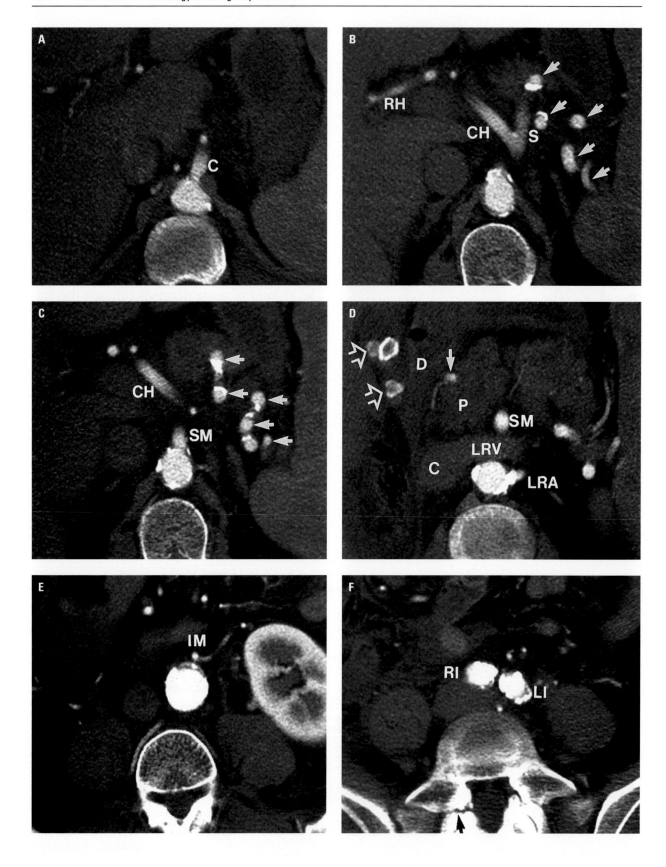

artery arises from the anterior surface of the aorta (Fig. 14.9C). One centimeter below this, the renal arteries arise from the lateral aspects of the aorta (Fig. 14.9D). Just above the aortic bifurcation, the small inferior mesenteric artery arises from the anterior wall of the aorta (Fig. 14.9E).

The IVC is formed by the confluence of the two common iliac veins at the L5 level, and it courses over the right common iliac artery and ascends to the right of the abdominal aorta. The IVC passes through the substance of the liver before passing through the diaphragm to drain into the right atrium. The size and shape of the IVC vary considerably based on intravascular volume, phase of respiration, and the presence or absence of IVC obstruction. The renal veins join the IVC at approximately the same level as the corresponding renal arteries. The right renal vein is shorter, whereas the left renal vein, which passes anterior to the aorta, is longer. The left renal vein receives the left gonadal vein.

Solid Organs

Liver and Biliary Tract
The liver fills much of the right upper quadrant of the abdomen, extending from the diaphragm to a point near or even below the right iliac crest. Its size and shape are quite variable. On conventional radiographs, the diagnosis of hepatomegaly should be reserved for instances in which the liver displaces adjacent structures. The size of the liver is readily measured by CT.

The liver is divided into lobes, segments, and subsegments based on its vascular anatomy. A line extended anteriorly and inferiorly from the middle hepatic vein separates the right and left hepatic lobes. The lobes are easy to separate in patients who have a well-defined interlobar fissure along the inferior margin of the liver, which then extends inferiorly as the gallbladder fossa. The large right lobe of the liver is divided into anterior and posterior segments by an imaginary line extended outward from the right hepatic vein to the lateral surface of the liver. The left hepatic lobe is typically much smaller than the right and is divided into lateral and medial segments by a line drawn from the left hepatic vein to the falciform ligament. Each of the four liver segments, which constitute the right and left lobes, is further divided into subsegments based on position above or below the portal venous confluence. The caudate lobe has a separate vascular supply and is a separate posteromedial lobe of the liver adjacent to the IVC. Couinaud and Bismuth designed a widely used system of numbered segments based on these anatomic subdivisions (Table 14.3; Fig. 14.10). Routine use of this system to describe hepatic pathology reduces ambiguity in communication and assists in surgical planning.

The gallbladder fossa lies at the inferior extent of the interlobar fissure of the liver. In the fasting state, the fully distended gallbladder has a thin wall, measuring no more than 3 mm in thickness (Figs. 11A and 11.B). The gallbladder's length is variable but rarely exceeds 10 cm. The gallbladder is circular in cross section.

Biliary anatomy can be evaluated either by US or CT scan (Fig. 14.12). In cross section, the hepatic ducts are usually located immediately anterior to the portal vein within the substance of the liver

Figure 14.9. Abdominal vascular anatomy. **A:** Origin of the celiac axis *(C)* at the inferior margin of the diaphragmatic hiatus. **B:** Division of the celiac axis into common hepatic *(CH)* and splenic *(S)* arteries. Note the splenic artery coursing in and out of the plane of section *(arrows)*. The right hepatic *(RH)* artery is visible in the porta hepatis. The third division of the celiac axis, the left gastric artery, is not visible on the section. **C:** Superior mesenteric *(SM)* artery origin 1.3 cm caudal to the celiac axis origin. The splenic artery is also visible *(arrows).CH* is the common hepatic artery. **D:** Origin of the left renal artery *(LRA)*. The right kidney is absent. The superior mesenteric *(SM)* artery passes anterior to the left renal vein *(LRV)*. The gastroduodenal artery *(solid arrow)* passes along the anterior margin of the pancreatic head. Several faceted rim-calcified gallstones *(open arrows)* are seen in the gallbladder. **E:** The inferior mesenteric *(IM)* artery originated from the anterior wall of the aorta on the image immediately cephalad to this one; on this image, the inferior mesenteric artery tracks to the left of midline. **F:** Aortic bifurcation at the L4-5 disc level. The irregularity of the common iliac artery walls and the aortic lumen is due to atherosclerosis. The aorta bifurcates into right *(RI)* and left *(LI)* common iliac arteries. There is a pars interarticularis defect on the right side of L5 *(arrow)*.

TABLE 14.3	Couinaud-Bismuth Segments and Corresponding Liver Anatomy		
Couinaud-Bismuth Segment	**Lobe**	**Segment**	**Subsegment**[a]
I	Caudate	—	—
II	Left	Lateral	Superior
III	Left	Lateral	Inferior
IVa	Left	Medial	Superior
IVb	Left	Medial	Inferior
V	Right	Anterior	Inferior
VI	Right	Posterior	Inferior
VII	Right	Posterior	Superior
VIII	Right	Anterior	Superior

[a]Superior or inferior to the transverse scissura (i.e., portal vein confluence).

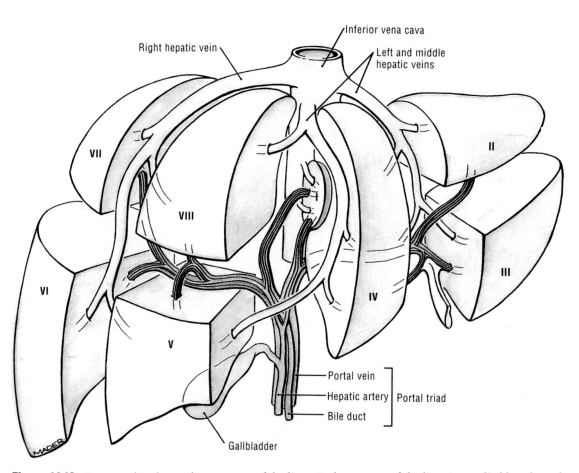

Figure 14.10. Segmental and vascular anatomy of the liver. Each segment of the liver is supplied by a branch of the hepatic artery, bile duct, and portal vein. The hepatic veins do not follow the structures of the portal triad and are considered intersegmental in that they drain portions of adjacent segments. (From Agur AMR. The abdomen. In: *Grant's Atlas of Anatomy.* 9th ed. Baltimore, MD: Lippincott Williams & Wilkins; 1991:115, with permission.)

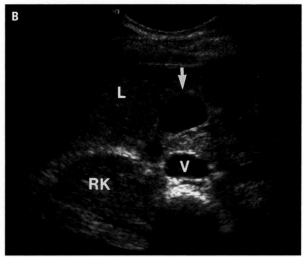

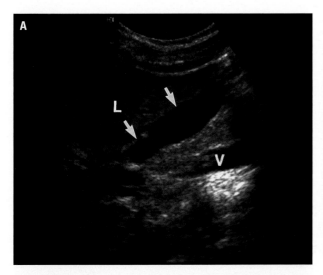

Figure 14.11. Normal gallbladder. Longitudinal (**A**) and transverse (**B**) ultrasound images of a normal gallbladder *(arrows)* within the gallbladder fossa immediately posterior to the liver *(L)*. *V,* inferior vena cava; *RK,* right kidney.

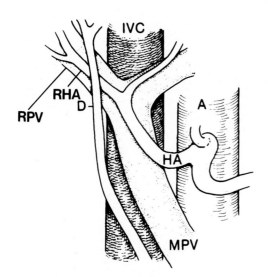

Figure 14.12. Schematic representation of the normal porta hepatis and their relationships to the inferior vena cava *(IVC)*. The structures of the porta hepatis bear a constant relationship to each other. The common hepatic duct *(D)* lies lateral to the proper hepatic artery *(HA)* and crosses anterior to the right hepatic artery *(RHA)* and right portal vein *(RPV)*. *MPV,* main portal vein; *A,* aorta. These relationships may be readily appreciated on both ultrasound and CT. (From Zeman RK, Simeone JF. The biliary ducts: anatomy, examination, technique and pathophysiologic considerations. In: Taveras JM, Ferrucci JT, eds. *Radiology: Diagnosis, Imaging, Intervention.* Vol 4. Philadelphia, PA: JB Lippincott; 1998:1–18. Modified from Zeman RK, Burrell MI. *Gallbladder and Bile Duct Imaging: a Clinical Radiologic Approach.* New York, NY: Churchill Livingstone; 1987, with permission.

(Fig. 14.13A). Caudally, the common hepatic duct (CHD) is seen anterolateral to the main portal vein. The hepatic artery lies anteromedial to the main portal vein. In cross section, both the CHD and hepatic artery appear as small, round structures, anterior to the portal vein. On the transverse view, the appearance of the CHD, hepatic artery, and portal vein has been likened to Mickey Mouse (Fig. 14.13B) and provides a frame of reference for longitudinal imaging of the CHD and common bile duct. A long segment of the bile duct may be demonstrated longitudinally, anterior to the portal vein (Fig. 14.13C). A portion of the hepatic artery is often seen in cross section between the bile duct and the portal vein. The size of the CHD varies with age and increases slightly after cholecystectomy. Generally, 6 mm is taken as the upper limit of the normal diameter of the CHD in adults. In adults older than 75 years, 10 mm is the upper limit of normal, whereas in children, 3 mm is the upper limit of normal. Distally, the common bile duct shows even greater variability in caliber and may be up to 3 mm larger than the CHD.

CT scans illustrate the biliary anatomy well. CT demonstration of the ducts may be limited by motion artifact. On CT, the gallbladder is filled with bile that has an attenuation value near that of water (0 to 20 Hounsfield units [HU]). The gallbladder wall is 1 to 3 mm in thickness, and it often enhances after the administration of IV

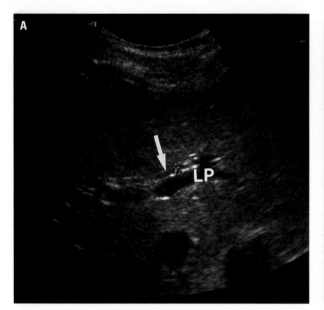

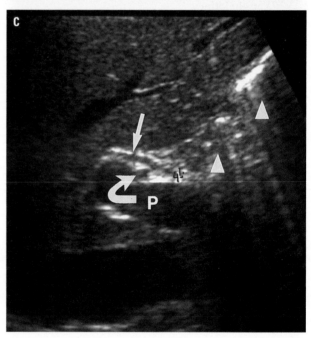

Figure 14.13. Ultrasound anatomy of the bile ducts. **A:** Transverse image through the porta hepatis at the left portal *(LP)* vein shows a normal caliber left hepatic duct *(arrow)* measuring 2 mm in diameter. Note that peripheral intrahepatic ducts are not visible. **B:** Transverse image through the porta hepatis as it exits the liver shows the "Mickey Mouse" appearance of the porta hepatis in a normal patient. The "head" is the portal vein *(open arrow)*, the "right" (lateral) ear represents the common hepatic duct *(straight arrow)*, and the "left" (medial) ear represents the hepatic artery *(curved arrow)*. Use of these landmarks can help in tracing the common duct through the porta hepatis. **C:** Longitudinal image through the extrahepatic bile duct shows the common duct *(electronic cursor and straight arrow)* measuring 1 mm in diameter. The main portal vein *(P)* is located posterior to the common duct. The right hepatic artery *(curved arrow)* is visible between the common duct and the main portal vein. Note the "dirty shadows" from a bowel loop located posterior and inferior to the liver *(arrowheads)*.

contrast material. CT usually demonstrates the common bile duct passing through the head of the pancreas.

Spleen

The spleen is located in the left upper quadrant of the abdomen along the lateral and posterior aspects of the left hemidiaphragm. The anterior medial border of the spleen abuts the stomach. Inferiorly, the posterior medial surface of the spleen is near the upper pole of the left kidney and the anterior surface is near the descending colon. The shape of the spleen is variable, but it is a crescentic, pliable organ that is much longer than it is thick. Clefts are common and may be as deep as 2 or 3 cm and are typically located along the upper surface of the spleen. Occasionally, small lobules of splenic tissue (accessory spleens) are encountered near the spleen, often near the hilum. The spleen is enhanced with IV contrast. Early after administration of the bolus of contrast material, the enhancement pattern is heterogeneous and may simulate splenic injury or other pathology (Fig. 14.14). After 60 seconds, the enhancement becomes homogeneous in a normal spleen.

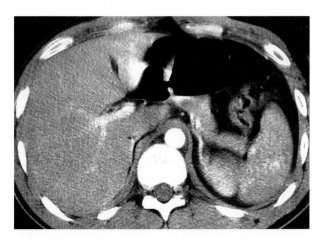

Figure 14.14. Early bolus effect in the spleen. CT image through the inferior portion of the spleen shows mottled central enhancement of the spleen with unenhancing parenchyma peripherally. This image was made 30 seconds after the beginning of the bolus of contrast material because of a technical error.

Pancreas

The pancreas is located deep in the epigastrium anterior to the lumbar vertebrae within the anterior pararenal space (Figs. 14.5B and 14.5C). The duodenum surrounds its head. The portal vein crosses anterior to its neck. A portion of the body and tail of the pancreas lies anterior to the splenic vein. The tip of the tail is often found adjacent to the splenic hilum near the anterior margin of the left kidney. The splenic artery follows a serpentine course superior and anterior to the pancreas. The normal pancreas is not visible on conventional radiography but is readily seen on CT scans, and it may be visible by US using an acoustic window between gas-filled bowel loops. The pancreatic duct is frequently visible on helical CT images, varying in diameter from 3 to 6 mm. The size of the pancreas is highly variable; thus, pancreatic pathology is detected by the presence of mass or heterogeneity in contrast enhancement rather than by measurement of the size of the pancreas.

Adrenal Glands

The adrenal glands are located cephalad and slightly anterior to the upper pole of each kidney (Fig. 14.5B). The adrenal glands are readily seen by CT and are well seen with US. The configuration of the adrenal glands is variable; typically, the right adrenal gland can be seen as an inverted "U", directed anteriorly and located between the medial aspect of the liver and the right crus of the diaphragm. The left adrenal most often has an inverted "V" configuration and is located between the fundus of the stomach and the left crus of the diaphragm. The limbs of the adrenal are variable in length but have a uniform thickness and shape. Adrenal masses are identified as nodular protrusions from the normal contour. An adrenal limb thicker than 10 mm is considered abnormal.

Urinary Tract

The kidneys are frequently visible on conventional radiographs because they are surrounded by perinephric fat. Overlying bowel contents may obscure them. Ninety percent of the time, the left kidney is higher than the right. Congenital absence of a kidney occurs in 1 in 700 individuals. When one kidney is absent or hypoplastic, the remaining kidney demonstrates compensatory hypertrophy. When visible, the adult renal shadow measures 12 to 14 cm in length, with the disparity in length between the kidneys not exceeding 1.5 to 2.0 cm.

The kidney consists of renal parenchyma surrounding a central renal pelvis. The parenchyma is divided into an outer cortex and an inner medulla, consisting of several renal pyramids whose apices project into the renal pelvis. Both CT and US are used to evaluate the kidneys. In the first 60 seconds after IV contrast medium injection, the enhancement of the cortex is greater than the enhancement of the medulla. After a 2-minute delay, the medulla may be more intensely enhanced than the cortex. Between 3 and 5 minutes after injection, contrast appears in the collecting system. The renal artery and vein pass anterior to the renal pelvis and divide into segmental branches supplying the renal parenchyma.

The ureters arise from the renal pelvis and extend through the medial aspect of the perirenal space and then continue caudally lateral to the great vessels. As they cross the pelvic brim, they track posterolaterally through the true pelvis to enter the trigone of the bladder from a posterolateral approach. The ureters are extraperitoneal along their entire course. Normal ureters can be identified on unenhanced CT scanning by tracing them on sequential, adjacent images from the renal pelvis. The ureters are readily visible when filled with opacified urine after IV administration of contrast material. The segments of the ureters that are best seen by US are the ureteropelvic junction and at the ureterovesicular junction. Ureteral peristalsis causes segmental variation in the caliber of the ureter through its course from the renal pelvis to the bladder.

Gastrointestinal Tract

The bowel gas normally present in the intestinal tract frequently aids in the recognition of GI pathology, both by conventional radiography and CT. However, bowel gas is undesirable for US because it causes shadows that obscure structures deep to the gas.

Gas is almost always present within the stomach. Gas migrates to the least dependent position within the stomach with a change in body position. On a supine radiograph, the gas is located in the body and/or antrum of the stomach (Fig. 14.15). In the erect position, the gas migrates into the gastric fundus. The stomach can be distinguished from the splenic flexure of the colon by the gastric rugal folds, which are outlined by gas in the stomach. The distance between the stomach bubble and the upper margin of the left hemidiaphragm on the erect radiograph increases due to mass effect of free intraperitoneal air. This is a useful tool in distinguishing between a normal stomach bubble and pneumoperitoneum under the left hemidiaphragm.

Gas is frequently present in the duodenal bulb in normal individuals. This gas bubble is located adjacent to the inferior edge of the liver in the right upper quadrant. The remainder of the duodenum is not typically gas filled. Gas is normally present in the small bowel in greater quantities in patients presenting with abdominal pain but in lesser quantities in ambulatory, asymptomatic patients. Normal gas-filled small bowel loops are typically less than 3 cm in diameter. Analysis of the pattern of small bowel gas is more important than the diameter of individual small bowel loops. On the erect radiograph, a few air–fluid levels may be apparent in the normal, nonobstructed small bowel.

In the normally functioning colon, liquid feces should not be present beyond the splenic flexure. On the supine radiograph, gas collects in the least dependent portions of the bowel, which include the transverse colon and portions of the ascending and descending colon. The cecum is often recognizable by the bubbly appearance of its liquid contents. The rectum is the most dependent part of the bowel and may empty normally. Thus, the absence of gas in the rectum is not a definitive indicator of bowel obstruction. On the erect radiograph, colonic gas will migrate upward into the hepatic and splenic flexures. Air–fluid levels are normally encountered in the fluid-filled ascending or transverse segments of the colon.

CT provides a more detailed evaluation of the bowel than conventional radiographs. The same principles of bowel dilatation that form the basis of conventional radiographic diagnosis should be used in evaluating the CT images. The small bowel and colon are further evaluated by assessment

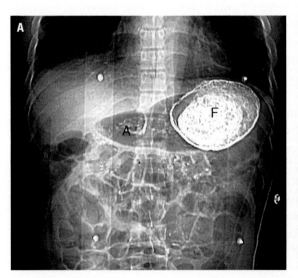
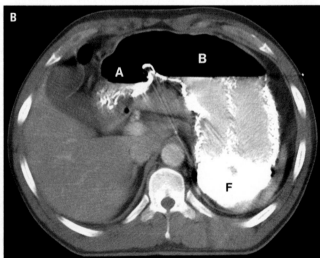

Figure 14.15. Stomach anatomy. **A:** Supine scout image for abdominal CT shows barium in the gastric fundus *(F)* and air in the gastric antrum *(A)*. **B:** CT image through the stomach shows dense barium in the gastric fundus, barium mixed with gastric fluid in the dependent portion of the body, and air in the nondependent portion of the gastric body *(B)* and gastric antrum *(A)*.

of the passage of liquid contrast material. The appearance of the small bowel is variable and depends on the degree of distention by gas or contrast material. The normal, nondistended small bowel wall is thick, but when completely distended by gas or contrast material, the wall measures no more than 3 mm in thickness. The colon is usually not well distended, so wall thickness is difficult to assess; however, when distended, the colon wall is typically less than 3 mm thick.

Using 2.5 mm MRCT technique and colonic distention with rectal contrast material, the appendix can be identified in most individuals. The appendix originates from the medial side of the apex of the cecum. The wall of the appendix is no more than 3 mm thick and no more than 6 mm in diameter. The normal appendix usually has no luminal contents but may contain a small amount of gas. GI contrast material administered before CT scanning may fill the normal appendix.

US has limited use in evaluation of the bowel, but it is useful in evaluating the appendix, particularly in thin patients. Using graded compression technique and a high-resolution transducer, the normal appendix may be identified originating from the cecal tip as a thin, blind-ending, nonperistaltic bowel segment (Fig. 14.16). The submucosa located centrally within the appendix is echogenic and is surrounded by the hypoechoic muscularis. By sonography, the normal appendix is less than 5 mm in diameter when compressed.

NONTRAUMATIC EMERGENCY CONDITIONS

Peritoneal Cavity

Pneumoperitoneum
Pneumoperitoneum most often results from recent abdominal laparotomy or laparoscopy; it usually resolves 3 to 7 days after the procedure but may be present for as long as 4 weeks. Spontaneous pneumoperitoneum is most often due to perforation of a gastric or duodenal ulcer, but it occurs less frequently from perforation of the remainder of the small bowel and intraperitoneal portions of the colon. Even less frequently, air migrates to the peritoneal cavity from the chest secondary to pneumomediastinum or pneumothorax through pores in the diaphragm. Rarely, pneumoperitoneum occurs as the result of perforation of the small bowel affected with pneumatosis intestinalis. CT is the most sensitive means to detect small amounts of free intraperitoneal air. Although unenhanced helical CT has been advocated as the initial diagnostic tool in the evaluation of acute abdominal pain, this approach is not widely used. Instead, chest and abdominal radiographs usually constitute the initial diagnostic examination (Fig. 14.17). The smallest collections of free air will be seen on a properly exposed horizontal beam (cross-table) lateral view as crescents of air located between the anterior surface of the liver and the diaphragm.

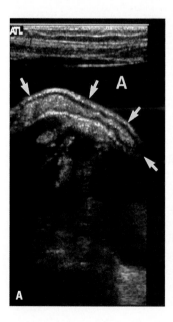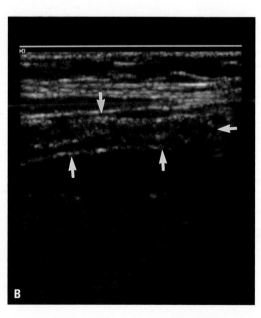

Figure 14.16. Ultrasound of the normal appendix. **A:** Longitudinal ultrasound image in a child with ascites *(A)* allows unusually clear visualization of the normal appendix *(arrows)*. Note the echogenic submucosa, the hypoechoic muscularis, and echogenic serosa. **B:** Longitudinal ultrasound image of a normal appendix *(arrows)* in a child shows similar ultrasonographic features, but the surrounding echogenic abdominal wall makes the normal appendix more difficult to see. (Case courtesy of Cynthia I. Caskey, MD.)

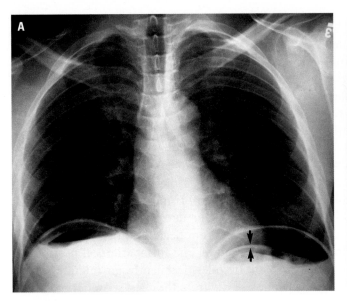
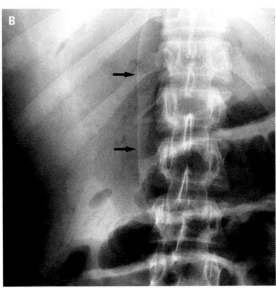

Figure 14.17. Pneumoperitoneum on erect radiograph. **A:** PA erect chest radiograph shows free intraperitoneal air beneath each hemidiaphragm. Note air outlining both sides of the stomach *(arrows)*. **B:** In the same patient, the close-up view AP supine abdominal radiograph shows the falciform ligament *(arrows)* outlined by free air.

In patients unable to stand, the left decubitus view should be obtained. As noted previously in the conventional abdominal radiography technique section, proper positioning and exposure is critical. On the decubitus view, air will be demonstrated in the right perihepatic space (Figs. 14.18 and 14.19). Occasionally, in patients with a very broad pelvis,

the decubitus view may show air collecting along the right parietal peritoneal margin in the pelvis (Fig. 14.18).

Although the upright or decubitus view readily demonstrates free intraperitoneal air, free air may be diagnosed on a supine radiograph alone. An "anterior-superior bubble" positioned in the

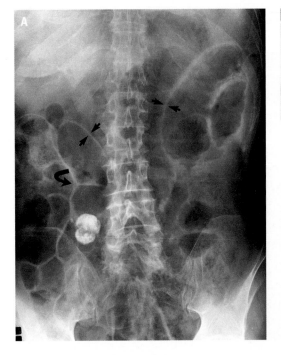
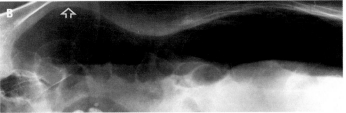

Figure 14.18. A: Supine view of the abdomen in a patient with massive pneumoperitoneum shows that both sides of several bowel loops are outlined by air in both the right and left upper quadrants *(arrows)*. The triangular gas bubble between adjacent bowel loops *(curved arrow)* is Rigler triangle. This may be the only sign of a less extensive pneumoperitoneum. **B:** Right side up decubitus view of the abdomen shows the possible locations for free intraperitoneal air in the right perihepatic space and in the right side of the pelvis *(open arrow)*. Note air outlining several small bowel loops and an air–ascites level within the peritoneal cavity.

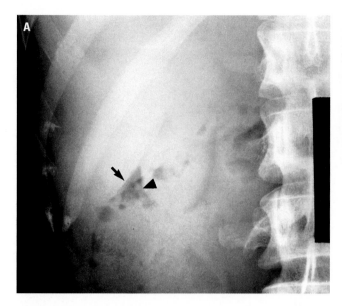

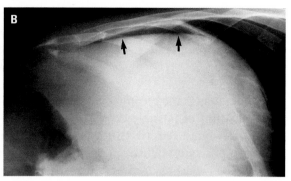

Figure 14.19. Pneumoperitoneum due to perforated duodenal ulcer. **A:** Supine radiograph shows free air between the liver edge *(arrow)* and the outer margin of the gallbladder fundus *(arrowhead)*. **B:** Right side up decubitus radiograph shows free intraperitoneal air in the right perihepatic space *(arrows)*.

medial half of the right upper quadrant of the abdomen below the hemidiaphragm is the most frequent juxtahepatic pattern of pneumoperitoneum (Fig. 14.17B). Other right upper quadrant signs include visualization of the falciform ligament as a thin linear density over the liver (Figs. 14.17B and 14.20); air within the hepatorenal recess (Morrison pouch) (Fig. 14.19A); extraluminal air outlining the serosal surface of bowel loops (Rigler sign) (Fig. 14.18); and a large, lucent, oval air collection in the midabdomen (football sign) (Fig. 14.20).

On CT, pneumoperitoneum collects in the recess between the rectus muscles and the anterolateral abdominal wall (Fig. 14.21). Air also collects between the liver and the anterior abdominal wall within the mesentery, lesser sac, or Morrison

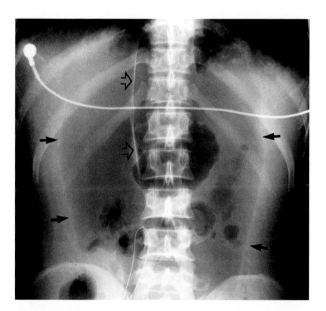

Figure 14.20. Massive pneumoperitoneum with demonstration of the falciform ligament *(open arrows)* outlined by air. The large collection of air in the midabdomen is described as a "football" sign *(solid arrows)*.

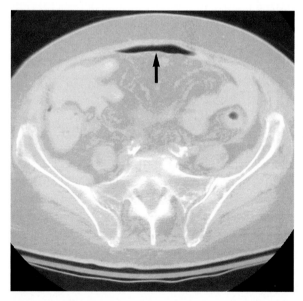

Figure 14.21. Pneumoperitoneum on CT. CT image through the midabdomen displayed at lung windows shows a collection of free intraperitoneal air *(arrow)* under the anterior abdominal wall in the least dependent part of the abdomen.

pouch. Findings can be subtle, with pneumoperitoneum manifesting as only a few trapped air bubbles in the mesentery. Wide window settings of more than 750 HU can help detect subtle air collections.

Radiography is the recommended initial test for the evaluation of possible bowel perforation. CT scanning is more sensitive for detection of small air collections and should be performed when well-exposed conventional radiographs are negative, but the patient's symptoms are suggestive of bowel perforation.

Ascites

The transudation or exudation of fluid into the peritoneal cavity is protean in etiology. Conventional radiography, US, or CT may demonstrate the presence of fluid within the peritoneal cavity. Although the attenuation value of a transudate is typically 0 to 30 HU and that of an exudate is greater than 30 HU, measurement of attenuation value is not an adequate test to distinguish transudate from exudate; biochemical analysis of the fluid is required for this purpose.

On conventional radiographs, ascites causes increased soft tissue density between the flank stripe and the colon. When present in large amounts, it causes the bowel to float to the middle of the abdomen, elevated from the pelvic floor, becoming centralized relative to the surrounding peripheral fluid density (Fig. 14.22). Large amounts of fluid give the abdomen a homogeneously gray, "ground-glass" appearance. Normal soft tissue shadows of the liver margin or renal or psoas shadows may be obliterated or obscured by ascites.

Peritonitis

In peritonitis, conventional radiographs show ascites and may show blurring of the flank stripe. CT signs of diffuse peritonitis include ascites, thickening and enhancement of the peritoneum, and inflammatory infiltration of the mesenteric and omental fat (Fig. 14.23). Similar findings are seen in patients with intraperitoneal carcinomatosis.

Intra-abdominal Abscess

Intra-abdominal abscess most frequently develops following abdominal surgery but also occurs as a complication of appendicitis, diverticulitis, Crohn disease, biliary sepsis, and other systemic infections. Most intra-abdominal abscesses occur in the

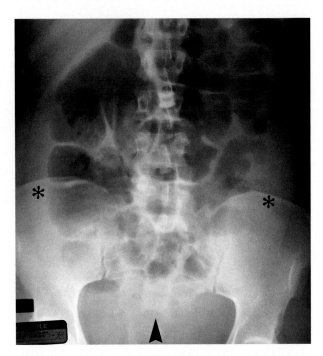

Figure 14.22. AP supine radiograph of the abdomen in a patient with ascites. Note the medial displacement of the air-filled loops of bowel including the ascending and descending colon, which are separated from the flank stripes by fluid in the paracolic gutters *(asterisks)*. Air-filled loops of bowel have floated out of the fluid-filled pelvis *(arrowhead)*.

liver, subphrenic spaces, and pelvis, but they may occur anywhere in the peritoneal cavity or extraperitoneal spaces. CT is the imaging modality of choice. Oral administration of contrast material is very important to opacify bowel loops, eliminating the possibility that an abscess will be mistaken for an unopacified bowel loop. Dilute barium solution should be given orally even when IV contrast is contraindicated.

Abdominal radiography is diagnostic of abscess in approximately one-half of cases. Abscesses may appear because of mass effect displacing adjacent structures (Fig. 14.24). Demonstration of an air–fluid level or cluster of small bubbles not caused by bowel gas is strongly suggestive of a gas-containing abscess.

The CT appearance of an intra-abdominal abscess depends on its location. Abscesses within parenchymal organs are usually round or oval (see Fig. 14.48). Those in the peritoneal cavity, particularly those adjacent to the liver and spleen, have a crescentic or lentiform shape, conforming to the shape of the perihepatic and perisplenic spaces

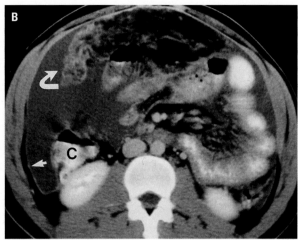

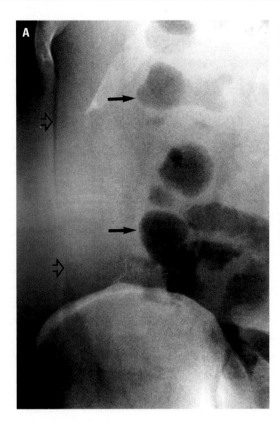

Figure 14.23. Ascites. **A:** Supine radiograph reveals increased opacity in the right paracolic gutter with increased distance between the flank stripe *(open arrows)* and the ascending colon *(solid arrows)*. **B:** Enhanced CT at umbilicus reveals thickening of the mesentery and omentum *(curved arrow)*. Ascites is present, displacing the ascending colon *(C)* from the abdominal wall, correlating with the appearance on the supine radiograph. The parietal peritoneum is thickened *(straight arrow)*.

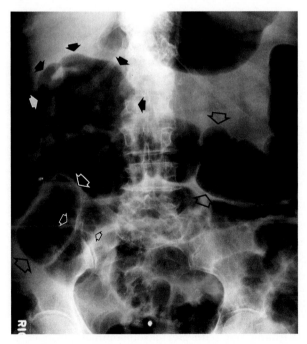

Figure 14.24. Subhepatic abscess. *Solid arrows* indicate a gas-filled subhepatic abscess. *Large open arrows* indicate distended colon. *Small open arrows* indicate dilated small intestine. The abscess produced peritonitis and resultant adynamic ileus.

(Fig. 14.25). Extraperitoneal abscess of the psoas muscles conforms to the shape of the muscle but may cause mass effect on adjacent structures (Fig. 14.26). Abscesses contain fluid with low attenuation near that of water. One-third contain small air bubbles or air–fluid levels. An enhancing rim of granulation tissue is characteristic, particularly as the abscess matures, but is present in only a minority of cases. Thickening of fascial planes and soft tissue strands infiltrating fat adjacent to the abscess are signs of inflammation that help distinguish an abscess from sterile fluid collections. However, when the characteristic features of abscess are absent, aspiration may be required to establish the diagnosis.

For patients too ill to be transported to the CT scanner, US is a useful modality for diagnosing an abscess. US is excellent for evaluation of the subphrenic and perihepatic spaces and the pelvis. On US, abscesses typically appear as rounded or oval collections of fluid containing internal echoes and debris. The walls may be well defined or irregular. Echogenic foci of gas, which may cause an acoustic shadow, are strong evidence that a mass seen by US is an abscess (see Fig. 14.48).

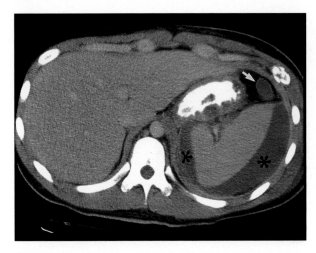

Figure 14.25. Postsurgical perisplenic abscess. Enhanced CT image below the left splenic hilum shows a thick-walled fluid collection in the perisplenic space *(asterisks)*. A smaller collection is seen anterior to the spleen *(arrow)*. The 400 mL of purulent material was aspirated.

Vascular

Abdominal Aortic Aneurysm
Abdominal aortic aneurysm (AAA) is diagnosed when the diameter of the abdominal aorta exceeds 3 cm, which is 50% larger than the upper limit of

normal aortic diameter of 2 cm. AAA of 5 cm in diameter or larger have a 25% risk of rupture over 5 years, whereas there is much less risk of rupture for smaller aneurysms. Rapid enlargement of an aneurysm by more than 1 cm per year and the development of pain are other important predictors of rupture. AAA may present as an asymptomatic pulsatile abdominal mass or may present with an acute crisis of hypotension, abdominal pain, and palpable aneurysm consistent with aortic rupture.

Conventional radiography often shows the calcified, atherosclerotic wall of a large AAA, but it is unable to demonstrate smaller aneurysms and is no longer used for initial evaluation of AAA (Fig. 14.27). Both US and CT are recommended for the initial evaluation of patients with suspected AAA. US has the advantage of being readily available and quickly performed. It is useful in confirming the presence of aneurysm and measuring its diameter (Fig. 14.28). It is limited in its ability to delineate the aneurysm and its relationship to adjacent visceral, renal, and iliac arteries. US cannot reliably demonstrate retroperitoneal hemorrhage, the most important indicator of ruptured AAA.

CT scanning without IV contrast may be used to confirm the presence and measure the size of an AAA. However, whenever possible, IV contrast

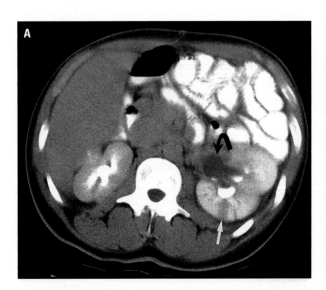
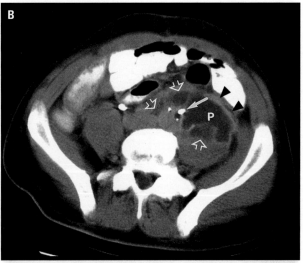

Figure 14.26. Left psoas abscess and left pyonephrosis. Young man with previous abdominal gunshot wound. **A:** Enhanced CT image through the left renal pelvis shows marked left hydronephrosis *(curved arrow)* and persistent nephrogram with focal hypoattenuation, indicating acute pyelonephritis *(straight arrow)*. **B:** Image in the pelvis demonstrates a 5.1-by-3.3-cm left psoas abscess *(P)* with an enhancing wall displacing the left ureter medially. Note the enhanced rim of the abscess *(arrowheads)* and the small loculi posteriorly and medially *(open arrows)*. Bullet fragments *(arrow)* are seen medial to the left ureter.

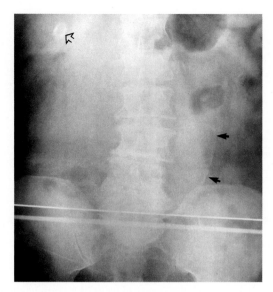

Figure 14.27. Ruptured abdominal aortic aneurysm (AAA). AP supine radiograph shows the atherosclerotic margin of a large AAA *(arrows)* in a patient presenting with an abdominal catastrophe. A rim-calcified gallstone is noted incidentally *(open arrow)*. This radiograph does not depict the associated retroperitoneal hemorrhage.

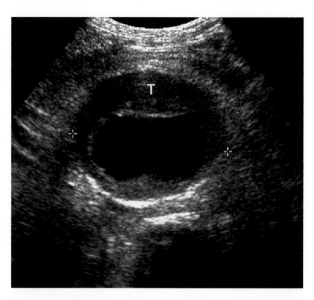

Figure 14.28. Abdominal aortic aneurysm (AAA). Transverse ultrasound image shows 6.8 cm in diameter AAA *(electronic cursors)*. Note the mural thrombus *(T)* surrounding the lumen.

material should be administered to provide additional information about the size and location of intraluminal thrombus and to demonstrate extravasation from a contained rupture (Fig. 14.29). CT is able to show the principal diagnostic sign

of a ruptured AAA, a periaortic retroperitoneal hematoma, which may extend into the perirenal or pararenal spaces. In the absence of retroperitoneal hemorrhage, signs of impending rupture may be detected, including "hyperdense crescent" sign, a high-attenuation crescent within the wall of the aorta; focal contour bulge; increased size; or the

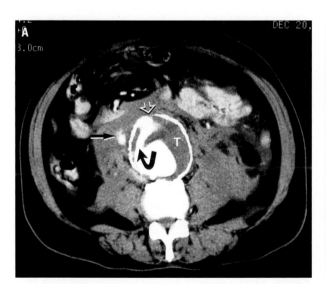

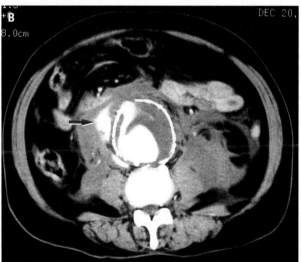

Figure 14.29. Ruptured abdominal aortic aneurysm. **A:** Enhanced CT image shows contrast material *(curved arrow)* leaking through mural thrombosis *(T)* and then through a gap *(open arrow)* in the calcified anterior wall of the aneurysm. Extravasated contrast material *(arrow)* is seen in the retroperitoneal hematoma on the right. **B:** Image at the same level made 3 minutes later shows an increased amount of extravasated contrast material *(arrow)*.

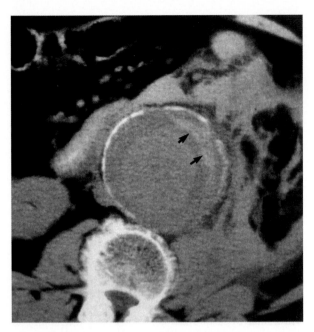

Figure 14.30. Elderly man with severe left lower quadrant pain from the previous day. This large abdominal aortic aneurysm has a calcified wall. Note the high-attenuation crescent inside the calcification (*arrows*), which indicates impending rupture. Abundant left retroperitoneal hematoma is further evidence of impending rupture.

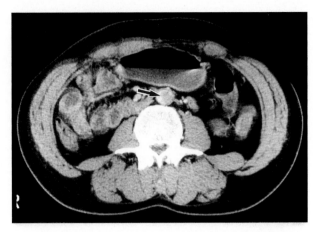

Figure 14.31. Acute aortic occlusion in a man presenting with an acute onset of bilateral cold, pulseless legs. Enhanced CT image of the distal aorta 2 cm above the bifurcation shows the upper margin of a completely occluding thrombus in the aorta (*arrow*). (Case courtesy of Steven Ashlock, MD.)

demonstration of a focal defect in an otherwise calcified aortic wall (Fig. 14.30).

In many clinical situations, dedicated helical CTA of the aorta using 1.0 mm collimation can accurately define the relationship of the aneurysm to the renal arteries. Such examination obviates standard angiography in the preoperative assessment of the aorta.

Acute Aortic Occlusion

Acute occlusion of the aorta causes pain, pallor, pulselessness, paresthesias, and paralysis of the lower extremities. Either embolism or in situ, thrombosis may cause the occlusion. Paresthesias and paralysis indicate limb ischemia, requiring urgent embolectomy or revascularization. CTA can identify the level of aortic occlusion and shows the extent of the blockage (Fig. 14.31).

Retroperitoneal Hemorrhage

Retroperitoneal hemorrhage may occur spontaneously in patients taking anticoagulant therapy (Fig. 14.32) as a complication of AAA or

iatrogenically after renal biopsy or translumbar aortography, by upward dissection of hematoma from transfemoral arterial puncture, or by rupture of retroperitoneal tumors. CT is the preferred modality for the detection and estimation of the size of hematomas within the retroperitoneum. For this purpose, IV contrast is not required, but contrast offers the advantage of demonstrating active

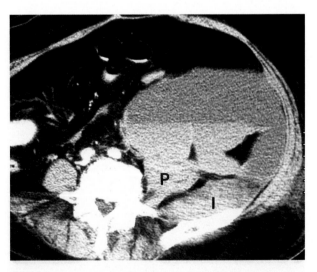

Figure 14.32. Massive retroperitoneal bleeding in a woman taking anticoagulant therapy. Enhanced CT image reveals large retroperitoneal hematoma with fluid–fluid levels dissecting through the left retroperitoneum. Note that the hematoma enlarges the left psoas (*P*) and left iliacus (*I*) muscles.

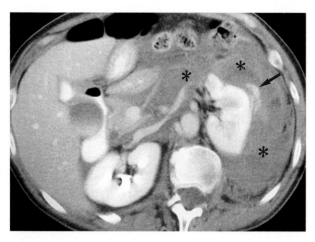

Figure 14.33. Spontaneous retroperitoneal hemorrhage in a woman taking anticoagulants. Enhanced CT image illustrates an area of active contrast extravasation *(arrow)* resulting in a massive left retroperitoneal hematoma *(asterisks)*, which extends across the midline.

arterial extravasation when it is present (Fig. 14.33). An acute hematoma is hyperdense (70 to 90 HU). In hematomas that result from excessive anticoagulation, fluid cell levels and heterogeneity within the hematoma may be seen.

Liver and Biliary Tract

Patients with abnormalities in the biliary system or liver usually present with one of two clinical syndromes: acute right upper quadrant pain or jaundice. Although it has many etiologies including right lower lobe pneumonia, acute right upper quadrant pain is most frequently caused by hepatobiliary disease.

Jaundice

Jaundice may be subdivided into hepatocellular jaundice ("medical jaundice") and mechanical biliary obstruction ("surgical jaundice"). Hepatocellular jaundice is most frequently caused by cirrhosis or hepatitis. Less frequently encountered causes include hemolytic anemia or Gilbert disease (benign elevation of unconjugated bilirubin). Obstructive jaundice is most often caused by carcinoma of the pancreas, carcinoma of the ampulla of Vater, cholangiocarcinoma of the bile ducts, choledocholithiasis, pancreatitis, and iatrogenic biliary strictures.

US is preferred for the initial evaluation of both acute right upper quadrant pain and suspected obstructive jaundice. US demonstrates gallstones and acute cholecystitis. US readily demonstrates both intrahepatic and extrahepatic biliary dilation, but CT is better able to define the underlying cause of biliary obstruction (Fig. 14.34). US is capable of detecting liver abscesses, although CT is more sensitive. CT is indicated when US is technically difficult due to patient body habitus or when bowel gas obscures visualization of the distal common bile duct. CT is the preferred modality when diffuse liver disease is the suspected clinical entity.

On US, intrahepatic obstructed bile ducts appear as dilated tubular structures immediately anterior to an accompanying portal vein branch. Ducts exceeding 2 mm in diameter and greater than 40% of the adjacent portal vein diameter are abnormally dilated (Fig. 14.35). The CHD can be identified in virtually every patient. Normally, the CHD does not exceed 6 mm in diameter, although it can enlarge up to 10 mm in diameter in elderly patients or patients with previous biliary tract disease. When the CHD exceeds 6 mm in diameter in a jaundiced patient, mechanical obstruction is the presumptive diagnosis. It is important to realize that it takes approximately 1 week for intrahepatic biliary ductal dilatation to develop after the onset of biliary obstruction. The CHD requires 3 days to become dilated. Because of this, the absence of bile duct dilatation does not exclude the possibility of mechanical biliary obstruction occurring early in the course of the disease.

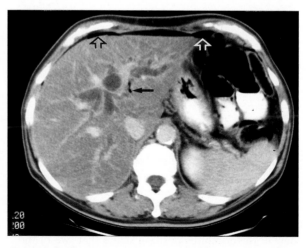

Figure 14.34. Intrahepatic biliary dilatation with air in the bile ducts *(solid arrow)* in a patient with pancreatic carcinoma. Note free intraperitoneal air along the anterior abdominal wall *(open arrows)*. (Case courtesy of Steven Ashlock, MD.)

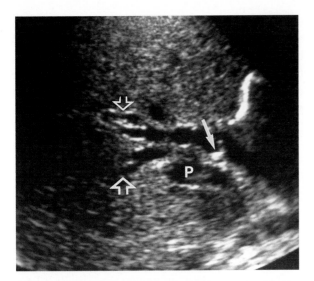

Figure 14.35. Obstructing common duct stone and intrahepatic biliary dilatation. Transverse image through the porta hepatis demonstrates dilated intrahepatic bile ducts *(open arrows)* measuring 4 mm in diameter. A shadowing, 5-mm echogenic common duct stone *(arrow)* is present. Note the portal vein *(P)* posterior to the common duct.

Acute Cholecystitis and Cholelithiasis

Gallstones are present in 5% of white women at age 20 years and in 25% by age 60. Men are less frequently affected. Most gallstones are composed of cholesterol and the remainder are pigmented stones made of calcium bilirubinate.

Gallstones present with one of three general US patterns: (1) fixed or mobile shadowing echogenic foci within the gallbladder (Fig. 14.36); (2) an echogenic focus in the gallbladder fossa with acoustic shadowing posterior to the echogenic focus but without a recognizable gallbladder (Fig. 14.37); and (3) nonshadowing, small echogenic foci within the gallbladder, which may be mobile or may be fixed to the gallbladder wall (Fig. 14.38). Demonstration of acoustic shadowing is an important diagnostic criterion. Accuracy of the US diagnosis of cholelithiasis is greater than 99% when shadowing echogenic foci are seen, but it declines to 80% when nonshadowing echogenic foci are demonstrated. Failure to visualize the gallbladder in a

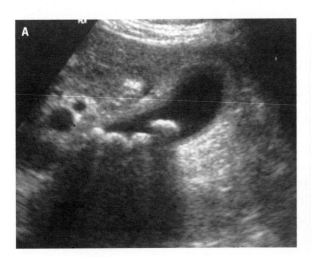

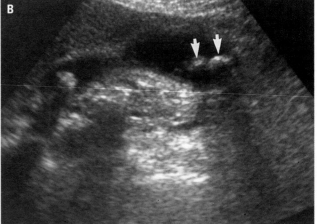

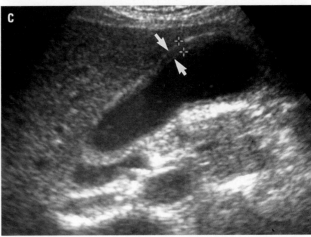

Figure 14.36. Acute cholecystitis with gallstones. **A:** Sagittal image of the gallbladder in the supine position shows four shadowing echogenic gallstones in the body and neck of the gallbladder. The largest stone measures 1.3 cm in maximum diameter. **B:** Sagittal view in the decubitus position shows that two of the stones *(arrows)* roll into the gallbladder fundus with the change in patient position. **C:** Image perpendicular to the gallbladder wall shows a thickened wall measuring 5 mm *(electronic cursors* and *arrows)*. (Case courtesy of Cynthia I. Caskey, MD.)

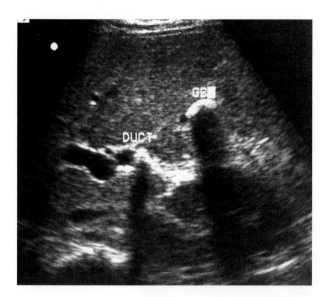

Figure 14.37. Stones in the gallbladder and right intrahepatic bile duct. Longitudinal ultrasound image showing a 1-cm stone within the right intrahepatic duct *(DUCT)*. More inferiorly, a curvilinear, shadowing echogenic focus 2 cm long represents one large or a collection of smaller stones within the gallbladder *(GB)*. (Case courtesy of Cynthia I. Caskey, MD.)

fasting patient may be a sign of cholelithiasis. In such a case, the patient has a contracted gallbladder containing one or more gallstones. However, air within the duodenum may mimic the finding of a contracted gallbladder. The two entities may be distinguished by demonstrating a clean acoustic shadow when gallstones are present. A "dirty shadow" with numerous reverberation artifacts is typical of bowel gas (Fig. 14.38).

Cholesterol or calcium bilirubinate crystals may precipitate out of bile, forming sludge. This frequently occurs in bedridden patients and patients receiving total parenteral nutrition. Sludge produces low-level echoes in the dependent portion of the gallbladder (Fig. 14.39). Over time, sludge may become increasingly echogenic and may be seen in the common bile duct (Fig. 14.39).

CT is less able to demonstrate gallstones than is US. Calcified stones composed of calcium bilirubinate are more readily detected by CT than the more common pure cholesterol stones. Stones have multiple appearances (Fig. 14.40): (1) large, rim-calcified stones with or without a central fissure containing fluid or gas (Mercedes Benz sign); (2) large, rim-calcified faceted stones; (3) small, dense calcium bilirubinate stones; and (4) small, low-attenuation, "pure" cholesterol stones. A false-negative CT examination may occur when stones are less than 5 mm in diameter due to volume averaging or when isodense stones are hidden in the surrounding bile. A false-positive CT examination occurs when the enhancing mucosa of a contracted or edematous gallbladder mimics a gallstone.

Acute calculus cholecystitis occurs when a gallstone obstructs the cystic duct, causing bile stasis and progressive distention of the gallbladder (hydrops). Inflammation, gallbladder wall necrosis,

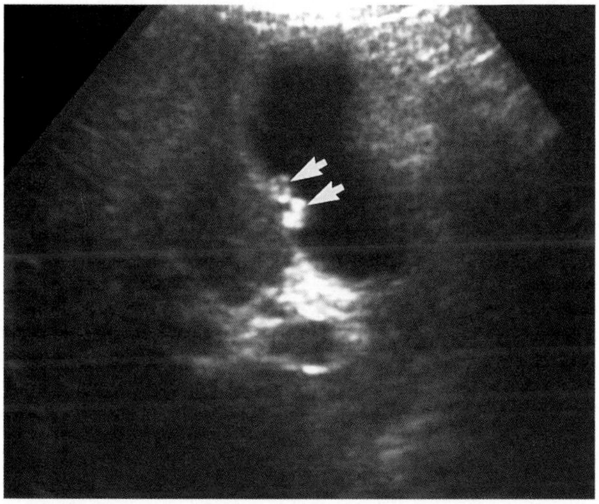

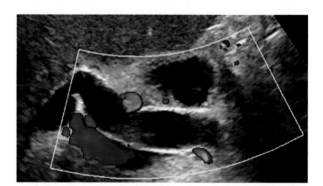

Figure 14.38. Longitudinal ultrasound view of the gallbladder shows two small 5- to 6-mm, nonshadowing gallstones *(arrows)* adherent to the gallbladder wall. (Case courtesy of Cynthia I. Caskey, MD.)

Figure 14.39. Gallbladder sludge in a patient with pancreatic carcinoma. Longitudinal, decubitus view of the gallbladder shows echogenic sludge filling the distended gallbladder and in large common bile duct. Common bile duct is grossly dilated coursing left. Dilated tubular structure in liver parenchyma is intrahepatic duct.

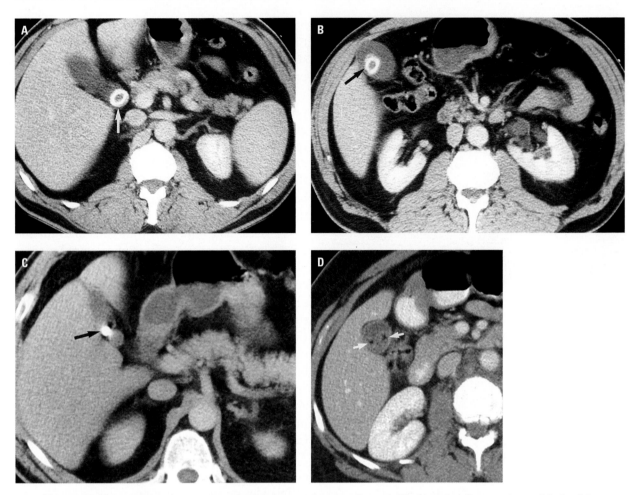

Figure 14.40. Gallstones. **A:** Enhanced CT image shows a rim-calcified, oval gallstone *(arrow)* lodged in the gallbladder neck. **B:** Image through the gallbladder fundus shows a large, faceted stone *(arrow)* in the gallbladder fundus in the same patient. **C:** Image through the gallbladder neck in a different patient shows a 9-mm, uniformly calcified stone *(arrow)* in the gallbladder neck. **D:** Image through the gallbladder fundus in a third patient shows gas-filled gallstones illustrating the "Mercedes Benz" sign *(arrows)*. All of these gallstones were incidental findings in patients imaged for trauma. No CT signs of acute cholecystitis are present.

and bacterial infection of the bile are secondary complications of cystic duct obstruction. The presence of gallstones and a positive sonographic Murphy sign are the two most reliable *gray scale* US criteria of acute cholecystitis. The sonographic Murphy sign is the detection of the point of maximum tenderness over the gallbladder. Operationally, the sign can be elicited by asking the patient to place the US transducer over the most painful part of the abdomen. The sign is present when the transducer shows the gallbladder at the point of maximum pain.

Additional US findings that help in the diagnosis of acute cholecystitis include the following:

1. Gallbladder wall thickening—the normal gallbladder measures 2 to 3 mm in thickness and is abnormal if it measures more than 3 mm. However, thickening is nonspecific and may be seen in ascites, cirrhosis, acute hepatitis, or hypoalbuminemia. Gallbladder wall thickness should be measured at a nondependent portion of the wall and only when the gallbladder is fully distended. Partial contraction of the gallbladder also thickens the wall (Fig. 14.36C).

2. Sonolucent halo surrounding the gallbladder—a hypoechoic, fluid-like rim surrounding the gallbladder represents pericholecystic fluid, associated with gallbladder wall edema.

3. Pericholecystic abscess—a hypoechoic mass with internal echoes adjacent to the stone-filled gallbladder is likely due to an abscess complicating acute cholecystitis.

4. Intraluminal or intramural air—small bubbles or a dense, bright band of reflectors in the gallbladder.
5. Hyperemic gallbladder wall—power Doppler sonographic demonstration of hyperemia in the gallbladder wall increases the accuracy of US diagnosis of acute cholecystitis. However, power Doppler sonography is highly susceptible to motion artifacts; thus, it requires correct application of technical parameters.

Chronic cholecystitis is characterized by a prolonged clinical course of abdominal pain and fatty food intolerance. Gallstones are usually present. The gallbladder wall is thickened by fibrosis rather than by the acute inflammation encountered in acute cholecystitis. The fibrotic gallbladder wall of chronic cholecystitis is not hypervascular, whereas the acutely inflamed gallbladder wall of acute cholecystitis is hypervascular. Therefore, acute cholecystitis may be distinguished from chronic cholecystitis by searching for gallbladder wall hypervascularity with power Doppler sonography.

Acalculous cholecystitis is usually seen in hospitalized patients after surgery or a debilitating illness and is not common in the emergency department population. With US, acalculous cholecystitis is evidenced by gallbladder wall thickening and distension sludge and often with pericholecystic fluid. False-positive studies occur with wall thickening in the absence of inflammation. Cholescintigraphy is used to establish the diagnosis.

Gangrenous cholecystitis is a rare but serious form of cholecystitis that may have a clinical presentation similar to acute cholecystitis. Sonographic clues to this diagnosis include the presence of air in or around the gallbladder, the presence of medium coarse echoes within the gallbladder lumen indicating intraluminal membranes (Fig. 14.41), and fluid collection or abscess adjacent to the gallbladder. This condition may lead to perforation of the gallbladder.

Emphysematous cholecystitis is an uncommon entity occurring more frequently in elderly men, particularly those with diabetes mellitus. Gallstones are usually absent. The underlying pathology is gallbladder ischemia leading to infection with gas-forming organisms. Gas may develop either in the gallbladder wall or in the lumen. At US, the demonstration of dirty acoustic shadows within the gallbladder, its wall, or the bile ducts is a clue to diagnosis. Intramural gas, typical of

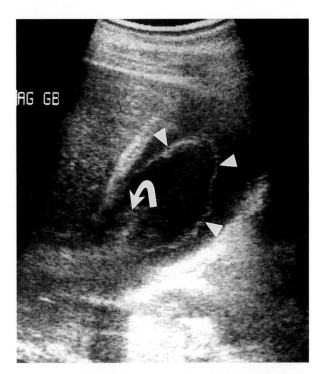

Figure 14.41. Gangrenous gallbladder. Longitudinal ultrasound view of the gallbladder reveals marked thickening of the gallbladder wall with intraluminal membranes *(arrowheads)*. Note gallstone in the gallbladder neck *(curved arrow)*. (Case courtesy of Cynthia I. Caskey, MD.)

emphysematous cholecystitis, is readily demonstrated by CT as a focus of low attenuation in the gallbladder wall (Fig. 14.42). Larger gas collections in the right upper quadrant are visible by conventional radiography.

CT criteria for acute cholecystitis include (1) gallbladder wall thickening greater than 3 mm and wall nodularity, (2) distention of the gallbladder greater than 5 cm in transverse or AP dimension, (3) stones in the gallbladder or cystic duct, (4) poor definition of the gallbladder wall at the interface with the liver, (5) thin rim of pericholecystic fluid, (6) inflammatory changes in the pericholecystic fat (Fig. 14.43), (7) increased density of the bile (greater than 20 HU), and (8) marked gallbladder wall enhancement.

Although conventional radiographs are not a primary imaging modality for right upper quadrant pain, signs of biliary and gallbladder pathology may be evident. Dense gallstones are readily detected (Fig. 14.27). Chronic obstruction of the biliary tree may result in chronic cholecystitis. On occasion, calcium carbonate crystals may precipitate within gallbladder sludge, resulting in a characteristic

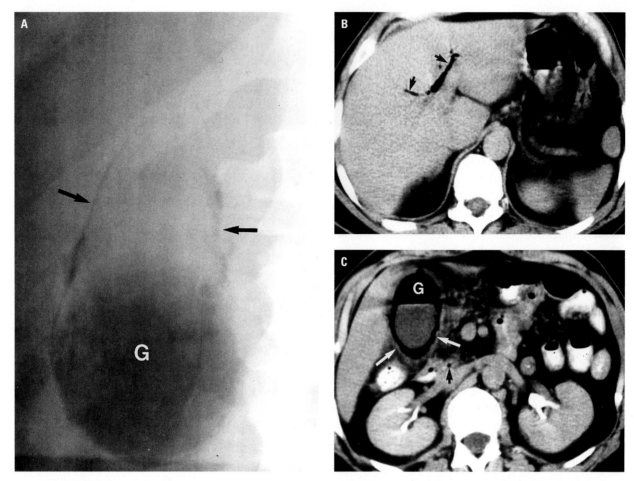

Figure 14.42. Emphysematous cholecystitis in a man with diabetes mellitus. **A:** Supine radiograph of the gallbladder reveals a bubble of air in the gallbladder fundus *(G)* associated with linear collections of air dissecting through the gallbladder wall *(arrows)*. **B:** Enhanced CT through the porta hepatis shows pneumobilia in the right and left hepatic ducts *(arrows)*. **C:** CT through the gallbladder shows the air–bile level in the gallbladder fundus *(G)* correlating with the radiographic appearance. Air is demonstrated within the wall of the gallbladder *(white arrows)* and in the common bile duct *(black arrow)*.

radiopaque substance within the gallbladder, called "milk-of-calcium" bile (Fig. 14.44). Intramural calcification may occur in the gallbladder wall as the result of chronic inflammation, producing the "porcelain gallbladder" visible by conventional radiography and CT (Fig. 14.45). Patients with porcelain gallbladder have an increased risk of gallbladder carcinoma. Selective mucosal calcification has an incidence of 7%; however, diffuse calcification has no definite increased risk.

Hepatobiliary scintigraphy (cholescintigraphy) is another accurate modality for diagnosing acute cholecystitis. It is a more expensive examination used primarily when US fails to demonstrate acute cholecystitis when there is high clinical suspicion. The test involves injection of a ^{99m}Tc-labeled IDA derivative, which is taken up by the liver and excreted in the bile. A positive study occurs when bile is excreted into the duodenum but does not fill the gallbladder (Fig. 14.46). False-positive examinations may occur when there is bile stasis, as is seen after prolonged fasting or with dehydration. False-positives are more frequent in gravely ill patients who have acalculous cholecystitis.

Choledocholithiasis

Choledocholithiasis is present in 10% to 15% of all patients with acute or chronic cholecystitis and is the most common cause of bile duct obstruction. Most of these stones form in the gallbladder and pass to the common bile duct, although some pigmented stones may form in the common bile duct,

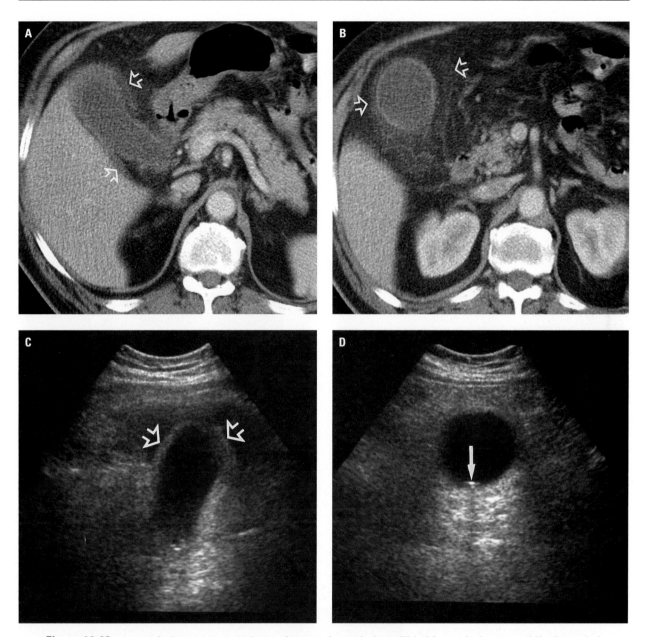

Figure 14.43. Acute cholecystitis. **A:** Enhanced image through the gallbladder neck shows a mildly distended gallbladder with a mildly thickened wall and some pericholecystic fluid *(open arrows)* between the gallbladder and the liver and external to the gallbladder. **B:** Image through the gallbladder fundus shows edema *(open arrows)* surrounding the mildly distended fundus of the gallbladder. **C:** Longitudinal gallbladder ultrasound view shows wall thickening *(open arrows)*. **D:** Transverse view through the fundus reveals a small shadowing, echogenic stone *(solid arrow)*.

particularly when biliary strictures and biliary stasis are present. Choledocholithiasis is present in 5% to 6% of patients who have undergone cholecystectomy. US or CT may demonstrate choledocholithiasis, but sensitivity is limited with either modality. Stones are typically located in the distal portion of the common bile duct near the ampulla of Vater; however, this area is frequently obscured by bowel

gas. On CT, direct demonstration of the distal common bile duct stone is the most reliable diagnostic criterion. Dense stones are relatively easy to detect, particularly when surrounded by anechoic bile (Fig. 14.47). Occasionally, a common duct stone has a low-attenuation value, similar to that of soft tissue or water. In this case, an abrupt change in the caliber of the common bile duct suggests the level of the

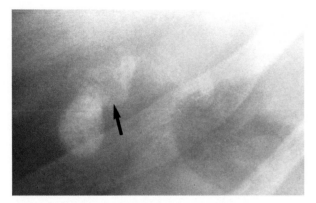

Figure 14.44. Milk-of-calcium bile. Close-up of an AP radiograph of the gallbladder illustrates milk-of-calcium bile with coated oval lucent stone in the proximal cystic duct *(arrow)*.

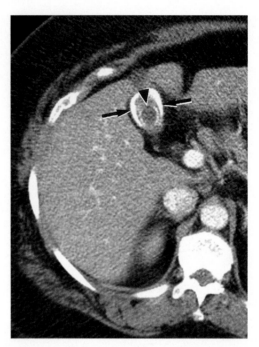

Figure 14.45. Porcelain gallbladder. Enhanced CT image of the gallbladder fundus shows calcification of the gallbladder wall *(arrows)* typical of porcelain gallbladder. Note the rim-calcified stone within the gallbladder *(arrowhead)*.

stone. However, this appearance is nonspecific and also occurs with tumor or pancreatic carcinoma. Magnetic resonance cholangiography or endoscopic retrograde cholangiopancreatography is required when CT and US fail to demonstrate a cause of biliary obstruction in a jaundiced patient.

Cholangitis (Ascending Cholangitis)
Cholangitis is a bacterial infection of the biliary tree in the presence of complete or partial biliary obstruction. Gram-negative enteric bacteria usually cause the infection. The classic clinical triad described by Charcot of right upper quadrant pain, fever, and jaundice is present in 60% to 70% of patients. The same clinical triad may be seen with cholecystitis and hepatitis. Diagnostic imaging is directed toward identification of the site and cause of biliary obstruction and to detect associated hepatic abnormality.

Figure 14.46. Hepatobiliary scintigraphy: Normal and acute cholecystitis. **Top row:** Anterior images obtained 15, 35, and 60 minutes after administration of ^{99m}Tc-labeled dimethyl iminodiacetic acid shows normal uptake by the liver, prompt excretion into the biliary tree, and progressive filling of the gallbladder *(solid arrows)*. Note the increasing activity within the small intestine *(open arrows)*. **Bottom row:** Similar anterior images in a patient with acute cholecystitis show prompt uptake and excretion of the radiopharmaceutical, but the gallbladder does not fill after 1 hour. Administration of morphine sulfate did not induce gallbladder filling. These findings are typical of acute cholecystitis. (Case courtesy of Lamk Lamki, MD.)

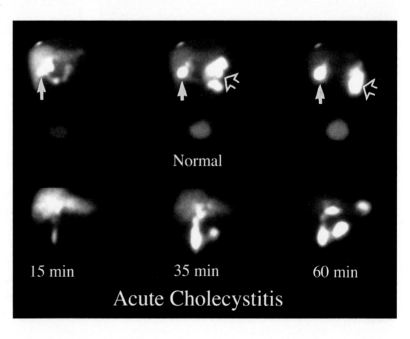

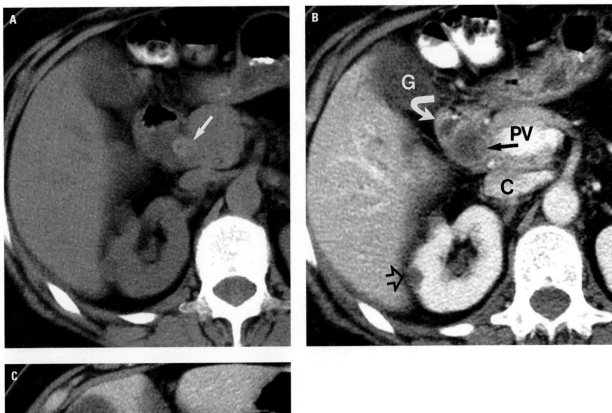

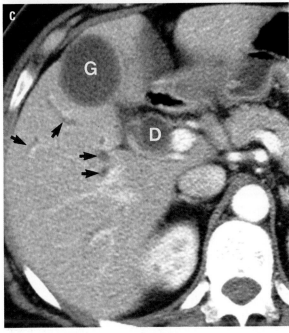

Figure 14.47. Common bile duct stone. **A:** Unenhanced CT image shows a rim-calcified stone lodged in the intrapancreatic portion of the common bile duct *(white arrow)*. **B:** Enhanced CT image at the same level shows that the stone *(black solid arrow)* is not conspicuous when the adjacent portal vein *(PV)*, inferior vena cava *(C)*, and duodenal wall *(white curved arrow)* become enhanced with contrast material. *G* is the gall bladder. Note the small peripheral Bosniak I renal cyst on the upper pole on the right kidney *(open arrow)*. **C:** Image cephalad to (**A** and **B**) through the gallbladder *(G)* demonstrates intrahepatic *(arrows)* and extrahepatic biliary duct *(D)* dilatation.

Hepatic Abscess and Other Focal Liver Lesions

Hepatic abscesses are either pyogenic or amebic. Liver abscesses are most commonly associated with biliary tract obstruction or cholangitis, but they may arise from underlying diverticulitis, pancreatic abscess, appendicitis, inflammatory bowel disease, or bacteremia from any cause. Pyogenic liver abscesses are caused by gram-negative enteric bacteria and enteric anaerobic bacteria. Amebic abscesses are due to fecal–oral transmission of *Entamoeba histolytica,* a protozoan that is endemic in many parts of the world.

Pyogenic and amebic abscesses have a similar CT and US appearance and, in individual cases, cannot be distinguished based on their imaging appearance. On CT scans, liver abscesses are usually solitary, round, or oval low-attenuation masses averaging 4 to 5 cm in diameter (Fig. 14.48). Approximately 10%

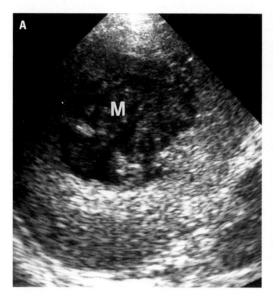

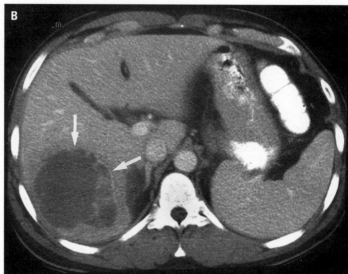

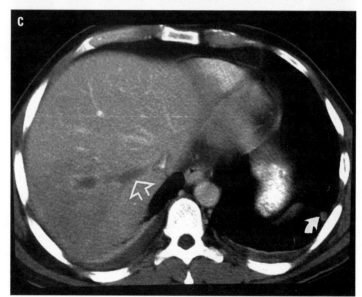

Figure 14.48. Liver abscess. **A:** Transverse ultrasound view reveals a complex cystic mass *(M)* in the right hepatic lobe. **B:** Enhanced CT through the porta hepatis reveals a large, heterogeneous cystic mass in the right lobe of the liver with a rim of contrast enhancement *(straight arrows)*. **C:** CT through the dome of the liver illustrates thrombosis of the right hepatic vein *(open arrow)* and a nodule *(short curved arrow)* representing a septic embolus in the left lower lobe. Minimal pleural effusion is present bilaterally.

of the time, liver abscesses are multilocular or multiple. The abscess margin has a variable morphology, ranging from relatively thin and well-defined to nodular and irregular. Most have an enhancing margin. Some have a rim of low-attenuation edema surrounding the enhancing margin. A liver abscess may have a central gas collection or an air–fluid level. Cystic or necrotic liver metastases may have a similar appearance.

The US appearance of hepatic abscesses is complex. They vary in shape and echogenicity. They are usually spherical or ovoid, but they may be flattened (Fig. 14.48). About 50% are anechoic, with the remainder being either hyperechoic or hypoechoic.

They may be filled with septa, fluid levels, or internal debris. Early in their course, hepatic abscesses are echogenic and poorly demarcated, but they become less echogenic and better demarcated as they mature. Compared to pyogenic abscesses, amebic abscesses are more likely to be round or oval and hypoechoic.

Abscesses must be distinguished from other focal liver lesions. On CT, hepatic cysts appear as well-circumscribed, thin-bordered, homogeneous, low-attenuation (less than 20 HU) masses without enhancement after IV administration of contrast material. They range in size from a few millimeters to several centimeters (Fig. 14.49). Hemangiomas

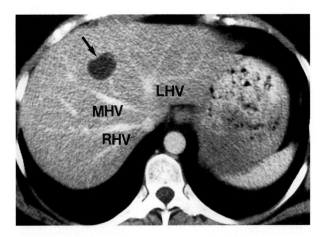

Figure 14.49. Hepatic cyst. Enhanced CT shows a well-defined 3.8-by-2.0-cm water attenuation cyst *(arrow)* in segment IV of the liver. *RHV*, right hepatic vein; *MVH*, middle hepatic vein; *LHV*, left hepatic vein.

of the liver are the most common benign neoplasms of the liver, occurring in 2% of the adult population. They appear as a well-defined, low-attenuation mass on unenhanced CT scans and have a distinctive progressive contrast enhancement pattern, which increases from arterial to delayed phases. Peripheral nodular or globular areas enhance initially, followed by enhancement from the periphery to the center. Complete opacification of the entire hemangioma requires between 3 minutes for smaller lesions and 20 minutes for larger lesions (Fig. 14.50).

On US, simple hepatic cysts are anechoic; have smooth, sharp margins; and show acoustic enhancement. Occasionally, they have multiple septa, have calcified walls, or contain internal hemorrhage or debris. Hepatic hemangiomas are typically homogeneous, hyperechoic lesions with well-defined margins; however, they may be hypoechoic or of mixed echogenicity (Fig. 14.51). Liver metastases have a variable appearance and may be cystic with hypoechoic fluid in the center—an appearance that is indistinguishable from an abscess. Because of the nonspecific, equivocal imaging appearance of focal liver lesions, percutaneous biopsy is often used for definitive diagnosis.

Alcoholic Liver Disease

The toxic effects of alcohol on the liver may be manifested as fatty liver, alcoholic hepatitis, or cirrhosis. These same pathologic conditions also occur as a result of other toxic insults to the liver.

Fatty Liver

Fatty liver (steatosis) is the excessive accumulation of triglycerides in hepatocytes. Alcoholic liver disease, diabetes mellitus, obesity, malnutrition, and chronic illness are common causes. The condition

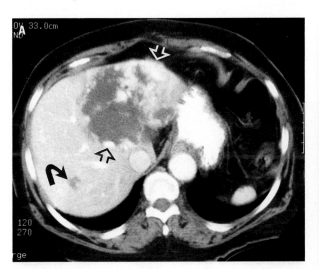
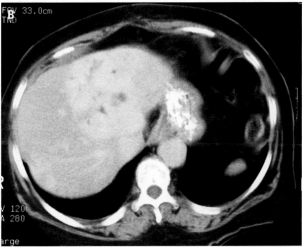

Figure 14.50. Cavernous hemangioma of the liver. **A:** Enhanced CT shows a large, 7 cm in diameter hemangioma filling most of the left lobe of the liver. Note the nodular appearance of contrast enhancement in the periphery of the mass *(open arrows)*. A small, 2 cm in diameter hemangioma is seen in segment VII *(curved arrow)*. **B:** Image at the same level made 7 minutes later shows that the central portions of the large hemangioma has filled in with contrast material. The hemangioma has the same attenuation value as the aorta and inferior vena cava. The smaller hemangioma had a similar pattern of contrast enhancement (not shown).

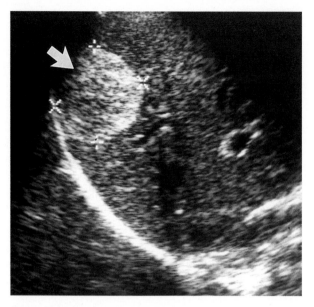

Figure 14.51. Cavernous hemangioma of the liver. Sagittal ultrasound image of the right lobe of the liver shows a 4.4-by-4.5-cm spherical echogenic mass located in the dome of the liver *(arrow* and *electronic cursors).* Note its homogeneously echogenic nature typical of a large cavernous hemangioma. Several other small hemangiomas were present elsewhere in the liver.

is easily diagnosed on unenhanced CT scans when the attenuation values of the liver are much lower than normal. Minor degrees of fatty liver may be diagnosed when the measured attenuation value of the liver is less than that of the spleen. Hepatic steatosis is more difficult to diagnose after IV contrast enhancement because of the time-dependent effects of IV contrast on the attenuation value of the liver and

spleen. As a general rule, the diagnosis is made when the attenuation of the liver is 20 to 30 HU less than the spleen on contrast redistribution phase images (Fig. 14.52) and when hepatic vessels appear denser than liver parenchyma.

Steatosis may be focal and may simulate the appearance of other focal lesions such as neoplasm or abscess. Focal fat accumulations are frequently segmental or wedge shaped with no mass effect or bulge in the hepatic contour (see Figs. 14.65 and 14.79). A common location of focal fatty replacement is adjacent to the fissure for the ligamentum teres. Importantly, hepatic and portal veins coursing through the low-attenuation area distinguish it from a space-occupying mass.

Hepatitis

Hepatitis is an acute or chronic inflammatory process affecting the entire liver that may be due to viral infection, alcohol ingestion, or other hepatotoxins, including drugs. Acute hepatitis is characterized by hepatocellular necrosis and degeneration. The chronic forms of hepatitis have the added features of periportal inflammation and architectural distortion of the liver. The CT appearance of hepatitis is nonspecific, including hepatomegaly, fatty liver, gallbladder wall thickening, and periportal edema. Lymphadenopathy adjacent to the liver may be seen in chronic hepatitis.

Cirrhosis

Cirrhosis is a generalized response to liver injury from various insults. It is a multistage process that progresses from inflammation to regeneration, and

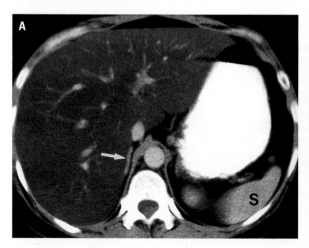
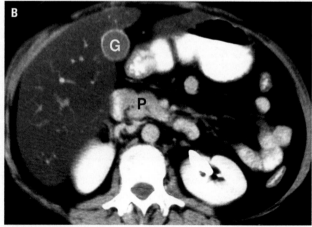

Figure 14.52. Fatty liver. Enhanced CT scans (**A** and **B**) show diffusely decreased attenuation of the liver relative to the spleen *(S),* pancreas *(P),* gallbladder *(G),* muscle, and right adrenal gland.

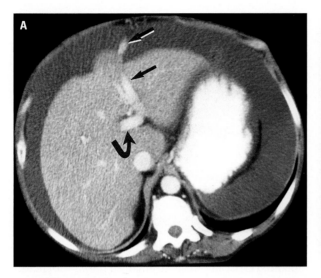
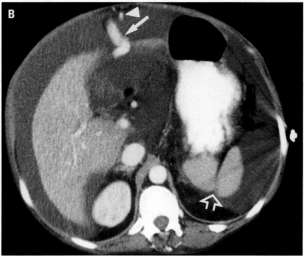

Figure 14.53. Cirrhosis of the liver. **A:** Enhanced CT image through the left portal vein shows mild nodularity of the liver contour. Note the recanalized paraumbilical vein *(straight arrows)* arising from the left portal vein *(curved arrow)*. **B:** Image through the right lobe of the liver demonstrates the large, tortuous paraumbilical vein *(straight arrow)* and a smaller collateral vein *(arrowhead)*. A deep congenital cleft is seen in the spleen *(open arrow)*.

finally, to fibrosis. Resultant changes in intrahepatic blood circulation lead to portal hypertension and cholestasis, leading to further injury to the liver with progressive fibrosis. The presence of fibrosis and the recognition of regenerating nodules are the key imaging features of cirrhosis.

Early in cirrhosis, CT scans show hepatomegaly, heterogeneity of liver parenchyma attenuation on unenhanced images, and heterogeneous enhancement on contrast-enhanced images. This heterogeneity is due to fibrosis and heterogeneous fatty infiltration. When the disease is more advanced, shrinkage of the liver (particularly the right lobe), prominence of the porta hepatis, and enlargement of the intrahepatic fissures are seen. The hepatic contour is usually nodular due to regenerating nodules. Fibrous septa form between the nodules, further contributing to heterogeneity of the hepatic parenchyma. Ascites typically occurs in association with cirrhosis (Fig. 14.53).

In these diffuse liver diseases, US is usually not helpful. In acute hepatitis, US shows the liver with decreased echogenicity with very echogenic periportal areas. In both fatty liver and cirrhosis, the liver is very echogenic, and the US beam has difficulty penetrating deeply into the liver. Abnormalities in the contour of the liver may be evident in cirrhosis.

Passive Congestion

When central venous pressures are elevated, as occurs in congestive heart failure and constrictive pericarditis, the sinusoids of the liver become congested and dilated and perisinusoidal edema develops. Diagnostic imaging is not required for this condition, but the CT appearance is striking. The liver shows diffusely mottled enhancement of the parenchyma associated with dilated IVC and hepatic veins. There may be reflux of contrast material into the hepatic veins. Associated cardiomegaly, pleural effusion, ascites, and periportal edema are all manifestations of the underlying elevated central venous pressure. Thrombosis of the hepatic veins in Budd-Chiari syndrome causes a mottled enhancement pattern in the liver without the other signs of systemic venous hypertension (Fig. 14.54).

Spleen

Splenomegaly

Pathologic enlargement of the spleen is an infrequent reason for emergency department visits. The etiologies are myriad and include portal hypertension, hematologic disorders, infiltration, infection, cysts, and neoplasms. On conventional radiographs, a splenic length greater than 15 cm indicates

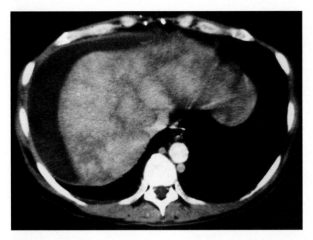

Figure 14.54. Budd-Chiari syndrome. Enhanced CT image through the hepatic veins shows mottled contrast enhancement throughout the liver due to hepatic venous obstruction. Note the large amount of ascites. Systemic venous hypertension due to congestive heart failure causes an identical enhancement pattern in the liver.

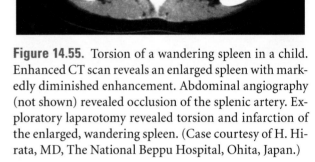

Figure 14.55. Torsion of a wandering spleen in a child. Enhanced CT scan reveals an enlarged spleen with markedly diminished enhancement. Abdominal angiography (not shown) revealed occlusion of the splenic artery. Exploratory laparotomy revealed torsion and infarction of the enlarged, wandering spleen. (Case courtesy of H. Hirata, MD, The National Beppu Hospital, Ohita, Japan.)

splenomegaly. Splenic volume may be estimated by measurements derived from CT scan, but this is too cumbersome for routine use. A useful qualitative measure of splenic enlargement is the convexity of its medial border.

Splenic Torsion and Infarction

Rarely, suspensory ligaments of the spleen may be lax, allowing the spleen to move freely within the abdomen. The most common clinical presentation of the "wandering" spleen is that of intermittent abdominal pain. An asymptomatic abdominal mass is a less common presentation. Least common, but most serious, is the patient presenting with acute abdominal pain due to torsion of the wandering spleen (Fig. 14.55).

Splenic infarction occurs secondary to thromboembolic disease, atherosclerosis, systemic lupus erythematosus, myeloproliferative disorders, pancreatitis, pancreatic masses, and sickle-cell anemia. Particularly if the infarcts are large, patients may present with acute left upper quadrant pain, fever, and symptoms of diaphragmatic irritation. Splenic infarcts appear as wedge-shaped, low-attenuation defects in the spleen, broader along the splenic capsule with their apices at the splenic hilum (Fig. 14.56). Patients with sickle-cell disease suffer multiple episodes of splenic infarction, eventually resulting in a shrunken spleen (Fig. 14.57).

Splenic Infection

Splenic infection is uncommon in the general population but is more prevalent in immunosuppressed patients with cancer, organ transplants, or acquired immunodeficiency syndrome (AIDS). *Mycobacterium tuberculosis*, *Mycobacterium avium-intracellulare*, and *Histoplasma capsulatum* are the organisms most frequently encountered.

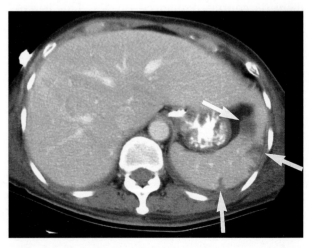

Figure 14.56. Splenic infarction. Enhanced CT image through the upper portion of the spleen shows multiple wedge-shaped areas of diminished enhancement in the spleen, representing multiple areas of embolic infarction *(arrows)*.

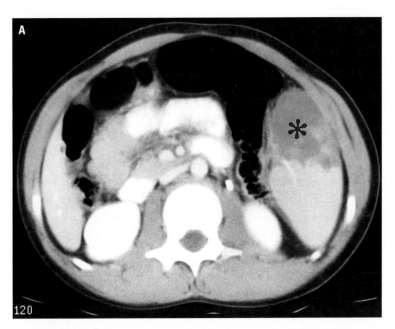
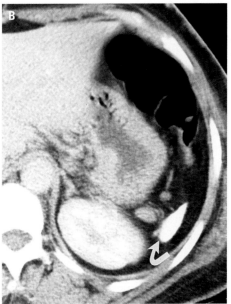

Figure 14.57. Splenic infarction in sickle-cell disease. **A:** Enhanced CT image below the splenic hilum in a 9-year-old boy shows an area of infarction *(asterisk)* in the anterior portion of the lower pole of the spleen. The spleen is markedly enlarged, seen on 25 contiguous, 7-mm images. **B:** Enhanced CT in a 43-year-old woman demonstrates a small, densely calcified, autoinfarcted spleen *(curved arrow)*. (Case in **A** courtesy of Steven Ashlock, MD.)

Splenic infection usually appears as small microabscesses throughout the spleen, often with similar lesions in the liver. Occasionally, a more well-defined, larger abscess will form. On CT, microabscesses typically appear as numerous, less than 1 cm diameter areas of low attenuation seen diffusely throughout the spleen (Fig. 14.58). The spleen may also be enlarged. On US, microabscesses appear as numerous hypoechoic nodules less than 5 mm in size, which are best seen with a 5-MHz linear array transducer.

Pancreas

Patients with pancreatic disease generally present to the emergency department with one of two clinical syndromes: abdominal pain or painless jaundice. Those presenting with abdominal pain may have acute pancreatitis; complications related to pancreatitis, including pancreatic abscess or pseudocyst; or chronic pancreatitis. Painless jaundice is the hallmark of pancreatic carcinoma. CT plays an important role in the initial evaluation of the pancreas. A specialized, thin-section, 2.5-mm CT pancreatic mass protocol

using precontrast images through the pancreas followed by arterial phase and portal venous phase helical images after IV administration of contrast material provides the highest diagnostic quality.

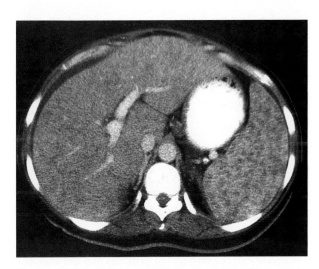

Figure 14.58. Splenic and hepatic microabscesses in an HIV-positive patient. Enhanced CT scan reveals numerous small hypodense lesions in the enlarged spleen and less distinct hypodense lesions throughout the liver. A small amount of ascites is present.

Acute Pancreatitis

The clinical presentation of acute pancreatitis varies from asymptomatic to complex intra-abdominal pathology. Acute pancreatitis typically presents with a rapid onset of upper abdominal pain, associated with variable degrees of abdominal tenderness. Pathologic features include interstitial edema and fat necrosis of the pancreatic parenchyma. More severe cases are characterized by necrosis of the pancreas and complications of pseudocyst or venous thrombosis.

Because of the variable clinical manifestations, the terminology used to describe acute pancreatitis is important. The terminology used here is based on that of the International Symposium on Acute Pancreatitis.

Mild acute pancreatitis is associated with minimal organ dysfunction and an uncomplicated recovery. Patients with mild acute pancreatitis usually require no cross-sectional imaging other than US screening for gallstones if the clinical presentation is typical of gallstone pancreatitis. When the clinical situation is uncertain, CT is the imaging modality of choice. On CT, diffuse or focal pancreatic enlargement, irregularity of pancreatic contour, focal areas of low attenuation, peripancreatic fat infiltration, or peripancreatic fluid collection are typical features (Fig. 14.59). On US, similar findings may be seen,

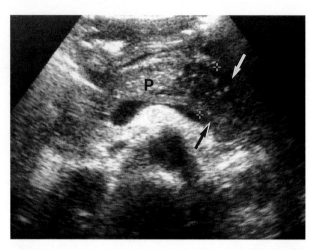

Figure 14.60. Acute distal pancreatitis. Transverse ultrasound image at the level of the splenic vein shows a heterogeneous hypoechoic texture of the distal pancreas *(arrows)* relative to the body of the pancreas *(P)*. A peripancreatic fluid collection was present at more caudal levels (not shown). (Case courtesy of Cynthia I. Caskey, MD.)

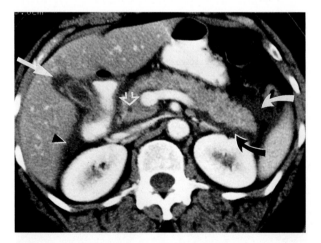

Figure 14.59. Mild pancreatitis. Enhanced CT image through the pancreas shows uniform parenchymal enhancement throughout the pancreas with a well-defined interface between the pancreas and the adjacent peripancreatic fluid *(curved arrows)*. Note the normal caliber common bile duct passing through the pancreatic head *(open arrow)*. Pericholecystic fluid surrounds the enhanced gallbladder wall *(solid straight arrow)* and minimal ascites in the hepatorenal recess *(arrowhead)*.

including focal or diffuse pancreatic enlargement, contour abnormalities, diffuse or focal hypoechoic areas, and fluid collections within or adjacent to the pancreas (Fig. 14.60). US is often limited due to adynamic ileus, which frequently occurs with acute pancreatitis. Patient distress, obesity, or fatty infiltration of the liver also limits US examination of the abdomen.

Severe acute pancreatitis is associated with organ failure and/or local complications, including pancreatic necrosis, pancreatic abscess, or pseudocyst. A thin-section, 5-mm helical CT scan before and after IV administration of contrast material is the best way to detect focal areas of pancreatic necrosis. US examination is often technically limited in its ability to visualize the entire pancreas and surrounding tissues. Magnetic resonance imaging (MRI) is excellent for evaluation of the biliary and pancreatic ductal systems and is more sensitive than CT or US in the detection of hemorrhage.

On CT, severe acute pancreatitis is characterized by swelling of the gland with blurring of the margin between pancreatic parenchyma and fat, particularly the ventral margin (Fig. 14.61). Edema and inflammation extend into the peripancreatic fat, collecting first on the left side of the anterior pararenal space but then dissecting throughout the entire anterior pararenal space, causing thickening of the anterior

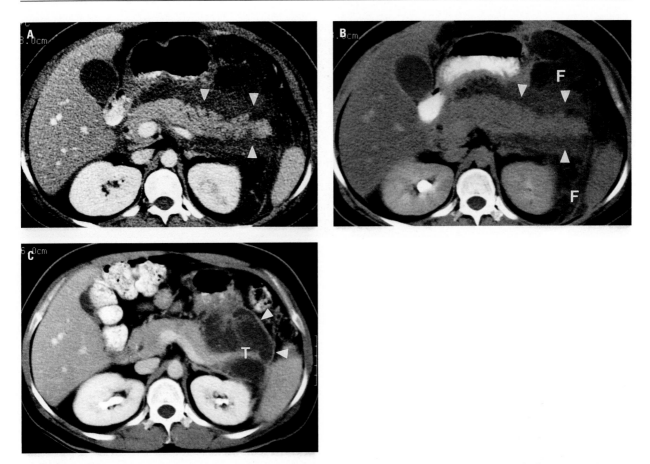

Figure 14.61. Severe acute pancreatitis. A: Thin-section pancreas protocol CT image through the pancreatic body and tail made soon after administration of the bolus of contrast material shows diminished enhancement in the tail with blurring of the interface between the pancreas and the adjacent peripancreatic fluid *(arrowheads)*. **B:** Delayed image at the same level demonstrates edema surrounding the pancreatic body and tail in the left anterior pararenal space *(arrowheads)*. Free fluid is present lateral to the left wall of the stomach and adjacent to the spleen *(F)*. **C:** Two months later, enhanced CT image at the same level demonstrates a pancreatic pseudocyst surrounding the tail of the pancreas *(T)*. An enhancing wall has formed along the left margin *(white arrowheads)*. Four months after the original examination, CT showed complete resolution of all peripancreatic fluid, including the pseudocyst.

renal fascia. Fluid also tracks posteriorly along the leaves of the posterior renal fascia, extending to the lateroconal fascia. Peripancreatic fluid may disrupt the parietal peritoneum, extend into the lesser peritoneal sac, and from there into the peritoneal cavity through the foramen of Winslow. Fluid may also track between the leaves of the adjacent gastrohepatic, gastrosplenic, and gastrocolic ligaments and into the transverse mesocolon and the root of the mesentery. Collections may also form within the pancreas itself. These acute fluid collections occur early in the course of acute pancreatitis, are located in or near the pancreas, and always lack a wall of granulation or fibrous tissue.

Pancreatic necrosis may be diffuse or focal and is typically associated with peripancreatic fat necrosis. The diagnosis is established on CT by diffuse or focal, well-marginated, nonenhancing zones of pancreatic parenchyma, larger than 3 cm in diameter or involving more than 30% of the total area of the pancreas (Fig. 14.62). Failure of enhancement is measured as less than or equal to 30 HU at peak enhancement on CT. Pancreatic necrosis, fluid collections in the pararenal spaces, and nonvisualization of the splenic or portal veins are ominous signs implying development of abscess and/or patient demise. These patients are likely to benefit from drainage of the necrotic tissues and/or fluid.

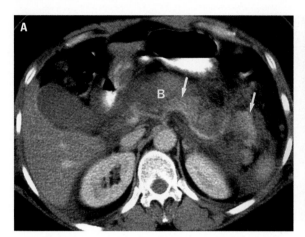
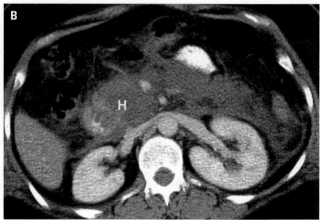

Figure 14.62. Acute pancreatic necrosis. **A:** Enhanced CT image through the pancreatic body and tail shows markedly diminished enhancement of the pancreatic parenchyma with focal areas of minimal enhancement in the body *(B)* and tail *(arrows)*. Peripancreatic fluid is seen in both the right and left anterior pararenal spaces. **B:** Image at the pancreatic head shows diminished enhancement of the entire head *(H)*. Diminished enhancement throughout most the pancreas indicates very severe acute pancreatitis with widespread necrosis.

Pancreatic pseudocyst is defined as a collection of pancreatic fluid enclosed by a wall of fibrous or granulation tissue, which develops secondary to acute pancreatitis, pancreatic trauma, or chronic pancreatitis. Pseudocysts may be seen by either CT or US. Small pseudocysts less than 6 cm in diameter may resolve spontaneously, but larger ones usually require drainage. On CT, pseudocysts are round or oval collections of low attenuation with a well-defined capsule (Figs. 14.61C and 14.63). The presence of focal or diffuse high attenuation within the pseudocysts suggests complicating infection or hemorrhage.

Pancreatic abscess is defined as a circumscribed intra-abdominal collection of pus in proximity to the pancreas with variable amounts of gas, a thickened wall, and no central enhancement, usually without pancreatic necrosis. The CT appearance is typical of abscesses elsewhere in the abdomen.

Chronic Pancreatitis

Chronic pancreatitis is characterized by recurrent attacks of pain, exocrine and endocrine pancreatic insufficiency, and, in the advanced stage, the formation of pancreatic calculi. Chronic pancreatitis is highly associated with alcohol abuse, but it also occurs in idiopathic and biliary forms. Occasionally, chronic pancreatitis results from recurrent episodes of acute pancreatitis, but it usually arises as a separate disease.

On conventional radiographs, chronic pancreatitis may be manifested by fine or coarse calcifications within the pancreas (Fig. 14.64). On CT, two-thirds of patients show pancreatic duct dilatation; half of patients have pancreatic atrophy and calcifications; and a third have fluid collections, focal pancreatic enlargement, and biliary ductal dilatation (Fig. 14.64). Peripancreatic fluid is unusual. Generalized enlargement is not typical.

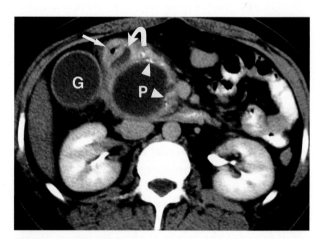

Figure 14.63. Pancreatic pseudocyst. Enhanced CT image through the pancreatic head shows a mature pancreatic pseudocyst *(P)*. Note the distended gallbladder *(G)*, the compressed duodenum *(straight arrow)*, and the distended common bile duct *(curved arrow)*. Several small pancreatic calcifications *(arrowheads)* are seen adjacent to the pseudocyst in this patient with chronic pancreatitis.

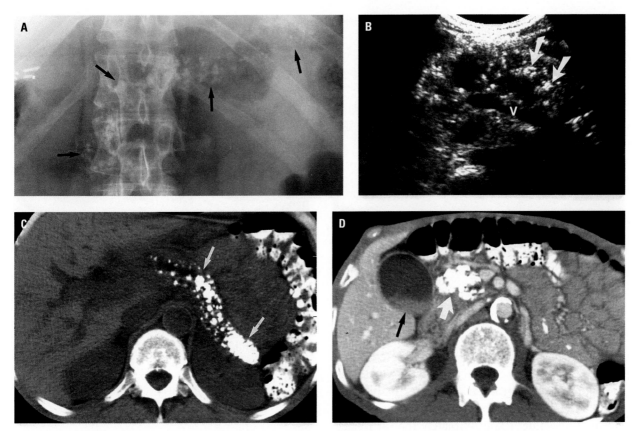

Figure 14.64. Chronic pancreatitis. **A:** Close-up of AP supine abdominal radiograph shows coarse calcifications along the entire course of the pancreas *(black arrows)*. **B:** In another patient, transverse ultrasound image of the pancreas shows that the entire pancreas is echogenic, with focally more echogenic areas representing pancreatic calcifications *(white arrows)*. The splenic vein *(V)* is visible posterior to the pancreas. **C:** In a third patient, unenhanced CT image through the pancreatic body reveals extensive coarse calcifications throughout the pancreas *(white arrows)*. Note atrophy of the pancreatic parenchyma. Dilatation of the main pancreatic duct was better depicted on other images. **D:** In the same patient as **C**, enhanced CT image at the head of the pancreas shows coarse calcifications in the head *(white arrow)*. Note sludge in the dependent portion of the distended gallbladder *(black arrow)*. (Case in **B** courtesy of Cynthia I. Caskey, MD.)

Pseudocysts may occur in chronic pancreatitis and have the same diagnostic criteria and appearance as described for acute pancreatitis. Those larger than 4 cm in diameter or developing outside the pancreas are less likely to regress spontaneously. Chronic pancreatitis is associated with splenic vein and portal vein obstruction.

Pancreatic Neoplasm

The jaundiced patient should be initially evaluated with US to search for evidence of biliary obstruction. At this time, a mass in the pancreas may be identified, but the absence of a mass does not exclude pancreatic carcinoma. When pancreatic carcinoma is the leading diagnostic possibility, the best initial diagnostic examination is a detailed pancreas protocol CT. Important imaging features of pancreatic adenocarcinoma include demonstration of a focal mass, particularly superimposed on an atrophic gland; identification of peripancreatic lymphadenopathy; demonstration of vascular invasion; and identification of biliary obstruction.

Adrenal

Diagnostic imaging is usually not required for the acute evaluation of patients with adrenal insufficiency. Instead, the diagnosis is established by clinical and biochemical findings. Incidental

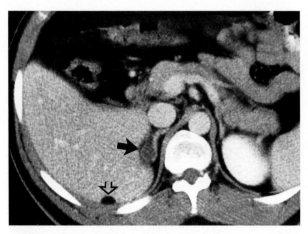

Figure 14.65. Adrenal adenoma. Enhanced CT image of the right adrenal gland shows a 1.5-cm diameter low-attenuation mass *(solid arrow)*. Note the focal area of fat on the posterior margin of the liver *(open arrow)*.

adrenal adenomas are frequently discovered by CT (Fig. 14.65). CT may be used to detect adrenal hemorrhage, which appears as unilateral or bilateral ovoid adrenal masses, about 3 cm in diameter. The attenuation value is approximately that of muscle and the areas of hemorrhage enhance poorly with IV contrast (Fig. 14.66).

CT scanning is important in the evaluation of pheochromocytoma. On CT, pheochromocytomas

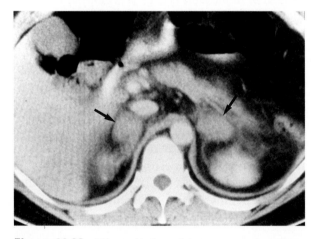

Figure 14.66. Bilateral adrenal hematomas in a man who had undergone splenectomy. Enhanced CT reveals ill-defined hematomas of both adrenal glands *(arrows)* associated with peri-adrenal stranding. (From Kawashima A, Sandler CM, Fishman EK, et al. Spectrum of CT findings in nonmalignant disease of the adrenal gland. *Radiographics.* 1998;18(2):393–412, with permission.)

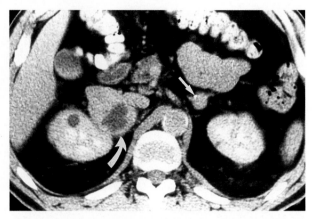

Figure 14.67. Bilateral pheochromocytomas in a man with a history of von Hippel-Lindau disease. Enhanced CT scan demonstrates a large, right adrenal mass with a cystic area *(curved arrow)* and a small, left adrenal mass with punctate calcification *(straight arrow)*. (From Kawashima A, Sandler CM, Fishman EK, et al. Spectrum of CT findings in nonmalignant disease of the adrenal gland. *Radiographics.* 1998;18(2):393–412, with permission.)

are usually round and 3 to 5 cm in diameter with heterogeneous contents of lipid-containing catecholamines as well as rapid washout of enhancement. When large, they often have areas of central necrosis (Fig. 14.67). IV administration of contrast material is not usually needed for detection of adrenal masses, but it aids in the diagnosis of extra-adrenal masses (paragangliomas). When IV contrast is needed, nonionic contrast medium is the preferred contrast material to reduce the risk of inducing a hypertensive crisis. Pheochromocytomas typically enhance intensely after administration of contrast material, and rapid washout of enhancement is characteristic.

Urinary Tract

Urolithiasis

Urolithiasis is a common health problem, affecting 2% to 5% of the population at some time in their life. One of the most important advances in emergency radiology in recent years is the development of unenhanced CT for the evaluation of renal colic and acute obstructive nephropathy. This technique was developed at Yale University by Smith and colleagues, who demonstrated that unenhanced CT

TABLE 14.4	Unenhanced Helical Computed Tomography Signs of Urolithiasis

Renal size—normal to enlarged

Intrarenal calculi

Intrarenal collecting system dilatation

Stranding of perinephric fat

Ureteral dilatation

Ureteral calculus

was more effective than intravenous urography (IVU) in precisely identifying ureteral stones and is equally effective as IVU in the determination of the presence or absence of ureteral obstruction. IVU allows assessment of renal function and provides a detailed image of the degree of renal-collecting system dilatation.

Central to the performance of this test is obtaining a standard renal stone protocol CT with a minimum of respiratory motion artifact. The urinary system is imaged from the middle of the T12 vertebral body to the middle of the symphysis pubis using 3-mm helical imaging.

Table 14.4 outlines the diagnostic information sought in the interpretation of each study. Identification of ureteral stone is the primary criterion. In contrast to conventional radiography, all urinary stones are radiopaque on CT. Those composed of uric acid, cystine, or xanthine crystals, which are nonopaque on radiography, measure at least 200 HU on CT and can be readily distinguished from adjacent soft tissues. Identification of a ureteral stone is best accomplished by sequentially tracing the ureter on each image. The search is facilitated by viewing images on a computer display in "stack mode" in which an electronic cursor can be used to mark the position of the ureter as the images are scrolled from top to bottom. Tracing the ureter is easy when there is abundant periureteral fat and ureteral dilatation, but the process is more difficult in patients with little retroperitoneal fat and no dilatation of the ureters. To evaluate for the presence of phleboliths above the pelvic brim, tracing the gonadal veins is helpful. To evaluate for stones versus phleboliths in the pelvis, it is helpful to follow the ureters back from the ureteropelvic junction.

Knowledge of the likely sites where stones become lodged can assist in analysis of the CT (Figs. 14.68 through 14.74). Stones may lodge in (1) the calyx of the kidney; (2) the ureteropelvic junction; (3) the midureter near the pelvic brim, where the ureter arches over the iliac vessels; (4) the ureterovesical junction as the ureter enters the muscular coat of the bladder (intramural ureter); and (5) the ureteral orifice. Seventy-five percent of stones are detected in the distal third of the ureters. In some cases, a calcification will be encountered along the expected course of the ureter when the

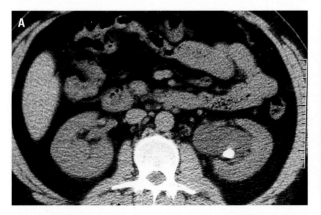
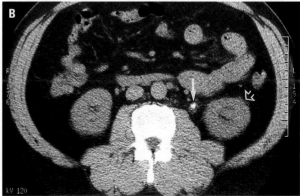

Figure 14.68. Obstructing proximal ureteral stone near the ureteropelvic junction (UPJ). **A:** Unenhanced CT image shows a 17-by-8-mm stone in the hydronephrotic left kidney. No perinephric stranding is present at this level. **B:** Seen 3 cm lower at the UPJ, a stone with a short-axis diameter of 5 mm is surrounded by a rim of soft tissue—the soft tissue rim sign *(solid arrow)*. Note minimal left perinephric stranding adjacent to the lower pole *(open arrow)*.

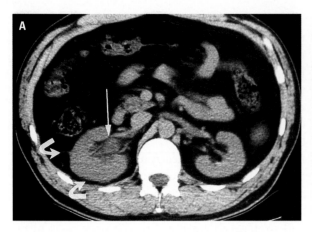

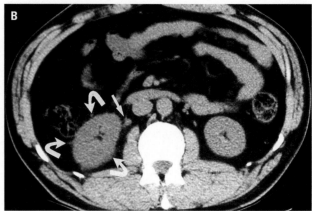

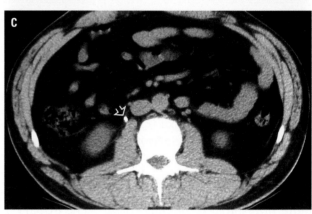

Figure 14.69. Obstructing proximal ureteral stone. **A:** Unenhanced CT image shows dilatation of the right renal pelvis *(straight arrow)* with mild perinephric stranding *(curved arrows)* and mild swelling of the right kidney. **B:** On the image taken 3.5 cm lower, note the mildly dilated right proximal ureter with both periureteric *(solid arrow)* and perinephric *(curved arrows)* stranding. **C:** On the image taken 1.5 cm lower, note the obstructing stone *(open arrow)* with a short-axis diameter of 4 mm. No soft tissue rim is present.

ureter cannot be traced. In these circumstances, demonstration of a soft tissue rim surrounding the calcification is a strong predictor of intraureteral location (Figs. 14.70 and 14.71). The absence of a rim sign does not exclude intraureteral location of

Figure 14.70. Obstructing midureteral stone with soft tissue rim sign. Unenhanced CT image through the midureter shows a stone *(black arrow)* with a short-axis diameter of 4 mm in the left midureter. Note the soft tissue rim surrounding the stone. Incidentally noted is a long retrocecal appendix containing a small appendicolith *(white arrow).*

the calcification because approximately one-third of all stones do not demonstrate the sign, particularly if they are large.

Dilatation of the intrarenal collecting system and ureter are frequently encountered signs of urinary tract obstruction. The presence of soft tissue strands in the perinephric fat is a nonspecific sign seen in urinary tract obstruction due to stone disease but also seen in pyelonephritis and renal vein thrombosis (Fig. 14.73).

The following diagnostic algorithm is proposed by Smith, Heneghan, and coworkers:

- A definite stone revealed within the lumen of the ureter on the symptomatic side: diagnosis established, no further imaging required.
- No ureteral stone identified, no ureteral dilatation nor perinephric stranding seen, no other abnormalities shown: ureteral stone disease is excluded; no further imaging.
- No ureteral stone revealed, both ureteral dilatation and perinephric stranding present on symptomatic side: recent stone passage or small ureteral stone that cannot be seen.
- Calcifications seen along the ureter but not clearly within the ureter, and one or more signs

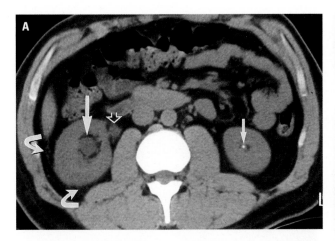
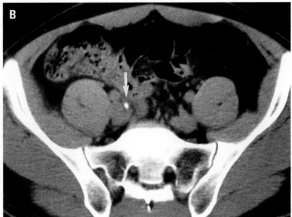

Figure 14.71. Obstructing ureteral stone at the pelvic brim and soft tissue rim sign. **A:** Unenhanced CT image through the lower pole of the right kidney shows right hydronephrosis *(long straight arrow)*, right renal swelling, and perinephric stranding *(curved arrows)*. Stranding is also seen around the ureteropelvic junction *(open arrow)*. Note the 2-mm renal stone *(short straight arrow)* in the left lower pole. **B:** In the image taken 12 cm lower, note the stone with a short-axis diameter of 4 mm lodged at the level of the pelvic brim *(short straight arrow)* where the ureter crosses the iliac vessels. A soft tissue rim sign is present.

of obstruction are present on the symptomatic side: if rim sign is present, ureteral stone is diagnosed; otherwise, the calcification is indeterminate.

■ No ureteral stone is revealed, but unilateral renal enlargement or moderate-to-severe perinephric fat stranding seen: suggest differential diagnosis of stone disease, pyelonephritis, and renal vein thrombosis.

■ CT examination is indeterminate: perform contrast-enhanced CT to evaluate for ureteral obstruction or other abnormalities.

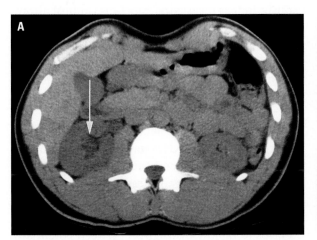
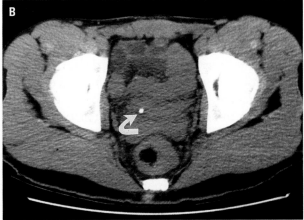

Figure 14.72. Obstructing ureterovesical junction (UVJ) stone. **A:** Unenhanced CT image demonstrates right hydronephrosis *(straight arrow)* with mild swelling of the right kidney. Note the 1-mm left renal stone lateral to the left renal hilum. Minimal perinephric stranding was seen in the lower pole (not shown). **B:** In the image taken 8 cm lower, there is a stone with a short-axis diameter of 5 mm lodged in the intramural portion of the right distal ureter *(curved arrow)*. A phlebolith might have a similar appearance. Because of the position of the stone, the lack of bladder distention, and the absence of surrounding fat, the presence of a soft tissue rim sign cannot be assessed. If the patient's symptoms had not been typical of a UVJ stone, a contrast-enhanced CT scan would have been appropriate to show that the stone was within the ureter.

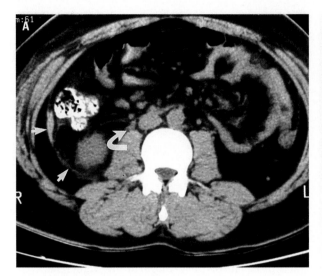 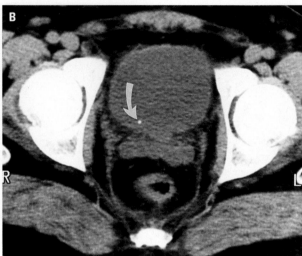

Figure 14.73. Obstructing stone in the ureteral orifice. **A:** Unenhanced CT image at the lower pole of the right kidney demonstrates moderate perinephric stranding and adjacent thickening of the right lateroconal fascia and posterior renal fascia *(straight arrows)*. Soft tissue strands surround the dilated right ureter *(curved arrow)*. Right hydronephrosis was evident at higher levels (not shown). **B:** At the trigone of the bladder, note a 3-mm short-axis diameter stone in the right ureteral orifice *(curved arrow)*. This is the usual position of the right ureteral orifice when it is not markedly swollen.

A supine abdominal radiograph (KUB) may be performed following the stone protocol CT. Comparison of the CT and KUB allows identification of small or faintly calcified stones on the conventional radiograph. The stone may then be followed by radiography rather than CT, which produces a relatively high radiation of 2 to 3 cGy compared to a KUB.

IVU has a limited role in the evaluation of acute renal obstruction secondary to stone disease. IVU assesses the severity of hydronephrosis, the delay in excretion of contrast material into the collecting system, and the time required for the contrast material to column down to an obstructing stone. Urography is limited to a few radiographs designed to answer the clinical question. Such series would include a 5-minute postinfusion AP radiograph of the kidneys, a 10-minute 14-by-17-inch KUB, and an oblique view of the affected side, with additional radiographs obtained in projections dictated by the initial examination. Delayed AP views obtained periodically for several hours may be required to demonstrate a column of contrast material terminating at an obstructing ureteral stone (Fig. 14.74).

When the position of the ureter is uncertain and the signs of urinary obstruction are equivocal, a contrast-enhanced CT of the urinary tract is helpful.

Demonstration of the course of the ureter clarifies whether a calcification in question is a ureteral stone or not.

The short-axis diameter of the stone should be reported because stone size predicts the likelihood of stone passage. At least 60% of all stones pass spontaneously. Stones measuring 1 to 2 mm almost always pass without intervention, whereas stones measuring 3 to 5 mm have a greater than 50% chance of spontaneous passage. Stones greater than 5 mm in size and more proximal stones are less likely to pass without intervention.

Renal Insufficiency and Renal Failure

US is the recommended modality for evaluating the patient with newly diagnosed renal insufficiency or renal failure. By demonstrating renal size, echogenicity, and resistive index and evaluating for hydronephrosis, cystic disease, and bladder distension, US helps to rapidly distinguish between potentially reversible and correctable causes of renal failure and irreversible end-stage renal disease.

Focused US examination of the kidneys should include longitudinal axis and transverse views of each kidney, visualizing upper, mid, and lower poles of each kidney; the cortices; and the renal pelvis. The length of each kidney should be measured. The echogenicity of the kidneys should be compared

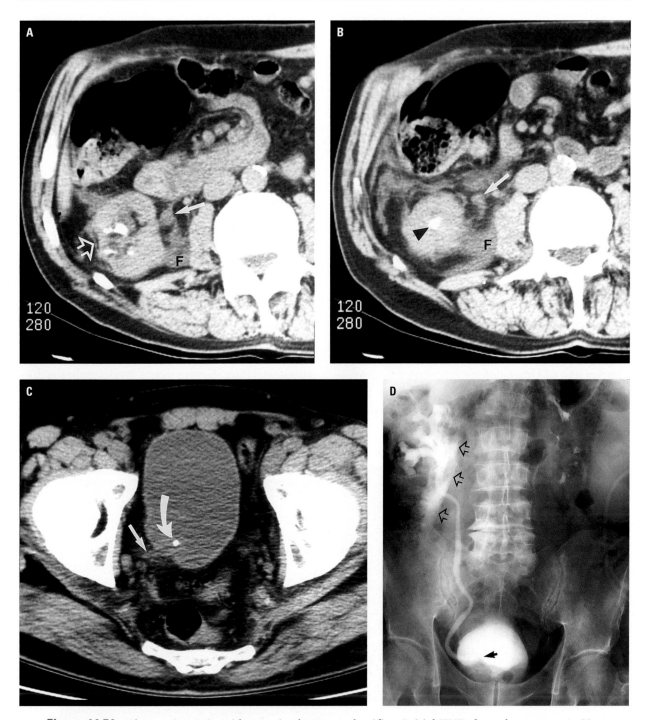

Figure 14.74. Obstructing uric acid stone in the ureteral orifice. Initial KUB showed no stone. **A:** Unenhanced CT image through the middle of the right kidney shows multiple uric acid stones, which have high attenuation on CT. The right ureter is dilated *(solid arrow)*. Note the marked perinephric fluid *(F)* and the area of parenchymal scarring laterally *(open arrow)*. **B:** In the lower pole, another stone is seen *(arrowhead)*. Note the marked perinephric fluid *(F)* and thickening of the adjacent retroperitoneal fasciae. The right ureter *(arrow)* is dilated. **C:** At the trigone of the bladder, note the 3-mm stone in the medially displaced right ureteral orifice *(curved arrow)*. Periureteral stranding is seen in the adjacent right distal ureter *(solid arrow)*. **D:** Subsequent intravenous urography shows moderate right hydronephrosis with contrast material extravasation arising from the renal pelvis and tracking inferiorly *(open arrows)*. The swollen right ureteral orifice has a pseudoureterocele appearance *(solid arrow)* correlating with the medial position of the impacted ureteral stone in **C**. Contrast material columns to the radiolucent stone. The left kidney and ureter are normal.

with the adjacent liver and spleen. Normally, the renal cortex is hypoechoic relative to the echogenic central echo complex, which consists of renal sinus fat, renal vessels, and the intrarenal collecting system. Hydronephrosis results in separation of the normally homogeneous central echo complex due to the presence of anechoic urine filling the intrarenal collecting system. If hydronephrosis is present and the kidneys are of normal size, regardless of whether echogenicity of the parenchyma is increased or not, acute obstructive uropathy is the likely cause and urgent decompression should be considered (Fig. 14.75). On the other hand, if hydronephrosis is present in the setting of small, echogenic kidneys, chronic renal failure is more likely and may not be reversible. In the absence of hydronephrosis, renal vascular and renal parenchymal diseases are the most likely causes of renal insufficiency.

Infection

The Society of Uroradiology recommends simplification of the terminology used to describe infections of the kidney. Only three diagnoses should be used: acute pyelonephritis (bacterial infection of an unobstructed kidney of variable severity), emphysematous pyelonephritis (a severe bacterial infection of the kidney associated with gas production, occurring almost exclusively in patients with diabetes mellitus), and pyonephrosis (bacterial infection of an obstructed kidney).

Acute pyelonephritis is defined clinically as flank pain, tenderness, and fever, accompanied by bacteriuria, pyuria, bacteremia, and sometimes hematuria. Pathologically, acute pyelonephritis refers to bacterial infection of the kidney with acute inflammation involving both the renal pelvis and renal parenchyma. Most cases of acute pyelonephritis are due to infection ascending from the lower urinary tract. In children, this infection is facilitated by vesicoureteral reflux, but in adults, reflux plays a much smaller role. Acute pyelonephritis represents a clinical and pathologic spectrum. Mild acute pyelonephritis has few imaging manifestations. Severe acute pyelonephritis has areas of hypoattenuation on enhanced CT scans, representing areas of focal renal ischemia with

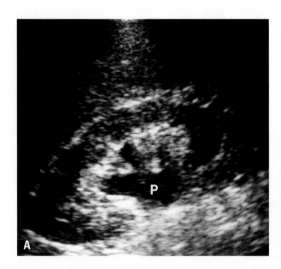

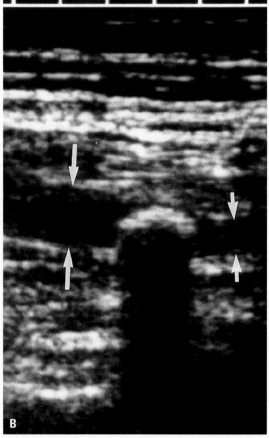

Figure 14.75. Obstructing midureteral stone. **A:** Longitudinal ultrasound image of the right kidney shows a pelvocaliectasis *(P)*, separating the central echo complex. Renal size and cortical echogenicity are normal. **B:** Image of the right midureter using a linear 7-MHz transducer shows an 8-mm ureteral stone causing proximal obstruction. The ureter proximal to the stone is dilated *(long arrows)* compared with the nondilated ureter distal to the stone *(short arrows)*. Note the sharply defined distal acoustic shadow. (Case courtesy of Cynthia I. Caskey, MD.)

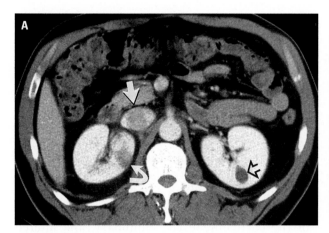
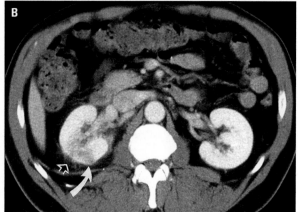

Figure 14.76. Acute pyelonephritis. Patient with right flank pain but no urinary calculus on unenhanced CT. **A:** Enhanced CT in the midportion of the kidneys shows a wedge-shaped area of low attenuation, typical of acute pyelonephritis *(curved arrow)*. Compare this with the simple cyst on the left *(open arrow)*. Note the pseudothrombus in the inferior vena cava *(solid straight arrow)* caused by opacified blood from the renal veins mixing with less opacified blood from the pelvis and lower extremities. **B:** More inferiorly, perinephric stranding *(open arrow)* and focal bulging of the renal contour *(curved arrow)* indicate another area of parenchymal infection.

renal tubule obstruction and interstitial inflammation (Fig. 14.76). These same areas may have prolonged staining with contrast material on delayed images. The kidney may swell focally in infected portions of the kidney or diffusely throughout the entire kidney. The combination of both parenchymal hypoenhancement (focal or diffuse) and swelling (focal or diffuse) indicates the most severe type of acute pyelonephritis (Fig. 14.77), which requires prolonged antibiotic therapy and carries a high risk of permanent damage to the affected tissue.

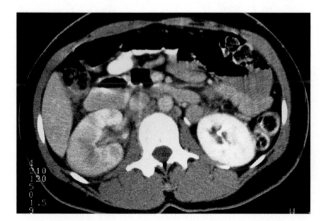

Figure 14.77. Severe acute pyelonephritis. Enhanced CT image at the right renal hilum shows a large, confluent area of hypoenhancement due to acute renal infection. The right kidney is swollen compared to the left.

To reduce ambiguity in radiology reports, the Society of Uroradiology recommends terminology for acute pyelonephritis that is based on the pathology and pathophysiology. All regions of hypoattenuating parenchyma demonstrated on CT scans are termed acute pyelonephritis. The severity of the condition should be characterized by the following modifiers:

■ Unilateral or bilateral
■ Focal (unifocal or multifocal) or diffuse
■ Focal swelling or no focal swelling
■ Kidney enlargement or no kidney enlargement
■ Complicated (renal or extrarenal abscess, gas production, obstruction) or not complicated

Note that complicated cases of acute pyelonephritis also have another radiologic diagnosis: abscess, emphysematous pyelonephritis, or pyonephrosis.

Severe tubulointerstitial inflammation may progress to form microabscesses, which may then coalesce to form a renal abscess. A mature abscess has a sharp margin with the adjacent renal parenchyma and has an enhancing rim.

Gas within the renal parenchyma indicates emphysematous pyelonephritis (Fig. 14.78). This is a serious complication encountered almost exclusively in diabetic patients. Virulent bacteria cause rapid tissue necrosis. The high-glucose environment of the diabetic kidney fosters gas production.

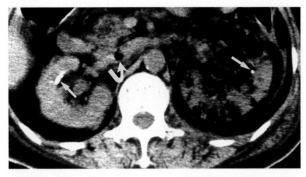

Figure 14.78. Emphysematous pyelonephritis in a woman with poorly controlled diabetes. Unenhanced CT scan shows enlarged left kidney with extensive gas in the renal parenchyma, collecting system, and perirenal space. Bilateral renal calculi are present *(straight arrows)*. Note the gas in the inferior vena cava *(curved arrow)*. (From Kawashima A, Sandler CM, Goldman SM, et al. CT of renal inflammatory disease. *Radiographics.* 1997;17(4):851–866, with permission.)

Pyonephrosis occurs when pus accumulates within the collecting system proximal to the level of ureteral obstruction. CT scans show the findings of acute pyelonephritis. The renal pelvis may thicken, and the collecting system may have higher attenuation on unenhanced scans due to pus within the urine (Fig. 14.79). However, these signs do not allow the distinction between uninfected and infected kidneys in all cases, and therefore cannot replace needle aspiration of the intrarenal collecting system. US may show echogenic material (pus and debris) in the dilated pyelocaliceal system (Fig. 14.80).

CT scanning is the preferred method for characterizing complications of acute pyelonephritis in adults. CT is recommended if a patient has not responded to antibiotic therapy after 72 hours or if the patient has a high risk for complication. US may depict focal or diffuse renal enlargement, loss of the corticomedullary boundary, and altered echogenicity in the parenchyma but is less sensitive than CT in depicting these signs of tubulointerstitial inflammation. Cortical renal scintigraphy is slightly more sensitive than CT in detecting focal abnormalities in patients with acute pyelonephritis and has found a role in the evaluation of pediatric patients.

Vascular Emergencies
Renal Infarction
Most patients presenting to the emergency department with renal colic, flank pain, and hematuria have urolithiasis. However, some patients with acute renal artery occlusion and renal vein thrombosis present with a similar clinical syndrome and fever.

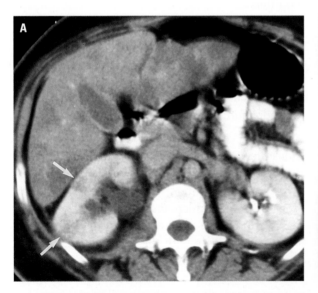
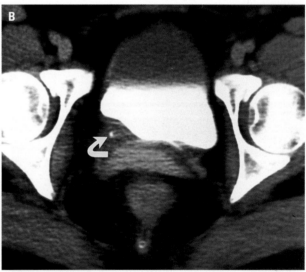

Figure 14.79. Pyonephrosis. Enhanced CT image through the right renal hilum (**A**) shows a hydronephrotic right kidney with delayed excretion of contrast material compared to the normal left kidney. The striated nephrogram *(straight arrows)* indicates parenchymal infection. An obstructing stone *(curved arrow)* is visible at the ureterovesical junction (**B**). The patient had gram-negative bacteremia due to the pyonephrosis. Multifocal areas of low attenuation seen in the liver represented multifocal fatty infiltration when the liver was biopsied.

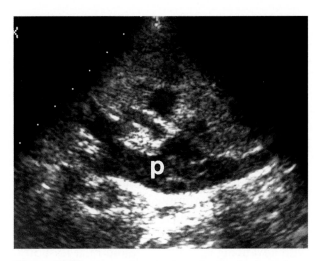

Figure 14.80. Pyonephrosis. Longitudinal renal ultrasound view reveals pelvocaliectasis with urine made echogenic by pus and debris filling the dilated renal pelvis *(P)*. (Case courtesy of Cynthia I. Caskey, MD.)

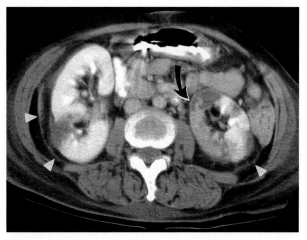

Figure 14.81. Bilateral embolic renal infarction. Image through the lower pole of the left kidney shows heterogeneous enhancement throughout the left lower pole. Multiple wedge-shaped areas of diminished enhancement are due to embolic infarction. Note enhancement along the outer margin of the left anterior infarct due to preserved capsular flow—the cortical rim sign *(curved arrow)*. The right kidney is malrotated and has a single infarction posteriorly. The renal fascia is thickened bilaterally *(arrowheads)*.

Others have less severe symptoms or may be asymptomatic. Renal vascular disorders should be considered when imaging studies fail to confirm the clinical impression of urolithiasis and in patients at high risk for renal vascular disorders, as discussed subsequently.

Acute occlusion of the main renal artery or its branches results in acute hemorrhagic infarction of the kidney. Embolism from the heart is the usual etiology. Less frequently, occlusion may be due to atherosclerosis, aneurysm, or vasculitis. Enhanced CT is the preferred modality to diagnose acute renal, arterial, and venous obstruction. US also has a role, particularly in patients who have a subacute presentation, in whom US is performed to determine the cause of renal insufficiency. T2-weighted MR urography and phase-contrast MR angiography are useful and do not use IV contrast. If MRI is contraindicated, then CTA is used when a vascular cause of renal failure is suspected.

Contrast-enhanced CT can reliably differentiate renal infarction from other causes of acute renal colic. Renal stone protocol CT will probably be normal in patients with renal infarction. With contrast enhancement, infarction of the entire kidney will be manifested by diminished enhancement of the entire kidney except for a thin, peripheral rim of capsular enhancement due to residual perfusion by collateral vessels. A segmental infarction will show a sharply demarcated nonenhancing area of renal parenchyma, which may have an enhancing

cortical rim (Figs. 14.81 and 14.82). The appearance may be similar to that of acute pyelonephritis.

On US, acute infarction may show a normal gray scale appearance. Segmental infarction may appear as a hypoechoic, wedge-shaped mass that is not distinguishable from acute pyelonephritis. However,

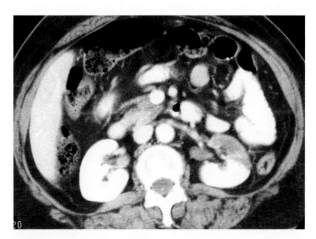

Figure 14.82. Segmental renal infarction. Enhanced CT image through the left renal hilum shows a well-demarcated area of decreased contrast enhancement in the anterior portion of the left kidney that corresponds to the anterior division of the left renal artery.

duplex and color Doppler will demonstrate the absence of flow to the entire kidney or a portion of the kidney.

Renal Vein Thrombosis

Patients with renal vein thrombosis may present with sudden total occlusion of the renal vein, resulting in hemorrhagic infarction of the kidney. If thrombosis develops more slowly, collateral vessels may allow normal renal nephrogram and preserve normal renal function. Renal vein thrombosis occurs in older children as the result of severe dehydration. In adults, it usually occurs as the result of a primary renal disorder such as amyloidosis, membranous glomerulonephritis or other causes of the nephrotic syndrome, or extrinsic compression of the renal vein due to tumor and trauma. Acute and sudden renal vein occlusion presents with flank pain and tenderness, fever, leukocytosis, and hematuria—a clinical presentation similar to acute pyelonephritis.

On contrast-enhanced CT, acute renal vein thrombosis is associated with an enlarged kidney and with prolonged visualization of the corticomedullary junction. If the condition is suspected before CT scanning is performed, a study focused on the renal vein may be diagnostic. The renal vein is localized before administration of contrast material. Imaging is performed 15 to 20 seconds after rapid administration of a bolus of contrast material, and an additional set of images is made approximately 60 seconds after administration of the bolus to image at the peak of vascular enhancement. Thrombus is seen as a low-attenuation filling defect in the renal vein (Fig. 14.83).

On US, nonspecific signs may be seen, including renal enlargement, edema, and hypoechoic parenchyma with loss of the normal corticomedullary differentiation. Doppler studies may identify thrombus within the renal vein.

Renal Cysts and Cystic Lesions

Renal cysts are not a reason for emergency visits, but they are a common incidental finding encountered in emergency radiology practice. Their inclusion here is prompted by the opportunity to identify cysts requiring further evaluation for early detection of neoplasm. Simple renal cysts occur with advancing age and are found in at least 50% of people older than age 50. On US, the diagnostic criteria for simple cyst include anechoic appearance; acoustic enhancement; sharp definition with barely perceptible, smooth far wall; and round or ovoid shape (Fig. 14.84). Cysts meeting these criteria require no further evaluation. Complex renal cysts have features that do not meet the strict criteria of simple cysts. Features of complex cysts include internal echoes, septations, calcifications, a perceptible wall, and mural nodularity. When encountered, complex renal cysts require further evaluation with contrast-enhanced CT (Figs. 14.85 and 14.89).

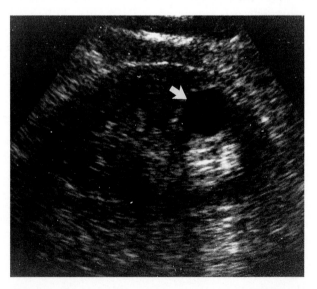

Figure 14.84. Bosniak I simple renal cyst. Longitudinal ultrasound image of the kidney shows an anechoic cyst in the lower pole of the kidney *(white arrow)*. Note the distal acoustic enhancement manifested as white echoes distal to the cyst.

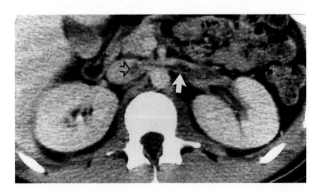

Figure 14.83. Renal vein thrombosis. Enhanced CT scan reveals a filling defect in the left renal vein *(white arrow)*. Clot extends into the inferior vena cava *(open black arrow)*. (Case courtesy of Stanford M. Goldman, MD.)

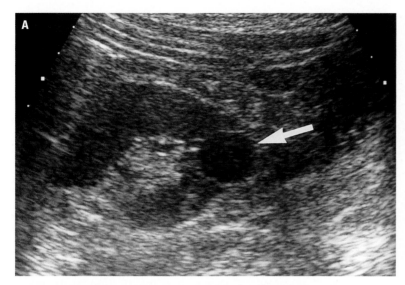
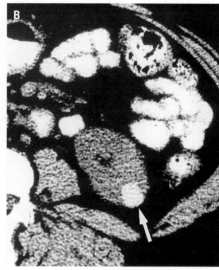

Figure 14.85. Bosniak II renal cyst, hyperdense on CT. **A:** Transverse ultrasound image of the left kidney shows a spherical hypoechoic mass with fine internal echoes *(arrow)* and faint distal acoustic enhancement. **B:** Unenhanced thin-section CT through the same region shows a well-defined, hyperdense mass on the margin of the posterior aspect of the left lower renal pole *(arrow)*. The lesion did not enhance after intravenous administration of contrast material (not shown). The ultrasound and CT findings are consistent with a hyperdense cyst.

On CT, cysts may be classified by the Bosniak system (Table 14.5; Figs. 14.84 through 14.89). Most cystic lesions are clearly benign and require no further imaging, but strict adherence to these criteria will facilitate appropriate evaluation of suspicious lesions.

Very small cysts (1.5 cm in diameter or less) are subject to volume-averaging artifacts and may not meet strict criteria as a Bosniak I or II cyst. Most radiologists do not recommend further evaluation of these lesions.

Renal Neoplasm

Definitive evaluation of solid renal masses is generally performed in the outpatient or inpatient setting and is not a usual part of emergency radiology practice. However, the serendipitous discovery of small renal neoplasms is important in any radiology practice.

The following diagnostic criteria aid, in the recognition of small renal neoplasms (Figs. 14.86, 14.88, and 14.89):

1. Mass that causes a bulge in the renal contour.
2. Attenuation value different from normal parenchyma. Small tumors are usually isodense and homogeneous, but larger tumors are hypodense and heterogeneous.

3. Reduced enhancement compared to normal renal parenchyma. Small tumors enhance homogeneously whereas larger tumors are more heterogeneous.
4. Unsharp margins between the mass and adjacent normal parenchyma. This finding is seen in only

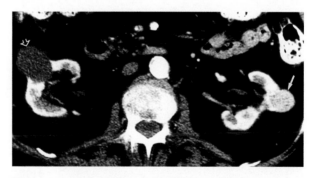

Figure 14.86. Bosniak I simple renal cyst *(white open arrow)* in right kidney and renal cell carcinoma *(white solid arrow)* in the left kidney. Enhanced CT scan obtained during the corticomedullary nephrographic phase reveals a well-defined, homogeneously enhancing mass *(solid arrow)* in the left kidney, measuring 78 HU. The lesion in the right kidney is a well-defined Bosniak I renal cyst *(open arrow)*. (From Kawashima A, Goldman SM, Sandler CM. The indeterminate renal mass. *Radiol Clin North Am.* 1996;34(5):997–1015, with permission.)

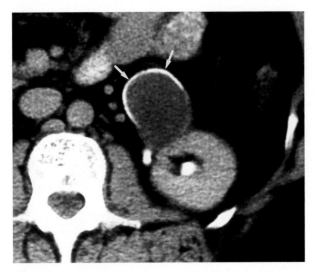

Figure 14.87. Benign calcified left renal cyst, Bosniak II-F. Contrast-enhanced CT scan through the left lower kidney shows a 3.5-by-4-cm, slightly thick-walled cystic mass with eggshell-like calcification *(arrows)*. The patient underwent partial nephrectomy, which showed no malignancy. (From Kawashima A, Goldman SM, Sandler CM. The indeterminate renal mass. *Radiol Clin North Am.* 1996;34(5):997–1015, with permission.)

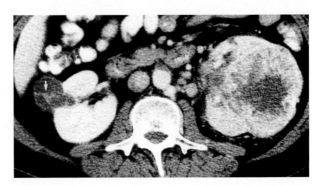

Figure 14.88. Bilateral renal cell carcinoma. Contrast-enhanced CT shows an exophytic Bosniak III cystic mass with an enhancing central septa in the right kidney *(white arrow)*. In the left kidney, there is a large, heterogeneously enhancing mass with central low attenuation (Bosniak IV). Both masses are renal cell carcinomas. (From Kawashima A, Goldman SM, Sandler CM. The indeterminate renal mass. *Radiol Clin North Am.* 1996;34(5):997–1015, with permission.)

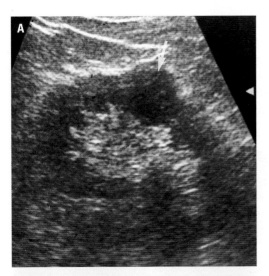

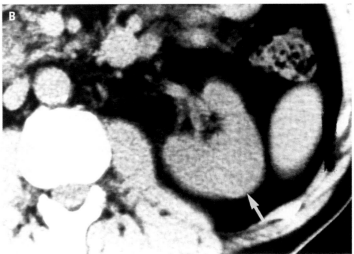

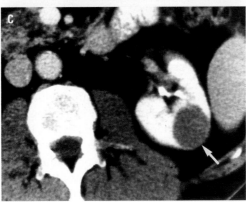

Figure 14.89. Renal cell carcinoma. **A:** Longitudinal ultrasound image of the left kidney demonstrates a 3-cm hypoechoic mass with no distal acoustic enhancement *(white arrow)*. **B:** Unenhanced CT image through the mid left kidney demonstrates no visible mass *(white arrow)*. **C:** Contrast-enhanced CT image at the same level demonstrates a well-defined mass with minimal enhancement *(white arrow)*. The CT appearance could be confused with a cystic mass, but the ultrasound shows that this is a solid tumor. (From Kawashima A, Goldman SM, Sandler CM. The indeterminate renal mass. *Radiol Clin North Am.* 1996;34(5):997–1015, with permission.)

TABLE 14.5	Bosniak Classification of Renal Cysts on Computed Tomography and Ultrasound		
Category	**Title**	**Imaging Findings**	**Management**
I	Simple benign cysts	Well marginated	Less than 1.5 cm; no further evaluation
		Thin, smooth walls	Greater than 1.5 cm, imaging follow-up, particularly in young patients
		Anechoic at sonography with acoustic enhancement	
		Not enhanced with intravenous administration CT	
		Water density (<20 HU)	
II	Benign cystic lesions that are minimally complicated	Thin septa	If identified on ultrasound, evaluate with CT scan. Lesions strictly fulfilling these criteria are benign and require no further evaluation.
		Small amount of calcification in the wall or septum	
		Hyperdense cyst (50–90 HU) due to high protein content	
		Criteria for inclusion:	
		3 cm or smaller in diameter	
		Round and sharply marginated with homogeneous attenuation using narrow window settings	
		No enhancement with intravenous contrast	
		Lesion must extend outside the kidney to demonstrate smoothness of the wall	
II-F	Probably benign cystic lesion requiring follow-up	Features similar to category II but:	Follow-up (usually at 6 and 12 months) or surgical exploration.
		Larger than 3 cm in diameter	
		Totally intrarenal	
III	More complicated cystic lesions with some radiologic features of malignancy	Thick, irregular calcification	Treated as small parenchymal neoplasm, usually radical nephrectomy.
		Irregular margins	
		Thickened, enhancing septa	
IV	Cystic carcinomas (clearly malignant)	Cystic lesions with thickened, irregular, and enhancing areas that are clearly malignant	Treat similarly to a solid neoplasm of the same stage.

a small fraction of small renal cell carcinomas. Most are well marginated.

5. If the lesion is cystic, enhancing thick and irregular walls, and thick septations.

Calcification is unusual in small renal cell carcinomas. Secondary signs—such as venous extension, metastases, lymphadenopathy, and adjacent organ invasion—are characteristic of larger, higher stage tumors. Thickening of the renal fascia and of bridging septa may be the result of edema and inflammation and do not necessarily indicate spread of tumor beyond the kidney. Renal cell carcinoma can usually be distinguished from a dromedary hump by diminished contrast enhancement in the carcinoma, compared with normal enhancement in the dromedary hump.

Angiomyolipoma, a benign renal neoplasm containing adipose tissue, smooth muscle, and thick-walled blood vessels, may be distinguished from a small renal cell carcinoma by the demonstration of fat within the angiomyolipoma.

In children, small renal masses are unusual. Wilms tumor is usually large at presentation. Leukemia presents with symmetric, diffuse renal enlargement with loss of corticomedullary differentiation.

Transitional cell carcinoma is less common than renal cell carcinoma. On occasion, it presents with renal colic and is a differential diagnostic consideration in cases of urinary colic where a urinary stone is not present.

Gastrointestinal Tract
Stomach
Bezoar

Bezoars are intragastric masses formed from ingested materials. They most commonly consist of vegetable or fruit products (phytobezoars), but they can also be composed of hair (trichobezoars) or accumulate as concretions of materials such as resins, gums, and antacids. They are most commonly seen in the setting of abnormal gastric motility or surgically altered anatomy. The operations commonly associated with bezoars include vagotomy or hemigastrectomy.

Radiographs usually show a mottled mass in the stomach, sometimes separated from the gastric wall by a rim of air (Fig. 14.90). On US, intense shadowing may be present due to air trapped in the bezoar. CT shows an irregular, heterogeneous mass surrounded by oral contrast material.

Gastric Volvulus

Acute gastric volvulus is a strangulating torsion of the stomach, resulting in gastric outlet obstruction. There are two types of volvulus: *organoaxial* and *mesenteroaxial*. Organoaxial volvulus occurs along the longitudinal axis of the stomach, which extends from the gastric cardia to the pylorus. Mesenteroaxial volvulus occurs along an axis that is perpendicular to the greater and lesser curvatures of the stomach. Laxity of the ligaments that suspend the stomach is the underlying cause. Volvulus is more frequent in patients with diaphragmatic abnormalities and paraesophageal hernias. On conventional radiographs, the stomach appears distended (Fig. 14.91). If mucosal ischemia has occurred, gas may enter the wall of the stomach. Pneumoperitoneum indicates perforation. On a

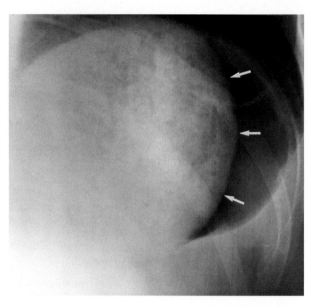

Figure 14.90. Gastric bezoar. Close-up of the stomach from a left side up decubitus abdominal radiograph shows a large, round mass containing mottled gas collections *(arrows)*. The bezoar is surrounded by air along its nondependent surface.

barium upper GI tract examination, contrast material will not enter the stomach but will terminate in a "beak" near the level of the twist. The appearance on CT is highly variable, depending on the points of torsion and the position of the stomach.

Gastric Outlet Obstruction

Hypertrophic pyloric stenosis (HPS) occurs most commonly in male infants from birth to 5 months, with a peak incidence at 3 to 6 weeks of age. US has become the diagnostic modality of choice. The examination should be performed with the stomach filled, but not overdistended, with water. A 5- to 7.5-MHz transducer should be used. Pyloric muscle thickness greater than 3 mm is abnormal (Fig. 14.92). The normal length of the pyloric canal is usually less than 1.2 cm. Peristalsis is often absent during the examination.

If US findings are equivocal, a barium upper GI tract examination can be performed. In pyloric stenosis, gastric emptying will be severely diminished or the stomach will not empty. Signs of pyloric stenosis include the "beak" sign (barium tapers to a beak as it nears the severely narrowed pyloric channel), the "string" sign (a thin coat of barium outlining the severely narrowed pyloric channel), the "double-track" sign (barium in the severely narrowed pyloric channel may cause the appearance of two or more

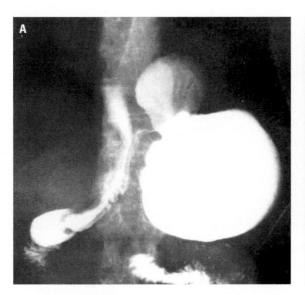
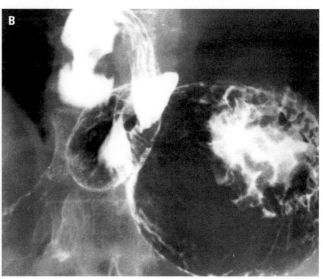

Figure 14.91. Gastric volvulus. **A:** AP radiograph from upper GI tract series illustrates organoaxial volvulus with partial diaphragmatic hernia *(arrow)*. Note the subdiaphragmatic location of the gastric fundus. **B:** Close-up AP radiograph from the upper GI tract shows partial gastric obstruction associated with diaphragmatic hernia and an upside-down configuration of the stomach due to mesenteroaxial volvulus. (From Balthazar EJ. Positional abnormalities of the stomach. In: Taveras JM, Ferrucci JY, eds. *Radiology: Diagnosis, Imaging, Intervention.* Vol 4. Philadelphia, PA: JB Lippincott; 1998:1–12, with permission.)

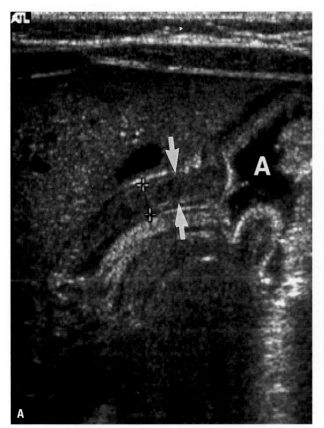
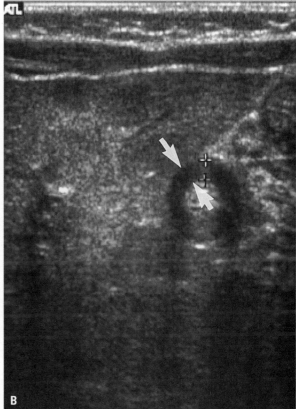

Figure 14.92. Infant with pyloric stenosis. Longitudinal (**A**) and transverse (**B**) images of the pylorus show an abnormally elongated pylorus with a thickened anterior wall measuring 3.6 mm from the lumen to the serosa *(electronic cursors* and *arrows)*. Water is present in the gastric antrum *(A)*.

lines, or tracks), and the "shoulder" sign (the hypertrophied pylorus impresses on the distal antrum, causing a mass effect) (Fig. 14.93).

Small Bowel

Foreign Bodies

Various foreign bodies, both radiopaque and radiolucent, can be swallowed (Fig. 14.94). Full evaluation requires conventional radiography of the entire GI tract from the pharynx to the rectum. Most small objects will pass through the GI tract without harm. However, sharp objects are often removed because of the risk of bowel perforation (Fig. 14.95).

Adynamic Ileus

Adynamic (paralytic) ileus is the retention of significant gas and fluid in the bowel secondary to severely diminished peristalsis. It is commonly seen after abdominal surgery and also occurs in association with peritonitis, electrolyte imbalances, particularly with hypokalemia, use of atropine-like medications and narcotics, shock, and gram-negative sepsis.

Conventional radiographs show proportionate dilatation of the stomach, small bowel, and colon (Fig. 14.96). The absence of a transition point differentiates adynamic ileus from obstruction.

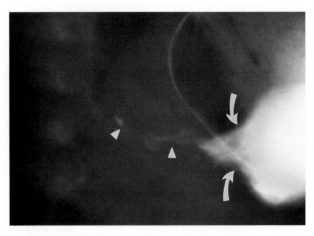

Figure 14.93. Pyloric stenosis in a 3-week-old infant. Coned-down view of the distal antrum and pylorus from an upper GI series shows an elongated pyloric channel with a very narrow lumen ("string sign") *(arrowheads)* that did not enlarge during fluoroscopic observation. Mass effect ("shoulder sign") *(curved arrows)* is noted on the distal antrum due to the thickened pyloric wall.

On upright and decubitus abdominal radiographs, air–fluid levels are identified. Typically, air–fluid levels in the small intestine will be on similar planes in each limb of a given bowel loop on both erect and decubitus radiographs. Although the

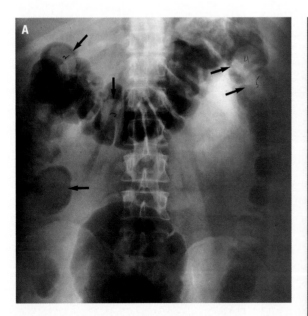 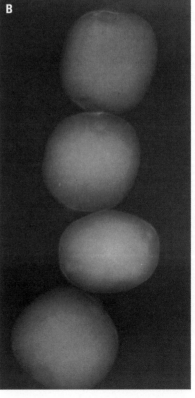

Figure 14.94. Drug-filled condoms in a drug smuggler. **A:** Conventional radiograph of the abdomen shows at least five soft tissue spheres numbered *1 to 5* within the colon *(arrows).* **B:** Radiograph of four evacuated specimens distinguishes them from fecal material because of their sharply defined spherical shape.

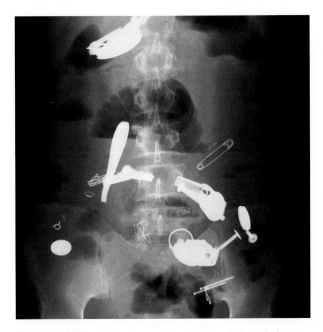

Figure 14.95. AP erect radiograph of the abdomen shows numerous radiopaque foreign bodies throughout the gastrointestinal tract, including a folded spoon in the gastric antrum and two wristwatches in the midabdomen.

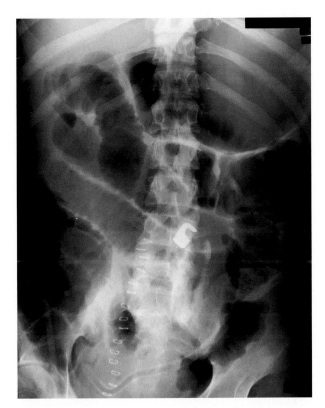

Figure 14.96. Adynamic ileus in a postoperative patient. The entire length of the GI tract is distended with air, including the stomach, small bowel, and colon. A spinal fixation hook overlies the L4 vertebral body.

location of the small bowel air–fluid levels alone may not distinguish ileus from a decompensated mechanical small bowel obstruction, the diagnosis of adynamic ileus can be reasonably established based on proportionate gastric and colonic distention. Cecal distention greater than 10 cm increases the risk of perforation.

Mechanical obstruction of the distal colon can be difficult to differentiate from colonic ileus. Provided that a digital rectal examination has not been performed, gas in the rectum helps exclude a distal colonic obstruction. A prone radiograph may show migration of gas into the rectum if no rectal gas is seen on the initial supine radiograph.

In focal adynamic ileus, a localized inflammatory process may result in distention of a single (sentinel) or a few adjacent loops of bowel such as in pancreatitis or acute cholecystitis. The affected sentinel bowel loop will be dilated, and air–fluid levels can be detected on upright or decubitus radiographs (Fig. 14.97).

Mechanical Small Bowel Obstruction

The most common cause of mechanical small bowel obstruction is adhesions from prior surgery. Other causes include internal or external hernias, masses, volvulus, strictures, and intussusception. However, in 35.5% of cases of obstruction, more than one cause is present. Conventional radiographs of the abdomen show small bowel loops distended with air and fluid. The dilatation of small bowel loops may be marked, making differentiation from colon difficult (Fig. 14.98). Small bowel is characterized by thin valvulae conniventes, which completely cross the lumen, and by central location of small bowel loops within the abdomen. However, colon is characterized by thicker colonic haustra, which do not completely cross the lumen, and by a more peripheral location within the abdomen (Fig. 14.99). The dilated small bowel loops may have a stacked ("stepladder") appearance on the supine radiograph and uneven, differential air–fluid levels on the erect radiograph (Fig. 14.100). Classically, mechanical small bowel is characterized by air–fluid levels on different planes within the same limbs of the same loop. When the small bowel is primarily fluid filled, small pockets of air trapped in the recesses between the valvulae conniventes produces the "string-of-pearls" sign on erect or decubitus radiographs (Fig. 14.101). If bowel loops proximal to the obstruction become completely fluid filled, no air bubbles

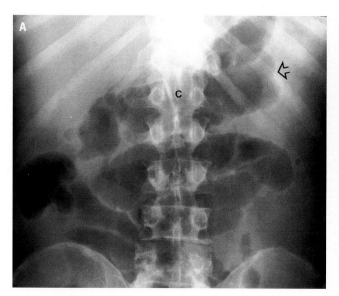
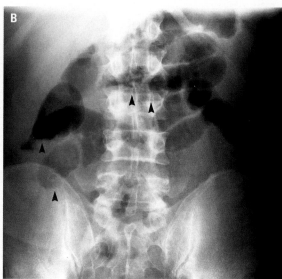

Figure 14.97. Focal ileus secondary to pancreatitis. Supine (**A**) and erect (**B**) abdominal radiographs demonstrate gaseous distention of several midabdominal small bowel loops with several air–fluid levels *(arrowheads)*. On the supine view (**A**), the transverse colon *(C)* is distended with gas up to an abrupt cutoff *(open arrow)*. This "colon cutoff sign" is the result of peripancreatic inflammation extending to the transverse mesocolon, inducing spasm in the transverse colon.

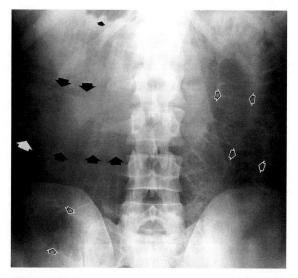
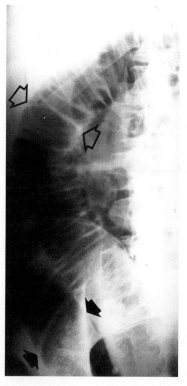

Figure 14.98. Complete mechanical small bowel obstruction. *Open arrows* indicate distended loops of small bowel containing primarily air. Note that the valvulae conniventes extend across the diameter of the distended loops. *Large solid arrows* indicate a dilated loop of small intestine that is primarily fluid filled. *Small solid arrow* indicates a haustral marking of the colon.

Figure 14.99. Mechanical small bowel obstruction. The abnormally distended small intestine *(open arrows)* can be identified by the thin, transverse linear densities, representing the valvulae conniventes that extend across the diameter of the small intestine. *Solid arrows* indicate the cecum, which can be identified because of its location and the absence of valvulae.

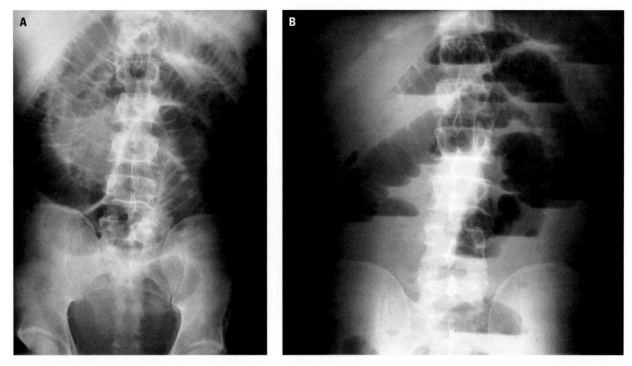

Figure 14.100. Mechanical small bowel obstruction. **A:** The supine radiograph shows multiple dilated loops of proximal small bowel. Little to no air is seen in the distal small bowel or colon. **B:** The upright radiograph shows air–fluid levels in the same loops.

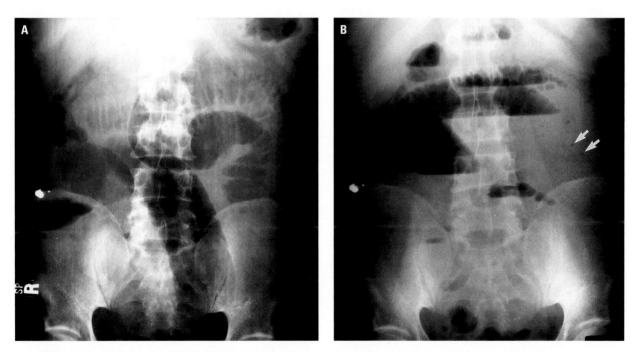

Figure 14.101. Mechanical small bowel obstruction with "string-of-pearls" appearance. When the distended small bowel loops are primarily filled with fluid and a lesser amount of gas, less gas will be seen on the supine radiograph (**A**), and a "string-of-pearls" appearance *(arrows)* may be seen on the upright radiograph (**B**) as the result of tiny collections of gas caught between adjacent valvulae conniventes in the bowel wall. A deformed bullet is present near the right iliac crest.

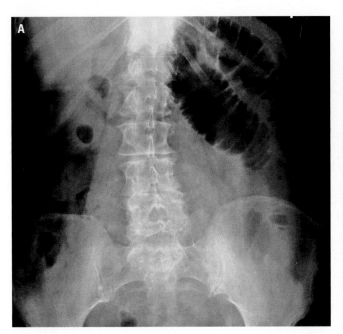
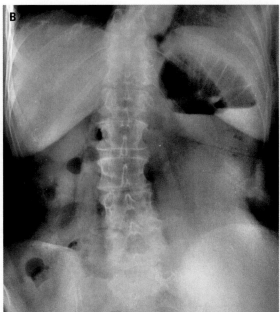

Figure 14.102. Closed-loop small bowel obstruction. **A:** Supine abdominal radiograph shows a single dilated small bowel loop in the left upper quadrant. Some residual gas and fecal material are seen in the right side of the colon. **B:** Erect abdominal radiograph demonstrates air–fluid levels in the obstructed, closed loop.

will be seen, and the abdomen can have a gasless, hazy appearance.

Closed loop obstruction of the small bowel occurs when a small bowel loop is obstructed at both its proximal and distal ends (Fig. 14.102). This condition is often associated with compromise of the vascular supply to the affected bowel loop. Closed loop obstruction may be due to adhesions, congenital bands, internal hernias, incisional hernias, or volvulus.

"Gallstone ileus" refers to a mechanical small bowel obstruction secondary to a gallstone that has eroded through the gallbladder wall and the wall of an adjacent small bowel loop. Peristalsis moves the gallstone distally in the small bowel until it becomes impacted, usually at the distal small bowel or terminal ileum (Fig. 14.103). Although the gallstone may not be identified on conventional radiographs, the essential finding is air in the biliary tree due to the abnormal communication between the gallbladder and the small bowel.

Hernias are a major cause for small bowel obstruction. Common hernias include inguinal, femoral, spigelian (Fig. 14.104), obturator, and postoperative ventral ("incisional") hernias (Fig. 14.105). Incarcerated (nonreducible) hernias can result in obstruction and/or bowel infarction. CT is valuable in identifying hernias and associated bowel obstruction or infarction.

CT has become the favored modality for evaluation of small bowel obstruction following the initial abdominal series (Fig. 14.106). CT is able to demonstrate the point and often the etiology of obstruction. CT has 95% accuracy in diagnosing the presence of a small bowel obstruction and 73% to 85% accuracy for identifying the cause of obstruction. Additionally, CT can demonstrate ischemic changes. When no cause of an obstruction is identified, then the presumptive cause is adhesions.

Intussusception

Intussusception most commonly occurs in children younger than 2 years of age, but it can occur in older children and, occasionally, in adults. Intussusception is the telescoping of a proximal segment of small bowel (intussusceptum) into a distal segment (intussuscipiens). In children, the most common type is ileocolic. Colocolic and ileoileal are uncommon. Typically, no cause is found in young children. A specific cause is often present in older children and adults. In older children, causes include polyps, duplication cysts, Meckel diverticulum, enlarged mesenteric nodes, and lymphoma. In adults,

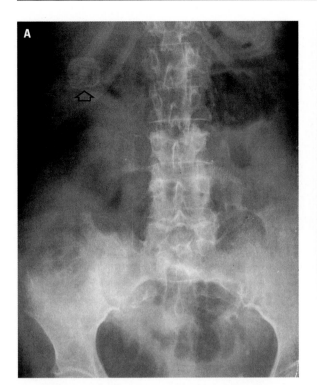
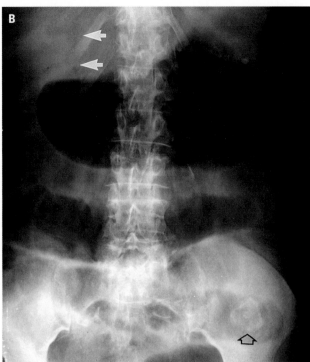

Figure 14.103. Gallstone ileus. **A:** Supine examination of the patient demonstrates a large solitary biliary calculus *(open arrow)*. **B:** In the supine examination of the abdomen of the same patient 1 year later, the stomach and proximal small intestine are dilated. On this examination, the biliary calculus that was previously located in the gallbladder is now seen in the left lower quadrant of the abdomen *(open arrow)*. Gas is present in the biliary ductal system *(solid arrows)*.

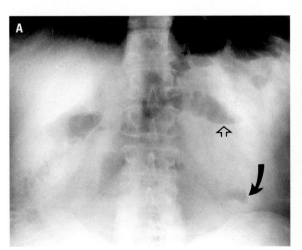
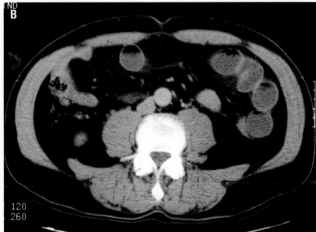

Figure 14.104. Spigelian hernia causing small bowel obstruction. **A:** Erect abdominal radiograph shows an air–fluid level in a distended small bowel loop in the midabdomen *(open arrow)* and a soft tissue mass containing a gas bubble in the left lower quadrant immediately cephalad to the left iliac crest *(curved arrow)*. **B:** Enhanced CT image through the midabdomen shows multiple dilated loops of small bowel with air–fluid levels. *(continued)*

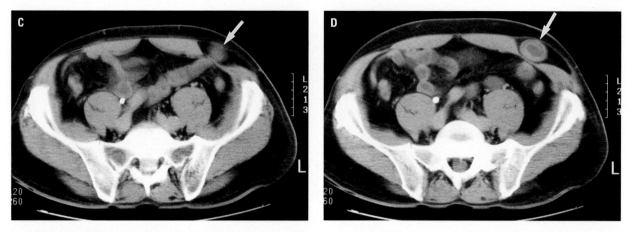

Figure 14.104. *(continued)* **C** and **D:** Two contiguous CT images through the upper pelvis demonstrate a loop of small bowel herniated through the linea semilunaris between the rectus and the transversus abdominis muscles (spigelian hernia, *arrow*).

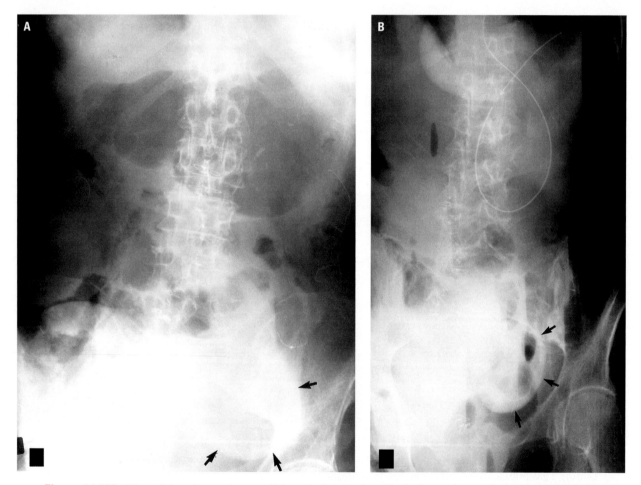

Figure 14.105. Ventral hernia causing small bowel obstruction. Both the supine radiograph (**A**) and the right lateral decubitus radiograph (**B**) identify a spherical soft tissue mass *(arrows)* overlying the left lower quadrant of the abdomen, which represents the patient's ventral hernia. Loops of distal small bowel trapped within this hernia cause the bowel obstruction. Note the air–fluid levels in **B**.

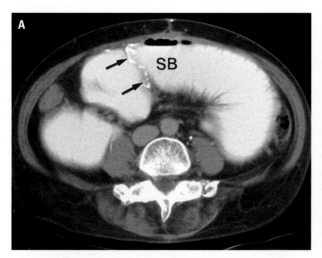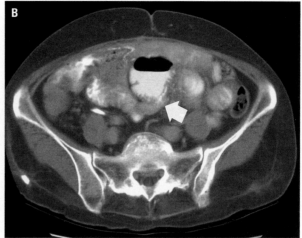

Figure 14.106. Small bowel obstruction due to adhesions in a patient with previous abdominal surgery. **A:** Enhanced CT image through the midabdomen shows markedly dilated loops of small bowel *(SB)* well opacified with dilute barium. Note the gastrointestinal staple line to the right of midline *(small arrows)*. **B:** CT image through the umbilicus shows the point of transition from dilated to normal-caliber small bowel located in the midline *(large arrow)*.

the cause is usually a tumor or previous abdominal surgery. Intussusception occurs more often in patients with a history of cystic fibrosis, Henoch-Schönlein purpura, or celiac disease.

Conventional abdominal radiographs may be normal, show findings consistent with a bowel obstruction, or show the invaginating bowel (intussusceptum) as a mass outlined by air within the surrounding bowel (intussuscipiens). When visible, the intussusceptum is most commonly seen in the cecum or transverse colon (Fig. 14.107). Clinical signs of peritonitis and/or radiographic signs of pneumoperitoneum contraindicate any form of enema study in suspected intussusception.

The diagnosis of intussusception in children is confirmed by either an opaque contrast or air enema. On a contrast enema, the intussusceptum may have the appearance of a mass-like or crescentic filling defect within the contrast column in the lumen of the intussuscipiens (Fig. 14.108). Contrast outlining the intussusceptum within the intussuscipiens may have a "spiral" appearance. With air enema, the appearance of the intussusception is similar to that seen with the hydrostatic contrast reduction technique. Extensive reflux of air into the small bowel usually indicates complete reduction, but the cecum should be evaluated for filling defects that may indicate incomplete reduction.

On CT, the intussusceptum and a surrounding rim of mesenteric fat can be identified within the lumen of the intussuscipiens (Fig. 14.109). Contrast material in the distal bowel may surround the intussusceptum. In adults, the lead point is usually a mass, which may be seen on CT.

US will show a mass with central echogenicity (mucosa) surrounded by multiple hypoechoic rings (muscular layers) but is occasionally falsely positive due to inflammation, hematoma, or volvulus mimicking intussusception.

Enteritis

Conventional radiographic findings of enteritis are nonspecific, with air–fluid levels and sometimes dilated large and small bowel (Fig. 14.110). The pattern can mimic an adynamic ileus, but if the dilatation is severe enough, it can mimic an obstruction. CT findings may show wall thickening and bowel dilatation.

Patients with AIDS often have symptoms referable to the GI tract. Barium studies are useful for mucosal detail but are performed infrequently. CT is advised in patients being evaluated for adenopathy or for workup for possible malignancy. AIDS patients can have varied pathology due to multiple simultaneous infections and because causative pathogens are definitively identified in only half of patients. In AIDS patients, cytomegalovirus can affect any part

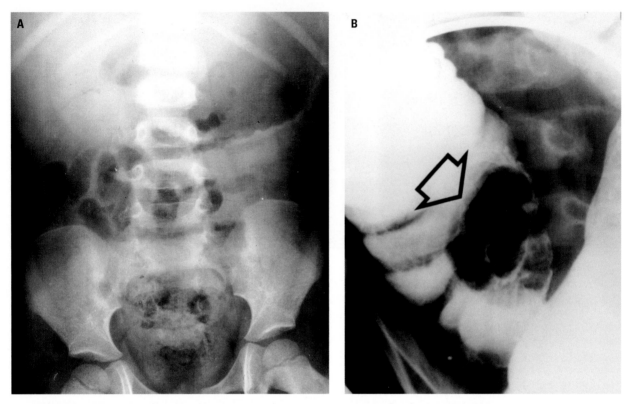

Figure 14.107. Ileocolic intussusception. **A:** In the supine examination of the abdomen, there is an absence of gas shadows in the right lower quadrant of the abdomen, and there is a soft tissue mass in the region of the cecum. **B:** At the time of barium enema, the intussusceptum *(arrow)* was seen in the midascending colon.

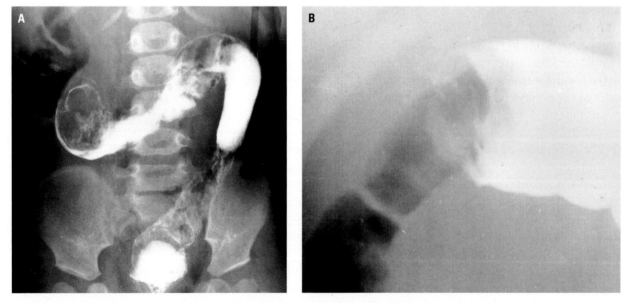

Figure 14.108. Acute ileocolic intussusception. **A:** There is complete obstruction in the proximal transverse colon by a large filling defect that is peripherally surrounded by a thin layer of barium that is located between the head and the sleeve of the invagination. **B:** In a radiograph made during the fluoroscopic examination, gas delineates the invaginated intussusceptum. Barium defines the lumen of the intussuscipiens, and the barium can be seen surrounding the head of the intussusceptum.

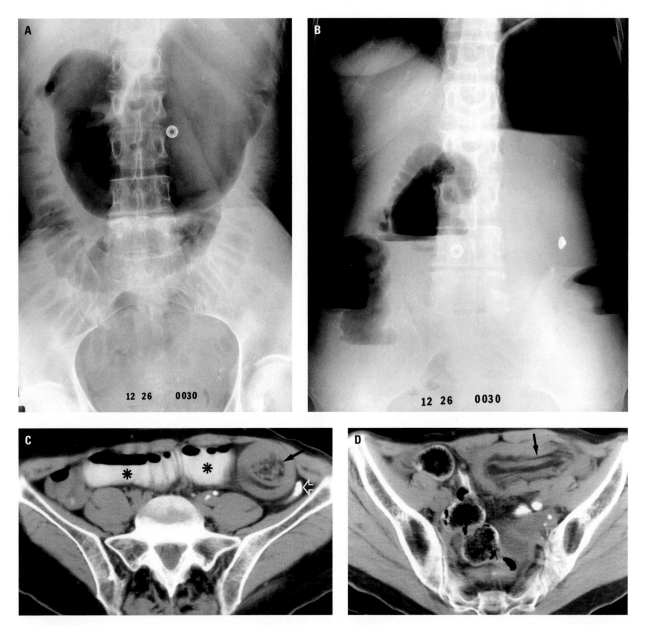

Figure 14.109. Ileoileal intussusception causing small bowel obstruction in an adult. **A** and **B:** Supine (**A**) and erect (**B**) radiographs of the abdomen show distention of the stomach and markedly dilated loops of small bowel containing air–fluid levels typical of small bowel obstruction. **C:** CT image through the upper pelvis after administration of oral and rectal contrast material but without intravenous contrast shows mesenteric fat trapped between the intussusceptum and markedly dilated intussuscipiens (*black arrow*) on the left side of the pelvis. The contrast medium-filled small bowel proximal to the intussusception is dilated (*asterisks*). The collapsed descending colon contains rectal contrast material (*open white arrow*). **D:** Image 5-cm lower demonstrates that the intussuscipiens has turned transversely so that the fat-containing layers of the intussusceptum (*black arrow*) are easily identified.

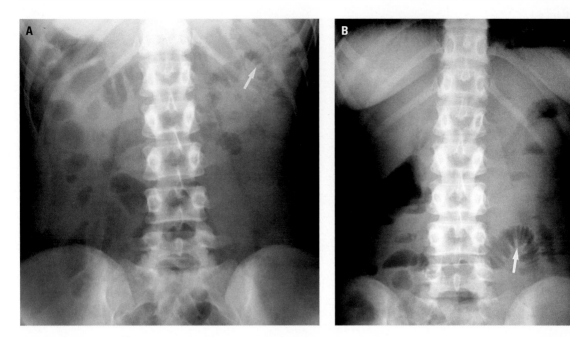

Figure 14.110. Viral gastroenteritis. Supine (**A**) and erect (**B**) radiographs of the abdomen show fold thickening in several jejunal loops on the left side of the abdomen *(arrows)*. A few air–fluid levels are present in these nondilated small bowel loops. Gas is present, scattered throughout the colon. The appearance is not typical of either mechanical obstruction or adynamic ileus. This abnormal, but non-specific, bowel gas pattern is frequently encountered with viral gastroenteritis.

of the GI tract from the esophagus to the rectum; in the small bowel, it causes nonspecific changes such as fold thickening (Fig. 14.111). *Cryptosporidium* primarily affects the small bowel and, usually, the proximal small bowel, causing thickened folds and bowel dilatation. *Giardia lamblia* commonly causes irregular fold thickening, usually in the proximal small bowel. *Entamoeba histolytica* usually affects the distal small bowel. *M. avium-intracellulare* usually affects the proximal small bowel, causing thickened folds, often with associated adenopathy that is characteristically of low density.

Crohn disease can affect any region of the small bowel, but the terminal ileum is the most commonly

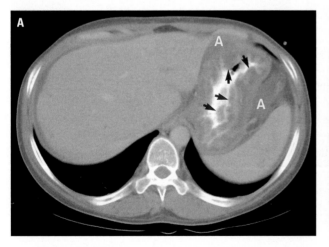
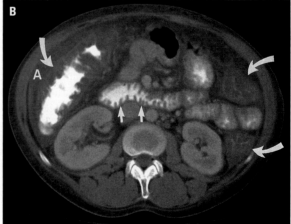

Figure 14.111. Gastrointestinal tract infection. Contrast-enhanced CT images through the stomach (**A**) and the third portion of duodenum (**B**) show marked thickening of the stomach wall with nodular gastric folds *(arrows)*. Fold thickening is also noted in the transverse duodenum *(straight arrows)* and throughout the colon *(curved arrows)*. A minimal amount of ascites *(A)* is present.

affected site. Characteristically, diseased segments will be separated by normal segments ("skip lesions"). Diseased segments show wall thickening, and the surrounding fat may have an increased, "hazy" density on CT (Figs. 14.112 and 14.113). Fistulae are common.

Small Bowel Ischemia/Acute Mesenteric Ischemia

Bowel ischemia results from decreased perfusion of the intestine. Acute small bowel ischemia usually affects patients older than 50 years of age who have a history of vascular disease and are at risk for embolic phenomena. The clinical signs and symptoms of ischemia include bloody diarrhea and poorly localized, often colicky abdominal pain. The clinical presentation is nonspecific and overlaps with pancreatitis, cholecystitis, or bowel obstruction. Symptoms can be mild despite extensive bowel infarction. The small bowel has poor collateral blood supply; thus, acute occlusion of the superior mesenteric artery is rapidly fatal after 12 hours and is associated

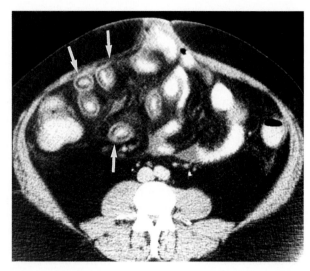

Figure 14.112. Crohn disease of the ileum. Enhanced CT image through the midabdomen shows thickening in several loops of ileum *(arrows)*. The low-attenuation bands in the bowel wall are the result of inflammation. An increased amount of fat separates these bowel loops—the "creeping fat" typical of Crohn disease.

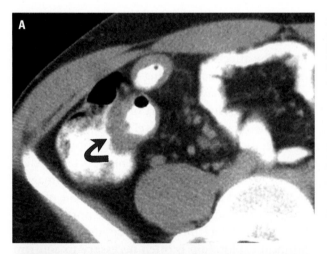

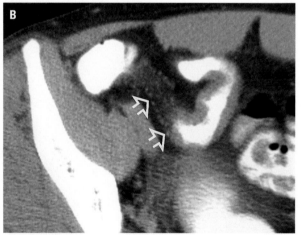

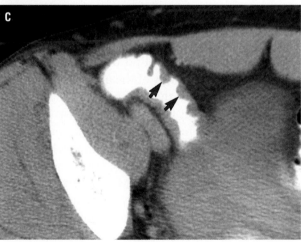

Figure 14.113. Crohn disease of the terminal ileum. Enhanced CT images of the ileocecal valve (**A**) and of the terminal ileum (**B** and **C**) demonstrate moderate thickening of the wall of the terminal ileum and ileocecal valve *(curved black arrow)*. Note the nodular mucosal fold thickening, particularly evident in **C** *(straight black arrows)*. Also note the infiltration of fat along the mesenteric border of the terminal ileum in **B** *(open white arrow)*.

with a mortality rate of at least 80%. Small bowel ischemia usually results from occlusion, dissection, or spasm of the superior mesenteric artery or its branches. Mesenteric venous thrombosis is a cause in only 5% to 13% of cases of small bowel ischemia.

Findings on conventional radiographs vary with how extensively the small bowel is involved and when in the course of the disease imaging is performed. Small bowel distention with air–fluid levels is often seen (Fig. 14.114). As time passes, the small bowel wall and valvulae conniventes become thickened. When gangrene develops, linear collections of air may be identified in the bowel wall. With perforation, free air may be seen on upright or left decubitus radiographs, and the patient will develop peritoneal signs on physical examination.

In bowel ischemia or infarction, CT can confirm air in the bowel wall (pneumatosis) and/or in the portal vein and can show bowel wall thickening

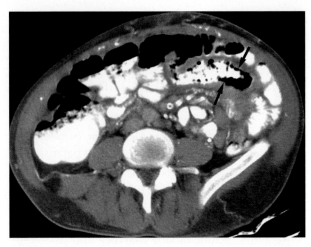

Figure 14.115. Small bowel infarction with pneumatosis intestinalis in a diabetic patient with severe vascular disease. Enhanced CT image through the upper pelvis shows a small bowel loop in the left midabdomen with marked wall thickening and air within the bowel wall *(arrows)*. Note the severe atherosclerosis in adjacent mesenteric arteries. At surgery, several loops of ischemic small bowel were excised.

(Fig. 14.115). Air in the bowel wall is most reliably diagnosed on CT when seen in the dependent bowel wall. The affected bowel may also be dilated, and it may be hyperemic, resulting in increased enhancement. CT also may show that the mesenteric fat may be infiltrated due to edema or hemorrhage. However, pneumatosis and bowel wall thickening are nonspecific signs. CTA will detect clot within the main trunk of the superior mesenteric artery. Detection of more distal emboli is improved with imaging in the arterial phase with a scan delay time of 35 to 40 seconds. Additional images in the portal venous phase may detect mesenteric venous thrombosis. Surgical exploration is often necessary to confirm the diagnosis of small bowel ischemia or infarction.

Meckel Diverticula

Meckel diverticula are blind outpouchings of the ileum that are remnants of the omphalomesenteric duct, which connects the embryonic yolk sac and the intestine. This entity has been described as following the "rule of 2's." The incidence is approximately 2%. Although most individuals are completely asymptomatic, patients who develop symptoms are usually younger than 2 years of age. Most diverticula occur within 2 ft of the ileocecal valve. Patients most commonly present with painless bleeding, secondary to ectopic gastric mucosa that may be present within

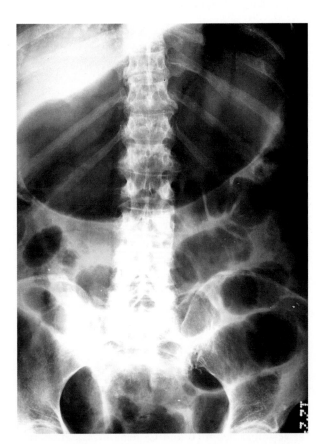

Figure 14.114. Occlusion of the superior mesenteric artery. On an AP supine radiograph, there is uniform dilatation of the small intestine. Minimal separation of the dilated small bowel loops is present. The marked distention of the stomach is not caused by thrombosis of the superior mesenteric artery.

the diverticulum. In addition, Meckel diverticula may become inflamed, resulting in clinical symptoms similar to acute appendicitis. When clinically symptomatic in adults, the most common manifestations are obstruction secondary to intussusception, with the diverticulum as the lead point; inflammation of the diverticulum; or volvulus.

Meckel diverticula can be demonstrated by scintigraphy when they contain ectopic gastric tissue. Small bowel series have limited sensitivity for detecting these diverticula. Enteroclysis has been reported to increase sensitivity. When inflammation is present, CT may be able to show the distended diverticulum containing an enterolith.

Colon

Obstruction

The most common cause of a large bowel obstruction is carcinoma. Colonic obstruction is also caused by volvulus, strictures, endometriosis, ischemia, fecal impaction, diverticulitis, intussusception, and adhesions.

On conventional radiographs, the large bowel is distended proximal to the site of obstruction (Fig. 14.116). Most commonly, the obstruction is on the left side of the colon. If the ileocecal valve is incompetent, small bowel loops will be dilated and air–fluid levels will be visible on an erect abdominal radiograph. As with adynamic ileus, the cecum can become significantly distended, and with a diameter greater than 10 cm, there is risk of perforation. In colonic obstruction secondary to tumor, the most common site of perforation is near the tumor. In colonic obstruction due to other causes, the most common site of perforation is the dilated cecum.

As discussed previously, the site of very distal large bowel obstruction may be difficult to identify. Air in the rectum on a prone cross-table lateral radiograph excludes complete obstruction proximal to the rectum.

Contrast studies need to be performed with caution in the setting of a colonic obstruction. Thick barium should not be given from above because inspissation of barium can convert a partial colonic obstruction to a complete obstruction. Usually an enema of water-soluble contrast material is administered to identify a point of obstruction (Fig. 14.117). Colon carcinoma usually has an "apple-core" appearance due to circumferential constriction of the bowel. However, diverticulitis can mimic this appearance.

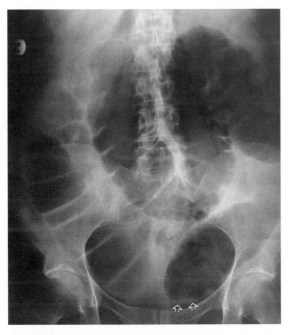

Figure 14.116. Colonic obstruction in a patient with carcinoma of the sigmoid colon. The entire length of colon is dilated and air filled down to the point of obstruction in the sigmoid colon (open arrows). Very little gas is seen in the small bowel, suggesting that the ileocecal valve is competent. (Case courtesy of Robert A. Novelline, MD.)

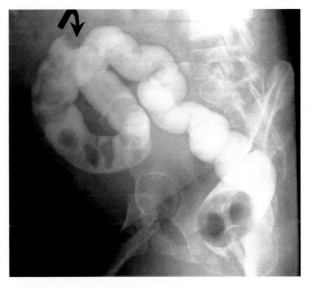

Figure 14.117. Obstructing colon carcinoma in the descending colon. Radiograph obtained in the left posterior oblique projection during a water-soluble contrast enema shows complete obstruction of the distal descending colon with a bilobed mass (curved arrow) at the superior end of the column of contrast material. The redundant sigmoid colon partially obscures the mass. Note the retained fecal material in the column of contrast material. A rectal balloon is in place.

Volvulus

Colonic volvulus causes approximately 10% of cases of clinically possible colonic obstruction. The most commonly involved sites are the cecum and sigmoid colon, with the transverse colon only rarely involved. For colonic volvulus to occur, the mesentery to the affected section of colon is abnormally long, allowing the affected colon to twist on itself.

Cecal volvulus usually occurs in patients between 30 and 60 years of age. In half of patients, the cecum inverts, with the tip of the cecum lying in the left upper quadrant, whereas in the other half, the cecum rotates on itself, with the tip of the cecum still located in the right lower quadrant.

On conventional radiographs, the small bowel will be distended because the volvulated cecum creates a complete mechanical small bowel obstruction. The cecum can be markedly distended, and one or two haustra may be seen. Because haustra are usually absent in the sigmoid colon, the presence of one or two haustra in the dilated colonic segment helps distinguish cecal from sigmoid volvulus. The distended cecum may be located anywhere in the abdomen and can assume a kidney shape. On a contrast enema study, the contrast column ends in a tapered point, indicating the site of torsion.

Sigmoid volvulus usually occurs in elderly, institutionalized mentally ill patients, or in young women with redundant sigmoid colon; it most commonly manifests as a chronic process with intermittent acute attacks. On conventional radiographs, the dilated sigmoid colon usually has an inverted "U" shape. The twisted sigmoid colon usually has no haustral markings and overlaps the left flank. The rounded part of the inverted "U" overlaps the inferior margin of the liver and lies high in the right upper quadrant. The central "wall" of the twisted sigmoid colon is thickened, consisting of the inner and outer walls of the two loops of colon that are immediately opposed to each other. The two loops usually arise from the left lower quadrant (Fig. 10.118).

Colitis

There are numerous causes of colitis and include infection, ischemia, and the idiopathic forms of ulcerative colitis and Crohn disease.

Conventional radiographs are useful for evaluating the severity and extent of acute colitis and for determining the presence of toxic megacolon and

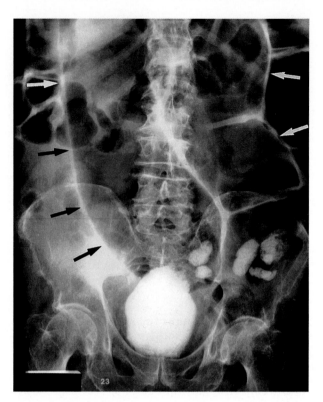

Figure 14.118. Sigmoid volvulus. Postevacuation radiograph following an attempted barium enema shows a markedly dilated, redundant loop of sigmoid colon that could not be filled with barium *(arrows)*. The central "wall" of the twisted sigmoid colon is thickened.

perforation. Toxic megacolon may result from any form of colitis. Radiographically, toxic megacolon is manifested by dilatation of the colon, particularly the transverse colon, with irregular mucosa. Mucosal islands mimic the appearance of polyps. Barium enema is contraindicated in patients with toxic megacolon because of the high risk of perforation.

All forms of colitis have similar appearances on conventional radiographs, contrast enema, and CT. However, the pattern of colonic involvement may help distinguish among the various entities (Fig. 14.119). *Pseudomembranous colitis*, caused by superinfection with *Clostridium difficile* secondary to antibiotic therapy, characteristically involves the entire colon but can involve just the right or transverse colon. Severe thickening of the wall of the colon typically produces marked "thumbprinting." Other forms of infectious colitis, including amebic colitis, can have a similar appearance. *Ischemic colitis* usually involves the left colon, causing wall thickening

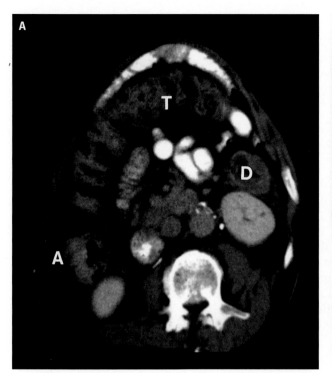

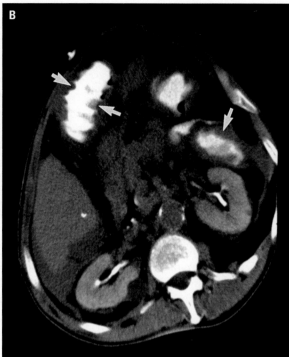

Figure 14.119. Pseudomembranous colitis. **A:** CT image through the midabdomen after administration of oral and intravenous contrast material demonstrates markedly thickened ascending colon *(A)*, transverse colon *(T)*, and descending colon *(D)*. **B:** Subsequent image at the lower costal margin after administration of rectal contrast material demonstrates marked wall thickening and a nodular mucosa in the transverse colon *(arrows)*. Ascites is seen in the paracolic gutter and around the tip of the liver.

and thumbprinting. *Ulcerative colitis* often causes loss of haustral folds. In advanced stages, the colon may appear foreshortened due to fibrosis. Almost all patients with ulcerative colitis have involvement of the rectum; the remainder of the colon may or may not be involved, but it is involved as one continuous segment. On CT, the wall is usually thickened from 6 to 10 mm and the layers of the wall can often be discriminated, with the muscularis mucosa and the outer muscularis propria layers being slightly hyperdense and the submucosa being hypodense, causing a characteristic "target" appearance (Fig. 14.120). In contrast, the diseased colon in patients with *Crohn disease* usually has a wall thickness of 11 mm or more, compared to patients with ulcerative colitis, and the involved segments of bowel may be separated by normal-appearing segments ("skip lesions") (Fig. 14.121). Fistulae and abscesses may be present. There may be proliferation of the adjacent mesenteric fat ("creeping fat"), and hazy increased density may extend into the mesenteric fat. Crohn disease

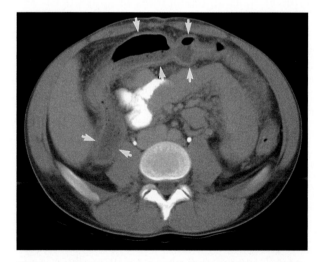

Figure 14.120. Ulcerative colitis and sclerosing cholangitis. Contrast-enhanced CT image through the midabdomen shows a thickened wall in the hepatic flexure and transverse colon *(arrows)*. Note the loss of normal haustra. The mesentery is diffusely infiltrated with soft tissue strands. Enlarged mesenteric lymph nodes are noted centrally.

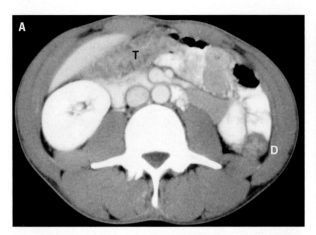
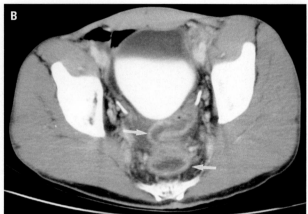

Figure 14.121. Crohn pancolitis. **A:** Enhanced CT through the midabdomen shows marked wall thickening and nodularity of the collapsed transverse colon *(T)* and descending colon *(D)*. The small bowel has a normal appearance. **B:** CT image through the rectum shows marked thickening of the rectal wall, which is highlighted by a fluid-filled lumen *(arrows)*. A small amount of fluid is present in the rectovesical space. The remainder of the colon (not shown) was similarly affected.

most commonly affects the terminal ileum, right colon, and rectum.

Appendicitis

Appendicitis is caused by obstruction of the appendiceal orifice by foreign bodies or tumor. The clinical signs and symptoms of appendicitis are usually typical. However, nearly a third of patients have atypical findings on clinical examination, which has led to the use of imaging to assist in diagnosis.

An appendicolith may be visible in the right lower quadrant on conventional radiographs. Appendicoliths are associated with a high incidence of perforation (Fig. 14.122). The radiograph may show a gasless abdomen, focal ileus, generalized ileus, or small bowel obstruction or may even appear relatively normal. When the inflamed appendix is retrocecal, its presence and the associated phlegmon displace the cecum medially from the flank stripe (Fig. 14.123). A retrocecal appendiceal abscess will produce a gas collection in the paracolic gutter. Periappendiceal inflammation may induce spasm in the cecum (Fig. 14.124).

US and CT have both been recommended for evaluating patients with possible appendicitis. US has a reported sensitivity of 90%. Proper evaluation

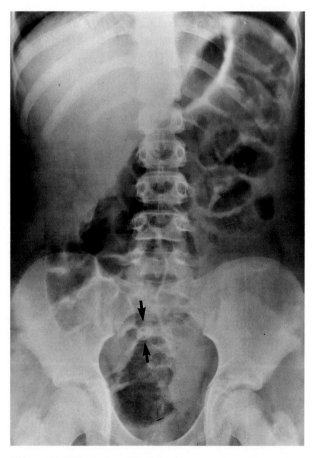

Figure 14.122. Appendicolith. *Arrows* point to an appendicolith overlying the sacrum.

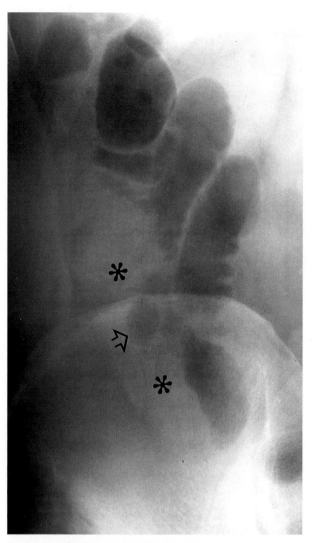

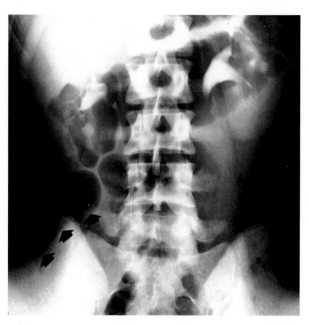

Figure 14.124. Inflammation associated with acute appendicitis has induced spasm in the cecum *(arrows)*. The intravenous urogram was performed because of an equivocal clinical presentation and microscopic hematuria. The urogram was negative. The inflamed appendix lay adjacent to the right ureter as it crossed the sacral ala.

Figure 14.123. Appendiceal abscess. Close-up of an AP abdominal radiograph reveals an extraluminal gas collection within the abscess *(open arrow)*. *Asterisks* overlie an inflammatory mass that displaces loops of bowel medially from the flank stripe.

by US requires technical expertise. The abnormal appendix is noncompressible, has an outer diameter of 7 mm, and may contain an appendicolith. Hypoechoic masses adjacent to the appendix raise the possibility of periappendiceal abscess (Fig. 14.125). Unfortunately, adequate imaging may not always be possible due to severe abdominal pain, muscle guarding, or obesity.

CT of the abdomen and pelvis has a sensitivity ranging from 87% to 98% and a specificity ranging from 83% to 97% for the detection of appendicitis depending on whether or not contrast is administered. A noncontrast CT technique is advantageous because it eliminates a delay in imaging required to adequately opacify the bowel with enteric contrast and eliminates the risk of an allergic reaction to IV contrast material and lowers the overall examination cost. However, multidetector helical CT is most accurate when oral and rectal contrast media are administered.

On CT, the normal appendix has a diameter of 6 mm or less and a wall thickness of 3 mm or less. The normal appendix appears empty, may contain gas or contrast material administered prior to the CT examination, but usually will not contain an appendicolith. The periappendiceal fat is of normal density. In mild appendicitis, the wall is thickened and the surrounding fat shows ill-defined increased density due to edema (Fig. 14.126). As the inflammation becomes more severe, adjacent structures show inflammatory changes (Fig. 14.127). The terminal ileum may become thickened and small bowel obstruction may develop. CT is useful in distinguishing abscess from phlegmon by

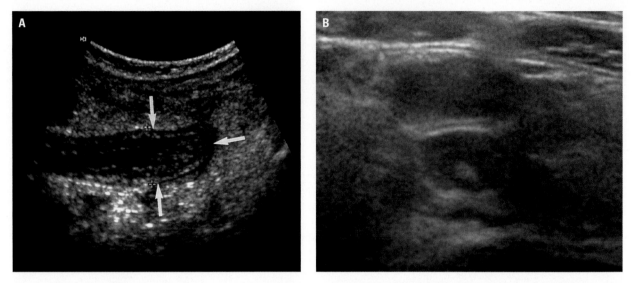

Figure 14.125. Appendicitis in a child. Longitudinal (**A**) and transverse (**B**) ultrasound images of the appendix in the right lower quadrant demonstrate an enlarged appendix. The lumen is distended, best seen on the transverse image as a sonolucent center. Echogenic focus in sonolucent center is appendicolith.

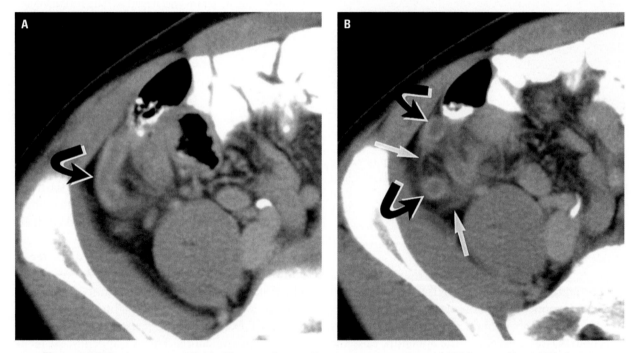

Figure 14.126. Acute appendicitis. Two contiguous 7-mm contrast-enhanced CT images (**A** and **B**) show a distended appendix *(curved arrows)* immediately beneath the right lateral abdominal wall. Note the mildly thickened, contrast-enhanced appendiceal wall and the periappendiceal inflammation *(straight arrows)*. No appendicolith is seen.

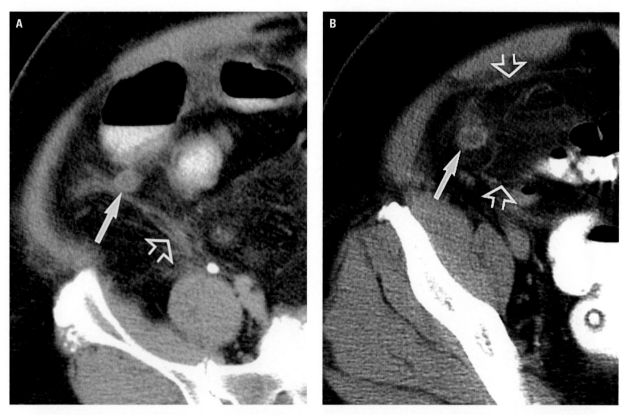

Figure 14.127. Acute appendicitis with periappendiceal inflammation. Enhanced CT images near the base (**A**) and tip (**B**) show a distended appendix with a thickened, contrast-enhanced wall (*straight arrows*). Note the abundant periappendiceal fat stranding on both images *(open arrows)*. At surgery, a grossly inflamed appendix was removed.

demonstrating the mass effect on the medial cecum and the enhancing, thickened wall typical of abscess. Periappendicular air is indicative of an abscess and can be detected either by CT or abdominal radiographs (Figs. 14.128 and 14.129).

The differential diagnosis for inflammatory changes in the right lower quadrant on CT includes cecal diverticulitis, infectious colitis, neutropenic typhlitis, Crohn disease, and epiploic appendagitis. In cecal diverticulitis, inflammatory changes are seen adjacent to the colon, usually above the level of the ileocecal valve. An abscess and free air may be seen with perforation (Fig. 14.130). In epiploic appendagitis, inflammation arises in the epiploic appendages, the fat-filled outpouchings arising from the surface of the colon, usually due to torsion of an appendage. Normally, these outpouchings are indistinguishable from surrounding mesenteric fat on CT. In epiploic appendagitis, a paracolic mass develops, with inflammatory edema greatest in the periphery of the lesion (Fig. 14.131).

Diverticulitis

Diverticula most often occur in the sigmoid colon and are asymptomatic until one of two complications develops: GI hemorrhage or diverticulitis. Diverticulitis occurs when the neck of a diverticulum becomes obstructed, which leads to inflammation and distention of the diverticulum, in much the same manner that appendicitis develops. Diverticulitis usually occurs in older patients and presents with either steady or cramping intermittent left lower quadrant pain and tenderness. However, because diverticula can occur anywhere in the colon, pain and tenderness are not limited to the left lower quadrant.

Conventional radiographic signs are variable. With severe inflammation, signs of a large bowel obstruction may be present. A soft tissue density with associated mass effect may be seen adjacent to the colon. Occasionally, an extraluminal air bubble is visible in a contained perforation that has not yet formed an abscess. With perforation that has not walled off to form an abscess,

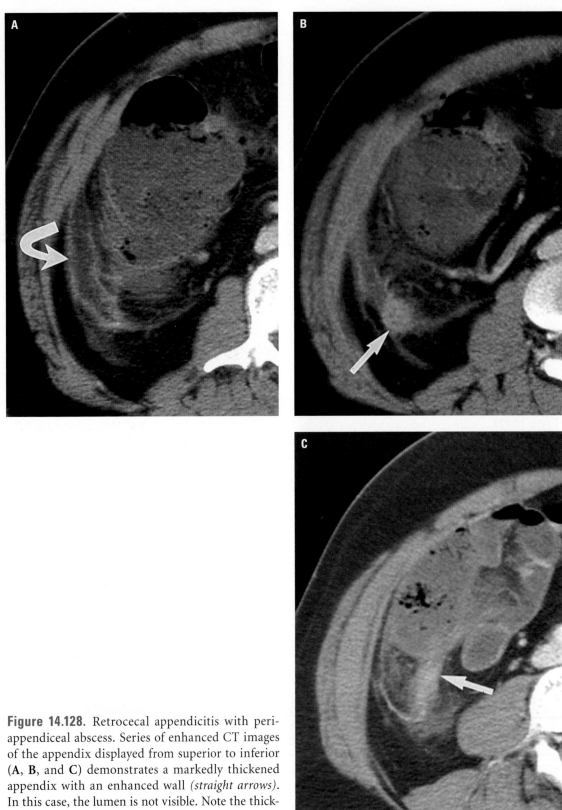

Figure 14.128. Retrocecal appendicitis with peri-appendiceal abscess. Series of enhanced CT images of the appendix displayed from superior to inferior (**A**, **B**, and **C**) demonstrates a markedly thickened appendix with an enhanced wall *(straight arrows)*. In this case, the lumen is not visible. Note the thick-walled abscess in the right paracolic gutter extending upward from the appendiceal tip *(curved arrow)*.

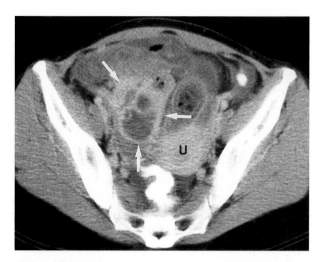

Figure 14.129. Periappendiceal abscess. Enhanced CT scan through the pelvis shows a rim-enhancing abscess in the right lower quadrant and midline of the pelvis *(arrows)*. The uterus *(U)* is displaced toward the left by the abscess.

the erect or left decubitus radiographs may show pneumoperitoneum.

CT has replaced contrast enema as the modality of choice for detection of diverticulitis because of its ability to evaluate the colonic wall

and the extracolonic soft tissues. The wall of the involved colon is usually thickened, and there is often inflammation of the pericolonic fat—sometimes described as mesenteric "stranding" (Fig. 14.132). Fluid may be identified at the base of the mesentery, and the mesenteric vasculature may be engorged and prominent. When present, extraluminal air may be abundant, but it can be as minimal as a single air bubble. Abscesses are seen as discrete, rounded fluid collections, occasionally containing air bubbles. Fistulae may be seen to adjacent organs. Despite the advantages CT has over contrast enema, differentiation of diverticulitis from colon carcinoma may be difficult.

Colonic Ischemia/Infarction

Colonic ischemia usually affects patients 60 years of age or older, who present with complaint of acute onset of lower abdominal pain and subsequent bloody diarrhea. Ischemic colitis occurs in watershed areas such as splenic flexure and rectosigmoid colon. The descending colon and sigmoid colon are most often involved, and the rectum is spared. Complete and sudden loss of arterial flow

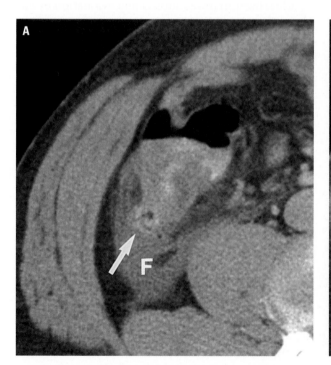
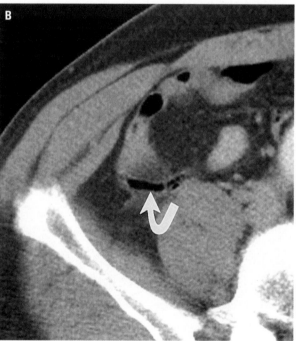

Figure 14.130. Cecal diverticulitis resembling acute appendicitis. **A:** Enhanced CT image through the cecum above the base of the appendix shows a cecal diverticulum along the posterolateral margin *(straight arrow)* filling with gastrointestinal contrast material. A fluid collection *(F)* surrounds the diverticulum. **B:** CT image more inferiorly demonstrates a normal sized, gas-filled appendix *(curved arrow)* with some surrounding fluid.

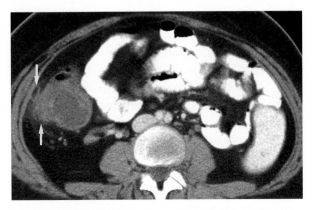

Figure 14.131. Epiploic appendagitis. Enhanced CT image through the midabdomen shows inflammatory stranding lateral *(arrows)* to the ascending colon with asymmetric thickening of the lateral wall. The colon is fluid filled.

to the colon results in bowel infarction, followed by perforation and peritonitis. Alternatively, decreased perfusion results in mucosal ulceration and subsequent fibrosis. With transient impairment of blood flow, the mucosa may slough, causing a bloody diarrhea, but symptoms often completely resolve. Processes that compromise colonic perfusion may cause ischemic colitis including heart failure, thromboembolic disease, diabetes, radiation therapy, or chronic obstruction.

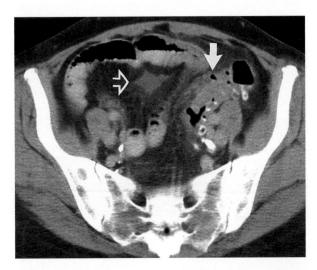

Figure 14.132. Sigmoid diverticulitis. Enhanced CT image through the sigmoid colon shows multiple sigmoid diverticula. One diverticulum is surrounded by particularly intense inflammatory stranding *(arrow)*. Note less severe stranding throughout the fat in the pelvis. A small collection of free fluid is seen between leaves of mesentery *(open arrow)*.

Conventional radiographs may show colonic dilatation with wall thickening and thumbprinting (Fig. 14.133). In severe cases, pneumatosis and portal venous gas may also be seen. Conversely, the affected portion of the colon may cause a functional obstruction, causing the proximal colon to dilate. Barium enema is contraindicated in acute ischemic colitis because of the risk of perforation. CT typically shows wall thickening and colonic dilatation (Fig. 14.133). In cross-sectional imaging, low-attenuation submucosal edema between mucosal and serosal layers creates at target sign. CT depicts pneumatosis well (Fig.14.134). If the right colon is affected, thrombi may be seen in the superior mesenteric artery or, less commonly, in the mesenteric vein.

Gastrointestinal Hemorrhage

Endoscopy is the primary diagnostic and therapeutic modality for GI hemorrhage. Diagnostic imaging plays a limited but important role.

Conventional radiographs are useful only in patients in whom bowel perforation is suspected in association with the GI bleeding. Barium studies are not indicated initially because the presence of residual barium limits subsequent evaluation by endoscopy or angiography.

Nuclear medicine bleeding scans are designed to detect hemorrhage and to localize the site of bleeding. If the bleeding source is not identified initially, the scintigram may be repeated for up to 24 hours after the initial injection of ^{99m}Tc-labeled red blood cells, which may help localize bleeding from slow or intermittent hemorrhage not apparent during the initial imaging session. A positive scan shows progressive accumulation of activity in the bowel (Fig. 14.135). Because the labeled red blood cells move within the bowel due to peristalsis, exact localization of the site of bleeding may not be possible. The results of scintigraphy help focus the angiographic evaluation to the most likely area of bleeding. Angiography is used to identify the source of hemorrhage in patients who have active bleeding, as indicated by hemodynamic instability or the need for ongoing blood transfusions. Once a source is identified, patients may be treated by embolization of the arterial supply of the hemorrhage or by infusion of a vasoconstricting agent. Although both the scintigraphy and angiography help to localize the site of hemorrhage, definitive diagnosis of the cause may require follow-up endoscopy or colonoscopy.

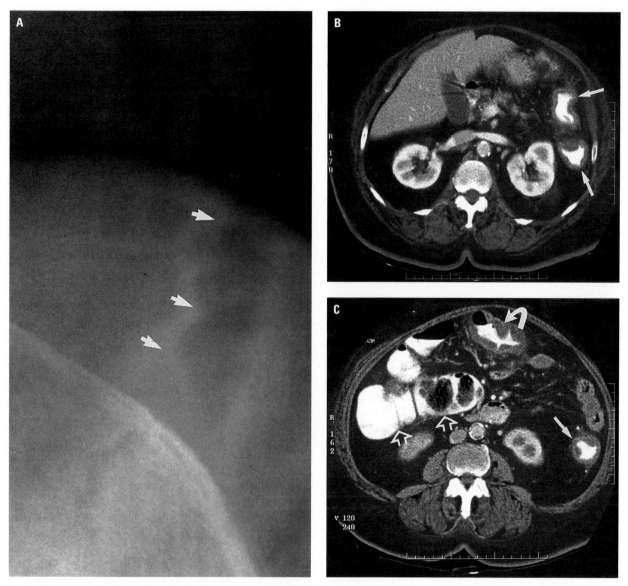

Figure 14.133. Ischemic colitis. **A:** Close-up of AP supine abdominal radiograph shows nodular thickening of the folds of the descending colon *(arrows)* just above the left iliac crest—"thumbprinting" *(solid straight arrows)*. **B:** Enhanced CT through the upper abdomen shows thickening of the colonic wall near the splenic flexure *(solid straight arrows)*. **C:** Image through the midabdomen shows wall thickening and nodular mucosal folds in the transverse colon *(curved arrow)* and mid-descending colon *(solid straight arrows)*. The ascending colon is normal *(open arrows)*. The sigmoid colon and rectum were not involved (not shown). The distribution of colitis is typical of an ischemic etiology.

Figure 14.134. Ischemic colitis in a patient with obstruction secondary to sigmoid cancer. Sagittal image of right abdomen shows dilated, fluid-filled cecum. Intramural air is seen diffusely in the wall of the colon, demonstrating pneumatosis. Note the low-attenuation lesions in the liver typical of metastasis.

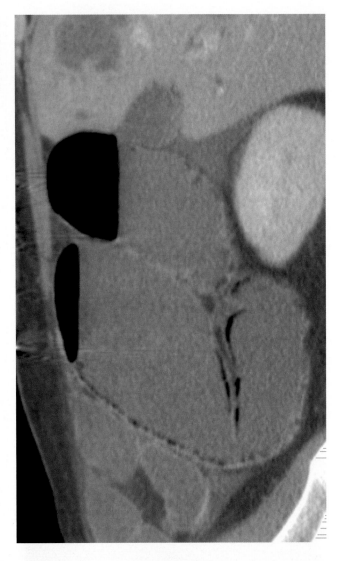

Figure 14.135. Gastrointestinal hemorrhage from the splenic flexure. A series of four anterior images obtained 5, 20, 30, and 40 minutes after administration of ^{99m}Tc-labeled red blood cells demonstrate a focus of activity in the splenic flexure on the 20-minute image *(curved arrow)*, which becomes larger on the 30-minute image and then moves with peristaltic activity along the descending colon to the sigmoid colon at 40 minutes *(curved arrows)*.

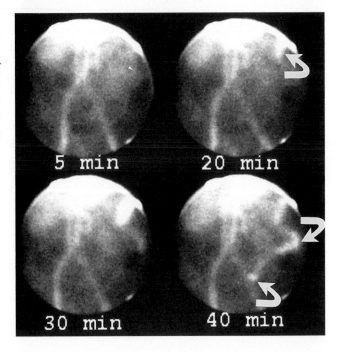

SUGGESTED READINGS

1. Ahn SH, Mayo-Smith WW, Murphy BL, et al. Acute nontraumatic abdominal pain in adult patients: abdominal radiography compared with CT evaluation. *Radiology.* 2002;225(1):159–164.

2. American College of Radiology. *2011 Practice Guidelines & Technical Standards.* Reston, VA: American College of Radiology; 2011.

3. American College of Radiology. *Appropriateness Criteria for Imaging and Treatment Decisions.* Reston, VA: American College of Radiology; 2011. *Gastrointestinal imaging, Urologic imaging, Cardiovascular imaging.*

4. Balfe DM, Molmenti EP, Bennett HF. Normal abdominal and pelvic anatomy. In: Lee JKT, Stanley RJ, Heiken JP, eds. *Computed Body Tomography with MRI Correlation.* Philadelphia, PA: Lippincott-Raven; 1998:573–635.

5. Bismuth H. Surgical anatomy and anatomical surgery of the liver. *World J Surg.* 1982;6(1):3–9.

6. Brown DF, Fischer RH, Novelline RA, et al. The role of abdominal computed tomography scanning in patients with non-traumatic abdominal symptoms. *Eur J Emerg Med.* 2002;9(4):330–333.

7. Couinaud C. *Le Foie: Etudes Anatomiques et Chirurgicales.* Paris, France: Masson, 1957.

8. Dalrymple NC, Verga M, Anderson KR, et al. The value of unenhanced helical computerized tomography in the management of acute flank pain. *J Urol.* 1998;159(3):735–740.

9. Kalish GM, Patel MD, Gunn ML, et al. Computed tomographic and magnetic resonance features of gynecological abnormalities in women presenting with acute or chronic abdominal pain. *Ultrasound Q.* 2007;23(3):167–175.

10. Mettler FA Jr, Guiberteau MJ. *Essentials of Nuclear Medicine Imaging.* 4th ed. Philadelphia, PA: WB Saunders; 1998.

11. Mularski RA, Sippel JM, Osborne ML. Pneumoperitoneum: a review of nonsurgical causes. *Crit Care Med.* 2000;28(7):2638–2644.

12. Pinto Leite N, Pereira JM, Cunha R, et al. CT evaluation of appendicitis and its complications: imaging techniques and key diagnostic findings. *AJR Am J Roentgenol.* 2005;185(2):406–417.

13. Rha SE, Ha HK, Lee SH, et al. CT and MR imaging findings of bowel ischemia from various primary causes. *Radiographics.* 2000;20(1):29–42.

14. Rosen MP, Sands DZ, Longmain HE III, et al. Impact of abdominal CT on the management of patients presenting to the emergency department with acute abdominal pain. *AJR Am J Roentgenol.* 2000;174(5):1391–1396.

15. Soyer P. Segmental anatomy of the liver: utility of a nomenclature accepted worldwide. *AJR Am J Roentgenol.* 1993;161(3):572–573.

CHAPTER 15

Abdomen: Traumatic Emergencies

Jorge A. Soto ■ O. Clark West ■ Amanda M. Jarolimek ■ John H. Harris Jr.

Multidetector computed tomography (MDCT) has become the principal diagnostic modality for evaluation of blunt abdominal trauma, replacing diagnostic peritoneal lavage (DPL) in most circumstances. Trauma centers designated by the American College of Surgeons as level I or level II are required to have computed tomography (CT) available at all times. Radiologists skilled in trauma imaging are valuable members of the trauma team, where they provide timely and expert interpretations of abdominal and pelvic CT. Many of the skills learned for general CT diagnosis apply to trauma patients, but a detailed understanding of the appearance of traumatic injuries, patterns of injury, the assessment of the hemodynamic status, and common image artifacts prepares the radiologist for excellence in trauma CT diagnosis.

Sonography has become popular for the initial assessment of blunt abdominal trauma in some centers, but turf battles over control of this modality have developed in a few centers. These differences aside, there is little doubt that sonographic detection of hemoperitoneum in a hemodynamically unstable patient affects the initial management of the patient. Sonography provides an exciting opportunity for emergency radiologists and ultrasound technologists to become integral members of the trauma team, responding to trauma alerts and participating in the initial assessment of trauma patients.

GENERAL CONSIDERATIONS

Injury Packages

Injuries sustained in motor vehicle collisions depend on multiple factors, including the size of the vehicle, the position of the victim in the vehicle, the type of accident (frontal impact, lateral impact, sideswipe, rear impact, or rollover), body habitus of the victim, and the use and type of restraint device.[1] Knowledge of the common patterns of injury in the lower chest, abdomen, and pelvis will aid the emergency radiologist in identifying injuries and assessing the significance of borderline findings. In all of the injury patterns discussed later, associated scalp, face, cranial, aortic, and extremity injuries are encountered but will be omitted for the sake of brevity. Unrestrained drivers involved in a frontal impact are at risk for injuries in the midline of the body, including sternal and rib fractures, pulmonary contusion and laceration, cardiac injury, and aorta and branch artery injuries. In the abdomen, lacerations of the spleen and liver and rupture of the small bowel are also encountered. Fractures of the pelvis and posterior dislocation of the hip complete the package.[1] Unrestrained drivers involved in a lateral impact on the left side of the vehicle sustain left-sided injuries, including left-sided rib fracture; left lung contusion and laceration; lacerations of the spleen, left kidney, or left lobe of the liver; and fractures of the

661

pelvis.[1] Passengers in a vehicle struck on the right side are prone to right-sided injuries, including right rib fractures, right lung contusions and lacerations, lacerations of the right lobe of the liver and right kidney, and pelvic fractures. Passengers are less prone to thoracic injuries and more prone to abdominal injuries than are drivers.[1]

Systematic Approach to Trauma: Computed Tomography Interpretation

As in general abdominal imaging, an ordered approach to trauma CT results in an interpretation that is both thorough and efficient. The "every organ on every slice" approach involves systematically looking at all of the images of the liver, spleen, pancreas, and so forth, until a mental checklist has been completed. To a large extent, such a general approach is applicable to CT of the trauma patient, but several life-threatening injuries should be added to the general approach. The following checklist is inspired by Halvorsen[2]:

- Life-threatening, trauma-specific
- Hemoperitoneum
- Pneumothorax (lung windows)
- Pneumoperitoneum (lung windows)
- Hemodynamic status
- Active arterial contrast extravasation
- Liver and right paracolic gutter
- Spleen and left paracolic gutter
- Upper abdominal organs, including duodenum and pancreas
- Retroperitoneum, including adrenals, kidneys, inferior vena cava, and aorta
- Bowel and mesentery
- Pelvis
- Muscles, including abdominal wall, psoas, iliacus, and buttocks
- Bones (bone windows)
- Lowest cut (thigh hematoma)

This approach places emphasis on immediate identification of life-threatening conditions requiring urgent treatment, followed by a detailed analysis designed to minimize missed injuries. The necessity of obtaining lung windows and bone windows, in addition to soft-tissue windows, must be emphasized. If a computer workstation is available, interpretation of multiple windows can be accomplished without printing multiple sets of films.

Computed Tomographic Signs in Blunt Abdominal Trauma

Jeffrey has defined several useful CT signs for assessing abdominal visceral injuries.[3] They are summarized below.

Sentinel Clot Sign
Clotted blood adjacent to the site of injury is of higher attenuation (45 to 70 Hounsfield units [HU]) than un-clotted blood (30 to 45 HU), which flows away from the site of injury (Fig. 15.1). When the source of intraperitoneal hemorrhage is not evident, the location of the highest attenuation blood clot is a clue to the most likely source.

Water Density Fluid Collections
Fluid collections with attenuation near that of water (0 to 15 HU) originate from rupture of the gallbladder, urinary bladder, small bowel, and cisterna chyli. When fluid of this density is encountered in the peritoneal cavity without an identifiable source, the safest assumption is that an undiagnosed bowel injury is present.

Hemodynamic Status
The size of the inferior vena cava (IVC) and, in children and young adults, the size of the aorta give valuable morphologic information that correlates with the patient's intravascular volume and cardiac output, as discussed later.

Active Arterial Contrast Extravasation
Termed "active arterial extravasation" by Jeffrey et al. and "vascular blush" by others, this sign represents arterial bleeding into extravascular tissues during the 1 to 3 minutes between the time of intravenous injection of contrast medium and the time the abdomen is imaged.[4–6] The extravasated arterial contrast material must be distinguished from extravasated oral contrast material and from a pseudoaneurysm of a vessel within the injured organ. Vascular extravasation typically appears as a poorly marginated, high-attenuation collection, often measuring over 100 HU, surrounded by a large hematoma. Extravasated gastrointestinal contrast material is not usually surrounded by a hematoma, and a pseudoaneurysm usually has a well-defined margin. Delayed scanning that is routinely done to evaluate the urinary tract can be extended to the area of active extravasation, allowing a qualitative assessment of the rapidity of hemorrhage.

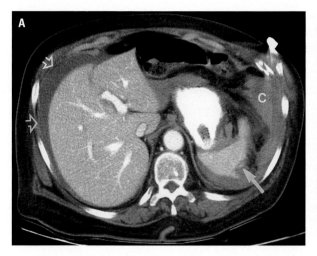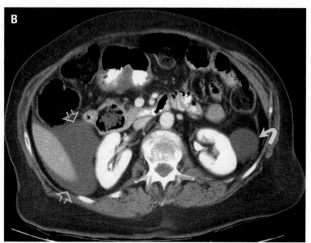

Figure 15.1. Grade II splenic laceration with sentinel clot. **A:** At the upper pole of the spleen, the lateral surface is lacerated *(solid arrow)*. A high-attenuation blood clot *(C)* floats in the nondependent portion of the perisplenic space—the sentinel clot sign. Low-attenuation fluid is present in the right perihepatic space *(open arrows)*. The electrocardiographic electrode over the left anterior chest causes a moderate streak artifact. **B:** In the hepatorenal recess, hemoperitoneum *(open arrows)* is only slightly higher in attenuation than the renal cyst lateral to the left kidney *(curved arrow)*. Intraperitoneal fluid in the hepatorenal recess typically wraps around the tip of the liver, distinguishing it from retroperitoneal fluid.

Jeffrey states that conservative management is generally not appropriate in the face of active arterial hemorrhage on CT, favoring urgent surgery or angiographic embolization.[3]

Staging Injuries for Nonoperative Management

Most blunt injuries to the liver, spleen, and kidneys can be managed nonoperatively. Most patients will stop bleeding with supportive care and others will respond to angiographic embolization, avoiding surgery.[7–9] CT is required for successful nonoperative management of liver, spleen, or kidney injuries to detect and determine the extent of the injury and to exclude other intraperitoneal or retroperitoneal injuries that require urgent surgery.[10,11] Describing the extent of injuries is facilitated by the use of a standardized staging system. Several systems have been proposed, generally based on the premise that larger and deeper lacerations, larger hematomas, and devitalized tissue are signs of more severe injuries with a worse prognosis and are more likely to require surgical management.[12–15] Staging systems are necessary to standardize nomenclature and establish a single classification system for comparative studies. However, no staging system is sufficient to predict precisely which patients will require surgery based on anatomic information alone. Instead, anatomic stage is one factor in a more complex equation. The presence of active arterial extravasation on CT has recently been recognized

as another important predictor of the need for surgery or angiographic embolization.[16] Important clinical factors include the patient's general medical condition, hemodynamic status, and need for ongoing fluid resuscitation or blood transfusion.[7,17]

The American Association for the Surgery of Trauma (AAST) has developed a series of organ injury scales. The staging parameters were originally developed for surgical description of injuries, but they have been used successfully for CT staging. Although imperfect, the AAST scales remain as the standard of communication among the trauma surgical community, and are therefore presented in this chapter. The use of these criteria for radiology reporting promotes detailed analysis of injuries and unambiguous communication of results. Other staging systems, such as the one described by Taylor and colleagues (Table 15.1), have been described but are not used extensively in practice.[18]

DIAGNOSTIC IMAGING TECHNIQUE

Computed Tomography

Technique

MDCT technology is optimal for assessment of blunt abdominal trauma. Helical (single detector) CT is acceptable, but it does not offer all the

TABLE 15.1	Grading Criteria for Abdominal and Retroperitoneal Injury

Level 0—Negative

No manifestation of injury to intra-abdominal or retroperitoneal organs (injury to osseous structures was not included).

Level 1—Indeterminate

Findings that could be caused by incidental pathologic conditions rather than trauma-related injury.

Possibility that the finding is a normal anatomic structure or variant.

Abnormality present, may be related to artifact.

Abnormality may be such a subtle manifestation that it does not meet diagnostic criteria for definite injury.

Level 2—Minor

Minimal injury to intra-abdominal or retroperitoneal organs (e.g., small laceration, subcapsular hematoma, or contusion involving 25% or less of organ).

Minimal hemoperitoneum: small amount of fluid in two or fewer intraperitoneal spaces, with trace or no fluid in the third intraperitoneal space.

Small mesenteric hematoma only; no associated hemoperitoneum; no bowel thickening or enhancement.

Level 3—Moderate

Moderate liver and/or splenic laceration or minor injury with moderate hemoperitoneum (involving greater than 25% but less than 50% of the organ).

Mesenteric hematoma with minimal/moderate hemoperitoneum, but no bowel thickening or enhancement.

Retroperitoneal: renal injury, fracture with small perirenal or subcapsular hematoma, extravasation from collecting system, partial devascularization, adrenal hematoma.

Moderate hemoperitoneum: fluid present in more than trace amounts in three or more intraperitoneal spaces.

Level 4—Severe

Extensive liver injury of 50% or greater of the organ volume or less extensive injury but with large hemoperitoneum.

Extensive splenic laceration/fracture 50% or greater or involving hilum, with perisplenic hematoma and presence of any hemoperitoneum.

Bowel injury: thickening of bowel wall, enhancement of bowel, contrast medium extravasation from bowel, or free air.

Pancreatic fracture, or intrapancreatic or peripancreatic hematoma with hemoperitoneum.

Vascular contrast medium extravasation associated with any grade of solid organ injury.

Retroperitoneal injury: renal fracture with disruption, large perirenal hematoma, pedicle injury.

Large hemoperitoneum: fluid distending intraperitoneal spaces, fluid anterosuperior to the bladder.[a]

[a]Criterion for hemoperitoneum modified from Kane et al. From Taylor CR, Degutis L, Lange R, et al. Computed tomography in the initial evaluation of hemodynamically stable patients with blunt abdominal trauma: impact of severity of injury scale and technical factors on efficacy. *J Trauma.* 1998;44(5):893–901.

capabilities available with MDCT and is more prone to respiratory motion artifacts. Administration of intravenous contrast medium is mandatory to detect all possible injuries. Unenhanced CT is performed rarely in trauma, limited to patients with a well-documented severe allergy to contrast material. Evaluation of vessels and solid organs is not complete unless intravenous contrast material is administered. Patient preparation is very important but must be accomplished efficiently. To minimize streak artifacts, metal objects within the scanning field should be removed or repositioned, including metal buckles on patient restraints, belts, electrocardiography electrodes (Fig. 15.1) and connecting cables, and metal or metal-reinforced backboards (Fig. 15.2). Some backboards cause such severe artifacts that the patient should be transferred to a more "CT friendly" wooden or plastic backboard. Once the patient is on the CT table, the patient's upper extremities should be raised above the head to avoid streak artifact. When upper extremity injuries preclude repositioning of the arms, placing the upper extremity close to the patient's side and enlarging the scanning field to include the upper extremity

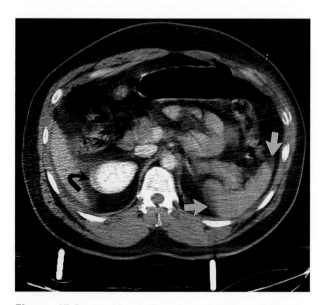

Figure 15.2. Streak artifact from backboard. At the splenic hilum and tip of the liver, severe streak artifact is so severe that the hemoperitoneum around the spleen is difficult to diagnose *(straight arrows)*. The patient's upper extremities at his side, the metal struts of the backboard, and respiratory motion cause the image degradation. Note the bright halo around the lateral portion of the right kidney, which simulates a subcapsular hematoma *(curved arrow)*.

reduces artifacts. Alert and cooperative patients should hold their breath during the imaging of the upper abdomen to minimize respiratory motion artifacts. However, successful breath holding is often not possible and scanning during shallow, quiet breathing is often necessary.

Intravenous catheters (18G or larger) should be placed in medially directed antecubital fossa or proximal forearm veins, so that these may be used for subsequent CT. Intravenous contrast (100 to 150 mL injected at a rate of 2 to 4 mL per second) is administered to all patients, and a 65- to 70-second delay is used for the portal venous phase acquisition. In addition, 5 to 7 minutes delayed images of the abdomen and pelvis are obtained selectively in those patients with injuries identified or suspected on the portal venous phase images.[19,20] Delayed scanning of the kidneys during this urographic phase of excretion of contrast material is essential to detect collecting system injuries. Delayed scans may also provide additional information about rapidly expanding hematomas and the rapidity of active extravasation of contrast material. Furthermore, delayed images help in characterizing extravascular collections of contrast-enhanced blood seen in the portal venous phase images. Importantly, these delayed phase images are acquired with a low radiation dose technique, reducing the tube current by 50% to 70% of that used for the portal venous phase series.[19] Arterial phase images (25- to 30-second delay) may be added in severely traumatized patients.

Although all the earlier studies were based on CT scanning performed with oral contrast media,[21-24] the need for oral contrast in the setting of blunt abdominal trauma has been questioned by trauma surgeons, emergency medicine physicians, and radiologists.[25-27] The main reasons are safety issues (risk for aspiration and subsequent complications), potential delay in diagnosis, and lack of proven substantial added diagnostic information for detection of significant bowel and mesenteric injuries. Extraluminal oral contrast is seen on CT in approximately 10% to 15% of patients with surgically proven significant bowel or mesenteric injuries.[21-24,28] In addition to its low sensitivity, it is exceedingly rare to find extraluminal oral contrast as the only confirmatory sign of bowel or mesenteric trauma on CT. Almost 100% of the patients have additional highly suspicious CT findings that should alert the radiologist to the presence of a significant injury. Axial images reconstructed at both

1 to 1.25 mm and 3.75 to 5 mm section thicknesses are provided for interpretation. Orthogonal (coronal and sagittal) reformations are generated for all patients for all series acquired, both with 2.5-mm thickness and 2.5-mm reconstruction interval.

Diagnostic Performance of Computed Tomography

CT has been shown to be as accurate as DPL in detecting blunt abdominal injuries.[29,30] In a prospective comparison of CT and DPL, sensitivity, specificity, and accuracy were 97%, 95%, and 96% for conventional CT and 100%, 85%, and 95% for DPL.[29] DPL involves placement of a catheter into the peritoneal cavity, aspiration of free fluid, instillation of normal saline, and aspiration of the lavage fluid. The fluid is analyzed for erythrocytes, white blood cells, amylase, bacteria, and bile, which are indicators of intraperitoneal injury. CT offers a number of advantages over DPL, including detailed anatomic evaluation of injuries, quantitation of associated hemorrhage, and detection of active arterial extravasation. CT staging is critical for successful nonoperative management of parenchymal organ injuries. CT excels at detection of retroperitoneal injuries, which are usually not detected by DPL or ultrasound. For these reason, CT has replaced DPL for evaluation of blunt trauma patients in most circumstances. In children, CT findings change the surgeon's initial diagnosis in 84% of patients and result in changes in the patient management plan in 44%.[31] Moreover, in a large, multi-institutional study of patients with suspected blunt abdominal trauma, CT had a negative predictive value of 99.63%.[32] Based on their results, the authors of this study concluded that following a negative abdominal CT study using a modern technology, trauma patients could be safely discharged from the emergency department without a period of either inpatient or outpatient observation.[32]

Focused Assessment with Sonography for Trauma

Technique

Focused assessment with sonography for trauma (FAST) is a limited abdominal ultrasound examination performed early in the evaluation of patients with suspected blunt abdominal trauma. The examination should be completed within a few minutes and is designed primarily to search for peritoneal fluid. Although parenchymal organ injuries may be detected, the search for such injuries should not delay the examination. A six-point study is best performed with a 3.5 MHz sector transducer. The small footprint of the sector transducer is advantageous in establishing an acoustic window through intercostal spaces, a technique usually required for patients in distress who are unable to hold a deep breath for subcostal scanning. Longitudinal and transverse images should be recorded in the following areas: (a) the right subphrenic space above the liver, (b) the hepatorenal recess (Morrison pouch), (c) the left subphrenic space above the spleen, (d) the perisplenic space at the inferior margin of the spleen, (e) the peritoneal recess of the pelvis, and (f) the pericardium.[33] Acoustic windows for this examination are usually found in the right midaxillary line either intercostally or subcostally, the left posterior axillary line either intercostally or subcostally, the midline 4 cm superior to the symphysis pubis, and the subxiphoid region.

Unclotted intraperitoneal blood is hypoechoic, typically with low-level internal echoes (Fig. 15.3). Clotted blood may be either isoechoic or hyperechoic and may be indistinguishable from the adjacent parenchyma of the liver or spleen. Failure to visualize a normal spleen is a sign that the spleen is injured. One must not make the erroneous mental leap from "I don't see much around the spleen," to "Therefore, nothing much is wrong with the spleen."

Advocates of FAST emphasize its ease of use and repeatability.[29] Indeed, to avoid missing injuries, FAST may need to be repeated serially, but literature demonstrating the value of this approach does not yet exist.

Diagnostic Performance of FAST

In a prospective study of severely injured patients, FAST had a sensitivity of 86%, a specificity of 99%, and an accuracy of 98% for the detection of abdominal injuries requiring surgery.[34] However, false-negative examinations were encountered with liver and spleen injuries, particularly those not associated with hemoperitoneum. Chiu and colleagues reported that of 52 abdominal injuries evaluated by both FAST and CT, 15 (29%) were evaluated as negative by FAST but were shown to include injuries to the liver or spleen without hemoperitoneum by CT.[35] Three patients required laparotomy to control bleeding. These data illustrate that a negative FAST should be interpreted as indicating the absence of hemoperitoneum, not the absence of intra-abdominal injury.[35]

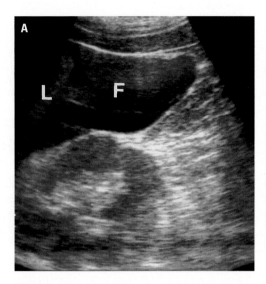
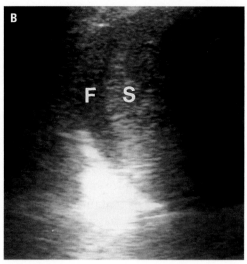

Figure 15.3. Hemoperitoneum. **A:** Longitudinal ultrasound image of the right upper quadrant obtained with a 3.5 MHz curved-array transducer demonstrates fluid *(F)* with low-level internal echoes in the hepatorenal recess adjacent to the tip of the liver *(L)*. **B:** In a different patient, echogenic fluid *(F)* is present between the diaphragm and the upper pole of the spleen *(S)*.

Because of its relatively low sensitivity, FAST should not be viewed as an equivalent replacement for either CT or DPL. A negative FAST should be viewed with some suspicion if the finding is not commensurate with the patient's clinical presentation. On the other hand, a positive FAST does not necessarily mandate laparotomy. Hemodynamically stable patients with a positive FAST should have their injuries staged with CT, affording them the benefit of nonoperative management whenever possible. FAST is not reliable for assessment of the retroperitoneum; CT performs far better in this role and is indicated when injury mechanism, in-jury patterns, or the presence of hematuria suggest a retroperitoneal injury.

BLUNT TRAUMATIC CONDITIONS

Peritoneal Cavity

Pneumoperitoneum

Pneumoperitoneum may be detected in the midabdomen beneath the anterior parietal peritoneum (Fig. 15.4) or in the upper abdomen over the anterior surface of the left lobe of the liver.

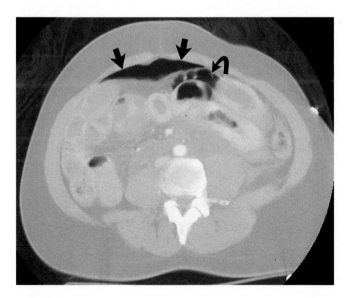

Figure 15.4. Pneumoperitoneum. In the midabdomen, a collection of free intraperitoneal air separates the parietal peritoneum of the anterior abdominal wall from the visceral peritoneum of the greater omentum *(straight arrows)*. Air within an adjacent jejunal loop *(curved arrow)* surrounds thickened valvulae conniventes, which clearly establishes its intraluminal location.

Bubbles of free air may be trapped between leaves of mesentery or in the peritoneal recesses. Lung windows are valuable in detecting pneumoperitoneum, which might be overlooked on soft tissue windows because free air may not be distinguishable from adjacent bowel gas at narrow window widths.

In trauma, extraluminal gas is a highly suggestive, but not pathognomonic, sign of bowel perforation.[36,37] Pneumoperitoneum is found on CT in 20% to 75% of patients with proven bowel perforations.[27,37–44] The amount of free intraperitoneal gas varies widely and can be massive, filling all peritoneal compartments, or very small, with only a few bubbles noted outside of the bowel lumen. In all blunt trauma patients with any CT finding that could potentially be associated with a hollow viscus injury, images should be reviewed with lung or bone window settings, in addition to the routine soft tissue settings. This approach facilitates the detection of small extraluminal gas collections. In addition, it is important to look for pneumoperitoneum in both the portal venous phase and delayed phase images because, occasionally, the pneumoperitoneum may appear only on the second acquisition. Many patients with surgically proven perforations do not have any evidence of pneumoperitoneum on CT. Various reasons may explain this circumstance: the perforation may be contained or may partially seal spontaneously, developing ileus may prevent passage of gas into the abdominal cavity, or small gas collections may rapidly be reabsorbed through the peritoneal lining. A few potential causes of a false-positive finding of pneumoperitoneum should also be considered and be ruled out before the diagnosis of bowel perforation is made on the basis of free intraperitoneal gas alone. Causes of pneumoperitoneum without bowel trauma include intraperitoneal rupture of the urinary bladder with an indwelling Foley catheter, massive pneumothorax (especially if there is a coexistent diaphragmatic rupture), barotrauma, benign pneumoperitoneum (e.g., as observed in some patients with systemic sclerosis), and the occasional DPL. Pseudopneumoperitoneum is another potential cause of a false-positive diagnosis of free intraperitoneal gas and bowel rupture. Pseudopneumoperitoneum—air confined between the inner layer of the abdominal wall and the parietal peritoneum—may be found in patients who suffer injuries to the

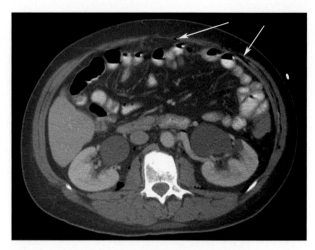

Figure 15.5. 58-year-old female patient with a pelvic fracture and a rectal wall tear, allowing leakage of gas into the extraperitoneal space of the pelvis. The axial CT image demonstrates gas in the retroperitoneum (surrounding the kidneys and descending colon) as well as in the extraperitoneal space of the anterior abdominal wall ("pseudopneumoperitoneum," *arrows*). The patient underwent repair of the rectal tear, but no laparotomy was performed.

extraperitoneal segments of the rectum, rib fractures, pneumothorax, or pneumomediastinum, with collections of extraluminal gas accumulating between the deep layers of the abdominal wall and the parietal peritoneum.[37] On CT, the appearance may closely resemble true pneumoperitoneum (Fig. 15.5). However, most patients with true pneumoperitoneum have collections of gas located deeper in the abdomen, often adjacent to the ruptured viscus, at the porta hepatis, or outlining the falciform ligament. If in doubt, delayed images or a decubitus series may help make this distinction.

Peritoneal Fluid

Blood collects in the peritoneal cavity following injuries to the liver, spleen, bowel, and mesentery. As discussed under General Considerations, a high-attenuation "sentinel" clot may be seen near the site of bleeding, with lower attenuation blood elsewhere in the peritoneal cavity. In the supine position, blood from the liver collects in the hepatorenal recess and travels down the right paracolic gutter into the pelvis. From the spleen, blood passes along the phrenocolic ligament to the left paracolic gutter and the pelvis (Fig. 15.6).[45] The volume of

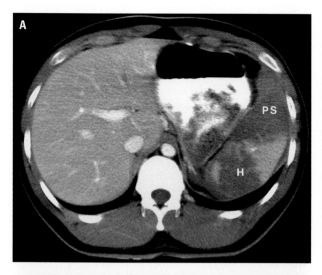

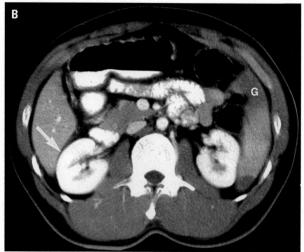

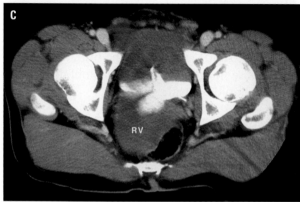

Figure 15.6. Grade IV splenic laceration with left-sided hemoperitoneum. **A:** Above the splenic hilum, the spleen is fragmented. Intraparenchymal hematoma *(H)* separates the fragments. Hemoperitoneum distends the perisplenic space *(PS)*. **B:** At the lower pole, the hemoperitoneum enters the upper portion of the left paracolic gutter *(G)*, but no hemoperitoneum is present in the hepatorenal recess *(arrow)*. **C:** In the pelvis, hemoperitoneum fills the rectovesical space *(RV)*.

hemoperitoneum may be estimated by searching for fluid in the perisplenic space, perihepatic space, hepatorenal recess, right and left paracolic gutters, and pelvis.[46] Small collections of fluid are confined to one space; moderate collections are seen in two or more spaces; and large collections involve all spaces. Although the volume of hemoperitoneum will have an effect on patient management decisions, a large hemoperitoneum does not mandate laparotomy.[10,17]

Hemoperitoneum typically has an attenuation value of 45 HU or greater. However, in a retrospective analysis of 42 patients, Levine and colleagues reported that 16% of patients with liver and spleen injuries had hemoperitoneum with attenuation values greater than 45 HU, 60% had hemoperitoneum with attenuation values between 20 and 45 HU, and 24% had hemoperitoneum with attenuation values less than 20 HU.[47] Thus, in some patients, hemoperitoneum may not be distinguishable from ascites, extravasated small intestinal fluid from bowel

perforation, or intraperitoneal urine from bladder rupture.

The finding on CT of free intraperitoneal fluid in blunt trauma patients with an absence of identifiable injury causes difficulty in interpretation for both radiologists and trauma surgeons, particularly in males. In reproductive age female patients, isolated free fluid in the pelvis can be explained by ruptured ovarian follicular cysts. In males, the question is often raised as to what is the clinical importance of this finding; that is, whether a change in management should result from the presence of free fluid alone. In the late 1990s, research suggested that the finding of free intraperitoneal fluid in the setting of blunt trauma, with the absence of identifiable injury to explain the finding, necessitated exploratory laparotomy.[48,49] More recent work has led to a more conservative approach, with some of these patients being admitted for observation without immediate surgical intervention.[32,50–53] With advances in CT technology, the sensitivity for detecting small amounts of free intraperitoneal fluid has improved, and the radiologist must use all the tools available to help guide further management.

Unexplained hemoperitoneum raises the likelihood of an underlying small bowel or mesenteric injury.[54] The attenuation of free blood in the peritoneal cavity is high (greater than 30 to 40 HU), as discussed previously. Drasin and colleagues showed that measuring the attenuation of the pocket(s) of free fluid may aid the radiologist and surgeon in determining the significance of the isolated free fluid in male patients.[55] In their study, isolated free fluid with low attenuation was found in 2.8% of male patients who suffered blunt trauma, and none was proven to have a surgically important bowel or mesenteric injury.[55] The mean attenuation of the pockets of fluid on the portal venous phase images

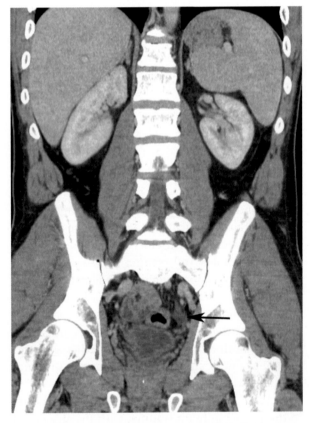

Figure 15.7. Isolated low attenuation free fluid. Coronal CT reformation demonstrates a small amount of low attenuation fluid (measured at 8 HU) in the pelvis *(arrow)*. No additional findings to indicate presence of a solid organ or hollow viscus injury were present. The patient was treated conservatively and had an uneventful hospital stay.

was 13.1 HU (Fig. 15.7), considerably lower than the mean attenuation of free fluid in the group of patients who did have an identifiable injury to explain the finding on CT (mean attenuation 45.6 HU). Similar results were subsequently reported by Yu and colleagues, who found that 4.8% of male blunt trauma patients may have a small amount of free fluid in the pelvis as the only finding on CT.[56] In this setting, the radiologist must carefully evaluate the CT images for findings that could explain the presence of low-attenuation fluid, such as intraperitoneal bladder rupture (urine) or biliary tract injury (bile). A trend for increased incidence of isolated free fluid can be seen in patients who receive higher volumes of fluid resuscitation.[61] Also, the radiologist plays an important role by reviewing the images from the trauma scan at the CT scanner, and if a suspicious finding (such as free peritoneal fluid) is noted on the initial portal venous phase images, the decision to obtain delayed images should be made.

Hemodynamic Status

CT provides an anatomic view of the patient's hemodynamic status, but the signs can be nonspecific and must be interpreted with knowledge of the patient's blood pressure, volume of resuscitation before CT, and estimated blood loss. A collapsed infrahepatic IVC on three or more consecutive images is a sign of intravascular volume depletion in a trauma patient who has received the usual 2 or more liters of crystalloid before CT scanning.[57] Flattening of both renal veins frequently accompanies the collapsed IVC. In children with shock, a hypoperfusion complex has been defined: diffuse dilatation of the intestine with fluid; abnormally intense contrast enhancement of the bowel wall, mesentery, kidneys, aorta, and IVC; and reduced diameter of the abdominal aorta and IVC (Fig. 15.8). The hypoperfusion complex in children is associated with a high mortality rate. A similar hypoperfusion complex has been described in adults but has a less grave prognosis.[58]

Conversely, distention of the IVC with the absence of the normal image-to-image respiratory variation in IVC caliber may be an indicator of intravascular volume expansion associated with rapid resuscitation.[59]

The size of the IVC is affected by many factors, including hemodynamic status, IVC obstruction from thrombus or extrinsic masses, developmental

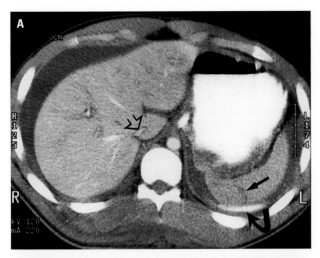

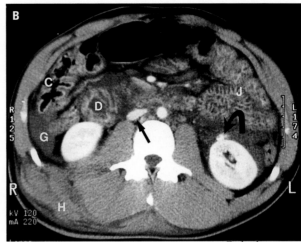

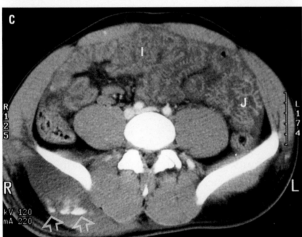

Figure 15.8. Splenic laceration with the hypoperfusion complex and active arterial extravasation in an 18-month-old infant. **A:** Image through the spleen demonstrates a grade II splenic laceration *(straight arrow)* with adjacent active arterial extravasation *(curved arrow)* and abundant hemoperitoneum surrounding the liver and spleen. Note the slit-like IVC *(open arrow)* as it passes through the liver. **B:** In the midabdomen, the duodenum *(D)*, jejunum *(J)*, and ascending colon *(C)* all have thickened walls and abnormally enhancing mucosa. Hemoperitoneum is seen in the right paracolic gutter *(G)*. Active arterial extravasation from the anterior surface of the left kidney *(curved arrow)* results in a perinephric hematoma. The IVC *(straight arrow)* is flattened and the adjacent aorta is relatively small. A large hematoma *(H)* is present in the right flank. **C:** In the upper pelvis, abnormal mucosal enhancement is noted in the jejunum *(J)* and, to a lesser degree, the ileum *(I)*. Active arterial extravasation is seen in the right buttocks *(open arrows)*. (Case courtesy of Steven Ashlock, MD)

anomalies, or portosystemic shunting. Flattening of the IVC is encountered in outpatients undergoing CT for nontrauma reasons.[60] However, in a hemorrhaging trauma patient, a flattened IVC indicates inadequate volume resuscitation. IVC flattening may precede clinical signs of shock. Recognition of intravascular volume depletion on CT should prompt aggressive volume resuscitation before the patient develops more overt signs of cardiovascular collapse.

Liver and Biliary Tract

Liver

The liver is the second most frequently injured solid organ, after the spleen. In our experience, blunt liver injuries occur slightly less frequently than splenic injuries. The widespread use of MDCT allows recognition of minor liver injuries that were not recognized in the past.[61] The right lobe is much more frequently injured than the left, with the

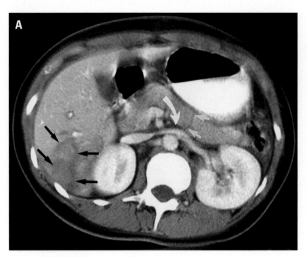 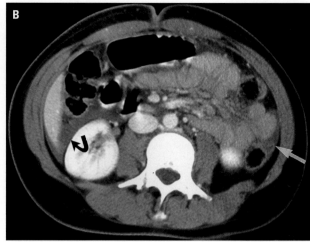

Figure 15.9. Grade III laceration of segments V and VI and complete pancreatic body laceration. **A:** Image through the right lobe of the liver shows a deep laceration extending to a portal vein branch in segment VI *(straight black arrows)*. A hairline fracture is seen through the entire thickness of the pancreatic body *(straight white arrows)*. Fluid between the pancreas and splenic vein *(curved white arrow)* indicates that this is a true pancreatic injury rather than a streak artifact over the pancreas. **B:** At the hepatorenal recess, hemoperitoneum *(curved black arrow)* surrounds the tip of the liver. Note a small amount of blood in the left paracolic gutter *(white arrow)*.

posterior segment of the right lobe most frequently injured.[62] Most liver injuries cause hemoperitoneum, but approximately one-fifth do not.[63] Liver injuries that do not produce hemoperitoneum will usually be missed by FAST, except in the unusual circumstance that a parenchymal laceration is seen directly by ultrasound. Liver injuries presenting without hemoperitoneum include minor liver injuries that do not cause significant bleeding, injuries that cause purely intraparenchymal hematoma, and injuries that disrupt the surface of the bare area of the liver and cause retroperitoneal hemorrhage.[64]

Based on their morphologic appearance, injuries to the liver parenchyma may be classified into descriptive categories: laceration, fracture, intraparenchymal hematoma, contusion, and subcapsular hematoma.

Lacerations are the most common type of liver injury.[62] Against a background of normally enhancing liver parenchyma, lacerations appear as linear or branching low-attenuation areas with sharp or jagged margins (Figs. 15.9–15.12).[65] Lacerations frequently travel along vascular planes (portal vein branches and hepatic veins) and fissures (for the ligamentum teres and ligamentum venosum), which are anatomic weak zones. Multiple parallel lacerations may be described as "bear claw"

lacerations. The depth of laceration and proximity to major vascular and biliary structures should be included in the radiology report. In particular, perihilar lacerations involving the first two or three divisions of portal venous branches are more likely

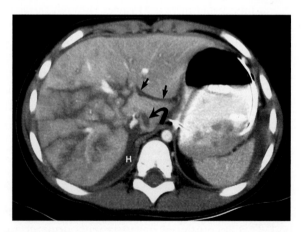

Figure 15.10. Grade V laceration of the entire right lobe of the liver. Multiple lacerations in a stellate pattern involve the entire right lobe of the liver, including the proximal portal vein branches and the intrahepatic IVC. Note retroperitoneal hematoma between the liver and the right hemidiaphragm *(H)* caused by lacerations involving the bare area. The fissure for the ligamentum venosum is filled with blood *(straight arrows)*. Laceration in the caudate lobe is an unusual finding *(curved arrow)*.

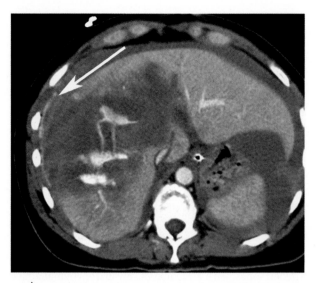

Figure 15.11. "Bear claw" liver laceration. Complex lacerations involving the left and right hepatic lobes, and extending to the porta hepatis.

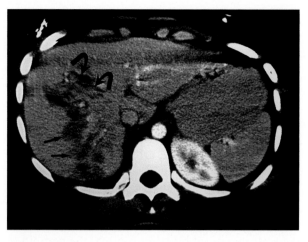

Figure 15.13. Hepatic contusion. The poorly defined area of low attenuation in the right lobe represents hepatic contusion *(straight arrows)*. More well-defined lacerations are seen anteriorly *(curved arrows)*.

to be associated with biliary tract injuries.[66] Lacerations extending to the proximal hepatic veins are important to identify because repair of hepatic vein injuries is technically difficult.[67]

The term "fracture" of the liver describes a through-and-through parenchymal laceration that may avulse a portion of the liver.

Intraparenchymal hematoma is a round or oval collection of blood retained within a liver laceration. A hepatic pseudoaneurysm or a focus of active arterial extravasation may be seen in the center of an intraparenchymal hematoma.

Hepatic contusion is an area of minimal intraparenchymal hemorrhage that appears as a low-attenuation zone without well-defined laceration (Fig. 15.13).

A subcapsular hematoma is a lentiform collection of blood beneath an intact liver capsule that deforms the contour of the liver. Most subcapsular hematomas are located along the anterolateral aspect of the right lobe (Fig. 15.14).[65] Respiratory motion artifact simulates the appearance of a subcapsular hematoma, as discussed later.

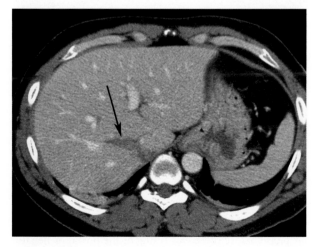

Figure 15.12. Grade II liver laceration *(arrow)* without associated hemoperitoneum.

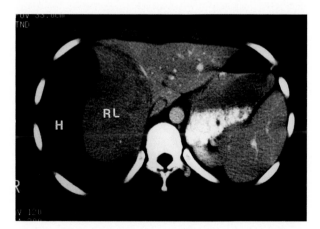

Figure 15.14. Large subcapsular hematoma of the liver. Above the porta hepatis, a large subcapsular hematoma *(H)* deforms the right lobe of the liver *(RL)*. Note that the right lobe has diminished parenchymal enhancement compared to the left, probably due to the pressure exerted by the hematoma. (Case courtesy of Steven Ashlock, MD)

Periportal low attenuation is often the result of hemorrhage along the portal vein. On occasion, it is the only sign of liver injury.[68] However, vigorous intravenous fluid administration or elevated central venous pressure—from tension pneumothorax or pericardial tamponade—may cause periportal low attenuation without liver injury.[59]

The detection of active arterial extravasation into the peritoneal cavity or within an intraparenchymal hematoma identifies patients who may need urgent endovascular or surgical treatment (Figs. 15.15 and 15.16). As with all extravascular collections of contrast-enhanced blood in trauma, the combined use of portal venous and delayed phase images is useful for characterizing contained lesions or true active extravasation.

Several pitfalls may complicate the interpretation of CT for liver injury. Respiratory motion artifact causes an indistinct gray margin around the right lobe of the liver, generally paralleling the contour of the liver (see Fig. 15.29). This appearance should not be confused with a subcapsular hematoma, which typically deforms the liver parenchyma. Respiratory motion artifact is the most common cause of false-positive diagnoses in abdominal trauma imaging.

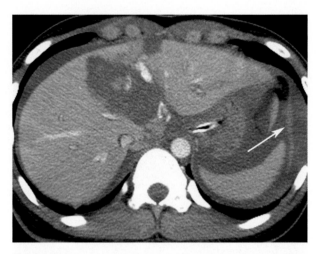

Figure 15.16. Massive liver laceration involving the right and left lobes, with large foci of intraparenchymal active extravasation as well as extravasation into the perisplenic space *(arrow)*. Note also abundant hemoperitoneum.

Unopacified hepatic veins may be mistaken for a liver laceration (Fig. 15.17). This pitfall occurs when scanning commences early in the contrast bolus, before the hepatic veins are opacified. A focal area of fat—frequently in proximity to the ligamentum venosum—should not be confused with a hepatic laceration.[69]

Image artifacts may simulate lacerations. Most problematic are beam-hardening artifacts from adjacent ribs and streak artifacts from air-contrast interfaces, electrocardiographic electrodes, or the upper extremities within the imaging field.

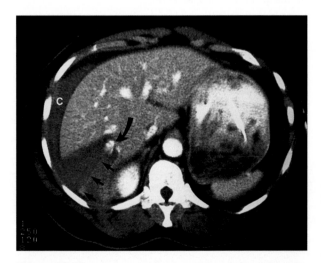

Figure 15.15. Grade III–IV laceration of the right lobe with active arterial extravasation. Above the porta hepatis, a deep laceration involving segment VII has a focus of active hemorrhage at its base *(curved arrow)*. Note the jet of active arterial extravasation extending to the periphery *(straight arrows)*. Relatively dense blood is seen adjacent to the liver—the sentinel clot sign *(C)*.

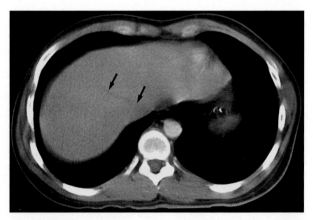

Figure 15.17. Unopacified middle hepatic vein simulating a liver laceration. This image was made in the early vascular phase before there was filling of the portal or hepatic veins. The middle hepatic vein *(arrows)* could be mistaken for a deep laceration.

TABLE 15.2	American Association for the Surgery of Trauma Liver Injury Scale (1994 revision)	
Grade[a]	**Injury description**	
I	Hematoma	Subcapsular, <10% surface area
	Laceration	Capsular tear, <1 cm parenchymal depth
II	Hematoma	Subcapsular, 10%–50% surface area
		Intraparenchymal, <10 cm in diameter
	Laceration	1–3 cm parenchymal depth, <10 cm in length
III	Hematoma	Subcapsular, >50% surface area or expanding
		Ruptured subcapsular or parenchymal hematoma
		Intraparenchymal hematoma >10 cm or expanding
	Laceration	>3 cm parenchymal depth
IV	Laceration	Parenchymal disruption involving 25%–75% of hepatic lobe or 1–3 Couinaud's segments within a single lobe
V	Laceration	Parenchymal disruption involving >75% of hepatic lobe or >3 Couinaud's segments within a single lobe
	Vascular	Juxtahepatic venous injuries (i.e., retrohepatic vena cava/central major hepatic veins)
VI	Vascular	Hepatic avulsion

[a]Advance one grade for multiple injuries, up to grade III. From Moore EE, Cogbill TH, Jurkovich GJ, et al. Organ injury scaling: spleen and liver (1994 revision). *J Trauma.* 1995;38(3):323–324, with permission.

The 1994 revision of the AAST liver injury scale uses the terms described earlier, except for hepatic fracture and hepatic contusion (Table 15.2). CT staging of liver injuries predicts patients likely to require surgery. However, a comparison study shows only partial agreement between CT and surgical-based staging.[70] CT is able to show intraparenchymal hematomas deep in the liver that are not visible at surgery, but CT also understages some lacerations.[70]

Gallbladder

Gallbladder injuries are unusual. They have been classified as disruption, which is laceration or perforation of the gallbladder by a penetrating wound or direct blow to the abdominal wall; avulsion (Fig. 15.18), which is tearing of the gallbladder away from the gallbladder fossa of the liver with the gallbladder held in place by the cystic duct and cystic artery; and contusion (Fig. 15.19), which is ecchymosis of the gallbladder wall, often with blood in the gallbladder lumen.[61] According

to Erb and colleagues, "The CT finding of an ill-defined contour of the gallbladder wall, intraluminal hemorrhage, or collapsed lumen, especially in the presence of pericholecystic fluid, suggests primary gallbladder injury in patients following blunt abdominal trauma. No combination of findings is believed specific for the type of gallbladder injury."[71]

Extrahepatic Bile Ducts

Injury to the extrahepatic bile ducts is uncommon and occurs at points of fixation, where the hepatic duct exits the liver and where the common bile duct enters the head of the pancreas.[72] Bile duct laceration may be partial or complete. The diagnosis is most often made at surgery and is probably not often recognized by CT. CT signs are nonspecific, including edema in the hepatoduodenal ligament, free intraperitoneal fluid, and associated liver or duodenal injuries.[45] Persistent peritoneal fluid on follow-up CT performed 3 to 7 days after injury may indicate bile leakage or continuing hemorrhage.[62]

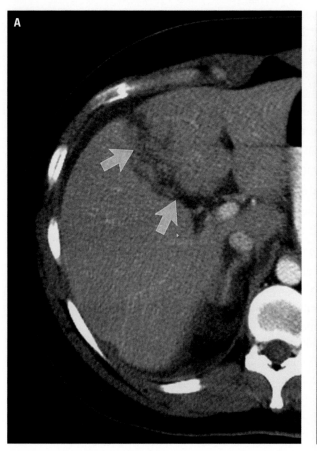

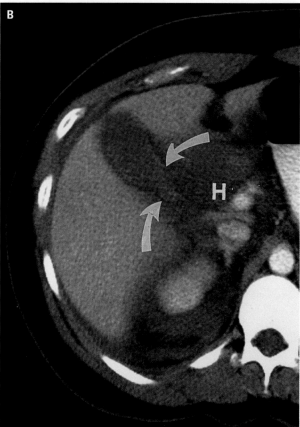

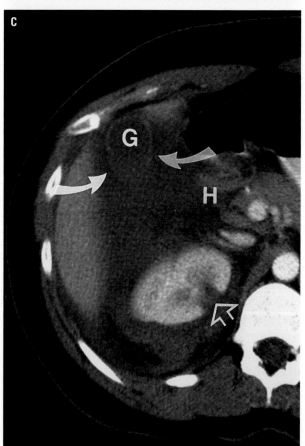

Figure 15.18. Gallbladder avulsion. **A:** At the porta hepatis, a grade III laceration runs along the interlobar fissure *(straight arrows)* cephalad to the gallbladder. **B:** In the gallbladder fossa, hematoma surrounds the gallbladder neck *(curved arrows)*. Hematoma *(H)* distends the hepatoduodenal ligament. **C:** More caudally, the fundus of the gallbladder *(G)* is surrounded by hematoma *(curved arrows)*. A grade II laceration of the right kidney *(open arrow)* causes right perinephric hematoma. The specific diagnosis of gallbladder avulsion is not possible by CT, but the hematoma surrounding the gallbladder and extending into the hepatoduodenal ligament suggest the diagnosis.

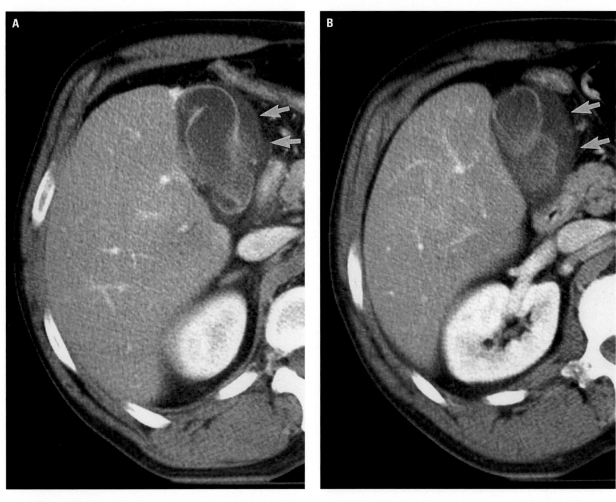

Figure 15.19. Gallbladder injury. **A:** In the body of the gallbladder, the enhancing mucosa is distorted by hematoma in the gallbladder wall *(arrows).* **B:** More caudally, the wall is markedly thickened *(arrows).* The enhancing mucosa could be confused with large gallstones.

Spleen

The spleen is the most commonly injured abdominal organ following blunt trauma. Although the stage of a splenic injury generally correlates with the need for surgical management, splenic injuries may be unpredictable. Apparently, low-stage splenic injuries develop delayed splenic hemorrhage in about 15% of cases.[16] Delayed splenic hemorrhage is defined as active hemorrhage from the injured spleen that occurs more than 48 hours after the initial injury.

Nonoperative management to preserve the immunologic function of the spleen is now preferred for most splenic injuries. The trend began among pediatric trauma surgeons who manage most patients without surgery and attempt to repair (splenorrhaphy) rather than remove the spleen when surgery is required. Nonoperative management is now widely accepted for adults, particularly those younger than age 55.[73] Embolization of an actively bleeding splenic injury is an alternative means of splenic salvage.[74]

Splenic injuries may be classified as contusions, lacerations, intraparenchymal hematomas, subcapsular hemorrhages, and vascular pedicle injuries.[75] On CT, splenic contusions appear as focal, poorly defined, nonlinear areas of decreased enhancement. Contusions should not be confused with heterogeneous enhancement caused by the early bolus effect in the spleen.

Lacerations are focal linear or branching areas of low attenuation within the enhancing splenic parenchyma (Figs. 15.20–15.22). Typically, lacerations extend to the splenic surface. On occasion, they extend to the vascular pedicle, a retroperitoneal bare area. Transverse lacerations are parallel to major

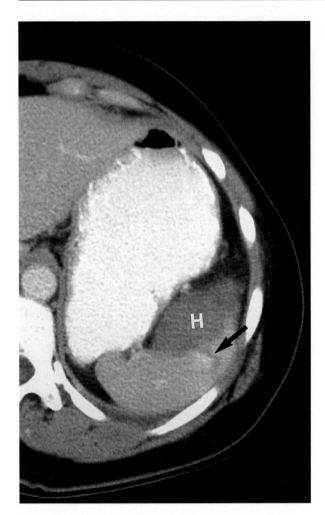

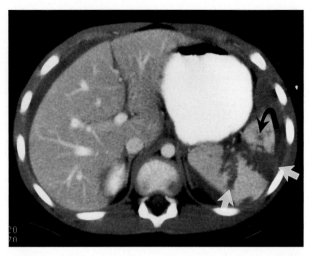

Figure 15.21. Grade III laceration of the spleen. In the midportion of the spleen, two lacerations intersect *(straight arrows)*. Contusion causes heterogeneous enhancement in the anterior fragment *(curved arrow)*. Hemoperitoneum is present. (Case courtesy of Steven Ashlock, MD)

contain a splenic pseudoaneurysm, which is a well-circumscribed focus of increased attenuation contained completely within the normally enhancing spleen (Fig. 15.25).[11]

Subcapsular hematoma is a crescentic low-attenuation area at the periphery of the spleen,

Figure 15.20. Splenic laceration with grade II subcapsular hematoma. In the upper portion of the spleen, a small laceration along the medial border *(arrow)* causes a moderate-sized subcapsular hematoma *(H)*. The subcapsular hematoma occupies 10% to 50% of the surface of the spleen, making this a grade II subcapsular hematoma.

trabecular vessels and are less likely to cause ongoing bleeding, whereas longitudinally oriented lacerations cross major trabecular vessels and are more likely to cause clinically important hemorrhage (Fig. 15.23).[73] Splenic fracture is a term applied to a deep splenic laceration resulting in complete separation of splenic fragments.

Intraparenchymal hematomas are lacerations that have filled with blood, appearing as rounded areas of low attenuation (Fig. 15.24). Clotted blood within an intraparenchymal hematoma may have relatively high-attenuation values (50 to 70 HU) (Fig. 15.25).[76] Intraparenchymal hematoma may

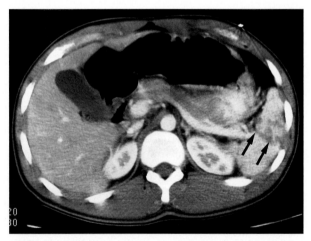

Figure 15.22. Transversely oriented grade IV splenic laceration without hemoperitoneum. At the splenic hilum, a transverse laceration *(arrows)* traverses the short axis of the spleen, involving the lateral peritoneal surface and the medial bare area at the hilum. This serious-appearing laceration has probably not injured a major trabecular vessel and has not caused hemoperitoneum. Such an injury is likely to be missed by focused assessment with sonography for trauma (FAST), unless the laceration is directly visualized. (Case courtesy of Steven Ashlock, MD)

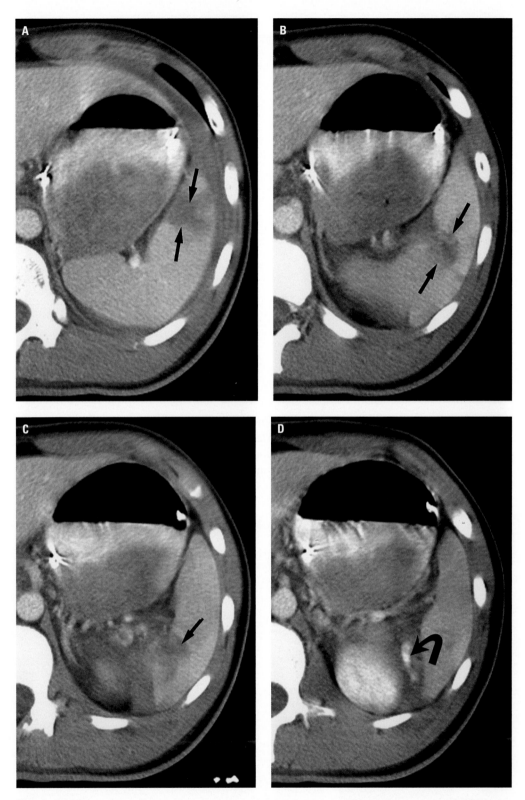

Figure 15.23. Longitudinally oriented grade III splenic laceration with active arterial extravasation. A series of four images from the top to the bottom of the spleen (**A–D**) demonstrates a laceration *(straight arrows)* extending along the medial border of the spleen from anterosuperior to posteroinferior, involving the hilum along its course. In the upper portion of the spleen, an intraparenchymal hematoma *(straight arrows)* is present. Near the lower pole (**D**), active arterial extravasation *(curved arrow)* is seen in the perisplenic space, indicating a need for angiographic embolization or attempts at surgical hemostasis. Longitudinally oriented lacerations cross trabecular vessels and are likely to bleed.

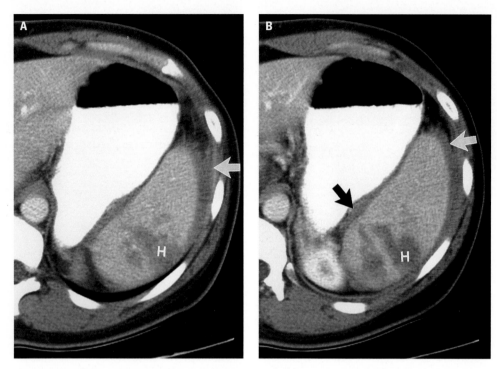

Figure 15.24. Grade III ruptured intraparenchymal hematoma. Two images above the splenic hilum (**A** and **B**) illustrate two parallel lacerations. One contains a globular collection of blood, forming an intraparenchymal hematoma *(H)*. The hematoma has ruptured into the perisplenic space with hemoperitoneum surrounding the spleen *(arrows)*.

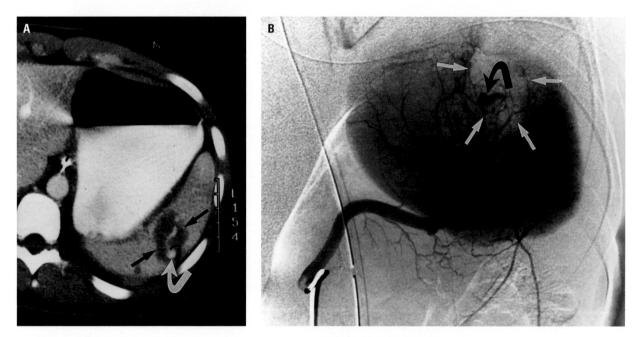

Figure 15.25. Grade II intraparenchymal hematoma with traumatic pseudoaneurysm. CT image above the splenic hilum (**A**) illustrates an oval intraparenchymal hematoma *(straight arrows)* with a central contrast-enhancing pseudoaneurysm *(curved arrow)*. Minimal hemoperitoneum is present at other levels. Angiographic image from a selective splenic arterial injection (**B**) shows branching splenic arteries and staining of the normal parenchyma. The intraparenchymal hematoma is seen as a hypovascular area *(straight arrows)*. The pseudoaneurysm is visible as the enlarged vessel at the center of the hematoma *(curved arrow)*. The angiographic appearance correlates well with the CT. This pseudoaneurysm was successfully embolized with a single coil in the feeding artery.

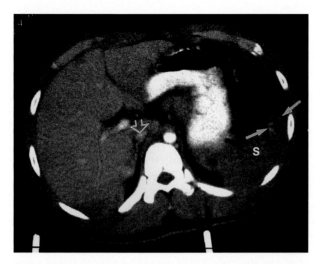

Figure 15.26. Splenic vascular pedicle injury in a patient in shock. Above the splenic hilum, an image made during the early portal venous phase of contrast enhancement shows a slit-like IVC *(straight open arrow)*. The spleen *(S)* is poorly enhancing. There is probably perisplenic or subcapsular fluid anteriorly *(straight solid arrows)*.

typically along the lateral margin. Subcapsular hematomas flatten and compress the contour of the spleen and are often associated with small underlying parenchymal lacerations.[76]

Vascular pedicle injuries represent either traumatic intimal dissection or avulsion of the splenic artery. In vascular pedicle injury, most or all of the spleen is nonenhancing, but there may be preserved perfusion to the upper pole of the spleen via short gastric arteries (Fig. 15.26). Avulsion of the splenic artery must be distinguished from hypoperfusion

related to shock or apparent hypoperfusion due to scanning before the contrast bolus has reached the spleen.[76]

Hemoperitoneum in the perisplenic space is high attenuation when splenic bleeding is the source (sentinel clot sign). On occasion, there may be a multilayered perisplenic clot caused by intermittent hemorrhage.[76] Also, given that the spleen is a highly vascular organ, CT images acquired with state-of-the-art technology often demonstrate extravascular collections of contrast-enhanced blood, which may be located within the splenic parenchyma (usually inside or adjacent to a laceration or contusion) or in the perisplenic space. As mentioned previously, characterization of these foci as active extravasation or vascular injuries (pseudoaneurysm or arteriovenous fistula) can be accomplished by carefully inspecting the portal venous phase and delayed phase images. Active bleeding typically appears as extravasation of contrast-enhanced blood, which results in collections with an attenuation (300 to 450 HU) that is much higher than clotted blood (40 to 80 HU).[77] On delayed images, the area of active extravasation characteristically increases in size, and the attenuation remains higher than that of blood inside the lumen of nearby vessels (blood pool) (Fig. 15.27). With MDCT, foci of active bleeding can be seen in up to 20% of patients with splenic injury.[78] Studies have concluded that the finding of active arterial bleeding on CT is an indication for immediate surgical management.[16,79,80] However, some institutions prefer endovascular therapy with embolization

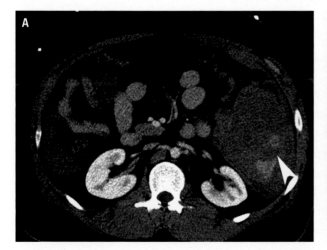
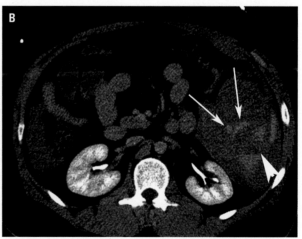

Figure 15.27. CT images obtained in the portal venous phase (**A**) and delayed phase (**B**) demonstrate a grade III splenic laceration (**A** and **B**, *arrowheads*) with associated perisplenic hematoma. The delayed phase image shows foci of active extravasation as irregular collections of contrast-enhanced blood (**B**, *arrows*).

for hemodynamically stable patients with active extravasation.

Vascular injuries include pseudoaneurysms and arteriovenous fistulae. These two lesions appear on CT as well circumscribed, contained foci of extravascular contrast-enhanced blood with an attenuation that is similar to adjacent contrast-enhanced arteries in all acquired phases and that remain similar in size and shape in all acquired phases. A splenic pseudoaneurysm is formed with a partial injury of the arterial wall, whereas a complete injury more typically results in active extravasation or vessel occlusion. Arteriovenous fistulae are much rarer and develop as a result of injury to both the artery and adjacent vein. Although the natural history of these lesions is not completely understood, the major potential complication of splenic pseudoaneurysms is rupture, with reported rates varying between 5% and 40%.[81] Therefore, the finding of a contained vascular injury appears to warrant intervention, usually with angiographic embolization.[82]

Active hemorrhage indicates an increased risk for ongoing bleeding and is a valuable sign in selecting patients for surgical or angiographic management.

Because nonoperative therapy is now contemplated in most patients with splenic injuries, an integral component of the comprehensive assessment by the trauma team and a key goal of the interpretation of the trauma CT scan by the radiologist is the detection of factors and findings that may predict failure of nonoperative management. CT findings that have been shown to impact the success of nonoperative management include AAST injury grade, amount of hemoperitoneum, evidence of ongoing hemorrhage, and presence of splenic vascular lesions. Presence of injuries classified as AAST grade III or higher and large volume hemoperitoneum (blood extending from the perisplenic space to the pelvis) increase the risk of failed nonoperative therapy.[83–85] In a 5-year retrospective review of CT performed in 150 adults with splenic injury, Federle and colleagues showed a strong correlation of the AAST grade (Table 15.3) with the need for surgery.[16] Most patients with grade I and II injuries were successfully managed nonoperatively. Almost one-half (43%) of the grade III injuries required surgery, and almost all of the grade IV and V injuries required surgery. Nearly all (93%) of the patients with active contrast extravasation were

TABLE 15.3	American Association for the Surgery of Trauma Splenic Injury Scale (1994 revision)	
Grade[a]		**Injury description**
I	Hematoma	Subcapsular, <10% surface area
	Laceration	Capsular tear, <1 cm parenchymal depth
II	Hematoma	Subcapsular, 10%–50% surface area
		Intraparenchymal, <5 cm in diameter
	Laceration	1–3 cm parenchymal depth, which does not involve a trabecular vessel
III	Hematoma	Subcapsular, >50% surface area or expanding
		Ruptured subcapsular or parenchymal hematoma
		Intraparenchymal hematoma >5 cm or expanding
	Laceration	Laceration >3 cm parenchymal depth or involving trabecular vessels
IV	Laceration	Laceration involving segmental or hilar vessels producing major devascularization (>25% of spleen)
V	Laceration	Completely shattered spleen
	Vascular	Hilar vascular injury which devascularizes spleen

[a]Advance one grade for multiple injuries up to grade III. From Moore EE, Cogbill TH, Jurkovich GJ, et al. Organ injury scaling: spleen and liver (1994 revision). *J Trauma*. 1995;38(3):323–324, with permission.

treated surgically. Along the same lines, Gavant and colleagues showed that active extravasation appearing as extra-splenic contrast extravasation, splenic pseudoaneurysm, or intraparenchymal hematoma predicted the need for surgery, even with grade I through grade III injuries.[11] In children, Benya and colleagues found that the staging system described by Mirvis and colleagues, which is similar to the AAST system, was useful in predicting nonsurgical success and the time required for injury healing—higher stage injuries required longer to heal.[13,86] A more recently updated version of the staging system proposed by Mirvis and colleagues, which includes identification with CT of contained vascular injury and active extravasation, has been shown to be more accurate for predicting the need for angiography or surgery as compared to the AAST scale.[87]

A number of pitfalls are encountered in imaging of the spleen. As in the liver, respiratory motion artifact should not be mistaken for subcapsular hematoma. Respiratory motion artifacts typically cause a gray halo paralleling the contour of the spleen (Fig. 15.28), whereas subcapsular hematoma is crescentic and deforms the contour of the spleen. Splenic lobulations or clefts most often appear medially along the upper margin of the spleen but can occur elsewhere. In some cases, clefts cannot be distinguished from splenic lacerations. Generally, well-defined linear low-attenuation areas along the medial aspect of the spleen are best considered clefts unless they are surrounded by hemoperitoneum or subcapsular hematoma (Fig. 15.29). An elongated left lobe of the liver may cause an interface with the upper pole of the spleen, which may be mistaken as a laceration of the upper pole of the spleen. Streak artifacts may also simulate splenic lacerations but are usually recognizable because they extend beyond the margins of the spleen. However, streak artifacts may degrade image

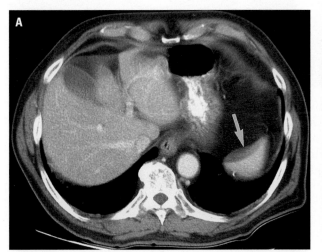

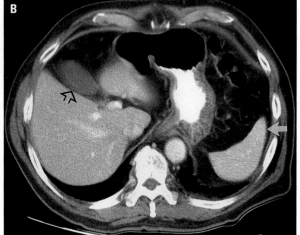

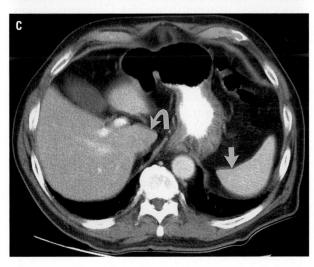

Figure 15.28. Respiratory motion artifact. Three contiguous images above the splenic hilum (**A–C**) demonstrate a gray halo surrounding portions of the spleen *(straight solid arrows)* that parallels the margin of the spleen in a pattern typical of respiratory motion artifact. A similar motion artifact is present along the caudate lobe of the liver *(curved solid arrow,* **C**) and along the margin of the gallbladder *(straight open arrow,* **B**).

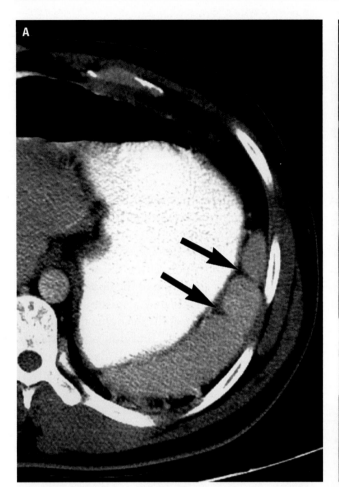
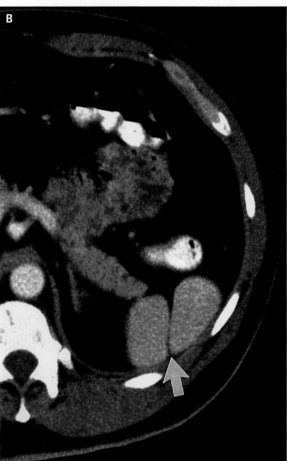

Figure 15.29. Splenic clefts. **A:** In the upper pole of the spleen, two parallel clefts *(arrows)* are in the typical location along the anterolateral margin. These well-defined clefts have no surrounding hemoperitoneum. **B:** In another patient, an image through the lower pole of the spleen demonstrates a less common location for a cleft *(arrow)* through the inferomedial portion of the spleen. Again, the well-defined cleft has no surrounding hemoperitoneum and should not be confused with a laceration.

quality so severely that laceration might be hidden by the superimposed artifact (Fig. 15.30). Premature scanning before the portal venous phase (before 60 to 70 seconds after the start of injection) may result in poor or heterogeneous enhancement of the spleen (Fig. 15.31). Delayed rescanning will show more homogeneous enhancement, but lacerations may be missed by failing to scan at the peak of parenchymal enhancement.[88]

Pancreas

Blunt pancreatic injury is uncommon, most often resulting from blows to the midabdomen from a steering wheel or bicycle handlebars. The pancreatic neck and body are the most common sites of pancreatic laceration. Lacerations of the pancreatic head are more likely to be complicated than are more distal pancreatic injuries. Common complications include hemorrhagic pancreatitis, sepsis, abscess, nonhemorrhagic pancreatitis, pseudocyst, and fistula.[89] Transection of the pancreatic duct is an important source of morbidity and increased mortality. Pancreatic laceration is usually associated with liver, spleen, or duodenal lacerations. Injuries to the pancreas are often difficult to diagnose. Only 70% of patients with pancreatic injury have an elevated serum amylase. DPL, ultrasound, and CT all miss some injuries and, when present, CT signs are often subtle.[89]

Pancreatic injuries may be classified as contusion, laceration, or transection. On CT, the injured pancreas may appear normal, particularly in the

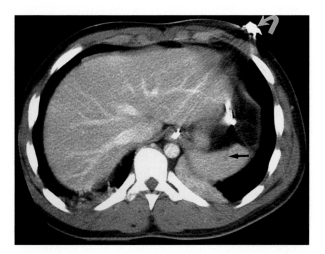

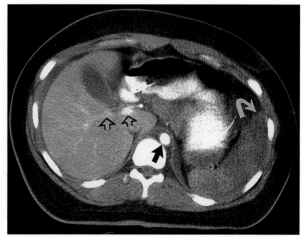

Figure 15.30. Streak artifact vs splenic laceration. Image through the upper pole of the spleen is degraded by considerable streak artifact from the electrocardiographic electrode on the anterolateral left chest wall *(curved arrow)* and the radiopaque nasogastric tube. One cannot determine with certainty whether the short linear low-attenuation area in the upper pole of the spleen *(straight arrow)* is a grade I laceration or a streak artifact. This case illustrates the importance of relocating electrocardiographic electrodes outside the scanning field.

Figure 15.31. Early bolus effect obscuring splenic laceration. Above the splenic hilum, this image was made early in the contrast bolus due to incorrect use of automatic scan triggering. The aorta *(straight solid arrow)* is intensely enhanced, whereas the portal vein *(open arrows)* is beginning to be enhanced. The spleen is poorly enhanced, but the irregular margin *(curved arrow)* may indicate perisplenic fluid. Hemoperitoneum is clearly present in the perihepatic space. The early bolus effect masked splenic lacerations later proven at surgery.

first 12 hours after injury.[90] Pancreatic contusion causes focal or diffuse swelling of the pancreas. Traumatic pancreatitis has an identical CT appearance. Laceration is characterized by a linear low-attenuation area in the enhancing pancreatic parenchyma (Figs. 15.32–15.34). Lacerations may involve a portion of the surface or may extend

through the entire pancreas, resulting in transection. The depth of laceration correlates with the likelihood of pancreatic ductal injury. Lacerations involving less than 50% of the thickness of the pancreas usually do not result in pancreatic ductal injury, whereas those involving more than 50% of the thickness, including those that completely

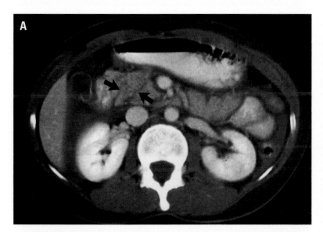

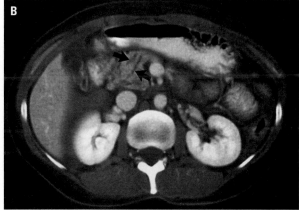

Figure 15.32. Pancreatic head lacerations. Two contiguous images through the pancreatic head (**A** and **B**) from the same patient as in Fig. 15.18 demonstrate a series of parallel lacerations *(arrows)* in the pancreatic head. Retroperitoneal hematoma is primarily from the actively hemorrhaging liver laceration. The distal pancreas appeared normal on other images.

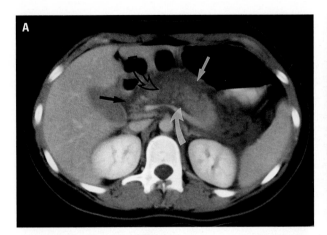
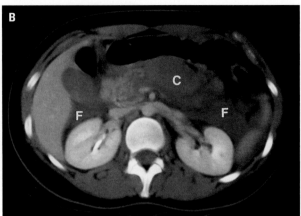

Figure 15.33. Transection of the pancreatic neck with acute peripancreatic fluid collection. **A:** At the level of the splenic vein, a jagged laceration extends through the entire thickness of the pancreatic neck *(curved open arrow)*. Fluid infiltrates the peripancreatic fat *(straight solid arrows)*. Fluid separates the posterior pancreas from the splenic vein *(curved solid arrow)*. **B:** At the renal veins, an acute peripancreatic fluid collection *(C)* is located caudal to the pancreatic laceration. Abundant retroperitoneal fluid *(F)* is located in both the right and left anterior pararenal spaces. (Case courtesy of Steven Ashlock, MD)

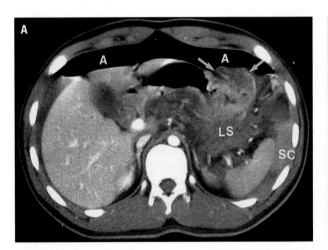
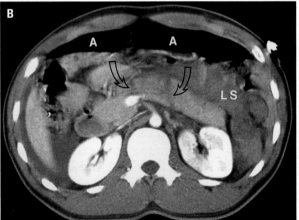

Figure 15.34. Pancreatic transection and stomach rupture. **A:** In the upper abdomen, abundant free intraperitoneal air *(A)* is interposed between the anterior abdominal wall and the liver on the right and the gastric fundus *(straight arrows)* on the left. No oral contrast material is present because the patient vomited every time oral contrast medium was administered. Fluid is present in the lesser sac *(LS)*. A large amount of peritoneal fluid is present throughout the abdomen and pelvis, with a sentinel clot *(SC)* in the perisplenic space, probably caused by bleeding associated with the perforated stomach. **B:** At the level of the body of the pancreas, two lacerations completely transect the neck and body of the pancreas *(curved open arrows)*. **C:** At the level of the splenic vein, the pancreas is completely transected *(curved open arrow)*.

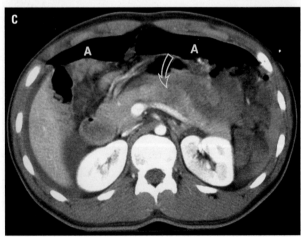

TABLE 15.4	American Association for the Surgery of Trauma Pancreatic Injury Scale	
Grade[a]	**Injury Description**[b]	
I	Hematoma	Minor contusion without duct injury
	Laceration	Superficial laceration without duct injury
II	Hematoma	Major contusion without duct injury or tissue loss
	Laceration	Major laceration without duct injury or tissue loss
III	Laceration	Distal transection or parenchymal injury with duct injury
IV	Laceration	Proximal[c] transection or parenchymal injury, **not** involving ampulla
V	Laceration	Massive disruption of pancreatic head

[a]Advance one grade for multiple injuries to the same organ.

[b]Based on most accurate assessment at autopsy, laparotomy, or radiologic study.

[c]Proximal pancreas is to the patient's right of the superior mesenteric vein. Wong YC, Wang LJ, Lin BC, et al. CT grading of blunt pancreatic injuries: prediction of ductal disruption and surgical correlation. *J Comput Assist Tomogr.* 1997;21(2):246–250.

transect the pancreas, usually cause ductal injury.[91] Indirect signs of pancreatic injury include fluid in the peripancreatic fat (Figs. 15.32 and 15.33), fluid around the superior mesenteric artery, fluid in the transverse mesocolon, fluid in the lesser peritoneal sac (Fig. 15.34), fluid separating the pancreas from the splenic vein (Fig. 15.33), and thickening of the left anterior renal fascia.[92]

Streak artifacts may simulate pancreatic lacerations. Unopacified duodenum or loop of jejunum adjacent to the pancreas with a well-defined low-attenuation plane between the pancreas and the bowel may give the false appearance of a pancreatic laceration.[45]

Wong and colleagues retrospectively reviewed 22 cases of blunt pancreatic injury and found that laceration was visible in 20 of the cases.[91] Complete transections and deep lacerations involved more than 50% of the pancreas and correlated with grade III and IV lacerations at surgery (Table 15.4). In a patient in whom the initial CT scan shows a normal pancreas and who subsequently develops abdominal pain, a follow-up CT scan within the first 24 to 48 hours after the injury may show an injury not evident initially.[89] Magnetic resonance cholangiopancreatography (MRCP) is a valuable method in patients with pancreatic trauma.[93] MRCP serves several purposes in this setting: accurate determination of involvement of the pancreatic duct by a laceration, characterization of questionable findings on initial CT, and follow-up of pancreatic lacerations and fluid collections, thereby decreasing the cumulative dose of ionizing radiation delivered to these often young patients. Endoscopic retrograde cholangiopancreatography may be needed for definitive diagnosis of pancreatic ductal injury, a condition that usually requires surgical management.[89]

Adrenal

Adrenal injuries are uncommon, but the widespread use of CT and awareness of the existence of these injuries results in their more frequent recognition.[94] The right adrenal is much more frequently injured than the left; occasionally, both adrenals are injured. The mechanism of injury may be compression of the adrenal between the liver and the spine. Transient compression of the IVC, resulting in elevated intraadrenal venous pressure, may also cause hemorrhage.

On CT, adrenal hemorrhage usually appears as a rounded or oval adrenal mass frequently surrounded by fat stranding (Fig. 15.35).[94] Uniform swelling of the gland with indistinct margins is a less common appearance. Amorphous, diffuse hemorrhage obliterating the gland represents a higher stage injury correlating with complete disruption of the gland at surgery (Fig. 15.36).[94] Thickening of the right crus

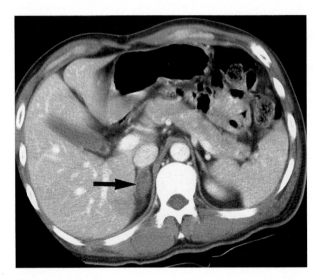

Figure 15.35. Right adrenal hematoma. Image through the lower limbs of the right adrenal shows a well-circumscribed, oval hematoma between the two lower adrenal limbs *(straight arrow)*. This is the most common appearance of an adrenal hematoma.

of the diaphragm or hemorrhage in the right posterior pararenal space next to the crus is a frequent associated finding.[94,95] Bilateral adrenal hemorrhage is unusual and puts the patient at risk for adrenal insufficiency (Fig. 15.37).

If only a little hemorrhage surrounds the injured adrenal, distinction from an adrenal neoplasm may not be possible. Follow-up CT showing resolution of the mass confirms prior hemorrhage.[94] Adrenal hemorrhage is of little clinical significance, particularly when it is unilateral.

Urinary Tract

Blunt renal injury is the third most common blunt abdominal injury after splenic and hepatic injuries. Gross or microscopic hematuria following abdominal trauma usually indicates renal injury.[96] The severity of hematuria may not directly reflect the extent of renal injury, but blunt renal injury almost never occurs without hematuria.[96]

In the past, intravenous urography (IVU) was used in patients with blunt trauma and suspected urinary tract injuries. A literature review based on studies that used IVU to detect renal injuries indicates that investigation of hematuria is warranted in patients with penetrating injury, gross hematuria, or microscopic hematuria with shock and in those suspected of having an associated major intra-abdominal injury.[97] The current widespread use of CT for evaluating blunt trauma patients has considerably decreased the emphasis on clinical

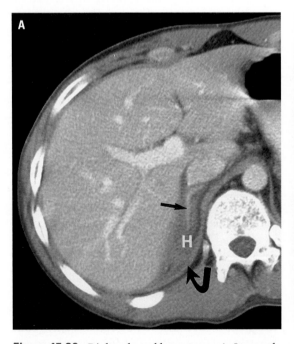
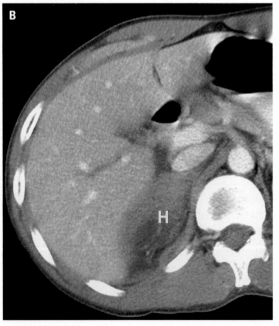

Figure 15.36. Right adrenal hematoma. **A:** Image through the lower limbs of the right adrenal shows the less common amorphous, diffuse hemorrhage *(H)* obscuring the gland *(straight arrow)*. Apparent thickening of the right crus of the diaphragm *(curved arrow)* may be caused by hemorrhage in the right posterior pararenal space. **B:** At a more caudal level, hematoma *(H)* fills the right retroperitoneum.

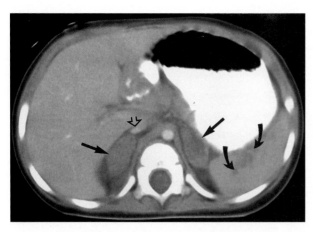

Figure 15.37. Bilateral adrenal hemorrhage in an infant. Image through the adrenal glands shows oval hematomas in each adrenal gland *(straight solid arrows)*. Because the adrenal hemorrhages are bilateral, adrenal insufficiency is a concern. A longitudinally oriented splenic laceration is seen medially *(curved solid arrows)* and is present on images both above and below this level. Note the slit-like IVC *(open arrow)* and small aorta, which indicate intravascular volume depletion.

and urinalysis findings to determine the need for evaluating the urinary tract with imaging. However, controversy remains regarding the need for abdominal CT in blunt abdominal trauma patients that have isolated microscopic hematuria and no additional finding to suggest intra-abdominal injury. A study that used CT to detect renal injury in 48 children showed that 17 (68%) of the 25 children with "significant" renal injuries had microscopic rather than gross hematuria.[98] Patients with suspected urinary tract injury who are evaluated with a screening CT of the abdomen and pelvis have their urinary tract imaged as part of that CT. As outlined previously under Technique, abdominal CT for trauma should include delayed images of the kidneys 5 to 10 minutes after initial injection of contrast material to demonstrate the "urographic" phase of excretion of contrast material into the calyces, renal pelvis, and ureters. Renal injuries may be classified as contusion, laceration, fracture, subcapsular hematoma, and vascular pedicle injuries. The AAST renal injury scale stages injuries based on the status of the renal pedicle, the extent and depth of parenchymal laceration, and the integrity of the renal collecting system (Table 15.5). Stern have correlated CT scan findings with the AAST system.[99] The following description is based on their formulation. Renal contusion (grade I) causes one or more focal regions of diminished parenchymal enhancement. Delayed images may show linear or patchy areas of retention of contrast material within the parenchyma. Acute subcapsular hematoma (grade I) appears as a crescentic high-attenuation collection of blood over the renal surface that often flattens the renal parenchyma

TABLE 15.5		American Association for the Surgery of Trauma Renal Injury Scale
Grade[a]		Injury Description[b]
I	Contusion	Microscopic or gross hematuria; urologic studies normal
	Hematoma	Subcapsular, nonexpanding without parenchymal laceration
II	Hematoma	Nonexpanding perirenal hematoma confined to the renal retroperitoneum
	Laceration	<1 cm parenchymal depth of renal cortex without urinary extravasation
III	Laceration	>1 cm parenchymal depth of renal cortex without collecting system rupture or urinary extravasation
IV	Laceration	Parenchymal laceration extending through the renal cortex, medulla, and collecting system
	Vascular	Main renal artery or vein injury with contained hemorrhage
V	Laceration	Completely shattered kidney
	Vascular	Avulsion of renal hilum, which devascularizes kidney

[a]Advance one grade for multiple injuries to the same organ.

[b]Based on the most accurate assessment at autopsy, laparotomy, or radiologic study. From Moore EE, Shackford SR, Pachter HL, et al. Organ injury scaling: spleen, liver, and kidney. *J Trauma.* 1989;29(12):1664–1666, with permission.

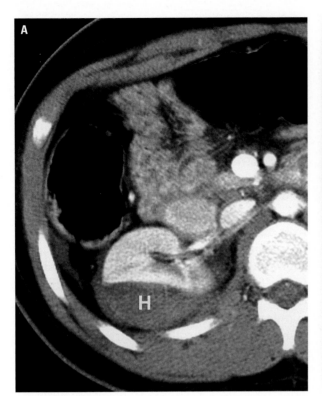
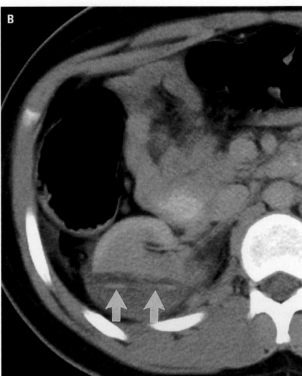

Figure 15.38. Subcapsular hematoma of the right kidney with active hemorrhage. In the interpolar region of the right kidney, an image at the peak of cortical contrast enhancement (**A**) shows a large subcapsular hematoma *(H)* compressing the posterior portion of the right kidney. On a delayed image at the same level (**B**), a horizontal line within the hematoma *(arrows)* represents extravasated contrast material.

(Fig. 15.38). As with the liver and spleen, a true subcapsular hematoma must be distinguished from respiratory motion artifact, causing a gray shadow around the kidney. Perinephric hematoma (grade II) fills portions of the perinephric space, sometimes causing considerable mass effect but may also have a subcapsular component that distorts the kidney (Fig. 15.39). Superficial laceration (grade II) is a small linear or wedge-shaped cortical defect often associated with focal perinephric or subcapsular hematoma (Fig. 15.40). A deep laceration (grade III) extends more than a centimeter into the renal parenchyma but does not injure the collecting systems sufficiently to cause urinary extravasation (Fig. 15.41). A moderate or large perinephric hematoma is usually present. Deep laceration with collecting system tear (grade IV) results in contrast extravasation on delayed CT scan (Fig. 15.42). Renal fracture (grades III and IV) is diagnosed when lacerations connect to cortical surfaces through the hilum (Fig. 15.42). Shattered kidney (grade V) is characterized by multiple deep lacerations that break the kidney into fragments

held together by vascular scaffolding. Typically, some portions of the renal parenchyma are enhanced, whereas other portions are infarcted. A large perinephric hematoma is usually present, and active arterial extravasation from disrupted renal artery branches may be present. Total renal infarction (grades IV and V) is caused by dissection or thrombosis of the main renal artery, resulting in diminished enhancement of most of the kidney. One-half of cases have residual enhancement of the outer renal cortex ("cortical rim sign") resulting from collateral supply from capsular arteries. The cortical rim sign may not be present initially but develops later. Grade IV injuries have contained hemorrhage, whereas grade V injuries are defined by avulsion of the renal hilum, which devascularizes the kidney and carries a high risk of ongoing hemorrhage.

Segmental renal infarction is not included in the AAST system. These limited vascular injuries are encountered much more frequently than main renal artery injuries and result in an infarction of the renal parenchyma supplied by the injured

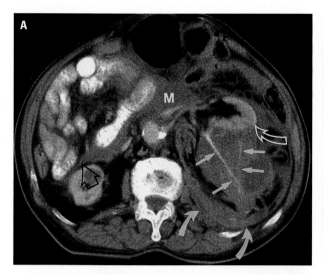 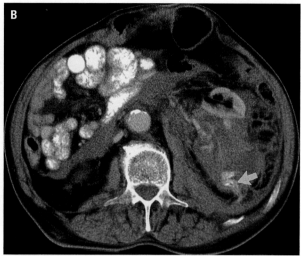

Figure 15.39. Large perinephric hematoma with active arterial extravasation. **A:** At the left renal hilum, two jets of active arterial extravasation shoot into the large posterior perinephric hematoma *(straight arrows)*. Hematoma is seen throughout the retroperitoneum, including the left posterior pararenal space *(curved closed arrows)*, the root of the mesentery *(M)*, and the right anterior pararenal space *(straight open arrow)*. The left kidney *(curved open arrow)* is markedly anteriorly displaced. **B:** At a lower level, the extravasated contrast material has pooled in the dependent portion of the left perinephric hematoma *(arrow)*.

segmental division of the renal artery (Fig. 15.43). The infarcted area shrinks over several weeks. Traumatic intimal dissection of the renal artery with partial arterial obstruction should be distinguished from occlusion of the main renal artery.

With partial obstruction, there is diminished but persistent parenchymal enhancement. Recognition of the hypoperfusion should lead to subsequent interventional radiological or surgical treatment of the dissection with preservation of the kidney.[100]

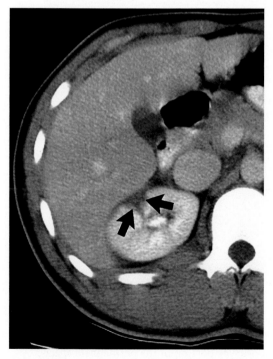 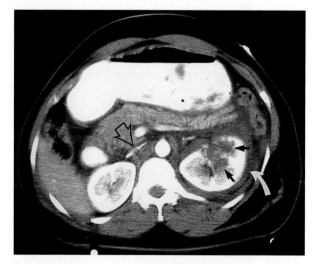

Figure 15.40. Superficial (grade II) wedge-shaped laceration in the upper pole of the right kidney *(arrows)*.

Figure 15.41. Deep (grade III) laceration of the left kidney. CT obtained in the cortical phase of contrast enhancement shows a deep laceration *(solid arrows)* in the lower pole of the left kidney. Perinephric hematoma is present *(curved arrow)*. No extravasation of urinary contrast material is present on delayed images (not shown). The slit-like IVC *(open arrow)* indicates that this adult patient is in shock.

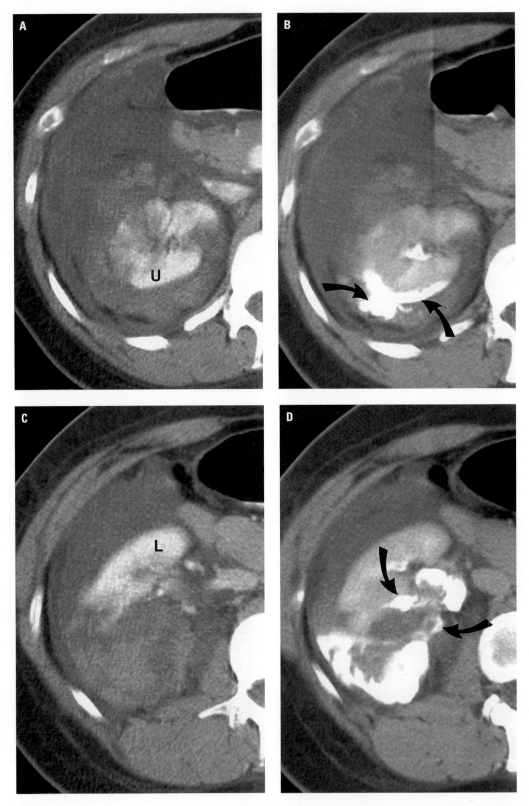

Figure 15.42. Renal fracture (grade V) with renal pelvis tearing and urine extravasation. **A:** Early image through the upper *(U)* pole of the right kidney shows multiple fracture lines surrounded by a large perinephric and pararenal fluid collection. **B:** Delayed image at the same level demonstrates urinary contrast material extravasation in the posterior portion of the perinephric space *(curved arrows).* **C:** The lower pole *(L)* fragment is displaced anteriorly. **D:** Delayed image at the same level shows urinary contrast material flowing out of the torn renal pelvis *(curved arrows).*

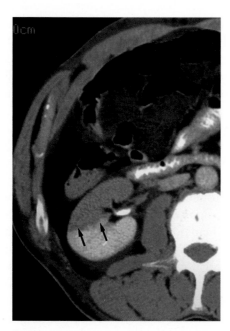

Figure 15.43. Segmental infarction of the lower pole of the right kidney. The parenchyma supplied by the anterior division of the right renal artery is nonenhanced *(arrows)* compared to the normally enhanced posterior parenchyma.

Nonoperative management is the rule for renal trauma. Extravasation of urine is not necessarily an indication for surgical intervention. Massive urine extravasation, active arterial hemorrhage, and very large perinephric hematomas with hemodynamic instability are the major indications for surgery.[96]

Non-iatrogenic ureteral injuries are rare and are usually caused by penetrating rather than blunt trauma. The ureteropelvic junction (UPJ) is most frequently injured, followed by the mid and lower ureter. CT accurately defines the location and extent of extravasation from the ureter. With UPJ or proximal ureteric injury, CT shows a large fluid collection, predominantly in the posteromedial perinephric space (Fig. 15.44).[101] The collection may surround the ipsilateral kidney. On unenhanced or early vascular-phase CT, the fluid collection contains an intermediate-attenuation (20 to 40 HU) mixture of blood and urine, whereas delayed scans show contrast extravasation. If the ureter is completely transected, the distal ureter will fail to opacify, but if the transection is incomplete, contrast material will fill the distal ureter.[101]

Gastrointestinal Tract

Although injuries to the hollow viscera and mesentery are rare, occurring in approximately 5% of patients who suffer severe blunt abdominal trauma and who require laparotomy,[102–106] one of the most essential tasks for a radiologist interpreting CT examinations of patients who suffered blunt trauma is to recognize the often subtle signs of bowel trauma. A delayed diagnosis of an injury to the bowel wall or mesentery that results in hollow viscus perforation leads to significant morbidity and mortality from

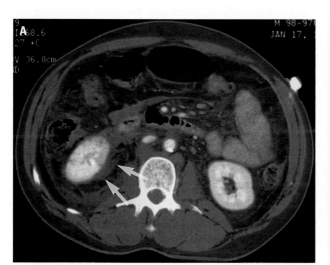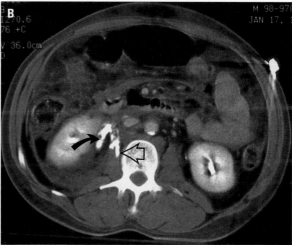

Figure 15.44. Ureteropelvic junction rupture. **A:** The lower pole of the right kidney is surrounded by perinephric fluid, particularly posteromedially *(straight arrows)*. **B:** The delayed image at the same level shows urine extravasation from the ureteropelvic junction into the posteromedial right perinephric space *(curved arrow)* and posterior to the ureter along the psoas muscle *(open arrow)*.

hemorrhage, peritonitis, or abdominal sepsis. Delays in diagnosis as short as 8 to 12 hours after the injury cause this increased morbidity and mortality.[107,108] Thus, early recognition with imaging is of critical importance.

Three basic mechanisms have been proposed as the cause of bowel and mesenteric injuries in blunt abdominal trauma: shearing injuries caused by deceleration, crush injuries from direct impacts, and burst injuries from sudden increases in intraluminal pressure.[109] At least one-half of hollow visceral injuries involve the small bowel, with colonic, duodenal, and gastric injuries occurring in decreasing order of frequency.[102,110] The proximal jejunum (distal to the ligament of Treitz) and the distal ileum (proximal to the ileocecal valve) are particularly susceptible to suffer injuries from blunt traumatic forces. The points of fixation at these two sites allow shearing forces to injure the more mobile loops.[111]

The clinical diagnosis of bowel trauma is a difficult one. Spillage of blood and intestinal contents into the abdominal cavity causes peritonitis and subsequent complications. Abdominal pain and guarding from peritoneal irritation are the main early clinical manifestations of bowel and mesenteric injuries. In alert and non-comatose patients, the presence of these clinical findings should raise the suspicion of a significant intra-abdominal injury. However, these are not specific and may not be present during the initial assessment after admission to the emergency department. Clinical signs of peritonitis may take hours before becoming unequivocally present. In addition, these patients often have significant neurological injuries to the head and spinal cord or receive medications that can mask pain and guarding, such that the physical examination of the abdomen is difficult or unreliable. As a result, the use of clinical assessment alone as the indication for laparotomy to treat bowel or mesenteric injuries is associated with a negative laparotomy rate that may be as high as 40%.[112,113] Thus, the diagnosis of bowel and mesenteric injuries from blunt trauma requires the use of various diagnostic tests, especially CT. At most institutions, DPL has been abandoned as a diagnostic examination. In some practices, ultrasonography (US) is used to triage blunt trauma patients. Positive findings, such as free intraperitoneal fluid, may trigger the request for a CT examination.

CT is 88% to 93% sensitive in detecting blunt bowel injuries.[24,114] Historically, limited sensitivity of CT in detecting injury to the bowel has been the

major argument against its universal acceptance for hemodynamically stable blunt abdominal trauma patients. Signs of bowel injury are frequently subtle, requiring meticulous attention to image quality and a thorough search of the bowel and mesentery on every CT examination.

The following are considered specific signs of bowel injury: transection of the wall with focal discontinuity, extraluminal oral contrast (in the rare occasions in which it is administered), pneumoperitoneum, and pneumoretroperitoneum. Specific signs of mesenteric trauma include mesenteric hematoma, intraperitoneal extravasation of intravenous contrast, and abrupt termination or unequivocal irregularity of the wall of mesenteric vessels. Other less specific (but more sensitive) CT signs of bowel trauma include focal wall thickening, abnormal bowel wall enhancement, and ill-defined increased attenuation ("stranding") of the mesentery and free intraperitoneal fluid. Studies that used different generation of scanners and relied on the multiple signs described in detail in this chapter report a sensitivity that varies between 70% and 95% and a specificity that varies between 92% and 100% for the diagnosis of bowel and mesenteric injuries.[37–43]

The most severe bowel injuries are seen directly on CT as frank perforations with a focal interruption in the continuity of the bowel wall and can be classifed as bowel lacerations. Although this sign is almost 100% specific, its sensitivity is low, as only approximately 7% of injuries present with this finding.[44] More often, traumatic bowel perforations are small and cannot be directly identified on CT. Diagnosis of small bowel perforations demands careful attention from the radiologist to detect subtle signs.

The most specific signs of bowel injury are pneumoperitoneum or retroperitoneal air, extravasation of oral contrast material (although its use in blunt trauma has declined considerably in recent years), and low-attenuation fluid between loops of bowel.[116]

Extraluminal gas is a highly suggestive, but not pathognomonic, sign of bowel perforation. Pneumoperitoneum as a sign of hollow viscus injury has been discussed in detail already in this chapter.

Stomach

Blunt injuries to the stomach are uncommon, but they are more common in children than in adults.[117,118] The anterior wall is the most common site of rupture, followed by the greater curvature, lesser curvature, and posterior wall. A history of repetitive vomiting of oral contrast material may be a clue to the diagnosis (Fig. 15.34).

Duodenum

Blunt duodenal injury is uncommon. The second and third portions of the duodenum are most frequently injured, and children are more likely to sustain this injury than adults.[119] Associated injuries to the liver, spleen, and pancreas are usually present.[120] In one retrospective surgical series, CT was diagnostic or suggestive in 60% of proven blunt duodenal injuries.[120] On CT, duodenal perforation is characterized by retroperitoneal gas near the duodenum, extravasated oral contrast material in the right anterior pararenal space, or a visible defect in the duodenal wall (Fig. 15.45).[114,121] In the absence of signs of perforation, focal thickening or a high-attenuation mass in the duodenal wall, possibly associated with retroperitoneal fluid, is suggestive of intramural hematoma.[75,121] Pneumoperitoneum from a perforation of the peritonealized surface of the duodenum occurs less commonly than retroperitoneal perforation.

False-positive diagnosis of duodenal injury may be suggested by unopacified small bowel loops adjacent to the duodenum; retroperitoneal hematoma from a nonduodenal source, particularly if the duodenum is collapsed and apparently thickened; or duodenal diverticulum simulating retroperitoneal air.[99]

Jejunum and Ileum

Unequivocal localized thickening of a small bowel loop or segment in the context of blunt trauma is usually an indication of a significant (surgically important) injury, such as a contusion, hematoma, ischemia secondary to mesenteric vascular trauma, or perforation (Figs. 15.46–15.49). Unequivocal focal abnormal enhancement (decreased or increased) of a segment of bowel is also a highly suspicious finding often associated with a significant injury (Fig. 15.50). The likelihood of focal wall thickening or focal abnormal enhancement representing a bowel injury that requires surgical intervention increases when found in association with pockets of fluid in the adjacent mesentery or free fluid in the peritoneal cavity.[122] Coronal and sagittal reformations are particularly useful for assessing the loops of small bowel and the associated mesentery for focal abnormalities. Focal full-thickness small bowel tears can be repaired by suture closure (enterorrhaphy); however, if multiple small bowel perforations are present, the affected loop(s) of small bowel are typically resected and primary anastomosis is performed.[123]

Diffuse bowel wall thickening is usually not a result of direct trauma. Instead, the underlying pathophysiology is more likely edema secondary to volume overload or, in the severely traumatized individual with continued bleeding, to profound hypotension

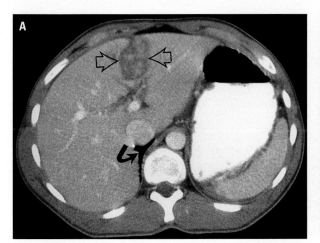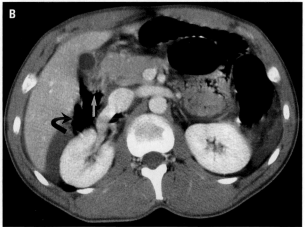

Figure 15.45. Perforation of the posterior wall of the second portion of the duodenum. **A:** An intraparenchymal hematoma *(open arrows)* extends from the surface of the left lobe to the left portal vein. A Y-shaped collection of retroperitoneal air is seen along the bare area of the liver posteromedial to the IVC *(curved arrow)*. At the second portion of the duodenum (**B**), the posterior wall of the duodenum has a visible defect *(straight arrow)* with retroperitoneal air abutting the defect *(curved arrow)*. Peritoneal fluid is present in the hepatorenal recess.

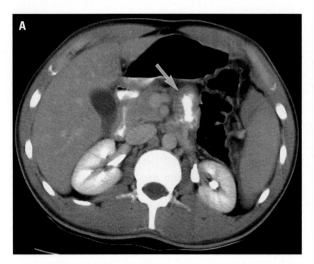
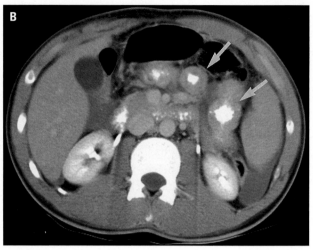

Figure 15.46. Jejunal contusion. **A:** On a delayed image at the lower pole of the spleen, the proximal jejunum near the ligament of Treitz is distended with contrast material and has a markedly thickened wall *(straight arrow)*. **B:** More caudally, other proximal jejunal loops also have marked wall thickening *(straight arrows)*. This patient has a grade II splenic laceration (not shown) causing hemoperitoneum. Bowel wall thickening is nonspecific but most likely is caused by contusion in this patient with left-sided injury.

with hypoperfusion complex ("shock bowel"), where there may be diffusely increased bowel wall enhancement.[58] Potential causes of increased bowel wall enhancement are leakage of contrast material due to increased vascular permeability during hypoperfusion,[55] preferential shift of blood flow to the mucosa, or slowing of transit time of blood through the mucosa during hypotension. Other findings characteristic of shock and hypoperfusion complex on CT include a flat IVC; increased enhancement of the adrenal glands; and bowel, pancreatic, and retroperitoneal edema. Diffuse bowel wall thickening and edema can also be caused by overhydration and fluid overload. In this situation, the liver may

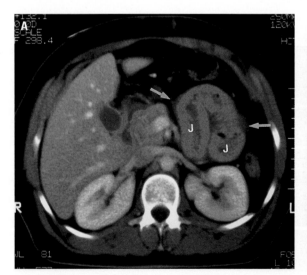
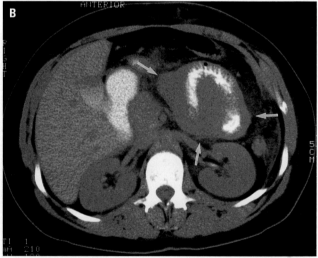

Figure 15.47. Jejunal perforation 7 cm distal to the ligament of Treitz. **A:** After administration of intravenous but not oral contrast material, a distended loop of proximal jejunum *(J)* has marked wall thickening and minimal mesenteric hematoma *(straight arrows)*. **B:** A second examination performed 13 hours later at the same level with oral contrast medium but without additional intravenous contrast material demonstrates marked increase in the mesenteric hematoma *(arrows)* surrounding the abnormal jejunal loop.

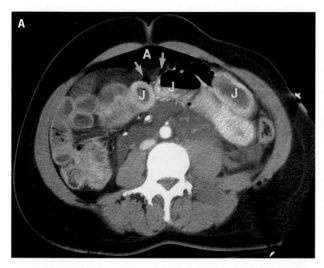
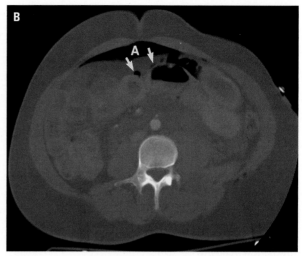

Figure 15.48. Jejunal perforation. **A:** In the midabdomen, there are several thickened jejunal loops *(J)*. Free intraperitoneal air is present beneath the anterior abdominal wall *(A)* and adjacent to jejunal loops *(arrows)*. **B:** A wide window image at the same level shows the gas bubbles to better advantage *(arrows)*.

demonstrate a heterogeneous pattern of enhancement ("nutmeg" appearance) and a concentric halo of low attenuation around the portal veins (periportal edema), whereas the other abdominal organs and vessels have a normal appearance.

Colon

Colonic injuries represent a small minority of traumatic bowel injuries and are seen in up to 5% of patients with blunt abdominal trauma.[124] On the

other hand, the colon is frequently affected in penetrating abdominal trauma from firearms and bladed weapons.[125]

Similar to the small bowel, the direct CT findings of blunt traumatic colonic perforation are free abdominal air, intramural air, focal wall discontinuity, and extravasation of oral contrast.[49] In the setting of colonic trauma, intraperitoneal air is

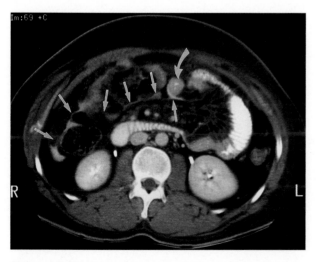

Figure 15.49. Hemorrhage from the small bowel. Delayed image in the midabdomen shows a thickened jejunal loop *(curved arrow)* with active arterial extravasation of contrast material tracking to the right paracolic gutter *(straight arrows)*.

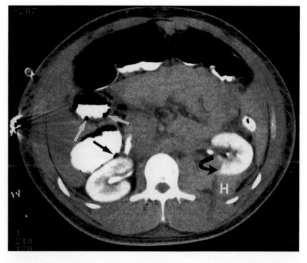

Figure 15.50. Infarction of the hepatic flexure due to mesenteric avulsion. CT with intravenous and oral contrast material performed 1 day after injury shows pneumatosis coli in the hepatic flexure of the colon. Gas bubbles are present in the dependent portions of the colonic wall *(straight arrows)*. Note the large left perinephric hematoma *(H)* resulting from the grade II renal laceration *(curved arrow)*.

most commonly identified. Retroperitoneal air may also be seen given the retroperitoneal course of both the ascending and descending colon; however, a duodenal source should also be considered. When retroperitoneal air is identified, it is most commonly seen in conjunction with intraperitoneal air rather than as an isolated finding. As previously discussed, alternative sources of retroperitoneal air such as pneumothoraces and pneumomediastinum should be considered, as air may dissect into the retroperitoneum due to the normal communications between these spaces. Conversely, air in the mediastinum may have its origin in the retroperitoneal space, for example, in the setting of retroperitoneal bowel perforation.

Given the relative insensitivity of direct signs of bowel injury, secondary signs of blunt colonic injury are crucial in aiding their detection. The indirect signs of colon injury are abnormal or focal bowel wall thickening or enhancement, stranding/infiltration of the adjacent mesentery or mesocolon, as well as free intraperitoneal fluid.[44] The bowel wall enhancement pattern and distribution are useful in suggesting the etiology of injury. Patchy or irregular increases in bowel wall enhancement after the administration of intravenous contrast material are suggestive, but not diagnostic, of full-thickness injury.[122] On the other hand, areas of decreased or absent contrast enhancement are indicative of ischemic bowel.

Mesentery and Omentum

Patients with evidence of bowel trauma on CT often have findings indicating presence of associated injuries to the mesentery. Mesenteric injuries can also be an isolated finding on CT. Specific findings of mesenteric trauma include intraperitoneal active extravasation of contrast-enhanced blood (Fig. 15.51), mesenteric hematoma (Figs. 15.51 and 15.52), infiltration of the mesentery, mesenteric rent with internal hernia (Fig. 15.53), and beading or abrupt termination of the mesenteric vessels.[44]

Active extravasation into the peritoneal cavity is uncommon, but the finding is almost 100% specific for presence of a significant injury that requires operative repair or, occasionally, endovascular therapy with coil embolization.[44] Nonoperative therapy with endovascular approaches can be attempted in patients with injuries to smaller vessels. The risk of inducing bowel ischemia must always be considered and, therefore, these patients should be observed carefully in the postprocedure period with clinical examination and liberal use of follow-up CT. A hematoma is a well-defined collection of blood within the mesentery of the small bowel, mesocolon, or omentum. Small isolated mesenteric hematomas are not always an indication for immediate surgery and can be treated with observation alone (Fig. 15.54). Larger hematomas occur in injuries to major mesenteric vessels, and therapeutic

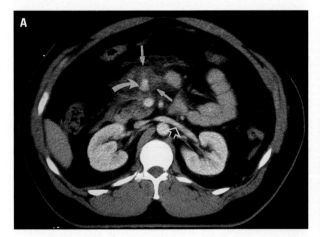
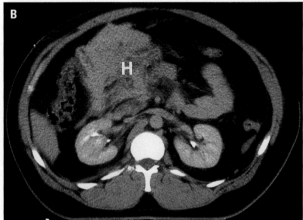

Figure 15.51. Expanding mesenteric hematoma. **A:** At the level of the left renal vein *(open arrow)* soon after administration of the bolus of contrast material, a mesenteric hematoma *(straight arrows)* surrounds a focus of active arterial extravasation *(curved arrow)*. **B:** Delayed image obtained 5 minutes later shows marked increase in the size of the mesenteric hematoma *(H)*, mandating urgent surgery to repair a bleeding mesenteric vessel.

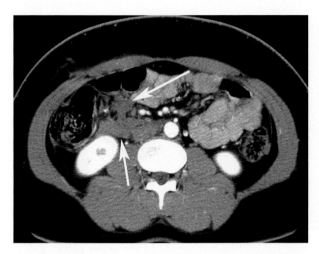

Figure 15.52. Focal hematoma in the root of the mesentery of the small bowel *(arrows)*. The size and location of this hematoma were considered highly suspicious for presence of an associated mesenteric vascular injury, which was confirmed at laparotomy.

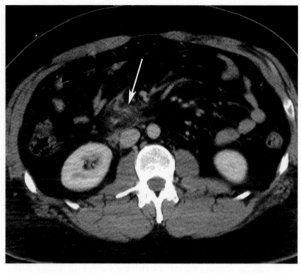

Figure 15.54. Small mesenteric hematoma. The CT examination demonstrates a focal small hematoma and stranding (bleeding) in the root of the mesentery. The patient was treated with observation only, and no intervention or further diagnostic procedure was performed.

laparotomy is usually required to avoid the risk of delayed bowel ischemia. The finding of a mesenteric hematoma on portal venous phase CT images should be further evaluated with delayed phase images. Enlargement or increased attenuation of the hematoma on the delayed phase are signs of associated active bleeding that necessitates immediate action. Isolated mesenteric injuries can also manifest on CT as focal, poorly defined haziness and fat stranding of the mesentery (Fig. 15.52). Abrupt

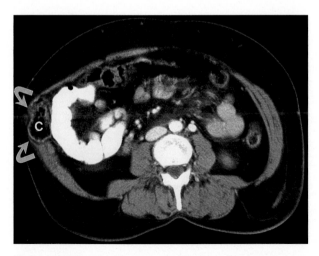

Figure 15.53. Mesenteric and abdominal wall hernia. In the midabdomen, the right lateral abdominal wall is torn *(curved arrows)*, with the ascending colon *(C)* herniating through the abdominal wall defect.

termination, focal dilatation, and irregular beading of the mesenteric arterial or venous branches in the setting of trauma are signs of significant vascular injury. Mesenteric vascular injuries are uncommon but are significant because they carry the risk of subsequent bowel ischemia. Therefore, operative repair is usually indicated. Mesenteric tears are difficult to detect on CT and may only become apparent when a segment of bowel migrates through the defect, causing an internal hernia. Closed loop bowel obstruction, volvulus, and strangulation can occur as a complication of a traumatic internal hernia.

Abdominal Wall Injuries

Abdominal wall injuries are easily overlooked if not specifically included in the CT search pattern. The most common are bruises, which appear on CT as skin thickening and soft tissue infiltration of subcutaneous fat (Fig. 15.55). Although bruises may occur at any point of impact, many are seen on the anterior abdominal wall at the points of contact with seat belts. Intramuscular hematomas are frequently seen in association with lumbar spine or pelvic fracture and present on CT as isodense swelling of muscle with loss of the normal intramuscular

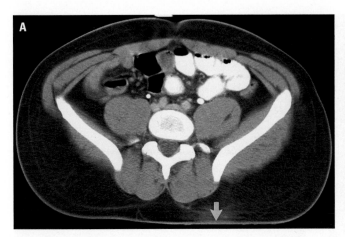
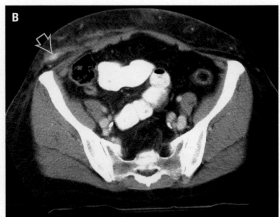

Figure 15.55. Abdominal wall tearing, bruises, and subcutaneous hemorrhage. **A:** In the upper pelvis, a bruise is seen over the left flank with thickening of the skin *(straight arrow)* and soft tissue infiltration of the subcutaneous fat. **B:** In the lower pelvis, more extensive infiltration of the anterior subcutaneous fat is present, particularly on the right side. A focus of active arterial extravasation *(open arrow)* is seen in the center of this subcutaneous hematoma.

fascial planes.[126] Tearing of the lateral abdominal wall or rectus abdominis muscle is an unusual occurrence that results in subcutaneous hematoma and, occasionally, in bowel herniation. Ongoing hemorrhage—identified as active extravasation of contrast material within the muscles—requires urgent attention to achieve hemostasis. Failure to recognize muscular injury as a source of internal hemorrhage may lead to exsanguination.

PENETRATING ABDOMINAL TRAUMA

Historically, almost all stab and gunshot wounds to the abdomen or flank required surgical exploration. In the past, the radiologist's role in the initial evaluation of penetrating injuries was limited to the interpretation of orthogonal (anteroposterior and lateral) radiographs and, occasionally, one-shot IVUs. With increased interest in nonoperative management of penetrating injuries, CT has become increasingly important in evaluating the extent of injury in selected hemodynamically stable patients.

Stab wounds are simply lacerations of variable length and depth. Wounds that penetrate the peritoneum are likely to involve the bowel and require surgical exploration. Wounds that are unequivocally superficial to the deep muscular fascia are treated with primary closure. Anterior stab wounds that

penetrate the deep fascia usually require further evaluation with laparoscopy or laparotomy because of the proximity of the peritoneum to the fascia and resultant likelihood of bowel laceration. In contrast, posterior stab wounds that penetrate the deep muscular fascia are often limited to paraspinal muscles and retroperitoneum and are not sufficiently deep to penetrate the peritoneum (Figs. 15.56); CT with intravenous, oral, and rectal contrast media ("triple-contrast CT") is effective in determining the depth

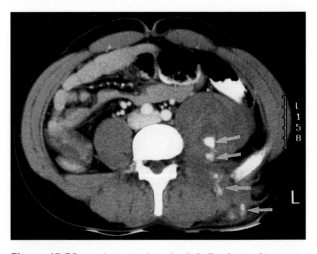

Figure 15.56. Stab wound to the left flank. In the upper pelvis, a knife tract contains foci of active arterial extravasation *(arrows)*. Note the marked enlargement of the left psoas muscle. (Case courtesy of Steven Ashlock, MD)

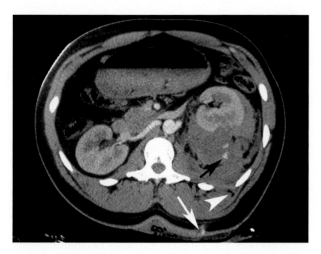

Figure 15.57. Stab injury to the left flank. The knife penetrated the muscles and fasciae and lacerated the posterior surface of the left kidney. There is a large perinephric hematoma with active extravasation of contrast-enhanced blood *(black arrow)*. The entry site is well demonstrated *(white arrow)* and the tract is delineated by gas bubbles *(white arrowhead)*.

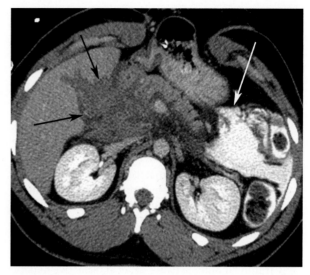

Figure 15.58. Abdominal gunshot injury. The CT scan was performed with rectal contrast. There is a large hematoma in the region of the hepatoduodenal ligament *(black arrows)*, with involvement of the head of the pancreas. There is also a focal accumulation of extracolonic contrast material *(white arrow)*. At laparotomy, a perforation of anterior distal transverse colon, a duodenal perforation, and lacerations of the liver and pancreas were found.

of wound relative to the deep muscle fascia.[127–130] In addition, CT can identify solid organ laceration, bowel perforation, urinary tract injury (Fig. 15.57), retroperitoneal hematoma, and hemoperitoneum, allowing informed decision making on the need for surgical exploration.[131,132]

In contrast to stab wounds, gunshot wounds are potentially complex injuries that depend on the type of weapon and projectile, local tissue factors, and the distance between the weapon and the victim.[99] For most handgun and shotgun wounds encountered in emergency radiology practice, CT is able to directly demonstrate the path of the bullet as it disrupts normal soft tissue planes, leaving hematoma, gas bubbles, and small metal fragments along its path (Fig. 15.58).[133,134]

In patients who suffered gunshot wounds, CT should be used only in selected patients who are hemodynamically stable. Right thoracoabdominal wounds may be managed nonoperatively if CT demonstrates that the bullet path is confined to the liver or right kidney without evidence of active hemorrhage.[134–137] Back and flank wounds may not require surgery if triple-contrast CT shows injuries confined to the muscles and retroperitoneal structures without penetration of the peritoneum or retroperitoneal portions of the bowel and without active hemorrhage or major injury to the urinary

tract.[134–137] Buttock and thigh wounds are candidates for nonoperative management if triple-contrast CT excludes bowel, urinary tract, or peritoneal penetration.[134] When clinical examination or radiographs indicate that the bullet may have crossed the bowel, laparoscopy or exploratory laparotomy is indicated, and CT should not be performed.

Penetrating wounds to the solid organs are staged using the AAST criteria discussed with blunt injuries. CT is often unable to detect the small perforations in bowel that result in only small amounts of peritoneal fluid without contrast material extravasation or pneumoperitoneum. If CT demonstrates the bullet path crossing the bowel or the presence of peritoneal fluid, surgical evaluation is indicated.

REFERENCES

1. Feliciano DV. Patterns of injury. In: Feliciano DV, Moore EE, Mattox KL, eds. *Trauma*. Stamford, CT: Appleton & Lange; 1996:85–103.
2. Halvorsen RA Jr, McCormick VD, Evans SJ. Computed tomography of abdominal trauma: a step-by-step approach. *Emerg Radiol*. 1994;1(6):283–291.

3. Jeffrey RB Jr. Cross-sectional imaging of the acute abdomen: overview of philosophy and technique. In: Jeffrey RB Jr, Ralls PW, eds. *CT and Sonography of the Acute Abdomen.* Philadelphia, PA: Lippincott-Raven, 1996:1–16.

4. Jeffrey RB Jr, Cardoza JD, Olcott EW. Detection of active intraabdominal arterial hemorrhage: value of dynamic contrast-enhanced CT. *Am J Roentgenol.* 1991;156(4):725–729.

5. Schurr MJ, Fabian TC, Gavant M, et al. Management of blunt splenic trauma: computed tomographic contrast blush predicts failure of nonoperative management. *J Trauma.* 1995;39(3):507–513.

6. Cox CS Jr, Geiger JD, Liu DC, et al. Pediatric blunt abdominal trauma: role of computed tomography vascular blush. *J Pediatr Surg.* 1997;32(8):1196–1200.

7. Ciraulo DL, Luk S, Palter M, et al. Selective hepatic arterial embolization of grade IV and V blunt hepatic injuries: an extension of resuscitation in the nonoperative management of traumatic hepatic injuries. *J Trauma.* 1998;45(2):353–359.

8. Goan YG, Huang MS, Lin JM. Nonoperative management for extensive hepatic and splenic injuries with significant hemoperitoneum in adults. *J Trauma.* 1998;45(2):360–365.

9. Akhrass R, Kim K, Brandt C. Computed tomography: an unreliable indicator of pancreatic trauma. *Am Surg.* 1996;62(8):647–651.

10. Pachter HL, Knudson MM, Esrig B, et al. Status of nonoperative management of blunt hepatic injuries in 1995: a multicenter experience with 404 patients. *J Trauma.* 1996;40(1):31–38.

11. Gavant ML, Schurr M, Flick PA, et al. Predicting clinical outcome of nonsurgical management of blunt splenic injury: using CT to reveal abnormalities of splenic vasculature. *AJR Am J Roentgenol.* 1997;168(1):207–212.

12. Mirvis SE, Whitley NO, Vainwright JR, et al. Blunt hepatic trauma in adults: CT-based classification and correlation with prognosis and treatment. *Radiology.* 1989;171(1):27–32.

13. Mirvis SE, Whitley NO, Gens DR. Blunt splenic trauma in adults: CT-based classification and correlation with prognosis and treatment. *Radiology.* 1989;171(1):33–39.

14. Moore EE, Shackford SR, Pachter HL, et al. Organ injury scaling: spleen, liver, and kidney. *J Trauma.* 1989;29(12):1664–1666.

15. Moore EE, Cogbill TH, Jurkovich GJ, et al. Organ injury scaling: spleen and liver (1994 revision). *J Trauma.* 1995;38(3):323–324.

16. Federle MP, Courcoulas AP, Powell M, et al. Blunt splenic injury in adults: clinical and CT criteria for management, with emphasis on active extravasation. *Radiology.* 1998;206(1):137–142.

17. Croce MA, Fabian TC, Menke PG, et al. Nonoperative management of blunt hepatic trauma is the treatment of choice for hemodynamically stable patients. Results of a prospective trial. *Ann Surg.* 1995;221(6):744–755.

18. Taylor CR, Degutis L, Lange R, et al. Computed tomography in the initial evaluation of hemodynamically stable patients with blunt abdominal trauma: impact of severity of injury scale and technical factors on efficacy. *J Trauma.* 1998;44(5):893–901.

19. Stuhlfaut JW, Lucey BC, Varghese JC, et al. Blunt abdominal trauma: utility of 5-minute delayed CT with a reduced radiation dose. *Radiology.* 2006;238(2):473–479.

20. Anderson SW, Varghese JC, Lucey BC. Blunt splenic trauma: delayed-phase CT for differentiation of active hemorrhage from contained vascular injury in patients. *Radiology.* 2007;243(1):88–95.

21. Levine CD, Gonzales RN, Wachsberg RH. CT findings in bowel and mesenteric injury. *J Comput Assist Tomogr.* 1997;21(6):974–979.

22. Hanks PW, Brody JM. Blunt injury to mesentery and small bowel: CT evaluation. *Radiol Clin North Am.* 2003;41(6):1171–1182.

23. Butela ST, Federle MP, Chang PJ, et al. Performance of CT in detection of bowel injury. *AJR Am J Roentgenol.* 2001;176(1):129–135.

24. Janzen DL, Zwirewich CV, Breen DJ, et al. Diagnostic accuracy of helical CT for detection of blunt bowel and mesenteric injuries. *Clin Radiol.* 1998;53(3):193–197.

25. Tsang BD, Panacek EA, Brant WE, et al. Effect of oral contrast administration for abdominal computed tomography in the evaluation of acute blunt trauma. *Ann Emerg Med.* 1997;30(1):7–13.

26. Stafford RE, McGonigal MD, Weigelt JA, et al. Oral contrast solution and computed tomography for blunt abdominal trauma: a randomized study. *Arch Surg.* 1999;134(6):622–627.

27. Clancy TV, Ragozzino MW, Ramshaw D, et al. Oral contrast is not necessary in the evaluation of blunt abdominal trauma by computed tomography. *Am J Surg.* 1993;166(6):680–685.

28. Jeffrey RB, Federle MP, Stein SM, et al. Case report. Intramural hematoma of the cecum following blunt trauma. *J Comput Assist Tomogr.* 1982;6(2):404–405.

29. Liu M, Lee CH, K. P'eng FK. Prospective comparison of diagnostic peritoneal lavage, computed tomographic scanning, and ultrasonography for the diagnosis of blunt abdominal trauma. *J Trauma.* 1993;35(2):267–270.

30. Catre MG. Diagnostic peritoneal lavage versus abdominal computed tomography in blunt abdominal trauma: a review of prospective studies. *Can J Surg.* 1995;38(2):117–122.

31. Neish AS, Taylor GA, Lund DP, et al. Effect of CT information on the diagnosis and management of acute abdominal injury in children. *Radiology.* 1998;206(2):327–331.

32. Livingston DH, Lavery RF, Passannante MR, et al. Admission or observation is not necessary after a negative abdominal computed tomographic scan in patients with suspected blunt abdominal trauma: results of a prospective, multi-institutional trial. *J Trauma.* 1998;44(2):273–282.

33. Fernandez L, McKenney MG, McKenney KL, et al. Ultrasound in blunt abdominal trauma. *J Trauma.* 1998;45(4):841–848.

34. McKenney KL, Nuñez DB Jr, McKenney MG, et al. Sonography as the primary screening technique for blunt abdominal trauma: experience with 899 patients. *AJR Am J Roentgenol.* 1998;170(4):979–985.

35. Chiu WC, Cushing BM, Rodriguez A, et al. Abdominal injuries without hemoperitoneum: a potential limitation of focused abdominal sonography for trauma (FAST). *J Trauma.* 1997;42(4):617–625.

36. Kane NM, Francis IR, Burney RE, et al. Traumatic pneumoperitoneum. Implications of computed tomography diagnosis. *Invest Radiol.* 1991;26(6):574–578.

37. Hamilton P, Rizoli S, McLellan B, et al. Significance of intra-abdominal extraluminal air detected by CT scan in blunt abdominal trauma. *J Trauma.* 1995;39(2):331–333.

38. Donohue JH, Federle MP, Griffiths BG, et al. Computed tomography in the diagnosis of blunt intestinal and mesenteric injuries. *J Trauma.* 1987;27(1):11–17.

39. Hagiwara A, Yukioka T, Satou M, et al. Early diagnosis of small intestinal rupture from blunt abdominal trauma using computed tomography: significance of the streaky density within the mesentery. *J Trauma.* 1995;38(4):630–633.

40. Sivit CJ, Eichelberger MR, Taylor GA. CT in children with rupture of the bowel caused by blunt trauma: diagnosis efficacy and comparison with hypoperfusion complex. *AJR Am J Roentgenol.* 1994;163(5):1195–1198.

41. Mirvis SE, Gens DR, Shanmuganathan K. Rupture of the bowel after blunt abdominal trauma: diagnosis with CT. *AJR Am J Roentgenol.* 1992;159(6):1217–1221.

42. Atri M, Hanson JM, Grinblat L, et al. Surgically important bowel and/or mesenteric injury in blunt trauma: accuracy of multidetector CT for evaluation. *Radiology.* 2008;249(2):524–533.

43. Stuhlfaut JW, Soto JA, Lucey BC, et al. Blunt abdominal trauma: performance of CT without oral contrast material. *Radiology.* 2004;233(3):689–694.

44. Brofman N, Atri M, Hanson JM, et al. Evaluation of bowel and mesenteric blunt trauma with multidetector CT. *Radiographics.* 2006;26(4):1119–1131.

45. Shuman WP. CT of blunt abdominal trauma in adults. *Radiology.* 1997;205(2):297–306.

46. Federle MP, Jeffrey RB Jr. Hemoperitoneum studied by computed tomography. *Radiology.* 1983;148(1):187–192.

47. Levine CD, Patel UJ, Silverman PM, et al. Low attenuation of acute traumatic hemoperitoneum on CT scans. *AJR Am J Roentgenol.* 1996;166(5): 1089–1093.

48. Cunningham MA, Tyroch AH, Kaups KL, et al. Does free fluid on abdominal computed tomographic scan after blunt trauma require laparotomy? *J Trauma.* 1998;44(4):599–603.

49. Breen DJ, Janzen DL, Zwirewich CV, et al. Blunt bowel and mesenteric injury: diagnostic performance of CT signs. *J Comput Assist Tomogr.* 1997;21(5):706–712.

50. Livingston DH, Lavery RF, Passannante MR, et al. Free fluid on abdominal computed tomography without solid organ injury after blunt abdominal injury does not mandate celiotomy. *Am J Surg.* 2001;182(1):6–9.

51. Brasel KJ, Olson CJ, Stafford RE, Johnston TJ. Incidence and significance of free fluid on abdominal computed tomographic scan in blunt trauma. *J Trauma.* 1998;44(5):889–892.

52. Rodriguez C, Barone JE, Wilbanks TO, et al. Isolated free fluid on computed tomographic scan in blunt abdominal trauma: a systematic review of incidence and management. *J Trauma.* 2002;53(1):79–85.

53. Fang JF, Chen RJ, Lin BC, et al. Small bowel perforation: is urgent surgery necessary? *J Trauma.* 1999;47(3):515–520.

54. Brody JM, Leighton DB, Murphy BL, et al. CT of blunt trauma bowel and mesenteric injury: typical findings and pitfalls in diagnosis. *Radiographics.* 2000;20(6):1525–1537.

55. Drasin TE, Anderson SW, Asandra A, et al. MDCT evaluation of blunt abdominal trauma: clinical significance of free intraperitoneal fluid in males with absence of identifiable injury. *AJR Am J Roentgenol.* 2008;191(6):1821–1826.

56. Yu J, Fulcher AS, Want DB, et al. Frequency and importance of small amount of isolated pelvic free fluid detected with multidetector CT in male patients with blunt trauma. *Radiology.* 2010;256(3):799–805.

57. Sivit CJ, Taylor GA, Bulas DI, et al. Posttraumatic shock in children: CT findings associated with hemodynamic instability. *Radiology.* 1992;182(3): 723–726.

58. Mirvis SE, Shanmuganathan K, Erb R. Diffuse small-bowel ischemia in hypotensive adults after blunt trauma (shock bowel): CT findings and clinical significance. *AJR Am J Roentgenol.* 1994;163(6):1375–1379.

59. Shanmuganathan K, Mirvis SE, Amoroso M. Periportal low density on CT in patients with blunt trauma: association with elevated venous pressure. *AJR Am J Roentgenol.* 1993;160(2):279–283.

60. Wachsberg R, Levine C, Baker S. Flattened inferior vena cava: a normal finding on unenhanced abdominal computed tomographic scan. *Emerg Radiol.* 1988;3(1):16–19.

61. Pachter HL, Liang HG, Hofstetter SR. Liver and biliary tract trauma. In: Feliciano DV, Moore EE, Mattox KL, eds. *Trauma.* Stamford, CT: Appleton & Lange; 1996:487–523.

62. Foley WD, Cates JD, Kellman GM, et al. Treatment of blunt hepatic injuries: role of CT. *Radiology.* 1987;164(3):635–638.

63. Sherbourne CD, Shanmuganathan K, Mirvis SE, et al. Visceral injury without hemoperitoneum: a limitation of screening abdominal sonography for trauma. *Emerg Radiol.* 1997;4(6):349–354.

64. Patten RM, Spear RP, Vincent LM, et al. Traumatic laceration of the liver limited to the bare area: CT findings in 25 patients. *AJR Am J Roentgenol.* 1993;160(5):1019–1022.

65. Shanmuganathan K, Mirvis SE. CT evaluation of the liver with acute blunt trauma. *Crit Rev Diagn Imaging.* 1995;36(2):73–113.

66. Stalker HP, Kaufman RA, Towbin R. Patterns of liver injury in childhood: CT analysis. *AJR Am J Roentgenol.* 1986;147(6):1199–1205.

67. Rovito PF. Atrial caval shunting in blunt hepatic vascular injury. *Ann Surg.* 1987;205(3):318–321.

68. Macrander SJ, Lawson TL, Foley WD, et al. Periportal tracking in hepatic trauma: CT features. *J Comput Assist Tomogr.* 1989;13(6):952–957.

69. Gay SB, Sistrom CL. Computed tomographic evaluation of blunt abdominal trauma. *Radiol Clin North Am.* 1992;30(2):367–388.

70. Croce MA, Fabian TC, Kudsk KA, et al. AAST organ injury scale: correlation of CT-graded liver injuries and operative findings. *J Trauma.* 1991;31(6):806–812.

71. Erb RE, Mirvis SE, Shanmuganathan K. Gallbladder injury secondary to blunt trauma: CT findings. *J Comput Assist Tomogr.* 1994;18(5):778–784.

72. Parks RW, Diamond T. Non-surgical trauma to the extrahepatic biliary tract. *Br J Surg.* 1995;82(10):1303–1310.

73. Esposito TJ, Gamelli RL. Injury to the spleen. In: Feliciano DV, Moore EE, Mattox KL, eds. *Trauma.* 3rd ed. Stamford, CT: Appleton & Lange; 1996:525–571.

74. Sclafani SJ, Weisberg A, Scalea TM, et al. Blunt splenic injuries: nonsurgical treatment with CT, arteriography, and transcatheter arterial embolization of the splenic artery. *Radiology.* 1991;181(1): 189–196.

75. Roberts JL. CT of abdominal and pelvic trauma. *Semin Ultrasound CT MR.* 1996;17(2):142–169.

76. Jeffrey RB Jr, Ralls PW. The spleen. In: Jeffrey RB Jr, Ralls PW, eds. *CT and Sonography of the Acute Abdomen.* 2nd ed. Philadelphia, PA: Lippincott-Raven; 1996:122–159.

77. Shanmuganathan K, Mirvis SE, Sover ER. Value of contrast-enhanced CT in detecting active hemorrhage in patients with blunt abdominal or pelvic trauma. *AJR Am J Roentgenol.* 1993;161(1):65–69.

78. Yao DC, Jeffrey RB Jr, Mirvis SE, et al. Using contrast-enhanced helical CT to visualize arterial extravasation after blunt abdominal trauma: incidence and organ distribution. *AJR Am J Roentgenol.* 2002;178(1):17–20.

79. Schurr MJ, Fabian TC, Gavant M, et al. Management of blunt splenic trauma: computed tomographic contrast blush predicts failure of nonoperative management. *J Trauma.* 1995;39(3):507–513.

80. Nwomeh BC, Nadler EP, Meza MP, et al. Contrast extravasation predicts the need for operative intervention in children with blunt splenic trauma. *J Trauma.* 2004;56(3);537–541.

81. Smith JA, Macleish DG, Collier NA. Aneurysms of the visceral arteries. *Aust N Z J Surg.* 1989;59(4):329–334.

82. Fu CY, Wu SC, Chen RJ, et al. Evaluation of need for operative intervention in blunt splenic injury: intraperitoneal contrast extravasation has an increased probability of requiring operative intervention. *World J Surg.* 2010;34(11):2745–2751.

83. Peitzman AB, Heil B, Rivera L, et al. Blunt splenic injury in adults: multi-institutional study of the Eastern Association for the Surgery of Trauma. *J Trauma.* 2000;49(2):177–189.

84. Bee TK, Croce MA, Miller PR, et al. Failures of splenic nonoperative management: is the glass half empty or half full? *J Trauma.* 2001;50(2):230–236.

85. Marmery H, Shanmuganathan K, Mirvis SE, et al. Correlation of multidetector CT findings with splenic arteriography and surgery: prospective study in 392 patients. *J Am Coll Surg.* 2008;206(5):685–693.

86. Benya EC, Bulas DI, Eichelberger MR, et al. Splenic injury from blunt abdominal trauma in children: follow-up evaluation with CT. *Radiology.* 1995;195(3):685–688.

87. Marmery H, Shanmuganathan K, Alexander MT, et al. Optimization of selection for nonoperative management of blunt splenic injury: comparison of MDCT grading systems. *AJR Am J Roentgenol.* 2007;189(6):1421–1427.

88. Ashlock SJ, Harris JH Jr, Kawashima A. Computed tomography of splenic trauma. *Emerg Radiol.* 1998;5(4):192–202.

89. Lane MJ, Mindelzun RE, Jeffrey RB. Diagnosis of pancreatic injury after blunt abdominal trauma. *Semin Ultrasound CT MR.* 1996;17(2):177–182.

90. Wilson RH, Moorehead RJ. Current management of trauma to the pancreas. *Br J Surg.* 1991;78(10):1196–1202.

91. Wong YC, Wang LJ, Lin BC, et al. CT grading of blunt pancreatic injuries: prediction of ductal disruption and surgical correlation. *J Comput Assist Tomogr.* 1997;21(2):246–250.

92. Sivit CJ, Eichelberger MR, Taylor GA, et al. Blunt pancreatic trauma in children: CT diagnosis. *AJR Am J Roentgenol.* 1992;158(5):1097–1100.

93. Soto JA, Alvarez O, Múnera F, et al. Traumatic disruption of the pancreatic duct: diagnosis with MR pancreatography. *AJR Am J Roentgenol.* 2001;176(1):175–178.

94. Burks DW, Mirvis SE, Shanmuganathan K. Acute adrenal injury after blunt abdominal trauma: CT findings. *AJR Am J Roentgenol.* 1992;158(3):503–507.

95. Gómez RG, McAninch JW, Carroll PR. Adrenal gland trauma: diagnosis and management. *J Trauma.* 1993;35(6):870–874.

96. Peterson NE. Genitourinary trauma. In: Feliciano DV, Moore EE, Mattox KL, eds. *Trauma.* 3rd ed. Stamford, CT: Appleton & Lange; 1996: 661–693.

97. American College of Radiology. Urologic imaging, series 2: renal trauma. In: *American College of Radiology Appropriateness Criteria for Imaging and Treatment Decisions.* Reston, VA: American College of Radiology; 1995:UR2 1.1–1.9.

98. Stein JP, Kaji DM, Eastham J, et al. Blunt renal trauma in the pediatric population: indications for radiographic evaluation. *Urology.* 1994;44(3):406–410.

99. Stern EJ. *Trauma Radiology Companion: Methods, Guidelines, and Imaging Fundamentals.* Philadelphia, PA: Lippincott-Raven; 1997:404, xii.

100. Jeffrey RB Jr, Ralls PW. The kidney and adrenal gland. In: Jeffrey RB Jr, Ralls PW, eds. *CT and Sonography of the Acute Abdomen.* Philadelphia, PA: Lippincott-Raven; 1996: 205–255.

101. Kawashima A, Sandler CM, Corriere JN Jr, et al. Ureteropelvic junction injuries secondary to blunt abdominal trauma. *Radiology.* 1997;205(2):487–492.

102. Dauterive AH, Flancbaum L, Cox EF. Blunt intestinal trauma. A modern-day review. *Ann Surg.* 1985;201(2):198–203.

103. Cox EF. Blunt abdominal trauma. A 5-year analysis of 870 patients requiring celiotomy. *Ann Surg.* 1984;199(4):467–474.

104. Buck GC III, Dalton ML, Neely WA. Diagnostic laparotomy for abdominal trauma. A university hospital experience. *Am Surg.* 1986;52(1):41–43.

105. Rizzo MJ, Federle MP, Griffiths BG. Bowel and mesenteric injury following blunt abdominal trauma: evaluation with CT. *Radiology.* 1989;173(1):143–148.

106. Davis JJ, Cohn I Jr, Nance FC. Diagnosis and management of blunt abdominal trauma. *Ann Surg.* 1976;183(6):672–678.

107. Killeen KL, Shanmuganathan K, Poletti PA, et al. Helical computed tomography of bowel and mesenteric injuries. *J Trauma.* 2001;51(1):26–36.

108. Scaglione M, de Lutio di Castelguidone E, Scialpi M, et al. Blunt trauma to the gastrointestinal tract and mesentery: is there a role for helical CT in the decision-making process? *Eur J Radiol.* 2004;50(1):67–73.

109. Hughes TM, Elton C. The pathophysiology and management of bowel and mesenteric injuries due to blunt trauma. *Injury.* 2002;33(4):295–302.

110. Kim HC, Shin HC, Park SJ, et al. Traumatic bowel perforation: analysis of CT findings according to the perforation site and the elapsed time since accident. *Clin imaging.* 2004;28(5):334–339.

111. Hawkins AE, Mirvis SE. Evaluation of bowel and mesenteric injury: role of multidetector CT. *Abdom Imaging.* 2003;28(4):505–514.

112. Fryer JP, Graham TL, Fong HM, et al. Diagnostic peritoneal lavage as an indicator for therapeutic surgery. *Can J Surg.* 1991;34(5):471–476.

113. Drost TF, Rosemurgy AS, Kearney RE, et al. Diagnostic peritoneal lavage. Limited indications due to evolving concepts in trauma care. *Am Surg.* 1991;57(2):126–128.

114. Mirvis SE, Gens DR, Shanmuganathan K. Rupture of the bowel after blunt abdominal trauma: diagnosis with CT. *AJR Am J Roentgenol.* 1992;159(6):1217–1221.

115. Sherck J, Shatney C. Significance of intraabdominal extraluminal air detected by CT scan in blunt abdominal trauma. *J Trauma.* 1996;40(4):674–675.

116. Jeffrey RB Jr, Ralls PW. The gastrointestinal tract. In: Jeffrey RB Jr, Ralls PW, eds. *CT and Sonography of the Acute Abdomen.* 2nd ed. Philadelphia, PA: Lippincott-Raven; 1996:256–314.

117. Semel L, Frittelli G. Gastric rupture from blunt abdominal trauma. *N Y State J Med.* 1981;81(6):938–939.

118. Brunsting LA, Morton JH. Gastric rupture from blunt abdominal trauma. *J Trauma.* 1987;27(8):887–891.

119. Allen GS, Moore FA, Cox CS Jr, et al. Hollow visceral injury and blunt trauma. *J Trauma.* 1998;45(1):69–75.

120. Allen GS, Moore FA, Cox CS Jr, et al. Delayed diagnosis of blunt duodenal injury: an avoidable complication. *J Am Coll Surg.* 1998;187(4):393–399.

121. Kunin JR, Korobkin M, Ellis JH, et al. Duodenal injuries caused by blunt abdominal trauma: value of CT in differentiating perforation from hematoma. *AJR Am J Roentgenol.* 1993;160(6):1221–1223.

122. Malhotra AK, Fabian TC, Katsis SB, et al. Blunt bowel and mesenteric injuries: the role of screening computed tomography. *J Trauma.* 2000;48(6):991–998.

123. Richardson JD. Treatment of small bowel injuries. In: Cameron JL, ed. *Current Surgical Therapy.* 9th ed. Philadelphia, PA: Mosby; 2008:998.

124. Cleary RK, Pomerantz RA, Lampman RM. Colon and rectal injuries. *Dis Colon Rectum.* 2006;49(8):1203–1222.

125. Pinedo-Onofre JA, Guevara-Torres L, Sánchez-Aguilar JM. Penetrating abdominal trauma [in Spanish]. *Cir Cir.* 2006;74(6):431–442.

126. Hill SA, Jackson MA, FitzGerald R. Abdominal wall haematoma mimicking visceral injury: the role of CT scanning. *Injury.* 1995;26(9):605–607.

127. Kirton OC, Wint D, Thrasher B, et al. Stab wounds to the back and flank in the hemodynamically stable patient: a decision algorithm based on contrast-enhanced computed tomography with colonic opacification. *Am J Surg.* 1997;173(3):189–193.

128. Velmahos GC, Constantinou C, Tillou A, et al. Abdominal computed tomographic scan for patients with gunshot wounds to the abdomen selected for nonoperative management. *J Trauma.* 2005;59(5):1155–1161.

129. Múnera F, Morales C, Soto JA, et al. Gunshot wounds of abdomen: evaluation of stable patients with triple-contrast helical CT. *Radiology.* 2004;231(2):399–405.

130. Shanmuganathan K, Mirvis SE, Chiu WC, et al. Penetrating torso trauma: triple-contrast helical CT in peritoneal violation and organ injury—a prospective study in 200 patients. *Radiology.* 2004;231(3):775–784.

131. Easter DW, Shackford SR, Mattrey RF. A prospective, randomized comparison of computed tomography with conventional diagnostic methods in the evaluation of penetrating injuries to the back and flank. *Arch Surg.* 1991;126(9):1115–1119.

132. McAllister E, Perez M, Albrink MH, et al. Is triple contrast computed tomographic scanning useful in the selective management of stab wounds to the back? *J Trauma.* 1994;37(3):401–403.

133. Hollerman JJ, Fackler ML, Coldwell DM, et al. Gunshot wounds: 2. Radiology. *AJR Am J Roentgenol.* 1990;155(4):691–702.

134. Grossman MD, May AK, Schwab CW, et al. Determining anatomic injury with computed tomography in selected torso gunshot wounds. *J Trauma.* 1998;45(3):446–456.

135. Renz BM, Feliciano DV. Gunshot wounds to the right thoracoabdomen: a prospective study of nonoperative management. *J Trauma.* 1994;37(5):737–744.

136. Demetriades D, Velmahos G, Cornwell E III, et al. Selective nonoperative management of gunshot wounds of the anterior abdomen. *Arch Surg.* 1997;132(2):178–183.

137. Ginzburg E, Carrillo EH, Kopelman T, et al. The role of computed tomography in selective management of gunshot wounds to the abdomen and flank. *J Trauma.* 1998;45(6):1005–1009.

CHAPTER 16

Gynecologic, Obstetric, and Scrotal Emergencies

Robert D. Harris ■ Roberta diFlorio Alexander ■ John H. Harris Jr.

Gynecologic, obstetric, and scrotal emergencies are among the most common urgent situations involving children or young adults: They frequently present with acute pain in otherwise healthy, young patients; they may be extremely anxiety producing to both the patient and clinician (because of the uncertainty of the diagnosis and the acuteness/severity of the medical condition); and they are often diagnosed with imaging, usually ultrasound (US). This is especially relevant due to recent concerns over the public health problem of medically related excessive radiation exposure that is occurring largely due to the increase in body and head computed tomography (CT) performed in emergency departments, placing the public at increased risk for developing cancer in 20 to 30 years in the future.

GENERAL CONSIDERATIONS

Gynecologic and obstetrical emergencies are two of the most common problems often encountered in teenage or premenopausal women presenting to the emergency ward or radiology department. In general terms, gynecologic emergencies usually present as a manifestation of pelvic pain and obstetrical emergencies, as vaginal bleeding in pregnancy.

The most frequently used imaging modality for obstetrical and gynecologic emergencies is pelvic US for four reasons: (1) it is widely available; (2) it is the most efficacious technique for visualizing the ovaries, uterus, fetus, and placenta; (3) it does so without adding to the burden of harmful ionizing radiation that accrues due to other imaging techniques; and (4) it can be obtained in real time in a short acquisition period. Conventional radiographs and CT, both of which use ionizing radiation to produce an image, have a more limited role, as the soft tissues of the pelvis are poorly delineated by the former technique, and limited contrast and spatial resolution of pelvic organs is a disadvantage in the latter modality. Magnetic resonance imaging (MRI) offers improved global anatomic visualization and contrast resolution compared with US, employs nonionizing radiation and is a problem-solving technique in some obstetrical and gynecologic emergencies. However, its cost, claustrophobic-associated limitations, longer duration of scanning, and limited availability preclude universal acceptance.

Conventional abdominal radiography is frequently the first-line imaging examination in the nonpregnant female patient with abdominal or pelvic pain. It may show dilated bowel loops or air–fluid levels in a patient with small bowel obstruction from pelvic adhesions, an appendicolith in acute appendicitis, or a radiopaque ureteral calculus in a patient with flank and pelvic discomfort. Other common causes for radiodensities or metallic foci are uterine/ovarian calcifications, pelvic phleboliths (calcified veins), fallopian tube clips from prior sterilization, and surgical clips from endoscopic surgery or herniorrhaphy. If additional diagnostic imaging is necessary, most patients will proceed to US (or, in some cases, CT) for further

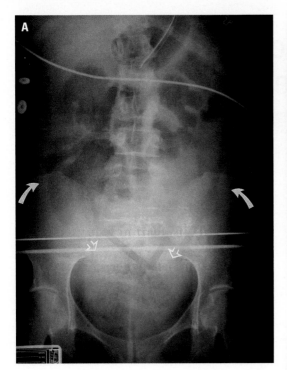

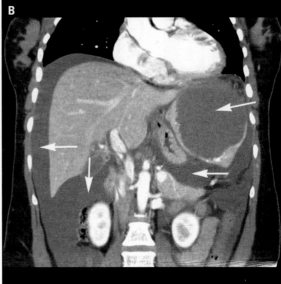

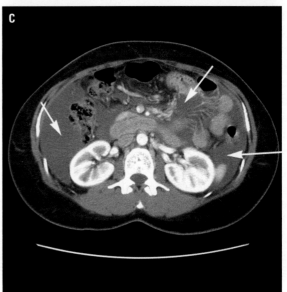

Figure 16.1. **A:** Hemoperitoneum due to ruptured ectopic pregnancy. Supine abdominal radiograph demonstrates a thickened peritoneal/flank stripe *(curved arrows)* and increased radiopacity in the pelvis *(open arrows)* due to a large amount of intraperitoneal blood. **B:** Coronal reconstructed CT showing large amount of hemoperitoneum in flanks, lesser sac, and Morrison pouch *(arrows)* from ruptured ectopic pregnancy. **C:** Axial CT in same patient showing large amount of free blood in the flanks and mesentery *(arrows)*.

diagnosis. Conventional radiographs or CT may reveal hemoperitoneum in patients with a ruptured ectopic pregnancy or hemorrhagic ovarian cyst (Fig. 16.1).

The indications for conventional radiography in a pregnant patient are much more restrictive due to the risks of exposing the fetus to ionizing radiation. Suspected renal colic (flank pain, hematuria, fever) or suspected bowel obstruction are the primary indications for a conventional radiograph, using shielding of nonimaged body parts and as low-dose radiation exposure as possible, in a gravid patient. First trimester radiography is to be avoided, if at all

possible, due to the extreme sensitivity of the early fetus or embryo.

The conventional teaching in radiology is that most urinary stones are radiopaque, but the actual figure varies and depends on the size of the stone and the radiographic technique as well. Obstetrical patients present special challenges. A third trimester fetus with a well-ossified skeleton may mask detection of upper tract calculi; also, there is the more common problem of differentiating pelvic phleboliths from distal ureteral calculi. Noncontrast helical CT, which has all but replaced intravenous urography in most medical centers, has not been used widely in obstetrical patients due to the significant radiation exposure concerns.

CT is generally not performed in obstetrical patients, unless there is an indication for pelvimetry. This pelvimetry technique has been well established without the use of any contrast material and requires only two or three images—low-dose images plus the scout localizer—similar to the frontal view of a routine radiograph. MRI has also been suggested as the modality for assessing cephalopelvic disproportion. Gynecologic patients may require CT for assessing complicated or extensive tubo-ovarian abscesses (TOAs) (Fig. 16.2). The imaging of cysts or ovarian masses too large to be completely visualized by US is usually by pelvic MRI with its excellent spatial and chemically based information. Most pelvic CT is obtained with oral contrast material (with the exception of the limited CT for appendicitis), but the need for intravenous contrast CT is less well established for true gynecologic and obstetrical emergencies. It is regarded as safe for the fetus; the only issue is maternal allergic reactions and renal function, as it is a well-documented nephrotoxic agent.

MRI has shown promise as an adjunctive imaging test in cases where US is equivocal or suboptimal, and there are extensive data supporting its use in fetal abnormalities, placenta previa or accreta,

and evaluating ovarian cysts and masses. MRI has also been helpful in the diagnosis of uterine incarceration, rare but potentially grave situation, with trapping of a retroverted uterus between pubis and sacrum. This condition—frequently associated with severe maternal pain, premature labor, and uterine rupture—is often missed with prenatal US and may be subsequently diagnosed with MRI (Fig. 16.3). However, US remains the preeminent imaging modality for most obstetrical and gynecologic emergencies.

GYNECOLOGIC IMAGING: MODALITIES

Ultrasound

US is the diagnostic "workhorse" for problems of the female pelvis. Radiographs may demonstrate a ureteral calculus or an appendicolith (calcificied stool in the appendix), and CT is useful to image a pelvic abscess from pelvic inflammatory disease (PID), but US is the modality of choice in most situations.

There are instances where conventional radiography may suggest the diagnosis, but in general, it only shows nonspecific signs. There may be a mass effect related to the bowel from a pelvic abscess in a patient with PID, but this may be difficult to differentiate from a distended bladder, abscess from other causes, or other soft tissue abnormality (i.e., tumor). Intrauterine contraceptive devices (IUDs) are generally radiopaque and well demonstrated with abdominal radiographs or CT. However, the usual clinical question of the exact location of the IUD (intrauterine vs. extrauterine) is difficult, if not impossible, to ascertain with conventional radiography (Fig. 16.4A) but is easily determined with CT or US. Rarely, IUDs may not be radiopaque, which presents difficulty in localization with conventional radiography. Mirena IUDs are not very radiopaque and can even be difficult to see on transvaginal (TV) pelvic US if they are not lined up precisely at the right geometry to the transducer (Fig. 16.4B,C).

Transabdominal US has been the traditional method to image the female pelvis and is still a useful first step in sonography. However, TVUS is state of the art in all centers because of better spatial and contrast resolution, and it is almost universally available on a 24-hour basis. Virtually, all emergent

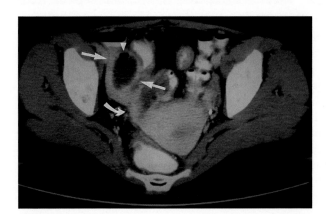

Figure 16.2. Tubo-ovarian abscess on CT. Contrast-enhanced (both intravenous and oral) scan shows an enlarged, thick-walled enhancing mass in right adnexa *(arrows)*, containing gas *(arrowhead)* and low-density *(fluid)* material. Also note the thickening of adjacent broad ligament *(curved arrow)*. This abscess was not visible on transvaginal ultrasound due to the location of the lesion beyond the range of the 5-MHz transducer.

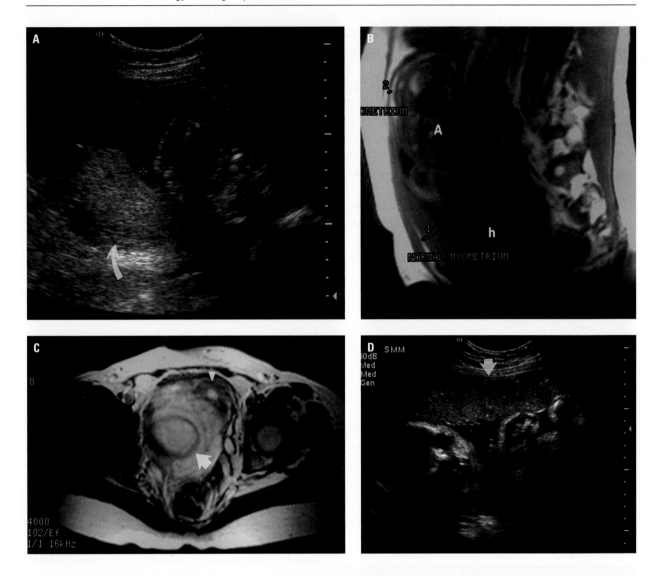

Figure 16.3. A: Incarcerated uterus missed on ultrasound. The patient presented at 28 weeks with preterm labor. On physical examination, the cervix was not seen. Ultrasound was performed, which also failed to reveal a definite cervix but showed the fetus in cephalic presentation and a posterior placenta *(curved arrow)*. *Electronic calipers* are measuring an amniotic fluid pocket. **B:** MRI obtained the same day to evaluate the cervix shows thinning of the anterior fundal myometrium *(2)*, which is actually the lower uterine segment, and the cervix is displaced anteriorly and elongated *(1)*. This longitudinal T1-weighted image shows that the anterior cervix is erroneously labeled "normal myometrium." *A*, fetal abdomen; *h*, fetal head. **C:** Axial T2-weighted image demonstrates markedly anterior cervix *(arrowhead)* stretched anterior to the fetal head *(arrow)*. **D:** Ultrasound 3 weeks later showing anterior placenta *(arrow)*. The uterus had spontaneously reduced itself.

pelvic sonograms require TV scanning. Translabial US, although occasionally useful when TV is contraindicated, is rarely used also. It may be useful in certain instances such as assessing placenta previa or if the patient is unable to tolerate a TV approach.

At most medical centers, TV scanning is the technique of choice. This obviates the need for a full bladder, and the image resolution is much improved compared to transabdominal or translabial US. Of course, if a more global view of the pelvis is needed, then one can perform transabdominal (i.e., transvesical) US if there is significant urine in the bladder to serve as an acoustic window.

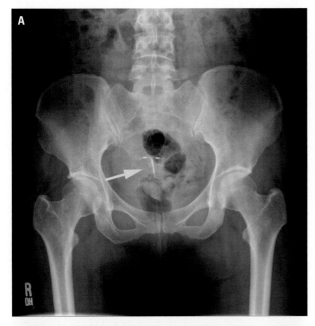

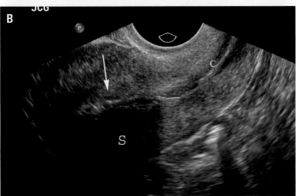

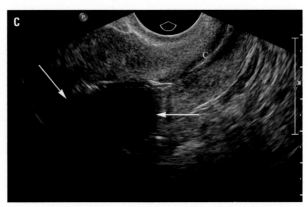

Figure 16.4. **A:** Radiographs of the abdomen showing an IUD in the pelvis *(arrow)*. This contraceptive device was a Mirena IUD and was found to be outside of the uterus at laparoscopy, but the exact location is not demonstrable on this radiograph. (Image courtesy of Petra Lewis, MD). IUD, intrauterine device. **B:** Sagittal transvaginal sonogram of the uterus in another patient containing a Mirena IUD *(arrow)*, a newer contraceptive device that secretes a small amount of progesterone continuously. It may be somewhat difficult to see at ultrasound if not properly aligned to the probe, but it usually has some degree of acoustical shadowing *(S)*. C, cervix. **C:** Sagittal transvaginal sonogram at a slightly different location and angle showing more discrete acoustic shadowing *(arrows)*. C, cervix.

Transabdominal US can be performed with a general purpose 2 to 6 MHz transducer and can provide a field of view as large as 18 to 20 cm. A 5 to 8 MHz transducer will provide better spatial resolution but will not penetrate much beyond 8 to 12 cm. Transabdominal US allows for better global visualization of the pelvis and may better image some large adnexal masses or high-riding ovaries, which may not be completely visualized with TV technique.

TV sonography is the preferred method of pelvic US and doesn't require full bladder, which optimizes transabdominal examination. Details of the TV technique will not be discussed in depth here; any basic US textbook will have this information. Placement of the TV probe is similar to a speculum exam, and the technique of introduction can be mastered relatively simply by an experienced physician or sonographer. (However, finding some pelvic structures can be quite challenging and will be addressed further on). The transducer, covered with sterile condom and gel, is placed into the vagina and oriented in the longitudinal plane, such that the bladder is visualized in the upper left of the image and posterior structures (rectum) are on the bottom right of the image. The conventional anteflexed uterus presents with the fundus oriented toward the left of the image just beneath the bladder (Fig. 16.5A,B). If the uterus is retroflexed, the fundus will be directed to the right inferior corner of the image. Rotating the transducer 90 degrees produces a more oblique coronal view traditionally labeled as transverse, referring to the plane of the transducer (Fig. 16.5C). By anteroposterior angulation of the probe, the uterus can be imaged in its entirety. Imaging of the adnexa is performed

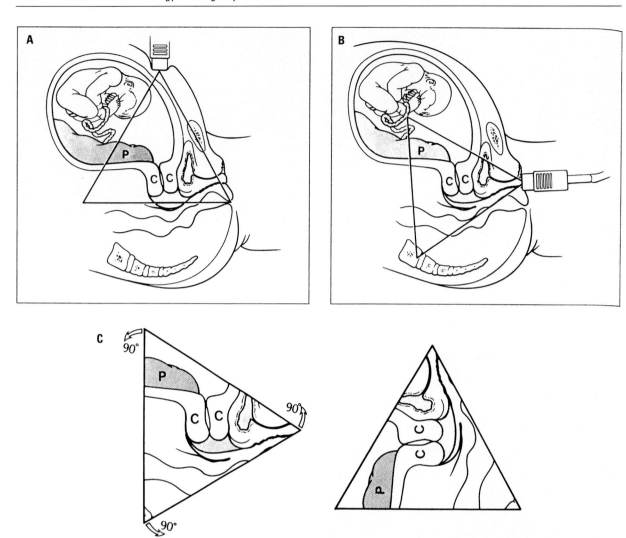

Figure 16.5. Schematic drawing of translabial sonography. **A:** A standard transabdominal approach is undertaken, and the length of the cervix is difficult to appreciate because the cervical canal *(C)* is parallel to the transducer. *P*, placenta. **B:** Translabial technique is performed, wherein the 3 MHz sector transducer in sterile covering is applied against the perineum at the vaginal introitus, and the ultrasound beam is perpendicular to the cervix. **C:** The anatomic image is rotated 90 degrees counterclockwise into the more conventional imaging orientation. (From Hertzberg BS, Bowie JD, Carroll BA, et al. Diagnosis of placenta previa during the third trimester: role of transperineal sonography. *AJR Am J Roentgenol.* 1992;159(1):83–87, with permission.)

by angling the probe to the patient's left or right. On occasion, the ovaries may be difficult to locate, particularly in postmenopausal women, and a useful landmark is the internal iliac vessels, which often reside just posterior and lateral to the ovary (Fig. 16.6). During real-time scanning, bowel loops will usually undergo peristalsis and so may be excluded as nonovarian tissue.

The transducer requirements for TVUS are unique and deserve mention. A higher frequency is used with TV than transabdominal sonography because the transducer is close to the cervix, uterus, and ovaries, so the overall depth coverage of the beam is not as important. The transducer is positioned in the vaginal fornices, and most state-of-the-art probes have almost 180 degrees of coverage and so can obtain a large field of view given the high frequency (6 to 10 cm). The method of emergent pelvic US performed in our radiology or emergency department is as follows: If the patient comes with a full bladder or a catheter in place, we commence with a transabdominal study

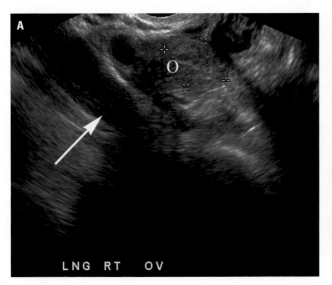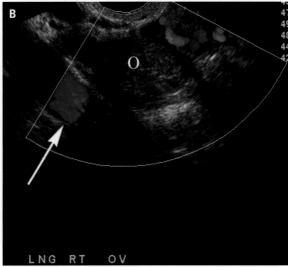

Figure 16.6. **A:** Sagittal transvaginal sonogram of the ovary, with a corpus luteum marked by *electronic calipers*, with the helpful "landmark" iliac vein located posterolateral to the ovary *(arrow)*. **B:** Color Doppler sonogram of the same structures show blue colorization of the iliac vein, as the blood flow is directed away from the transducer, toward the patient's feet. *O*, ovary.

(through the full bladder) and progress (if necessary) to a TV study. In some cases of fetal demise or placental abruption, the transabdominal study suffices. We then have the patient void or empty the bladder through a catheter and proceed to TV technique. In most cases of gynecologic or obstetrical emergencies, the study is incomplete without TV scanning. If the patient arrives with an empty or partially distended bladder, she is asked to void and we proceed directly to TV scanning.

Computed Tomography and Magnetic Resonance Imaging

CT and MRI are usually secondary imaging tests in patients with a gynecologic or obstetrical emergency. CT is best performed 1 to 2 hours after administration of oral contrast material (300 to 600 mL) to opacify the bowel, taking contiguous 5-mm thick images to cover the entire pelvis. Helical scanning allows the entire pelvis to be scanned in 5 to 15 seconds and is generally acquired with a pitch of 1 to 2 (pitch = table speed ÷ slice collimation). Intravenous contrast is occasionally indicated and can be helpful in suspected pelvic abscesses or acute appendicitis or even to delineate the blood vessels from nonvascular structures. MRI usually includes T1-gradient echo and fast T2-weighted sequences in multiple imaging planes. Occasionally, short T1 inversion recovery (STIR) or specialized gradient-echo pulse sequences may be helpful. Gadolinium is the generic intravenous contrast agent used in MRI, but its use is rarely indicated in emergent pelvic imaging and is relatively contraindicated in obstetrical imaging. The role of fetal MRI, a recently developed technique with very selective indications (fetal central nervous system [CNS] anomalies, placenta accreta), will not be discussed here due to space limitations and the fact that it is rarely an emergent study.

Normal Imaging Anatomy

The uterus, on US, appears as an oval or elliptical organ that resides posterior to the bladder and anterior to the rectum. Its size is dependent on the age and childbearing status of the patient. In premenarche, the uterus is small, ranging from 3 to 4 cm in maximum length. For the menstrual years in nulliparous women, it reaches 6 to 8 cm, and in multiparous women, it may enlarge from 8 to 10 cm. Postmenopausal women have a smaller uterus that measures 4 to 6 cm.[9] The uterus is composed of an echogenic endometrial stripe (Fig. 16.7A) that varies in thickness relative to the point in the menstrual cycle, reflecting the hormonal status, and

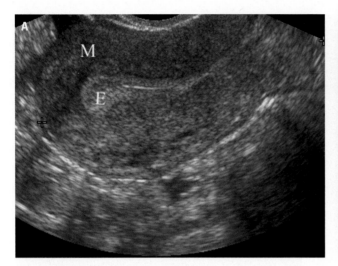
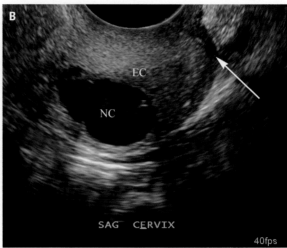

Figure 16.7. Longitudinal view of the uterus and cervix. **A:** The uterus is characterized by the bright or echogenic endometrium *(E)* and the more hypoechoic myometrium *(M)*. **B:** The cervix is defined by the external os *(arrow)* and in this example, prominent Nabothian cysts *(NC)*, a common finding of no clinical significance. The endocervical *(EC)* mucosa is not well delineated on this exam.

is generally 3 to 15 mm thick in premenopausal women—thicker in the secretory phase (latter half of menstrual cycle). The myometrium consists of the inner zone or junctional zone, which is slightly hypoechoic compared with the outer myometrium, which is of a medium-level homogeneous echo texture. However, this distinction is not often visible on US imaging and is better seen on pelvic MRI. The cervix is a smooth muscular structure that resembles a small "barrel" and can best be imaged in the longitudinal plane (Fig. 16.7B).

Ovarian size also depends on patient age and menstrual status, with premenarchal ovaries measuring 2 to 6 mL (volume = length × width × height × 0.52); those of menstruating women, 8 to 18 mL (often with small follicles); and those of postmenopausal women, less than 6 to 8 mL.[8] Ovaries may be difficult to recognize in prepubertal and postmenopausal patients because of the lack of follicles, which are usually apparent in the menstruating years (Fig. 16.8). The sonographic appearance of ovarian stroma is homogeneous and similar in echogenicity to the myometrium. The fallopian tubes are thin, elongated (7 to 12 cm), paired structures coursing from the uterine cornua (or horn) to lie next to the ovary, but they are not generally visualized on US unless they are distended with fluid, blood, or an ectopic pregnancy (Fig. 16.9). Most of the paraovarian structures visualized by US are bowel loops, which can be seen to undergo peristalsis during real-time

scanning—one of the reasons that physicians should be physically present for the US examination in the emergent setting.

US is extremely operator dependent, and virtually, any two-dimensional plane of scanning is possible with experience and knowledge of pelvic anatomy. The operator must have the flexibility to go beyond the standard transverse and sagittal planes, as much patient anatomy does not adhere to the traditional anatomy textbooks. Traditionally, transabdominal images are obtained in the transverse and longitudinal planes, with oblique images added as necessary. The uterus typically sits in the midline or just off midline in the true pelvis, with paired ovaries laterally adjacent to the fundus, but these are notorious for lying outside of the classic ovarian fossa. Occasionally, ovaries may reside on a long mesosalpinx, and they may rest behind the uterus (in the cul-de-sac) or out toward the pelvic sidewall or even up in the false pelvis.

TV technique (as described earlier) is more difficult to learn than transabdominal scanning, as the few customary anatomic landmarks are limited, and hands-on scanning experience is essential to become familiar with the variations in pelvic anatomy and the subtle probe mechanics for obtaining an excellent TV image. The longitudinal view is relatively straightforward anatomically, but the transverse view is semiaxial or semicoronal in the anatomic planes. All permutations in between are possible,

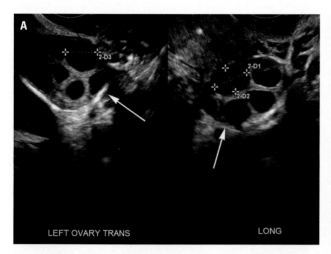 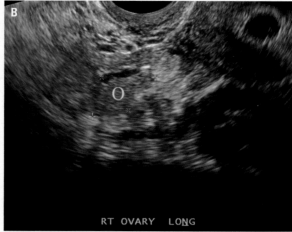

Figure 16.8. **A:** A dual transverse and longitudinal image of the normal left ovary *(arrows)* in a 33-year-old female undergoing infertility evaluation. There are seven small follicles, the largest is 12 mm and measured with the *electronic calipers.* In postmenopausal patients, the absence of follicles renders the ovaries often difficult to visualize from adjacent structures. **B:** Postmenopausal left ovary, longitudinal sonogram, in a 63-year-old patient referred with right pelvic pain. Note the difficulty delineating the quiescent ovary from the surrounding fat. *O,* ovary.

and oblique imaging is quite helpful for demonstrating the uterus and ovaries, which are rarely midline (or in the same anatomic plane) structures as in the anatomy textbooks. It is essential to become familiar with the TV probe used because the angle of the

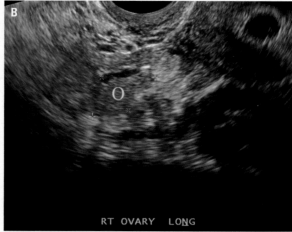

Figure 16.9. Dilated fallopian tube, or hydrosalpinx *(arrows)*, in the cul-de-sac in a 21-year-old college student recovering from pelvic inflammatory disease, with the resultant tubal inflammation. The characteristic fimbria *(arrowheads)* are well seen due to outlining with serous fluid in the tubal lumen.

beam is variable, and side-, end-, and oblique-fire transducer options are all possibilities.

The location and appearance of the uterus and ovary are variable on CT (and anatomically) and are not particularly well defined due to their soft tissue density being similar to that of bowel. If bowel is not opacified with contrast material, it may be difficult to distinguish from the uterus and adnexal structures. In general, CT is not indicated in the acute gynecologic emergency, and US is the primary imaging modality. On occasion, MRI may be indicated because of its larger, more global visualization of the female pelvis. The pelvic organs have a characteristic appearance on T2-weighted images (T2WIs). The uterus is depicted as a high-signal endometrium, an inner myometrium (or junctional zone) of lower signal, and an outer myometrium of intermediate signal (Fig. 16.10). The ovaries are characterized by the high T2 signal follicles that are present in the menstruating years that help to identify the ovaries; the ovarian stroma is of low-to-medium signal intensity on T2WIs (Fig. 16.11).

GYNECOLOGIC EMERGENCIES

The problem of acute pelvic pain (defined as <48 hours duration) in young to middle-aged women is a common clinical dilemma. The most

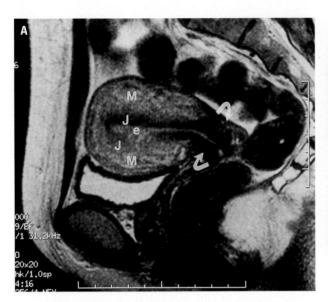

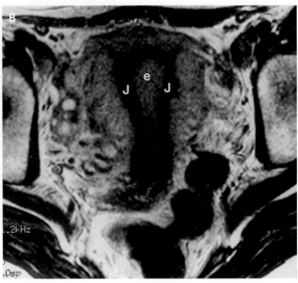

Figure 16.10. A: Normal uterus on T2-weighted sagittal image. Note the three layers of signal intensity: A bright, thin endometrium *(e)*; a darker junctional or inner zone of myometrium *(J)*, and an outer layer of myometrium *(M)* of medium signal intensity. Note the dark signal of the cervical stroma *(curved arrows)*. **B:** Normal axial view of anteverted uterus on axial T2-weighted images (same patient as in **A**). The darker junctional zone *(J)* is even more apparent on this image. *e*, endometrium.

frequent causes are ovarian cyst (enlargement or rupture) or torsion, PID, ectopic pregnancy, endometriosis, or less likely in the acute emergency setting, an ovarian or uterine neoplasm. A negative US is useful in excluding significant pathology in most cases. All patients of childbearing age should ideally have a pregnancy test, preferably a serum human chorionic gonadotropin (B-hCG), before being evaluated with US or other imaging, as the quantitative levels of the pregnancy test largely influences the interpretation of the sonographic findings. Briefly stated, if the B-hCG is more than 2,000 mIU and the patient has a normal pregnancy, then a gestational sac should be identified in the endometrial cavity. If not present, then there is a concern for a nonviable pregnancy, either an ectopic or a spontaneous miscarriage.

Ovarian Cysts and Neoplasms

The functioning (premenopausal) ovary frequently contains follicles (arbitrarily defined as smaller than 2.5 cm), functional or small physiologic cysts (defined as larger than 2.5 cm), or corpus luteum cysts. Theca lutein cysts (associated with high hCG levels, i.e., from a molar pregnancy) are much less frequent but are often quite large (10 to 20 cm) and typically bilateral (40% to 60%). A simple cyst is defined by four sonographic criteria: It is anechoic; has a smooth, well defined, thin wall; has enhanced through transmission; and is unilocular. Bleeding into a cyst causes homogeneous, low-level echoes,

Figure 16.11. Axial T2-weighted image of normal ovaries *(curved arrows)* in a premenopausal woman. The ovarian follicles are hyperintense to fat and the ovarian stroma. The right ovary is normal in size, and only a portion of the left ovary is seen on this image.

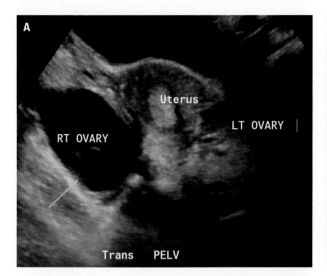 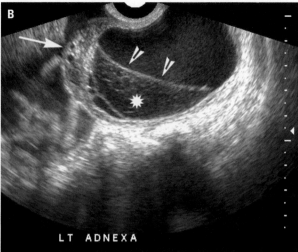

Figure 16.12. Hemorrhagic ovarian cyst. **A:** Transabdominal sonogram in transverse view reveals a large hemorrhagic cyst in the right ovary *(arrow)* in this 26-year-old, with 2 days of right-sided pelvic pain. **B:** Transvaginal transverse sonogram in a 34-year-old female with acute onset of left adnexal pain. Note the complex appearance to the hemorrhage, with small crescent of normal ovarian tissue at the margin *(arrow)*, the thick septation *(arrowheads)*, and the more complex echogenic fluid or clot *(asterisk)* in one of the compartments consistent with the different stages of evolving hematoma.

and the characteristic "snowstorm" or "spider's web" appearance (Fig. 16.12). It must be noted, however, that endometriomas may also frequently present with this sonographic appearance or may be more homogeneous in echo texture (Fig. 16.13). Hemorrhagic cysts can also have these thicker septations or loculations.

If a cyst contains mural nodules or papillary projections, thick walls, or solid echogenic foci, a neoplasm must be considered a strong possibility. Coarse calcifications or multiple strongly echogenic foci in an ovarian mass suggest a dermoid, as do echogenic, irregular foci superimposed on a low-level, homogeneously echogenic background. However, these calcifications should not be confused with the more common finding of multiple peripheral, tiny echogenic foci present in the ovaries (up to 37%), which most likely represent the echogenic walls of superficial epithelial inclusion cysts, which are too small to resolve at US (Fig. 16.14).

Most ovarian tumors are not acutely symptomatic until they enlarge enough to compress or displace adjacent structures (bladder, rectum, intestines), allow for ovarian torsion, or metastasize. Much interest has developed in attempting to differentiate benign from malignant ovarian masses with US, and most sonographic experts feel

that differentiation is possible in 80% to 90% of cases. Specific sonographic morphology, and not spectral or color Doppler blood flow analysis, is the predominant means for discrimination: More simple-appearing cysts tend to be benign, and the more complex or solid masses have a higher chance of malignancy. Of course, the presence of ascites should always heighten suspicion of ovarian malignancy, given the absence of a pelvic infection or ovarian torsion.

Ovarian Torsion

Ovarian torsion occurs most commonly in patients with a benign adnexal cyst or mass, which predisposes to twisting of the ovarian pedicle along its long axis. The usual clinical presentation is pelvic pain, nausea, vomiting, and/or fever. However, the diagnosis is often difficult, as the presentation is often atypical, both clinically and sonographically, and US remains the workhorse imaging modality. It often allows for differentiation of the other entities in the differential, from acute appendicitis, ovarian cyst or rupture, to PID. Most often, ovarian torsion at sonography is depicted as a large cystic or complex cystic mass, often midline, with diminished blood

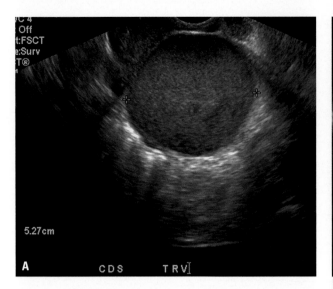

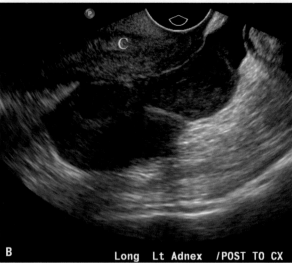

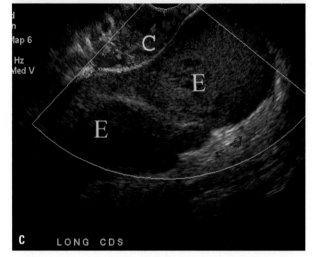

Figure 16.13. Endometrioma. **A:** Transverse transvaginal image of homogeneously low-level echogenic cystic mass *(electronic calipers)* in the cul-de-sac, proven to be endometriosis at surgery in a 36-year-old woman. **B:** Transvaginal sagittal image of the cul-de-sac in same patient shows tubular endometrioma behind the cervix *(C)*. **C:** Color Doppler image in same orientation as Figure 16.13B shows the endometrioma *(arrows)* to be avascular in nature, consistent with old hemorrhage. *E*, endometrium; *C*, cervix.

Figure 16.14. Transvaginal image of an ovary in a 43-year-old infertility patient. Multiple small echogenic foci *(arrows)* seen representing the bright walls of tiny cysts that are too small to be visualized, superficial inclusion cysts.

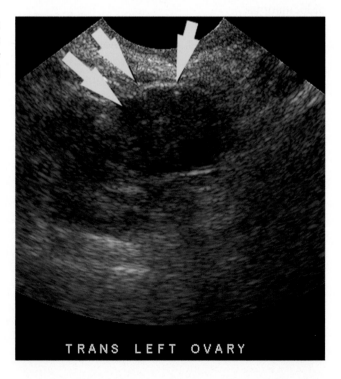

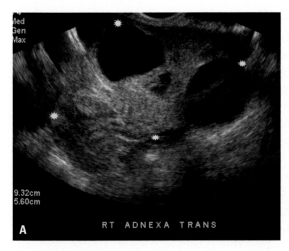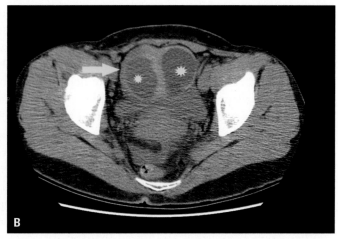

Figure 16.15. **A:** Transverse transvaginal US reveals a very large right ovary in a 41-year-old woman with acute onset of pelvic pain, with several moderate sized cysts, between *yellow asterisks.* Ovary volume was approximately 150 mL (normal 10 to 18 mL). **B:** CT in same patient shows a loculated cystic *(asterisks)* mass *(arrow)* in midline, anterior to uterus, representing a torsed ovary, in this case originating from the right side. Surgically proven torsion.

flow (Fig. 16.15). The differential diagnosis for torsion includes causes of complex cystic adnexal masses: Ectopic pregnancy, TOA, endometrioma, or teratoma (Fig. 16.16). In theory, torsion should result in decreased blood flow to the ovary, but because the ovary has a dual blood supply, the results on color flow Doppler sonography are variable. The chronicity and completeness of the torsion are also factors in the sonographic appearance, with some cases of intermittent torsion-detorsion (ITD) being very problematic to diagnose, depending on which part of the ITD cycle the patient is in when examined with US. According to Vijayaraghan and Fleischer, a positive whirlpool sign in the twisted vascular pedicle of the ovary is the most definitive sign of ovarian torsion. Absence of blood flow in the twisted pedicle

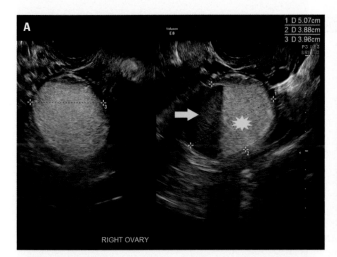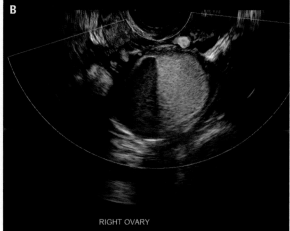

Figure 16.16. Ovarian teratoma. **A:** A transverse (**left side of image**) and longitudinal (**right side**) image of a teratoma in a 46-year-old asymptomatic woman. The two contrasting echogenicities are nonspecific, with fluid-filled levels, probably representing sebaceous material in the brighter layer *(asterisk)*, and more serous fluid in the darker layer *(arrow)*. This could also represent a hemorrhagic cyst or endometrioma, but it is unchanged more than 2 years, which is atypical for heme products. **B:** Color Doppler image shows no blood flow to this lesion, as is typical for teratomas.

and visualization of the flow in the artery alone are predictive of nonviability of the ovary.

One study evaluated 20 patients with surgically proven ovarian torsion. Sonographic findings varied with age: Prepubertal girls usually demonstrated large, extrapelvic cystic, or complex cystic masses, whereas pubertal females most often had a solid adnexal mass. Color Doppler flow was variable and did not correlate with morphology or age of patient. Other authors report that if torsion is complete, venous blood flow will be absent with preservation of abnormal arterial flow (high-resistive index or low-peak systolic flow) (Fig. 16.17). In another study, Fleischer et al. showed that specific signs on color Doppler US were predictive of ovarian viability: Lack of central venous ovarian flow represented infarction of the ovary, and the presence of venous flow indicated an ovary that was salvageable. However, a more recent study of 10 surgically proven cases of ovarian torsion with color Doppler analysis reported that color flow was normal in 60%. They showed that when color Doppler blood flow is abnormal, the time to diagnosis is less and the hospital stay significantly shortened. In ovulation induction (OI) patients, however, the sensitivity fell to 25% for abnormal color Doppler flow. In this population, it seems, abnormal color Doppler US is even less accurate and caution is undertaken when evaluating this subset of patients in the emergent setting.

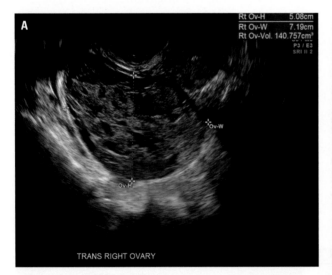

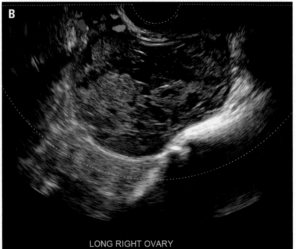

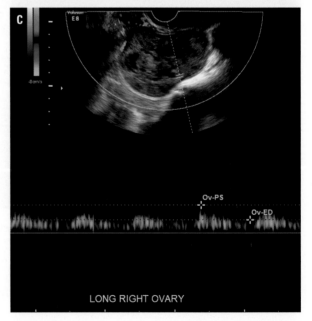

Figure 16.17. A: Transvaginal transverse view shows an enlarged right ovary *(electronic calipers)* in this young woman who presents with 3 days of right-sided, acute pelvic pain. Gray scale US reveals a very enlarged ovary measuring 140 mL. **B:** Color Doppler image shows a paucity of blood flow to the affected ovary. **C:** Spectral Doppler reveals a scant amount of arterial flow, but no venous flow was documented despite extensive Doppler interrogation. Surgery revealed intermittent torsion-detorsion scenario.

Pelvic Inflammatory Disease

PID is diagnosed clinically and with positive cultures in most patients without requiring imaging. US or, less often, CT is important in medically refractory or complicated cases. PID is a disease predominantly seen in the young, sexually active female who is infected with common sexually transmitted pathogens (*Chlamydia* and gonococcus most commonly), initially infecting the cervix and uterus and then propagating proximally to fallopian tubes and ovaries. Clinically, the patients may have few or no symptoms, yet the sonographic findings may be striking or vice versa. Patients with TOA often have fewer signs of acute illness than those without TOA.[16] On US, the characteristic finding of PID is a dilated, thick-walled tubular structure with incomplete septa (characteristic mucosal folds) containing internal echoes in the adnexa (pyosalpinx), or a thickened, echogenic tubular structure in the adnexal region (Fig. 16.18). In the subacute or chronic stage of disease, one may

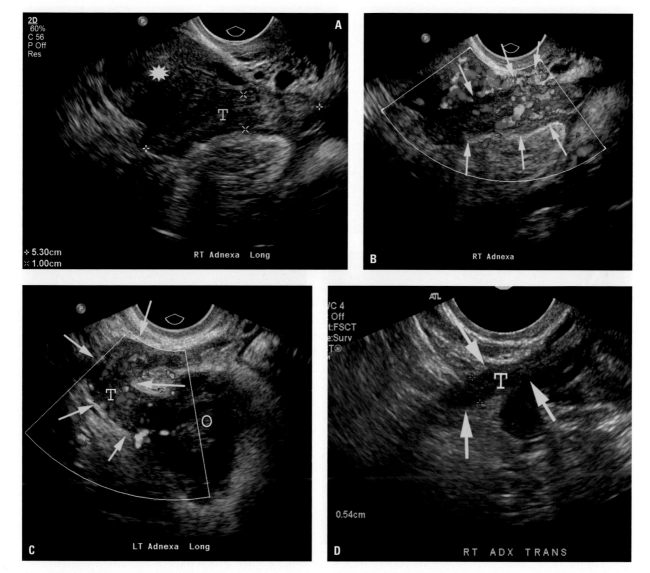

Figure 16.18. PID with bilateral salpingitis. **A:** Sagittal view of the right adnexa in a 27-year-old woman with 8 days of crampy pelvic pain. Note thick-walled, echogenic right fallopian tube *(T)*. Portion of uterus *(asterisk)* seen. PID, pelvic inflammatory disease. **B:** Color Doppler image of same tube shows marked hyperemia *(arrows)* indicating acute inflammation. **C:** Color Doppler longitudinal image of left tube and ovary shows hyperemic *(arrows)*, thickened tube *(T)* and adjacent ovary *(O)*. **D:** After 5 weeks of medical therapy, the image of the right adnexal region in transverse plane reveals marked improvement in the right fallopian tube *(T)*, *between arrows*. Note the decreased width of more normal tube.

encounter a hydrosalpinx (a thin-walled tubular structure without internal echoes) or a "string of beads" sign. A thicker wall correlates well with more acute disease.[17] Bilateral adnexal involvement is common with PID. If left untreated, the infection often extends to ovaries and paraovarian tissues as a large cystic or complex cystic mass—the TOA (Fig. 16.19). In a recent study of 25 cases of surgically proven TOA, 23 had an adnexal mass of 5 to 10 cm and most consisted of complex cystic and solid components. Exuberant color Doppler flow was shown in the borders and septa of the masses, contrasting this entity from ovarian torsion. An adequate clinical or sexual history also usually allows one to differentiate between these two entities. Other pathology included in

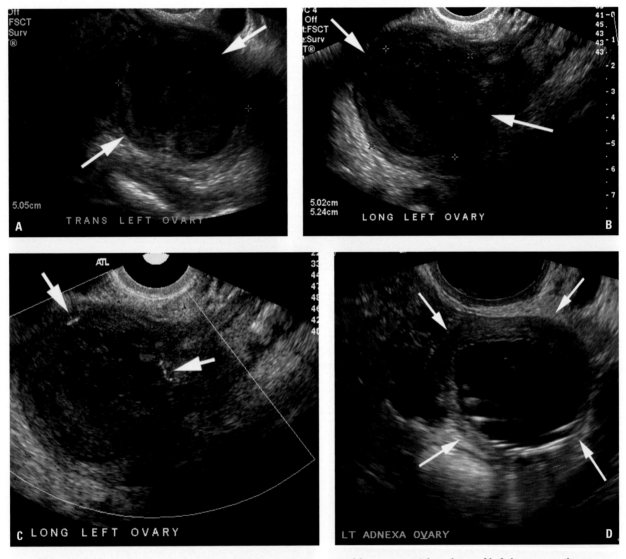

Figure 16.19. Tubo-ovarian abscess (TOA). **A:** A 42-year-old woman with 4 days of left lower quadrant pain, diarrhea, and fever. The transverse transvaginal image shows a moderate, mixed echogenic mass in the left ovary (*arrows*). **B:** Longitudinal image of the left ovary shows an enlarged, heterogeneous mass (*arrows*) with differential diagnosis of TOA, endometrioma, hemorrhagic cyst, or teratoma. **C:** Longitudinal color Doppler image of left ovary reveals mildly increase blood flow at periphery of abscess (*arrows*) but no central flow. **D:** After appropriate antibiotic therapy, the TOA has evolved into a more complex cystic mass (*arrows*).

the differential diagnosis, with a negative urine or serum hCG, are ovarian cystic neoplasms, endometrioma, appendiceal mucocele, and periovarian fluid collections.

OBSTETRIC EMERGENCIES

Obstetric emergencies are life-threatening conditions that occur during pregnancy and are unique in that the goal of treatment is to obtain the best outcome for two patients—the fetus and the mother. Fetal well-being is dependent on maternal well-being, and optimizing maternal care usually ensures the best outcome for the fetus. Imaging is constrained by the need to minimize ionizing radiation. Fortunately, US uses nonionizing radiation and is virtually without risk to fetus or mother. Ultrasound may theoretically cause thermal or mechanical injury to the fetus and therefore should be kept to a minimum. At this time there is no clinical evidence of fetal injury from diagnostic

ultrasound. MRI also uses nonionizing radiation and may be used in stable patients, particularly to better visualize abnormalities of the placenta.

Normal Early Pregnancy

The sonographic landmarks for a normal early intrauterine pregnancy (IUP) have been well established for both transabdominal and TV technique. TV sonography (TVUS) is more sensitive for findings of IUP in the first trimester. The first sign of an IUP that can be seen by TVUS is the gestational sac, occurring approximately 4.5 weeks after the last menstrual period (LMP). The gestational sac is a round or oval fluid-filled cavity with surrounding echogenic, decidualized endometrium that is eccentrically positioned within the uterine cavity. A gestational sac as small as 2 to 3 mm can frequently be seen as the first sign of an IUP (Fig. 16.20A). However, endometrial edema (pseudogestational sac) or decidual cysts

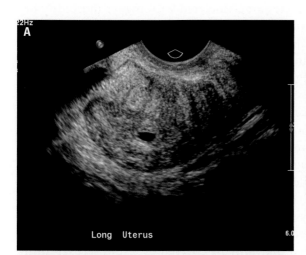

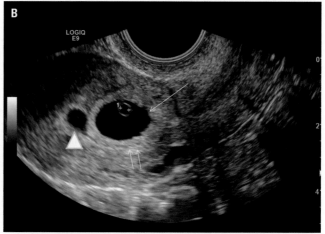

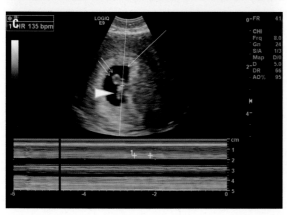

Figure 16.20. A: Sagittal TVUS image: Early intrauterine pregnancy of 4.5 weeks gestational age with 4 mm gestational sac in the endometrial cavity. **B:** Sagittal TVUS of uterus: Early IUP at 5.5 weeks gestational age showing a yolk sac *(calipers)* within the gestational sac *(arrow)* that is eccentrically positioned within the endometrial cavity. There is surrounding echogenic decidual reaction *(double arrow)* and a small, likely physiologic subchorionic hematoma *(arrowhead)* of doubtful clinical significance. **C:** Early IUP, 7 weeks gestational age showing gestational sac *(arrow)*, yolk sac *(double arrow)*, and embryo *(arrowhead)* with embryonic cardiac activity at a rate of 135 bpm.

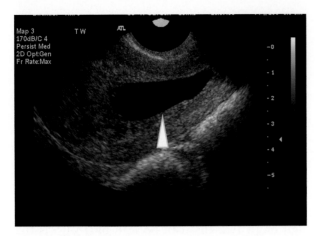

Figure 16.21. "Pseudogestational sac." TVUS longitudinal image through uterus demonstrates fluid collecting centrally within the endometrial canal *(arrowhead)* due to endometrial edema in the setting of an ectopic pregnancy. The central rather than eccentric position of the fluid collection and the lack of a strong echogenic decidual reaction are signs of an ectopic pregnancy.

secondary to an ectopic pregnancy may appear similar to a gestational sac (Fig. 16.21). Therefore, the first reliable sign of an IUP is the yolk sac, which should be visible by TVUS when the gestational sac reaches a mean sac diameter of 8 mm at approximately 5 to 5.5 weeks (Fig. 16.20B). A yolk sac is a cystic echogenic structure within the gestational sac, and a yolk sac that is abnormal in size or appearance may be a very early sign of an abnormal pregnancy (Fig. 16.22). When the gesta-

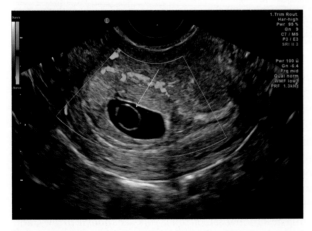

Figure 16.22. Abnormally enlarged yolk sac *(arrow)* measuring greater than 5 mm in diameter associated with early demise.

tional sac reaches a mean sac diameter of 16 mm by TVUS, an embryo should be seen, and once the embryo is 5 mm in length, there should be embryonic cardiac activity (Fig. 16.20C). Normal embryonic heart rates should be above 100 beats per minute (bpm) after 6 weeks gestational age, and if less than 90 bpm, follow-up US is recommended to ensure a viable pregnancy.

Ectopic Pregnancy

Ruptured ectopic pregnancy is a significant cause of obstetric morbidity and mortality and is the cause of 10% to 15% of all maternal deaths. Approximately 1% to 2% of all pregnancies are ectopic in location. The most common location for ectopic pregnancy is in the fallopian tube, occurring in 95% to 97% of cases. Most tubal ectopic pregnancies occur in the ampullary portion of the tube, whereas the interstitial or uterine portion of the fallopian tube is the least common site of a tubal ectopic. Interstitial ectopic pregnancies are associated with higher morbidity because the interstitial segment of the fallopian tube dilates more readily and accommodates a larger embryo before presenting with pain and bleeding (Fig. 16.23C). Uncommon locations for ectopic pregnancy include the cervix, cesarean section scar, ovary, and abdominal cavity. Cervical ectopic implantation is rare; however, cervical ectopics are associated with higher risk of severe bleeding because the cervix does not contain contractile tissue to control hemorrhage (Fig. 16.23D). Cesarean section scar ectopic pregnancies are associated with increased risk of uterine rupture because the pregnancy implants into scar tissue that may only be covered by a thin serosal lining without intervening myometrium.

Risk factors for ectopic pregnancy include a history of PID or pelvic surgery, IUD, and assisted reproduction (thought in part to be related to altered tubal motility secondary to hormones). The classic clinical triad of patients with ectopic pregnancy is pelvic pain, vaginal bleeding, and palpable adnexal mass. However, this is only present in about 30% of patients. The most common presenting symptom is pelvic pain, often without associated bleeding. Therefore, any pregnant patient with pelvic pain should be evaluated for an ectopic pregnancy.

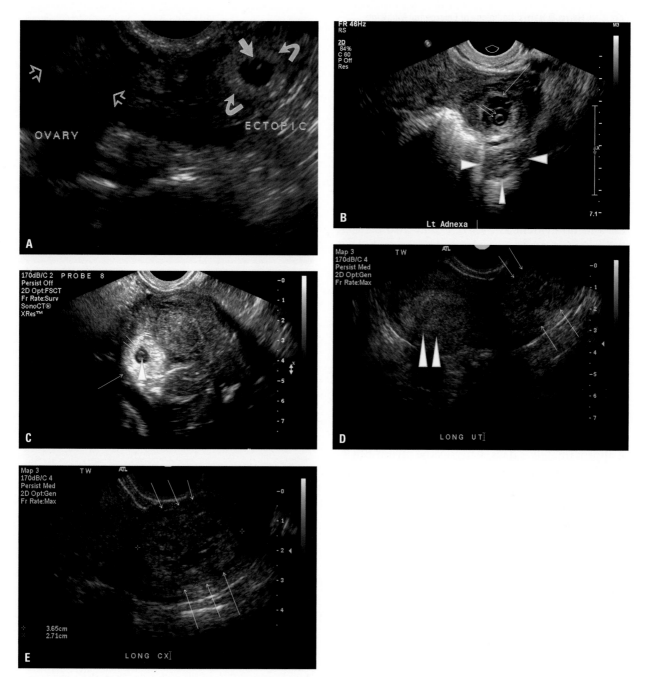

Figure 16.23 **A:** Ectopic pregnancy. Transvaginal sagittal view of the right adnexa demonstrates an ectopic gestational sac *(curved arrows)* containing a yolk sac *(straight arrow)* in the fallopian tube. Right ovary is seen to the left of the image *(open arrows)*. This ectopic pregnancy was treated successfully with methotrexate. **B:** Tubal ectopic. TVUS transverse image through left adnexa showing classic tubal ectopic pregnancy with extrauterine complex cystic mass containing gestational sac *(arrow)* and yolk sac *(double arrow)* in the left adnexa adjacent to the left ovary *(arrowheads)*. Note that the echogenic rim of the tubal ectopic is more echogenic than the adjacent ovarian parenchyma. **C:** Interstitial ectopic. TVUS transverse image through upper uterine fundus shows echogenic ring *(arrow)*, gestational sac *(double arrow)*, and yolk sac *(arrowhead)* of ectopic pregnancy within the interstitial portion of the fallopian tube. Sonographic signs of an interstitial ectopic implantation seen in this case include extremely eccentric location of gestational sac within the uterus and lack of discrete rim of myometrium around the early pregnancy. Patient presented with marked hemoperitoneum but was discharged home in stable condition after treatment. **D:** Cervical ectopic. Longitudinal TVUS image through the uterus demonstrates no evidence of a gestational sac or early IUP in the upper uterus where only echogenic endometrium is seen *(arrowheads)*. There is a complex mass within the cervical canal that represents ectopic cervical implantation *(arrows)*. **E:** Cervical ectopic pregnancy. TVUS longitudinal image through cervical canal shows complex cystic mass *(arrows)* consistent with cervical ectopic.

The classic sonographic appearance of an ectopic pregnancy is an empty uterine cavity with an extrauterine gestational sac containing a yolk sac or embryo (Fig. 16.23A). This classic appearance is seen in approximately 30% of cases. When there is no discrete intrauterine or extrauterine pregnancy in a patient with a positive pregnancy test, there is significant concern for an ectopic pregnancy that cannot be directly visualized sonographically. Nonetheless, a patient with a positive pregnancy test and no evidence of an IUP may also be seen in the setting of a miscarriage or a very early IUP that is not yet visible by US. Sonographic findings must therefore be correlated with a quantitative serum B-hCG. When the B-hCG is above the discriminatory level of 1,500 to 2,000 mIU, a gestational sac should be seen within the uterus. This discriminatory level should be used with caution, as studies have demonstrated that up to 30% of patients with BhCG above the threshold level and without evidence of an IUP have been shown to progress to normal IUP on a follow-up US. In a normal pregnancy, the BhCG has a doubling time of approximately 2 days, whereas the serum BhCG doubles more slowly in an ectopic pregnancy. Therefore, if a patient is clinically stable, it is possible to follow the pregnancy with serial BhCG and a repeat US in several days.

The presence of an IUP significantly decreases the possibility of an ectopic pregnancy as the incidence of a heterotopic pregnancy (both an intrauterine and extrauterine pregnancy) is 1 per 3,000 to 1 per 8,000. This, however, is not the case in patients who have undergone assisted reproduction, in whom the risk of a heterotopic pregnancy is approximately 1 per 100. Therefore, in this group of patients with a higher pretest clinical probability of heterotopic pregnancy, a careful sonographic evaluation for an ectopic pregnancy is necessary even in the presence of an IUP.

An ectopic pregnancy is most commonly visualized as a complex adnexal mass with variable morphology ranging from complex cystic to solid. The appearance of an echogenic tubal ring that is separate from the ovary is seen in approximately 70% to 80% of ectopic pregnancies. There is associated marked peripheral vascularity due to trophoblastic tissue seen by Doppler US and referred to as the "ring of fire" (Fig. 16.24). A tubal ectopic pregnancy is often adjacent to the ovary, and it may be difficult to differentiate

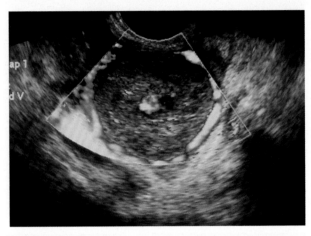

Figure 16.24. "Ring of fire" appearance in an ectopic pregnancy. Power Doppler image demonstrates the prominent peripheral vascularity and relatively hypovascular central portion. This mass, which appeared solid and separate from the right ovary, is to be distinguished from a hemorrhagic corpus luteal cyst, which has similar color Doppler features but is located within the ovary.

an exophytic intraovarian corpus luteum with marked peripheral flow from an extraovarian ectopic pregnancy. Doppler studies have not been shown to reliably discriminate the mural flow of a corpus luteum from the peripheral vascularity of an ectopic pregnancy. However, the echogenicity of the rim of an ectopic pregnancy can be a discriminating feature, as several studies have shown that the echogenic rim of the tubal ectopic is likely to be more echogenic than the adjacent ovarian parenchyma (Fig. 16.23D) and more echogenic than the rim of the corpus luteum. A recent study has also shown that the echogenic tubal ring of an ectopic pregnancy is more echogenic than the endometrium in 32% of cases, and this feature was not present in any of the corpora lutea in the study.

Complex free fluid in the pelvis is a strong predictor of ectopic pregnancy, usually representing hemoperitoneum secondary to rupture. Echogenic free fluid may be the only finding in a patient with an ectopic pregnancy and may obscure the adnexal mass. Echogenic free fluid, even if present as an isolated finding in a patient with a positive BhCG, has a positive predictive value (PPV) for ectopic pregnancy of nearly 90% (Fig. 16.24).

Placenta Previa

Placenta previa is the abnormal implantation of placental tissue in the lower uterine segment that partially or completely covers the internal os of the cervix. It occurs in 0.5% of pregnancies and risk factors include prior cesarean section where scarring may prevent normal placental remodeling, advanced maternal age, and smoking. Placenta previa is classified as complete when the internal os is completely covered by placental tissue, marginal when the placental edge is at the margin of the cervix, and low lying when the placental edge is within 2 cm of the cervical os (Fig. 16.25).

The relationship of the placenta to the cervix changes throughout pregnancy, and approximately 90% of cases seen in the second trimester will convert to a normal location in the third trimester. This conversion is usually seen with low lying and marginal placenta previa. The remodeling of the placenta is likely due to a combination of rapid growth of the lower uterine segment in the third trimester and preferential growth of the placenta in the upper uterine segment, where there is better vascular perfusion. If placenta previa persists in the third trimester, cervical effacement and progressive thinning of the lower uterine segment can rupture placental vessels and can cause maternal hemorrhage and fetal decompensation. Placenta previa usually presents with painless vaginal bleeding in the third trimester and is the most common cause of bleeding throughout pregnancy.

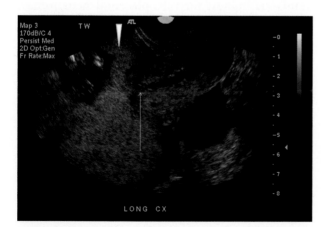

Figure 16.25. Complete placenta previa. TVUS longitudinal image through cervix shows extension of echogenic posterior placenta *(arrowhead)* completely covering the internal cervical os *(arrow)*.

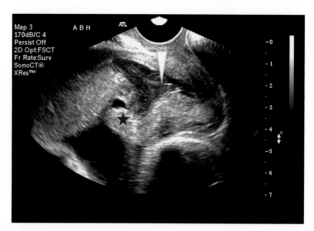

Figure 16.26. Marginal placenta previa with subchorionic hematoma. Patient presented with vaginal bleeding in the third trimester. TVUS longitudinal image through a shortened cervix with funneling of the internal os. There is extension of an anterior placenta *(arrow)* over the anterior cervix with associated hypoechoic subchorionic hematoma *(arrowhead)* beneath the marginal previa and filling the dilated upper cervical canal. The placental edge abuts the internal os but does not cover the posterior margin of the cervix *(star)*. TVUS, transvaginal ultrasound.

Sonographically, placenta previa is seen as echogenic placental tissue approaching or covering the cervical os (Fig. 16.26). When the patient presents with bleeding, US may show a hematoma between the placenta and the underlying cervix (Fig. 16.27). Alternatively, an echogenic subchorionic hematoma adjacent to the placental edge may be mistaken for placental tissue and thought to represent placenta previa. Unlike the vascular placenta, a hematoma should not have any evidence of internal vascularity. The position of the placenta is assessed in all transabdominal second trimester screening exams, and if there is concern for lowlying placenta, a TVUS should be obtained, as it has been shown to be more specific in the diagnosis of placenta previa.

Placenta Accreta

Placenta previa and history of cesarean section are associated with increased risk for placenta accreta spectrum. Placenta accreta, increta, and percreta refer to abnormal implantation of the placenta onto the uterine myometrium, invasion through the

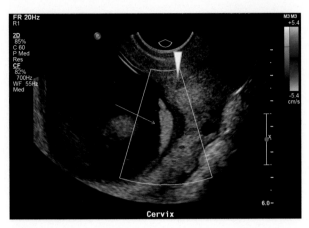

Figure 16.27. A and B: Amniotic clot secondary to previous subchorionic hemorrhage. TVUS longitudinal (**A**) and transverse (**B**) images through the lower uterine segment and cervix show echogenic material *(arrow)* overlying the internal os *(arrowhead)*. Doppler interrogation did not reveal any evidence of internal vascularity. Real-time evaluation showed the clot to be mobile and variable in contour. Therefore, this is not consistent with placenta previa. Patient had a previous large subchorionic hemorrhage, which dissected through the chorion and amnion to enter the amniotic cavity.

myometrium, and invasion beyond the uterine serosa, respectively. The prevalence of placenta accreta is 10 times higher than it was 50 years ago due to the increasing rate of cesarean section delivery. Placental lacunae are one of the most sensitive signs for placenta accreta consisting of irregularly shaped anechoic vascular spaces within the placenta that show turbulent flow on Doppler imaging. There may be absence of the normal hypoechoic retroplacental space; however, this finding is seen with some frequency in normal patients and, as an isolated finding, is not reliable. MRI may be used to confirm the diagnosis if US is equivocal. MRI may show focal interruptions of the myometrial signal and may show placental invasion of adjacent structures such as the bladder (Fig. 16.28).

Placental Hematoma and Abruption

Placental hematomas may be classified as subchorionic, retroplacental, and rarely, preplacental in location. They occur on the fetal (subchorionic and preplacental) or maternal (retroplacental) side of the placenta. The clinical significance of placental hematomas is variable and related to location,

gestational age at the time of diagnosis, symptoms, and size of the hematoma. Differences in outcome are likely due to different underlying mechanisms for the placental hemorrhage. The most common etiologies are felt to be vascular and inflammatory in nature. Underlying vascular disease leading to placental hemorrhage may have a similar pathophysiology to preeclampsia in which there is defective trophoblast invasion and incomplete transformation of the maternal spiral arteries from high-resistance uterine spiral arteries to low-resistance uteroplacental arteries. The increased resistance of the decidual arteries seen in hypertensive conditions, such as preeclampsia, likely predisposes the vessels to rupture and hemorrhage.

Subchorionic hematomas are the most common location of placental hemorrhage accounting for approximately 80% of all placental hematomas and are more commonly seen before 20 weeks. Subchorionic hematomas are associated with preterm delivery and adverse outcome if they are diagnosed at an early gestational age and are very large in size, greater than 50% the size of the gestational sac (Fig. 16.29). They almost always involve the margin of the placenta and are usually due to a venous bleed. Blood dissects between the chorion and the placenta in a collection that is usually crescentic in shape reflecting the low pressure, venous nature of the bleed. The collection may be contiguous with the marginal origin of the bleed or may be seen some distance from the placental margin (Fig. 16.30).

Retroplacental hematomas represent approximately 16% of all hematomas and are more commonly seen after 20 weeks. The frequency of fetal demise is highest for retroplacental hematomas. They are usually due to rupture of spiral arteries with blood collecting between the placenta and the underlying maternal decidua. They may be visualized as rounded collections beneath the placenta that exert mass effect on the overlying placenta reflecting the high pressure, arterial nature of the bleed.

Preplacental hematomas are quite rare. They may represent subchorionic hematomas that begin at the margin of the placenta and dissect between the placenta and chorionic membrane. Alternatively, preplacental bleeds may be subamniotic in location, occurring in the potential space between the amnion and chorion. When the hematoma is subamniotic in location, it is usually limited by the umbilical cord. Large subamniotic bleeds may compress the

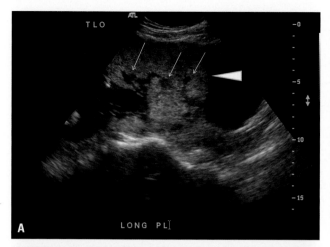

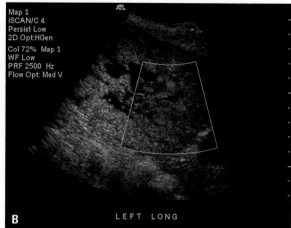

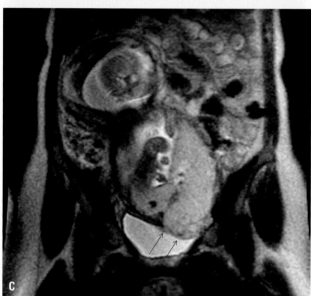

Figure 16.28. A: Placenta percreta. Longitudinal transabdominal ultrasound through the lower uterine segment at 22 weeks gestational age in a patient with a history of two previous cesarean sections. There is placenta previa and absence of the retroplacental complex between the lower uterine segment and the bladder wall *(arrowhead)*. There are multiple anechoic lacunae within the placenta *(arrows)*. **B:** Placenta percreta. Color Doppler ultrasound shows flow within multiple placental lacunae. **C:** Placenta percreta. Coronal T2-weighted MRI images obtained at 23 weeks gestational age confirms extension of anterior placenta into bladder with disruption of outer myometrium *(arrows)*. (From Elsevier, with permission.)

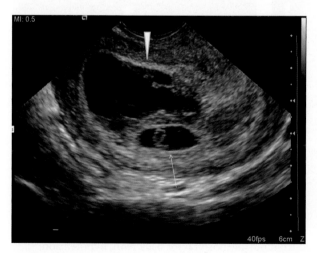

Figure 16.29. Large subchorionic hematoma at 5.5 weeks. The subchorionic hematoma *(arrowhead)* is at least twice the size of the gestational sac *(arrow)* containing a yolk sac. Although a large hematoma at this early gestational age can be associated with an adverse outcome, this patient had a normal term delivery and normal healthy neonate.

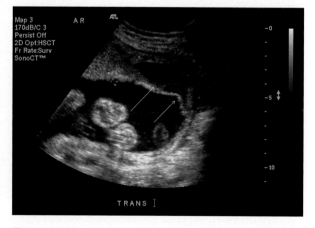

Figure 16.30. Subchorionic hematoma. Transabdominal transverse ultrasound image at 18 weeks gestational age shows a crescentic hypoechoic collection at the margin of the placenta *(arrows)*. Patient was not symptomatic, and this was an incidental finding during a second trimester screening ultrasound.

adjacent umbilical cord and vessels, thereby compromising fetal oxygenation. There is felt to be some association between short umbilical cords and subamniotic bleeds thought to be related to high tension on the shortened cord with fetal movement.

Placental abruption is a subset of placental hematomas defined as a symptomatic premature separation of a normally implanted placenta from the uterine wall after 20 weeks gestational age. Symptoms include vaginal bleeding and a painful tense uterus due to uterine contractions. Abruption occurs in 1% of all pregnancies and is one of the most serious complications of pregnancy. Placental abruption accounts for 10% to 25% of all perinatal deaths and may cause life-threatening maternal hemorrhage and associated coagulopathy. Abruption is usually caused by rupture of the decidual spiral arteries presenting as a retroplacental hemorrhage. However, abruption may also appear as a hematoma at the placental margin, known as a marginal abruption, or may dissect below the chorionic membrane to collect at a site distant to the origin of the bleed.

Bleeding occurs when retroplacental blood ruptures through the margins of the placenta and into the cervical canal. This occurs in 60% to 80% of cases, although in the remainder of cases, the blood does not egress through the cervix but remains contained in the placental membranes. These so-called concealed hematomas may be associated with significant mass effect compressing the adjacent placental vessels and compromising fetal circulation, possibly leading to fetal demise. Concealed hematomas may also be seen in patients who present in shock with severe fetal distress but without any vaginal bleeding. In these patients, circulatory collapse is due to contained hemorrhage and superimposed disseminated intravascular coagulation (DIC) secondary to thromboplastin released from the sequestered hematoma that triggers the maternal clotting cascade (Fig. 16.31).

At this time, sonography is the only practical method for evaluating acute abruption, although MRI has been studied in this setting and may become a valuable tool in a subset of stable patients as a predictor of outcome. Unfortunately, sonographic findings are present only 25% to 50% of the time and therefore should not be relied on for diagnosis or management. Of some concern is a study suggesting that abruptions associated with positive US findings have worse outcomes, and there is speculation that this may be due to more aggressive management when abruption is confirmed sonographically.

The sonographic appearance of placental hemorrhage is variable depending on location and age.

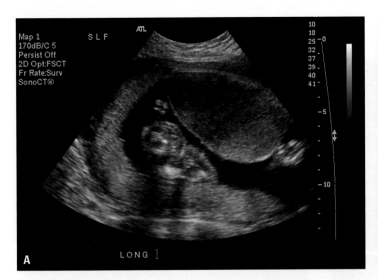
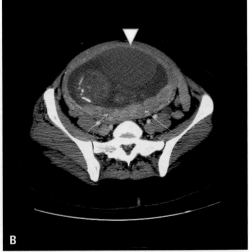

Figure 16.31. A: Placental abruption. Patient transferred from outside hospital for back pain, hypotension, and decreased hematocrit at 22 weeks gestational age. In transit, patient was in shock and was transfused six units of red blood cells. Transabdominal ultrasound obtained on admission showed 10 × 10 cm marginal contained subchorionic hematoma. No vaginal bleeding. Normal fetal biophysical profile and umbilical artery Doppler. **B:** CT obtained after ultrasound to exclude additional source of bleeding. CT shows marginal abruption (*arrowhead*) that was seen on US anteriorly and placenta (*arrows*) posteriorly without evidence for additional bleeding source. Patient was discharged home in stable condition and lost to follow-up.

Acute hemorrhage is more likely to be echogenic relative to the placenta, becoming isoechoic in the subacute phase at 3 to 7 days, and then hypoechoic to anechoic after 1 to 2 weeks (Fig. 16.32). It may not be possible to differentiate an isoechoic hematoma from the adjacent placenta, and the only sign of hemorrhage in this setting may be an apparently enlarged placenta measuring greater than 5.5 cm in thickness (Fig. 16.32A). It is important to differentiate a retroplacental collection secondary to hemorrhage from the normal hypoechoic retroplacental complex, uterine fibroids, or focal myometrial contractions. Hematomas do not have internal blood flow, whereas there should be Doppler signal in the veins of the retroplacental complex, and some flow is usually seen within a fibroid. Uterine contractions should resolve over time.

A recent study has shown MRI to have an extremely high sensitivity of 100% for the diagnosis of placental abruption with T1 and diffusion-weighted sequences shown to be most accurate for identification of placental hematoma. In patients who are hemodynamically stable, MRI may better delineate the extent of hemorrhage and allow larger hematomas to be monitored more closely.

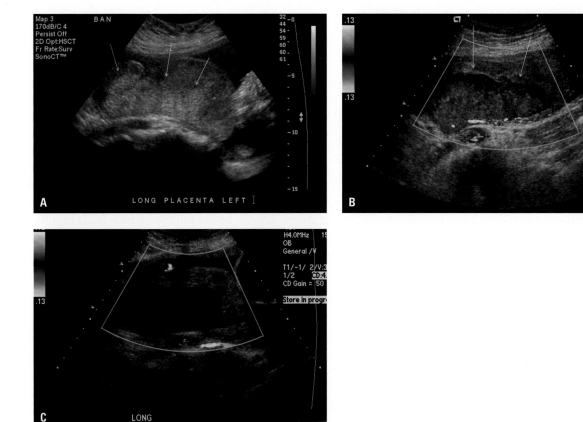

Figure 16.32. A: Abruption secondary to retroperitoneal hematoma. Patient referred from outside institution for poor growth at 24 weeks gestational age. Patient was hypertensive but no evidence of preeclampsia. Initial transabdominal ultrasound showed a thickened placenta measuring 6.5 cm. No discrete hematoma was seen, although in retrospect, there is a minimally more echogenic region of the posterior placenta *(arrows)* that was shown to be the site of the retroplacental hematoma on subsequent ultrasounds. Nonetheless, in this setting, a thickened placenta is highly suspicious for acute placental hematoma. **B:** Retroplacental abruption. Follow-up transabdominal ultrasound obtained at 25 weeks gestational age shows a discrete hypoechoic retroplacental hematoma *(arrows)* with expected progressive sonographic appearance. **C:** Retroplacental hematoma. Transabdominal ultrasound obtained later shows more anechoic appearance of the hematoma and no evidence of internal vascularity. No fetal growth over several weeks; abnormal umbilical artery Doppler and eventual nonreassuring fetal stress test led to delivery by cesarean section at 29 weeks gestational age.

Uterine Incarceration

Approximately 15% of women have a retroverted uterus; however, with pregnancy, the retroverted uterine fundus usually repositions into an anteverted location as it ascends into the abdomen with expansion of the developing fetus. If the gravid uterus remains retroverted after 16 weeks, the uterine fundus is lodged beneath the sacral promontory, and the uterus becomes trapped or incarcerated within the pelvis. The enlarging retroverted gravid uterus compresses and elongates the anterior cervix against the symphysis pubis. This may compress the urethra and bladder neck leading to bladder outlet obstruction. Most patients are asymptomatic; however, patients may present with abdominal pain, urinary retention, and gastrointestinal symptoms. If diagnosed before 20 weeks, it may be possible to reposition the uterus. After 20 weeks, patients are usually monitored for preterm labor and delivered by cesarean section.

This condition is rare, occurring in 1 in 3,000 pregnancies. Uterine incarceration may occur when the retroverted fundus is fixed within the pelvis due to adhesions from previous surgery or endometriosis. Uterine and pelvic malformations, fibroids, and pelvic tumors may also contribute to uterine incarceration. Complications of bladder atony or rupture, uterine rupture, and preterm labor may occur.

The diagnosis may be quite elusive by physical exam and imaging. Sonographically, the elongated, anteriorly displaced cervix is often misinterpreted as the anterior myometrium, and the posterior pregnancy may appear to be ectopic in location, possibly intra-abdominal. A fundal placenta will project inferiorly in the retroverted uterus, and therefore, may be mistaken for placenta previa. MRI is recommended to clarify the anatomy and may better demonstrate the elongated, anteriorly displaced cervix (Fig. 16.32).

Uterine Rupture

Uterine rupture is defined as separation of all layers of the uterine wall, including the serosa, with abnormal communication between the uterine cavity and the peritoneal cavity. More than 90% of cases of uterine rupture are associated with prior cesarean delivery due to weakening of the uterine wall at the site of the previous incision. This catastrophic condition may also be seen in the setting of previous myomectomy, uterine malformations, and in pregnant patients after major trauma.

Uterine rupture may have a variable clinical presentation ranging from vague symptoms, such as uterine tenderness and nonreassuring fetal heart rate, to acute maternal hypovolemic shock. US has been reported to inconsistently demonstrate the myometrial defect but can reveal the extrauterine location of the fetus and associated peritoneal hematoma. US can be done at the bedside fairly rapidly in this emergent condition. CT and MRI will show similar findings but will better delineate the site of rupture within the uterine wall (Fig. 16.33). Uterine dehiscence is defined as incomplete rupture of the

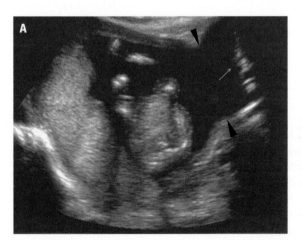 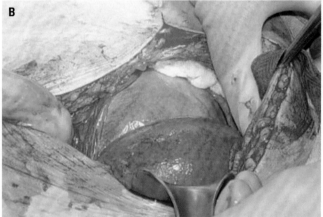

Figure 16.33. A: Uterine dehiscence. Transabdominal longitudinal ultrasound through the lower uterine segment demonstrates a large defect *(arrowheads)* in the anterior uterus through which the amniotic sac and cord *(arrow)* are protruding. Patient had a history of prior cesarean section. **B:** Uterine dehiscence. Amniotic sac protruding through uterine defect at the time of surgery. (From Fielding JR, Brown DL, Thurmond AS. *Gynecologic Imaging.* Philadelphia, PA: Elsevier Saunders; 2011, with permission.)

uterine wall involving endometrium and myometrium with an intact serosal layer. Ultrasound may show fetal parts and amniotic fluid extending beyond the margins of the uterus and contained by a thin serosal layer (Fig 16.33).

IMAGING OF SCROTAL EMERGENCIES

The scrotum is an intelligently designed sac to allow the crucial male reproductive apparatus to work well and vital endocrinologic tissues to be active at temperatures that are cooler than the body core. However, its superficial location and lack of protective organs/tissues render it extremely vulnerable to trauma, whereas the same characteristics lend themselves to unsurpassed imaging, especially with high-resolution US. US is paramount for the diagnosis of most scrotal pathology, especially in determining testicular viability after trauma or torsion, detecting infection of the epididymis and testis, and evaluating scrotal "lumps and bumps." Nuclear medicine, which historically had a major imaging role for the acute scrotum, has been relegated to a more limited role for evaluating testicular torsion in rare instances. Scrotal MRI infrequently serves as an adjunct to evaluating testicular rupture or for evaluation of possible subtle testicular tumors and will not be further discussed due to its very limited role in emergent scrotal imaging.

Preparation of the patient with scrotal symptoms in a quiet, dark room is important for a successful US exam. The testicles of an injured patient should be examined in a nonthreatening, relaxed environment as possible. Younger patients, especially, have considerable anxiety regarding their scrotum, injured or not, so multiple observers should be discouraged. The scrotum is draped on a rolled-up towel placed between the patient's adducted thighs, and warm gel is liberally applied over the scrotum (Fig. 16.34). The penis is elevated onto the abdominal wall and covered with a towel or drape so as not to interfere with the examination. A 7.5-to-12 MHz linear transducer is most appropriate, as it provides a large enough field of view to compare the two testes in dual mode, yet it provides the necessary fine resolution to detect subtle abnormalities. Sonography is performed in serial longitudinal and transverse images, with the asymptomatic side optimally examined first. The normal testis should serve as a reference for determining the optimal amount of gray scale and color gain and output: The gain is maximized by holding

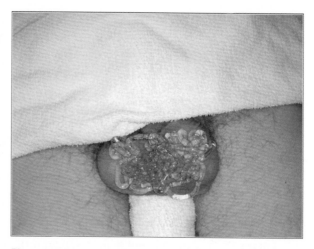

Figure 16.34. A simple technique proposed for scanning the scrotum. The penis is elevated and covered with a towel and a rolled-up towel placed between the adducted thighs. Copious gel is then applied to the scrotum to allow for high-resolution imaging, a form of "water bath," if you will that reduces poor contact imaging artifacts.

the transducer in the air until artifactual echoes are seen; the gain is then reduced to the setting, whereby the artifactual color signals disappear. The color Doppler velocity scale or pulse repetition frequency should be normally set at 5 to 10 cm per second, as most intraparenchymal flow is toward the lower end of the velocity range setting. Decreases in flow settings may need to be made in pediatric patients to maximize the low flow state frequently present while reducing any artifactual noise.

Normal Imaging Anatomy

The normal scrotum is composed of layers of skin, subcutaneous fat, and dartos fascia; the latter is continuous with the layers of superficial fascia in the groin and abdomen. The dartos fascia continues into a median raphe, which divides the scrotum into two compartments (hemiscrotum). These individual layers of connective tissue and skin are indistinguishable from each other with sonography but are often nonspecifically thickened in infection, inflammation, or torsion (Fig. 16.35).

The testis is an ovoid structure of homogeneous echogenicity, with the size varying with age. It is covered by a thick capsule of fibrous tissue, the tunica albuginea. This structure is not sonographically visible except in certain rare pathologic conditions. The accepted range of testicular volume (length × width × height × 0.52) is less than 2 cm³

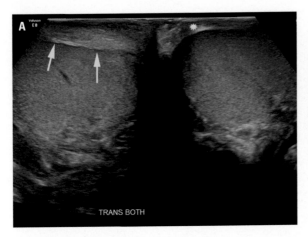
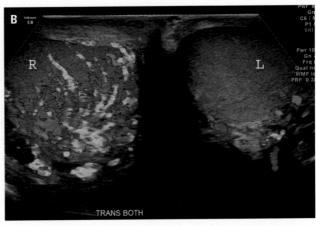

Figure 16.35. Skin thickening from scrotal inflammatory disease. **A:** A dual transverse image ("buddy image") of the testes and skin shows mild right hemiscrotal skin thickening *(arrows).* Note the thin skin around the left hemiscrotum *(asterisk).* **B:** Color Doppler buddy view, same patient, reveals the markedly hypervascular findings representing acute orchitis on the right side. *R,* right; *L,* left.

in boys younger than age 11, 2 to 10 cm³ in prepubertal boys, and 10 to 25 cm³ in young men and adults. The testis normally atrophies slowly after middle age.

The testicular mediastinum is an echogenic line that runs longitudinally in the posterolateral aspect of the testis (Fig. 16.36). This represents the conflu-

ence of the collecting tubules into an invagination of the tunica albuginea to form the rete testis, which in turn converge to form the efferent ductules that then coalesce into the proximal or head of the epididymis. The epididymis, isoechoic to slightly hyperechoic to the testis, is a convoluted, tubular structure that lies posterolateral to the testis and has

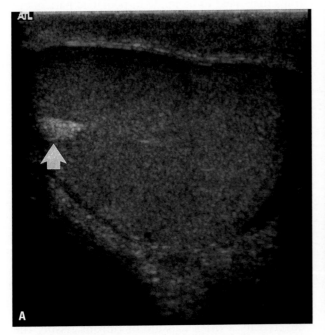
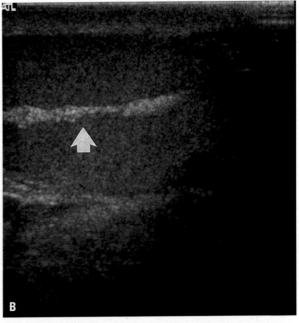

Figure 16.36. Normal mediastinum of the testis. **A:** Transverse sonogram of the right testis demonstrates a triangular echogenic area *(arrow)* in the posterolateral aspect; this represents the confluence of collecting tubules, which is slightly more echoic compared with the remaining testicular parenchyma. **B:** Sagittal view of the same testis shows the mediastinum *(arrow)* to be a longitudinal echogenic band.

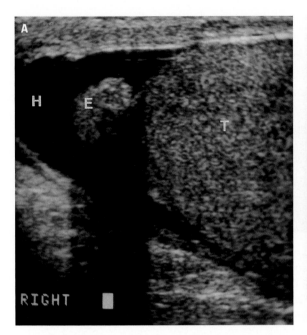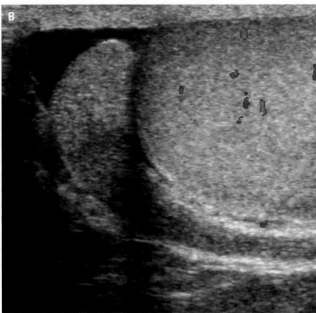

Figure 16.37. **A:** Longitudinal view of the normal head of the epididymis *(E)*. A small hydrocele *(H)* outlines the epididymis and the superior pole of the testis *(T)*. **B:** Normal color flow image of epididymis shows the relatively hypovascular nature of the epididymis, but this can be variable.

a superiorly positioned globular head (globus major) (Fig. 16.37), a narrow body (unless the patient has had a vasectomy), and a caudally placed tail (globus minor). From the epididymal tail, the vas deferens continues superiorly into the spermatic cord, along with the important arterial and venous supply of the testis (Fig. 16.38). Sonographic analysis of the spermatic cord is a recent phenomenon, which has generated much recent interest for the diagnosis of testicular/spermatic cord torsion.

The epididymis has a larger head (Fig. 16.39A) and a smaller body and tail; the latter two structures are

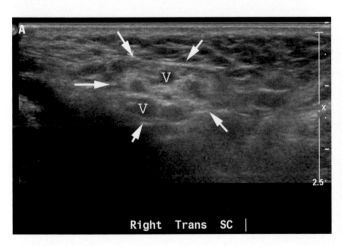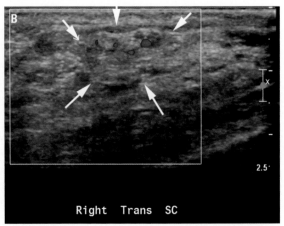

Figure 16.38. Spermatic cord normal sonographic appearance. **A:** Transverse view of the spermatic cord in the right supratesticular area shows several hypoechoic small dots that correspond to the vas and spermatic vessels *(V)*. A faintly hyperechoic, poorly defined fascia surrounds the spermatic cord *(arrows)*. **B:** Color Doppler transverse image of same structure shows some hypoechoic dots to represent vessels, and the thin fascia layer surrounding the cord is not well defined *(arrows)*.

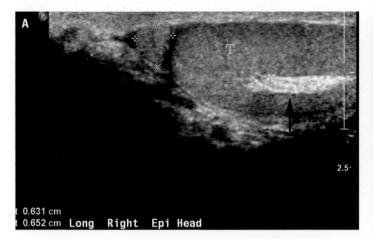
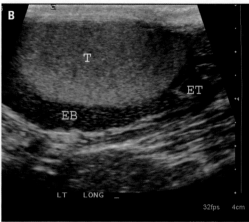

Figure 16.39. A: Normal epididymis. Note the rounded appearance of the normal epididymis *(electronic calipers)* in this 18-year-old referred for a palpable lesion (not in epididymis). The normal testis *(T)* is noted and mediastinum *(arrow)* is prominent but also normal. **B:** Thickened epididymis status post (S/P) vasectomy. Note the prominent body *(EB)* and tail *(ET)* of the "corrugated" appearing epididymis in this longitudinal image of the left testis *(T)* and epididymis. This is seen normally in up to 60% to 70% of postvasectomy patients referred for ultrasound.

not well demonstrated with US unless inflamed or enlarged or in postvasectomy patients (Fig. 16.39B). Epididymal cysts, also called spermatoceles, are quite common (in the head more often than the tail [Fig. 16.40]), are generally of no clinical significance, and result from the proposed blockage of the efferent ductules or the vas deferens. The blood supply is from the deferential artery, and newer equipment readily shows blood flow with color or power Doppler imaging in the head or tail.

The blood supply of the testis originates from three arteries: The testicular artery, which provides most of the parenchymal flow to the testis; the deferential artery, which perfuses the vas deferens and epididymis tail; and the cremasteric artery, which supplies branches to the tunica vaginalis. All three arteries have rich anastomoses over the tunica vaginalis and testis. The testicular artery gives rise to capsular arteries over the periphery of the testis, which in turn gives off centripetal branches that course toward the mediastinum in the fibrous septa between the seminiferous tubules (Fig. 16.41). These arteries may then branch into smaller centrifugal arteries that loop back to the periphery in the testicular parenchyma. Normal intratesticular blood flow is of low impedance (high diastolic flow) and low-peak systolic flow (5 to 10 cm per second). The testicular venous drainage is through the pampiniform plexus—an abundant supply of small venules

and veins that constitute a large portion of the spermatic cord.

Surrounding much of the testis is a fused sac, the tunica vaginalis, which constitutes a potential space, much like the pleura surrounding the lung. It

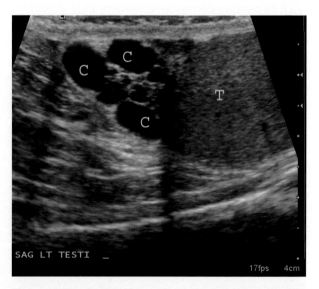

Figure 16.40. Epididymal cysts. Longitudinal image of left testis *(T)* and epididymal head shows multiple small epididymal cysts *(C)* or spermatoceles. These are most often of no clinical significance, although they often present with a painless scrotal mass, so may be clinically mistaken for a testicular neoplasm by anxious patients or providers.

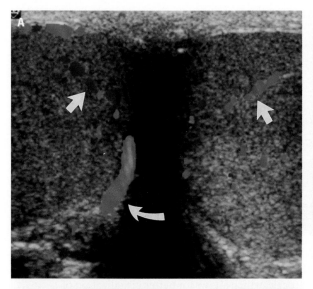

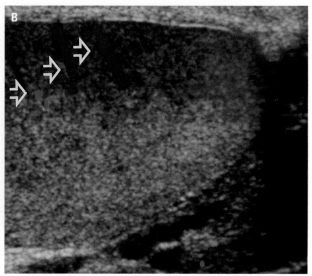

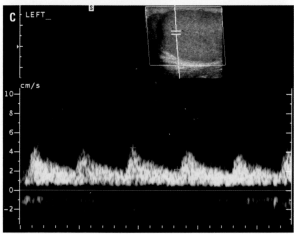

Figure 16.41. Normal testicular blood flow. **A:** Transverse color Doppler sonogram of both testes shows the normal capsular artery on the right *(curved arrow)* and prominent centripetal arteries bilaterally *(straight arrows)*. **B:** Sagittal ultrasound demonstrates the parallel orientation of the centripetal or mediastinal arteries *(open arrows)* in a normal testis. The amount of color flow present is normal, but this varies somewhat from patient to patient and should be relatively symmetrical in the same patient. **C:** Normal spectral Doppler of testicular centripetal artery shows low-velocity, low-resistance flow. The peak systolic flow is 4.3 cm per second.

is composed of parietal and visceral layers and normally leaves only a small "bare" area of the posterior testis uncovered. Adjacent to the superior pole of the testis are small extratesticular structures known as the testicular appendages (appendix testis and appendix epididymis), which are remnants of the embryologic Müllerian duct (Fig. 16.42). These are generally visible only in the setting of a significant hydrocele and will be discussed subsequently as a cause of acute scrotal pain.

The Painful, Nontraumatized Scrotum

Four conditions account for most scrotal pathology encountered in the emergency department: Testicular torsion, epididymo-orchitis (EO), testicular appendage torsion, and traumatic testicular rupture.

All four are characterized by the sudden onset of severe lower abdominal or scrotal pain, nausea, vomiting, and fever. It is imperative to establish the diagnosis of these emergent entities promptly, as their management and prognosis varies dramatically. US serves as the crucial method to make this diagnosis.

Testicular Torsion

Testicular torsion is a surgical emergency that results from abnormal embryologic fusion of the tunica vaginalis with the scrotal wall, commonly referred to as the "bell-clapper" deformity. Testicular torsion accounts for 20% of acute scrotal pathology in adults and approximately 40% to 50% in children (most often younger than 1 year of age and adolescents). Physical examination is notoriously poor in diagnosing torsion, particularly in young infants or

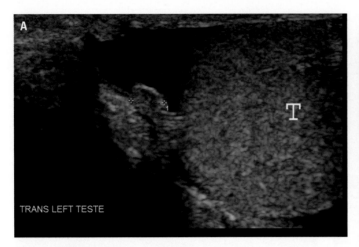
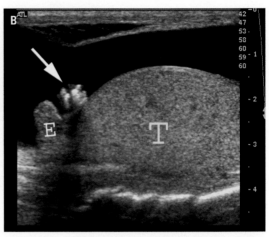

Figure 16.42. Testicular appendage. **A:** Transverse view of left testis *(T)* and appendage *(between yellow calipers)* in a patient referred in for a palpable scrotal mass, which turned out to be a large epididymal cyst. Note the presence of a moderate hydrocele, which allows for better visualization of the testicular appendage. **B:** Longitudinal image of the left hemiscrotum in another patient shows punctuate calcifications in the appendage *(arrow)*, representing prior inflammatory or ischemic changes. This is an unusual finding but makes the appendage sonographically distinct. *E*, epididymis; *T*, testis.

children. Other entities that may mimic torsion are EO, acute hydrocele, strangulated hernia, abscess, testicular hemorrhage (from a tumor), and Henoch-Schönlein purpura.

The pain due to testicular torsion is often sudden, as opposed to insidious or variable for epididymitis or testicular appendage torsion. Torsion often leads to testicular infarction, and a salvageable testis after torsion depends on the duration and extent of infarction. Most torsed testes (more than 80%) are salvageable with surgery up to 6 hours after onset of pain; from 6 to 12 hours, the salvage rate declines to 70%; and after 12 hours, fewer than 20% of testes are viable. A diffusely hypoechoic testis in the setting of acute torsion invariably represents a nonsalvageable structure at surgery.

Color or power Doppler US is imperative when evaluating possible torsion. On gray scale US imaging, the findings of acute torsion (after 1 to 24 hours) are nonspecific; the testicle is often mildly to moderately enlarged, slightly hypoechoic, and inhomogeneous (Fig. 16.43A). In the subacute phase (1 to 5 days), the hypoechoic nature and enlargement may become more pronounced. Rarely, the testis may be isoechoic compared to the contralateral side, or very uncommonly, it may become hyperechoic from acute infarction with hemorrhage. Chronic (more than 7 days) or missed

torsion is characterized by mixed echogenicity in a normal to smaller sized testis. Skin thickening is often present as an associated but nonspecific finding. All these findings may be seen in many other conditions affecting the testicle: Infection, inflammation, or trauma. Volume measurement of the testicles is mandatory at our institution, especially useful in suspected cases of torsion (same formula for the prolate ellipse already mentioned for the ovary).

Color flow Doppler has revolutionized the diagnosis of testicular ischemia or torsion. Several studies have shown sensitivities of 73% to 100%, specificities of 80% to 100%, and accuracy of 95% to 97%. The normal testis should be used as a control for the demonstration of the low arterial flow (5 to 10 cm per second) of intratesticular arteries. Once color Doppler flow is optimized on the normal testis, the symptomatic testis is then examined.

The absence of intratesticular flow is the sine qua non for testicular ischemia (Fig. 16.43B), although marked asymmetry of flow is also very suggestive (Fig. 16.43C). The presence of capsular arterial flow may persist in the setting of torsion, reflecting perfusion by anastomoses of the cremasteric or deferential arteries, which may not be completely occluded by the torsion. A diffusely

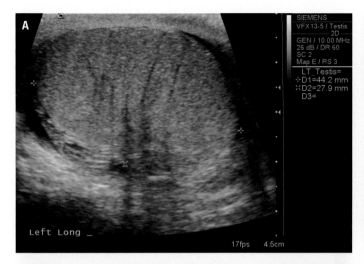

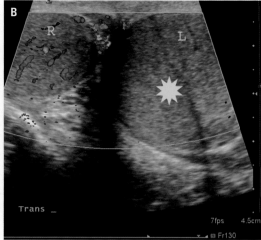

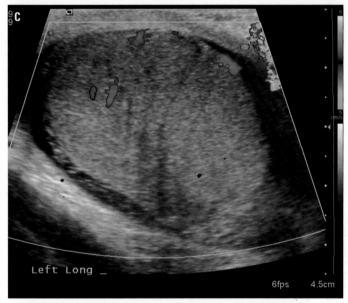

Figure 16.43. Early testicular torsion, salvageable. **A:** Longitudinal view of the left testis shows moderate testicular enlargement (volume = 22.2 mL vs. 11 mL for asymptomatic right side) and mild heterogeneity and striations. **B:** Color Doppler "buddy" transverse image of both testicles reveals normal blood flow to right side *(R)* and absence of flow *(asterisk)* to the enlarged, ischemic left *(L)* testes. At surgery, the left testis was twisted 540 degrees but was salvaged. **C:** Torsed left testis, same patient, showing reduced blood flow on color Doppler. Note the large areas of the testis that showed no or little blood flow during the examination. The patient had presented with 16 hours of severe pain, nausea, and vomiting before surgery.

hypoechoic testis with little or no flow is seldom salvageable (Fig. 16.44).

The prepubertal scrotum presents challenges, as normal blood flow may be difficult to detect even with low Doppler scale settings (Fig. 16.45). The accuracy of color flow Doppler for diagnosing torsion in children is clearly less than in adults. The use of testicular scintigraphy may confirm or exclude the diagnosis when the US is equivocal in infants or children. Power Doppler (a more sensitive Doppler technique for detecting smaller vessels and slower blood flow) may be useful for documenting torsion in neonates or prepubertal children when color Doppler is inadequate.

The diagnosis of spontaneous detorsion may be suggested when increased testicular or paratesticular flow is demonstrated in the clinical setting of

torsion, but these findings may also be seen in cases of epididymitis and/or orchitis, so accurate clinical history is paramount. Partial or early torsion may present as diminished but present blood flow compared with the asymptomatic testis, and the interpreting physician must be alert to avoid false-negative studies for incomplete torsion.

More recently, spermatic cord and epididymal torsion has been reported to be more accurate in some instances of torsion, especially if intratesticular blood flow is preserved in the acute setting (Fig. 16.46). Vijayaraghavan reported 61 cases of complete torsion that demonstrated the "whirlpool sign" of the spermatic cord with a sensitivity of 100%. Arce et al. reported a small series of six patients with spermatic cord torsion who demonstrated a rotated spermatic cord on the side of

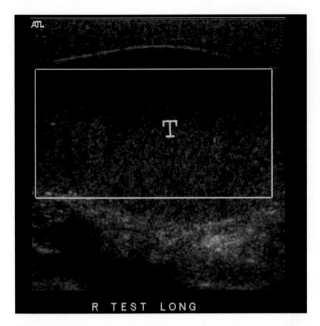

Figure 16.44. A longitudinal color Doppler view of the right testis shows a diffusely avascular, very hypoechoic testis that was not viable at surgery. The *green rectangle* is the color box, which should show dots and dashes of color that represent blood flow if present. Note the mild skin thickening. *T*, testis.

torsion. All of these cases had preserved but mildly diminished (relative to asymptomatic side) blood flow in the testes on color Doppler US. Documentation of the spermatic cord orientation has not garnered much attention in the US literature, but the existent data is compelling, and this part of the scrotal US exam is now included in the suspected torsion cases at our medical center.

Torsion of Testicular Appendage

Torsion of the testicular appendages is the most common cause of acute scrotal pain in children and frequently misdiagnosed as testicular torsion. Torsion of the appendages is more common than testicular torsion, is self-limiting, and is treated conservatively. The classic clinical appearance is the "blue dot" sign, a small bluish discoloration of the scrotal skin just superficial to the infarcted appendage, but as in many "classical signs," is prevalent in less than 50% of cases. The most common finding on US is an enlarged, hypoechoic, or heterogeneous nodule representing the infarcted appendage adjacent to the epididymis, also called

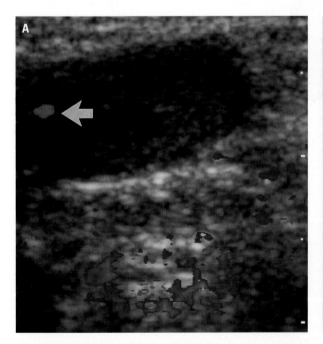

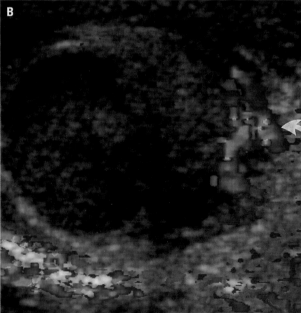

Figure 16.45. A: Normal testicular blood flow in a 22-month-old boy. Note the paucity of color flow *(arrow)*, even with a low color flow setting (6.4 cm per second), at this young age. **B:** Contralateral infarcted testis (missed torsion) demonstrates enlarged, hypoechoic echo pattern with hyperemic paratesticular flow *(curved arrow)*. This testicle was nonviable at surgery. The lack of color flow in **A** shows the frequent difficulty in using intratesticular flow for diagnosing torsion in infants and young children.

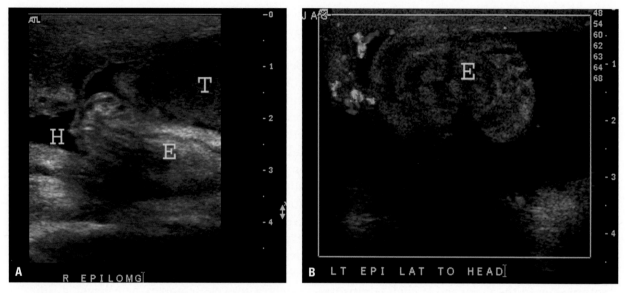

Figure 16.46. **A:** Longitudinal image of the right epididymis *(E)* and testis *(T)* and a small hydrocele *(H)* shows a thickened and twisted epididymis that suggests acute torsion. **B:** Transverse view of the left epididymis in another patient with acute testicular torsion, lateral to the testis (not shown). Note the enlarged, twisted appearance of the epididymis without demonstrable blood flow. There is exuberant blood flow in the extratesticular vessels *(color dots)*. *E,* epydidymis.

the "Mickey Mouse" sign (Fig. 16.47). However, more recent work stated that the upper pole extratesticular nodule was seen in only in 31% of 29 children (age 7 months to 14 years). Secondary inflammatory signs of hydrocele (76%), enlarged epididymis (76%), scrotal wall edema (55%), and swollen testicle (31%) were common findings. The inflammatory signs alone were present in almost half of the patients (lacking the extratesticular nodule). Caution must be taken not to make the erroneous diagnosis of epididymitis under these circumstances.

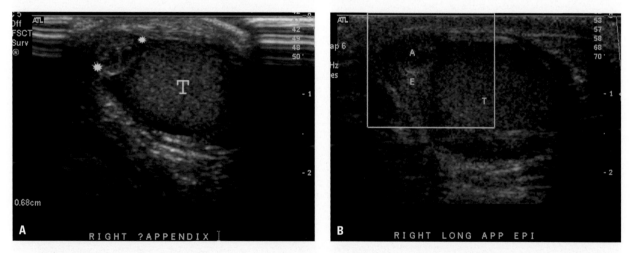

Figure 16.47. Torsion of the testicular appendage. **A:** Longitudinal image of the right testis *(T)* reveals a separate structure *(between asterisks)* that was also distinct from the epididymis (not shown) that is slightly hyperechoic, enlarged, and heterogeneous and corresponded to the painful testicular appendage on physical exam. **B:** Longitudinal color Doppler image of the right side showing the avascular, enlarged testicular appendage *(A)* nestled between the epididymis *(E)* and testis *(T)*.

Epididymitis/Orchitis

Inflammatory or infectious disease is the most common affliction of the adult scrotum. The epididymis is almost always involved; the testis less frequently so and almost never alone. EO generally results from a retrograde infection of the lower urinary tract, with the most frequent pathogens in patients older than age 35 being *Escherichia coli*, *Proteus mirabilis*, and *Pseudomonas* species. Younger patients tend to be infected with sexually transmitted gonococcus and *Chlamydia* organisms. Viral agents are much less prevalent (mumps, influenza) but have a significant rate of complications in the adult population. The peak incidence of epididymitis is between the fifth and sixth decades of life. A recent study of the acute scrotum showed the mean age of epididymitis to be 41 years versus 14 years for testicular torsion, and the mean duration of symptoms before imaging of epididymitis of 4.5 days versus 19 hours for torsion. The onset of symptoms is variable, it may be acute or more insidious, and is often accompanied by urethral discharge, dysuria, pyuria, and fever.

The diagnosis of EO may be made clinically, but sonographic findings increase the accuracy, and color Doppler sonography adds increased sensitivity and specificity. The normal epididymis is isoechoic to slightly hyperechoic to the testis with demonstrable but not hypervascular blood flow on color imaging. The inflamed epididymis is often enlarged and hypoechoic acutely (Fig. 16.48) and occasionally transforms into a hyperechoic or heterogeneous structure in chronic epididymitis. The testis, if involved, becomes enlarged and hypoechoic in the acute phase but may be normal sized to slightly enlarged and hyperechoic in the chronic state. Color Doppler will often show hyperemia (increased number or concentration of vessels). Some expert sonologists feel that the presence of easily detectible, increased venous flow on spectral Doppler US suggests acute orchitis. A hydrocele or, more rarely, a pyocele (complex or echogenic fluid) is usually present, and the scrotal skin is often thickened (Fig. 16.49).

Tuberculous epididymitis is characterized by predominant enlargement of the epididymal tail (as opposed to diffuse swelling or enlargement of the head) and more heterogeneous echo texture due to calcifications and sinus tracts.

Extension of epididymal infection or inflammation to the testis results in orchitis in approximately

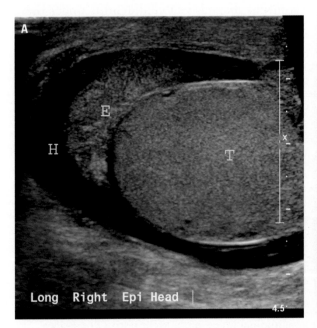
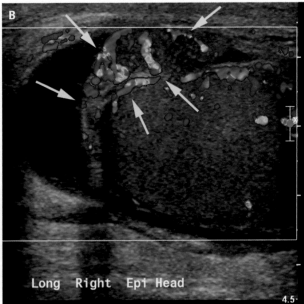

Figure 16.48. Acute epididymitis. **A:** Longitudinal image of the right testis *(T)* and epididymal head *(E)* reveals an enlarged, slightly hypoechoic epididymis in a 63-year-old male with several days of right-sided scrotal pain. Note made of moderate reactive hydrocele *(H)*. **B:** Longitudinal color Doppler image showing the extremely hypervascular epididymis *(arrows)* representing inflammation and normal vascularity of the testis. The epididymis should normally never be more vascular than the testis.

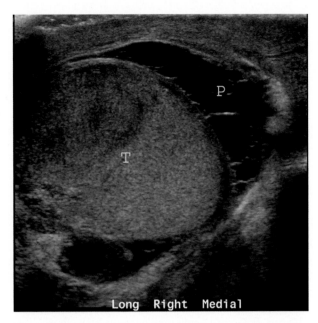

Figure 16.49. Pyocele. Longitudinal view of right hemiscrotum. Complex fluid collection *(P)* around testis *(T)* characterized by multiple thin and thick septa, and this complicated, chronic infection was treated with multiple antibiotics with only partial relief. Patient was to undergo surgery for chronic epididymitis.

20% of cases. In our experience, the testicle shows abnormal hyperemia on color flow Doppler more frequently than demonstrating morphologic changes, such as edematous hypoechoic areas, which may be focal or diffuse (Fig. 16.50). If the

infection is severe, the intratesticular arterial flow may be diminished or absent and lead to testicular infarction. Distinction from testicular torsion may be difficult in such cases, and evaluation of the spermatic cord may help distinguish the two entities. If an infection goes untreated, an epididymal or testicular abscess may develop, which warrants surgical debridement for definitive therapy (Fig. 16.51).

The Enlarged Scrotum

The enlarged scrotum is most often caused by a hydrocele, a varicocele, or an inguinal hernia extending into the scrotum. Normal amounts of fluid (1 to 5 mL) exist between the visceral and parietal layers of the tunica vaginalis in 85% of asymptomatic patients. This fluid surrounds the anterolateral portions of the testis, as the tunica is normally fused posteriorly (the bare area). Accumulation of an abnormal amount of fluid is the most frequent painless cause of scrotal swelling. Hydroceles may be acquired or congenital; the former related to trauma, torsion, infection, or neoplasm. The latter group arises from a persistent processus vaginalis, which allows open communication between the peritoneum and the scrotal sac, which usually obliterates by 18 months of age.

Sonography is invaluable for evaluating the testicle when physical examination is hampered by the presence of a large hydrocele. Anechoic fluid serves

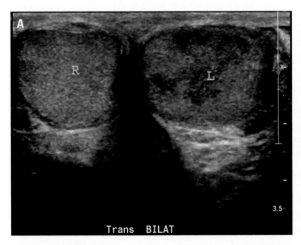
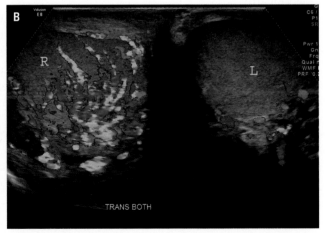

Figure 16.50. Orchitis. **A:** Transverse "buddy" view of the testes (*R*, right; *L*, left) shows patchy areas of hypoechoic architecture of the left testis, which was involved with orchitis. **B:** Transverse color Doppler "buddy" view of another patient with right orchitis shows marked hyperemia of the affected right side. *R*, right; *L*, left.

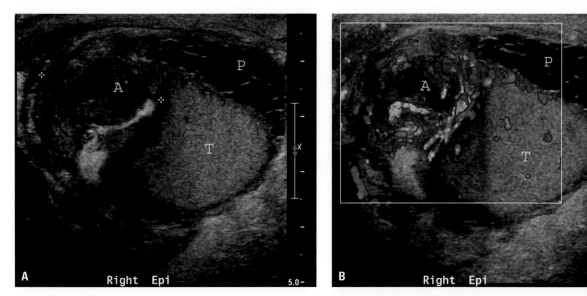

Figure 16.51. Epididymal abscess. **A:** Longitudinal color Doppler sonogram shows an early abscess *(A)* developing in the markedly enlarged, heterogeneous epididymis. **B:** Color Doppler image, same view, shows marked peripheral vascularity around the evolving abscess *(A)*. *T,* testis; *P*, pyocele.

as an excellent acoustic window for visualization of the testis. Low-level echoes may represent high protein levels, fibrin bodies, or cholesterol crystals in a hydrocele in an asymptomatic patient. In the setting of an infection of the scrotum, fluid containing internal echoes or septations indicates a pyocele (Fig. 16.49). Hematoceles also present as complex fluid collections, often with thicker and irregular septations—the "spider web" appearance—in the extratesticular space and are most commonly associated with trauma or neoplasms or sometimes coagulopathy.

A varicocele is a dilatation of the pampiniform plexus (paratesticular veins) more than 2 mm in diameter, most often around the upper pole of the testis or head of the epididymis. Valsalva maneuver or upright positioning significantly increase their caliber (Fig. 16.52). Varicoceles are generally not cause for emergency visits, but they may rarely present as an acutely painful scrotum. More often, they present as a chronic condition, predominantly on the left side. The onset of a new varicocele can be an indication of a tumor, hydronephrosis, or venous thrombosis—the secondary (compressive or obstructive) causes of varicoceles. Primary varicoceles are the result of incompetent valves of the spermatic vein and are a major cause of male infertility.

Scrotal hernias occur when a large defect is present in the lower abdominal wall or inguinal canal, allowing descent of intra-abdominal contents into the scrotum (Fig. 16.53). Most of these are clinically diagnosed, but ultrasonography is helpful in unusual cases. Hernia contents include small bowel, colon, and/or omentum. Peristalsis may enable differentiation from other paratesticular masses. If peristalsis is absent, the presence of very echogenic material is consistent with the diagnosis of omental or peritoneal fat. Scanning cephalad through the inguinal canal should allow visualization of the extension of the hernia contents from the peritoneal cavity. MRI has proven useful in difficult patients with technical issues such as obesity, prior surgery, or severe pain that preclude accurate sonographic evaluation.

The Traumatized Scrotum

The question of paramount importance in major scrotal trauma is testicular rupture. The clinical diagnosis is usually made more difficult by the presence of swelling and pain. Blunt trauma accounts for approximately 85% of cases and penetrating trauma the remainder. If the tunica albuginea is violated or ruptured, the seminiferous tubules will extrude into

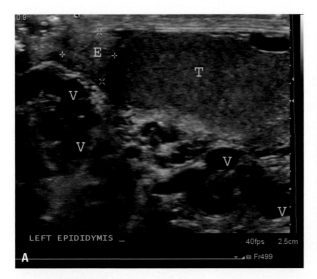
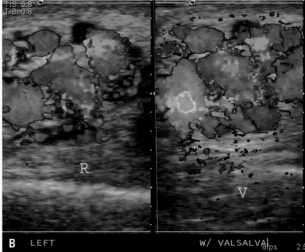

Figure 16.52. A: Longitudinal sonogram of a 14-year-old boy with large left varicocele *(V)*. The dilated, serpentine veins surround the testes and appear as a "pack of worms" in real-time imaging. *T*, testis; *E*, epididymis. **B:** Color Doppler sonogram at rest *(R)* and with Valsalva *(V)* maneuver shows a modest increase in size of the varicocele with increased intra-abdominal pressure.

the tunica vaginalis, and emergency surgery is indicated to repair the testicular capsule. Testicular viability is related to prompt diagnosis and treatment: 90% are salvageable if surgery is undertaken within 72 hours, whereas the rescue rate is less than 50% if treatment is delayed past 3 days. The presence of a large scrotal hematoma (extratesticular) is another indication for surgical exploration because this

bleeding may compress and occlude arterial flow, leading to testicular ischemia or infarction.

Sonography is the primary imaging technique in scrotal trauma, as it has been shown to be accurate in assessing the parenchymal disruption as well as extratesticular hematoma. Features of focal architectural disruption or alterations in echogenicity often indicate acute hemorrhage or infarction but

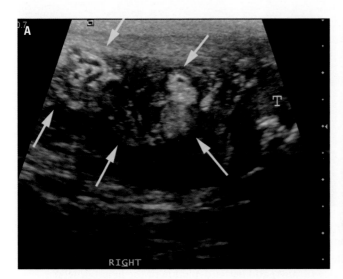
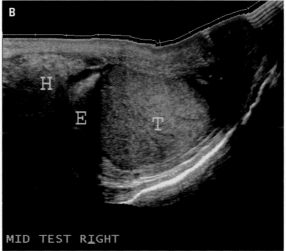

Figure 16.53. Scrotal hernia. **A:** Mixed hyperechoic mass *(arrows)* above the testicle *(T)* is consistent with intraperitoneal fat and omentum herniating into the scrotal sac on the right longitudinal image. **B:** Panoramic view of the right testis *(T)* in the longitudinal plane shows the hernia *(H)* descending into the scrotum on the right side. *E*, epididymis.

may be present with an intact tunica. An irregular or ill-defined outline of the testis may be a sign of testicular rupture (Fig. 16.54), although a clearly defined fracture line is visible in fewer than 20% of patients on US. Care must be taken not to confuse testicular rupture with the presence of a complex extratesticular hemorrhage (Fig. 16.55). Color Doppler and spectral flow may be helpful in delineating the differences between these two entities: Hematomas will be avascular, whereas the testis will have prominent intraparenchymal flow (if viable).

Penetrating trauma occurs most often due to bullet wounds, and intrascrotal foreign bodies are readily recognized with US. MRI may be helpful in sonographically equivocal or difficult cases, as testicular rupture may be more evident with the larger, more global field of views and multiplanar capabilities afforded by MRI.

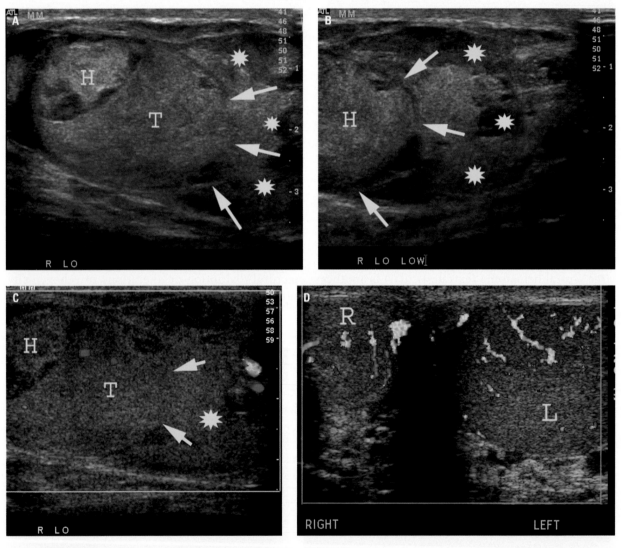

Figure 16.54. Testicular rupture from a motorcycle accident in a 40-year-old. **A:** Longitudinal sonogram of the right testis *(T)* shows an intratesticular hematoma *(H)*, a ruptured inferior pole *(arrows)* with loss of definition of the tunica, and a large extratesticular hematoma and extruded tubules *(asterisks)*. **B:** Longitudinal view of the lower pole of the testis shows loss of tunica *(arrows)* and better depiction of the heterogeneous, largely hypoechoic extratesticular collection, reflecting the extratesticular hematoma *(H)* and seminiferous tubules *(asterisks)*. **C:** Color Doppler sonogram of same area as **A** and **B** shows the avascular nature of the extratesticular hematoma and tubules *(asterisks)*. *T*, viable testis; *H*, intratesticular hematoma. *Arrows* depict the ruptured tunica. **D:** Transverse "buddy" view of both testes with color Doppler performed 6 months later shows significant right testis atrophy. *R*, right; *L*, left.

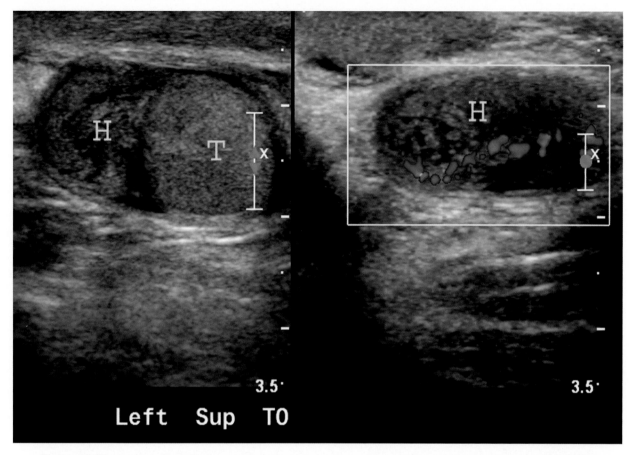

Figure 16.55. Traumatic epididymal hematoma in an 8-year-old. Transverse dual image views (**left side**) of left testis *(T)* and epididymis reveal a large extracapsular hematoma *(H)*. Note the intact tunica of the testis. Color Doppler image reveals perfusion of the intact epididymis *(color dots/dashes)* and the avascular hematoma *(H)* surrounding it. Nonsurgical therapy was instituted, and the patient recovered with good results.

SUGGESTED READINGS

1. Levine D, Barnes PD, Robertson RR, et al. Fast MR imaging of fetal central nervous system abnormalities. *Radiology.* 2003;229(1):51–61.
2. Brenner DJ, Hall EJ. Computed tomography—an increasing source of radiation exposure. *N Engl J Med.* 2007;357(22):2277–2284.
3. Smith-Bindman R. Is computed tomography safe? *N Engl J Med.* 2010;363(1):1–4.
4. Karmazyn B, Steinberg R, Livne P, et al. Duplex sonographic findings in children with torsion of the testicular appendages: overlap with epididymitis and epididymoorchitis. *J Pediatr Surg.* 2006;41(3):500–504.
5. Abul F, Al-Sayer H, Arun N. The acute scrotum: a review of 40 cases. *Med Princ Pract.* 2005;14(3):177–181.
6. Harris RD, Holtzman SR, Poppe AM. Clinical outcome in female patients with pelvic pain and normal pelvic US findings. *Radiology.* 2000;216(2):440–443.
7. Vijayaraghavan SB. Sonographic whirlpool sign in ovarian torsion. *J Ultrasound Med.* 2004;23(12):1643–1649.
8. Arce JD, Cortes M, Vargas JC. Sonographic diagnosis of acute spermatic cord torsion. Rotation of the cord: a key to the diagnosis. *Pediatr Radiol.* 2002;32(7):485–491.
9. Vijayaraghavan SB. Sonographic differential diagnosis of acute scrotum: real-time whirlpool sign, a key sign of torsion. *J Ultrasound Med.* 2006;25(5):563–574.
10. Varras M, Polyzos D, Perouli E, et al. Tubo-ovarian abscesses: spectrum of sonographic findings with surgical and pathological correlations. *Clin Exp Obstet Gynecol.* 2003;30(2–3):117–121.

11. Peña JE, Ufberg D, Cooney N, et al. Usefulness of Doppler sonography in the diagnosis of ovarian torsion. *Fertil Steril.* 2000;73(5):1047–1050.

12. Timor-Tritsch IE, Lerner JP, Monteagudo A, et al. Transvaginal sonographic markers of tubal inflammatory disease. *Ultrasound Obstet Gynecol.* 1998;12(1):56–66.

13. Dogra V, Bhatt S. Acute painful scrotum. *Radiol Clin North Am.* 2004;42(2):349–363.

14. Lazebnik N, Lazebnik RS. The role of ultrasound in pregnancy-related emergencies. *Radiol Clin North Am.* 2004;42(2):315–327.

15. Dogra V, Paspulati RM, Bhatt S. First trimester bleeding evaluation. *Ultrasound Q.* 2005;21(2):69–85.

16. Redline RW. Placental pathology: a systematic approach with clinical correlations. *Placenta.* 2008; 29(suppl A):S86–S91.

17. Tikkanen M. Etiology, clinical manifestations, and prediction of placental abruption. *Acta Obstet Gynecol Scand.* 2010;89(6):732–740.

18. Leite J, Ross P, Rossi AC, et al. Prognosis of very large first-trimester hematomas. *J Ultrasound Med.* 2006;25(11):1441–1445.

19. Oyelese Y, Ananth CV. Placental abruption. *Obstet Gynecol.* 2006;108(4):1005–1016.

20. Masselli G, Brunelli R, Di Tola M, et al. MR Imaging in the evaluation of placental abruption: correlation with sonographic findings. *Radiology.* 2011; 259(1):222–230.

21. Lee EJ, Kwon HC, Joo HJ, et al. Diagnosis of ovarian torsion with color Doppler sonography: depiction of twisted vascular pedicle. *J Ultrasound Med.* 1998;17(2):83–89.

CHAPTER 17

Pelvis, Including Lower Urinary Tract Trauma

John H. Harris Jr.

GENERAL CONSIDERATIONS

In this chapter, the pelvis is considered to include the bony pelvis and its extraperitoneal soft tissues. Injuries involving the pelvis and its contents result in some of the most challenging and serious diagnostic problems to confront the radiologist, emergency physician, and traumatologist. Radiographically, this is particularly true for two reasons. First, the pelvis is the single area of the body that defies the radiologic dictum of obtaining radiographs in both frontal and lateral projections. Second, the soft tissue injuries frequently associated with pelvic skeletal injury are radiographically much less striking than the skeletal injury but are of far greater clinical significance.

The principal cause of death associated with pelvic trauma is hemorrhage, estimated to be as high as 60% in patients with major pelvic trauma.[1,2] Interventional angiography has resulted in a significant reduction in this mortality rate.[3,4]

Rupture of the bladder or urethral injury occurs in approximately 20% of patients with significant pelvic ring disruption (PRD). However, bladder and urethral injuries should be suspected in all patients with major pelvic trauma.[5–7]

The proper evaluation of urethral injuries requires a retrograde urethrogram (RUG) as the initial diagnostic procedure in all male patients with a PRD who are unable to void spontaneously.[8–15] If the RUG is negative, a cystogram should be performed next. There is no justification for the insertion of a Foley catheter before performing an RUG in male patients with PRD. All male patients suspected of having a urethral injury, either on a clinical basis or because of radiographically demonstrated PRD, must have an RUG prior to insertion of a Foley catheter.

RADIOGRAPHIC EXAMINATION

The routine radiographic examination of the pelvis is the anteroposterior (AP) view (Fig. 17.1). This projection must include the iliac crests, each hip joint, and the proximal portion of each femur.

Blood and/or urine in the extraperitoneal, perivesical space alters the radiographic appearance of the normal soft tissue structures commonly visible on the AP radiograph of the pelvis (Fig. 17.2).

The caudad ("inlet") and cephalad ("outlet") angled AP projections (Fig. 17.3) of the pelvis are particularly useful in the assessment of PRD because each presents a different perspective of fracture fragment alignment. When possible, oblique projections provide invaluable assistance in conceptualizing complex types of PRD (Fig. 17.4). The nearly universal application of multiplanar computed tomography (MPCT) in the initial assessment of patients with PRD accurately depicts the orientation of components of PRD, as illustrated subsequently in this chapter.

The os pubis and the ischia are canted anteroposteriorly approximately 30 degrees. Consequently, the AP radiograph of the pelvis more correctly represents an oblique view of the anterior pelvic arch. It is therefore quite possible to overlook minimally displaced fractures of this portion of the pelvis in the straight AP radiograph.

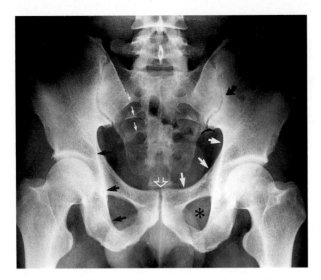

Figure 17.1. AP radiograph of a normal adult pelvis. The principal skeletal anatomic landmarks include the SI joint *(curved arrow)*, sacral arcuate lines *(small white arrows)*, ilioischial line *(black arrows)*, iliopectineal line *(large white arrows)*, pubic symphysis formed by the pubic bodies *(open arrow)* and obturator foramen *(asterisk)* formed by the superior pubic ramus, pubic body, inferior pubic ramus, and ischium. The contiguous margins of the sacrum and ilium should be on the same plane or form a continuous arc (∩).

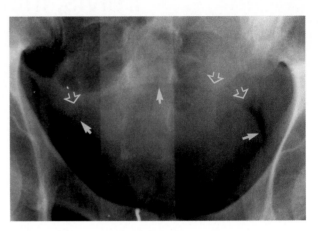

Figure 17.2. Pelvic soft tissue structures commonly visible on the AP radiograph of the pelvis include the urinary bladder *(white arrows)* made visible by the contrasting lucency of the extraperitoneal perivesical fat, and the pelvic peritoneal reflection *(open arrows)*, which contains the pelvic ileum separated from the bladder by the thin lucency of intraperitoneal fat.

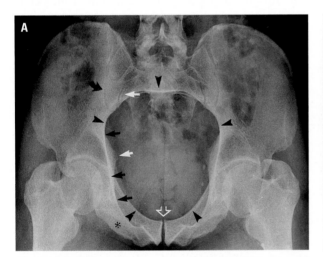

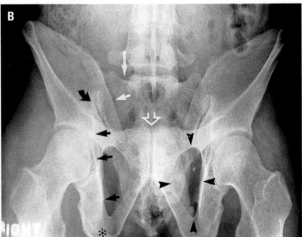

Figure 17.3. Inlet **(A)** and outlet **(B)** radiographs of the pelvis. The inlet view **(A)** is obtained with the patient supine and the central x-ray beam centered midway between the umbilicus and the pubic symphysis and angled 35 degrees caudally. This projection shows the pelvic ring (plane of the inlet to the true pelvis *[arrowheads]*), the anterior *(curved arrow)* and posterior *(short white arrow)* margins of the SI joints, the ilioischial line (an arc of the quadrilateral plate forming the medial wall of the acetabulum and extending caudally to the ischial tuberosity as the inferior portion of the posterior column of the acetabulum) *(black arrows)*, the ischial tuberosity *(asterisk)*, the ischial spine *(white arrow)*, and the symmetry of the pubic symphysis *(open arrow)* between the pubic bodies. The outlet view **(B)** is obtained with the central x-ray beam centered on the superior margin of the pubic symphysis and angled 35 degrees rostrally. This projection shows the superior portion of the sacrum, including the ala *(long white arrow)*, the anterior *(curved arrow)* and posterior *(short white arrow)* margins of the SI joint *(curved arrow)*, the ilioischial line *(black arrows)* and pubic symphysis *(open arrow)* in different perspective, and the margins of the obturator foramen *(arrowheads)*.

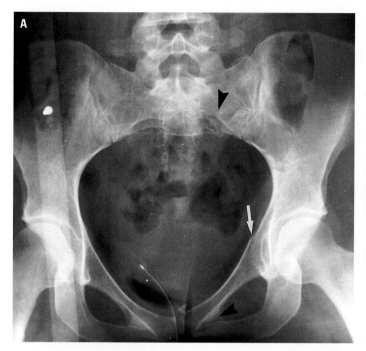
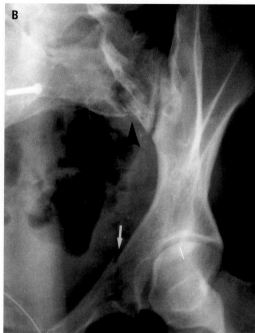

Figure 17.4. The subtle superior pubic ramus component *(arrow)* of the minimally displaced Malgaigne pelvic ring disruption *(arrowheads,* **A**) was confirmed on the left anterior oblique projection *(arrow,* **B**), which also shows the left sacral alar component *(arrowhead)* to better advantage.

The routine radiographic examination of the sacrum and coccyx (Fig. 17.5) alone must include a straight AP projection and a true lateral radiograph of the sacrum and coccyx. However, in the context of PRD, computed tomography (CT) best demonstrates sacral and sacroiliac (SI) anatomy and traumatic pathology.

CT is indicated in all types of major pelvic injuries demonstrated on the initial conventional radiographic examination of the pelvis (obtained in the Trauma Bay), for the reasons stated earlier. When a PRD is demonstrated, axial CT images of the pelvis should be obtained from above the level of the iliac crests to the acetabula in consecutive 5-mm slices and from the acetabula to below the ischial tuberosities in consecutive 3-mm slices.

Although urethral and/or urinary bladder injuries occur in fewer than 20% of patients with pelvic trauma, approximately 73% of lower urinary tract injuries are the result of blunt pelvic trauma. Therefore, particularly in all male patients with PRD, evaluation of the lower urinary tract by RUG is essential before Foley catheterization. "Diagnostic" or blind attempts to catheterize male patients with PRD fail the accepted standard of care because of the inherent possibility of iatrogenic urethral trauma, initiation or reactivation of urethral hemorrhage, extending an existing urethral injury, converting a tear into a complete transection, or introducing infection.

The RUG is performed by the insertion of a 7-mL balloon catheter into the urethra under sterile conditions. Following inflation of the balloon to approximately 4 to 5 mL, the catheter is slowly withdrawn until the balloon "falls" into the fossa navicularis. At that time, the balloon is maximally inflated. Before injection of contrast material, a gentle tug on the catheter should determine that the balloon is securely positioned in the fossa. Before the contrast medium is injected, the patient should be in a slight degree of obliquity so that the urethra can be visualized along its entire length. The application of gentle traction to the catheter will assist in elongating the urethra. In this position, 15 to 20 mL of contrast material is introduced in a steady, continuous flow with the radiographic exposure obtained after the introduction of 15 to 17 mL. The resultant radiograph must show the entire urethra as well as contrast in the urinary bladder. If not, the RUG must be repeated.

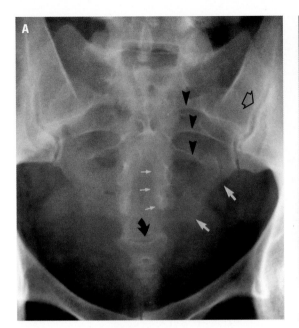

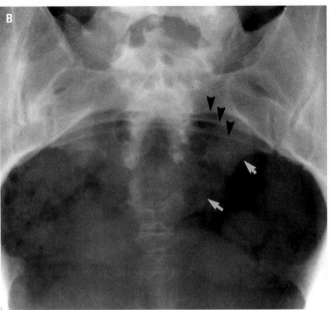

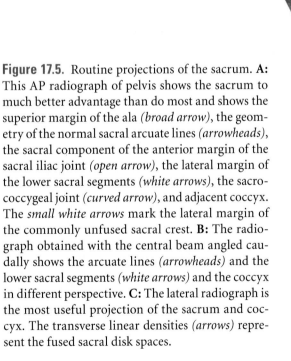

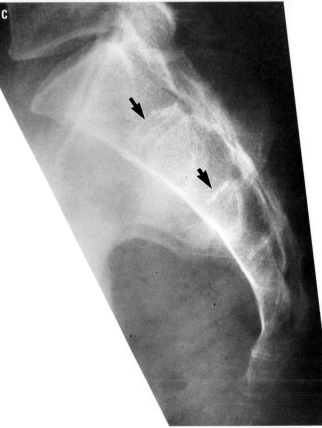

Figure 17.5. Routine projections of the sacrum. **A:** This AP radiograph of pelvis shows the sacrum to much better advantage than do most and shows the superior margin of the ala *(broad arrow)*, the geometry of the normal sacral arcuate lines *(arrowheads)*, the sacral component of the anterior margin of the sacral iliac joint *(open arrow)*, the lateral margin of the lower sacral segments *(white arrows)*, the sacrococcygeal joint *(curved arrow)*, and adjacent coccyx. The *small white arrows* mark the lateral margin of the commonly unfused sacral crest. **B:** The radiograph obtained with the central beam angled caudally shows the arcuate lines *(arrowheads)* and the lower sacral segments *(white arrows)* and the coccyx in different perspective. **C:** The lateral radiograph is the most useful projection of the sacrum and coccyx. The transverse linear densities *(arrows)* represent the fused sacral disk spaces.

With a normal RUG, the catheter balloon may be deflated, the catheter safely advanced into the bladder, and a cystogram performed. The cystogram should include an AP radiograph of the bladder after the introduction of approximately 150 mL of contrast medium and after maximum distention of the bladder with approximately 350 to 400 mL or to the limit of the patient's pain tolerance. An AP and each oblique radiograph of the completely filled bladder and an AP radiograph of the drained bladder complete the cystogram. Corriere and Sandler have reported a 4% incidence of extraperitoneal bladder rupture detected only on the postevacuation radiograph.[16] Obviously, this "routine" protocol should be modified or terminated with the demonstration of a bladder injury. Demonstration of any type of urethral injury, including the type I periurethral hematoma, mandates further evaluation by a urologist.

Retrograde cystography is also indicated in any patient with gross hematuria and a radiographically intact pelvis following blunt abdominopelvic trauma. The working clinical hypothesis in these circumstances is that the urethra is intact (patient voided) and the bladder is ruptured (gross hematuria).

The RUG and retrograde cystogram can and should be performed in the trauma center without fluoroscopic guidance.

Opacification of the urinary bladder by intravenously administered contrast material for abdominal CT is not considered adequate to exclude a bladder injury because of inadequate distention of the bladder by the contrast material. If the abdominal CT is done first, a retrograde cystogram may be performed with the patient on the CT gurney and the distended bladder reexamined by CT. The CT cystogram must also include postdrainage CT of the bladder.

Retrograde urethrography is not applicable to female patients because the anatomy of the short female urethra prevents the creation of a watertight system necessary to delineate the urethral lumen. Furthermore, the presence of a female urethral injury is established by the presence of blood in the vagina because the urethrovaginal membrane is so thin that it is usually torn in association with urethral injury.

Pelvic angiography is valuable in the identification of arterial bleeding sites that are amenable to percutaneous transcatheter embolization.[3,4,17]

However, although only 6% to 18% of patients with unstable PRD sustain pelvic arterial injuries that warrant embolization, unexplained hemodynamic instability should be the specific indication for pelvic angiography.[18]

RADIOGRAPHIC ANATOMY

It is important to be familiar with changes in the radiographic appearance of the pelvis related to normal growth and development. This is so that (1) normal anatomy may not be misinterpreted as signs of trauma and (2) the basis of avulsive injuries of the adolescent pelvis may be understood and recognized.

The radiographic appearance of the pelvis of a normal child is seen in Figure 17.6. The triradiate cartilage (TRC), the site of union of the pubis, ischium, and ilium, usually fuses concomitant with puberty. The ischiopubic synchondrosis may fuse between the ages of 5 and 12 years.[19] This synchondrosis varies greatly in radiographic appearance during the fusion process, not only from child to

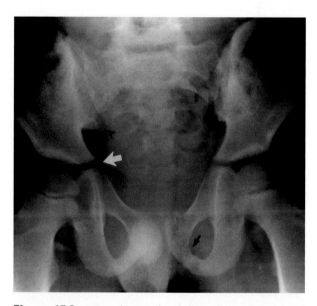

Figure 17.6. AP radiograph of the pelvis of a normal 8-year-old child. Normally in children, the SI joints *(open arrow)* appear abnormally wide because of incomplete ossification of the contiguous surfaces of the SI joints. The triradiate cartilages *(white arrow)* are physiologically open until ages 13 to 16 years. Also, by this age, the ischiopubic synchondroses *(black arrow)* are fused.

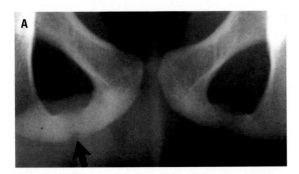

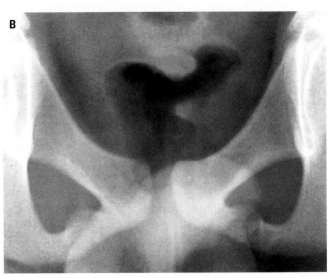

Figure 17.7. A and B: Examples of the variability of the radiographic appearance of the ischiopubic synchondrosis in children of different ages. In the younger child (**A**), the right synchondrosis *(arrow)* could be misinterpreted as either an acute incomplete or a healing fracture.

child (Fig. 17.7) but also from side to side in the same child (Fig. 17.8). The appearance of this synchondrosis rarely suggests an acute fracture but very commonly simulates a healing one (Fig. 17.8). By age 14 years, the TRC is nearly fused and the ischiopubic synchondroses are fused (Fig. 17.9).

The pelvis of adolescents and young adults contains several apophyses that may be mistaken for acute fractures or that may be the site of acute avulsive injuries. These include apophyses of the iliac crest, the anterosuperior and inferior iliac spines, the ischial tuberosity (Fig. 17.10), and the inferior margin of the pubic bodies (Fig. 17.10B), all of which ossify with puberty and fuse between the ages 20 and 25 years.[20] The anterosuperior iliac spine apophysis is the site of origin of the sartorius muscle; the anteroinferior iliac spine apophysis, the rectus femur muscle; and the ischial apophysis, the hamstring muscles.

An inconsistent secondary ossification center may constitute the superior aspect of the posterior acetabular lip either unilaterally or bilaterally. These centers, which usually appear between the ages of 14 and 18 years and fuse in early adulthood, may persist ununited throughout adult life as the os acetabuli and simulate a posterior acetabular lip fracture (Fig. 17.11). As with ununited secondary ossification centers elsewhere, dense cortication of the margins of the separate center and smooth sclerotic contiguous surfaces of the adjacent portions of the pelvis and ununited center (Fig. 17.11) should easily distinguish these ununited secondary ossification centers from an acute fracture fragment.

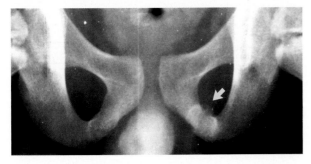

Figure 17.8. Disparity in the radiographic appearance of the ischiopubic synchondroses *(arrow)* in an asymptomatic child. There was no history of antecedent trauma to the pelvis, and the bulbous configuration of the left ischiopubic synchondrosis is entirely normal.

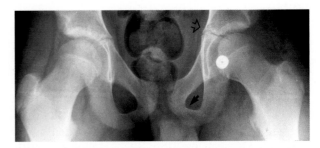

Figure 17.9. Normal appearance of the inferior portion of the pelvis of a 14-year-old child. The triradiate cartilages *(open arrow)* are almost completely fused, whereas the ischiopubic synchondroses *(black arrow)* are fused.

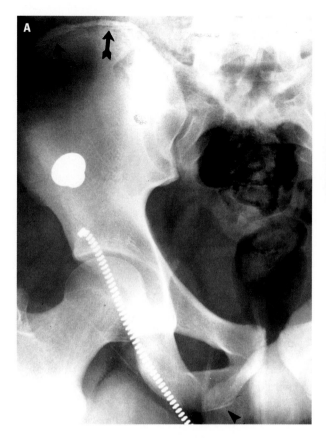

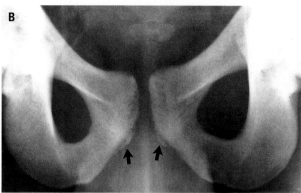

Figure 17.10. Partially fused apophyseal centers of the iliac crest *(arrows)* and ischial tuberosity *(arrowhead)* (**A**) and of the pubic symphysis *(arrows)* (**B**).

In the straight AP radiograph of the adult, the pelvic ring is the round or oval plane of the inlet of the true pelvis and includes the sacral promontory, the inferior margins of the SI joints, the iliopectineal line extending to the superior margin of the superior pubic rami, and the superior margin of the pubic symphysis. The pelvic ring is divided into an anterior and a posterior arch by an imaginary line connecting the ischial spines (Fig. 17.12). The ilioischial line (Figs. 17.1 and 17.3) is not a single bony margin but is composed, superiorly, of the arc of the quadrilateral plate tangent to the x-ray beam and, inferiorly, by the internal cortex of the ischium extending to its tuberosity. The ilioischial line extends obliquely downward lateral to the iliopectineal line. The quadrilateral plate comprises the lateral surface of the true pelvis (birth canal) and, as such, constitutes the medial wall of the acetabulum.

The teardrop shadow of the pelvis (Fig. 17.13) is a composite U-shaped shadow located at the

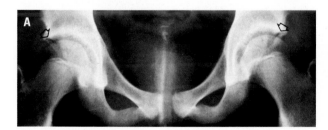

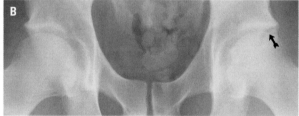

Figure 17.11. **A:** Frontal examination of the hips of a patient without symptoms referable to the pelvis. *Open arrows* indicate secondary ossification centers of the posterior lip of each acetabulum. **B:** The frontal projection of the hips of an adult demonstrates a persistent ununited secondary ossification center (os acetabuli) on the left. The radiographic characteristics of the contiguous surfaces of the os acetabuli and the posterior acetabular rim *(arrow)* should distinguish this normal variant from an acute posterior lip fracture.

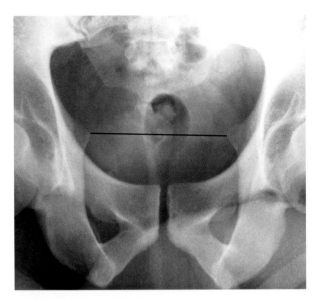

Figure 17.12. Although not a component of the pelvic inlet, the ischial spines are the reference points used to divide the pelvic ring into its anterior and posterior arches.

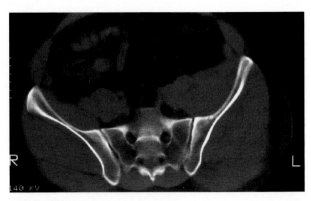

Figure 17.14. Axial computed tomography of the normal sacrum and the SI joints of an adult.

anteroinferior portion of the acetabular fossa and constitutes the anterior margin of the acetabular notch. It consists of cortical and medullary bone principally of the ischium with a small medial component from the superior pubic ramus.[21]

The SI joints are oblique structures with the sacral alar component anterior to the iliac wing

component. Consequently, the iliac and sacral alar margin of the anterior edge of the SI joint is usually clearly recognizable throughout its vertical extent. The posterior margin of the SI joint, which lies medial to the anterior margin, is much less well seen on the AP radiograph of the pelvis and is frequently identified only by the posterior margin of the iliac wing component (Fig. 17.3). Oblique views intended to demonstrate the SI joints en face usually only demonstrate the anterior aspect of the joint space. The SI joints are optimally demonstrated on axial CT images (Fig. 17.14). An important anatomic relationship is formed by the inferior cortical margins of the contiguous sacral alar and iliac surfaces of the anterior margins of the SI joints, which normally should be on the same plane or constitute a continuous imaginary arc (Fig. 17.1).

The sacral arcuate lines (Fig. 17.15), sometimes incorrectly referred to as "struts," reflect the normal

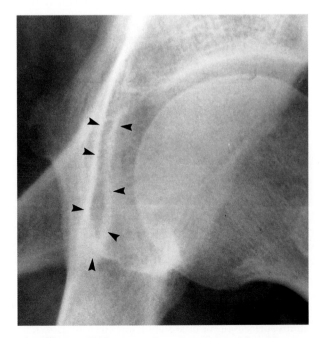

Figure 17.13. Pelvic "teardrop" *(arrowheads)*.

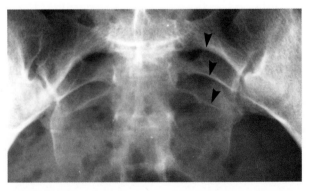

Figure 17.15. Normal sacral arcuate lines, sometimes improperly referred to as "struts" *(arrowheads)*. These bilaterally symmetrical, arched, linear-appearing densities represent the arc of the sacral foramina tangent to the central x-ray beam.

anatomy of the sacral foramina. The arcuate lines do not represent a specific cortical edge. Rather, they represent the arc of the superior surface of the sacral foramen that happens to be tangent to the x-ray beam. As described by Jackson et al., the sacral arcuate lines appear as rather sharply defined, superiorly convex curvilinear densities that are broad superomedially and taper gently and smoothly as they extend inferolaterally.[22] The arcuate lines are normally equidistant from each other and are bilaterally symmetrical. Usually, the arcuate lines of only the upper three foramina are visible on the straight AP radiograph of the pelvis.

RADIOGRAPHIC MANIFESTATIONS OF TRAUMA

Pelvic Injuries

Many classifications of pelvic fractures have been proposed. An early classification of pelvic fractures is Kane's modification of the Key-Conwell classification (Table 17.1).[23] A simplified and more inclusive version of the Kane classification of pelvic injuries prepared by the author is found in Table 17.2. The term "injuries" is preferred to "fractures" because

some pelvic injuries are ligamentous disruptions and not fractures (e.g., pubic symphysis separation or SI joint diastasis).

The most widely accepted classification of PRD by orthopedic surgeons is that proposed by Pennal et al.[24] and modified by Tile (Table 17.3).[25,26] More recently, Young et al.[27] have proposed a classification of "pelvic injury" based on pattern of fragment distribution, similar to that of Pennal and Tile, that attempts to relate arterial bleeding to the fracture fragment pattern (Table 17.4).

The classifications of Kane, Pennal, and Tile are predicated on the mechanism of injury as deduced from the position of the fragments of the PRD on the initial AP radiograph (e.g., anteroposterior compression [APC], lateral compression [LC], and vertical shear [VS]). Pennal et al.[24] noted, in proposing this basis for classification of pelvic fractures, that in fully one-third of the patients, the position of the fragments was consistent with more than one of the mechanisms of injury. Further, these classifications—either of pelvic fractures[23] or PRD[24-27]—fail to take into account the work of Chenoweth et al.,[28] Gertzbein and Chenoweth,[29] and Bucholz,[30] which conclusively demonstrate "that an injury at one site of the pelvic ring must be associated with another on the other side of the ring."[28] Furthermore,

TABLE 17.1	Kane's Modification of Key-Conwell Classification of Pelvic Fractures
Type	**Description**
I	Breaks of individual bones not involving the pelvic ring. Includes avulsion fractures of a single ramus, and isolated fractures of the iliac wing, sacrum, or coccyx.
II	Single breaks in the pelvic ring, occurring through both ipsilateral rami, one SI joint, or subluxation of the symphysis pubis. By definition, there can be no displacement; otherwise, a second break in the ring must also be present.
III	Double breaks in the pelvic ring. Includes three subtypes: 1. Malgaigne variants, also called double vertical or dimetric fractures. 2. Bilateral double ramus fractures, referred to as either straddle fractures or butterfly pattern. 3. Severe multiple or crushing fractures.
IV	Acetabular fractures. Includes three subtypes: 1. Rim fractures. 2. Central acetabular fractures. 3. Ischioacetabular fractures.

From Kane WJ. Fractures of the pelvis. In: Rockwood CA, Green DP, eds. *Fractures in Adults.* 2nd ed. Philadelphia, PA: JB Lippincott; 1984:1093–1209 with permission.

TABLE 17.2	Classification of Pelvic Injuries (Harris)

I. Injuries of isolated pelvic bones without disruption of pelvic ring
  A. Avulsion injuries
    1. Anterosuperior iliac spine
    2. Anterorinferior iliac spine
    3. Ischial tuberosity apophysis
    4. (Lesser trochanter apophysis, femur)
  B. Fractures of isolated bones, for example,
    1. Iliac wing (Duverney), pelvic teardrop
    2. Lower sacral segments
    3. Coccyx

II. Pelvic ring disruption
    1. Malgaigne—ipsilateral anterior and posterior arch disruption
    2. "Bucket-handle"—contralateral anterior and posterior arch disruption
    3. "Open-book"
    4. Other combinations of anterior and posterior arch disruption not identified by eponym

III. Insufficiency fracture

IV. Stress fracture

V. Acetabular fracture

TABLE 17.3	Tile Classification of Pelvic Disruption

Type A
Stable

  A1—Fractures of pelvis not involving the ring
  A2—Stable, minimally displaced fractures of the ring

Type B
Rotationally unstable, vertically stable

  B1—Open-book
  B2—Lateral compression; ipsilateral
  B3—Lateral compression; contralateral (bucket-handle)

Type C
Rotationally and vertically unstable

  C1—Unilateral
  C2—Bilateral
  C3—Associated with an acetabular fracture

From Tile M. Pelvis ring fractures: should they be fixed? *J Bone Joint Surg Br.* 1988;70:1, with permission.

TABLE 17.4	Injury Classification According to the Young System

Category	Distinguishing Characteristics[a]
LC	Transverse fracture of pubic rami, ipsilateral, or contralateral to posterior injury I—Sacral compression on side of impact II—Crescent (iliac wing) fracture on side of impact III—LC-I or LC-II injury on side of impact; contralateral open-book (APC) injury
APC	Symphyseal diastasis and/or longitudinal rami fractures I—Slight widening of pubic symphysis and/or anterior SI joint; stretched but intact anterior SI, sacrotuberous, and sacrospinous ligaments; intact posterior SI ligaments II—Widened anterior SI joint; disrupted anterior SI, sacrotuberous, and sacrospinous ligaments; intact posterior SI ligaments III—Complete SI joint disruption with lateral displacement; disrupted anterior SI, sacrotuberous, and sacrospinous ligaments; disrupted posterior ligaments
VS	Symphyseal diastasis or vertical displacement anteriorly and posteriorly, usually through the SI joint, occasionally through the iliac wing and/or sacrum
CM	Combination of other injury patterns, with LC/VS being the most common

[a]LC, lateral compression; APC, anteroposterior compression; SI, sacroiliac; VS, vertical shear; CM, combined mechanisms.
From Young JW, Burgess AR, Brumback RJ, et al. Pelvic fractures: value of plain radiography in early assessment and management. *Radiology.* 1986;160(2):445–451 with permission.

our own experience in the review of 300 initial AP radiographs of patients with PRD confirms that disruption of the anterior pelvic arch by either fracture or pubic symphysis diastasis must be associated with disruption of the posterior arch by either fracture or SI joint diastasis. Consequently, because of the animal and clinical research cited earlier, it is apparent that with the exception of the "insufficiency fracture," stress fracture, or an anterior pelvic arch fracture in a child with unfused TRC, the type II fractures found in Kane's modification of the Key-Conwell classification of pelvic fractures (Table 17.1) (e.g., "single breaks in the pelvic ring, occurring through both ipsilateral rami, one SI joint, or subluxation of the pubic symphysis") simply do not exist following major blunt pelvic trauma.

Although the mechanism of injury classification of PRD has relevance in patient management, it is of little value in the identification of sites of PRD, which is the primary responsibility of the radiologist. Therefore, to facilitate recognition of PRD, we propose a classification of pelvic injuries that reflects the actual pathology of the injury and is based on the investigations of Chenoweth et al.,[28] Gertzbein and Chenoweth,[29] Bucholz,[30] and our own experience. This classification of pelvic injuries, which includes PRD, appears in Table 17.2. Pelvic injuries are discussed in the sequence contained in Table 17.2.

Injuries of Isolated Pelvic Bones Without Disruptions of the Pelvic Ring
Avulsion Injuries
Avulsion injuries of pelvic apophyses are the result of sudden, maximum muscular effort, such as those requiring rapid acceleration (e.g., short-distance runners) or abrupt changes of speed or direction (e.g., football, basketball, soccer, lacrosse players). The athlete usually experiences a sudden sharp pain in the area of the avulsion and a "popping" or "snapping" sensation and is abruptly incapacitated, frequently falling.

Avulsion of the apophysis of the anterosuperior iliac spine (Fig. 17.16) is the result of violent

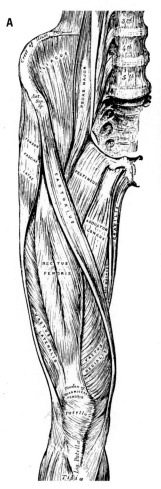
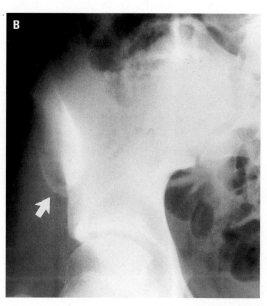

Figure 17.16. Avulsion of the apophysis of the anterosuperior iliac spine. The anatomic drawing (**A**) indicates the origin of the sartorius muscle from the anterior superior iliac spine. The radiograph (**B**) illustrates the common location of the thin, faintly dense, avulsed anterosuperior iliac spine apophysis *(arrow)*.

contraction of the sartorius muscle. This apophysis is a thin piece of bone that is commonly difficult or impossible to see with routine pelvic radiographic technique. The history of the injury is so characteristic that if the avulsed anterior superior iliac spine apophysis is not visible on the routine AP pelvic radiograph, oblique views of the involved hemipelvis should be obtained with reduced ("soft tissue") radiographic technique.

The anteroinferior iliac spine apophysis is avulsed by the intact rectus femoris muscle (Fig. 17.17). This apophysis may be a large, obvious, separate piece of bone or a minimally displaced, small, and subtle fragment (Fig. 17.18). Rarely, both superior and inferior anterior iliac spine apophyses will be avulsed simultaneously (Fig. 17.19). The location and radiographic characteristics of a healed anteroinferior iliac spine avulsion (Fig. 17.20), coupled with a history of childhood "hip" injury, should distinguish this benign, posttraumatic finding from a primary bone neoplasm.

The hamstring muscles arise from the ischial tuberosity and in the adolescent athlete, violent contraction of these muscles results in avulsion of the ischial tuberosity apophysis (Fig. 17.21) rather than in the hamstring "pull" or "tear"

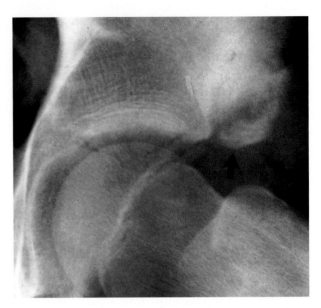

Figure 17.17.   Avulsed anteroinferior iliac spine apophysis *(arrows)*.

commonly seen in more mature athletes. The older the adolescent and the larger the ischial tuberosity apophysis, the easier it will be to identify this injury (Fig. 17.21). When the avulsed apophysis is small and only faintly ossified, as

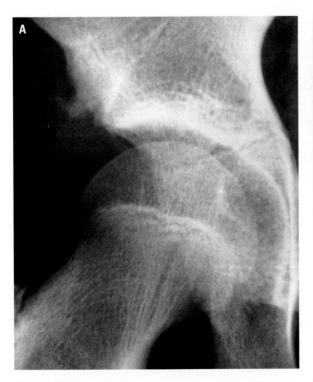
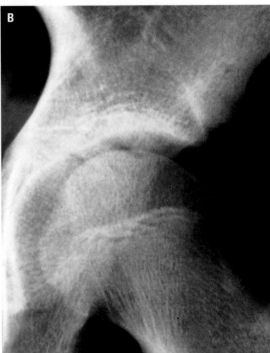

Figure 17.18.   Minimally displaced avulsion of the anteroinferior iliac spine apophysis *(arrow,* **A**). The contralateral normal anterior iliac spine apophysis in this same patient is seen in **B** for comparison.

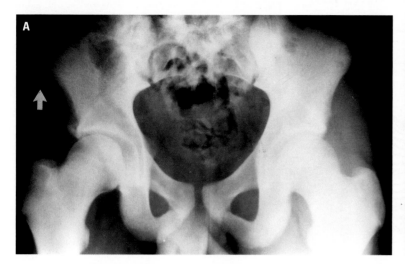

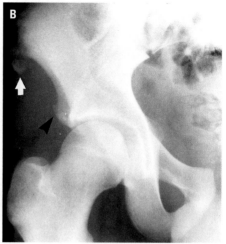

Figure 17.19. Simultaneous avulsion of the right superior *(arrow)* and inferior *(arrowhead)* iliac spine apophyses. Comparison of the inferior iliac spine apophyses in the AP radiograph of the pelvis **(A)** establishes the abnormal appearance on the right side. The avulsed anterosuperior spine apophysis is better demonstrated by using slightly underexposed ("soft tissue") technique **(B)**.

occurs in younger children, the avulsed fragment may be difficult (Fig. 17.22A) or nearly impossible (Fig. 17.22B) to identify radiographically. In the latter circumstance, the diagnosis may be made by recognizing the subtle difference in the appearance of the injured and normal ischial tuberosity (Fig. 17.22B) coupled with the clinical correlation or by magnetic resonance imaging (MRI).

Avulsion of the apophysis of the lesser trochanter of the femur, although not an injury of the pelvis per se, is included here because of the similarity of the clinical presentation and the geographic proximity to the avulsive injuries of the pelvis. As the site of insertion of the iliopsoas muscle, the avulsed lesser trochanteric apophysis will be retracted proximally (Fig. 17.23).

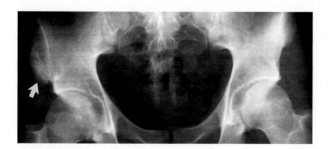

Figure 17.20. Healed avulsion of the anteroinferior iliac spine apophysis *(arrow)*.

Fractures of Isolated Bones of the Pelvis without Pelvic Disruption

The isolated iliac wing fracture (Duverney) that does not disrupt the integrity of the pelvic ring may be comminuted and readily detectable on the straight AP pelvic radiograph (Fig. 17.24) or may be so subtle as to require oblique projections (Fig. 17.25) for identification.

Isolated fractures of the lower sacral and the coccygeal segments are usually the result of a direct blow, as occurs in a fall when the patient lands in a sitting position. The sacral concavity precludes visualization of all sacral segments on a single straight AP radiograph of the pelvis. For adequate examination of the sacrum by plain radiography, frontal projections obtained with the x-ray tube angled cranially and caudally (Fig. 17.26) are required. These projections of the sacrum are very similar to those seen on the inlet and outlet views of the pelvis. However, isolated sacral (and coccygeal) fractures are best evaluated on the lateral projection of the sacrum and coccyx. Because the median sacral crest, which represents the fused sacral spinous processes, is extremely variable in appearance on the lateral radiograph, the detection of sacral fractures is best achieved by recognizing disruption of the anterior and posterior cortices of the fused sacral segments (Fig. 17.27). The presence of a presacral hematoma provides valuable supportive evidence of an acute sacral fracture.

(text continues on page 768)

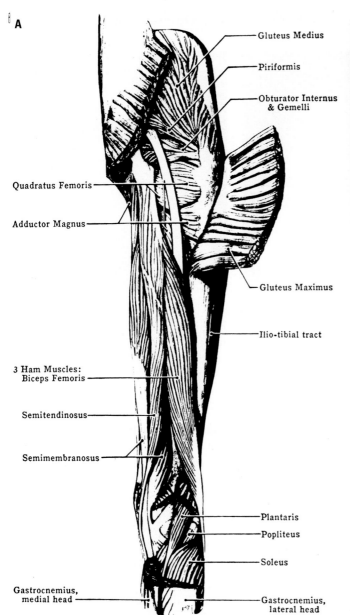

Gluteus Medius

Piriformis

Obturator Internus & Gemelli

Quadratus Femoris

Adductor Magnus

Gluteus Maximus

Ilio-tibial tract

3 Ham Muscles: Biceps Femoris

Semitendinosus

Semimembranosus

Plantaris

Popliteus

Soleus

Gastrocnemius, medial head

Gastrocnemius, lateral head

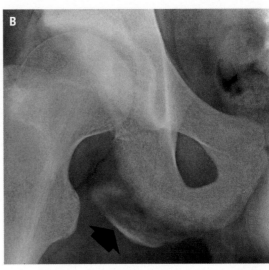

Figure 17.21. A: Anatomic drawing of the muscles of the posterior aspect of the thigh, indicating the site of origin of the hamstring muscles from the ischial tuberosity. **B:** Radiographic appearance of avulsion of a mature iliac spine apophysis *(arrow)*.

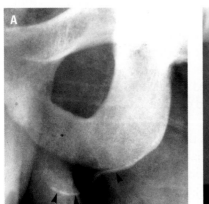
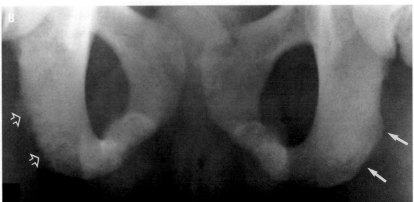

Figure 17.22. A: Partial avulsion *(arrowheads)* of an immature ischial tuberosity apophysis. **B:** The only indication that an extremely immature right ischial tuberosity apophysis has been avulsed is the irregularity of the surface of the right tuberosity *(open arrows)* compared with that of the normal left *(arrows)*.

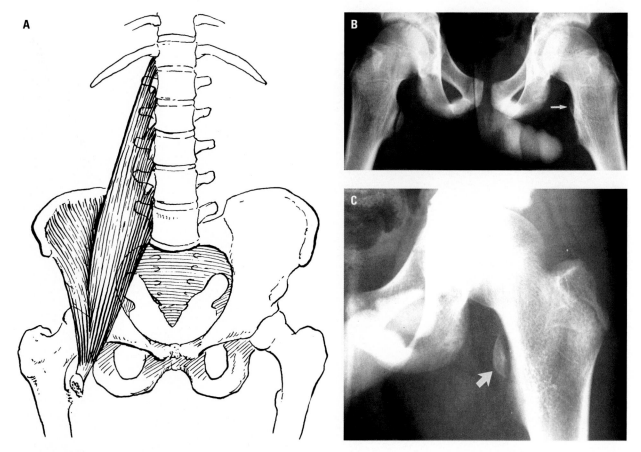

Figure 17.23. **A:** Schematic representation of avulsion of the apophysis of the lesser trochanter of the femur by the iliopsoas muscle. **B:** In the frontal radiograph, the rostrally retracted apophysis *(arrow)* is largely obscured by the femoral neck. **C:** With external rotation of the femur, the displaced apophysis *(arrow)* is clearly visible.

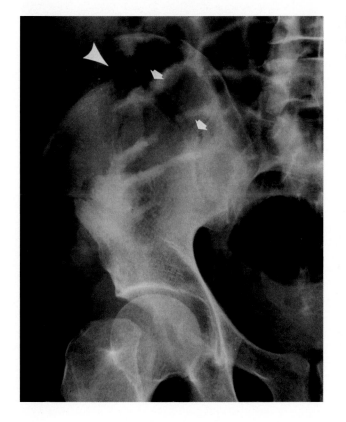

Figure 17.24. Severely comminuted, displaced fracture confined to the iliac wing *(arrow and arrowheads)* that does not disrupt the pelvic ring.

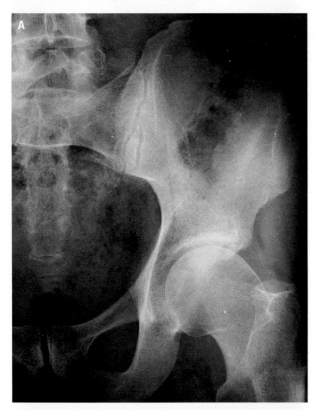

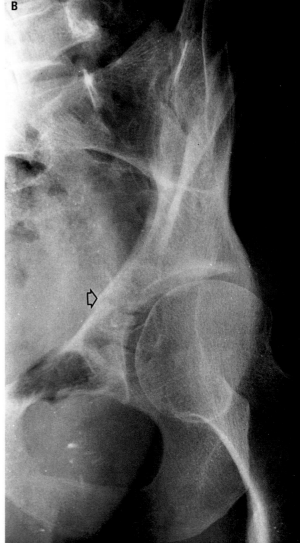

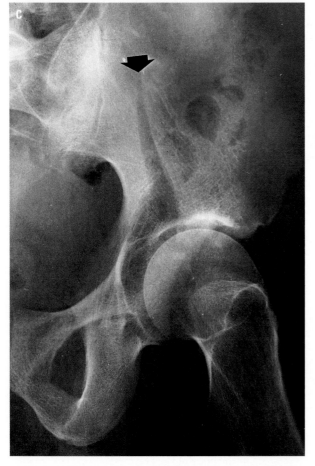

Figure 17.25. The iliac wing fracture line is barely perceptible in the routine frontal projection (**A**). Disruption of the iliopectineal line *(open arrow)* is visible in the anteriorly rotated oblique projection (**B**). Only in the posteriorly rotated oblique projection (**C**) is the extent of the fracture line and separation of the fragments *(arrow)* clearly visualized.

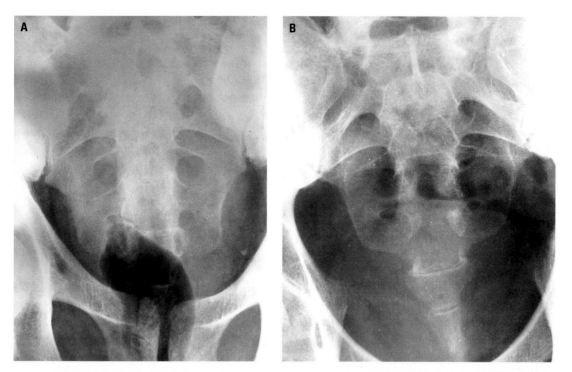

Figure 17.26. The cranially angled frontal projection of the sacrum (**A**) demonstrates the upper sacral segments very clearly, whereas the caudally angled frontal projection (**B**) demonstrates the lower sacral and coccygeal segments.

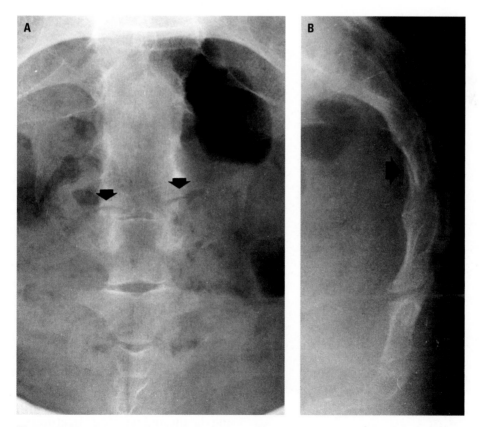

Figure 17.27. In the frontal projection of the sacrum (**A**), segments of the fracture line are indicated by the *arrows*. Because of the proximity of the fracture line to the intersegmental space, the fracture line could be interpreted as a portion of the intersegmental line. In the lateral projection (**B**), however, the fracture in the body of the fourth sacral segment is unambiguously evident *(arrow)*.

The clinical diagnosis is much more reliable than the radiographic diagnosis of sacrococcygeal dislocation and coccygeal fracture. This is because of the normal great variability of the relationship of the coccyx to the last sacral segment and because of the size and configuration of the coccygeal segments.

Pelvic Ring Disruption

PRD is defined as interruption of the normal contour of the perimeter of the plane of the inlet of the true pelvis at two or more sites on opposite sides of the pelvic ring by either fracture or pubic symphyseal or SI joint diastasis. In adults, one or more sites of interruption must occur on opposite sides of the pelvic ring, commonly described as occurring in the anterior and posterior pelvic arches (Fig. 17.12).[28–30] Two caveats pertain to this fundamental tenet. The first is that the pelvic ring may be disrupted at a single site in pediatric patients until fusion of the TRC (Fig. 17.28).[31] The second relates to the coincidence of PRD and acetabular fractures. In our group of 300

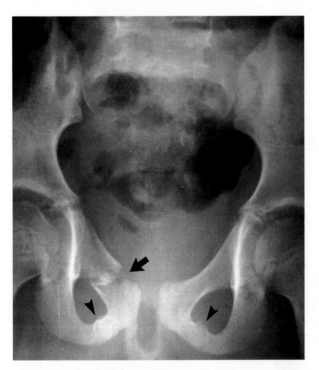

Figure 17.28. The comminuted, slightly displaced fracture of the superior pubic ramus *(arrow)* is the only site of PRD in this 6-year-old child. The bulging ischiopubic synchondroses *(arrowheads)* are normal for a child of this age, and neither should be misinterpreted as a fracture site.

patients with PRD, 41 (13.6%) sustained concurrent acetabular fractures. However, in no instance did the acetabular fracture constitute any component of the PRD. This seeming contradiction—that is, that acetabular fractures are not included as a component of PRD when, indeed, acetabular fractures do interrupt the continuity of the perimeter of the inlet to the true pelvis—is directly related to the definition of PRD, which requires interruption of the continuity of the pelvic ring at two or more sites on opposite sides of the ring. Acetabular fractures fail this definition by involving only one side of the pelvic ring.

The concept of a concomitant PRD and acetabular fracture is illustrated in Figure 17.29. The PRD consists of the comminuted fracture of the left pubic body and inferior ramus coupled with the left sacral alar fracture. The minimally displaced transverse left acetabular fracture is clearly neither the anterior nor the posterior component of the PRD.

As noted earlier, many classifications of pelvic injuries and PRD have been proposed. With respect to PRD, the classifications of Tile[26] (Table 17.3) and of Young et al.[27,32] are probably the most widely accepted. The Tile classification is based on stability or instability of the PRD, which in most instances is a clinical rather than a radiologic diagnosis. The Young classification is based on that of Pennal et al.[24] and Tile and Pennal[33] in which the mechanism of injury—for example, LC, APC, and VS—is determined by the position of the disrupted ring components on the initial AP radiograph. The Young (Table 17.4) classification further divides the LC and APC injuries into subgroups I, II, and III, depending on the degree of ring disruption. Because Pennal found that the pattern or distribution of disrupted ring components could be ascribed to two or more of the mechanisms of injury in approximately one-third of the patients, it seems reasonable that the same would apply to the Young classification. Although the Tile and Young classifications (Tables 17.3 and 17.4, respectively) are of unquestioned value in patient management decisions, neither directly addresses the primary responsibility of the radiologist in the emergency center, namely, the accurate diagnosis of PRD, which is based on detecting the site and type (e.g., fracture or joint diastasis) of the ring disruptions.

Prompted by the fact that 72% of sacral alar fractures were unrecognized by the faculty radiologists of our institution,[22] which meant that PRDs

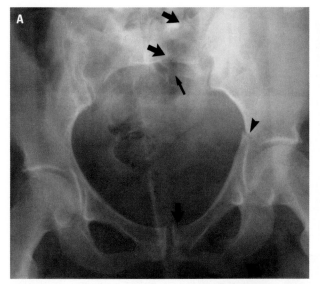

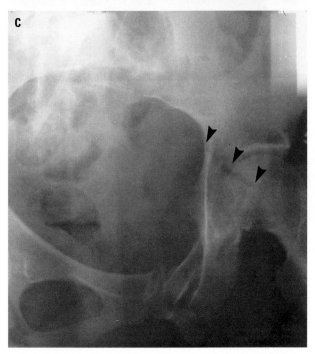

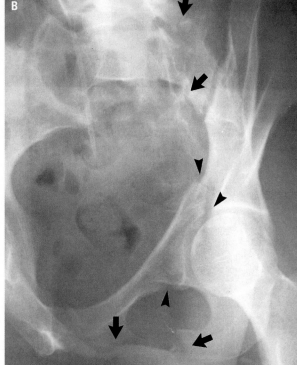

Figure 17.29. Malgaigne PRD with concomitant acetabular fracture in frontal (**A**), left (**B**), and right (**C**) anterior oblique projections. The Malgaigne injury consists of fractures of the left anterior pelvic arch *(arrows)* and the left sacral ala *(arrows, **A and B**)*. *Arrowheads* indicate the transverse left acetabular fracture (**A–C**).

were misdiagnosed in the same degree and stimulated by the work of Chenoweth et al.,[28] the work of Gertzbein and Chenoweth,[29] and the autopsy findings of Bucholz[30] and frustrated by the radiologic diagnostic shortcomings of the Pennal and the Tile classifications of PRD, members of our department retrospectively reviewed the initial AP pelvic radiographs of 300 consecutive adult patients admitted to Hermann Hospital with PRD between January 1983 and December 1987 in the hope of developing a system of pattern recognition of PRD that would enhance and facilitate the plain radiograph diagnosis of

PRD. The changes in contour, spatial relationships, and symmetry of the sacral arcuate lines caused by acute trauma (Fig. 17.30) as described by Jackson et al.[22] were invaluable in the recognition of sacral alar fractures. Although we were well aware that the type of PRD (e.g., fracture or joint diastasis) is of great clinical significance, the type of ring disruption was considered immaterial for the purely diagnostic purposes of this study. Our method consisted of recording the sites of disruption on a schematic representation of the pelvic ring divided into anterior and posterior arches at the level of the ischial

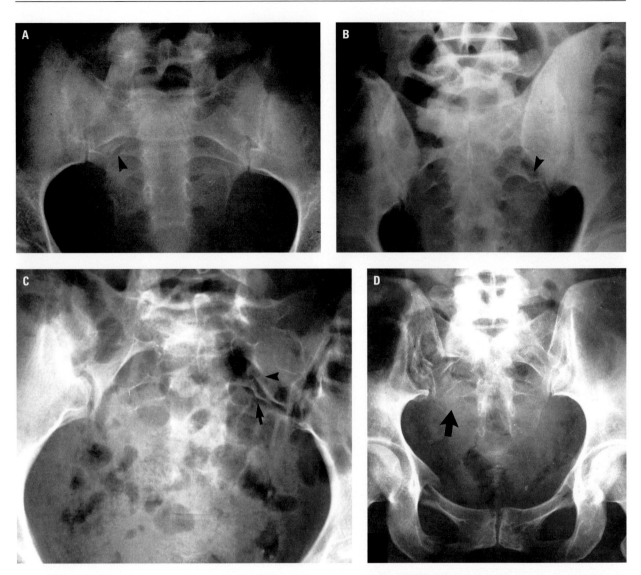

Figure 17.30. Some examples of subtle alterations in the appearance of the sacral arcuate lines caused by alar fractures. The arcuate line(s) may be obviously fractured (*arrowhead*, **A**), angulated (*arrowhead*, **B**), displaced and crowded (*arrowhead*, **A and C**), and/or angulated (*arrow*, **C**), or asymmetric (*arrow*, **A and D**).

spines (Fig. 17.12). Ipsilateral superior and inferior pubic rami fractures were considered a single site of disruption, as was pubic diastasis with associated fracture. In the posterior pelvic arch, SI joint diastasis, fracture diastasis, or iliac or sacral alar fractures on the same side were considered a single site of ring disruption.

Inlet and outlet views, which may be obtained easily and quickly in the emergency center, are very helpful in confirming the presence of minimally displaced disruptions involving the anterior pelvic arch or of sacral alar fractures obscured by intestinal content (Fig. 17.31). CT, if immediately available and if the patient's condition will permit, provides

very distinct delineation of fractures not visualized on the plain radiographs and very clearly delineates the extent of sacral fractures (Fig. 17.31).

Abnormal prominence or bulging of the obturator internus muscle or its aponeurosis (Fig. 17.32) caused by underlying hemorrhage may be the most striking sign of a subtle superior pubic ramus fracture component of a minimally displaced PRD.[34]

Our analysis of PRDs in the 300 AP pelvic radiographs resulted in the emergence of five distinct patterns of disruption, which we arbitrarily designated as types I through IV (Fig. 17.33). We hasten to disclaim any attempt to propose yet another classification of PRD. As with midfacial fractures where

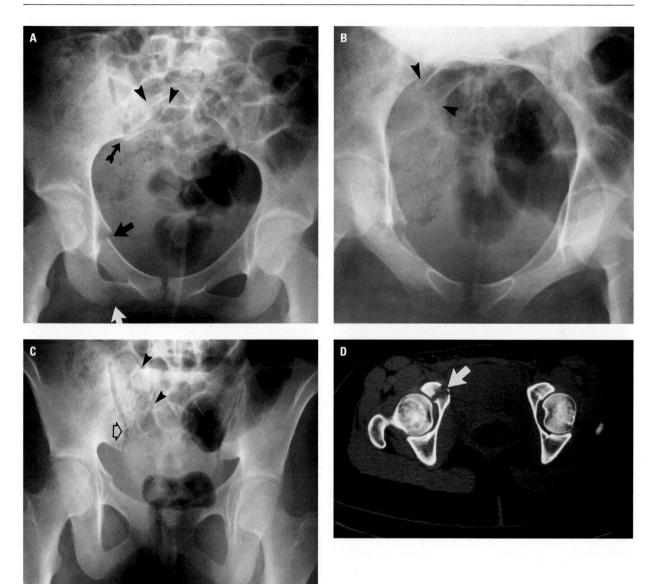

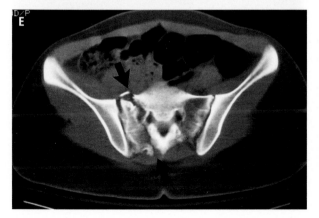

Figure 17.31. Minimally displaced Malgaigne (type I) PRD. *Arrows* indicate the right anterior arch fractures. The slightly diastatic right SI joint *(feathered arrow)* and the abnormal right sacral arcuate lines *(arrowheads)* that are obscured by intestinal content constitute the posterior arch component in the frontal pelvic radiograph (**A**). The inlet view (**B**) clearly demonstrates the right sacral alar fracture *(arrowheads)*, and the outlet view (**C**) confirms the right SI joint diastasis *(open arrow)* and right alar fracture *(arrowheads)*. Axial CT demonstrates the magnitude of separation of the fragments of the fracture at the junction of the superior pubic ramus and ischium *(arrow,* **D**) as well as the extent of the right sacral alar fracture *(arrows,* **E**).

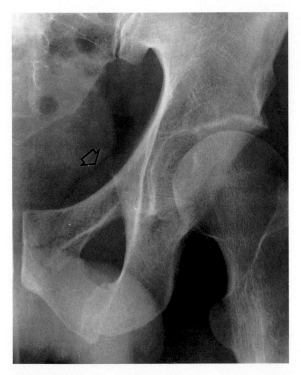

Figure 17.32. Bulging aponeurosis *(open arrow)* of the obturator internus muscle is an indirect sign of a subtle superior pubic ramus fracture.

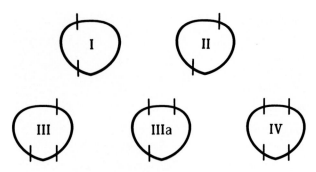

Figure 17.33. Schematic representation of patterns of pelvic ring disruption.

injury detection is greatly facilitated if the observer knows the patterns of fracture distribution, so with PRD an awareness of the sites of disruption facilitates PRD detection, particularly when the injuries are subtle.

The type I pattern of PRD (39%) (Fig. 17.34) consisted of ipsilateral anterior and posterior arch disruptions (e.g., the Malgaigne injury).[35] If the only anterior arch disruption was pubic symphysis diastasis associated with a single site of posterior arch

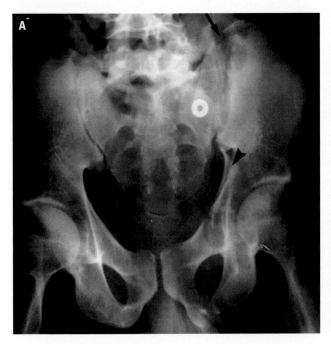
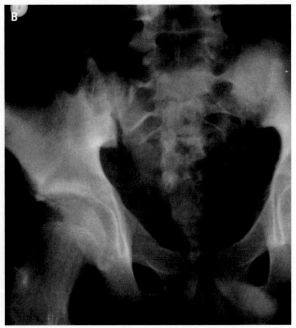

Figure 17.34. Malgaigne (type I) PRD. **A:** The obvious example consists of a comminuted left anterior arch fracture *(arrowheads)* and posterior left SI joint fracture diastasis *(arrows)*. In this example, the large left hemipelvic fragment, including the hip joint, is rostrally displaced as described by Malgaigne. **B:** A much more subtle Malgaigne injury, consisting of ipsilateral, minimally displaced fractures of the right superior pubic ramus and body *(arrowheads)* and a right SI fracture separation *(arrow)*. The sacral alar fracture is evidenced by angulation, asymmetry, and crowding of the right alar arcuate lines.

disruption, this pattern of injury was included in the Malgaigne (type I) group (Fig. 17.35).

The type II pattern (13.5%) (Fig. 17.36) consisted of contralateral anterior and posterior sites of disruption (e.g., the "bucket-handle" injury). The anterior component of the type II PRD must be fracture of the margins of the obturator foramen on the side opposite the posterior disruption. A concomitant bucket-handle and acetabular fracture is clearly depicted by three-dimensional (3-D) CT (Fig. 17.37). Figure 17.38 illustrates a subtle bucket-handle fracture coexistent with an obvious central acetabular fracture. This PRD is an excellent illustration of the application of the "opposite-side" concept of PRD in the identification of PRD and the significance of subtle alterations in the sacral arcuate lines in the detection and recognition of sacral alar fractures. The right anterior pubic arch fractures are obvious. The opposite-side concept demands careful examination of the posterior pelvic arch for the second component of the PRD. Recognition of

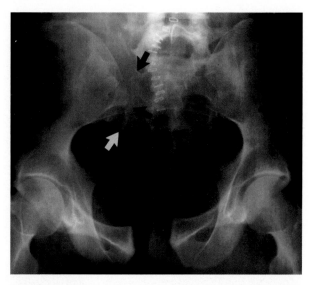

Figure 17.35. "Open-book" (type I) PRD. The pubic symphyseal diastasis is associated with a distracted right sacral alar fracture *(arrows)*. Because the pubic diastasis is midline, the pattern of pubic symphyseal diastasis and unilateral posterior arch disruption was arbitrarily assigned to the type I PRD injury pattern.

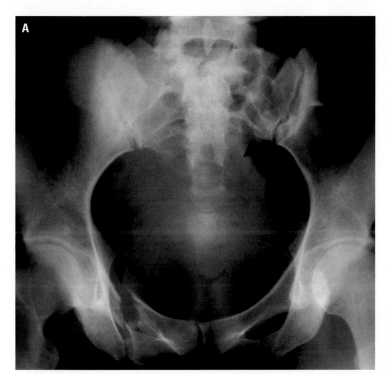

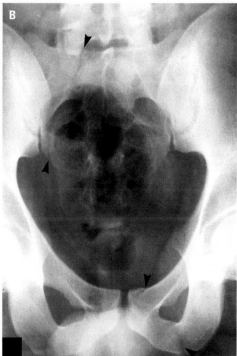

Figure 17.36. "Bucket-handle" (type II) PRD. **A:** The typical configuration of contralateral anterior and posterior sites of PRD *(arrowheads)* is clearly evident. The right sacral alar fracture is evidenced by disruption, angulation, and crowding of the arcuate lines. **B:** A much more subtle bucket-handle PRD in a different patient, consisting of left anterior arch and right sacral alar fractures *(arrowheads)*.

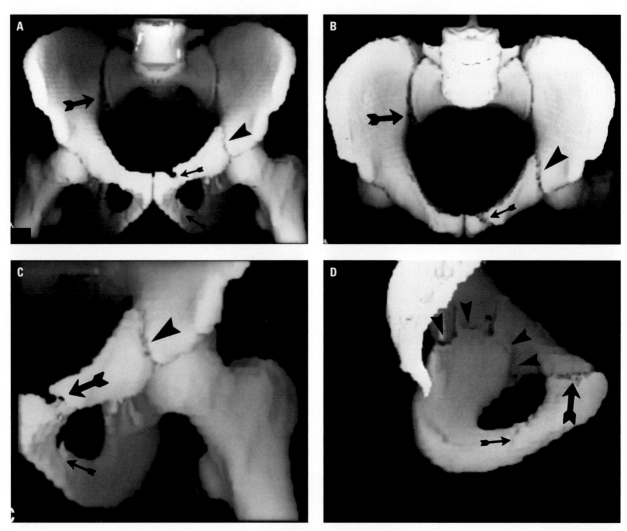

Figure 17.37. Concomitant bucket-handle (type II) PRD consisting of left anterior arch fracture and right SI joint diastasis *(arrows)* and left acetabular fracture *(arrowheads)* demonstrated by 3-D CT. The relationship of the PRD and left acetabular fracture is clearly seen in the straight AP **(A)** and inlet **(B)** 3-D CT images. The AP 3-D CT image of the left hip **(C)** clearly depicts the distinction between the anterior component of the PRD *(arrows)* and the anterior extent of the transverse acetabular fracture *(arrowhead)*. **D** is a 3-D CT image of the internal surface of the left hemipelvis that demonstrates the anterior component of the PRD *(arrows)* and the distribution of the transverse acetabular fracture *(arrowheads)* through the extent of the quadrilateral plate.

the subtle changes of the left sacral arcuate lines identifies and establishes the contralateral posterior component of the type II PRD.

The classic "open-book" type of PRD is the result of blunt APC of the pelvis, which typically results in pubic symphyseal separation and lateral rotation of the hemipelvis (Fig. 17.39). This type of PRD derives its name from the similarity of the appearance of the pubic symphyseal diastasis to that of a partially open book. The typical pathology is

ligamentous, consisting of separation of the pubic symphysis and one (Fig. 17.39) or both (Fig. 17.40) SI joints. With respect to the SI joints, the vector force causes disruption of the anterior SI ligaments and reciprocal compression of the posterior ligaments. Consequently, even though the pubic symphyseal diastasis is usually readily apparent, the SI joint separation may be subtle and only detected or confirmed by CT (Figs. 17.40A and B). The mechanism of injury of the open-book PRD commonly

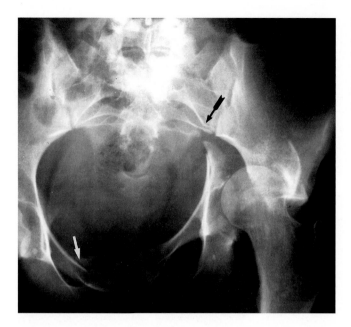

Figure 17.38. Subtle bucket-handle (type II) PRD and concomitant displaced central acetabular fracture. The right anterior pelvic arch fractures *(arrows)* are obvious. Very subtle alterations in contour and continuity of the left arcuate lines *(arrow)* establish the left sacral alar fracture.

includes an element of vertical shear, resulting in cephalic as well as lateral displacement of the involved hemipelvis (Figs. 17.41 and 17.42). In this instance, not only will the SI joint be opened anteriorly but also the iliac component of the joint will be displaced upward with respect to its sacral counterpart, thereby disrupting the continuity of the inferior margins of the SI joint and the posterior SI ligaments. When such discontinuity is

minimal, it may be easily overlooked. Application of the opposite-side concept of sites of disruption of the pelvic ring should force a diligent search for subtle other sites of PRD.

There is no relation between the degree of pubic symphyseal separation and lower urinary tract injury. This is particularly true with respect to urethral injury, where even minor separation may be associated with any type of urethral injury

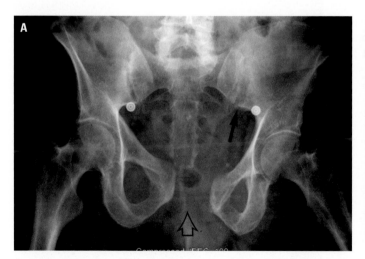
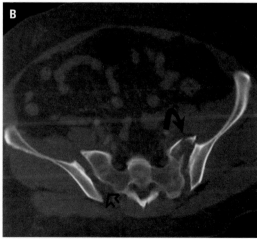

Figure 17.39. Open-book PRD. The AP radiograph of the pelvis (**A**) shows the pubic symphysis diastasis *(open arrow)* and separation of the left SI joint *(arrow)*. CT of the pelvis (**B**) demonstrates the right SI diastasis *(open arrow)* not apparent on the AP radiograph, as well as a left sacral alar fracture *(curved arrow)*, also not apparent on the AP radiograph.

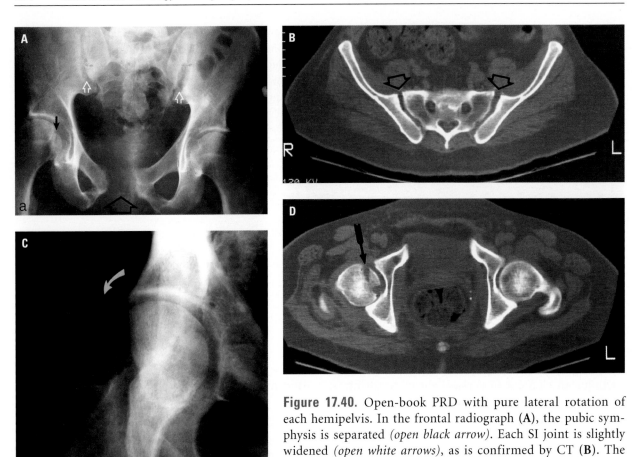

Figure 17.40. Open-book PRD with pure lateral rotation of each hemipelvis. In the frontal radiograph (**A**), the pubic symphysis is separated *(open black arrow)*. Each SI joint is slightly widened *(open white arrows)*, as is confirmed by CT (**B**). The patient also sustained a concomitant right posterior acetabular lip fracture *(curved arrow, **C**)* and a right femoral head fracture *(arrows, **A** and **D**)*.

Figure 17.41. Open-book PRD with vertical shear. Cephalad displacement of the right hemipelvis is indicated by pubic symphyseal asymmetry *(open arrow)* and minor upward displacement of the iliac component *(closed arrow)* in relation to the sacral component *(arrowhead)* of the SI joint. Compare this relationship with the comparable normal anatomy on the left.

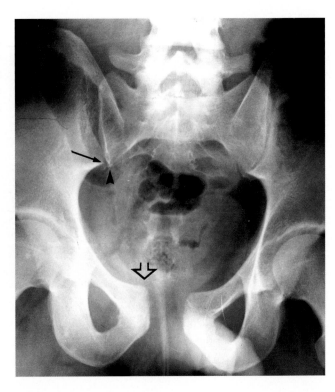

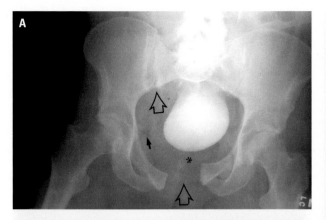

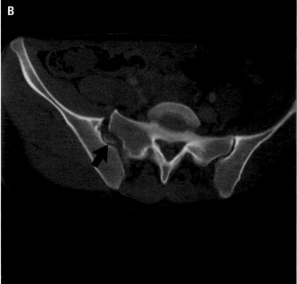

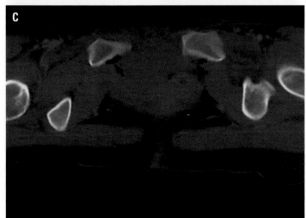

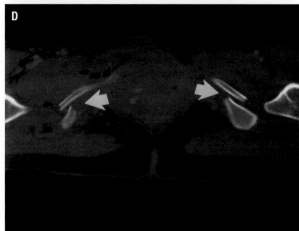

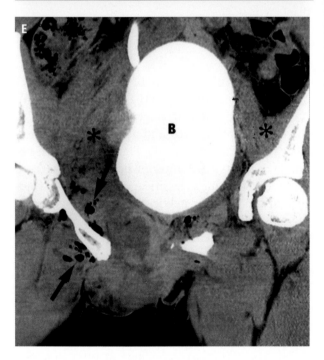

Figure 17.42. Open-book PRD with large extraperitoneal, perivesical hematoma and subcutaneous emphysema. The soft tissue open-book PRD (*open arrows*) is clearly evident on the AP radiograph. The *asterisk*, with an intact urinary bladder, indicates the perivesicle hematoma. The *solid arrow* indicates right-sided extrapelvic air (**A**). Axial CT images of the pelvis (**B–D**) indicate a concomitant right sacral fracture (**B**, *arrow*) and extensive pelvis and extra pelvic subcutaneous emphysema (**C**, *arrows*). (**D**) Inferior pubic rami fractures (*arrows*). The postinfusion cystogram (**E**) shows the hourglass configuration of the urinary bladder (*B*), the perivesicle hematoma (*asterisks*), and the intrapelvic and extrapelvic subcutaneous emphysema (*arrows*).

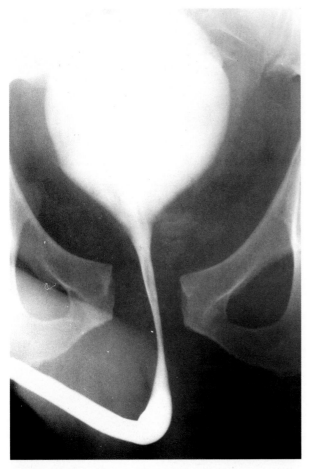

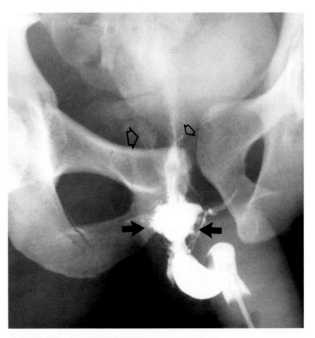

Figure 17.44. Minimal pubic symphyseal separation and a concomitant type III urethral injury demonstrated by retrograde urethrography. The type III urethral injury is characterized by the contrast medium extravasated through the posterior urethral tear both above *(open arrows)* and below *(closed arrows)* the urogenital diaphragm indicating disruption of the urogenital diaphragm.

Figure 17.43. Open-book PRD with moderate pubic diastasis associated with a large periurethral hematoma (type I urethral injury) that attenuated and narrowed the urethral lumen by tamponade on retrograde urethrography.

(Figs. 17.43 and 17.44). Conversely, the urethra is frequently intact in the presence of a clinically or radiographically unstable open-book PRD (Fig. 17.45).

The open-book PRD may present in any of the ring disruption configurations shown in Figure 17.33. The open-book PRD, because of the frequently associated extensive pelvic soft tissue injuries, is the most serious and complex of all PRDs.

The type III pattern (7%) of PRD consisted of two sites of disruption of the anterior pelvic arch and one site of disruption posteriorly. This pattern of PRD sites appeared in different variations but always with two sites of disruption anteriorly and only one posteriorly. One variety included fractures of each side of the anterior pelvic arch in

conjunction with a fracture of the posterior aspect of the iliac wing adjacent to the SI joint (Fig. 17.46). A second consisted of fractures of each side of the anterior pelvic arch and a sacral alar fracture (Fig. 17.47). Parenthetically, Figure 17.47 is an example of the type of anterior pelvic arch fracture referred to in Kane's classification as "isolated fracture of the anterior pelvic arch." This inaccurate diagnosis is the result of failure to recognize alterations of the sacral arcuate lines as representing the posterior pelvic arch sacral alar fracture. A third variation of the type III pattern of PRD is seen in Figure 17.48 in which the anterior component includes a unilateral arch fracture and pubic symphyseal separation in conjunction with a SI joint separation posteriorly.

The type IIIa pattern (8.5%) of PRD sites was the opposite of that just described as type III, namely, a single site of disruption in the anterior arch and two in the posterior pelvic arch. An "all-bone" variety of the type IIIa pattern is seen in Figure 17.49. An example of a type IIIa pattern

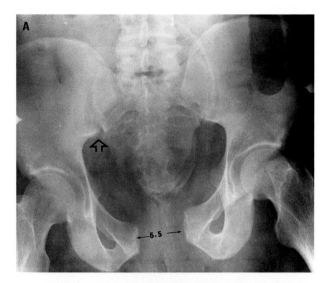

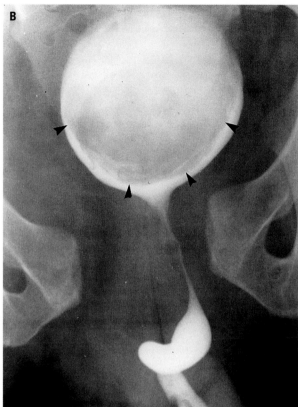

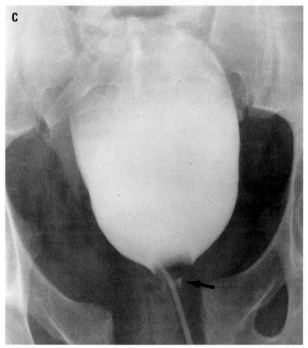

Figure 17.45. Pubic symphysis diastasis without urethral injury. The AP radiograph of the pelvis (**A**) shows an open-book PRD with 5.5-cm diastasis of the pubic symphysis and widening of the SI joint *(open arrow)* in a male patient. The retrograde urethrogram (**B**) demonstrates an intact urethra but a large blood clot *(arrowheads)* in the bladder, which resulted from the tear *(arrow)* at the base of the bladder demonstrated on the cystogram (**C**).

in which all sites of disruption are ligamentous injuries (e.g., pubic symphyseal and bilateral SI diastasis) is seen in Figure 17.40. The value of CT, and particularly of 3-D CT, as the definitive imaging study not only in the detection of the full extent of subtle PRDs but also of the spatial relationships of the PRD fragments, is demonstrated in type IIIa PRDs (Fig. 17.50).

The pattern of PRD characterized by two sites of disruption in both the anterior and the posterior arch was designated type IV (22%). As with all the other patterns of PRD sites, the disruption could be represented either by a fracture or by separation or fracture separation of the pubic symphysis or SI joint on CT. Figures 17.51 and 17.52 are some examples of type IV PRD. Figure 17.51 is an "all-fracture" variety with fractures of each side of the anterior arch and bilateral sacral alar fractures. In Figure 17.52, the anterior sites of disruption include pubic symphysis separation and fractures of the left anterior pelvic arch. The posterior sites include a right iliac wing fracture and left SI joint separation.

The importance of CT and 3-D CT in identification of the sites of PRD and of the spatial

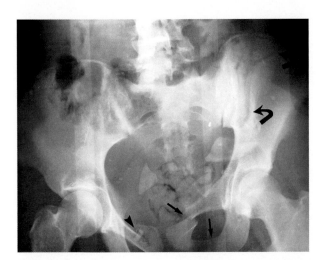

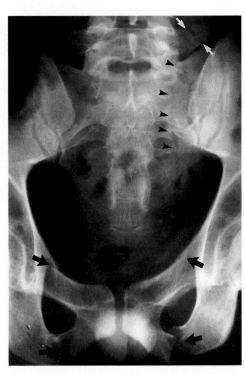

Figure 17.46. Type III pattern of PRD. The right pubic body fracture *(arrowhead)* and the left superior and inferior pubic rami fractures *(straight arrows)* constitute the anterior components, whereas the comminuted fracture of the left iliac wing *(curved arrows)* adjacent to the SI joint constitutes the posterior arch component.

Figure 17.47. Type III PRD characterized by bilateral anterior pelvic arch fractures *(black arrows)* and left sacral alar fracture *(arrowheads)*. Failure to recognize the subtle signs of the posterior arch disruption (alar fracture) gave rise to the incorrect concept of a "double vertical" fracture. The left transverse process of L5 is also fractured *(white arrows)*.

Figure 17.48. Type III pattern of PRD in which the two anterior sites of disruption include a right arch fracture *(arrowheads)* and pubic diastasis *(open arrow)*, and the single posterior site is a left SI joint fracture-separation *(closed arrows)*.

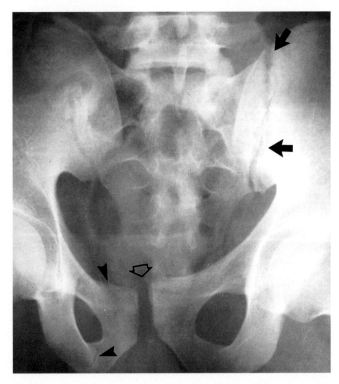

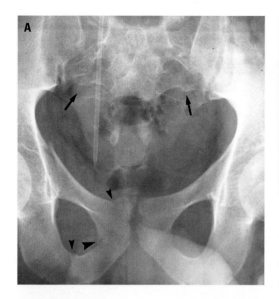

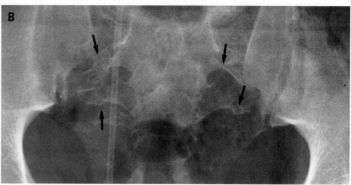

Figure 17.49. A and B: All-bone variety of type IIIa PRD. The minimally displaced fractures of the right anterior pelvic arch *(arrowheads)* represent the single site of anterior pelvic arch disruption. The two sites of posterior arch disruption are the bilateral alar fractures *(arrows)*.

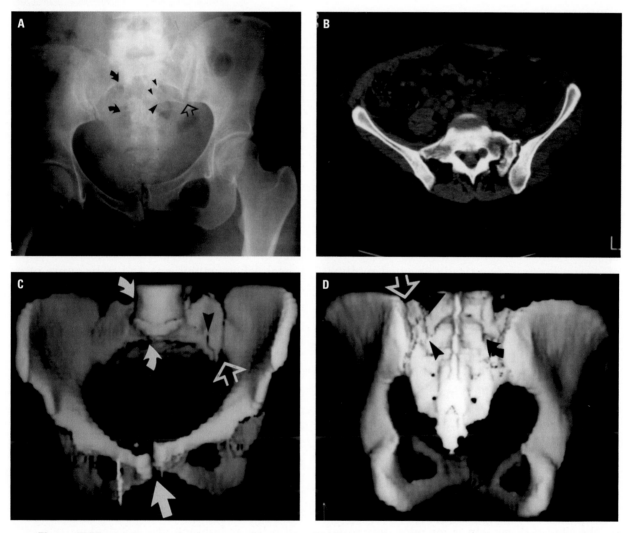

Figure 17.50. Subtle, mixed soft tissue and bone type IIIa PRD confirmed by CT. **A:** In the frontal radiograph of the pelvis, the pubic symphyseal separation *(straight arrow)* is the only site of anterior arch disruption. Posteriorly, the left sacral alar fracture *(arrowheads)* and SI joint diastasis *(open arrow)* are obvious. The second site of posterior disruption involves the right sacral ala *(curved arrows)* and is very subtle. **B:** The left sacral fracture and SI joint diastasis are clearly evident in the axial CT image. **C:** The frontal 3-D CT image demonstrates all sites of disruption and very clearly depicts the abnormal spatial relationships at the diastatic left SI joint. **D:** In the posterior 3-D CT image, the comminuted right sacral fracture *(curved arrow)* is readily apparent.

Figure 17.51. Type IV PRD consisting of bilateral anterior pelvic arch fractures *(curved arrows)* and bilateral sacral alar fractures *(arrowheads)*. Failure to recognize the sacral alar fractures could lead to the erroneous impression that the patient had sustained a "double vertical" or "straddle" fracture limited only to the anterior pelvic arch.

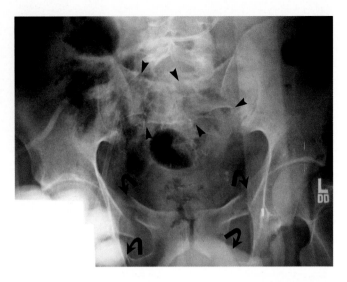

relationships of the PRD components is again emphasized by the type IV PRD illustrated in Figure 17.53. The AP, inlet, and outlet radiographs of the pelvis indicate all of the sites of pelvic disruption except for the right SI joint separation that is clearly depicted on both the axial and 3-D CT images. The 3-D images eliminate ambiguity relative to the spatial relationships of the disrupted pelvic ring components.

In this analysis of PRD, we encountered a few instances of PRD in which the posterior arch site of disruption was a vertically oriented midline fracture of the sacrum. This fracture site may be difficult to identify if its fragments are only minimally displaced (Fig. 17.54). Figure 17.55 is an example of a midline sacral fracture and pubic symphysis separation. This combination of injuries does not fall into any of the five PRD types described earlier. The PRD in which the posterior arch component is a single midline sacral fracture falls into either the type I pattern if the anterior component is a unilateral anterior arch fracture or the type III pattern if bilateral anterior arch fractures are present.

As stated at the outset of this discussion of PRD, the concept of determining the type of PRD based on the sites of disruption is intended only to facilitate the identification of PRD. This system also forces the observer to acknowledge the basic tenet of PRD, namely, that if the anterior pelvic arch is disrupted by major blunt trauma, the posterior pelvic arch will be disrupted in at least one site. This system also emphasizes the significance of alterations in the

sacral arcuate lines as being indicative of sacral alar fractures.

Massive PRD, most commonly of the open-book variety, with or without rostral displacement, may be associated with a perineal laceration that is frequently clinically unrecognized because of the difficulty in examining the perineum by direct inspection. A perineal laceration is usually associated with extraperitoneal emphysema within the pelvis (Fig. 17.56). It is critically important for the radiologist to recognize extraperitoneal pelvic emphysema and to be aware of its clinical significance. Perineal laceration usually mandates a diverting colostomy that should be performed very early in the definitive management of the patient.

The stability of PRD is, in most instances, a clinical assessment rather than a radiographic determination. Tile[26] has defined radiologic criterion of PRD instability as rostral displacement of the iliac component of the SI joint greater than 1.5 cm (Fig. 17.57). If the PRD components are grossly displaced (Fig. 17.58), the radiographic determination of instability is obvious. The inherent difficulty in assessing PRD stability (or instability) radiographically is that the initial pelvic radiograph may not demonstrate PRD instability when the pelvis is, indeed, unstable (Figs. 17.59 and 17.60).

The stability of the pelvis is contingent on the integrity of its skeletal and ligamentous components. Clearly, a PRD may be unstable because of marked displacement of pelvic fracture fragments

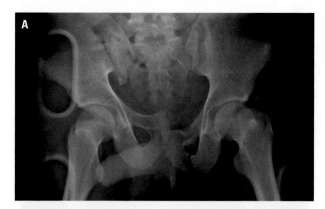

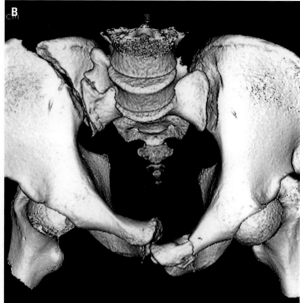

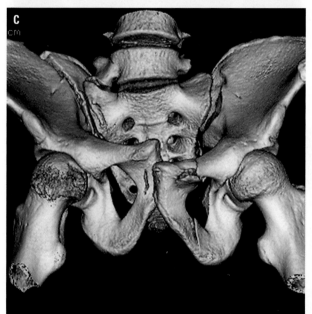

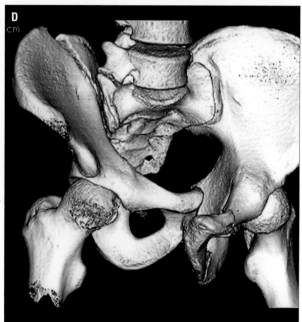

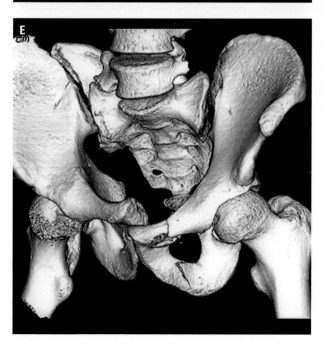

Figure 17.52. Mixed osseous and soft tissue Type IV pelvic ring disruption. The anteroposterior radiograph of the pelvis (**A**) shows two anterior ring sites of disruption—pubic symphysis diastasis and left anterior obturator ring fractures and two posterior sites, right iliac wing fracture and left SI joint disruption. The 3-D CT inlet view (**B**) confirms the findings on the conventional radiograph. The 3-D CT outlet view (**C**) seems to indicate a left iliac wing fracture rather than a left superior iliac joint diastasis. The right and left 3-D CT oblique projections (**D and E**) respectively, however, confirm that the left SI joint is diastatic and without a left wing fracture.

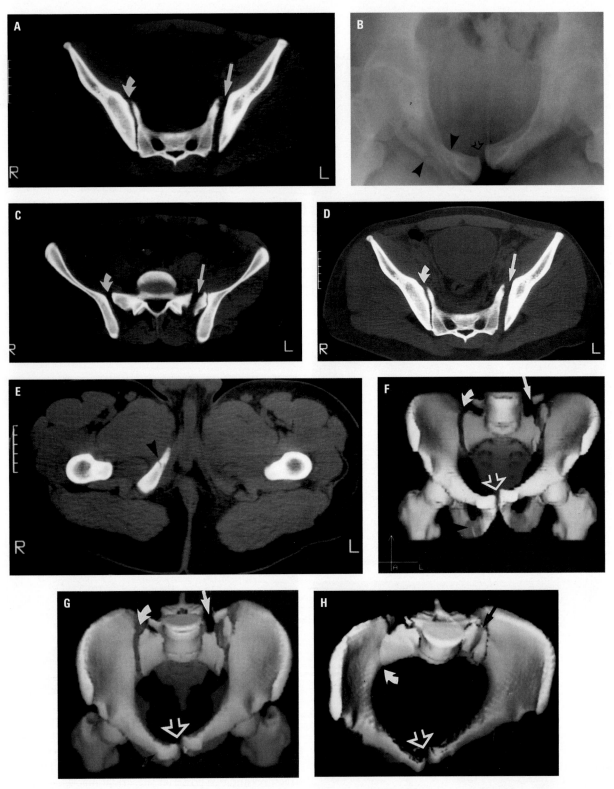

Figure 17.53. The value and role of 3-D CT in imaging PRD are well demonstrated in this subtle type IV injury. The very subtle right anterior pelvic arch fracture *(arrowheads)*, not visible on the AP radiograph of the pelvis (**A**), is well established on the inlet view (**B**). The second anterior arch site of disruption, the pubic diastasis *(open arrow)*, is evident on both AP (**A**) and inlet (**B**) views. Of the two posterior sites of disruption, the left SI joint separation-alar fracture *(straight arrows)* is easily recognized, but the right SI joint separation *(curved arrow)* could easily be overlooked. Axial CT clearly demonstrates the bilateral SI joint diastasis and the left sacral alar fracture (**C and D**) and confirms the right inferior pubic ramus fracture *(arrowhead,* **E**). The 3-D CT images in frontal (**F**), inlet (**G**), and exaggerated inlet (**H**) projections clearly depict all sites of pelvic ring disruption and demonstrate the posterior sites, their pathology, and the spatial relations of their components without ambiguity.

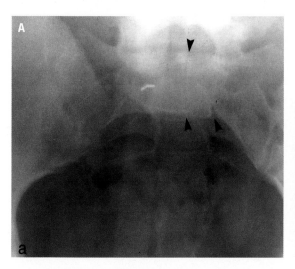
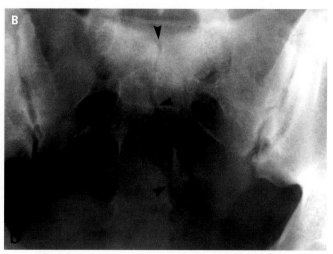

Figure 17.54. The midline sacral fracture *(arrowheads)* is barely perceptible in the straight AP projection of the pelvis (**A**) but is clearly evident in the rostrally angled AP of the sacrum (**B**).

(Fig. 17.58). Pelvic ring stability related primarily to ligamentous disruption is much more difficult to assess radiographically, contrary to the commonly held belief that pubic diastasis greater than 2.5 cm is a radiographic sign of skeletal instability.[36–38] Knowledge of the anatomy of the major pelvic ligaments and an understanding of the ligamentous pathophysiology caused by the vector forces of APC and VS, which are the usual causes of open-book PRD, constitute the basis of the more logical radiographic signs of instability related to the SI joint and defined by Tile.[26]

The sacrospinous, sacrotuberous, anterior and posterior SI, SI interosseous ligaments and the arcuate ligament of the pubic symphysis all contribute to pelvic stability (Figs. 17.61–17.64). The anterior SI ligaments, being relatively thin, and the sacrospinous ligaments, because of their short and anteriorly directed orientation, are not

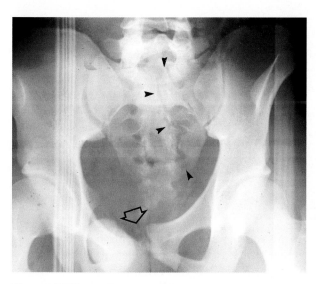

Figure 17.55. Midline sacral fractures *(arrowheads)* associated with pubic symphysis separation *(open arrow)*.

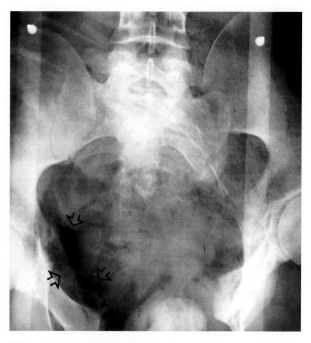

Figure 17.56. The massive extraperitoneal perivesical emphysema *(open arrows)* is indicative of a peroneal laceration in this patient with a markedly displaced open-book PRD.

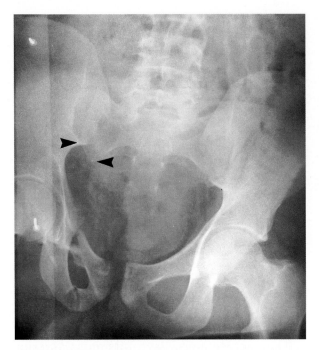

Figure 17.57. Unstable Malgaigne (type I) PRD. The large right hemipelvic fragment containing the hip joint meets the definition of a Malgaigne PRD. Posterior or rostral displacement of the separate fragment greater than 1.5 cm measured at the inferior margin of the SI joint *(arrowheads)* meets the Tile[26] criterion of instability.

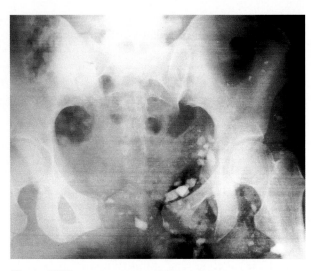

Figure 17.58. Radiographically unstable open-book pelvic ring disruption with both lateral and rostral rotation of the entire left hemipelvis. Perivesical subcutaneous emphysema indicates a peroneal laceration. The irregular densities are gravel and road dirt.

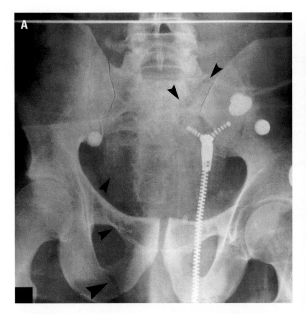

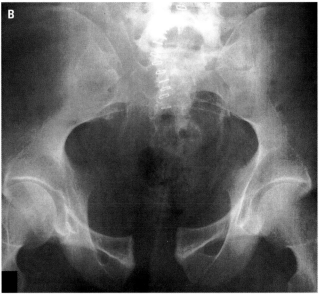

Figure 17.59. **A:** The initial AP radiograph of the pelvis of this patient wearing military antishock trousers (MAST) reveals a minimally displaced pelvic ring disruption *(arrowheads)* that, by radiologic criteria, is stable. **B:** After removal of the MAST suit postoperatively, the pelvic instability is obvious.

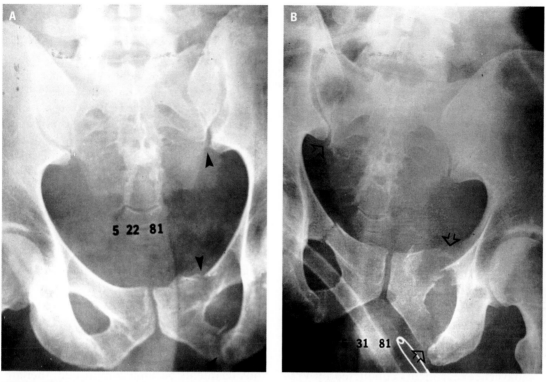

Figure 17.60. Radiographically falsely stable PRD. **A:** The initial AP radiograph of the pelvis demonstrates a minimally displaced left Malgaigne PRD disruption *(arrowheads)*. There is nothing on this examination to suggest that the pelvic ring is unstable. **B:** On the frontal examination obtained approximately 9 days later, there has been a marked shift in the position of the right hemipelvis as a result of instability of the left anterior pelvic arch fractures and the right SI joint diastasis *(open arrows)*.

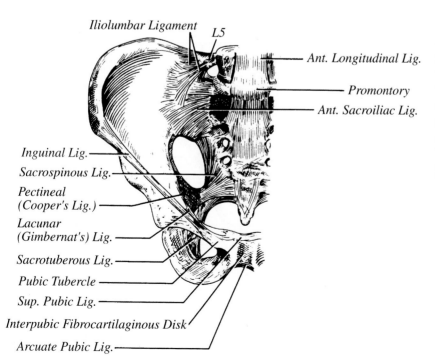

Figure 17.61. Schematic representation of the major pelvic ligaments as seen from the front. Of these, the sacrospinous and sacrotuberous are the most important. *ant.*, anterior; *lig.*, ligament; *sup.*, superior. (From Pansky B. *Review of Gross Anatomy.* 4th ed. New York, NY: Macmillan; 1979, with permission.)

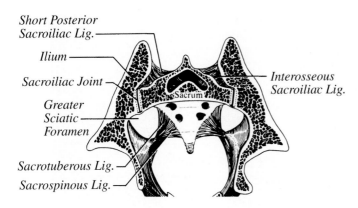

Short Posterior Sacroiliac Lig.

Ilium

Sacroiliac Joint

Greater Sciatic Foramen

Sacrotuberous Lig.

Sacrospinous Lig.

Sacrum

Interosseous Sacroiliac Lig.

Figure 17.62. Schematic representation of the pelvic inlet as seen earlier to illustrate the locations of the short posterior SI and the interosseous SI ligaments, which are extremely important in pelvic stability. Obviously, in an open-book type of pelvic ring disruption, those ligaments will be compressed rather than disrupted unless there is a concomitant vertical shear component to the mechanism of injury. *lig.*, ligament (From Pansky B. *Review of Gross Anatomy.* 4th ed. New York, NY: Macmillan; 1979, with permission.)

major factors in pelvic ring stability. Conversely, the long, thick sacrotuberous ligaments, the very densely intertwined long posterior SI ligaments, and the short dense interosseous ligaments between the upper three sacral segments and the iliac wing are the major structures related to pelvic stability. These observations were confirmed by the cadaveric experiments conducted by Vrahas et al.,[39] which demonstrated that the posterior SI and pubic symphyseal ligaments contribute the most to ligamentous stability. The role of the ligaments in pelvic stability becomes clear in an analysis of the pathophysiology resulting in pelvic ring instability, particularly as defined by Tile.[26] The arcuate ligament of the pubic symphysis is illustrated in Figure 17.65.

Pure APC causes lateral rotation of each hemipelvis, which, in turn, disrupts the pubic symphysis and places the more anterior of the pelvic ligaments under tension. Depending on the magnitude of the lateral displacement, the sacrospinous and the anterior SI ligaments may be attenuated or partially or completely disrupted. Reciprocally, lateral rotation anteriorly results in compression posteriorly, and the interosseous, posterior SI, and sacrotuberous ligaments become compressed, thereby maintaining posterior stability (Figs. 17.39 and 17.40). Predominant APC of such proportions as to cause massive posterior, posteromedial, or posterolateral

Sacrospinous Lig.

Sacrotuberous Lig.

Figure 17.63. Midsagittal schematic representation of the pelvis, demonstrating the short, directly anterior orientation of the sacrospinous ligament compared with the longer and more vertically oriented sacrotuberous ligament. *lig.*, ligament (From Thorek P. *Anatomy in Surgery.* 2nd ed. Philadelphia, PA: JB Lippincott; 1962, with permission.)

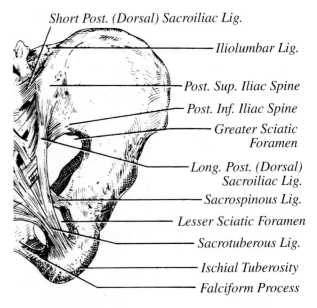

Short Post. (Dorsal) Sacroiliac Lig.

Iliolumbar Lig.

Post. Sup. Iliac Spine

Post. Inf. Iliac Spine

Greater Sciatic Foramen

Long. Post. (Dorsal) Sacroiliac Lig.

Sacrospinous Lig.

Lesser Sciatic Foramen

Sacrotuberous Lig.

Ischial Tuberosity

Falciform Process

Figure 17.64. Schematic representation of the major posterior pelvic ligaments illustrates the great tensile strength afforded by their mass and interwined relationships. *Lig.*, ligament; *Post.*, posterior; *Sup.*, superior; *Inf.*, inferior. (From Pansky B. *Review of Gross Anatomy.* 4th ed. New York, NY: Macmillan; 1979, with permission.)

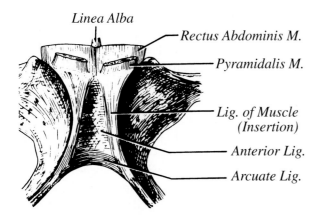

Figure 17.65. Schematic representation of the pubic symphysis and its arcuate ligament. (From Pansky B. *Review of Gross Anatomy.* 4th ed. New York, NY: Macmillan; 1979, with permission.)

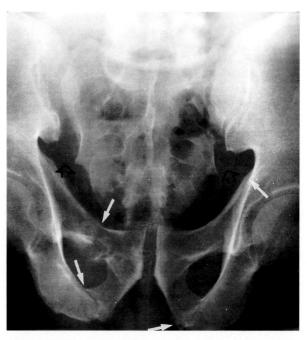

Figure 17.66. The marked bilateral rostral and lateral SI joint diastasis (*open arrows*) indicates disruption of the anterior, posterior, and interosseous SI ligaments and an unstable PRD. The sacrospinous ligaments are probably torn; the sacrotuberous ligaments are probably not torn because of their essentially vertical orientation and because the relationship between the sacrum and the ischial tuberosities remains essentially unaltered. The anterior arch fractures (*arrows*) are minimally displaced.

(Fig. 17.66) displacement of one or both hemipelvis will disrupt the posterior ligaments.

Simultaneous APC and VS or a VS mechanism of injury place the major posterior ligaments under tension, leading to their disruption and pelvic instability. Tile[26] has reported that a disruption between the inferior cortical margins of the SI joints greater than 1.5 cm is radiographic indication of disruption of the posterior ligaments and an unstable pelvic injury (Figs. 17.41 and 17.66).

Associated Pelvic Soft Tissue Injuries

Extraperitoneal hemorrhage and lower urinary tract injuries are frequent components of pelvic injuries, particularly PRD. These soft tissue injuries may be of greater clinical significance than the skeletal injury itself. Pelvic hemorrhage, which is usually venous from the pelvic floor or oozing from the fracture site, is clinically silent until the signs of major blood loss become manifest. As much as 2,000 mL of blood—enough to produce clinical shock in an adult—may accumulate within the extraperitoneal perivesical space without clinical evidence of the source of hemorrhage. Signs of extraperitoneal perivesical fluid collection of blood, urine, or both are, however, evident on the plain AP radiograph of the pelvis and may be quantified at least as minimal and focal, moderate, or massive.[34]

Although lower urinary tract injury is typically clinically silent, urethral lacerations are suggested by inability to void or blood on the external meatus; urinary bladder rupture is suggested by gross hematuria.

Extraperitoneal Perivesical Effusion
Even though current standard of care requires all patients with radiographic or clinical evidence of PRD to have CT as soon as clinically feasible, it is also the generally accepted standard of care that patients with major abdominopelvic trauma have, as part of their initial assessment, an AP radiograph of the pelvis. Therefore, it is useful to be able to recognize signs of perivesical, extraperitoneal fluid on the initial pelvic radiograph.

The radiographic signs of extraperitoneal perivesical effusion are determined by the anatomy of this potential space and the radiographically discernible structures within it (Figs. 17.2 and 17.67). The extraperitoneal perivesical space is a caudal extension of the extraperitoneal fat of the flank stripe and is bounded superiorly by the pelvic

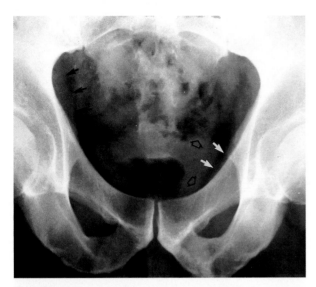

Figure 17.67. The belly of the obturator internus muscle *(closed black arrows)*, its aponeurosis *(white arrows)*, and the urinary bladder *(open black arrows)* are commonly made visible on the AP radiograph of the pelvis by the lucency of the adjacent extraperitoneal perivesical fat.

peritoneal reflection, laterally by the levator ani and obturator internus muscles, anteriorly by the pubic symphysis, posteriorly by the sacrum, and inferiorly by the urogenital diaphragm (Figs. 17.68 through 17.70).

Anterosuperiorly, the extraperitoneal perivesical space is continuous with the space of Retzius of the anterior abdominal wall (Fig. 17.71). It is important to be aware of the location of the space of Retzius because extraperitoneal contrast in that space may suggest intraperitoneal bladder rupture simply based on the location of the contrast (Fig. 17.72). The shaggy, ill-defined character and the absence of contrast-outlined loops of bowel should readily distinguish the extraperitoneal space of Retzius contrast (Fig. 17.73) from intraperitoneal contrast. The perivesical space is filled with loose adipose tissue that is continuous with the extraperitoneal fat of the flank stripe. The extraperitoneal and intraperitoneal spaces, as they appear on axial CT of the pelvis, are schematically represented in Figure 17.74, and, in a patient with large hemoperitoneum, in Figure 17.75.

The signs of an extraperitoneal perivesical effusion (blood or urine) seen on the AP radiograph of the pelvis include a homogeneous soft tissue density that, if unilateral, obliterates the shadow of the ipsilateral obturator internus muscle and displaces the bladder in the opposite direction (Fig. 17.76). A moderate-sized extraperitoneal perivesical effusion obliterates all soft tissue anatomy within the pelvis and displaces the pelvic ileal loops out of the pelvis (Fig. 17.77). A larger perivesical effusion

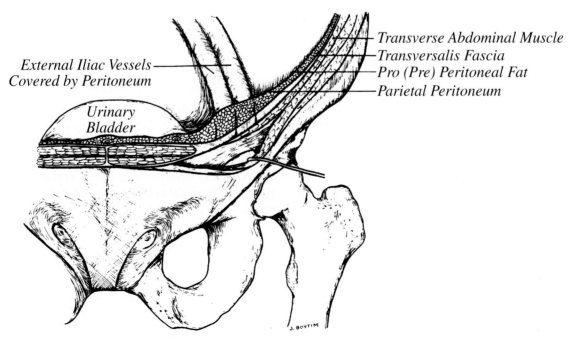

Figure 17.68. Schematic representation of the extraperitoneal (properitoneal or preperitoneal) fat extending continuously into the extraperitoneal perivesical space.

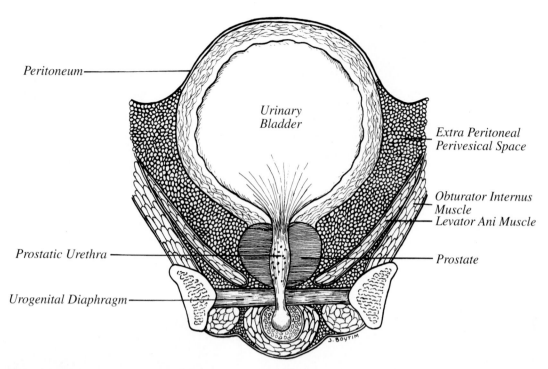

Figure 17.69. Schematic representation of the gross anatomy of the pelvis, seen in frontal projection, demonstrates the extraperitoneal perivesical space, bounded superiorly by the pelvic peritoneum, laterally by the lateral pelvic wall, and inferiorly by the urogenital diaphragm. Note the relationship of the prosthetic urethra to the superior layer of the diaphragm.

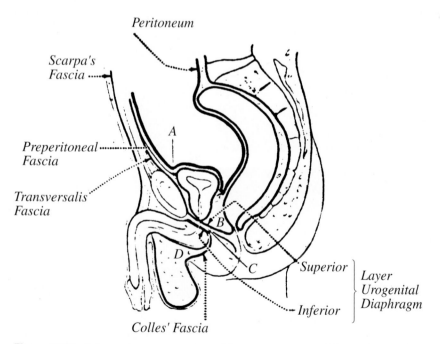

Figure 17.70. Schematic representation of the gross anatomy of the midsagittal plane of the male pelvis. The perivesical space (*A*) referred to in Figure 17.68 is seen to be bounded anteriorly by the pubic symphysis and posteriorly by the anterior wall of the rectum. The urinary bladder and the prostate lie above the urogenital diaphragm (*B and C*). The membranous portion of the urethra lies between the superior and inferior layers of this diaphragm. (From Holyoke EA. Some anatomical considerations of pelvic injuries and their complications. *Nebr State Med J.* 1958;43(5):195–198, with permission.)

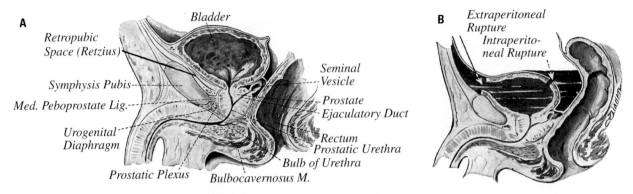

Figure 17.71. Midsagittal schematic drawing of the lower abdomen and pelvis showing the space of Retzius (**A**). Schematic (**B**) shows urine from an extraperitoneal bladder rupture extending into the space of Retzius. *M.*, muscle. (From Thorek P. *Anatomy in Surgery.* 2nd ed. Philadelphia, PA: JB Lippincott; 1962, with permission.)

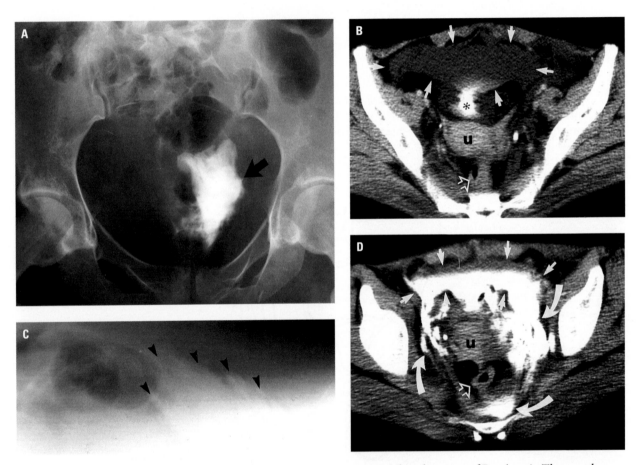

Figure 17.72. Extraperitoneal bladder rupture with contrast material in the space of Retzius. **A:** The postdrainage AP radiograph of the pelvis shows a small collection of contrast material *(arrow)* in the extraperitoneal perivesical space. **B:** The CT scan obtained shortly after **A** shows the collapsed bladder *(asterisk)* with contrast material leaking into the dependent portion of the urine-filled space of Retzius *(arrows)*. **C:** A cross-table radiograph of the lower abdomen and pelvis shows the shaggy margins of contrast *(arrowheads)* extending from the pelvis into the space of Retzius. **D:** The delayed axial pelvic CT shows the space of Retzius nearly filled with contrast *(arrows)* and contrast extending posteriorly in the extraperitoneal space *(curved arrows)* to the presacral space. In **B and D**, the anteriorly projecting uterus *(u)* and broad ligaments and the rectum *(open arrow)*, surrounded by intraperitoneal fat, are clearly visible.

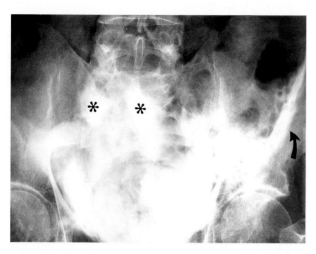

Figure 17.73. Extraperitoneal bladder rupture with contrast material extending into the space of Retzius of the anterior abdominal wall *(asterisks)* and into the flank stripe *(curved arrow)* of the lateral abdominal wall.

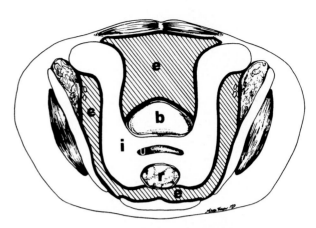

Figure 17.74. Schematic representation of the peritoneal and extraperitoneal spaces of the pelvis as seen on an axial CT image. The extraperitoneal space is indicated by *e*, the intraperitoneal space by *i*, the urinary bladder by *b*, the uterus by *u*, and the rectum by *r*. (From Sivit CJ, Frazier AA, Eichelberger MR. Pelvic and retroperitoneal spaces; CT of pediatric blunt abdominal trauma. *Emerg Radiol.* 1997;4:150–166, with permission.)

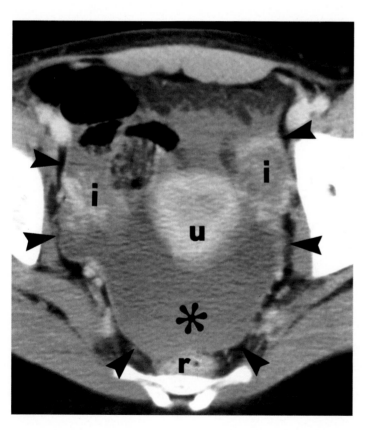

Figure 17.75. Axial CT demonstration of hemoperitoneum. Blood *(asterisk)* in the pelvic peritoneal space bounded by the pelvic peritoneum *(arrowheads)* surrounds the peritoneum-covered uterus *(u)*, invaginating into the peritoneal space and displaces the rectum *(r)* posteriorly. Intraperitoneal bowel loops *(i)* are bilaterally adjacent to the uterus.

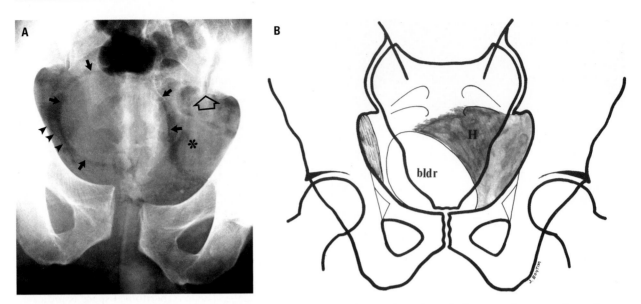

Figure 17.76. A: Displacement of the urinary bladder *(closed arrows)* to the right by a small extraperitoneal perivesical hematoma *(asterisk)* that also obliterates the left obturator internus muscle shadow. The obturator internus muscle is visible on the right *(arrowheads)*. Separation of the pubic symphysis and the left SI joint *(open arrow)* constitutes a Malgaigne injury. **B:** Schematic representation of the effect of a small, unilateral, extraperitoneal perivesical effusion. *bldr*, bladder; *H*, hematoma.

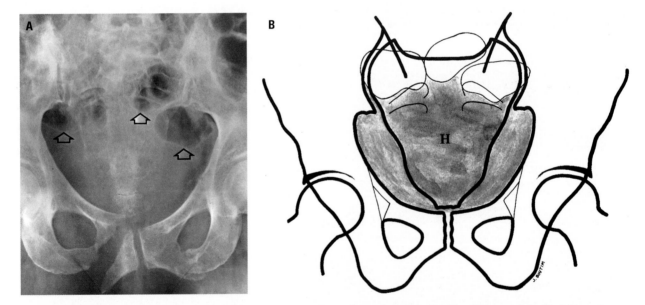

Figure 17.77. A: The homogeneous soft tissue density throughout the pelvis that has obliterated the bladder and the obturator muscle shadows and displaced the pelvic ileal loops *(open arrows)* upward represents a moderate extraperitoneal perivesical effusion. An oblique fracture through the right os pubis and minimally displaced fractures of the left anterior pelvic arch, together with right SI joint diastasis, represent a type III pattern of PRD. **B:** Schematic representation of the effect of a moderate extraperitoneal perivesical effusion *(H)*.

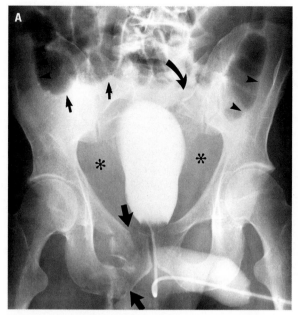

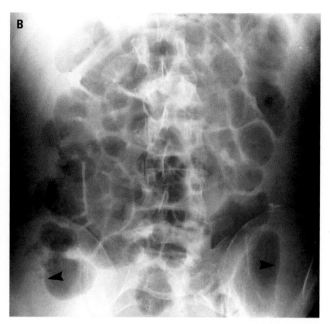

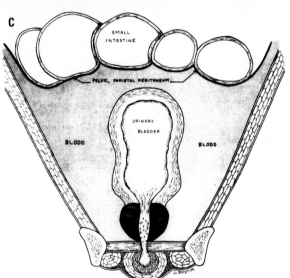

Figure 17.78. Massive extraperitoneal effusion with retrograde extension into the flank stripes. **A:** The cystogram of a patient with a bucket-handle PRD *(large* and *curved arrows)* shows a large extraperitoneal effusion *(asterisks)* throughout the pelvis that obliterates the normal soft tissue anatomy, symmetrically compresses and elongates the bladder, elevates the pelvic ileal loops *(small arrows)* out of the pelvis, and extends into the inferior portion of the flank stripes *(arrowheads).* **B:** The AP radiograph of the abdomen shows the flank stripes obliterated by the extraperitoneal effusion *(arrowheads).* **C:** Schematic representation of the pathologic spaces of the findings seen in **A and B.**

not only will obliterate all of the extraperitoneal pelvic soft tissue anatomy and displace the pelvic ileal loops out of the pelvis but also will extend rostrally in a retrograde fashion into the flank stripe, obliterating its lucency and displacing the parietal peritoneum (medial border of the flank stripe) medially (Fig. 17.78).[34,40] Conversely, fluid within the peritoneal space contained by the pelvic peritoneal reflection will appear as a homogeneous soft tissue density, sharply defined laterally and inferiorly by the peritoneum, with gas-filled pelvic ileal loops displaced out of their normal position within the pouch of Douglas (Fig. 17.79) while the extraperitoneal pelvic soft tissue anatomy remains normal. Displacement of the pelvic ileal loops pertains in supine examinations of the abdomen and pelvis because the pelvic peritoneal space is the most dependent portion of the peritoneal space, even in recumbency.

The pelvic intraperitoneal and extraperitoneal anatomy as seen on axial CT is illustrated in Figures 17.67 and 17.72 through 17.75.

Lower Urinary Tract Injury

Injury to the bladder and posterior urethra occurs from 5%[5,12,41] to 17%[13,42] of patients with pelvic trauma. Although there is usually a direct relationship between the displacement of anterior

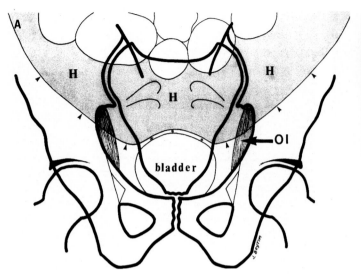

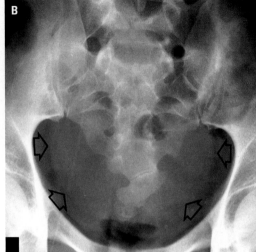

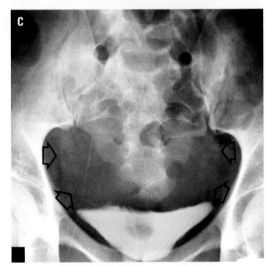

Figure 17.79. Hemoperitoneum. The schematic representation of fluid in the peritoneum (**A**) illustrates the blood *(shaded arrow, H)* within the pouch of pelvic peritoneal space to be sharply defined laterally and inferiorly *(arrowheads)* by the pelvic peritoneum reflection and displacing the pelvic ileal loops upward out of their normal position in the pelvis. The extraperitoneal soft tissue structures (urinary bladder and obturator internus muscle *[OI]*) remain visible. (Compare with Fig. 17.77C schematic.) The AP view of the pelvis (**B**) of a patient with massive rupture of the liver demonstrates a sharply defined *(open arrows)*, homogeneous density with pelvic ileal loops displaced over the upper sacral segments. Although this density could represent a distended urinary bladder, the cystogram (**C**) clearly establishes the density to be intraperitoneal and consistent with blood in the pelvic peritoneal space. (Compare with Fig. 17.77.)

pelvic arch fracture fragments or pubic symphysis diastasis and lower urinary tract injury, it is sufficiently important to emphasize, by repetition, that significant urinary tract damage may also exist in the face of even minimal pelvic skeletal change. Lower urinary tract injuries, in civilian practice, are most commonly the result of blunt trauma. Gunshot and stabbing wounds account for the small percentage of penetrating injuries that involve the bladder. Although there is a slightly greater frequency of bladder injuries in men than in women,[43] there is a marked predilection for urethral injuries in men.[44] Urethral injuries in women (Fig. 17.80) are rare.[45]

Because the most common etiology of urethral and bladder injury is PRD and because the clinical signs of lower urinary tract injury are so clinically

inconspicuous, Conolly and Hedberg[6] and Holdsworth[5] believe that every patient sustaining PRD should be considered to have a lower urinary tract injury until proven otherwise. Conolly and Hedberg[6] state that "every patient with a major fracture of the pelvis should be investigated for complications that may well kill him" (i.e., hemorrhage or lower urinary tract injury).

The indications for radiologic evaluation of the urethra and bladder in male patients and of the urinary bladder in female patients include PRD, microscopic hematuria of more than 10 red blood cells per high-power field,[46] gross hematuria, or blood on the external meatus. Gross hematuria in the presence of an intact pelvis, particularly in a patient sustaining lower abdominal or pelvic trauma from a seat belt, must be considered

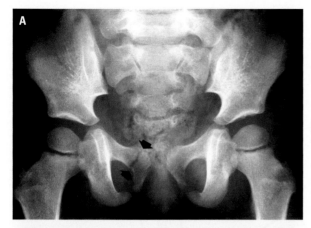

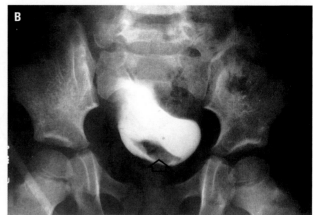

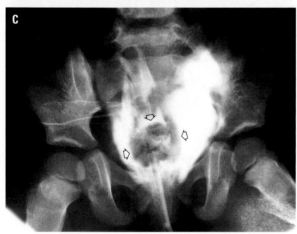

Figure 17.80. Transection of the posterior urethra in a 6-year-old girl, associated with a minimally displaced PRD. The only visible skeletal injury in the AP radiograph of the pelvis (**A**) is the innocuous-appearing fracture of the right os pubis *(arrows)*. The antegrade urogram (**B**) demonstrates elevation of the bladder and a large defect at its base *(open arrow)*. Gross extraperitoneal rupture of the urethrovesical junction is demonstrated by cystography (**C**), where the *open arrows* represent the urinary bladder.

indicative of a urinary bladder rupture and requires retrograde urethrocystography in men and a cystogram in women.

Lower urinary tract injuries occur commonly in severely injured patients.[47] Obviously, in such patients, evaluation of the lower urinary tract must assume a lower priority to lifesaving measures. However, even in these patients, prompt evaluation of the urethra and bladder is advocated in order to reduce morbidity and mortality.[42,48] In less severely injured patients in whom bladder or urethral injuries are suspected, radiographic examination of the lower urinary tract should be part of the initial, immediate patient evaluation.

Although McCort[49] has advocated performing the RUG and cystogram under fluoroscopic guidance, as stated earlier in this chapter, these studies can, and should, be performed in the trauma center and should therefore be an integral part of the early assessment of patients with suspected lower urinary tract injury. The technique of RUG and cystography has also been previously described in this chapter.

Urethral Injuries

Urethral injuries are most commonly the result of blunt pelvic trauma and may be divided into those involving the anterior urethra (inferior to the urogenital diaphragm) or those involving the posterior urethra (superior to the urogenital diaphragm). Anterior urethral injuries are most commonly associated with the "straddle" injury, such as occurs when a male patient slips off of the pedals of a bicycle, striking the perineum on the crossbar. The clinical and physical findings suggestive of an anterior urethral injury are generally readily apparent, and the urethra should be investigated by retrograde urethrography.

Posterior urethral injuries are usually the result of blunt pelvic trauma and have been classified as types I, II, and III by Colapinto and McCullum.[43,50] Recently, Kawashima et al.[51] described a type IV

A   B

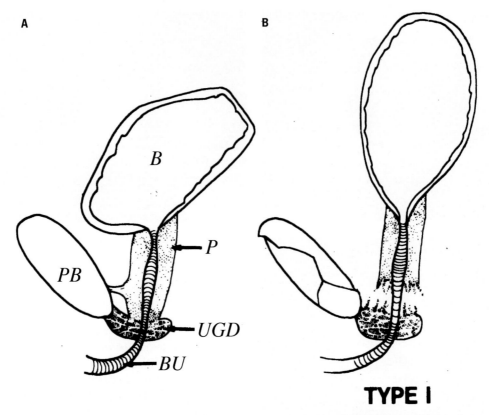

TYPE I

Figure 17.81. **A:** Schematic representation of normal male posterior urethrovesical anatomy in which *B* is the urinary bladder; *P*, the prostate; *UGD*, the urogenital diaphragm; *BU*, the bulbous urethra; and *PB*, the pubic bone. **B:** Type I urethral injury with disruption of the prostate just above the UGD and of the puboprostatic ligament but with an intact posterior urethra. (Modified from Dunnick NR, Sandler CM, Amis ES Jr, et al, eds. *Textbook of Uroradiology.* Baltimore, MD: Williams & Wilkins; 1997:317.)

urethral injury. The type I urethral injury is both a pathologic and radiologic misnomer in that the urethra itself is intact. Hemorrhage from disruption of periurethral tissues surrounds the urethra causing its attenuation and circumferential narrowing (Fig. 17.81).

On retrograde urethrography, the tamponade effect of the periurethral hematoma may be so profound as to preclude filling of the posterior urethra (Fig. 17.82A) or, if less severe, may result in elongated, circumferential narrowing of the posterior urethral lumen (Fig. 17.82B). In either event, the distal end of the narrowed column of contrast in the urethra is smooth and gently tapering over a relatively short distance, and there is no extravasation of contrast material outside the urethral lumen.

The type II urethral injury (Fig. 17.83) is laceration (Fig. 17.84) of the posterior urethra, usually at the junction of the prostatic and membranous urethra above the intact urogenital diaphragm. With transection of the urethra, the bladder and prostate are retracted upward, resulting in a defect where the prostate is normally palpable on digital rectal examination. Regardless of the magnitude of urethral injury, the type II injury is characterized by extravasation of contrast medium into the extraperitoneal perivesical space above the intact urogenital diaphragm.

The type III urethral injury (Fig. 17.85), pathologically, consists of disruption of the posterior urethra through its membranous portion, associated with disruption of the urogenital diaphragm. Radiographically, the type III urethral injury is characterized by extravasation of contrast material above and below the urogenital diaphragm (Fig. 17.86).

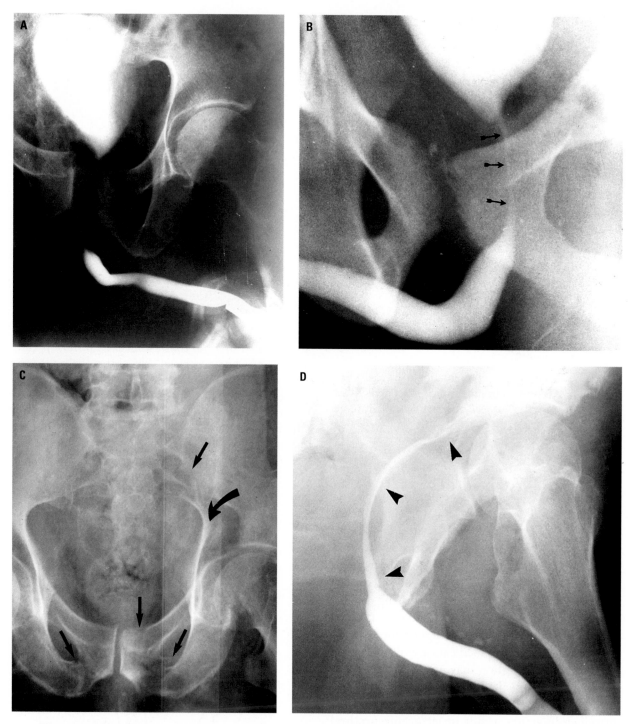

Figure 17.82. Type I urethral injury. **A:** The tamponade effect of the periurethral hematoma completely occluded the posterior urethra, preventing its opacification. Distention of the penile urethra, the short symmetrical tapering of the proximal end of the column of contrast, and the absence of extraluminal contrast are sufficient signs to diagnose a type I urethral injury. Bladder opacification was from an antegrade urogram. **B:** The attenuated, elongated, symmetrically narrowed intact posterior urethra *(arrows)*, without extraluminal contrast, is characteristic of a periurethral hematoma. **C and D:** In a third patient, in whom the AP radiograph of the pelvis (**C**) shows a minimally displaced type III PRD *(arrows)* and concomitant left central acetabular fracture *(curved arrow)*, a large periurethral hematoma has resulted in a long type I urethral injury *(arrowheads,* **D**).

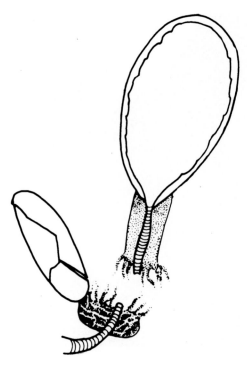

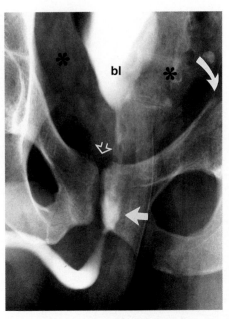

Figure 17.83. Schematic representation of a type II urethral injury. (Modified from Dunnick NR, Sandler CM, Amis ES Jr, et al, eds. *Textbook of Uroradiology.* Baltimore, MD: Williams & Wilkins; 1997:317.)

Figure 17.84. Type II urethral injury characterized by extravasated urethral contrast material *(arrow)* is confined to the extraperitoneal pelvic space above the urogenital diaphragm. The anterior components of the PRD, pubic symphysis separation *(open arrow)* and the fracture of the superior pubic ramus *(curved arrow)*, are only minimally displaced. A large bilateral extraperitoneal hematoma *(asterisks)* has elevated and symmetrically compressed the bladder *(bl)* into a teardrop configuration.

The type IV urethral injury described by Kawashima et al.[51] is a tear of the urethra at the urethrovesical junction. Because of the surrounding prostatic tissue, the type IV urethral injury appears as a longitudinal slit in the prostatic urethra on RUG. Extension of the tear into the base of the bladder usually results in extravasation of contrast material into the extraperitoneal space (Fig. 17.87).

Attempts to pass a Foley catheter in male patients with possible urethral injury without prior RUG fail the current standard of medical care. Blind or "diagnostic" catheterization may initiate or reactivate bleeding from an existing urethral laceration, extend a urethral laceration to complete transection, introduce infection, result in iatrogenic urethral injury (Fig. 17.88), or result in the catheter being inflated extraluminally (Fig. 17.89).[8,13–15]

In the rare circumstance in which it is necessary to evaluate the urethra of a male patient in whom a Foley catheter has already been inserted, McLaughlin and Pfister[52] and McCort[49] recommend performing an RUG by introducing contrast medium into the urethra through a pediatric feeding catheter introduced into the urethra alongside the existing Foley catheter (Fig. 17.90).

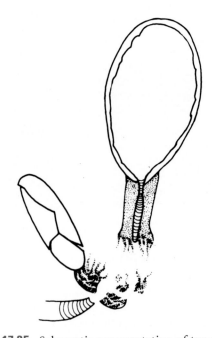

Figure 17.85. Schematic representation of type III urethral injury. (Modified from Dunnick NR, Sandler CM, Amis ES Jr, et al, eds. *Textbook of Uroradiology.* Baltimore, MD: Williams & Wilkins; 1997:317.)

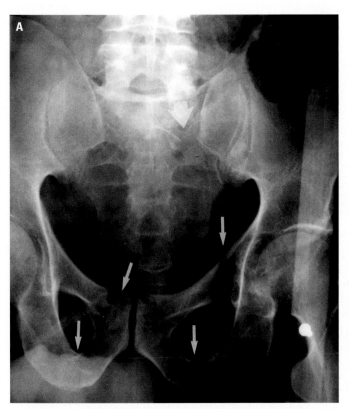

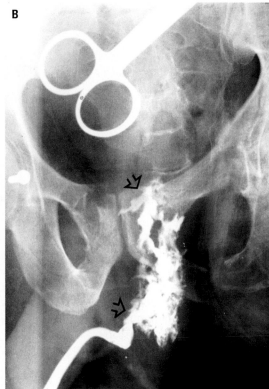

Figure 17.86. Type III urethral injury in a patient with a minimally displaced PRD. The purpose of this figure emphasizes that the degree of displacement of PRD fragments has negative predictive value regarding the presence or type of urethral injury. The AP radiograph of the pelvis **(A)** indicates minimal displacement of the sites of PRD *(arrows)*. The retrograde urethrogram **(B)** demonstrates contrast both above and below *(open arrows)* the urogenital diaphragm (i.e., a type III urethral injury).

Bladder Injuries

The most common cause of bladder injury is blunt lower abdominal or pelvic trauma. Approximately 8% of patients with pelvic fractures sustain bladder injuries,[53,54] but approximately 95% of bladder injury is associated with PRD.[54] Other types of pelvic fractures (e.g., the Duverney fracture, insufficiency, and stress fractures) are not associated with bladder injury. Severely displaced (Fig. 17.91) or central acetabular fractures with major protrusion of the acetabular fragments or the femoral head (Fig. 17.92) into the true pelvis may be a cause of bladder injury.

The incidence of intraperitoneal and extraperitoneal rupture of the bladder is approximately equal,[12,43,48,54] with a greater incidence of intraperitoneal rupture in the absence of pelvic fracture.[9] The latter circumstance is most commonly the result of abrupt compression of a distended bladder by a lap seat belt. The association of a restrained patient in an abrupt deceleration injury with hematuria or

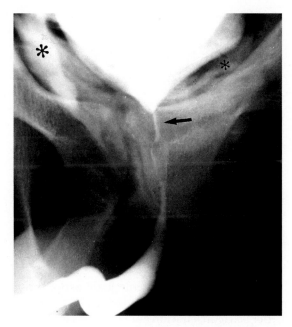

Figure 17.87. Type IV urethral injury *(arrow)* and extraperitoneal perivesical extravasation of contrast material *(asterisks)*.

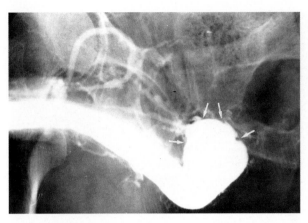

Figure 17.88. Iatrogenic urethral injury. Attempts to insert a Foley and a filiform catheter were unsuccessful in this patient with PRD. After transfer, the retrograde urethrogram demonstrated complete obstruction of the posterior urethra and several mucosal irregularities *(arrows)* of the distended bulbous urethra. Distention of the urethra has resulted in retrograde flow of contrast material into venous and lymphatic channels of the penile shaft.

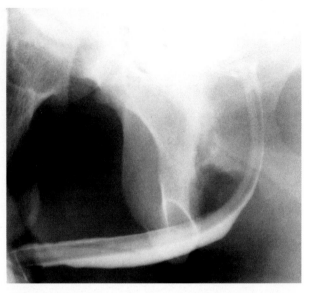

Figure 17.90. Intact urethra demonstrated by retrograde urethrography performed around an indwelling Foley catheter.

blood on the external meatus and a radiographically intact pelvis occurs so commonly with traumatic rupture of the bladder that bladder rupture must be the working diagnosis until proven otherwise. Twenty percent of patients with pelvic fracture

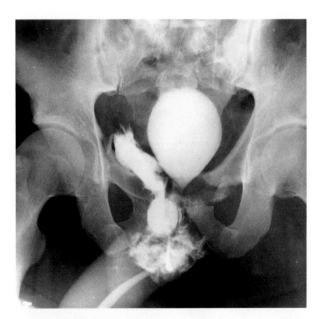

Figure 17.89. Retrograde urethrogram performed following attempted catheterization of a patient with severe anterior pelvic arch fractures of PRD. The Foley catheter passed through the urethral tear and lodged in the periurethral soft tissues, causing the round defect to the right of the midline.

and extraperitoneal rupture of the bladder also have associated posterior urethral laceration.[9] As many as one-third of patients with extraperitoneal rupture of the bladder may also have clinically unrecognizable intraperitoneal injury.[55]

Bladder injuries have been described as contusion, extraperitoneal rupture, intraperitoneal rupture, or combined extraperitoneal–intraperitoneal rupture.[12] Sandler[56] has modified this traditional classification of bladder injuries based on the radiographic appearance to include type I, bladder contusions; type II, intraperitoneal rupture; type III, interstitial rupture; type IVa, simple extraperitoneal rupture; type IVb, complex extraperitoneal rupture; and type V, combined. Bladder contusion (type I) and interstitial rupture (type III) are rarely recognizable by cystography. Intraperitoneal bladder rupture has significantly higher morbidity and mortality rates than extraperitoneal rupture because of urine-induced chemical peritonitis.[57]

The radiologic evaluation of bladder injury is optimally and preferably performed in the trauma center by retrograde cystography through a Foley catheter. In male patients, the cystogram must be preceded by demonstration of an intact urethra by RUG. In female patients, Foley catheterization may be attempted initially because injuries to the short, mobile female urethra caused by blunt trauma are rare.[58–61] The previously described

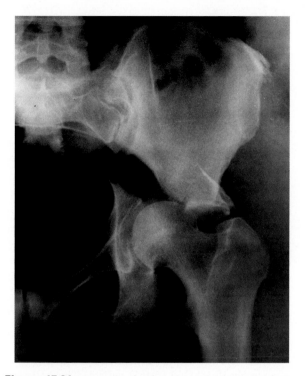

Figure 17.91. Severely displaced transverse acetabular fracture. The location of the proximal margin of the inferior acetabular fragment should prompt the consideration of injury to the urinary bladder or a major branch of the internal iliac artery.

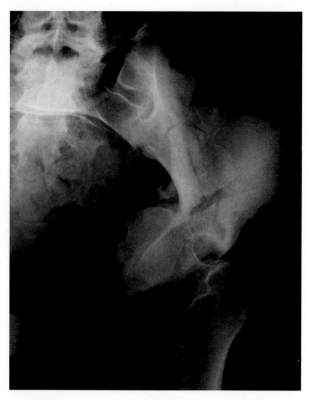

Figure 17.92. Central acetabular fracture with gross intrapelvic protrusion of the femoral head. Fracture comminution extends into the iliac wing.

protocol regarding cystography must be followed in order to exclude small flap-like tears of the bladder wall that will be closed by compression of the distended bladder and become patent only when the bladder is drained (Fig. 17.93). Obviously, the cystogram protocol should be either terminated or modified for specific indications, such as the demonstration of extraluminal contrast material. As stated earlier, opacification of the bladder by intravenously administered contrast medium for intravenous urography or abdominal/abdominopelvic CT does not constitute an adequate cystogram to exclude bladder rupture.[62,63]

Extraperitoneal rupture of the bladder is characterized by streaky collections of contrast medium confined to the extraperitoneal perivesical space (Figs. 17.72, 17.73, and 17.93 through 17.96).

Intraperitoneal rupture of the bladder is characterized by the presence of intravenously or cystographically administered contrast medium

within the peritoneal space outlining the paracolic gutters, the pelvic peritoneal recess, and surrounding loops of bowel (Figs. 17.97 and 17.98). Usually, intraperitoneal bladder rupture is readily apparent by demonstration of intraperitoneal contrast on the initial cystogram. However, this is not always the case, and in the absence of any other explanation for hematuria, a delayed radiograph of the abdomen and pelvis (Fig. 17.99) or subsequent abdominopelvic CT will demonstrate the intraperitoneal contrast. Because there is no direct relation between the degree of displacement of pelvic ring fragments and urethral injury, minimally displaced PRD and/or lateral displacement of the anterior arch components of PRD do not militate against the possibility of traumatic bladder rupture (Fig. 17.99).

Concomitant extraperitoneal and intraperitoneal bladder rupture is demonstrable by both radiography and CT (Fig. 17.100).

In infants and young children, the urinary bladder is more an abdominal than a pelvic organ and,

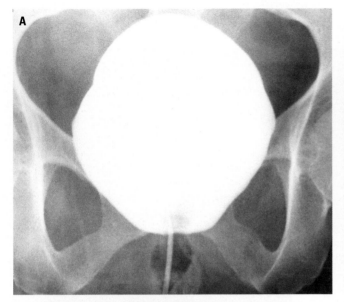

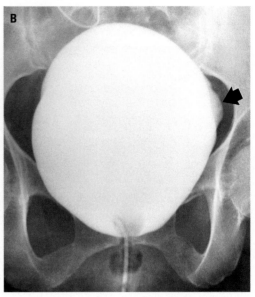

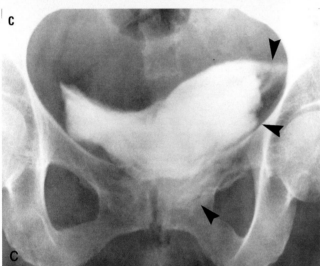

Figure 17.93. Flap-like bladder rupture seen only on postevacuation radiograph. The importance of strict adherence to the established protocol for trauma-indicated cystography is clearly illustrated in this patient. The radiograph of the incompletely filled (150 to 200 mL) bladder (**A**) is negative. Maximum distention of the bladder (350 to 400 mL) (**B**) demonstrated a smooth outpouching from the left lateral bladder wall (*arrow*) that could represent simply a diverticulum or intrastitial rupture. There is no extravasation of contrast medium on this study. In the postevacuation radiograph (**C**), however, extraperitoneal extravasation (*arrowheads*) is obvious.

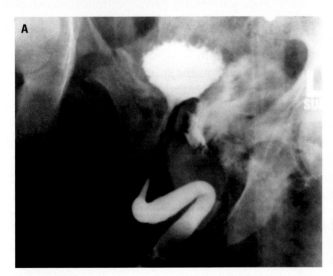

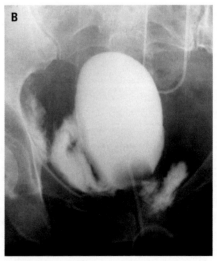

Figure 17.94. Extraperitoneal rupture of the bladder. The shaggy, ill-defined, streaky characteristics of the contrast medium in the perivesical space is typical of extraperitoneal rupture of the bladder demonstrated by retrograde urethrography (**A**) in a male patient and by cystography (**B**) in a female patient. In the latter instance, the elongated configuration of the urinary bladder reflects the presence of a large accumulation of urine, and possibly blood, in the extraperitoneal perivesical space.

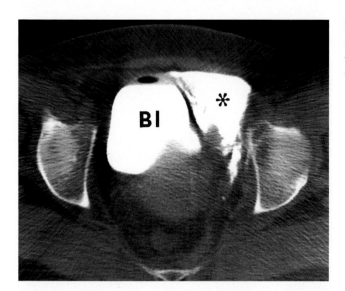

Figure 17.95. Extraperitoneal bladder rupture. The axial CT of the pelvis shows an extraperitoneal perivesical collection of contrast material *(asterisk)* lateral to the urinary bladder *(Bl)*.

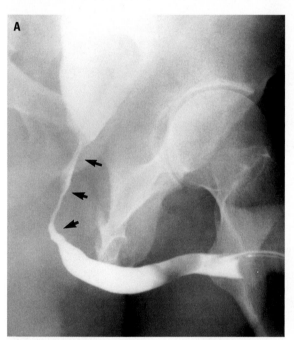

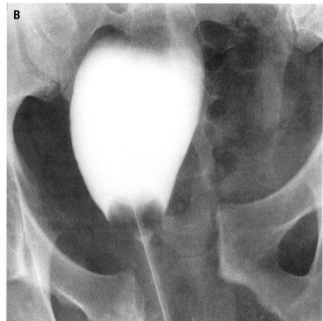

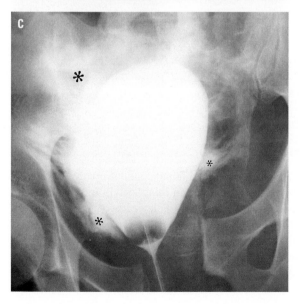

Figure 17.96. Extraperitoneal bladder rupture demonstrated only with maximum distention of the bladder. **A:** This adult male patient with an open-book PRD had a type I urethral injury *(arrows)* on the retrograde urethrogram. **B:** On the cystogram of the partially filled bladder, there was no extravasation of contrast material. **C:** The extraperitoneal bladder rupture *(asterisks)* was demonstrated only after maximal distention of the bladder with approximately 400 mL of contrast material.

Figure 17.97. Intraperitoneal rupture of the bladder. Contrast medium is seen between loops of intestine. The sharp definition of the lateral margins of the contrast medium in the paracolic gutters and outlining the surfaces of the liver and the relative homogeneity of the collections of contrast as well as the sharp definitions of the contrast outlining loops of bowel are absolutely characteristic of intraperitoneal bladder rupture.

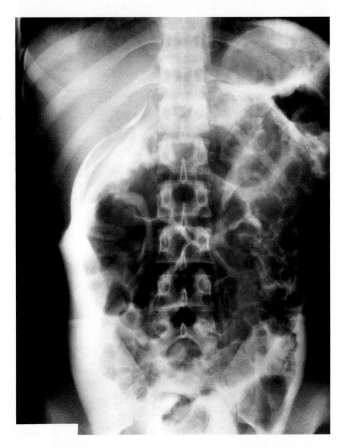

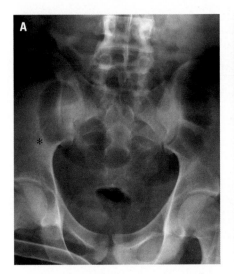
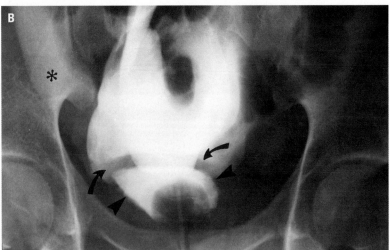

Figure 17.98. Intraperitoneal bladder rupture, without PRD, in a restrained female patient involved in a motor vehicle accident. **A:** The AP radiograph of the abdomen demonstrates an intact pelvis and fluid in the right paracolic gutter *(asterisk)*. **B:** The cystogram reveals the balloon of a Foley catheter in a small bladder *(arrowheads)*, a lucent stripe between the bladder lumen and the peritoneal space *(curved arrows)* that represents the bladder wall and areolar tissue normally interposed between the bladder and the pelvic peritoneal reflection, as well as the characteristic appearance of contrast within the peritoneal space (pouch of Douglas). Contrast in the right paracolic gutter *(asterisk)* is interposed between the lucency of the fat of the flank stripe and the gas within the cecum.

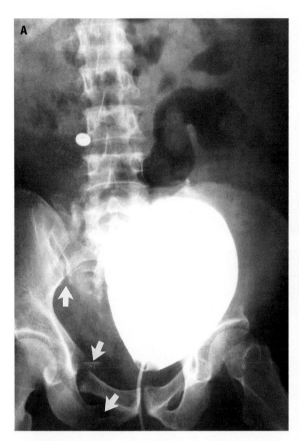
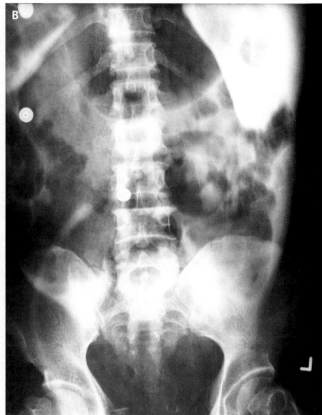

Figure 17.99. Intraperitoneal bladder rupture demonstrated only on a delayed AP radiograph of the abdomen in a patient with a minimally displaced left Malgaigne PRD *(arrows)*. **A:** The cystogram demonstrates displacement of the bladder to the left by a large right pelvic hematoma. There is no evidence of either extraperitoneal or intraperitoneal extravasation. **B:** A delayed AP radiograph of the abdomen demonstrates the characteristic appearance of intraperitoneal contrast, even with the loss of definition caused by patient respiratory motion.

as such, is susceptible to intraperitoneal rupture by blunt (Fig. 17.101) or penetrating trauma.

Extraperitoneal Perivesical Hemorrhage

It is impossible to distinguish extraperitoneal perivesical blood from urine by conventional radiography. Therefore, all the radiographic signs of extraperitoneal effusion previously described and illustrated (Figs. 17.76 through 17.78) apply to the presence of extraperitoneal blood. Obviously, the demonstration of an intact lower urinary tract by RUG and cystography indicates that the extraperitoneal collection must be blood. Extravasation of lower urinary tract contrast material into the extraperitoneal space does not exclude concomitant hemorrhage. The only definitive CT sign of bleeding into the extraperitoneal space is the presence of

frank extravasation of intravenously administered contrast material.

Although pelvic hemorrhage remains the most important cause of death with major PRD, that mortality rate has decreased as the result of measures taken at the scene of injury or in the trauma center, such as external pelvic fixation or percutaneous pelvic angiography and embolization. The clinical significance of extraperitoneal hemorrhage associated with PRD has prompted a recent classification of PRD that attempts to predict the patient at risk for massive pelvic hemorrhage[18] on the basis of a modification of the Pennal[24] classification. A more comprehensive study[64] attempts to develop a classification of PRD, again based on the Pennal classification,[24] from which the pattern of organ injury and resuscitation (including hemorrhage)

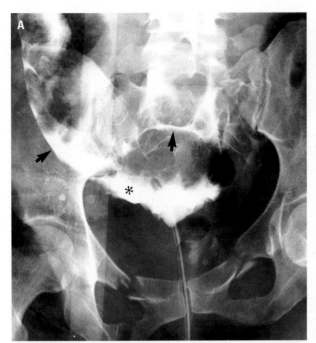

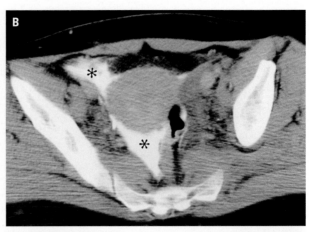

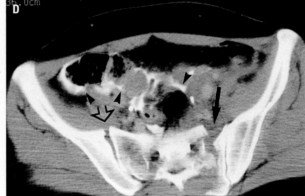

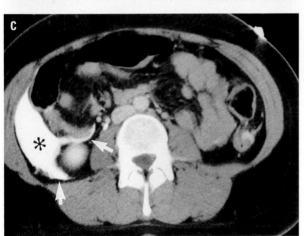

Figure 17.100. Concomitant extraperitoneal and intraperitoneal bladder rupture. The postdrainage AP radiograph of the pelvis (**A**) shows both extraperitoneal (*asterisk*) and intraperitoneal (*arrows*) bladder rupture. The CT images of the pelvis (**B**) and lower abdomen demonstrate contrast in the perivesical extraperitoneal space (*asterisks*) and (**C**) the right flank stripe (*asterisk*) and the anterior and posterior pararenal spaces (*arrows*), respectively. The CT image of the upper pelvis (**D**) shows intraperitoneal contrast surrounding loops of bowel (*arrowheads*). The right SI joint is slightly diastatic (*open arrow*), and there is a posteriorly displaced fracture of the left sacral ala (*arrow*).

requirements could be predicted. Each of these studies is based on the initial AP, inlet, and outlet radiographs obtained in the trauma center. Each classification is compromised by the inherent limitation of the Pennal classification in which approximately one-third of the patterns of PRD meet the criteria of two or more of the Pennal patterns (e.g., APC, LC, and VS). A second caveat is that while statistical analyses and percentages of

predictability provide valuable information to cohorts of patients, each patient with major blunt abdominal, pelvic, or abdominopelvic trauma and PRD must be assessed and managed on an individual basis.

The sources of extraperitoneal perivesical hemorrhage are identified earlier as being from the extensive venous system of the pelvic floor, oozing from pelvic fractures, and from arterial sources.

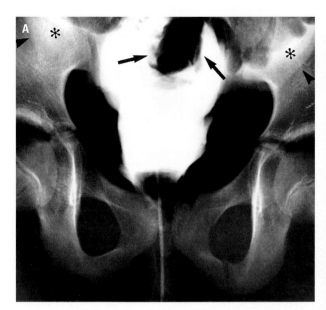

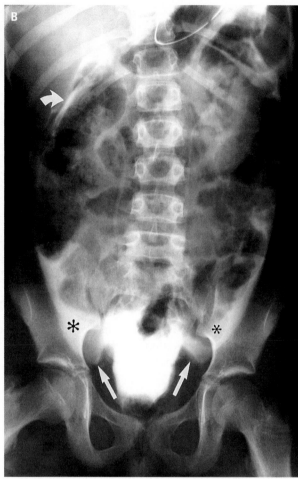

Figure 17.101. Intraperitoneal bladder rupture in a child. **A:** The cystogram shows contrast in the peritoneal space outlining loops of pelvic ileum *(arrows)* and in the paracolic gutters *(asterisks)*. The sharp lateral contrast within the gutters *(arrowheads)* represents the parietal peritoneum. **B:** On the delayed abdominal radiograph, the intraperitoneal contrast outlines the lateral pelvic peritoneal reflection *(white arrows)*, the paracolic gutters *(asterisks)*, loops of bowel, and the inferior surface of the liver *(curved arrow)*.

Abdominopelvic angiography should be considered in any patient with PRD who is hemodynamically unstable without an otherwise recognizable source of blood loss.

The hypogastric (internal iliac) artery is the source of the major blood supply to the true pelvis via its branches—the iliolumbar, sacral, gluteal, pudendal, vesical, and obturator arteries. Of these, the superior gluteal artery is the major source of arterial bleeding associated with posterior pelvic arch fractures,[65] and the obturator artery is the major source of arterial bleeding caused by anterior arch fractures.

The plain radiograph signs of extraperitoneal perivesical fluid (including blood) are described and illustrated earlier. As in other sites of skeletal injury, a focal hematoma may be the most obvious radiographic sign of a subtle pelvic fracture or diastasis. This is a particularly useful sign of occult superior pubic ramus fracture when

subperiosteal hemorrhage causes the aponeurosis of the obturator internus muscle to become abnormally prominent (Figs. 17.32, 17.102, and 17.103).

Insufficiency Fracture

Insufficiency and stress fractures[66] are the only fractures of the pelvic ring occurring in adults, other than the acetabular fracture, in which there is a single site of fracture.

The insufficiency fracture characteristically occurs in elderly osteoporotic women following relatively minor trauma, such as a fall from a chair or out of bed. The most common sites of insufficiency fracture in the pelvis include the sacral ala, the iliac wing,[67] and the pubic bones. Insufficiency fractures of the os pubis characteristically cause minimal comminution of the pubic body unilaterally or bilaterally. The fracture may be manifested only by subtle cortical disruption, change in contour, or multiple short

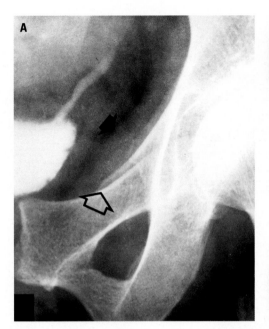
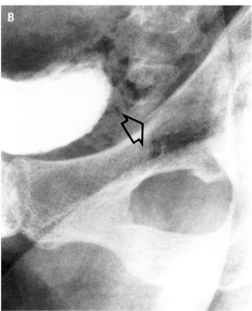

Figure 17.102. The subtle superior ramus fracture *(open arrow)* in the AP (**A**) and left anterior oblique (**B**) projections is confirmed by bulging of the obturator internus muscle, which is representative of a subperiosteal hematoma.

linear densities representing comminution of the pubic body (Fig. 17.104) or by a minimally displaced fracture of either the superior (Fig. 17.105) or inferior pubic ramus. In the pubic body, the insufficiency fracture may resemble a lytic metastatic locus.[68] Ob-

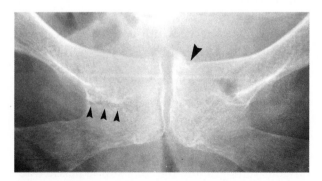

Figure 17.103. Marked bulging of the right obturator internus muscle and its aponeurosis *(arrowheads)* by subperiosteal hematoma is the most obvious radiographic sign of the right superior pubic ramus fracture, indicated only by angulation at the fracture site *(arrow)*.

scure insufficiency fractures of the sacral ala or iliac wing may require CT for their identification.

Stress Fracture

Stress fractures of the pelvis are uncommon and are usually the result of muscle or ligamentous pull rather than chronic inappropriate weight bearing. Keats[69] considers the insufficiency fracture of the pelvis a type of stress fracture. Stress fractures associated with the traditional history of repeated, unusual weight bearing have been reported in military inductees[70,71] and marathon runners.[72] Such stress fractures most commonly involve the os pubis, particularly the pubic body, and the sacrum.

Figure 17.104. Insufficiency fractures *(arrowheads)* of each pubic body.

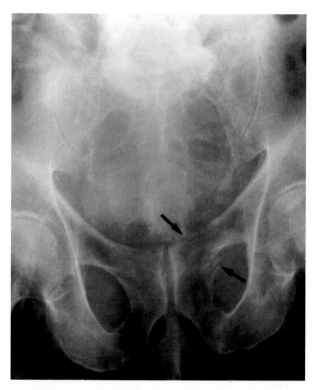

Figure 17.105. Insufficiency fracture of the left pubic body *(arrows)*.

NONTRAUMATIC CONDITIONS

Infection

Paget Disease

Paget disease may involve one (Fig. 17.106) or all (Fig. 17.107) the bones of the hips and pelvis and is typically manifested by demineralization, corti-

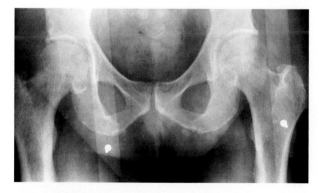

Figure 17.106. Paget disease involving the right femur is characterized by cortical thickening and trabecular prominence (compare with the left femur).

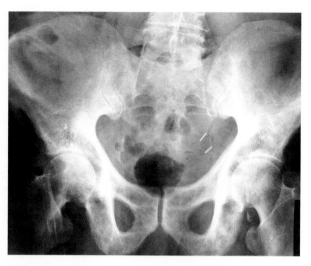

Figure 17.107. Biphasic Paget disease involving all the bones of the pelvis and each femoral head.

cal thickening, and trabecular prominence. When biphasic (Fig. 17.107), Paget disease may simulate blastic (prostatic) metastasis.

Neoplastic Disease

Benign neoplasms involving the bones of the pelvis may be symptomatic and prompt an emergency center visit. Osteoid osteoma and solitary osteochondroma are examples in point—the osteoid osteoma because of pain, and the solitary osteochondroma because of a mass.

Osteoid osteoma clinically occurs in adolescents and young adults, usually younger than the age of 30 years, and typically produces dull, persistent pain that is worse at night and that is usually relieved by aspirin. Although osteoid osteoma may occur in many locations, a common site is the junction of the femoral neck and shaft near the lesser trochanter. Osteoid osteoma is typically limited to the cortex but may involve the intramedullary portion of bone. The cortical lesion is typically an area of dense sclerotic cortical thickening with a central lucid nidus (Fig. 17.108). The nidus, which may be very subtle on the plain radiograph, becomes readily apparent by plain radiograph tomography or CT. Scintigraphy is also an effective method of establishing or confirming the diagnosis. Because the nidus is highly vascular, it will demonstrate even greater concentration of the radiopharmaceutical than does the surrounding sclerotic bone. This difference in radioactivity has been termed the "double-density" sign.[73]

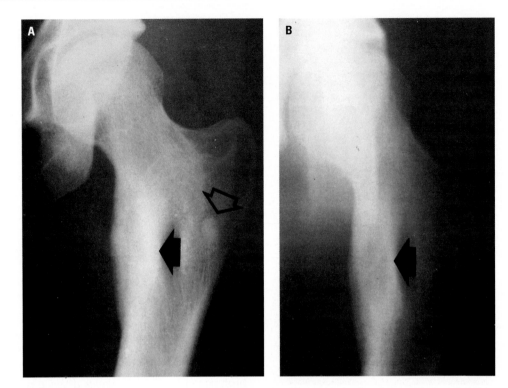

Figure 17.108. Osteoid osteoma of the femur *(closed arrow)*. In the plain radiograph (**A**), a large but focal area of increased density caused by both cortical and endosteal proliferation is present. The cortical new bone formation is smooth and sharply delineated, indicating a nonaggressive process. The frontal tomogram (**B**) demonstrates an oval central lucent nidus *(closed arrow)*. These findings are typical of an osteoid osteoma in this 21-year-old woman who complained of pain in her hip, which was worse at night and relieved by aspirin over several weeks' duration. The smaller, discrete density *(open arrow)* in the frontal radiograph (**A**) is a bone island.

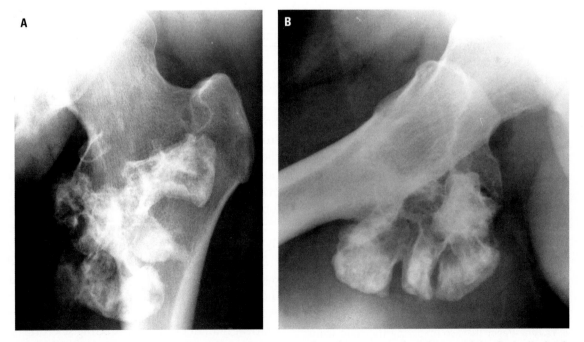

Figure 17.109. Characteristic radiographic appearance of a solitary osteochondroma of the femur in both frontal (**A**) and frog leg (**B**) projections.

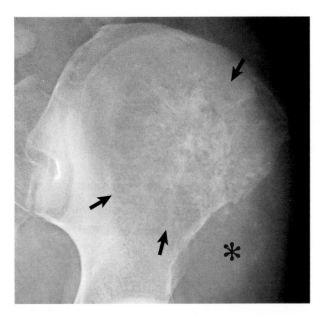

Figure 17.110. Chondrosarcoma of the left iliac wing *(arrows)* with a large soft tissue component *(asterisk).*

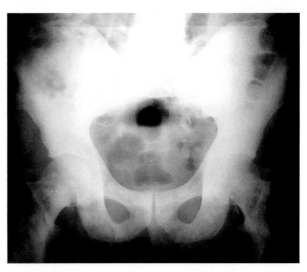

Figure 17.112. Osteoblastic metastasis from carcinoma of the prostate.

Solitary osteochondroma (osteocartilaginous exostosis) is a cartilage-capped bony excrescence. It is a common lesion usually encountered in the second or third decade and typically arises from the cortex adjacent to the metaphysis of a long tubular bone,

particularly the proximal humerus, proximal and distal femur, and distal radius.[74] The characteristic radiographic appearance of an osteochondroma is seen in Figure 17.109.

Primary malignant neoplasms may involve the bones of the pelvis or hip. These may be localized, such as chondrosarcoma (Fig. 17.110), or generalized, such as primary round cell diseases, including multiple myeloma or one of the non-Hodgkin lymphomas (reticulum cell sarcoma, Fig. 17.111).

Metastatic neoplasia may be osteoblastic (Fig. 17.112) or osteolytic (Fig. 17.113). Either may lead to a pathologic fracture (Fig. 17.114).

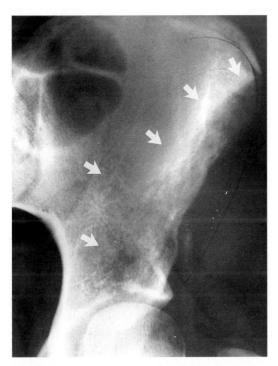

Figure 17.111. The permeative appearance of the left iliac wing, extending from the supraacetabular region to the anterior superior iliac spine *(arrows)*, represents histologically proven reticulum cell sarcoma.

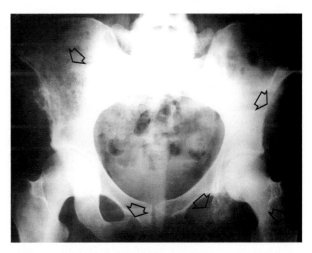

Figure 17.113. Osteolytic metastasis *(open arrows)* from primary breast carcinoma.

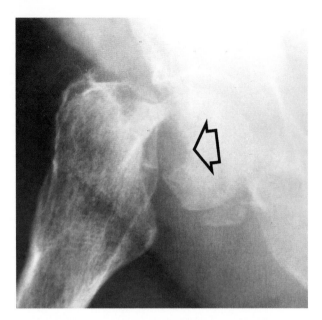

Figure 17.114. Pathologic fracture in the neck of the right femur, secondary to primary breast carcinoma. The characteristic margins of the fracture fragments *(open arrow)* and the lytic defect with loss of trabecular pattern in the femoral neck fragment are typical signs of a metastatic lesion through which a fracture has occurred.

REFERENCES

1. Braunstein FW, Skudder PA, McCarroll JR, et al. Concealed hemorrhage due to pelvic trauma. *J Trauma.* 1964;4:832–838.
2. Rothenberger DA, Fischer RP, Strate RG, et al. The mortality associated with pelvic fractures. *Surgery.* 1978;84(3):356–361.
3. Margolies MN, Ring EJ, Waltman AC, et al. Arteriography in the management of hemorrhage from pelvic fractures. *N Engl J Med.* 1972;287(7):317–321.
4. Matalon TS, Athanasoulis CA, Margolies MN, et al. Hemorrhage with pelvic fractures: efficacy of transcatheter embolization. *AJR Am J Roentgenol.* 1979;133(5):859–864.
5. Holdsworth FW. Injury to the genito-urinary tract associated with fractures of the pelvis. *Proc R Soc Med.* 1963;56:1044–1046.
6. Conolly WB, Hedberg EA. Observations on fractures of the pelvis. *J Trauma.* 1969;9(2):104–111.
7. Wilson RF, Smith JB, McCarroll KA. Trauma to the urinary tract. In: Wilson RF, Wall AJ, eds. *Management of Trauma: Pitfalls and Practice.* 2nd ed. Baltimore, MD: Williams & Wilkins; 1996:611.
8. Weens HS, Newman JH, Florence TJ. Trauma of the lower urinary tract; a roentgenologic study. *N Engl J Med.* 1946;234:357–364.
9. Mitchell JP. Trauma to the urinary tract. *N Engl J Med.* 1973;288(2):90–92.
10. Mitchell JP. Trauma to the urethra. *Injury.* 1975;7(2):84–88.
11. Rieser C. Diagnostic evaluation of suspected genitourinary tract injury. *JAMA.* 1967;199(10):714–719.
12. Brosman SA, Fay R. Diagnosis and management of bladder trauma. *J Trauma.* 1973;13(8):687–694.
13. Dunnick NR, Sandler CM, Amis ES, et al, eds. *Textbook of Uroradiology.* 2nd ed. Baltimore, MD: Williams & Wilkins; 1997:316.
14. McAninch JW. Genitourinary trauma. In: Moore EE, Mattox KL, Feliciano DV, eds. *Trauma.* 2nd ed. Norwalk, CT: Appleton & Lange; 1991:582.
15. Wilson RF, Smith JB, McCarroll KA. Trauma to the urinary tract. In: Wilson RF, Walt AJ, eds. *Management of Trauma: Pitfalls and Practice.* 2nd ed. Baltimore, MD: Williams & Wilkins; 1996:614.
16. Corriere JN Jr, Sandler CM. Management of the ruptured bladder: seven years of experience with 111 cases. *J Trauma.* 1986;26(9):830–833.
17. Ring EJ, Athanasoulis C, Waltman AC, et al. Arteriographic management of hemorrhage following pelvic fracture. *Radiology.* 1973;109(1):65–70.
18. Cryer HM, Miller FB, Evers BM, et al. Pelvis fracture classification: correlation with hemorrhage. *J Trauma.* 1988;28:973–980.
19. Caffey J. *Pediatric X-ray Diagnosis.* 5th ed. Chicago, IL: Year Book; 1973.
20. Clemente CD, ed. *Gray's Anatomy.* 30th ed. Philadelphia, PA: Lea & Febiger; 1984.
21. Bowerman JW, Sena JM, Chang R. The teardrop shadow of the pelvis: anatomy and clinical significance. *Radiology.* 1982;143(3):659–662.
22. Jackson H, Kam J, Harris JH Jr, et al. The sacral arcuate lines in upper sacral fractures. *Radiology.* 1982;145(1):35–39.
23. Kane WJ. Fractures of the pelvis. In: Rockwood CA, Green DP, eds. *Fractures in Adults.* 2nd ed. Philadelphia, PA: JB Lippincott; 1984:1093–1209.
24. Pennal GF, Tile M, Waddell JP, et al. Pelvic disruption: assessment and classification. *Clin Orthop Relat Res.* 1980;151:12–21.
25. Tile M. *Fractures of the Pelvis and Acetabulum.* Baltimore, MD: Williams & Wilkins; 1984.
26. Tile M. Pelvis ring fractures: should they be fixed? *J Bone Joint Surg Br.* 1988;70(1):1–12.
27. Young JW, Burgess AR, Brumback RJ, et al. Pelvic fractures: value of plain radiography in early assessment and management. *Radiology.* 1986;160(2):445–451.
28. Chenoweth DR, Cruickshank B, Gertzbein SD, et al. A clinical and experimental investigation of occult injuries of the pelvic ring. *Injury.* 1980;12(1):59–65.
29. Gertzbein SD, Chenoweth DR. Occult injuries of the pelvic ring. *Clin Orthop Relat Res.* 1977;128:202–207.

30. Bucholz RW. The pathological anatomy of Malgaigne fracture-dislocations of the pelvis. *J Bone Joint Surg Am.* 1981;63(3):400–404.

31. Canale ST, Beaty JH. Pelvic and hip fractures. In: Rockwood CA Jr, Wilkins KE, Beaty JH, eds. *Fractures in Children.* 4th ed. Philadelphia, PA: JB Lippincott Co; 1996:1117–1118.

32. Young JW, Burgess AR. *Radiologic Management of Pelvic Ring fractures: Systematic Radiographic Diagnosis.* Baltimore, MD: Urban & Schwarzenberg; 1987.

33. Tile M, Pennal GF. Pelvic disruption: principles of management. *Clin Orthop Relat Res.* 1980;151:56–64.

34. Harris JH Jr, Loh CK, Perlman HC, et al. The roentgen diagnosis of pelvic extraperitoneal effusion. *Radiology.* 1977;125(2):343–350.

35. Malgaigne JF. *Traité des Fractures et des Luxations.* Paris, France: JB Bailliere; 1855.

36. Wild JJ Jr, Hanson GW, Tullos HS. Unstable fractures of the pelvis treated by external fixation. *J Bone Joint Surg Am.* 1982;64(7):1010–1020.

37. Edeiken-Monroe BS, Browner BD, Jackson H. The role of standard roentgenograms in the evaluation of instability of pelvic ring disruption. *Clin Orthop Relat Res.* 1989;240:63–76.

38. Bucholz RW. Pathomechanics of pelvic ring disruptions. *Adv Orthop Surg.* 1987:167–169.

39. Vrahas M, Hern TC, Diangelo D, et al. Ligamentous contributions to pelvic stability. *Orthopedics.* 1995;18(3):271–274.

40. Levene G, Kaufman SA. The diagnostic significance of roentgenologic soft tissue shadows in the pelvis. *AJR Am J Roentgenol.* 1958;79(4):697–704.

41. Kusmierski S, Tobik S. Some problems in surgical management of ruptured urethra in fracture of pelvis. *J Urol.* 1965;93:604–606.

42. Flaherty JJ, Kelley R, Burnett B, et al. Relationship of pelvic bone fracture patterns to injuries of urethra and bladder. *J Urol.* 1968;99(3):297–300.

43. Cass AS, Ireland GW. Bladder trauma associated with pelvic fractures in severely injured patients. *J Trauma.* 1973;13(3):205–212.

44. MacMahon R, Hosking D, Ramsey EW. Management of blunt injury to the lower urinary tract. *Can J Surg.* 1983;26(5):415–418.

45. Wilson RF, Smith JB, McCarroll KA. Trauma to the urinary tract. In: Wilson RF, Walt AJ, eds. *Management of Trauma: Pitfalls and Practice.* 2nd ed. Baltimore, MD: Williams & Wilkins; 1996:612.

46. Palmer JK, Benson GS, Corriere JN Jr. Diagnosis and initial management of urological injuries associated with 200 consecutive pelvic fractures. *J Urol.* 1983;130(4):712–714.

47. Cass AS. Urethral injury in the multiple-injured patient. *J Trauma.* 1989;24(10):901–906.

48. del Villar RG, Ireland GW, Cass AS. Management of bladder and urethral injury in conjunction with the immediate surgical treatment of the acute severe trauma patient. *J Urol.* 1972;108(4):581–585.

49. McCort JJ. *Trauma Radiology.* New York, NY: Churchill Livingstone; 1990.

50. Colapinto V, McCallum RW. Injury to the male posterior urethra in fractured pelvis: a new classification. *J Urol.* 1977;118(4):575–580.

51. Kawashima A, Sandler CM, Corriere JN Jr, et al. Type IV urethral injuries: retrograde urethrographic findings in six cases. *AJR Am J Roentgenol.* 1999;172(suppl):213.

52. McLaughlin AP III, Pfister RC. Double catheter technique for evaluation of urethral injury and differentiating urethral from bladder rupture. *Radiology.* 1974;110(3):716–719.

53. Cass AS. Diagnostic studies in bladder rupture. Indications and techniques. *Urol Clin North Am.* 1989;16(2):267–273.

54. Brick SH, Friedman AC. Imaging in pelvic trauma. In: Friedman AC, Radecki PD, Lev-Toaff AS, Hilpert PA, eds. *Clinical Pelvic Imaging, CT, Ultrasound, and MRI.* St. Louis, MO: Mosby; 1990:409.

55. Levine JI, Crampton RS. Major abdominal injuries associated with pelvic fractures. *Surg Gynecol Obstet.* 1963;116:223–226.

56. Dunnick NR, Sandler CM, et al, eds. *Textbook of Uroradiology.* 2nd ed. Baltimore, MD: Williams & Wilkins; 1997:313–316.

57. Corriere JN Jr, Harris JD. The management of urologic injuries in blunt pelvic trauma. *Radiol Clin North Am.* 1981;19(1):187–193.

58. Perry JF Jr, McClellan RJ. Autopsy findings in 127 patients following fatal traffic accidents. *Surg Gynecol Obstet.* 1964;119:586–590.

59. Bonavita J, Pollack HM. Injuries to the genitourinary tract. In: Grainger RG, Allison DJ, eds. *Diagnostic Radiology.* 2nd ed. Edinburgh: Churchill Livingstone; 1992:1339.

60. Netto NR Jr, Ikari O, Zuppo VP. Traumatic rupture of female urethra. *Urology.* 1983;22(6):601–603.

61. Bredael JJ, Kramer SA, Cleeve LK, et al. Traumatic rupture of the female urethra. *J Urol.* 1979;122(4):560–561.

62. Carroll PR, McAninch JW. Major bladder trauma: the accuracy of cystography. *J Urol.* 1983;130(5):887–888.

63. Mee SL, McAninch JW, Federle MP. Computerized tomography in bladder rupture: diagnostic limitations. *J Urol.* 1987;137(2):207–209.

64. Dalal SA, Burgess AR, Siegel JH, et al. Pelvic fracture in multiple trauma: classification by mechanism is key to pattern of organ injury, resuscitative requirements, and outcome. *J Trauma.* 1989;29(7):981–1000.

65. Smith K, Ben-Menachem Y, Duke JH Jr, et al. The superior gluteal: an artery at risk in blunt pelvic trauma. *J Trauma*. 1976;16:273–279.

66. Gaucher A, Pere P, Bannwarth B. Insufficiency fractures of the pelvis. *Clin Nucl Med*. 1986;11(7):518.

67. Davies AM, Evans NS, Struthers GR. Parasymphyseal and associated insufficiency fractures of the pelvis and sacrum. *Br J Radiol*. 1988;61(722):103–108.

68. Hauge MD, Cooper KL, Litin SC. Insufficiency fractures of the pelvis that simulate metastatic disease. *Mayo Clin Proc*. 1988;63(8):807–812.

69. Keats T. *Radiology of Muscular Skeletal Stress Injury*. Chicago, IL: Year Book; 1990.

70. Meurman KO. Stress fracture of the pubic arch in military recruits. *Br J Radiol*. 1980;53(630):521–524.

71. Ozburn MS, Nichols JW. Pubic ramus and adductor insertion stress fractures in female basic trainees. *Mil Med*. 1981;146(5):332–334.

72. Noakes TD, Smith JA, Lindenberd G, et al. Pelvic stress fractures in long distance runners. *Am J Sports Med*. 1986;13:120–123.

73. Helms CA. *Fundamentals of Skeletal Radiology*. Philadelphia, PA: WB Saunders; 1989.

74. Resnick D. Tumors and tumor-like lesions of bone. In: Resnick DN, Niwayama G, eds. *Diagnosis of Bone and Joint Disorders*. Philadelphia, PA: WB Saunders; 1981.

SUGGESTED READINGS

1. Brandser E. The pelvis. In: Rogers LF, ed. *Radiology of Skeletal*. 3rd ed. Philadelphia, PA: Churchill Livingstone; 2002:930–978.

2. Resnick CS. Pelvis and acetabular fractures. In: Mirvis SE, Shanmuganathan K, eds. *Imaging in Trauma and Critical Care*. 2nd ed. Philadelphia, PA: WB Saunders; 2003:559–566.

3. Schultz RJ. *The Language of Fractures*. 2nd ed. Baltimore, MD: Williams & Wilkins; 1990:152–164.

4. Starr AJ, Malekzadeh AS. Fractures of the pelvic ring. In: Bucholz RW, Heckman JD, Court-Brown C, eds. *Rockwood and Green's Fractures in Adults*. 6th ed. Philadelphia, PA: Lippincott Williams & Wilkins; 2006:1583–1664.

5. Kellam JF, Browner BD. Fractures of the pelvic ring. In: Browner BD, Jupiter JB, Levine AM, et al, eds. *Skeletal Trauma*. 2nd ed. Philadelphia, PA: WB Saunders; 1998:1117–1180.

6. Manaster BJ, May DA, Disler DG. *The Requisites: Musculoskeletal Imaging*. 3rd ed. Philadelphia, PA: Mosby; 2007:183–189.

7. Greenspan A. *Orthopedic Imaging: A Practical Approach*. 4th ed. Philadelphia, PA: Lippincott Williams & Wilkins; 2004:215–226.

8. Chew FS. *Musculoskeletal Imaging*. Philadelphia, PA: Lippincott Williams & Wilkins; 2003:97–103.

Anthony J. Wilson ■ John H. Harris Jr.

Fractures of the acetabulum are generally considered to be different than other pelvis fractures because they involve the hip joint, the largest weight-bearing joint in the body. Unlike pelvic ring injuries, isolated acetabular fractures are not usually life threatening. However, they can have significant long-term sequelae. These sequelae can be minimized by anatomic reduction and stabilization. For many years, orthopedic surgeons have used the classification system of Letournel and Judet for acetabular fracture evaluation and surgical planning. Because surgical approaches and fixation methods vary with the classification, accurate classification of these fractures is important for worthwhile communication between radiologist and orthopedist.

Traditionally, the mainstay of classification has been pelvic radiographs. The standard workup has consisted of three projections: an anteroposterior (AP) view and two oblique views, with all three covering the entire pelvis. Orthopedists usually refer to the oblique views as "Judet views." The anterior and posterior oblique projections of each hip demonstrated on the Judet views are known as the "obturator" and "iliac" obliques, respectively. In more recent years, computed tomography (CT) has also become a popular method for preoperative planning. There have been differences of opinion between different observers concerning the need for multiplanar and 3-D reformations and their value. Some observers have suggested that multiplanar reformations of CT should replace the radiographs and recent studies have supported this concept. A clear understanding of both the standard radiographs and axial and reformatted CT images is important in accurately classifying acetabular fractures.

THE COLUMN PRINCIPLE

In his 1993 book, Letournel described the acetabular column principle. This principle considers the hemipelvis to be an inverted "Y" with a "C" shaped acetabular articular surface positioned between the limbs of the "Y" (Fig. 18.1). The transmission of weight-bearing loads from the lower extremity to the spine is via the anterior and posterior limbs of the "Y," known as the anterior and posterior columns, respectively. Immediately adjacent to these columns are the anterior and posterior walls of the acetabulum. The classification system of Letournel and Judet simply analyzes the patterns of involvement of the columns and walls.

RADIOGRAPHIC EVALUATION

On the AP radiograph, cortical lines can be found, which are markers for the columns and walls (Figs. 18.2 and 18.3). The marker for the anterior column is an anterior cortical line, extending from ilium to pubis, known as the iliopectineal line. The marker for the posterior column is a posterior cortical line extending from ilium to ischium, known as the ilioischial line (Fig. 18.2). Two oblique cortical lines can usually be found projecting through the

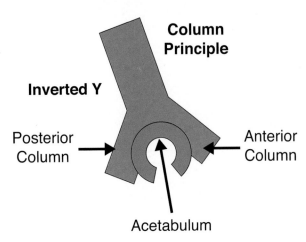

Figure 18.1. The column principle of Letournel and Judet.

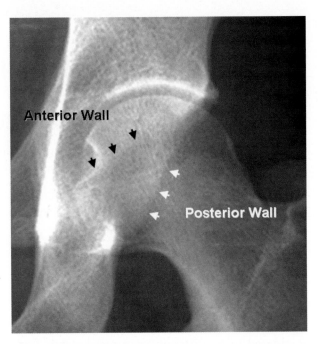

Figure 18.3. The location on an anteroposterior radiograph of the anterior and posterior walls of the acetabulum.

femoral head. The more lateral and slightly more vertical of these lines is the edge of the posterior acetabular wall. The more medial and slightly more horizontal line is the edge of the anterior wall (Fig. 18.3). The posterior wall should always be visible on a good quality AP radiograph, but the anterior wall is not always so well defined.

COMPUTED TOMOGRAPHIC EVALUATION

It is essential to carefully evaluate each axial CT slice for subtle injuries. However, the most helpful axial CT image for classifying acetabular fractures is the one that passes through the roof or "tectum" of the acetabulum (Fig. 18.4). The orientation of the

fracture on this image is the most important clue to the correct classification and extensions of the fracture into the iliac wing; posterior column, anterior column, and/or obturator ring will give further clues to the correct classification.

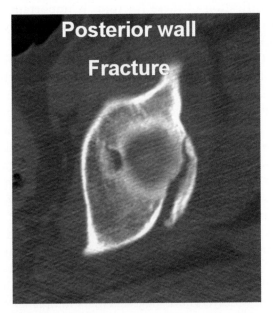

Figure 18.4. Axial CT scan through the acetabular tectum, showing the oblique orientation of a posterior wall fracture.

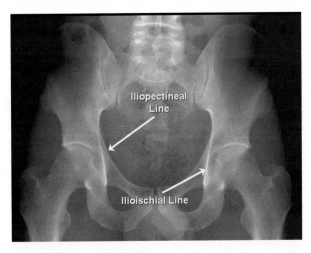

Figure 18.2. The radiographic markers for the anterior and posterior columns.

CLASSIFICATION

Letournel and Judet described five basic or "elemental" patterns of acetabular fractures and five combined patterns. Four of the basic fracture patterns divide the acetabulum into anterior and posterior sections. Each of these four elemental fractures involves only a single column or wall. A fifth elemental fracture divides the acetabulum transversely into superior and inferior components and extends across both of the columns. Thus, the five elemental patterns are anterior column, posterior column, anterior wall, posterior wall, and transverse (Fig. 18.5). All of the combined patterns include two or more of these elements. The five combined patterns are posterior column with posterior wall, both columns, transverse with posterior wall, transverse with "T" extension, and anterior column with posterior hemitransverse (Fig. 18.6).

Although at first this classification sounds complicated and difficult to remember, it can be simplified by listing the different fracture types into three categories: column fractures, wall fractures, and transverse fractures (Fig. 18.7). Most of the combined patterns fall into more than one of these categories. An additional factor that helps with sorting out the patterns is the fact that some of the patterns are distinctly uncommon. Studies have shown that posterior wall fractures, both-column fracture, and transverse fracture variants account for well more than 90% of all acetabular fractures. Thus, if the observer can separate these three patterns, classification of most acetabular fractures becomes easy.

Separating these three fracture patterns is not difficult as long as the observer follows a few simple principles. Isolated posterior wall fractures are unlikely to be confused with the other two common patterns because of the posterior wall fracture's simplicity, different location, and different orientation. The problem then becomes how do you separate both-column pattern from the transverse varieties, as all of these fractures involve both of the acetabular columns? The distinction between these two is also straightforward. All column fractures divide the acetabulum vertically into anterior and posterior components and appear as coronal fractures of an axial CT image of the acetabular tectum (Fig. 18.8). All transverse fractures divide the acetabulum horizontally into superior and inferior components and appear as sagittal fractures on an axial CT image of the acetabular tectum (Fig. 18.9). Additionally, both-column fracture start in the iliac wing and extend inferiorly through the iliopectineal

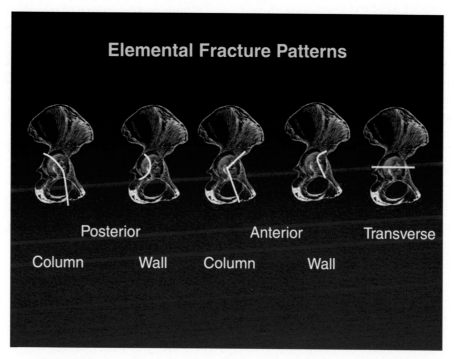

Figure 18.5. The five elemental fracture patterns of Letournel and Judet.

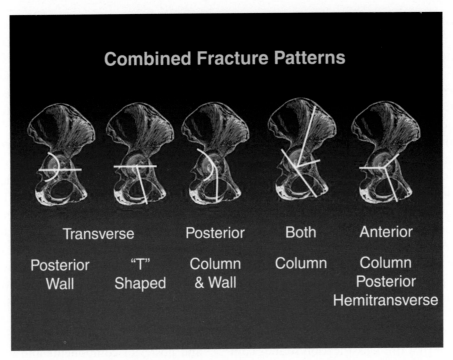

Figure 18.6. The five combined fracture patterns of Letournel and Judet.

line, ilioischial line, and ischiopubic ramus. All transverse fractures also extend through both the iliopectineal and ilioischial lines, and although the T-shaped variant includes an ischiopubic ramus fracture, there is no transverse pattern that extends upward into the iliac wing.

On the initial evaluation, the observer should determine if the iliopectineal line, the ilioischial line, or both lines are disrupted. If both are disrupted, the choice lies between a transverse variant and both-column fracture (Figs. 18.10 and 18.11). If the fracture extends up into the ilium, both-column fracture is most likely. However, the final proof can be obtained from the orientation of the fracture on an axial CT image of the acetabular tectum (Figs. 18.4, 18.8, 18.9, and 18.12).

Acetabular wall fractures, whether isolated or combined, will appear as oblique fracture lines on the tectal CT image (Fig. 18.4). Posterior wall fractures, although usually visible and diagnosable on AP radiographs, are more clearly demonstrated by an obturator oblique view (Fig. 18.13).

Combined fracture patterns such as transverse/ posterior wall or anterior column/posterior hemi-transverse will show combinations of the earlier fracture orientations on the tectal CT image.

In summary, if the observer identifies the fracture lines to determine any involvement of the iliac wing, iliopectineal line, ilioischial line, and/or ischiopubic ramus (Fig. 18.14) and then checks the orientation of the fracture on the tectal CT (Fig. 18.12), the classification should be clear.

Figure 18.7. The fracture patterns separated into three simple groups.

Three Fracture Groups

Transverse	Column	Wall
Transverse	Ant Column	Anterior Wall
Trans/ Post Wall	Post Column	Posterior Wall
"T"-Shaped	AC/Post Hemi Tr	Trans/ Post Wall
	Post Col/Wall	Post Col/Wall
	Both Column	

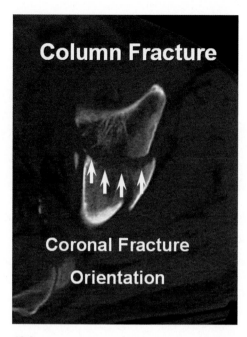

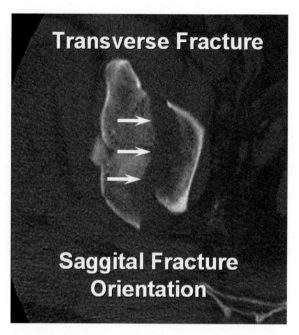

Figure 18.8. Axial CT scan through the acetabular tectum, showing the coronal orientation of a both column fracture.

Figure 18.9. CT scan through the acetabular tectum, showing the sagittal orientation of a transverse fracture.

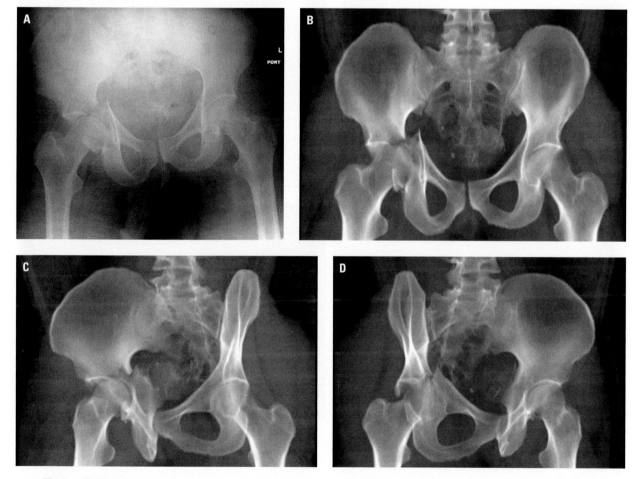

Figure 18.10. Transverse fracture, with disruption of both the iliopectineal and ilioischial lines. Conventional radiograph (**A**) compared to simulated radiographs created by 3-D reformation of CT data including AP (**B**), iliac oblique (**C**), and obturator oblique (**D**).

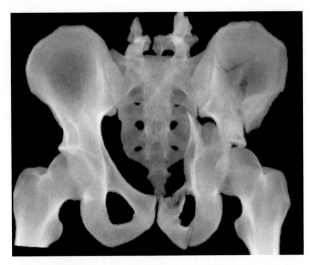

Figure 18.11. Both column fracture. 3D reformation of CT data with soft tissue structures removed.

Acetabular Fractures
Tectal CT Orientation

Coronal	Sagittal	Oblique
Column	Transverse	Wall

Figure 18.12. Diagrammatic representation of the orientation of column, transverse, and wall fractures on an axial CT scan through the acetabular tectum.

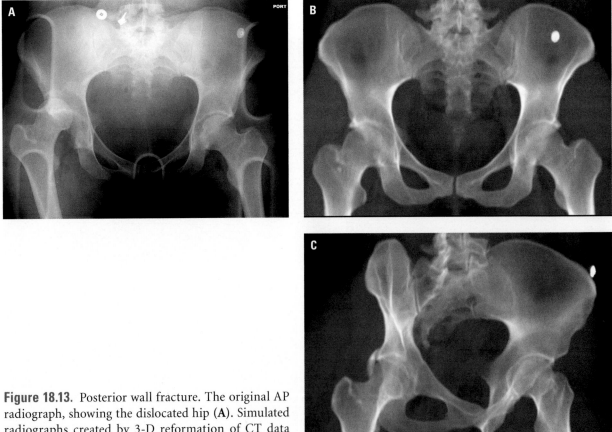

Figure 18.13. Posterior wall fracture. The original AP radiograph, showing the dislocated hip (**A**). Simulated radiographs created by 3-D reformation of CT data including AP (**B**) and obturator oblique view (**C**).

The Commonest Fracture Patterns

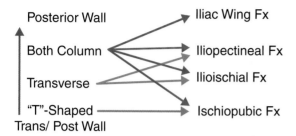

Figure 18.14. Summary diagram of the five most common fracture patterns, with locations of fracture lines. *Fx*, fracture.

Computed Tomography-Based Classification of Acetabular Fractures

Analysis of the data obtained from the CT scans of the 112 acetabular fractures revealed that all the fractures studied fell into one of four general categories, as shown in Table 18.1. These were category 0, those limited to the wall only; category I, those involving a single column (either anterior or posterior); category II, those involving both the anterior and posterior columns simultaneously, except for the floating acetabulum; and category III, those in which the acetabulum was completely separated from the axial skeleton anteriorly and posteriorly, such as the floating acetabulum.

Wall fractures were designated as category 0 to preserve categories I and II for single- and two-column fractures, respectively. When a wall fracture (category 0) occurred in conjunction with a single- or a two-column fracture, the injury was described as category I or II with associated anterior or posterior wall component.

Most acetabular column fractures are comminuted, particularly those involving both columns. The column category designations in this classification system are based solely on the number of columns fractured and presence and direction of fracture extension, if any, regardless of the degree of comminution. In category II, the subgroup designations indicate the direction (superior, inferior, or both) of fracture extension because fracture extension is an important feature of surgical planning. The degree of comminution is irrelevant regarding the determination of surgical approach. Therefore, the degree of comminution was purposely excluded regarding fracture category designation.

Category 0: Wall Fracture

The walls, as seen on axial CT scans of the acetabulum, are illustrated in Figure 18.15. Wall fractures are those limited to the posterior and posterosuperior (common) or anterior (uncommon) wall component of the columns. Wall fractures may occur as isolated injuries (Fig. 18.16 A–C) or in conjunction with any other category of acetabular fracture.

TABLE 18.1	Frequency of Fracture Types	
Category	**Definition**	**Frequency (%)**
0	Wall only or possible component of another type	21
I	Single column	21
II	Two column (horizontal)	48
Subcategory	Extension (%)	
A	None (27)	
B	Superior (5)	
C	Inferior (11)	
D	Superior and inferior (5)	
III	Floating acetabulum: articulating surface not attached to axial skeleton anteriorly or posteriorly	10
Total		100

From Harris JH, Lee JS, Coupe KJ, et al. Acetabular fractures revisited: part I, redefinition of the Letournel anterior column. *AJR.* 2004;182(6):1363–1366, with permission.

Figure 18.15. Schematic representation shows midacetabular CT scan. Line a–a¹ establishes the anterior (AC) and posterior (PC) columns. Anterior (AW) and posterior (PW) walls lie lateral to line b–b¹. (From Harris JH, Lee JS, Coupe KJ, et al. Acetabular fractures revisited: part I, redefinition of the Letournel anterior column. *AJR*. 2004;182(6):1363–1366, with permission.)

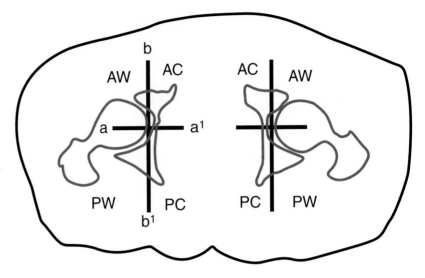

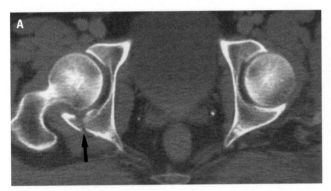

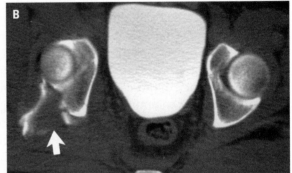

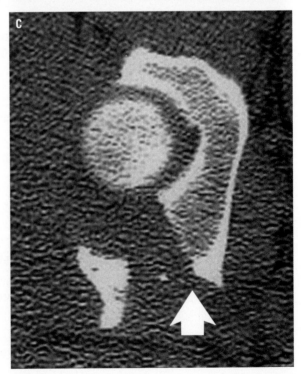

Figure 18.16. Type 0: Wall fractures in three patients. **A:** Axial CT scan of midpelvis shows minimally displaced posterior wall fracture *(arrow)*. **B:** Axial CT scan shows comminuted displaced posterior wall fracture *(arrow)*. **C:** Axial CT scan shows posterior wall fracture with fracture line at wall column junction *(arrow)*. (From Harris JH, Lee JS, Coupe KJ, et al. Acetabular fractures revisited: part I, redefinition of the Letournel anterior column. *AJR*. 2004;182(6):1363–1366, with permission.)

Category I: Single-Column Fracture

A single-column fracture is limited to only the anterior (Fig. 18.17A–D) or the posterior column (Fig. 18.17E–F). Clearly, a single column does not transverse the acetabulum. Single-column fractures may also extend superiorly or inferiorly from the acetabulum.

Category II: Two-Column Fracture

The proposed two-column category is a major departure from, and simplification of, the Letournel classification. This broad category includes all fractures that simultaneously involve both the anterior and posterior columns, with the exception of the floating acetabulum, regardless of their pathologic anatomy. This category, therefore, includes the following Letournel fracture types: pure transverse, T-shaped and its varieties, transverse and posterior wall, and anterior column and hemitransverse. None of these is specifically identified in the Letournel system as involving both columns. This category also includes the large variety of unnamed acetabular fractures that involve both columns but are not included in the Letournel classification.

Fractures in category II fall into subcategories based on fracture extension beyond the acetabulum as follows:

■ Subcategory IIA includes those two-column acetabular fractures in which the fracture is limited to the acetabulum without extension beyond the acetabulum (Fig. 18.18A–B). This category of acetabular fractures includes the Letournel pure transverse regardless of whether the fracture is horizontal or obliquely horizontal and regardless of its location through the acetabulum such as supratectal, tectal, infratectal, or through the middle or inferior portions of the acetabulum; transverse and posterior fractures; and fractures of the anterior column

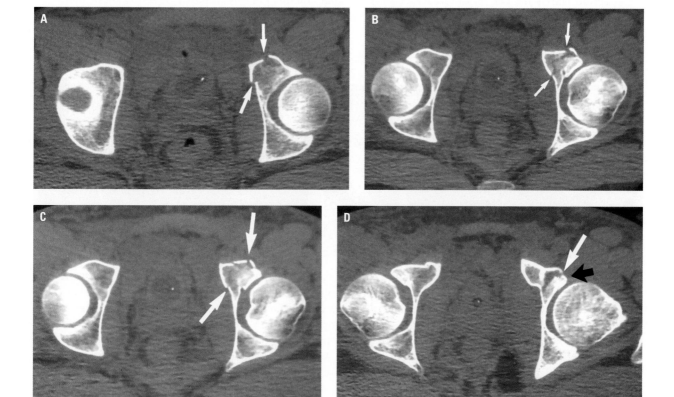

Figure 18.17. Type I: Single-column fracture. **A:** Axial CT scan of midpelvis shows minimally displaced left anterior column fracture *(arrows)*. **B:** Axial CT scan of midpelvis shows comminuted, minimally displaced left anterior column fracture *(arrows)*. **C:** Subjacent caudal axial CT scan shows caudal extension of comminuted anterior column fracture *(arrows)*. **D:** Further subjacent caudal axial CT scan shows extension of anterior column fracture *(white arrow)* in anterior wall *(black arrow)*. *(continued)*

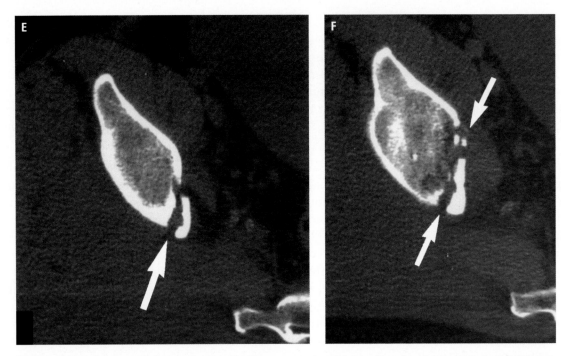

Figure 18.17. *(continued)* **E:** Axial CT scan shows posterior column fracture *(arrow).* **F:** Axial CT scan obtained more caudal than E of third patient shows comminution of posterior column fracture *(arrows).* (From Harris JH, Lee JS, Coupe KJ, et al. Acetabular fractures revisited: part I, redefinition of the Letournel anterior column. *AJR.* 2004;182(6):1363–1366, with permission.)

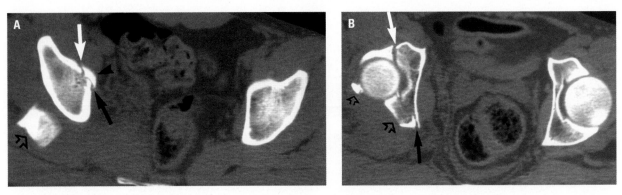

Figure 18.18. Type IIA: Two-column fracture without extension but with associated posterior wall fracture. **A:** Supraacetabular axial CT scan shows anterior column fracture *(white arrow),* iliopectineal line *(arrowhead),* and posterior column fracture *(solid black arrow). Open arrow* indicates superiorly displaced posterior wall fragment. **B:** Type IIA: Axial CT scan obtained more caudal than **A** of the same patient shows anterior *(white arrow)* and posterior *(solid black arrow)* column fractures. *Open arrows* indicate associated posterior wall fracture. (From Harris JH, Lee JS, Coupe KJ, et al. Acetabular fractures revisited: part I, redefinition of the Letournel anterior column. *AJR.* 2004;182(6):1363–1366, with permission.)

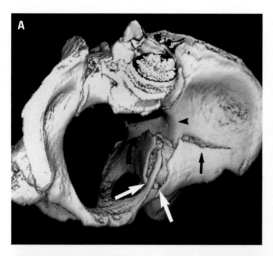
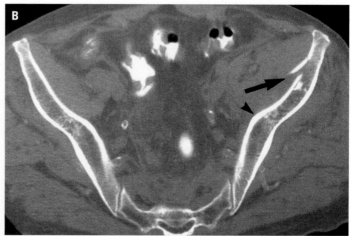
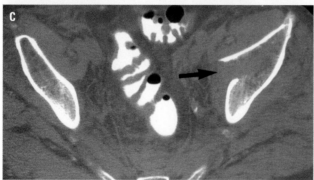
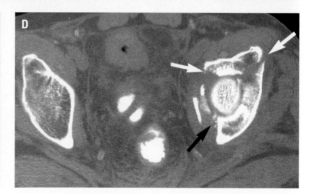

Figure 18.19. Type IIB: Two-column fracture with superior extension to iliac wing. **A:** 3-D reformatted CT scan shows anterior *(white arrows)* and posterior *(curved arrow)* column fractures. *Arrowhead* indicates iliopectineal line. *Straight black arrow* indicates superior extension of acetabular fracture to iliac wing. **B:** Axial CT scan of false pelvis shows superior extension of fracture *(arrow)* above iliopectineal line *(arrowhead)* into iliac wing. **C:** Type IIB: Axial CT scan of false pelvis shows fracture *(arrow)* at the level of iliopectineal line. **D:** Type IIB: Axial CT scan shows comminuted anterior column fracture with associated anterior wall component *(white arrows)* and posterior column fracture *(black arrow)*. (From Harris JH, Lee JS, Coupe KJ, et al. Acetabular fractures revisited: part I, redefinition of the Letournel anterior column. *AJR.* 2004;182(6):1363–1366, with permission.)

or wall associated with a hemitransverse fracture posteriorly.

■ Subcategory IIB includes those two-column acetabular fractures in which a fracture component extends superiorly above the iliopectineal line into the iliac wing (Fig. 18.19A–D).

■ Subcategory IIC includes those two-column acetabular fractures in which a fracture component extends into either the ischium, to the junction of the ischium and inferior pubic ramus (Letournel T-shaped and variants), or to the inferior pubic ramus (Fig. 18.20A–C).

■ Subcategory IID includes those acetabular fractures with both superior and inferior extensions

beyond the acetabulum (Fig. 18.21A–D). The Letournel classification does not include this variety of acetabular fracture.

Category III: Floating Acetabulum (Letournel "Associated Both-Column Fracture")

The essential feature of the floating acetabulum that distinguishes it from all other two-column fractures is that the articulating surface of the acetabulum is separated from the axial skeleton both anteriorly and posteriorly (Fig. 18.22A–E). The Letournel classification does not include this fracture but does include the "associated both-column fracture," the

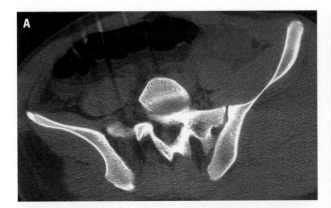

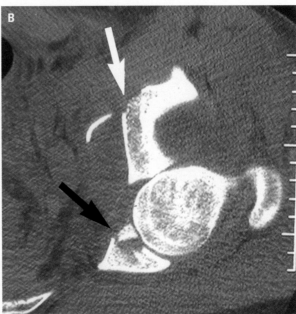

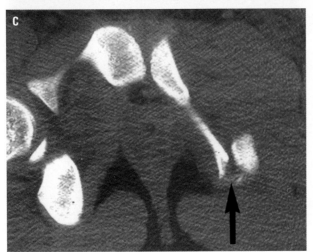

Figure 18.20. Type IIC: Two-column acetabular fracture with inferior extension. **A:** Axial CT scan of false pelvis shows each iliac wing intact, thereby excluding superior fracture extension. **B:** Axial CT scan shows comminuted and displaced anterior *(white arrow)* and posterior *(black arrow)* column fractures. **C:** Axial CT scan through level of pelvic outlet shows fracture *(arrow)* of left ischial tuberosity. (From Harris JH, Lee JS, Coupe KJ, et al. Acetabular fractures revisited: part I, redefinition of the Letournel anterior column. *AJR.* 2004;182(6):1363–1366, with permission.)

definition of which is ambiguous. This ambiguity is further extended by the implication contained in its name that the associated both-column fracture is the only acetabular fracture that involves both columns. Because the acetabular articulating surface is uniquely separated from the axial skeleton, we believe, as does Tile, this fracture merits category designation to itself, which is another departure from the Letournel system.

The floating acetabulum (category III) fracture is characterized by fracture lines that extend transversely through the posterior column and separate the acetabulum from the axial skeleton posteriorly, and fractures of the pubic rami, body, or both that separate the articulating surface from the axial skeleton anteriorly.

The distinction between the category IID (two column with superior and inferior extensions) and the category III (floating acetabulum) is frequently difficult because of their complexity and similar appearance on axial CT. Although a complete fracture through the posterior column disrupts the osseous continuity between the acetabulum and the axial skeleton, an incomplete posterior column fracture does not, thereby excluding a category III fracture.

The relationship of the Letournel fracture types to the proposed classification is shown in Figure 18.23 and the frequency of the various fracture types in Table 18.1.

Although based on the axial CT appearance of acetabular fractures, the proposed classification has direct application to 3-D reformatted images as well.

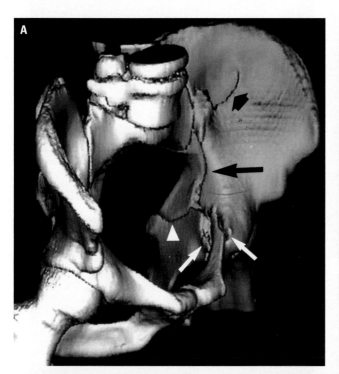

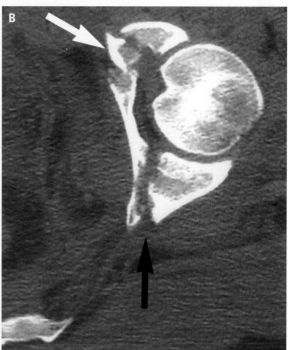

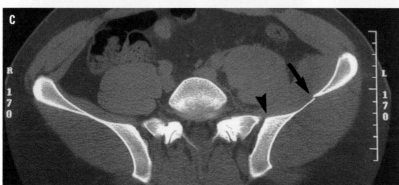

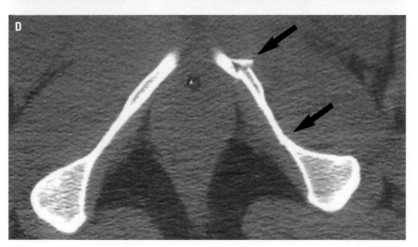

Figure 18.21. Type IID: Two-column acetabular fracture with superior and inferior extension. **A:** 3-D reformatted CT scan shows anterior *(white arrows)* and posterior *(long black arrow)* column fractures, superior extension above iliopectineal line *(short black arrow)*, and inferior extension *(white arrowhead)*. **B:** Midpelvic axial CT scan shows left anterior *(white arrow)* and posterior *(black arrow)* column fractures. **C:** Axial CT scan obtained rostral to iliopectineal line *(black arrowhead)* shows superior fracture extension to iliac wing *(black arrow)*. **D:** Axial CT scan obtained through inferior pubic rami shows inferior fracture extension to left inferior pubic ramus *(black arrows)*. (From Harris JH, Lee JS, Coupe KJ, et al. Acetabular fractures revisited: part I, redefinition of the Letournel anterior column. *AJR.* 2004;182(6):1363–1366, with permission.)

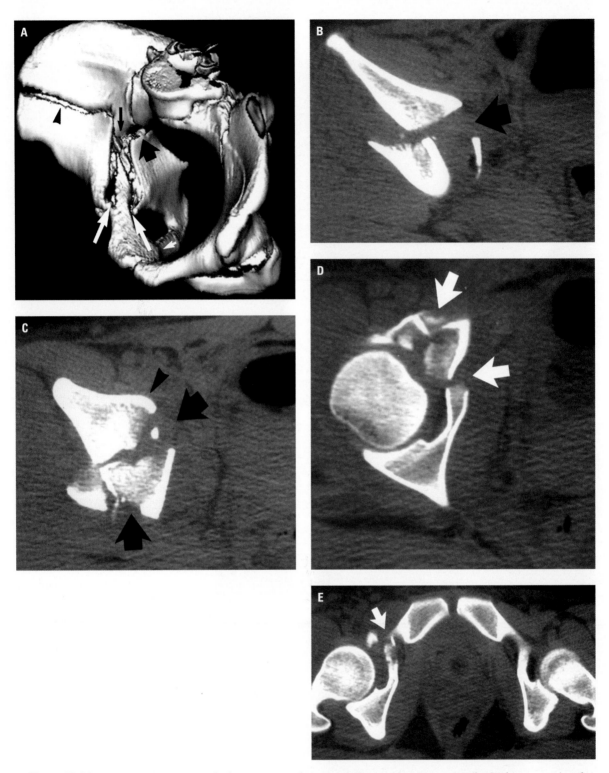

Figure 18.22. Type III: Floating acetabulum. **A:** 3-D reformatted CT scan shows anterior *(long white arrows)* and inferior pubic ramus fractures *(short white arrow)*, which, together, separate acetabulum from axial skeleton anteriorly; posterior column fracture *(long black arrow)*, which separates acetabulum from axial skeleton posteriorly; superior fracture extension to right iliac wing *(arrowhead)*; and inferior fracture extension *(short black arrow)*. **B:** Axial CT scan obtained through level of iliopectineal line shows right superior fracture extension *(black arrow)*. **C:** Axial CT scan shows comminuted displaced right posterior column fracture *(black arrows)*. *Black arrowhead* indicates iliopectineal line. **D:** Midpelvic axial CT scan shows comminuted, displaced anterior column fracture *(white arrows)*. **E:** Axial CT scan obtained through level of inferior pubic rami shows comminuted, displaced fracture of right inferior pubic ramus *(white arrow)*. (From Harris JH, Lee JS, Coupe KJ, et al. Acetabular fractures revisited: part I, redefinition of the Letournel anterior column. *AJR*. 2004;182(6):1363–1366, with permission.)

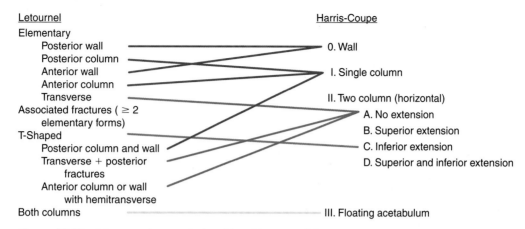

Figure 18.23. Diagram shows relationship of Letournel fracture types to Harris-Coupe categories. (From Harris JH, Lee JS, Coupe KJ, et al. Acetabular fractures revisited: part I, redefinition of the Letournel anterior column. *AJR.* 2004;182(6):1363–1366, with permission.)

SUGGESTED READINGS

1. Brandser E. The pelvis. In: Rogers LF, ed. *Radiology of Skeletal Trauma.* 3rd ed. Philadelphia, PA: Churchill Livingstone; 2002:979–1002.
2. Chapin RW. Acetabular fractures. In: Jeffery RB, Manaster BJ, Gurney JW, et al, eds. *Diagnostic Imaging: Emergency.* Salt Lake City, UT: Amirsys, Inc; 2007:I-4-126–I-4-130.
3. Chew FS. *Musculoskeletal Imaging.* Philadelphia, PA: Lippincott Williams & Wilkins; 2003: 105–109.
4. Letournel E. *Fractures of the Acetabulum.* Heidelberg, Germany: Springer-Verlag; 1993.
5. Reiley MC. Fractures of the acetabulum. In: Bucholz RW, Heckman JD, Court-Brown C, eds. *Rockwood and Green's Fractures in Adults.* 6th ed. Philadelphia, PA: Lippincott Williams & Wilkins; 2006:1665–1714.
6. Resnik CS. Pelvic and acetabular fractures. In: Mirvis SE, Shanmuganathan K, eds. *Imaging in Trauma and Critical Care.* Philadelphia, PA: Saunders; 2003:559–574.
7. Stern EJ. *Trauma Radiology Companion.* Philadelphia, PA: Lippincott-Raven; 1997;297–308.

CHAPTER 19

Hips and Proximal Femora

John H. Harris Jr.

GENERAL CONSIDERATIONS

The hip is a ball and socket joint consisting of the acetabulum and the head of the femur. The articulating (lunate) surface of the acetabulum is incomplete medially (acetabular notch) and is thickest superiorly to accommodate the pressure of the body weight when erect. This radiographically dense segment portion of the lunate surface must not be misinterpreted as the reactive sclerosis of degenerative joint disease.

The femoral head, which occupies the acetabular fossa, has a shallow concavity (fovea centralis) on its superomedial surface to which the ligamentum teres is attached. The ligamentum teres carries a small artery, the artery of the ligamentum teres, which supplies only approximately 10% of the blood supply to the femoral head. This has an important relationship to subcapital femoral neck fractures that is discussed and illustrated in the body of this chapter.

The femoral neck including the intertrochanteric crest and the proximal femoral shaft are, anatomically, not considered part of the hip. However, because fractures of these segments of the proximal femur are clinically referred to as "hip fractures," they are included in this chapter.

It is necessary to realize that the "frog leg lateral" of the hip is not the true lateral projection of the proximal femur but is simply an externally rotated view. The "groin" or cross-lateral projection of the proximal femur is the only true lateral orthogonal view of the hip. This important fact is illustrated in the body of this chapter.

The capital femoral epiphysis appears during the first year of life, the apophysis of the greater trochanter appears before the fifth year, and that of the lesser trochanter during the 13th year. All of these centers unite with the femur during the 18th to 20th years.

A homily aptly describes the relationship of the femoral head to the femoral neck. The femoral head rests symmetrically on the femoral neck like a scoop of ice cream squarely placed in an ice cream cone. In both the anteroposterior (AP) and lateral radiographs, the sweep of the cortex extending from the neck to the head is smooth and symmetrical (Fig. 19.1). Before the fusion of the head with the neck, the capital femoral epiphysis sits squarely on the metaphysis of the femoral neck. Asymmetry of the head with respect to the neck, even if seen in only one projection, is an abnormal finding and represents either slipped capital femoral epiphysis (SCFE) in an adolescent or a subcapital fracture in an adult.

The routine examination of the hip includes AP (Fig. 19.1A), lateral (Fig. 19.1B), and externally rotated (Fig. 19.1C) projections. The AP view of the hip must include a clear depiction of the greater trochanter (Fig. 19.1D). Distinction must be made between true lateral and frog leg lateral projections of the hip. The true (horizontal beam, cross-table, groin) lateral projection is obtained with the patient supine and the injured lower extremity in full extension. The opposite, uninvolved hip and knee are flexed approximately 90 degrees each, and the ipsilateral foot is supported off the radiographic table

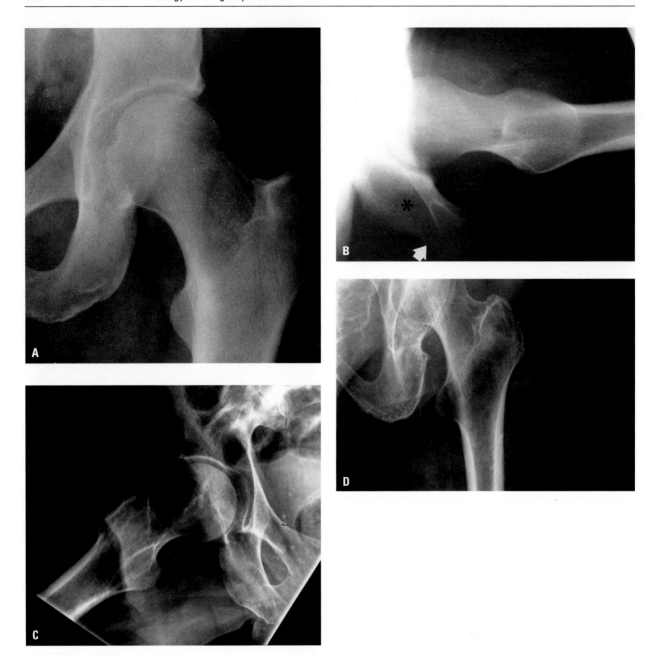

Figure 19.1. AP and lateral radiographs of the hip. **A:** On the frontal projection, linear lucencies *(open arrows)* representing fascial planes covering the gluteus minimus *(superior open arrow)* and the iliopsoas *(inferior open arrow)* muscles are frequently mistakenly thought to outline the hip joint capsule. The capsule is deep to each of these muscles. **B:** On the groin lateral projection, the angle subtended by the intersection of the long axis of the femoral neck and the proximal femoral shaft should be approximately 120 degrees, with the apex posteriorly directed. The horizontal beam lateral projection can always be oriented properly using the ischium *(asterisk)* and its tuberosity *(white arrow)* as landmarks. **C:** Frog leg projection: The frog leg projection results in an approximately 45-degree oblique view of the proximal femur. It is *not* a lateral view as suggested by the misnomer "frog leg lateral." **D:** The frontal view of the proximal femur must include a true depiction of the greater trochanter.

by a low stool or box. The x-ray tube is then positioned so that the beam is parallel to the table top, with the central ray directed mediolaterally parallel to and in the same vertical plane as the inguinal crease. The cassette is firmly positioned against the flank between the iliac crest and the 12th rib on the injured side perpendicular to the central ray. This beam cassette geometry results in the true lateral radiograph of the hip (Fig. 19.1B), which is essential for the complete evaluation of injuries of the proximal portion of the femur.

The "frog leg lateral" projection, on the other hand, is actually an oblique projection of the proximal portion of the femur and is obtained with the patient supine and the femur abducted and externally rotated. The x-ray tube is vertically positioned with respect to the patient (and the radiographic table) and centered over the hip joint. The resultant radiograph depicts the femur in midposition between true AP and true lateral positions. The frog leg radiograph is inappropriate in the evaluation of the patient with an acute injury of the hip because of the manipulation of the hip necessary to achieve this view and because neither the femoral neck-shaft angle nor the greater trochanter can be adequately evaluated.

In the frontal projection of the hip (Fig. 19.2), the lateral weight-bearing portion of the acetabular roof is thicker and more densely sclerotic than the other radiographically visible portions of the acetabular concavity. The transition from the weight-bearing portion of the roof to the adjacent surface of the fossa is normally abrupt and represents the free margin of the lunate surface. The posterior acetabular rim, which is usually visible through the density of the femoral head, appears as a thin, faint, occasionally slightly undulating linear density that extends inferomedially from the lateral free margin of the acetabular roof. The anterior acetabular rim, which is less often visible, is medial to the posterior rim and has a similar oblique orientation. The inferior portion of the acetabular fossa, with the exception of the teardrop shadow, is not visible radiographically because of the acetabular notch.

The femoral head arises from a single ossification center that appears at the end of the first year of life (Fig. 19.3) and fuses with the femoral neck at approximately age 18 years. The fused physeal scar identifies the anatomic neck of the femur.

In the straight frontal, externally rotated oblique, and groin lateral projections, the femoral head is normally symmetrically situated on the femoral neck. The convexity of the subchondral cortex of the head is normally congruent with the concavity of the lunate surface of the acetabulum. The fovea centralis (Fig. 19.2) is a short concavity located in

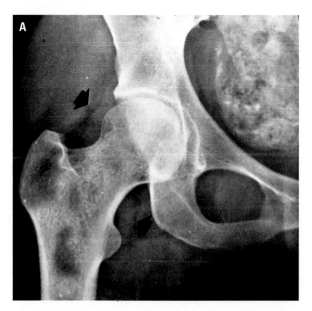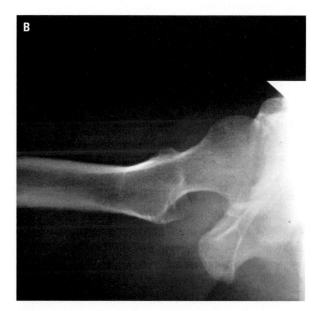

Figure 19.2. Normal adult hip in AP (**A**) and horizontal beam groin lateral (**B**) projections. On the AP radiograph (**A**), the *superolateral arrow* indicates the fascial plane covering the gluteus minimus muscle; the *inferomedial arrow*, the iliopsoas muscle.

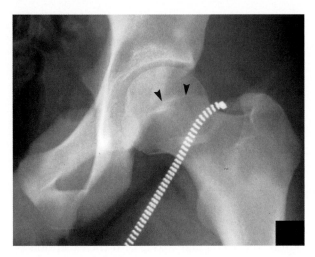

Figure 19.3. AP projection of an adolescent hip. The thin curvilinear density *(arrowheads)* is the "scar" of the fused proximal femoral physis.

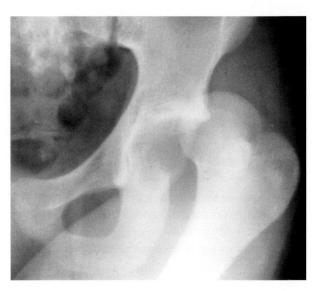

Figure 19.4. Posterior dislocation of the left hip without associated fracture.

the convexity of the femoral head into which inserts the ligamentum teres (ligament of the head of the femur). This ligament generally contains a small artery that provides approximately 10% of the blood supply of the femoral head.

HIP TRAUMA

Hip Dislocation

The most common mechanism of injury in dislocation of the hip is abrupt deceleration such as occurs in a motor vehicle accident in which the knee strikes the dashboard with the force of impact transmitted along the femoral shaft to the femoral head. If, at the moment of impact, the thigh is adducted, the femoral head may be dislocated posterolaterally, without (Fig. 19.4) or with (Fig. 19.5) fracture of the posterior acetabular lip. Because the mechanism of injury of posterior dislocation of the hip also usually includes an element of superior displacement, the femoral head will come to rest in some degree of superior displacement with respect to the acetabular fossa. Its posterior location is established on the horizontal beam lateral projection (Fig. 19.4). Anterior dislocation of the hip represents 10% to 15% of traumatic hip dislocations.[1–4] In anterior dislocation, the femur may be displaced anteriorly and medially toward the superior pubic ramus (Fig. 19.6) or toward the obturator foramen (Fig. 19.7).[5] In this instance, an impaction of the femoral head on the dense, blunt anteroinferior arc of the anterior acetabular rim may produce a Hill-Sachs type of fracture of the femoral head (Fig. 19.7B). Medial displacement of the femoral head with respect to the acetabulum, in the frontal projection (Fig. 19.6A), is characteristic of anterior dislocation and distinguishes it from the typical superolateral position of the posteriorly dislocated hip. The anterior dislocation will be confirmed in the horizontal beam lateral radiograph (Fig. 19.6B).

The configuration of the posterior rim of the acetabulum resembles the blade of a hatchet or axe. Consequently, as described and illustrated, the thin edge of the rim is subject to fracture (Figs. 19.5 and 19.8) with posterior hip dislocation. When, because of the direction of the dislocating force, the posterior acetabular rim functions as a cutting edge, the impacting force is dissipated on the femoral head, resulting in capital femoral epiphyseal separation in adolescents (Fig. 19.9) or fracture of the femoral head in adults (Figs. 19.10 and 19.11). The cardinal signs of femoral head fracture on the initial examination include a flat segment of the femoral head without its normal subchondral cortex and separate fracture fragment(s) within the acetabular fossa (Figs. 19.10 and 19.11). The role of computed tomography (CT) and 3-D CT in evaluation of injuries of the hip is illustrated in a patient with

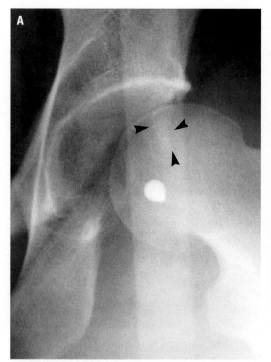

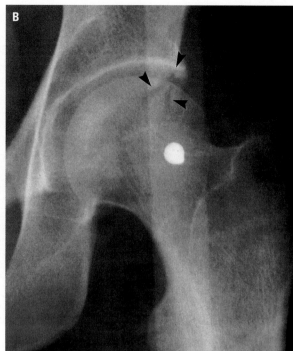

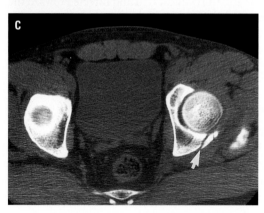

Figure 19.5. Posterior fracture dislocation. **A:** On the AP radiograph, the dislocation of the femoral head should be obvious because of the gross incongruity of its cortical margins with that of the acetabulum. A faint, vertical density *(arrowheads)* represents a minimally displaced posterior rim fragment. **B:** The fracture line *(arrowheads)* is more evident on the postreduction radiograph. **C:** The posterior rim fracture *(arrow)* is confirmed on CT.

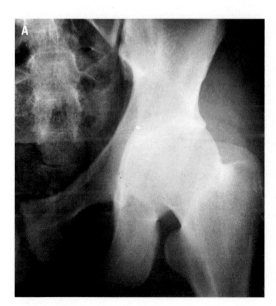

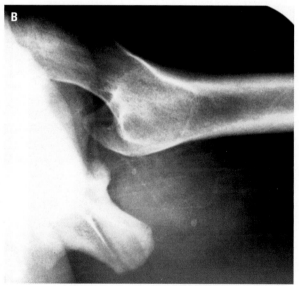

Figure 19.6. Anterior dislocation of the hip in which the femoral head is displaced medially and toward the superior pubic ramus (**A**). The anterior dislocation is confirmed in the horizontal beam lateral projection (**B**).

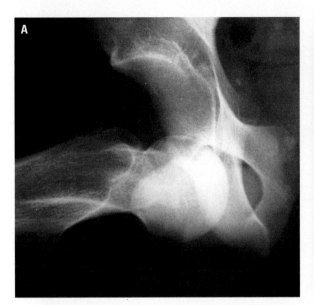
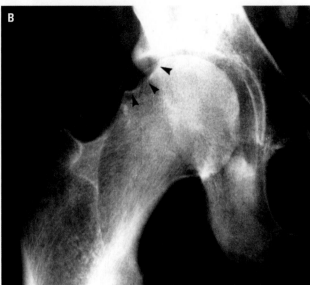

Figure 19.7. "Obturator" variety of anterior hip dislocation with associated compression fracture of the femoral head. **A:** In the frontal projection, the femoral head is anteriorly dislocated and directed toward the obturator foramen. With the femoral head in this position relative to the acetabulum, it is entirely reasonable to suspect the possibility of a femoral head compression fracture. **B:** In the postreduction radiograph, the femoral head compression fracture *(arrowheads)* is clearly evident.

bilateral posterior dislocations of the hip and bilateral femoral head fractures (Fig. 19.12) in which the 3-D CT images provide unambiguous spatial orientation and relationships of the intra-articular fragments and the dislocated femora with respect to the acetabular fossae.

Proximal Femoral Fractures

Fractures of the proximal end of the femur may be classified based on their relationship to the hip joint capsule—that is, intracapsular (subcapital, transcervical, and basicervical) or extracapsular

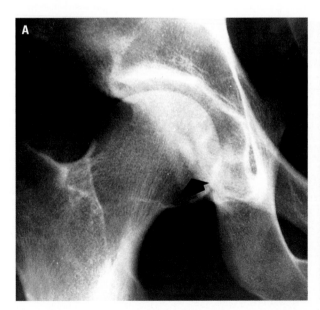
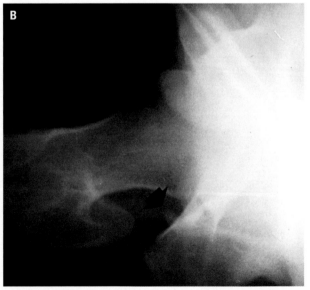

Figure 19.8. Isolated fracture of the posterior acetabular lip. *Arrows* indicate the posterior lip fragment in both frontal (**A**) and horizontal beam lateral (**B**) projections. There is no evidence of associated dislocation.

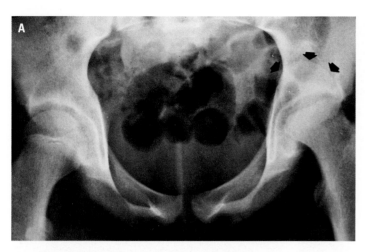

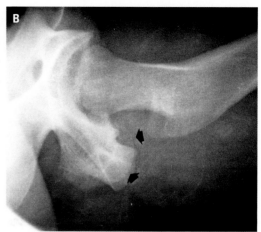

Figure 19.9. Capital femoral epiphyseal separation–posterior dislocation. **A:** In the frontal projection, the capital femoral epiphysis is indicated by the *arrows*. The femoral neck has remained within the acetabulum, and its metaphyseal plate relates to the acetabular fossa. **B:** In the horizontal beam lateral radiograph, the *arrows* indicate the posteriorly dislocated capital femoral epiphysis.

(intertrochanteric, subtrochanteric, and trochanteric)[6]—or based on the geographic location of the fracture, that is, femoral neck (subcapital, transcervical, and basicervical), intertrochanteric (subclassified based on number of fragments), trochanteric, and subtrochanteric.[7–9] Intracapsular fractures have a significantly higher incidence (10% to 35%)[6,9,10] of aseptic

(avascular) necrosis of the femoral head than extracapsular fractures. Posttraumatic avascular necrosis of the femoral head is greatest in fractures in which there is displacement of the fragments. Extracapsular fractures, on the other hand, usually heal well but are more likely to be unstable, particularly the three- and four-part intertrochanteric fractures.

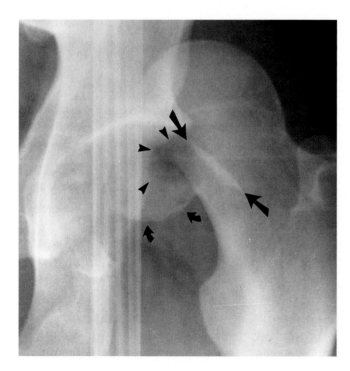

Figure 19.10. Concomitant posterior column (rim) and femoral head *(curved arrows)* fractures associated with posterior dislocation of the hip. *Straight arrows* indicate the rim fragment, and *arrowheads* indicate its defect in the posterior acetabular rim.

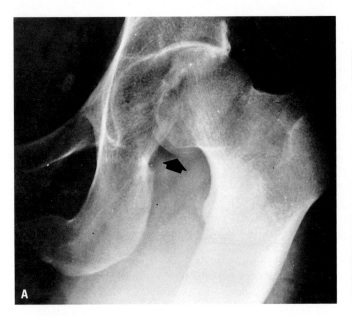
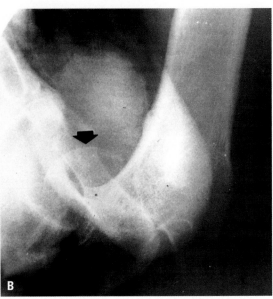

Figure 19.11. Posterior dislocation of the left hip with a large femoral head fragment. In the frontal projection (**A**), the dislocation is obvious. The faint crescentic density *(arrow)* inferior to the femoral head is a separate femoral head fragment confirmed to be within the acetabulum in the horizontal beam lateral radiograph (**B**).

The hip joint capsule extends anteriorly from the anteroinferior iliac spine and the iliopectineal eminence of the innominate bone to the intertrochanteric line of the femur. The hip capsule is attached posteriorly to the acetabulum approximately 5 to 6 mm above its rim, distally to the femoral neck well above the intertrochanteric crest, and inferomedially to the femoral neck above the lesser trochanter (Fig. 19.13). The trochanters are extracapsular.

The normal radiographic skeletal and soft tissue anatomy of the hip is repeated (Figs. 19.1 and 19.14) here for ease of comparison. Contrary to an often repeated imprecision, the soft tissue linear lucencies, superolateral and inferomedial to the femoral head and neck (Fig. 19.1A), do not indicate the hip joint capsule. Rather, they represent areolar tissue in the fascial plane covering the gluteus minimus muscle superiorly and the tendon of the iliopsoas muscle inferiorly. A large intrasynovial fluid collection may displace the lucent stripes or make them convex. However, it must be clearly understood that normal fascial planes about the hip joint do not exclude intrasynovial pathology. This is particularly true in the instance of young children who refuse to bear weight on one leg and in whom septic arthritis (pyarthrosis)

is clinically suspected. This circumstance requires scintigraphy CT or Magnetic resonance imaging (MRI) for further evaluation. This recommendation must be transmitted to the referring physician.

Intracapsular proximal femoral fractures include the subcapital, transcervical, and basicervical. Subcapital fractures are commonly extremely subtle and, in AP projection, may be manifested only by superimposition of the rim of the base of the femoral head upon the femoral neck (Fig. 19.15). Typically in subcapital fractures, the femoral head rotates clockwise on the right and counterclockwise on the left within the acetabulum. The rotational displacement of the head results in impaction at the medial end of the fracture line and flattened normal neck–head relationship laterally (Fig. 19.16A–D), whereas the inferior neck–head anatomy appears normal with intact cortex (Fig. 19.17A). In the horizontal beam lateral projection, displacement of the femoral head, which is usually posterior with respect to the neck, in association with disruption of the anterior cortex (Fig. 19.17B) confirms the diagnosis. Impaction of the femoral head on the neck will produce an indistinct broad band of relative increased density in the subcapital region

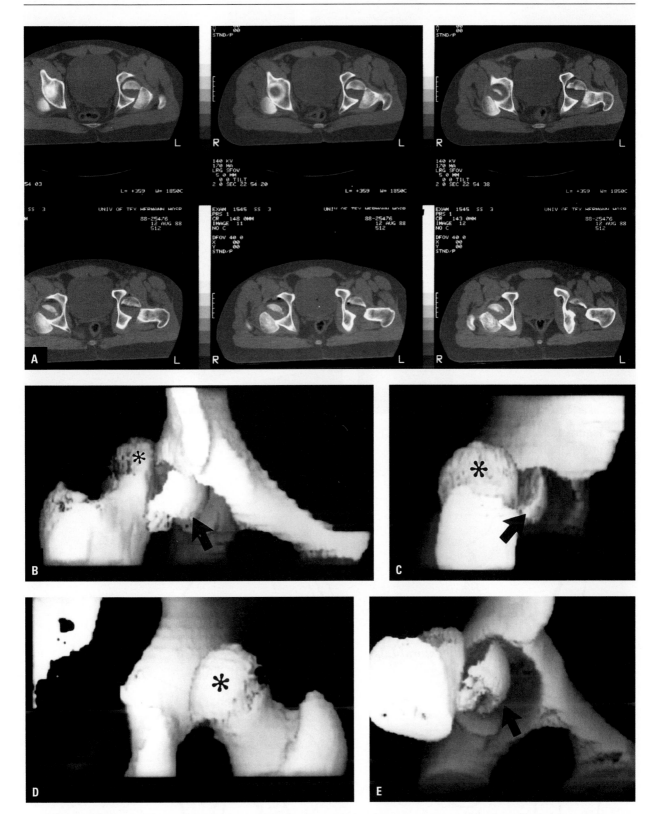

Figure 19.12. Bilateral posterior femoral head fracture dislocations demonstrated with axial CT (**A**) and 3-D CT (**B–I**). The frontal (**B**), lateral (**C**), posterior (**D**), and inferosuperior (**E**) 3-D CT projections all clearly depict the size and location of the femoral head fractures. **E:** Location of the large right intra-acetabular femoral head fragment *(arrow)* and the spatial relationships of the dislocated femoral head *(asterisk)* to the acetabulum. *(continued)*

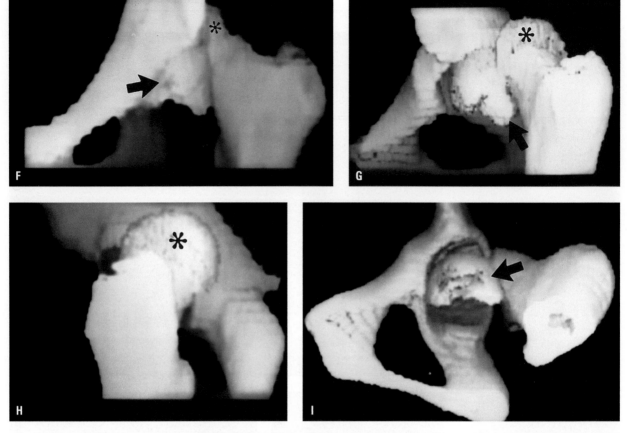

Figure 19.12. *(continued)* Similar 3-D CT projections of the left hip (**F–I**) provide an unambiguous, precise representation of this injury.

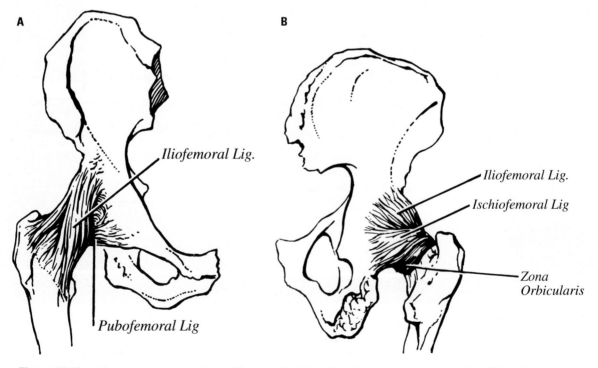

Figure 19.13. Schematic representation of the capsule of the hip joint as seen from anterior (**A**) and posterior (**B**) perspectives. (From O'Rahilly R. *Basic Human Anatomy*. Philadelphia, PA: WB Saunders; 1983, used with permission.)

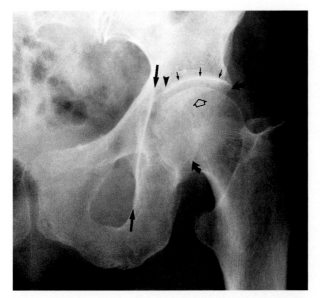

Figure 19.14. AP projection of the hip, demonstrating the weight-bearing portion of the acetabular roof *(small arrows)*, which terminates normally and abruptly at the margin of the lunate surface *(arrowhead)*. The lateral oblique density is the margin of the posterior acetabular lip *(curved arrows)* and the more medially situated density, the anterior acetabular lip *(open arrow)*. *Large arrows* indicate the ilioischial line.

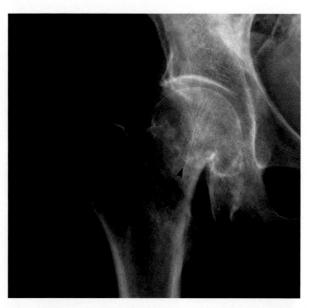

Figure 19.15. Subtle subcapital fracture. The impacted femoral head cortex *(arrowheads)* is superimposed on the proximal femoral neck. The fracture line occurs at the neck–head junction.

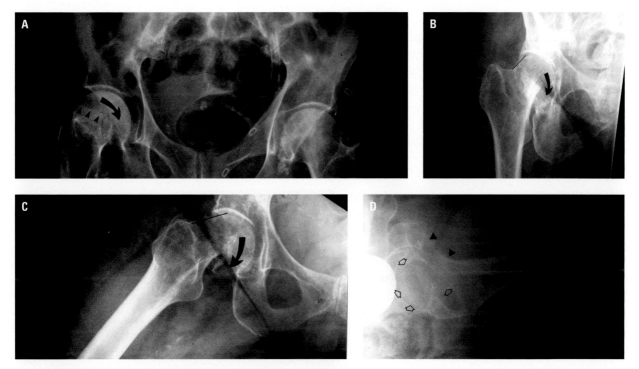

Figure 19.16. Displaced right subcapital fracture. In the AP radiograph of the hips and pelvis (**A**), the right femoral head has rotated in a clockwise direction within the acetabulum. The proximal end of the neck component *(arrowheads)* is visible through the head component. The anteroposterior radiograph of the right hip (**B**) shows the clockwise rotation of the head *(curved arrow)* and flattening of the lateral neck–head relationship *(black line)*. Flattening of the normal head–neck relationship *(black line)* is seen to better advantage in the externally rotated projection (**C**). The groin lateral projection (**D**) shows posterior displacement/rotation of the femoral head fragment *(open arrows)*. *Arrowheads* indicate the anterior cortex of the femoral neck.

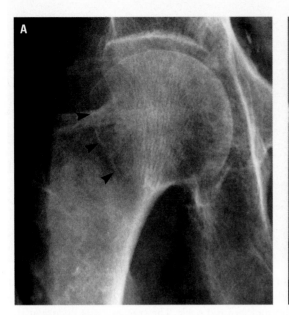
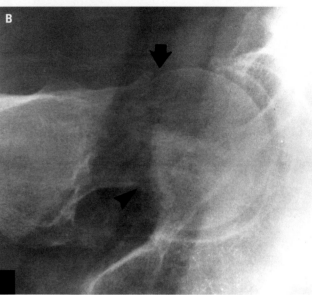

Figure 19.17. Minimally displaced subcapital fracture of the femoral neck. **A:** In the frontal projection, the only suggestion of the presence of a fracture is impaction of the superior cortex of the neck into the base of the femoral head as evidenced by superimposition of the base of the head *(arrowheads)* on the neck. **B:** In the horizontal beam lateral projection, the femoral head is rotated posteriorly with impaction posteriorly *(arrowhead)* and with separation of the fragments anteriorly *(arrow)*.

(Fig. 19.18), which may be the most obvious sign of a subcapital fracture. A subcapital fracture, when impacted in essentially anatomic position, may permit ambulation and relatively painless full range of passive motion, thereby rendering both the clinical diagnosis and the radiologic diagnosis in the AP projection equivocal (Fig. 19.19A). In the lateral radiograph (Fig. 19.19B), posterior

rotation of the head fragment makes the head asymmetrical with respect to the neck, and the anterior cortex of each fragment may be on the same plane. This obviously abnormal femoral head–neck relationship, coupled with disruption of the anterior subcapital cortex, should establish the diagnosis. The infrequent, displaced subcapital fracture is usually obvious in the AP

Figure 19.18. The faint, poorly marginated band of increased density at the base of the femoral head *(arrowheads)* represents the zone of impaction of this subcapital fracture. The impaction is also evident by the disruption and angulation at the junction of the superior neck cortex with the femoral head *(arrow)*.

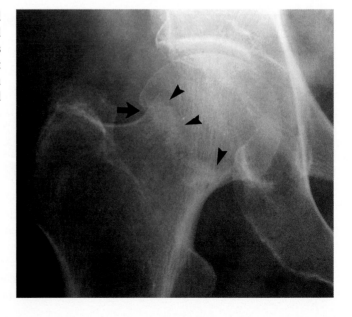

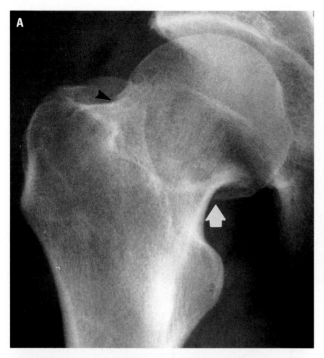

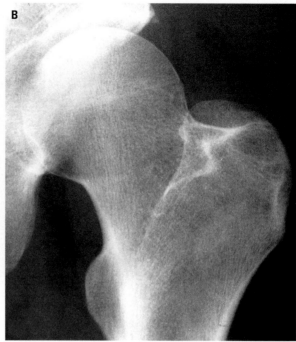

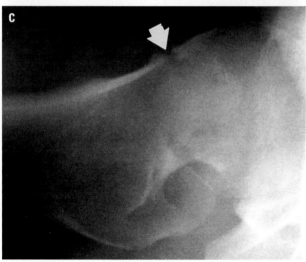

Figure 19.19. Minimally displaced, impacted subcapital fracture of the right femur (**A**). A casual observation of the frontal projection of the injured side (**A**) might be interpreted as normal. However, in comparing the injured side with the uninvolved left hip (**B**), it is evident that the right femoral neck is foreshortened with disruption of the superior cortex at the junction of the neck and head *(arrowhead)* and with impaction of the femoral neck and head inferiorly *(arrow)*. In the horizontal beam lateral projection of the right hip (**C**), the fracture is obvious, evidenced by posterior rotation of the head fragment. Consequently, the anterior cortex of the neck and the femoral head are on the same plane, which is disrupted at the fracture site *(arrow)*.

radiograph (Fig. 19.20) and is associated with 66%[11,12] to 88%[13] incidence of aseptic necrosis of the head fragment secondary to disruption of its major blood supply (Fig. 19.20C,D).

Transcervical fractures occur in the femoral neck between the subcapital area and the intertrochanteric crest. Transcervical fractures are usually readily apparent in the frontal projection of the hip and are typically associated with a varus deformity at the fracture site resulting from rotation of the proximal fragment within the acetabulum and abduction, proximal displacement, and external rotation of the distal fragment (Figs. 19.21 and

19.22). Basicervical fractures are those situated at the base of the femoral neck just proximal to the intertrochanteric crest.

Of the extracapsular fractures, the intertrochanteric fractures are by far the most common. Intertrochanteric fractures are designated according to the number of separate fragments, with the two-part (i.e., a proximal and a distal fragment only) being the simplest and the four-part (i.e., proximal, distal, and each trochanter a separate fragment) being the most complex and unstable. Of the intertrochanteric fractures, the two-part is the type most likely to be radiographically obscure, particularly when the

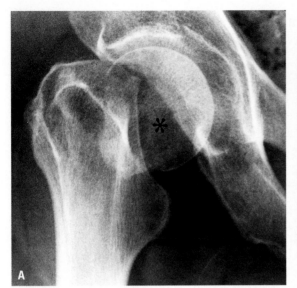

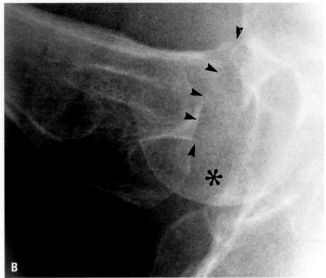

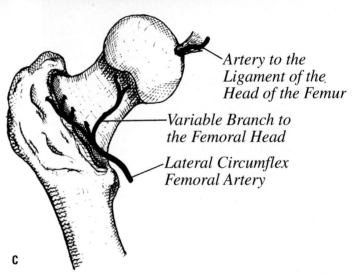

Artery to the
Ligament of the
Head of the Femur

Variable Branch to
the Femoral Head

Lateral Circumflex
Femoral Artery

C

Posterosuperior
Branches to the
Femoral Head

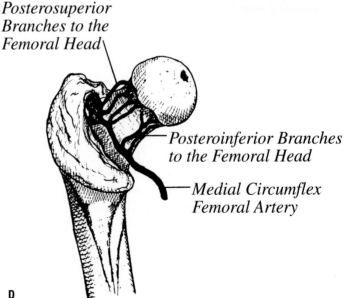

Posteroinferior Branches
to the Femoral Head

Medial Circumflex
Femoral Artery

D

Figure 19.20. The purpose of presenting this obvious displaced subcapital fracture is to emphasize by illustration the basis of the approximately two-third incidence of avascular necrosis of the femoral head with displaced subcapital fractures. **A** and **B** show the displaced, posteriorly rotated femoral head fragment *(asterisk)*. The lateral projection (**B**) confirms the fracture site at the junction *(arrowheads)* of the femoral head and neck. The anatomic drawings (**C** and **D**) show the major blood supply to the femoral neck and head to come from the lateral (**C**) and medial (**D**) femoral circumflex arteries. Parenthetically, the artery of the ligamentum teres supplies only approximately 10% of the femoral head circulation.

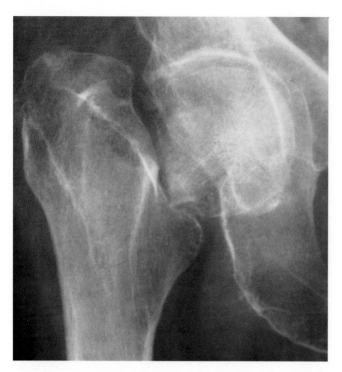

Figure 19.21. Transcervical fracture of the femoral neck. In the frontal projection, the varus deformity at the fracture site is the result of clockwise rotation of the head within the acetabulum combined with lateral and proximal displacement and external rotation of the distal fragment. The varus deformity and the rotational displacement of the distal femoral fragment explain the appearance of the injured lower extremity, clinically.

fragments are only minimally displaced (Fig. 19.23). The displaced two-part intertrochanteric fracture (Fig. 19.24) is easily recognized. The three-part intertrochanteric fracture consists of a proximal and distal fragment and either the lesser trochanter (Fig. 19.25) or the greater trochanter (Fig. 19.26) constituting the third fragment. The lesser trochanteric fragment is a very important component of intertrochanteric fractures because it typically includes a large portion of the posterior cortex of the femoral neck. The latter is an important factor in the instability of three- and four-part intertrochanteric fractures. The magnitude of the posterior cortical component of the lesser trochanteric fragment is easily appreciated in

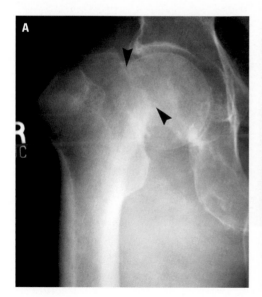
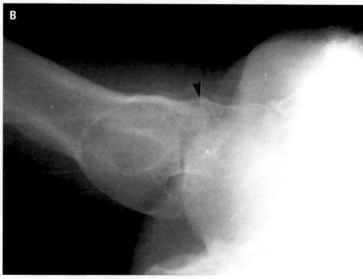

Figure 19.22. Impacted, displaced transcervical femoral neck fracture in AP (**A**) and lateral (**B**) projections. The transcervical location of the fracture *(arrowheads)* is clearly evident.

Figure 19.23. Minimally displaced two-part intertrochanteric fracture. The subtle fracture line is indicated by *arrowheads*.

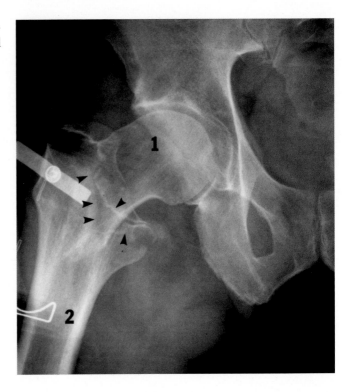

Figure 19.25. The alignment of the four-part intertrochanteric fragments may assume many configurations (Figs. 19.27 to 19.30), but all have in common the four separate fragments and a definite varus configuration at the major fracture site. Occasionally, even the four-part intertrochanteric fragments may be minimally displaced and difficult to recognize (Figs. 19.31 and 19.32).

Basicervical fractures occur, as the name implies, at the base of the femoral neck adjacent to the intertrochanteric crest (Fig. 19.33). By definition, basicervical fractures do not involve either femoral

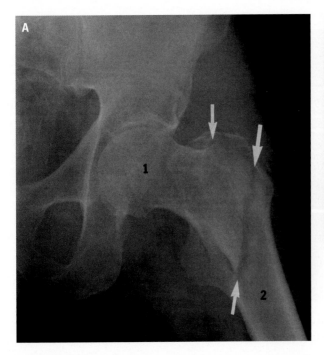

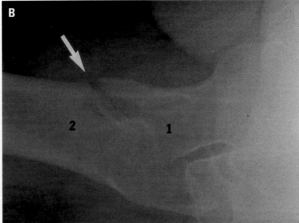

Figure 19.24. Two-part intertrochanteric fracture in groin lateral (**A**) and frontal (**B**) projections. The fracture line is indicated by *arrows*.

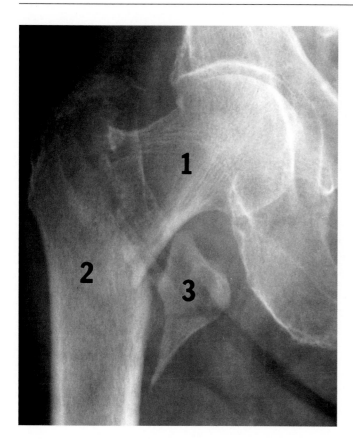

Figure 19.25. Displaced three-part intertrochanteric fracture in which the lesser trochanter *(3)* is a separate fragment.

trochanter. Occasionally, a basicervical fracture line will extend inferiorly to include the lesser trochanter (Fig. 19.34). Transcervical (Fig. 19.21) and minimally displaced intertrochanteric fractures (Fig. 19.23) may resemble, but should be distinguished from, the basicervical fracture.

Subtrochanteric fractures are distinguished from intertrochanteric fractures by a fracture of the proximal femoral shaft distal to the intertrochanteric line (Figs. 19.35 and 19.36). As with the intertrochanteric fractures, the subtrochanteric fractures may have three or four major

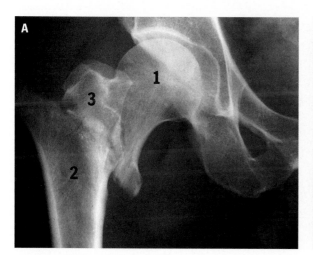
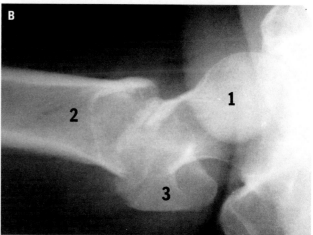

Figure 19.26. Three-part intertrochanteric fracture in which the greater trochanter *(3)* is a separate fragment.

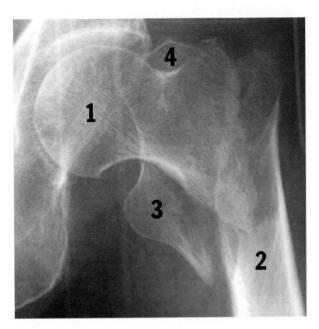

Figure 19.27. Four-part intertrochanteric fracture. In this unstable fracture, the femoral head and neck (*1*), the femoral shaft (*2*), and the lesser (*3*) and greater (*4*) trochanters each constitutes a separate fragment.

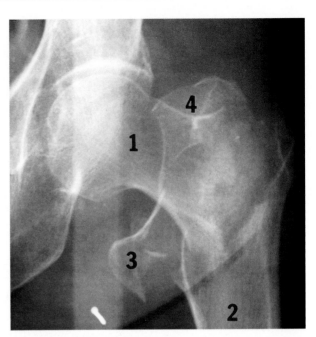

Figure 19.28. Four-part intertrochanteric fracture.

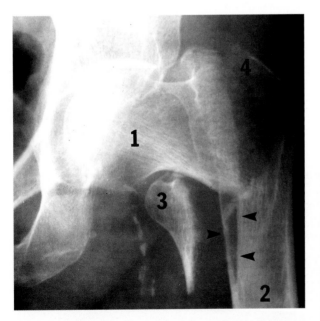

Figure 19.29. Displaced four-part intertrochanteric fracture. In this example, most of the greater trochanter stayed with the proximal fragment (*1*), with a smaller separate greater trochanteric fragment (*4*) interposed between *1* and *2*. The large defect (*arrowheads*) in the posteromedial aspect of the distal fragment (*2*) caused by the lesser trochanteric fragment (*3*) is clearly evident.

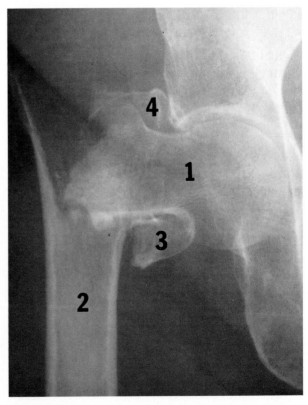

Figure 19.30. Severely displaced four-part intertrochanteric fracture with a marked varus deformity.

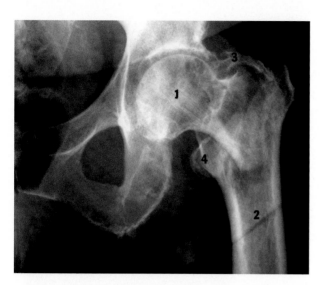

Figure 19.31. Four-part intertrochanteric fracture.

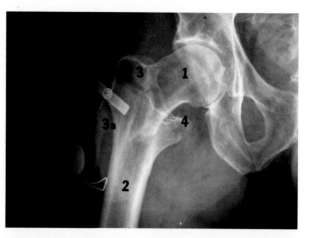

Figure 19.32. Four-part intertrochanteric fracture. This fracture is unusual in that the greater trochanteric fragment is comminuted (*3* and *3a*) and that the lesser trochanteric fragment *(4)* is small and minimally displaced. The proximal and distal fragments are *1* and *2*, respectively.

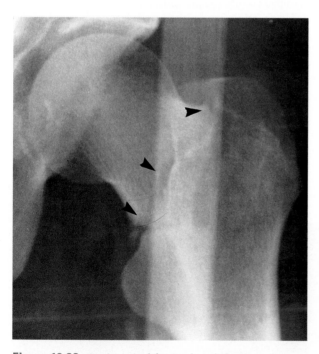

Figure 19.33. Basicervical femoral neck fracture *(arrowheads)*.

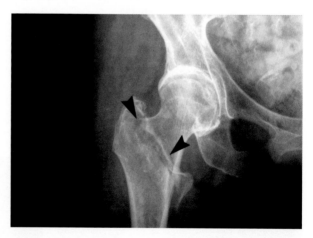

Figure 19.34. Basicervical femoral neck fracture. The fracture line *(arrowheads)* occurs at the base of the femoral neck, just proximal to the trochanteric crest. In this patient, the lesser trochanter constitutes a separate fragment.

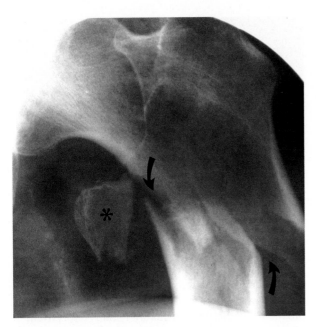

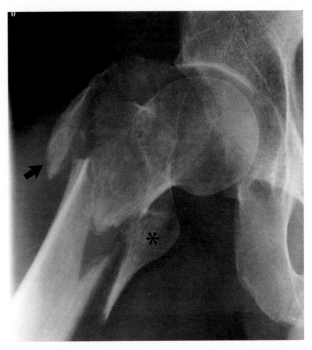

Figure 19.35. Subtrochanteric fracture in which the lesser trochanter *(asterisk)* constitutes a separate fragment. The principal comminuted fracture line *(curved arrows)* is located in the proximal femoral shaft just distal to the intertrochanteric crest.

Figure 19.36. Comminuted, impacted subtrochanteric fracture. In this example, the major proximal fragment is impacted into the proximal end of the distal fragment. The impaction has resulted in the lateral portion of the base of the greater trochanter *(arrow)* constituting a separate fragment. The lesser trochanter *(asterisk)* is also a very large separate fragment.

fragments and are typically more severely comminuted and displaced (Fig. 19.37).

Transcervical (Fig. 19.21) and minimally displaced intertrochanteric fractures may resemble, but should be distinguished from, the basicervical fracture (Fig. 19.33).

Isolated fractures of the greater trochanter occur more commonly in osteoporotic women than in men and are the result of a fall directly to the greater trochanter. The fall is usually considered relatively trivial, such as a slip while walking or a fall from a chair or bed. Both the clinical and radiographic diagnoses require a high index of

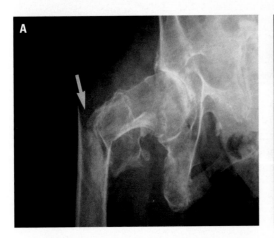

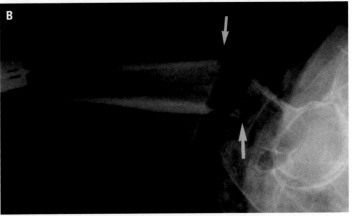

Figure 19.37. Subtrochanteric femoral fracture in AP (**A**) and groin lateral (**B**) projections. The comminuted fracture line *(arrows)* is in the proximal femoral shaft distal to the trochanteric crest. On the groin lateral projection (**B**), the normal femoral shaft–neck angle is completely reversed due to anterior angulation at the fracture site.

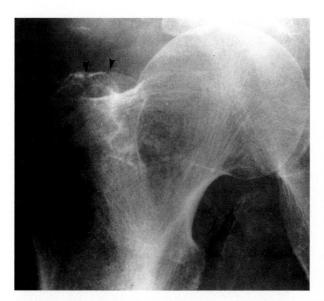

Figure 19.38. Comminuted, minimally impacted fracture of the superolateral cortex of the greater trochanter *(arrowheads).*

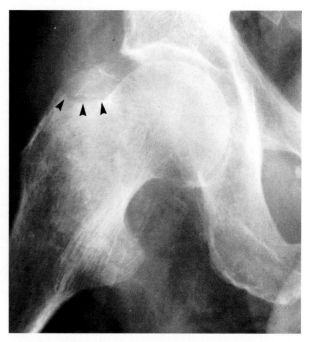

Figure 19.39. Transverse, minimally displaced fracture of the greater trochanter *(arrowheads).*

suspicion for this fracture because, although the patient complains of "pain in the hip," both active and passive ranges of motion are usually relatively pain free. Radiologically, the greater trochanteric fracture may be equally enigmatic because the patient is usually referred with the working diagnosis of hip fracture, but the radiographs are negative for any evidence of the usual or typical variety of proximal femoral fractures. Additionally, the radiographic technique usually required for adequate visualization of the hip and the femoral neck will overexpose the greater trochanter, further compounding the recognition of greater fractures. The radiologic diagnosis of a greater trochanteric fracture may require reducing radiographic technique, obtaining oblique views of the trochanter, or manipulation of the window and level settings of the digital images. The most subtle of isolated fractures of the greater trochanter is impaction of its lateral cortex (Figs. 19.38 and 19.39). Because the superolateral cortex of the greater trochanter is normally irregular, computed tomography or MRI may be required to establish the diagnosis. More obvious isolated fractures of the greater trochanter include displaced fractures of the trochanter itself (Fig. 19.40) or through its base (Fig. 19.41), which may be best appreciated in the lateral projection. In nonosteoporotic patients, forceful direct trauma to the greater trochanter usually results in

a transverse fracture of the trochanter (Fig. 19.42) or of its base, which may be comminuted and displaced (Fig. 19.43).

An MRI should be strongly considered for further evaluation of the hip of elderly patients who

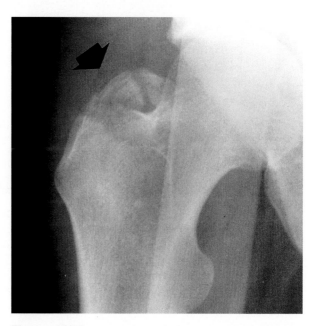

Figure 19.40. Comminuted fracture of the greater trochanter *(arrow).*

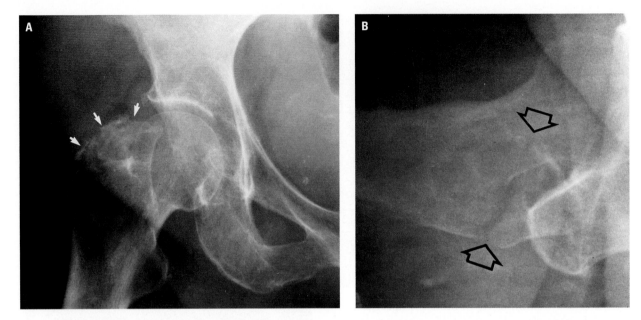

Figure 19.41. Comminuted, minimally displaced fracture of the base of the greater trochanter. Comminution of the greater trochanter *(arrows)* is evident in the frontal projection (**A**), but the true extent of the principal fracture line through the base of the greater trochanter *(open arrows)* is evident only in the horizontal beam lateral projection (**B**).

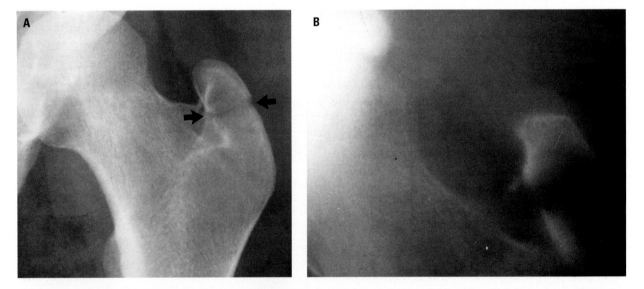

Figure 19.42. Minimally displaced, transverse fracture of the greater trochanter *(arrows)* in a young adult (**A**). The tomograph (**B**) confirms the absence of comminution, which is typical of greater trochanteric fractures in patients with normal bone mineralization.

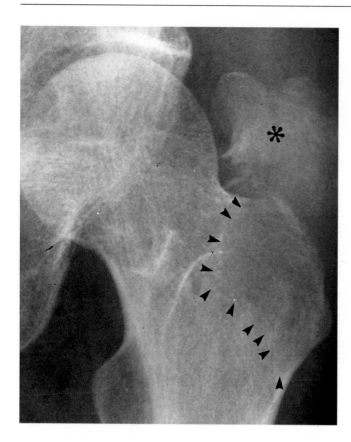

Figure 19.43. Comminuted, displaced fracture of the base of the greater trochanter. The greater trochanteric fragments *(asterisk)* have been retracted proximally. *Arrowheads* indicate the anterior margin of the fracture defect at the base of the greater trochanter.

complain of hip pain following minor trauma such as a fall from standing or slipping off a chair and in whom the radiographic examination is negative.[14] The MRI can detect occult fractures not demonstrated by conventional radiography or CT or soft tissue injury for which appropriate treatment can be instituted. For similar reasons, an MRI plays a critical role in sports-related injuries and in assessment of insufficiency and stress fractures of the pelvis and hip.[15,16]

NONTRAUMATIC CONDITIONS

Infection

The nontraumatic emergencies of the pelvis that do not involve the musculoskeletal system are discussed in Chapters 14 and 16. The following are but a few examples of the nontraumatic conditions of the pelvis or hips that might prompt an emergency center visit.

Septic arthritis (pyarthrosis) of the hip may be manifested radiographically by widening of the

space between the femoral head and the acetabular roof and bulging of the joint capsule as reflected in change in contour or the gluteus minimus and iliopsoas fascial stripes (Fig. 19.44). More commonly, however, these signs will be absent or equivocal, in which event, either scintigraphy or MRI is indicated.

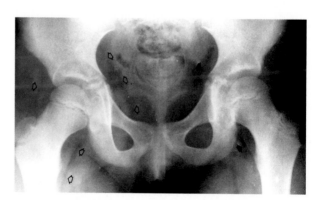

Figure 19.44. Prominence of the soft tissue shadows about the right hip, including bulging of the obturator internus muscle and its aponeurosis *(open arrows)*, indicates distention of the joint capsule. The contralateral normal soft tissue shadows are indicated by *closed arrows*.

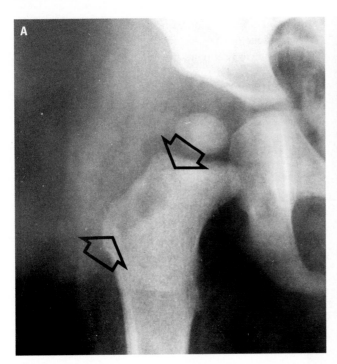

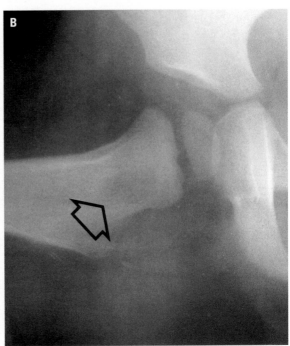

Figure 19.45. *Open arrows* indicate ill-defined, poorly marginated radiolucent defects in the femoral neck that are caused by acute osteomyelitis.

Skeletal changes of acute osteomyelitis (Fig. 19.45) usually do not appear until some time between 2 and 3 weeks after infection.

Slipped Capital Femoral Epiphysis

The SCFE typically occurs in boys between the ages of 12 and 16 years and is uncommon in children younger than the age of 10 years. It is usually an insidious process extending more than a period of several weeks and is associated with progressive discomfort and a limp. The pain associated with an SCFE may be experienced in the hip but is commonly referred to the knee. Therefore, it is imperative that the hip be examined clinically and, if indicated, radiographically in every child with unexplained pain in the knee.

The proximal femoral epiphysis usually slips posteriorly and medially, resulting in a varus deformity (Fig. 19.46), although the epiphysis may shift in either direction alone. The earliest radiographic signs of SCFE are subtle. Depending on the direction of movement of the epiphysis, the abnormal radiographic findings may be visible in only one projection. Straight AP and horizontal beam lateral projections should be obtained initially. If these are negative, an AP radiograph in the frog leg position is indicated because in this position the femoral head and neck are seen in the plane midway between that projected in the straight AP and the true lateral radiograph. The most reliable radiographic sign of SCFE is, obviously, asymmetry of the epiphysis with respect to the femoral neck in at least one of the three projections of the hip. The asymmetry is further reflected by the lateral cortex of the head and neck being on essentially the same plane on the AP radiograph (Fig. 19.46C,D) and by the anterior cortex of each being on the same plane in the frog leg projection. The typical appearance of an old-fused, minimally displaced SCFE is seen in Figure 19.47. Figure 19.48 is an example of a frank SCFE. The mottled density of the metaphysis is consistent with early avascular necrosis.

Calcifying Peritendinitis

Calcification occurring in the joint capsule or surrounding tendons or in the bursae is variously referred to as calcifying peritendinitis, peritendinitis calcarea, or calcific bursitis.[17] The etiology

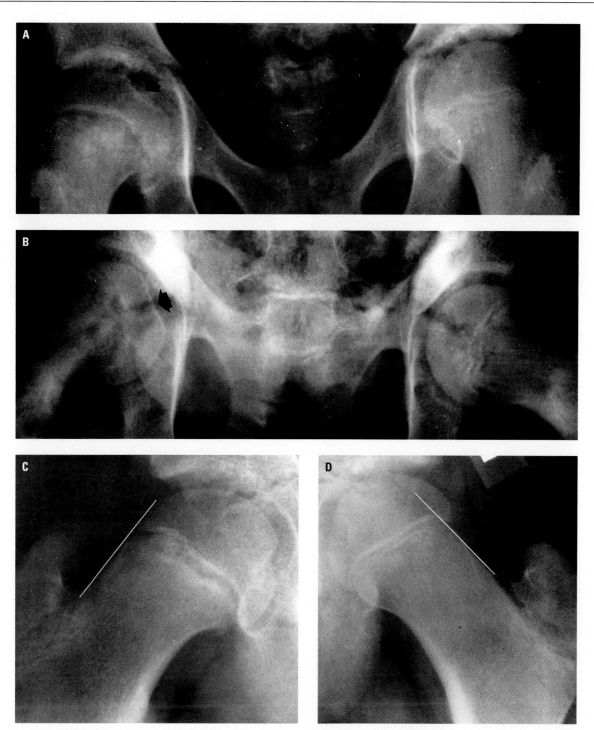

Figure 19.46. Right slipped capital femoral epiphysis (SCFE). **A:** In the AP projection, the slippage appears minimal and could conceivably be overlooked. However, the capital femoral epiphysis is medially displaced with respect to the metaphysis, resulting in the lateral cortex of the femoral neck and of the epiphysis being on the same plane *(open arrow)*. Additionally, the capital femoral epiphysis is flattened *(arrow)*, and the right hip joint space is widened. **B:** In the frog leg projection, the medial and posterior displacement and flattening of the capital femoral epiphysis are obvious *(arrow)*. **C:** In a different patient, the subtle SCFE is indicated by the superior cortex of the femoral neck and epiphysis being on the same plane *(white line)*. **D:** The AP radiograph of the opposite (normal) hip of the same patient shows the normal femoral neck–capital epiphyseal relationship *(white line)*.

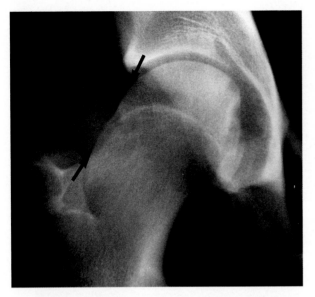

Figure 19.47. Old, healed, minimal slipped capital femoral epiphysis. The lateral cortex of the femoral head and neck are on the same plane *(arrows)*, resulting in a buccaneer's pistol grip deformity of the femoral head and neck.

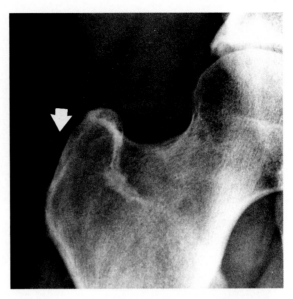

Figure 19.49. Calcifying trochanteric bursitis. The faint amorphous calcification *(arrow)* separated from the lateral cortex of the greater trochanter coincides with the location of the trochanteric bursa.

of these soft tissue calcifications not related to arthritis may be secondary to previous trauma, but its etiology is generally unknown. Typically, there is no relationship between the presence of these soft tissue calcifications and acute symptoms.

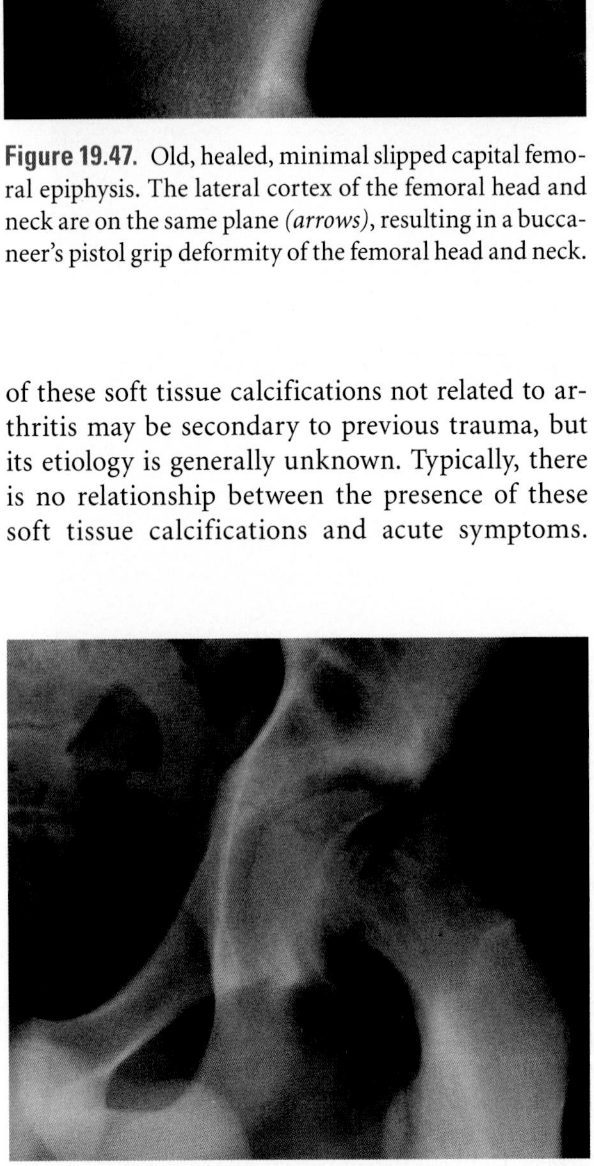

Calcifying peritendinitis about the hip joint is infrequent. When present, it has been described as being above the femoral head lateral to the joint capsule.[18] Calcific bursitis about the hip is also uncommon, but the hip bursa most commonly involved is the trochanteric bursa that separates the tendon of the gluteus medius muscle from the lateral cortex of the greater trochanter on which it inserts. Trochanteric bursal calcification is usually amorphous, poorly marginated, and clearly separate from the lateral cortex of the greater trochanter (Fig. 19.49).

Paget Disease

Paget disease may involve one (Fig. 19.50) or all (Fig. 19.51) the bones of the hips and pelvis and is typically manifested by demineralization, cortical thickening, and trabecular prominence. When biphasic (Fig. 19.51), Paget disease may simulate blastic (prostatic) metastasis.

Neoplastic Disease

Benign neoplasms involving the bones of the pelvis may be symptomatic and prompt an emergency center visit. Osteoid osteoma and solitary

Figure 19.48. Frank slipped capital femoral epiphysis. The capital femoral epiphysis is displaced medially, inferiorly, and posteriorly. Inhomogeneity of the density of the femoral neck metaphysis is consistent with early avascular necrosis.

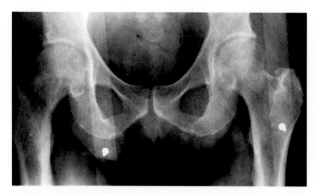

Figure 19.50. Paget disease involving the right femur is characterized by cortical thickening and trabecular prominence (compare with the left femur).

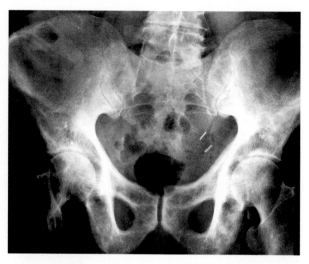

Figure 19.51. Biphasic Paget disease involving all the bones of the pelvis and each femoral head.

osteochondroma are examples in point—the osteoid osteoma because of pain, and the solitary osteochondroma because of a mass.

Osteoid osteoma clinically occurs in adolescents and young adults, usually younger than the age of 30, and typically produces dull, persistent pain that is worse at night and that is usually relieved by aspirin. Although osteoid osteoma may occur in many locations, a common site is the junction of the femoral neck and shaft near the lesser trochanter. Osteoid osteoma is typically limited to the cortex but may involve the intramedullary portion of the bone. The cortical lesion is typically an area of dense sclerotic cortical thickening with a central lucid nidus (Fig. 19.52). The

nidus, which may be very subtle on the plain radiograph, becomes readily apparent by CT. Scintigraphy is also an effective method of establishing or confirming the diagnosis. Because the nidus is highly vascular, it will demonstrate even greater concentration of the radiopharmaceutical than does the surrounding sclerotic bone. This difference in radioactivity has been termed the "double-density" sign.[19]

Solitary osteochondroma (osteocartilaginous exostosis) is a cartilage-capped bony excrescence. It is a common lesion usually encountered in the

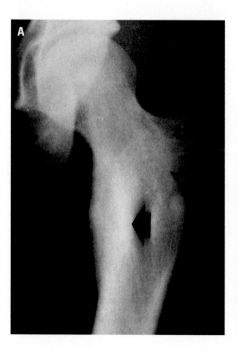

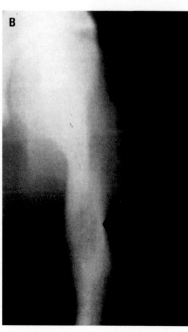

Figure 19.52. Osteoid osteoma of the femur *(closed arrow).* In the plain radiograph (**A**), a large but focal area of increased density caused by both cortical and endosteal proliferation is present. The cortical new bone formation is smooth and sharply delineated, indicating a nonaggressive process. The frontal tomogram (**B**) demonstrates an oval central lucent nidus *(closed arrow).* These findings are typical of an osteoid osteoma in this 21-year-old woman who complained of pain in her hip, which was worse at night and relieved by aspirin over several weeks duration. The smaller, discrete density *(open arrow)* in the frontal radiograph (**A**) is a bone island.

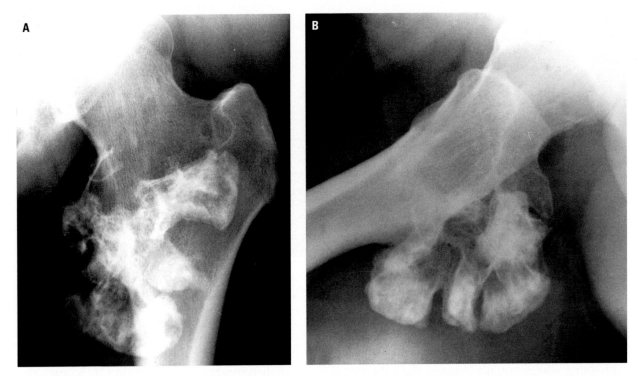

Figure 19.53. Characteristic radiographic appearance of a solitary osteochondroma of the femur in both frontal (**A**) and frog leg (**B**) projections.

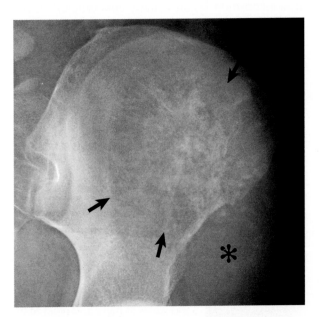

Figure 19.54. Chondrosarcoma of the left iliac wing *(arrows)* with a large soft tissue component *(asterisk)*.

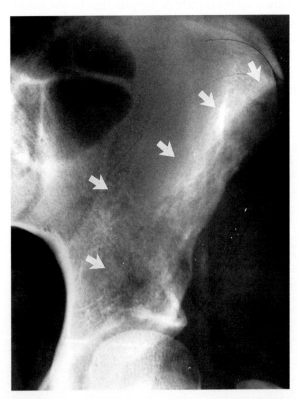

Figure 19.55. The permeative appearance of the left iliac wing, extending from the supraacetabular region to the anterior superior iliac spine *(arrows)*, represents histologically proven reticulum cell sarcoma.

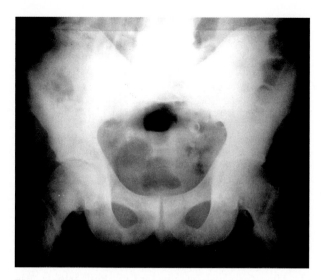

Figure 19.56. Osteoblastic metastasis from carcinoma of the prostate.

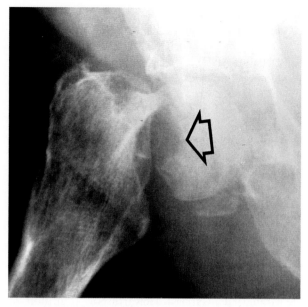

Figure 19.58. Pathologic fracture in the neck of the right femur secondary to primary breast carcinoma. The characteristic margins of the fracture fragments *(open arrow)* and the lytic defect with loss of trabecular pattern in the femoral neck fragment are typical signs of a metastatic lesion through which a fracture has occurred.

second or third decade and typically arises from the cortex adjacent to the metaphysis of a long tubular bone, particularly the proximal humerus, proximal and distal femur, and distal radius.[20] The characteristic radiographic appearance of an osteochondroma is seen in Figure 19.53.

Primary malignant neoplasms may involve the bones of the pelvis or hip. These may be localized, such as chondrosarcoma (Fig. 19.54), or generalized, such as primary round cell diseases including multiple myeloma or one of the non-Hodgkin lymphomas (reticulum cell sarcoma, Fig. 19.55).

Metastatic neoplasia may be osteoblastic (Fig. 19.56) or osteolytic (Fig. 19.57). Either may lead to a pathologic fracture (Fig. 19.58).

REFERENCES

1. DePalma AF. *The Management of Fractures and Dislocations.* Philadelphia, PA: WB Saunders; 1970.
2. Berquist TH, Coventry MB. The pelvis and hips. In: Berquist TH, ed. *Imaging of Orthopedic Trauma.* 2nd ed. New York, NY: Raven Press; 1992:264.
3. DeLee JC. Fractures and dislocations of the hip. In: Rockwood CA Jr, Green DP, Bucholz RW, eds. *Fractures in Adults.* 4th ed. Philadelphia, PA: JB Lippincott Co; 1996:1763.
4. Epstein HC. *Traumatic Dislocation of the Hip.* Baltimore, MD: Williams & Wilkins; 1980.
5. DeLee JC, Evans JA, Thomas J. Anterior dislocation of the hip and associated femoral head fractures. *J Bone Joint Surg Am.* 1980;62:960–963.
6. Weissman BN, Sledge CB. *Orthopaedic Radiology.* Philadelphia, PA: WB Saunders; 1986.
7. Thaggard A III, Harle TS, Carlson V. Bony pelvis and hip. Fractures and dislocations of bony pelvis and hip. *Semin Roentgenol.* 1978;13(2):111–128.
8. Mounts RJ, Schloss CD. Injuries to the bony pelvis and hip. *Radiol Clin North Am.* 1966;4(2):307–322.
9. Berquist TH, Coventry MB. The pelvis and hips. In: Berquist TH, ed. *Imaging of Orthopedic Trauma and Surgery.* Philadelphia, PA: WB Saunders; 1968.

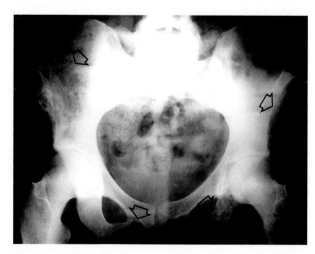

Figure 19.57. Osteolytic metastasis *(open arrows)* from primary breast carcinoma.

10. Swiontkowski MF. Intracapsular hip fractures. In: Browner BD, Jupiter JB, Levine AM, et al, eds. *Skeletal Trauma*. Philadelphia, PA: WB Saunders; 1992.

11. DePalma AF. *The Management of Fractures and Dislocations: An Atlas*. Philadelphia, PA: WB Saunders; 1970:1280.

12. Catto M. A histologic study of avascular necrosis of the femoral head after transcervical fracture. *J Bone Joint Surg Br*. 1965;47:749–776.

13. Sevitt S. Avascular necrosis and revascularization of the femoral head after intercapsular fractures. *J Bone Joint Surg Br*. 1964;46:270–296.

14. Bogost GA, Crues JV. Posttraumatic hip pain: The role of magnetic resonance imaging in the emergency setting. *Emergency Radiology*. 1998;5(6):368–374.

15. Kneeland JB. MR imaging of sports injuries of the hip. *Magn Reson Imaging Clin North Am*. 1999;7(1):105–115.

16. Grangier C, Garcia J, Howarth NR, et al. Role of MRI in the diagnosis of insufficiency fractures of the sacrum and acetabular roof. *Skeletal Radiol*. 1997;26(9):517–524.

17. Shanks SC, Kerly P, eds. *A Textbook of X-ray Diagnosis*. 4th ed. London, United Kingdom: HK Lewis; 1969.

18. Jones GB. Proceedings and reports of universities, colleges, councils and associations. *J Bone Joint Surg Br*. 1965;47:376.

19. Helms CA. *Fundamentals of Skeletal Radiology*. Philadelphia, PA: WB Saunders; 1989.

20. Resnick D. Tumors and tumor-like lesions of bone. In: Resnick DN, Niwayama G, eds. *Diagnosis of Bone and Joint Disorders*. Philadelphia, PA: WB Saunders; 1981.

SUGGESTED READINGS

1. Ashman CJ, Yu JS. The hip and femoral shaft. In: Rogers LF, ed. *Radiology of Skeletal Trauma*. 3rd ed. Philadelphia, PA: Churchill Livingstone; 2002:1030–1109.

2. Koval KJ, Cantu RV. Intertrochanteric fractures. In: Bucholz RW, Heckman JD, Court-Brown C, eds. *Rockwood and Green's Fractures in Adults*. 6th ed. Philadelphia, PA: Lippincott Williams & Wilkins; 2006:1793–1826.

3. Leighton RK. Fractures of the neck of the femur. In: Bucholz RW, Heckman JD, Court-Brown C, eds. *Rockwood and Green's Fractures in Adults*. 6th ed. Philadelphia, PA: Lippincott Williams & Wilkins; 2006:1753–1792.

4. Leung K. Subtrochanteric fractures. In: Bucholz RW, Heckman JD, Court-Brown C, eds. *Rockwood and Green's Fractures in Adults*. 6th ed. Philadelphia, PA: Lippincott Williams & Wilkins; 2006: 1827–184.

5. Manaster BJ, May DA, Disler DG. *The Requisites: Musculoskeletal Imaging*. 3rd ed. Philadelphia, PA: MOSBY Elsevier; 2007:194–201.

6. Miller TT, Schweitzer ME, eds. *Diagnostic Musculoskeletal Imaging*. New York, NY: McGraw-Hill; 2005:217–222.

7. Pope TE, Bloem HL, Beltran J, et al, eds. Pelvis-hip: Technical aspects, normal anatomy, common variants. In: *Imaging of the Musculoskeletal System*. Philadelphia, PA: Saunders/Elsevier; 2008: 405–433.

8. Pope TE, Bloem HL, Beltran J, et al, eds. Acute osseous injury to the hip and proximal femur. In: *Imaging of the Musculoskeletal System*. Philadelphia, PA: Saunders/Elsevier; 2008:470–498.

9. Salter RB. *Textbook of Disorders and Injuries of the Musculoskeletal System*. 3rd ed. Philadelphia, PA: Lippincott Williams & Wilkins; 1999:632–642.

10. Stoller DW, Tirman PFJ, Bredella MA, et al. *Diagnostic Imaging: Orthopaedics*. Salt Lake City, UT: Amiris Inc; 2006:4-46–4-62.

11. Tornetta P III. Hip dislocations and fractures of the femoral head. In: Bucholz RW, Heckman JD, Court-Brown C, eds. *Rockwood and Green's Fractures in Adults*. 6th ed. Philadelphia, PA: Lippincott Williams & Wilkins; 2006:1715–1752.

CHAPTER 20

Knee

Ne Siang Chew ■ Philip Robinson ■ John H. Harris Jr.

GENERAL CONSIDERATIONS

The knee is probably more commonly injured than any other joint of the body and is the most vulnerable joint from the standpoint of athletic injury. Extensive soft tissue damage may exist without a recognizable radiographic sign. Thus, a normal-appearing radiographic examination of the knee does not exclude the possibility of significant injury to the ligaments surrounding, or within, the knee joint. Magnetic resonance imaging (MRI) is the imaging modality of choice in the diagnosis of acute (and chronic) soft tissue, chondral, and occult skeletal injuries of the knee. However, because the definitive evaluation and management of patients with soft tissue and occult skeletal injuries of the knee are not within the purview of emergent care and because MRI is currently not a generally accepted part of the emergency imaging of the appendicular skeleton, the reader is referred to the cited references.

The use of multidetector computed tomography (MDCT) is useful in the search of undisplaced fractures and is now an integral in the evaluation of traumatized knees, especially in the depiction of complex fracture anatomy. MDCT provides fast-volume imaging, multiplanar reconstructions (MPRs) with near isotropic viewing, three-dimensional (3-D) images, and thick-slice (wedge) MPRs, which offer surgeons a detailed road map for preoperative planning. Computed tomography (CT) has also allowed for grading of trauma in knees especially in tibial plateau type fractures (Schatzker classification), permitting patients to be managed more effectively. The potential benefits and disadvantages of MDCT over plain radiography are summarized in Table 20.1.

In children, particularly, pain caused by an abnormality of the hip may be referred to the knee. It is important that the hip be specifically examined when a child complains of knee pain that seems to be disproportionate to the clinical and radiographic evaluation of the knee or if a young child refuses to bear weight on one leg. In adults, a nontraumatic swollen, hot, tender knee should prompt consideration of bacterial pyarthrosis.

GENERAL ANATOMY OF THE KNEE JOINT

Key radiologic anatomy pertinent to interpretation of trauma radiographs is summarized in the next paragraphs.

The Femur

The distal femur is composed of two bulbous bony projections: The medial and lateral femoral condyles. On the sagittal projection or lateral radiograph, the medial condyle can be discerned from the lateral condyle by its morphology (Figs. 20.1 and 20.2); the medial condyle is larger and has a convex articular surface. Both femoral condyles contain condylopatellar sulci, minor indentations that divide the condyles in a sagittal oblique plane.

| TABLE 20.1 | Benefits and Disadvantages of the Use of Multidetector Computed Tomography over Plain Radiography in the Traumatized Knee |

Benefits	Disadvantages
■ Fast image acquisition ■ High spatial resolution ■ Reconstruction in multiple planes allow for more accurate surgical road mapping ■ Imaging through splints and casts do not degrade image quality ■ Positioning of knee not as crucial as radiography; pain can hinder satisfactory positioning for radiography ■ Modern CT scanners can image soft tissue structures such as the anterior cruciate ligament	■ Radiation exposure using CT (CT average effective dose = 1 mSV vs. 0.06 mSV for plain radiography)

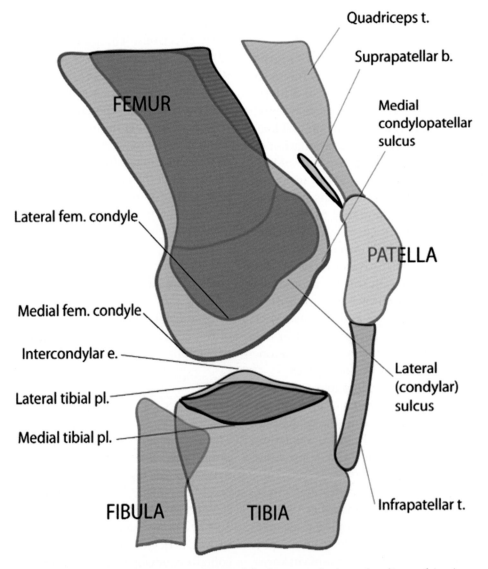

Figure 20.1. Recognizing the structures of the knee on the lateral radiographic view. *b*, bursa; *e*, eminence; *fem*, femoral; *t*, tendon; *pl*, plateau.

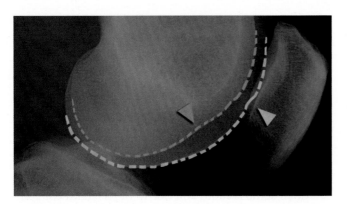

Figure 20.2. A magnified lateral view of the knee. The *yellow dotted line* outlines the larger, more convex medial femoral condyle. The medial condylopatellar sulcus is denoted by the *yellow arrowhead*. The *blue dotted line* outlines the lateral femoral condyle. The lateral condylopatellar sulcus is denoted by the *blue arrowhead*.

The medial condylopatellar sulcus divides the condyle into an anterior one-third and a posterior two-third segment. The lateral condylopatellar sulcus divides the condyle into two approximate halves. Aside from these minor indentations, the condyles should be smooth.

The medial and lateral condyles are separated inferiorly by the intercondylar notch (Figs. 20.3 and 20.4).

The Tibia

On the lateral projection, the medial tibial plateau is concave medially with a pointed dorsal corner (Fig. 20.5; see also Figs. 20.3 and 20.4 for accompanying frontal projection). The lateral tibial plateau is relatively flat with a rounded dorsal corner. Disruption to these contours should raise the suspicion for a fracture.

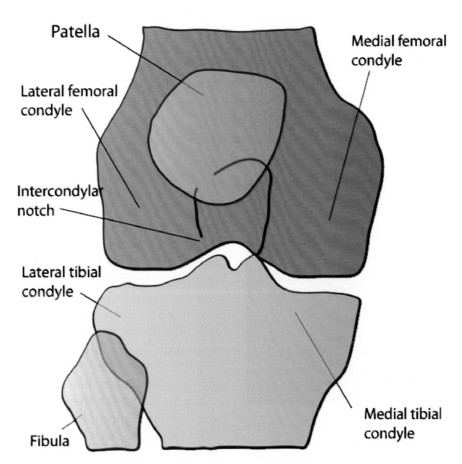

Figure 20.3. Recognizing the normal structures on the frontal/anteroposterior (AP) projection of the knee.

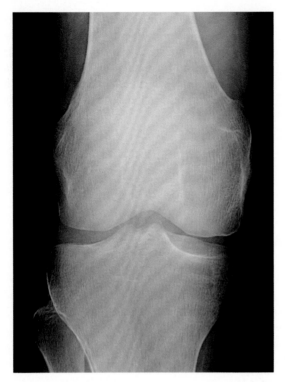

Figure 20.4. Normal frontal/anteroposterior (AP) radiographic appearance of an adult knee.

The medial and lateral tibial plateaus are separated by an intercondylar eminence (Fig. 20.6). The intercondylar eminence is devoid of cartilage and mainly serves as a footprint for ligamentous attachments. It is a triangular area with a base anteriorly and an

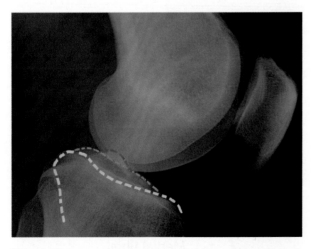

Figure 20.5. A magnified view of the lateral radiograph of the knee. The *purple dotted line* denotes the lateral tibial spine, the *blue dotted line* denotes the lateral tibial condyle, and the *yellow dotted line* denotes the medial tibial plateau.

apex posteriorly. Posteriorly near the apex arise two bony projections: The slightly anterior medial and a posterior lateral tibial spines/tubercles/eminences (Fig. 20.6). The anterior intercondylar eminence serves as the root attachments for the anterior medial and lateral menisci and footprint for the anterior cruciate ligament (ACL). The posterior intercondylar eminence functions as root attachments for the posterior medial and lateral menisci and the footprint for the posterior cruciate ligament (PCL). The medial tibial spine is more anterior than its lateral counterpart and can be discerned on the lateral radiograph.

The ACL inserts between the medial and lateral tibial spines, 10 to 14 mm behind the anterior border of the tibia (Fig. 20.7). Presence of an anteriorly placed bony fragment in the intercondylar notch is suspicious for distal ACL avulsion (Fig. 20.7C). The PCL attaches in a depression between the two tibial plateaus dorsally. Focal discontinuity of the posterior tibial plateau articular surface should suggest distal PCL avulsion (Fig. 20.8).

The anterior tibial tubercle is a bony protuberance located on the anterior aspect of the proximal tibia. It acts as the distal attachment for the infrapatellar tendon.

Gerdy tubercle is a bony protuberance at the anterior lateral tibial condyle, serving as the distal attachment for the iliotibial band (ITB).

The Fibula

The proximal fibula comprises a head and styloid process that act as attachment sites for posterolateral corner structures of the knee (Fig. 20.9). The styloid process is the pointed aspect of the fibula head. Knowledge of anatomical ligamentous attachment landmarks can help the reader discern the type of ligamentous injury that has occurred. The posterosuperior medial facet of the fibular styloid process is occupied by the popliteofibular ligament attachment. The fibular styloid process/fibular head apex serves as the distal attachment for the arcuate, fabellofibular, and popliteofibular ligaments, collectively known as the arcuate complex. The arcuate ligament is deep to that of the fabellofibular ligament. The fabellofibular ligament insertion lies medial to the direct arm of the short head of biceps femoris (not shown). The lateral collateral ligament and long head of biceps femoris are further lateral and are attached to the lateral margin of the fibular head.

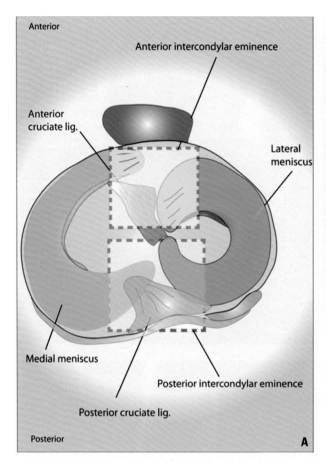

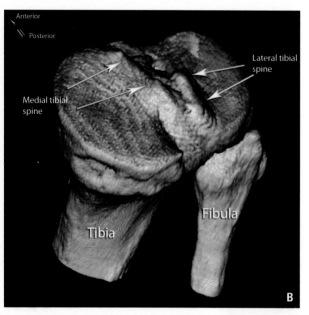

Figure 20.6. **A:** An axial section through the menisci and intercondylar eminences. The intercondylar eminences are devoid of cartilage and serve as root attachments for the menisci and footprints to the ACL and PCL. *lig*, ligament. **B:** 3-D reconstruction of the tibia and fibula. The medial and lateral tibial spines are depicted. Note the more anterior medial tibial spine.

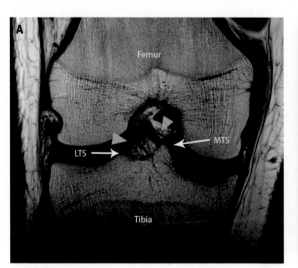

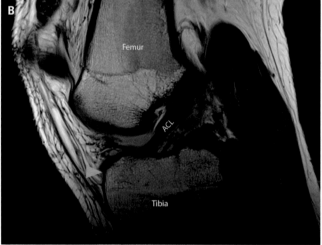

Figure 20.7. **A:** A 3-Tesla coronal T1 MRI demonstrates the distal insertion of the ACL. The ACL inserts between the *yellow arrowheads*, between the lateral tibial spine *(LTS)* and the medial tibial spine *(MTS)*. **B:** A 3-Tesla sagittal PD (proton density) MRI image depicting the normal location of the distal anterior cruciate ligament *(ACL)* insertion, located 10 to 14 mm posterior to the anterior tibial border *(yellow triangle)*. *(continued)*

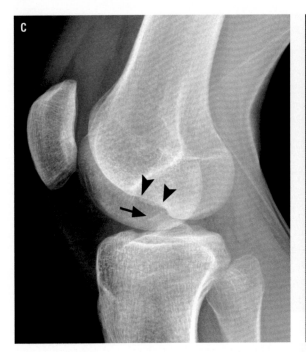

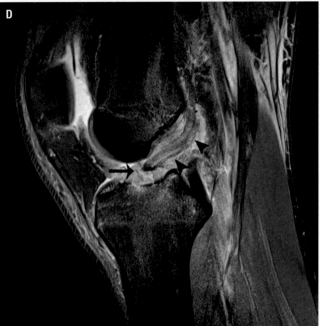

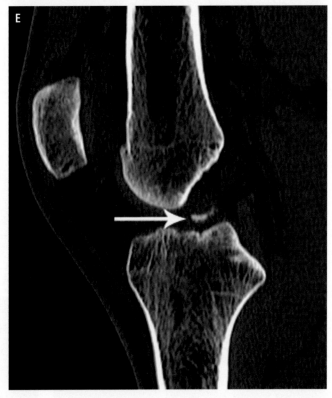

Figure 20.7. *(continued)* **C:** Presence of an anteriorly placed bony fragment *(black arrow)* in the intercondylar notch in a rugby player with an effusion in the setting of acute trauma. The *arrowheads* demonstrate a deepened lateral sulcus (deep notch sign), compatible with pivot-shift type injury mechanism, relating to an ACL injury. **D:** A sagittal T2 fat-saturated MRI of the same patient shows an avulsion of the ACL footprint. The *black arrow* points to avulsed cortex of the intercondylar eminence, attached to the distal fibers of the ACL. The ACL, depicted by *black arrowheads*, is redundant. **E:** A corresponding sagittal reformatted CT shows the avulsed bony footprint of the ACL.

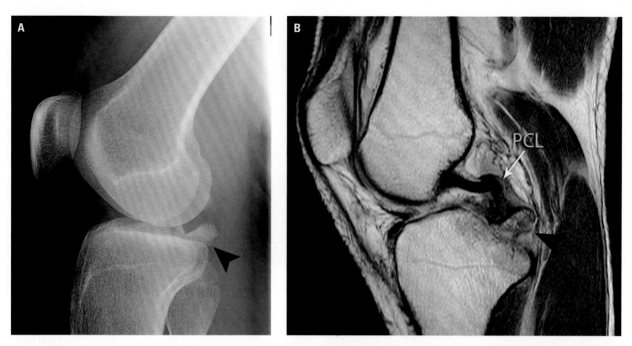

Figure 20.8. A: Discontinuity of the posterior tibial plateau secondary to a distal posterior cruciate ligament (PCL) avulsion injury in a football player. **B:** Corresponding sagittal T1 image of the same patient demonstrating a bony avulsion *(black arrowhead)* of the distal PCL footprint.

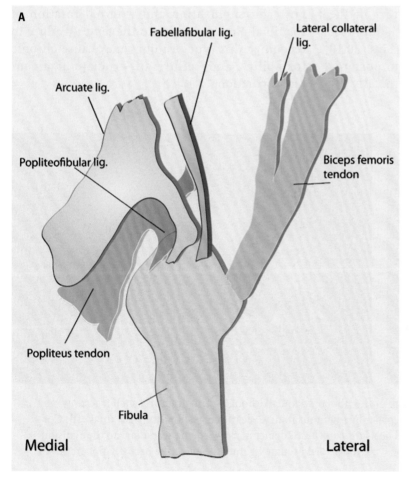

Figure 20.9. A: Ligamentous attachments to the fibula. The popliteofibular ligament attaches to the posterosuperior facet of the fibula. The fibula apex acts as the attachment for the arcuate and fabellofibular ligaments. The lateral collateral ligament and long head of biceps femoris are attached further laterally at the lateral margin of the fibula head. *(continued)*

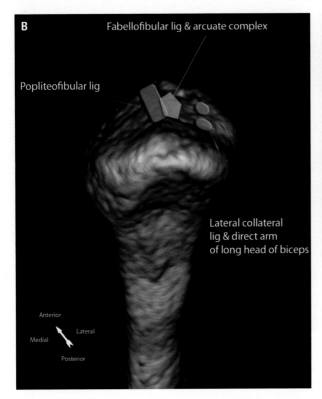

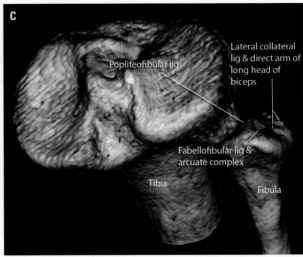

Figure 20.9. *(continued)* **B:** Individual attachments of the posterolateral corner structures on the fibular styloid and head. **C:** A para-axial representation of the relationship between the posterolateral corner ligamentous attachments. *lig,* ligament.

Identification of an avulsion fracture of the fibular head is important because it may reflect injury to the arcuate complex (Figs. 20.10 and 20.11). Such injuries may lead to posterolateral instability, characterized clinically by posterior subluxation and external rotation of the tibial plateau relative to the femur. Failure to recognize this type of injury may cause chronic instability and failure of cruciate ligament reconstruction.

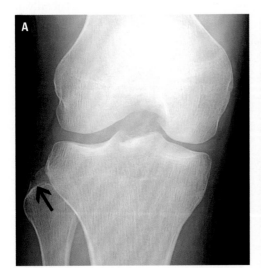

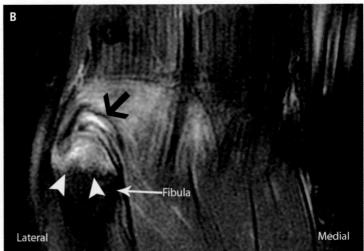

Figure 20.10. **A:** Tiny avulsion fracture of the fibular styloid. Although a tiny fracture, such fractures may herald more significant posterolateral corner ligamentous injury. See the corresponding MRI image. **B:** Corresponding coronal STIR MRI image: The *white arrowheads* depict marrow edema secondary to the avulsion. The *black arrow* points to an edematous, partially torn arcuate ligament. Notice the arched appearance of the arcuate ligament.

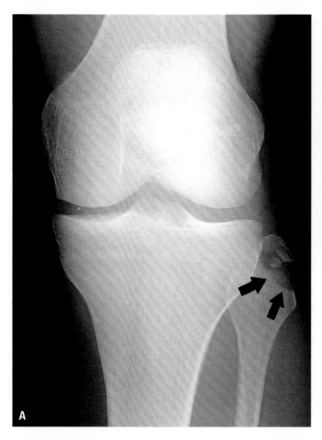

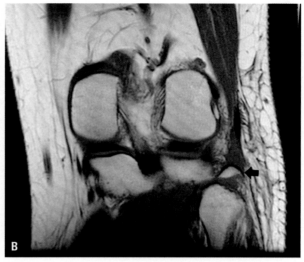

Figure 20.11. A: The *black arrows* depict an avulsion of the fibula head. Notice that compared to Figure 20.10, the site of the avulsion is more inferolateral, a feature that may indicate a lateral collateral ligament and biceps femoris avulsion. See the corresponding MRI image. **B:** Coronal T1 MRI image with a *black arrow* identifying the avulsed fibular head, which is still attached to the combined biceps femoris and lateral collateral ligament.

The Proximal Tibiofibular Joint

The proximal tibiofibular joint is the articulation of the lateral tibial condyle and the fibula head, located posterolaterally in relation to the tibia. Bound by a joint capsule and connected via anterior and posterior ligaments, the relationship between the tibia and fibula should be constant. Overcoverage or undercoverage of the fibula head on anteroposterior (AP) radiographs should raise the suspicion of proximal tibiofibular joint dislocation. A useful landmark in identifying the correct position of the fibula head and in excluding proximal tibiofibular joint dislocation or subluxation is the posterior tibial groove. The posterior tibial groove, located posteromedially within the lateral tibial condyle, can be recognized by following the lateral tibial spine inferiorly along the posterior aspect of the tibia on the lateral radiograph. Radiographically, this can be seen as an oblique radiodense line. On lateral projections, this line should intersect the fibula head (Fig. 20.12). Anterior and lateral deviation of the fibula head on lateral and AP radiographs respectively signify anterolateral dislocation, whereas posterior and medial deviation of the fibula on lateral and AP radiographs respectively indicate posteromedial dislocation.

The Patella

The patella (Figs. 20.1 to 20.4 and 20.13) is the largest sesamoid bone in the human body, lying within the substance of the quadriceps mechanism. This flat, triangular structure, with a distal apex, articulates with the trochlear groove of the femur.

The patella has two main surfaces or facets: The medial and lateral facets, separated by a central ridge. Knowledge of patella facetal morphology can aid orientation. There are three main variations of patella morphology, that is, Wiberg types I to III (Table 20.2).

The most common patella morphology is the Wiberg type II patella (Fig. 20.13). On the axial plane, the lateral facet is generally flatter, wider, and deeper than its medial counterpart. The medial

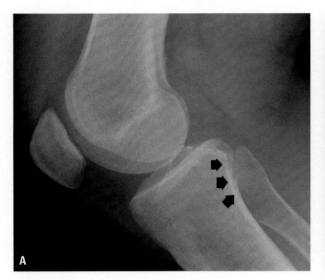
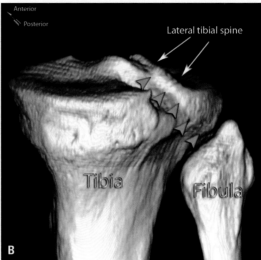

Figure 20.12. **A:** The normal posterior tibial groove. Follow the *dotted yellow line*, denoting the lateral tibial spine proximally, which becomes the posterior tibial groove, demonstrated by the *short bold black arrows*. The posterior tibial groove is the radiodense line, which in normality should intersect the fibula head. Any deviation, together with a relevant clinical history, should raise suspicion of a dislocation injury. **B:** 3-D paracoronal depiction of the posterior tibial groove *(purple arrowheads)*.

facet can be easily recognized; it contains a vertical bridge that divides it from a smaller, more medial "odd" facet. The odd facet only contacts the femoral condyle in flexion.

With the knee slightly flexed, the craniocaudal patella tendon length should be equal to the length of the craniocaudal length of the patella (Insall-Salvati ratio) (Fig. 20.14A). Variation in this ratio of up to 0.2 is acceptable but beyond this, one should suspect injury to the extensor mechanism, especially when there is a relevant clinical history and soft tissue swelling. In particular, if the apparent patella tendon length is 20% more than that of the bony patella (patella alta, high-riding patella) (Fig. 20.14B), a patella tendon rupture should be assumed. Conversely, for the reversed scenario with patella baja (low-riding patella), then a quadriceps tendon rupture is suspected.

RADIOGRAPHIC ANATOMY ACCORDING TO PROJECTION

The radiographic anatomy of the normal adult knee is seen in Figure 20.15. In the frontal projection (Fig. 20.15A), the patella is obscured by the density of the superimposed intercondylar portion

of the femur. Therefore, the AP projection of the knee usually has little significance in the evaluation of the patella. The medial and lateral intercondylar spines are well seen within the concavity of the intercondylar notch of the femur (Fig. 20.3). On a properly positioned frontal projection of the knee made with the central beam passing approximately 1 cm inferior to the inferior pole of the patella, the medial and lateral compartments of the joint space and the contiguous surfaces of the femoral condyles and the tibial plateau are clearly demonstrated.

TABLE 20.2	Patella Morphology According to Wiberg
Patella Morphology	**What Does It Mean?**
Wiberg type I	Medial facet is of similar length to the lateral facet
Wiberg type II	Medial facet is slightly shorter than the lateral facet
Wiberg type III	Medial facet is very much shorter than the lateral facet

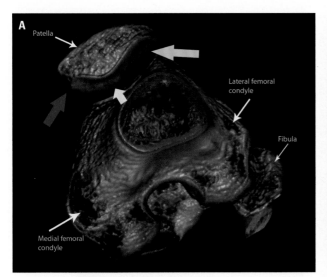
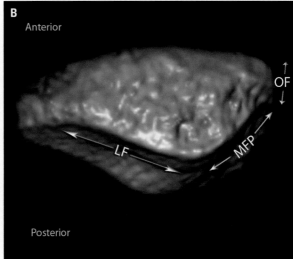

Figure 20.13. **A:** An axial 3-D CT reconstruction of a Wiberg type II patella. The *yellow arrow* points to the lateral facet, the *short white arrow* points to the median ridge, and the *purple arrow* points to the vertical bridge that divides the medial facet. **B:** An axial 3-D CT view of the patella and its facets of a 70-year-old female patient. The patella morphology corresponds to a Wiberg type II classification. *LF*, lateral facet; *MFP*, medial facet proper; *OF*, odd facet.

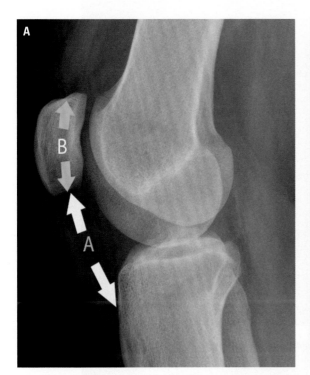
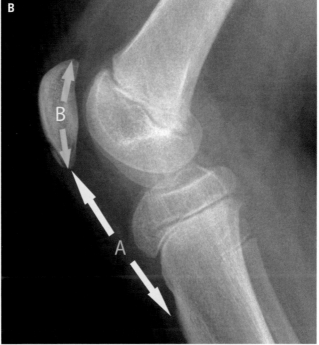

Figure 20.14. **A:** The Insall-Salvati ratio, which is the ratio of the craniocaudal patella tendon length *(A)* to the patella length *(B)*, should be 1.0 ± 0.2. **B:** Patella alta in a patient with cerebral palsy, with no history of trauma. Inferior fragmentation of the patella is thought to be related to chronic traction/stress. The Insall-Salvati ratio is much greater than 1.2.

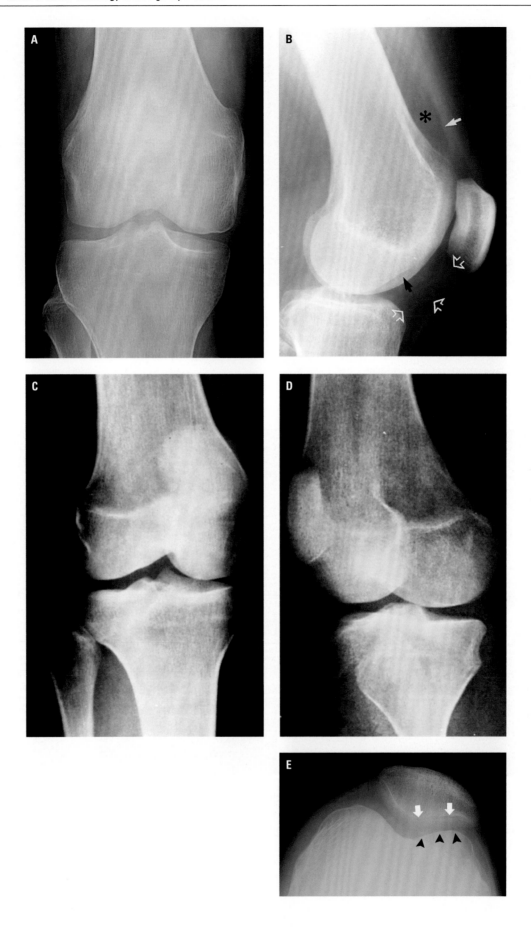

In the true lateral projection (Fig. 20.15B), the articulating surface of the femoral condyles should be closely superimposed and the patellofemoral space clearly evident. The suprapatellar recess of the joint space should be easily identified on a properly exposed lateral radiograph. The infrapatellar portion of the joint space, lying anterior and inferior to the femoral condyles, should be visible as a rectangular area of relative radiolucency (Hoffa fat pad).

External (Fig. 20.15C) and internal (Fig. 20.15D) oblique projections provide a perspective of the femoral condyles and tibial tuberosities not visible on the straight frontal and lateral projections. Additionally, the patella is partially projected free of the femur, making possible the evaluation of its medial and lateral margins.

The axial (tangential, "sunrise") view of the patella is seen in Figure 20.15E. In this projection, the patellofemoral compartment and the posterior surface of the patella are well delineated. The medial femoral condyle is larger and more prominent than the lateral, and the slope of the smaller medial facet of the posterior surface of the patella is steeper than that of the larger lateral facet. This is the anatomic basis for the fact that dislocation of the patella practically always occurs laterally. The axial projection may be obtained with the patient either prone or supine. In either event, the leg is flexed on the thigh approximately 45 degrees, and the central x-ray beam is directed posterior to the patella through the patellofemoral compartment.

RADIOGRAPHIC EXAMINATION

The number of radiographic projections deemed necessary to make a definitive diagnosis in knee trauma varies according to institutions. Verma et al. attests to the use of a single lateral radiograph for fracture screening; this being 100% sensitive in depicting knee fractures with a 100% negative predictive value. In many American institutions, the routine radiographic examination of the knee consists of a frontal/AP, lateral, and each oblique projections (Fig. 20.15). Although the Ottawa study recommends only an AP, lateral, and one oblique projection as the routine radiographic examination, some authors advocate a four-view examination for the acutely injured knee in light of the potential patient inconvenience, administrative, and legal costs that could result from a missed fracture on the three-film examination. In the United Kingdom, however, it is common practice to perform two orthogonal views (AP and lateral) in the initial assessment of knee trauma. This practice is compatible with Eisenberg et al.'s recommendations derived from a prospective large veteran association study. Eisenberg concluded that AP and lateral views were optimum for diagnosis for compensable service-related disabilities, including fractures. In our institution, if patients are still symptomatic and non-weight-bearing on reassessment, further cross-sectional imaging either with MRI or CT is performed.

If injury to the patella is suspected, an axial (tangential) view of the patella (Fig. 20.15E) should be obtained at the time of the initial radiographic examination. The axial projection of the patella may be obtained with the patient either prone or supine. When clinically necessary, it is possible, with gentle-controlled positioning, to flex the knee sufficiently to obtain an axial view of the patella.

The open-joint ("tunnel") projection (Fig. 20.16) is designed to provide optimum visualization of the intercondylar eminences and the intercondylar notch. It frequently provides the best visualization of foci of osteochondritis dissecans and of loose bodies (osteochondromatosis) within the joint space.

CT with 3-D reformation is useful in confirming a suspected fracture or to unambiguously demonstrate the extent and spatial relationships of a comminuted fracture of the proximal tibia or distal femur.

Figure 20.15. A: Normal adult knee in the frontal AP projection. B: Normal adult knee seen in lateral projection. Lateral radiograph of a normal adult knee. The positioning is nearly perfect, as judged by the superimposition of the femoral condyles. The slight concavity (black arrow) is the lateral (condylar) sulcus. The normal lucency of the suprapatellar recess (asterisk) identifies the deep surface of the quadriceps tendon (white arrow). The infrapatellar space (open arrows) is also normally lucent. C: Normal adult knee seen in externally oblique projection. D: Normal adult knee seen in internally rotated oblique projection. E: Axial ("sunrise") view of the normal patella. The lateral femoral condyle (black arrowheads) and the long lateral facet (white arrows) of the patella are less steep than their medial counterparts.

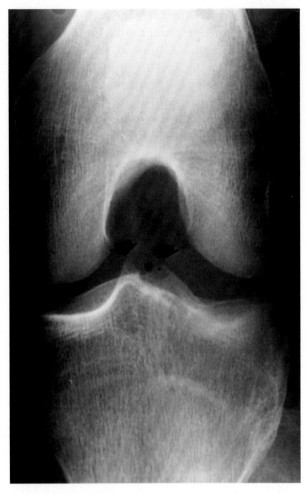

Figure 20.16. Intercondylar ("tunnel," "open joint") projection of the knee. *Arrows* indicate the intercondylar spines.

TABLE 20.3	**Radiographic and Computed Tomography Manifestation of Knee Joint Trauma**

Primary Signs

■ Fracture line—lucent (if fracture fragment separation) or sclerotic (if depressed, overlapping or impacted fracture)

Secondary Signs

■ Subcutaneous emphysema
■ Joint effusion, especially with presence of a fat–blood density interface (lipohemarthrosis).

RADIOGRAPHIC MANIFESTATIONS OF TRAUMA

General Radiographic Signs

The primary and secondary radiographic signs that accompany trauma of the knee are summarized in the Table 20.3.

We discuss the secondary signs and their origins in the next paragraphs.

Subcutaneous emphysema (Fig. 20.17) appears as irregularly distributed focal areas of decreased density in the soft tissues. The morphology of a knee joint effusion is illustrated in Figures 20.18 and 20.19 (compare with a normal suprapatellar recess/bursa in Fig. 20.15). The suprapatellar recess/bursa is a potential space bounded anteriorly by the suprapatellar fat pad and posteriorly by the prefemoral fat pad. These fat pads, containing fat, are lucent on plain radiographs. Normally, the suprapatellar recess/bursa measures less than 5 mm in AP diameter. When filled with fluid (effusion) or blood (hemarthrosis), a radiodense suprapatellar recess becomes evident, effacing both anterior suprapatellar and posterior prefemoral fat pads. The anatomy and plain radiographic findings of a knee joint effusion are illustrated in an MRI of a patient with an ACL rupture and small resultant knee joint effusion, depicted in Figure 20.18B. The principal effect of an effusion that causes distention of the knee joint capsule is to displace the quadriceps femoris muscle, the suprapatellar tendon, and the patella anteriorly. In addition, a large effusion usually causes the patella to be rotated around its coronal axis so that it is canted antero-inferiorly (Fig. 20.19).

The presence of liquid fat and blood (lipohemarthrosis) within the joint capsule produces a fat–fluid density interface (Fig. 20.20) that resembles an air–fluid level. This sign described by Nelson is seen only in the horizontal beam cross-table lateral radiograph made with the patient supine and is extremely valuable in the identification of minimally displaced intra-articular fractures of the distal femur and proximal tibia. Such fractures permit the flow of blood and liquid marrow fat from the medullary cavity into the joint space (Fig. 20.20B). Fractures of the patella have also been associated with lipohemarthrosis. Lipohemarthrosis and pneumo-hemarthrosis have very similar radiographic characteristics. However, the greater lucency of air within

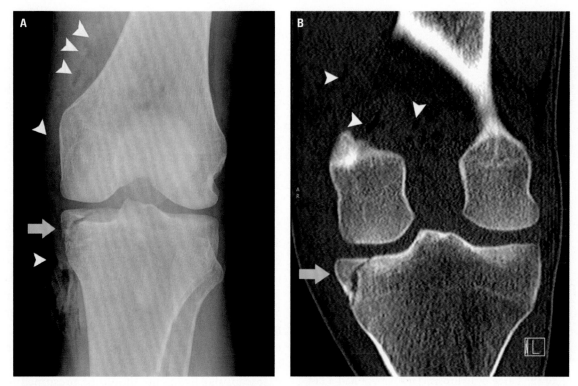

Figure 20.17. **A:** An open fracture of the medial tibial plateau (Schatzker III configuration), denoted by the *yellow arrow* with subcutaneous emphysema. The mottled, varying size lucent areas *(white arrowheads)* in the soft tissues medial to the knee represent subcutaneous emphysema. **B:** Accompanying coronal CT image of the medial tibial plateau fracture. Note the soft tissue emphysema demonstrated by the *white arrowheads*. The *yellow arrow* shows the medial tibial plateau fracture.

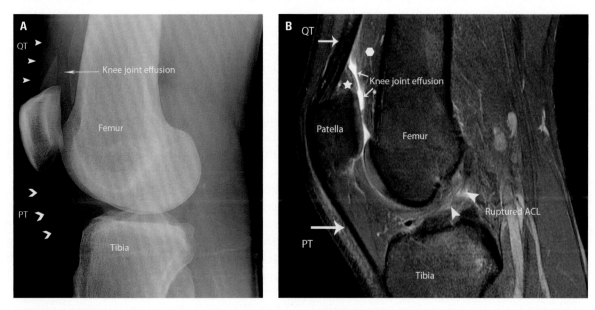

Figure 20.18. **A:** Soft tissue anatomy depicted on lateral plain radiographic projection. *Arrowheads* and *chevrons* indicate the anterior margins of the suprapatellar and patellar tendons, respectively. There is a small knee joint effusion located posterior to the suprapatellar fat pad *(yellow triangle)* and anterior to the prefemoral fat pad *(light blue structure)*. **B:** Corresponding soft tissue anatomy in the same patient (as in **A**) with an ACL rupture. The *white star* denotes the anterior suprapatellar fat pad, whereas the *hexagon* represents the posterior prefemoral fat pad. There is a small knee joint effusion. *QT*, quadriceps tendon; *PT*, patellar tendon.

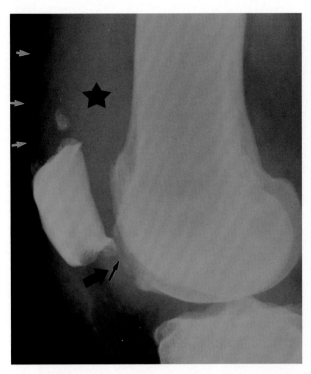

Figure 20.19. Large pyarthrosis. This patient had a hot, tender, swollen knee. The suprapatellar recess is completely filled with a soft tissue density *(black star)*, which could represent a sterile effusion, blood, or pus. The suprapatellar portion of the thigh is abnormally and anteriorly convex *(white arrows)*. The soft tissue density effusion has distended the suprapatellar recess and blended imperceptibly with the deep surface of the quadriceps tendon, rendering it invisible. The patella is displaced and canted anteriorly with respect to the femoral condyles. The unusual feature of this pyarthrosis is that the effusion is seen in the infrapatellar portion of the joint space *(thick solid black arrows)*. Osteomyelitis has eroded the subchondral cortex of the lateral condyle *(thin black arrow)* and the subcortical trabeculae.

the joint space combined with the presence of subcutaneous emphysema should help distinguish a pneumohemarthrosis (Fig. 20.21) from a lipohemarthrosis (Fig. 20.20A).

Knee Dislocation

Although knee dislocation with complete disruption of the femorotibial articulation is rare, (representing 0.02% to 0.2% of orthopedic injuries), it is a true orthopedic emergency due to the risk of neurovascular injury. Up to one-third of knee dislocations are associated with vascular injury. Vascular injury to the popliteal artery in this setting may be limb

threatening. Being rigidly tethered superiorly at the adductor magnus hiatus and inferiorly by the gastrocnemius-soleus arch, the popliteal artery has little room for displacement. The popliteal artery is, hence, vulnerable to traction and subsequent tear, shear, laceration, or thrombosis during knee injury. Where clinically suspected, MDCT angiography is a reliable and useful one-stop-shop procedure in the detection and characterization of both arterial and osseous injuries.

Dislocations of the knee (Fig. 20.22) are rare and are defined by the relationship of the tibia to the femur. Dislocations of the knee are considered an orthopedic emergency because of the potential compromise of the popliteal artery. Dislocation of the knee is commonly associated with avulsion fracture(s) of the articulating surface of the tibia. Subluxation of the knee may be anterior, posterior, lateral (Fig. 20.23A,B), or medial (Fig. 20.23C). Because the bones of the knee are so broad, rupture of both cruciate ligaments, the joint capsule, and the extracapsular ligaments should be presumed in all cases of complete knee dislocation.

Patella Dislocation

Patella dislocation mainly affects the young and active, with women in their 20s being at high risk. Dislocation of the patella invariably occurs laterally and is predisposed by various structural and biomechanical factors.

The extensor apparatus of the knee can be compared to that of a belt in a pulley system. The pulley is represented by the trochlea, whereas the belt by the quadriceps tendon-patella-patella tendon complex. For such a system to work, the belt and pulley have to be aligned on the same frontal plane. Pathoanatomy including trochlear dysplasia, patella alta, and excessive lateral distance between the tibial tubercle and trochlear groove (TTTG) contribute to lateral patella dislocation and instability. Trochlear dysplasia is a condition where the trochlear groove is shallow with abnormal trochlear morphology. Patella alta or a high-riding patella (Fig. 20.14B), located high above the trochlear fossa, occurs when the patella tendon is elongated. An excessive TTTG distance indicates lateralization of the tibial tubercle, so when the knee is flexed, the patella is pulled laterally.

Displacement of the patella may infrequently be incomplete (subluxation) (Fig. 20.24). When completely dislocated, the patella slips over the margin

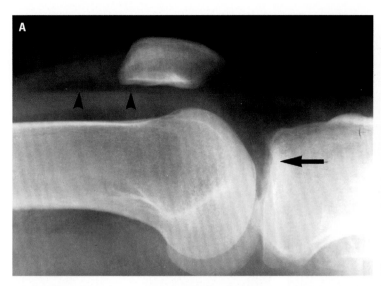
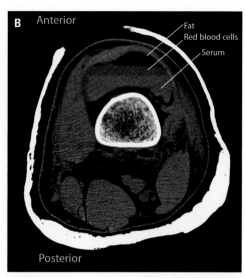

Figure 20.20. A: Lipohemarthrosis. The lucent soft tissue interface *(arrowheads)* on this horizontal beam cross-table lateral radiograph represents a fat–blood interface indicative of an intra-articular fracture which, in this patient, is a subtle, impacted, depressed fracture medial tibial tubercles *(arrow)*. **B:** An axial CT image of a different patient's knee joint with lipohemarthrosis. CT depicts three levels, corresponding to fat, red blood cells, and serum, in order of increasing gravity. Note the surrounding plaster of Paris *(white surround)*.

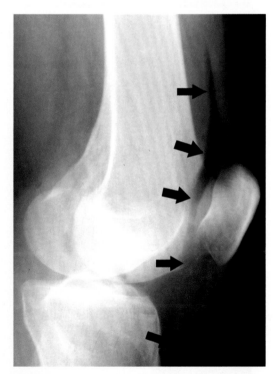
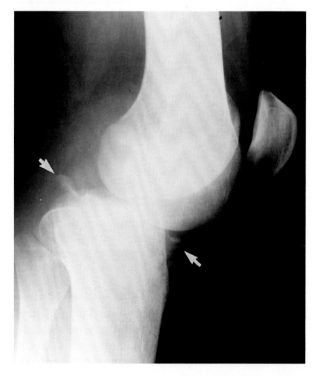

Figure 20.21. Pneumohemarthrosis *(arrows)* in the lateral radiograph of the left knee. The air–fluid level follows the contour of the blood within the joint space, and the lucency of the air is greater than that of a lipohemarthrosis (compare with Fig. 20.20).

Figure 20.22. Posterior dislocation of the knee associated with anterior and posterior osteochondral tibial fragments *(arrows)*.

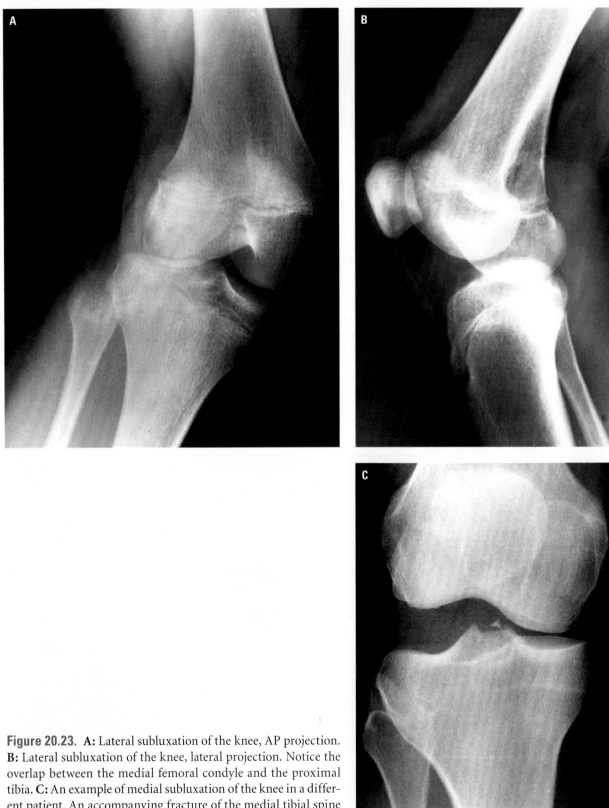

Figure 20.23. **A:** Lateral subluxation of the knee, AP projection. **B:** Lateral subluxation of the knee, lateral projection. Notice the overlap between the medial femoral condyle and the proximal tibia. **C:** An example of medial subluxation of the knee in a different patient. An accompanying fracture of the medial tibial spine is also present.

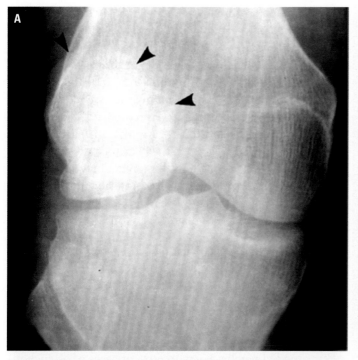

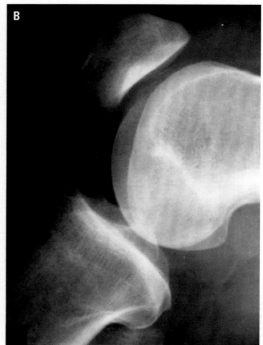

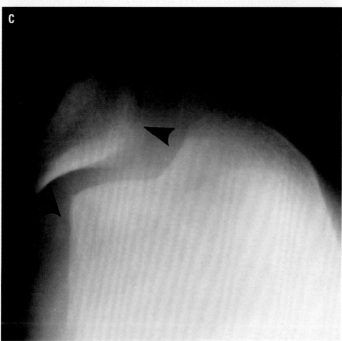

Figure 20.24. A: Lateral subluxation of the patella *(arrowheads)* is suggested in frontal projection. **B:** Lateral patellar subluxation. The lateral radiograph provides no additional useful information. **C:** Lateral patellar subluxation. The subluxation *(arrowheads)* is clearly evident in the axial "sun-rise" projection.

of the lateral femoral condyle (Fig. 20.25). In many cases, patients may be unaware of the lateral patella dislocation as it usually resolves spontaneously.

The mechanism of lateral patella dislocation can be simplified into two steps (Fig. 20.26). First, the dislocation stage—as the patella translates laterally, the osteochondral injury/fracture to the retropatellar cartilage *(yellow triangle)* and/or to the articular anterolateral femoral condyle *(star)* may arise. The patella may either rest parallel to the lateral surface of the condyle (Fig. 20.25) being fixed at this position or it may relocate back into the trochlear groove. The second or relocation/recoil stage, should it occur, may involve the medial patella facet impacting against the nonarticular lateral femoral condyle. The latter may give rise to osteochondral

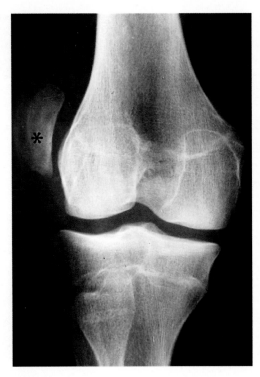

Figure 20.25. Complete lateral dislocation of the patella *(asterisk).*

injury/fracture to the medial patella facet and/or osseous injury to the nonarticular anterolateral femoral condyle (Fig. 20.26, *stars*).

An osteochondral injury/fracture is characterized by separation of a piece of articular cartilage with subchondral bone. Only the osseous portion of the osteochondral injury/fracture is detected radiographically (Fig. 20.27A). An MRI may demonstrate a donor site (Fig. 20.27B). In patella dislocation injuries, the osteochondral fragment may be small and is commonly located in the anterior portion of the joint space. The significance of the osteochondral fragment is that it may act as a loose body within the joint space and may cause impaired motion, frank locking, or degenerative disease of the knee.

The incidence of osteochondral injuries is more commonly detected than previously observed due to the increased use of MRI. Forty percent of patients have osteochondral injuries involving the lateral femoral condyle and more than 66% involving the medial patella. Forty to 60% of cases of osteochondral injuries are underdiagnosed on radiographs. Osteochondral fractures may remain elusive on

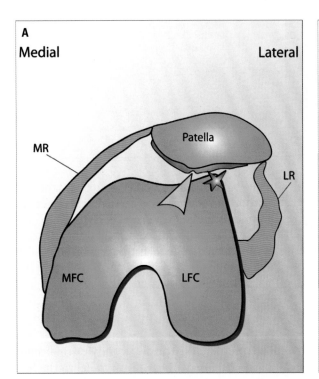

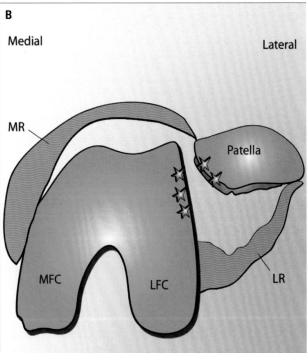

Figure 20.26. **A:** First stage of lateral patella dislocation: As the patella translates laterally, the osteochondral injury to the retropatellar cartilage *(yellow triangle)* and/or to the articular anterolateral femoral condyle *(star)* may occur. **B:** The second stage of dislocation: Relocation. As the patella swings back into the trochlear groove, the medial patella facet may impact against the nonarticular lateral femoral condyle, causing osteochondral and osseous injuries, respectively. *MFC,* medial femoral condyle; *LFC,* lateral femoral condyle; *MR,* medial retinaculum; *LR,* lateral retinaculum.

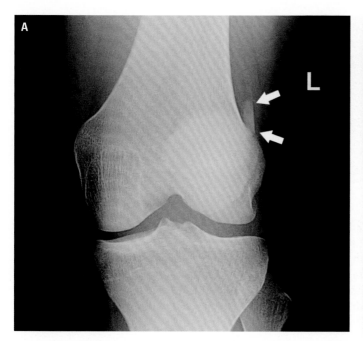
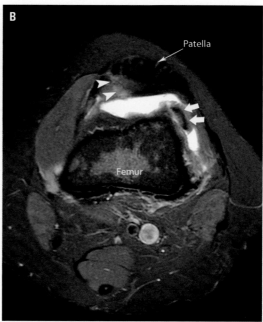

Figure 20.27. A: Osteochondral fragment *(arrows)* located at the lateral suprapatellar pouch in the frontal projection. **B:** Corresponding axial proton density fat-saturated (PDFS) MRI of the same patient shows the osteochondral fragment *(arrows)* in the lateral suprapatellar pouch. The donor site is the medial retropatellar facet *(arrowheads)*.

plain radiographs if only a small fragment of subchondral bone is sheared off. Although it is possible to detect intra-articular osteochondral lesions using CT, a MRI is the modality of choice with a sensitivity of more than 90%. Plain radiographic signs of lateral patellar dislocation include loss of the subchondral cortex of the medial facet (Fig. 20.28) or the medial margin of the patella. Patellar dislocations or subluxations rarely occur medially, but medial displacement of the patella may also be associated with an osteochondral fracture (Fig. 20.29).

Special Signs/Fractures in Relation to Knee Trauma

In this section, several relatively small and benign appearing fractures that in fact portend significant soft tissue injury involving the major stabilizing structures of the joint (ligamentous, tendinous, and capsular) are described. Great care should be placed in identification of such abnormalities as their detection could change management significantly. An MRI should be the next imaging investigation when such fractures are encountered due to their associations with considerable soft tissue injury.

The Segond Fracture

The Segond fracture is a capsular avulsion arising from the lateral tibial rim, posterior to Gerdy tubercle, also designated the *lateral capsular sign* (Fig. 20.30). Although sometimes a minute fracture, Segond fractures often herald more significant ligamentous injury associated with a high incidence of ACL (92%) and meniscal injuries. Anterolateral rotational instability—that is, anterior rotational subluxation of the lateral tibial condyle in relation to the lateral femoral condyle, with the tibia internally rotated on the axis of the PCL—must be considered present until proven otherwise. This fracture results from forced internal rotation of tibia with the knee in flexion, leading to avulsion of the distal ITB, middle third lateral capsular ligament (LCL), and the anterior oblique band (AOB) of the fibular collateral ligament complex (FCL); these structures are intimately interconnected. Previously, Segond fractures were only thought to represent avulsion of the meniscotibial portion of the middle LCL. In our experience, the most commonly observed pathology leading to a Segond fracture is capsular avulsion. Figure 20.31 summarizes the anatomical relationship between these structures.

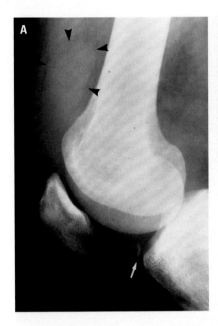

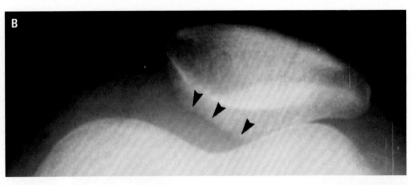

Figure 20.28. **A:** The lateral radiograph demonstrates a small osteochondral fragment *(arrow)* and a moderate effusion within the suprapatellar recess *(arrowheads).* **B:** Corresponding axial projection shows that the patella remains laterally subluxed following manipulation. The segment of the medial surface of the patella devoid of cortex *(arrowheads)* is the donor site of the osteochondral fragment seen in **A.**

The ITB is the distal extension and combination of the fascia lata and the tendon of the tensor fascia lata. It comprises two layers: its tendinous *superficial* layer, which inserts distally at Gerdy tubercle, on the anterior lateral tibia and the *deep* layer, which attaches to the intermuscular septum of the distal femur.

The mid-third LCL is a thickening of the lateral capsule of the knee, thought to be semiequivalent to the deep medial collateral ligament (MCL) of the knee. It comprises the meniscofemoral and meniscotibial ligaments, attaching the meniscus

to the femur and tibia, respectively. Proximally, it is identified as thickening of the lateral capsule, extending from the lateral gastrocnemius tendon attachment to anterior to the popliteus tendon origin on the femur. Distally, it attaches to the tibia, posterior to Gerdy tubercle.

The FCL comprises two bands: a straight band, which runs to the fibula head, and an oblique band, which runs obliquely to insert at the lateral tibial rim—this is known as the AOB. It blends with the posterior fibers of the ITB.

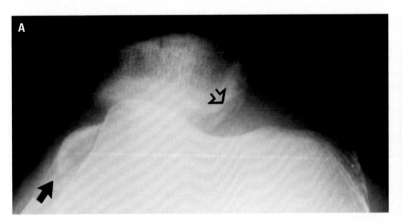

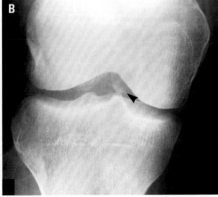

Figure 20.29. **A:** Medial dislocation of the patella. On the axial view, the patella is medially displaced but not dislocated. The evidence that the patella was medially dislocated is the large fragment *(solid arrow)* medial to the medial condyle on the femur and the lateral marginal fragment *(open arrow)* of the patella. **B:** Signs of medial dislocation of the patella. An osteochondral fragment is present, medial to the medial intercondylar spine on the AP radiograph *(arrowhead).*

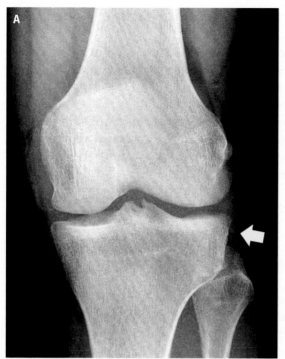

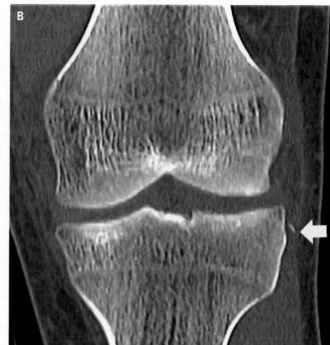

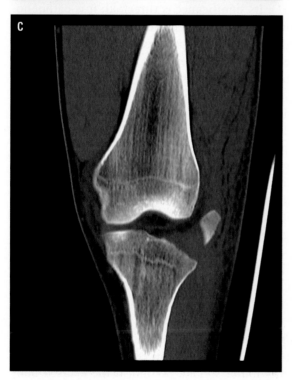

Figure 20.30. **A:** Segond fracture. The small separate fragment *(arrow)* is retracted proximally. **B:** Segond fracture. Accompanying coronal CT reformat shows the tiny avulsed lateral tibial rim. **C:** Segond fracture. Coronal CT image of another patient demonstrates a larger bony fragment avulsed from the lateral tibial rim.

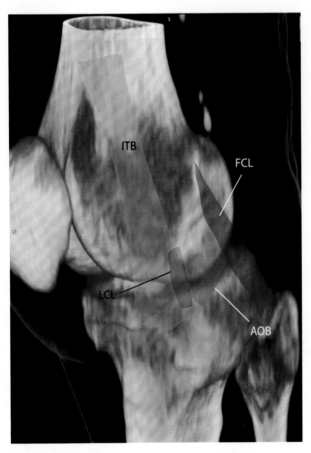

Figure 20.31. The anatomical basis of the Segond fracture, depicted with a 3-D sagittal representation of the lateral femorotibial compartment. A Segond fracture is an avulsion of the lateral tibial rim, the common attachment of the distal iliotibial band *(ITB),* middle third lateral capsular ligament *(LCL),* and the anterior oblique band *(AOB)* of the fibular collateral ligament *(FCL).*

Segond fractures may be acute or chronic. When acute, the avulsed fragment is identified several millimeters below the joint line, and its donor site may be evident on radiographs. When chronic, the avulsed fragment may reattach to the tibia, forming an osteophyte-like bony excrescence. This should be differentiated from an osteophyte that occurs at the level of the joint line.

Another mimicker of the Segond fracture is the fibular head avulsion by biceps femoris or the fibular collateral ligament, which both insert to the fibular head. This is distinguishable anatomically from the Segond fracture as these fractures are more laterally and distally placed (Fig. 20.11).

The Reverse Segond Fracture

The reverse Segond fracture is a mirror-image fracture of the described Segond fracture, characterized by avulsion fracture at the tibial insertion of the deep capsular component of the MCL of the knee. In contradistinction to the Segond fracture, the proposed mechanism of injury is external rotation with valgus overload. The importance of detecting this injury is its reported associations with disruption of the PCL (midsubstance tear and footprint avulsion) and medial meniscal tear.

The Arcuate Complex Avulsion Fracture

The avulsion fracture of the fibular head, also designated the *arcuate sign,* is manifested by an elliptical fragment with its long axis horizontally orientated on an AP radiograph (Figs. 20.10 and 20.11). Its significance is threefold; it is pathognomonic of significant posterolateral corner injury, suggests presence of posterolateral instability of the knee, and is associated with anterior and posterior cruciate ligamentous injury. Underrecognition of posterolateral instability may lead to failed ACL or PCL reconstruction.

Two patterns of arcuate signs have been described. Depending on anatomical location of the fracture fragment, size, and severity, the injured posterolateral corner structures involved can be implied or identified. Identification of the type of injury is important as it influences the treatment plan. First, if the bony fragment is small (a few millimeters), displaced just superior and medial to the fibular styloid, the injury is likely to involve the more medial posterolateral corner structures, namely the popliteofibular ligament (PFL) and arcuate ligament (Fig. 20.10). Avulsion of the fibular styloid may or may not be demonstrated on plain radiographs. MRI may add by demonstrating the fracture or marrow edema or both localized to the fibular styloid. Second, if the avulsed bony fragment is large (1.5 to 2.5 cm), more proximally displaced (2 to 4 cm from the fibular head), the conjoined tendon is involved (Fig. 20.11). The more displaced fracture fragment is likely to be related to the greater pulling strength of the conjoined tendon. On MRI, the fibular head edema is also more diffuse, involving the lateral aspect or whole of the fibular head.

Other stabilizing structures of the knee including the ACL, PCL, LCL, medial and lateral collateral ligaments, ITB, popliteus muscle, menisci, and peroneal nerve may also be injured along with the arcuate complex. Hence, presence of an arcuate complex fracture should prompt MRI evaluation.

The Deep Notch Sign

The lateral femoral condylopatellar sulcus is a shallow notch that is smooth and symmetrical, with a normal depth of no more than 1.5 mm. Deepening of the lateral sulcus with increased density and irregularity occurs when it impacts the posterior lateral margin of the lateral tibial plateau during an ACL injury (Fig. 20.7C).

FRACTURES BY ANATOMICAL LOCATION

Fractures of the Patella

The patella is anatomically predisposed to fractures due to its subcutaneous anterior location, accounting for 1% of all skeletal injuries treated in hospital. The common patellar fractures are transverse- and stellate-type fractures, both of which are most commonly the result of a direct blow to the patella. Fractures are usually clearly evident on routine views of the knee, particularly the lateral projection.

A common pitfall in the diagnosis of a patellar fracture is the presence of a bipartite patella (Fig. 20.32) misconstrued as a fracture. The patella normally develops from a single ossification center. Occasionally, it may arise from two centers that are separated by a transverse lucent defect in the middle third of the patella. These centers typically fuse, and the transverse defect present in infancy and childhood is obliterated in adulthood. The superior lateral corner of the patella may arise from a secondary ossification center that remains as a discrete separate ossicle. Features that help differentiate a true patella fracture and a bipartite patella are summarized in the Table 20.4.

Marginal fractures of the patella refer to fractures of its medial and lateral borders. They are uncommon compared with other types of patellar fractures and usually result from patellar dislocation or from a direct blow to the edge of the patella. Marginal fractures may be visible on the oblique projections

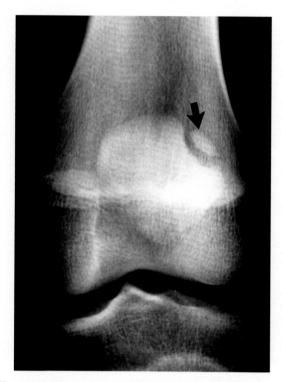

Figure 20.32. Bipartite patella: The ununited secondary ossification center *(arrow)* is characteristically located in the superolateral aspect of the patella and has smoothly corticated margins.

of the knee or the axial projection of the patella but best demonstrated on CT (Fig. 20.33).

Fractures of the inferior pole of the patella (Fig. 20.34) are also not common. The most common mechanism of acute injury is thought to be

TABLE 20.4	Differentiating a True Patella Fracture from a Bipartite Patella
True Patella Fracture	**Bipartite Patella**
Unilateral	Invariably bilateral. If there is clinical doubt, compare with contralateral patella
Margins of a fracture are usually serrated, ill-defined, and irregular.	Margins of the separate ossicle are sclerotic and well-defined.
Parent bone and fracture fragment are not usually parallel.	Parent bone and ossicle surfaces are smooth, contiguous, and parallel.
	Typically located superior laterally.

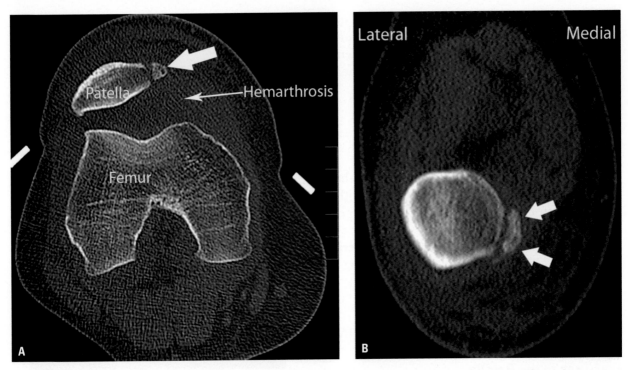

Figure 20.33. **A:** Fracture of the medial margin of the patella *(large arrow)* depicted on axial CT section, following a dislocation injury in a 33-year-old during a rugby match. **B:** Fracture of the medial margin of the patella *(large arrows)* depicted on coronal reformatted CT in the same patient as **A**.

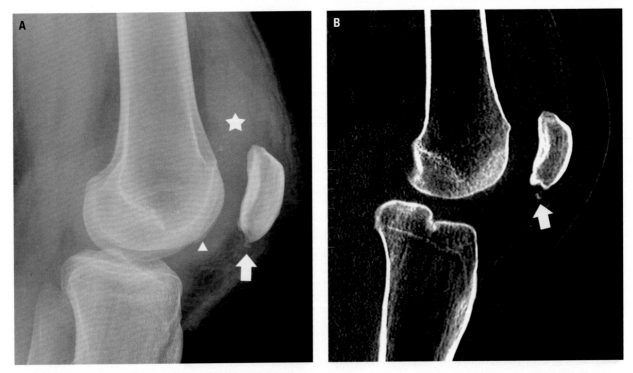

Figure 20.34. **A:** Tiny inferior patella pole fracture *(large arrow)* with associated hemarthrosis within the suprapatellar recess *(star)* and Hoffa fat pad *(triangle)*. **B:** Corresponding sagittal CT reformat in the same patient **A**. The inferior patella pole fracture is denoted by the *large arrow*.

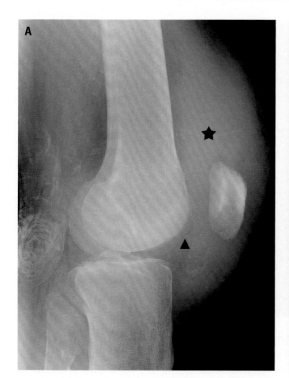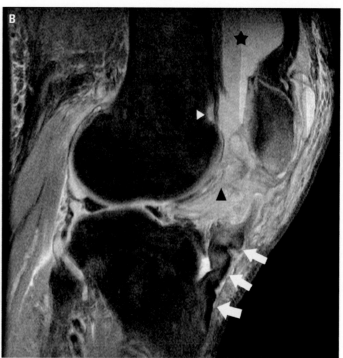

Figure 20.35. A: Rupture of the infrapatellar tendon, resulting in the "high-riding" patella in the lateral projections. Hemarthrosis in the suprapatellar recess *(star)* and in Hoffa fat pad *(triangle)*. **B:** An accompanying sagittal T2 FS MRI image shows a complete full-thickness proximal infrapatellar tendon rupture, resulting in a torn, sagging, and redundant infrapatellar tendon *(white arrows)*, hemarthrosis in the suprapatellar recess *(black star)* and Hoffa fat pad *(black triangle)*. The *white triangle* points to a further fracture of the anterior distal femoral metaphysis, not seen on the plain radiograph.

dislocation or subluxation of the patella. Radiographically, inferior patellar pole fractures may consist of a single large fragment or small, radiographically subtle avulsion fragments. Disruption of the infrapatellar tendon results in a "high-riding patella," best appreciated on the lateral projection of the knee (Fig. 20.35). Avulsion of the insertion of the infrapatellar tendon from its insertion on the tibial tubercle (Fig. 20.36) also results in high-riding patella.

Supracondylar Fractures

Supracondylar fractures of the distal femur are uncommon. These fractures occur at the transition site between the distal femoral diaphysis and metaphysis. Owing to the morphologically weaker metaphyseal flares of the distal femur, fractures frequently commence at this site.

Supracondylar fractures have a bimodal distribution. In the elderly (more commonly female), low impact trauma on a background of osteoporosis is implicated. In the young (more commonly men), these fractures are due to high impact trauma. In Figure 20.37, a supracondylar fracture of the lateral surface of the lateral condyle involves the origin of the lateral collateral ligament.

Tibial Fractures

Tibial Avulsion Fractures

Although most ACL tears involve the midsubstance of the ligament, avulsion of its tibial attachment may occur, particularly in children. Patients often give a history of an aching flexed knee with signs of anterior instability. The causation varies between children and adults. In children, the pathomechanism is forced flexion of the

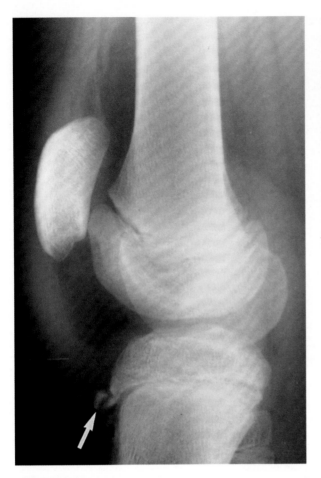

Figure 20.36. High-riding patella due to avulsion of the insertion of the infrapatellar tendon on the anterior tubercle *(arrow)* of a child.

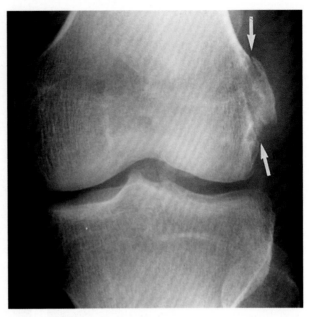

Figure 20.37. Supracondylar fracture of the lateral cortex of the lateral condyle *(arrows)*. This fracture involves the lateral collateral ligament origin and is likely to destabilize the ligament.

knee and tibial internal rotation. This pattern of injury is not associated with other knee injuries. In adults, the pathomechanism is severe hyperextension (e.g., following a motor vehicle accident). This pattern of injury is associated with other injuries (e.g., MCL injury).

In the child, prior to physeal fusion, the unossified tibial eminence is weaker than that of the intrinsic strength of the ACL. In the event of an injury, the ACL fails at the chondroosseous transition, near the tibial spine, giving rise to a bony avulsion, which may be perceived on plain radiographs.

Contrary to previous published data, the ACL does not attach to the medial tibial spine per se but inserts between the medial and lateral tibial spines, 10 to 14 mm behind the anterior border of the tibia (Fig. 20.7). Figure 20.6 illustrates the site of attachment of the anterior and posterior cruciate ligaments on the proximal end of the tibia. A dis-

placed fracture of the tibial eminence may cause loss of biomechanical function of the ACL, leading to instability.

Telltale signs of avulsion fractures of the intercondylar eminence include presence of bony fragment in the intercondylar notch with cortical irregularity of the tibial spine. A MRI correlation is recommended to identify that the fragment originates from the tibia and to assess the integrity of the ACL. Associations including meniscal (injured in 40% to 70% of cases, affecting the medial meniscus mainly) and MCL injuries should also be assessed on MRI.

There are four types of intercondylar eminence fractures based on the modified Meyers and McKeever classification (Fig. 20.38). The type of fracture is important in determining whether the injury can be treated closed or requires open reduction and internal fixation.

Radiographically, the type I intercondylar eminence fracture is incomplete and only minimally elevated (Fig. 20.39); the type II fragment is more clearly elevated anteriorly but not completely separated posteriorly in a hinge configuration (Fig. 20.40); and the type III fragment is completely displaced from the proximal tibia, devoid of bony apposition, and may be rotated as much as 90 degrees so that

Figure 20.38. Fractures of the intercondylar spine according to the modified Meyers and McKeever classification. *ACL,* anterior cruciate ligament.

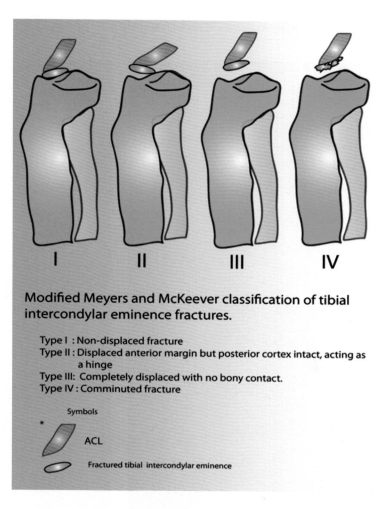

Modified Meyers and McKeever classification of tibial intercondylar eminence fractures.

Type I : Non-displaced fracture
Type II : Displaced anterior margin but posterior cortex intact, acting as a hinge
Type III: Completely displaced with no bony contact.
Type IV : Comminuted fracture

Symbols

ACL

Fractured tibial intercondylar eminence

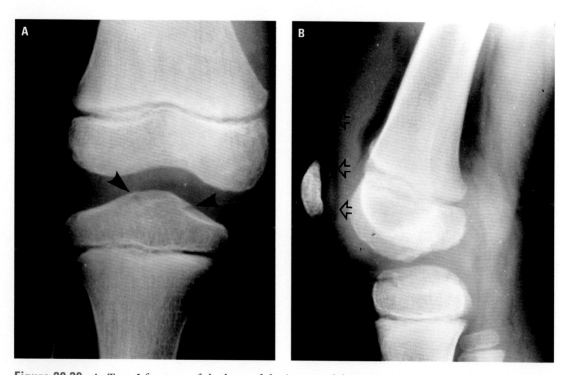

Figure 20.39. A: Type I fracture of the base of the intercondylar eminence *(arrowheads)* in the frontal projection. **B:** Type I fracture of the base of the intercondylar eminence *(arrowheads)* in the lateral projection with associated lipohemarthrosis *(open arrows)*.

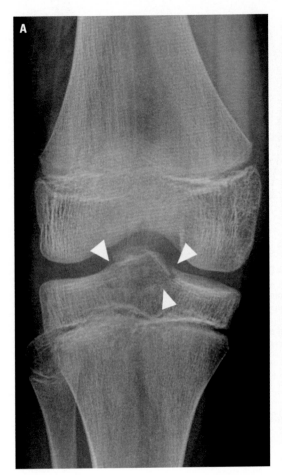

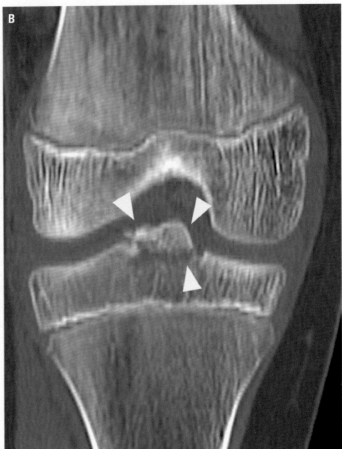

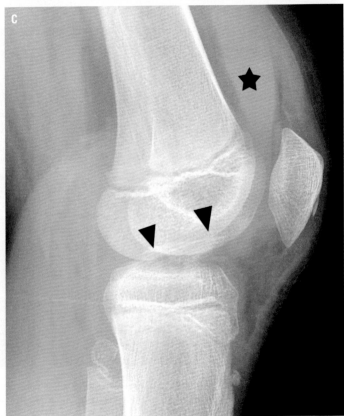

Figure 20.40. A: Type II fracture of the base of the intercondylar eminence *(arrowheads)* in the frontal projection. **B:** Corresponding coronal reformatted CT shows the type II fracture of the base of the intercondylar eminence *(arrowheads)* in detail. **C:** Same patient: Lateral projection demonstrates the type II fractured intercondylar eminence *(black arrowheads)* being lifted off but hinged posteriorly. Associated lipohemarthrosis *(black star)*.

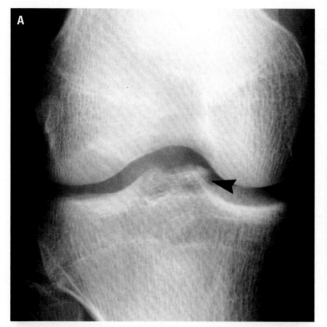

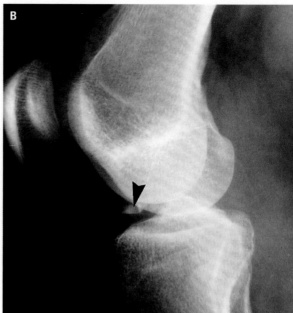

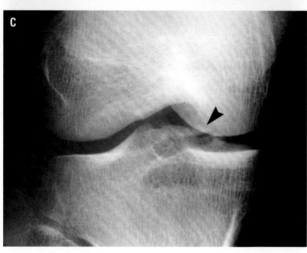

Figure 20.41. A: Type IV comminuted fracture of the medial intercondylar spine *(arrowhead)* in frontal projection. **B:** Type IV comminuted fracture of the medial intercondylar spine *(arrowhead)* in the lateral projection; the fragments are clearly completely separated from the proximal tibia. **C:** Type IV comminuted fracture of the medial intercondylar spine *(arrowhead)* in the oblique projections.

the articulating surface of the separate fragment is posteriorly directed. Type IV fractures (Fig. 20.41) are comminuted.

Arthroscopic fixation is the current treatment for types II, III, and IV tibial eminence fractures.

Isolated fractures of the lateral intercondylar spine (Fig. 20.42) do not involve either cruciate ligament.

Proximal Tibial Fractures

In children, Salter-Harris physeal injuries may involve either the proximal tibia (Fig. 20.43) or distal femur (Figs. 20.44 and 20.45).

In adults, proximal tibial fractures may be very subtle (Fig. 20.46) and may be either detected only on oblique projections, inferred by the presence of a lipohemarthrosis, or detected by CT (Fig. 20.46) or MRI. In our institution, CT is the imaging modality of choice as it is quick and accurate method of assessment of proximal tibial fractures.

Eighty percent of tibial plateau fractures involve the lateral plateau and occur mainly in patients older than 50 years of age. This is due to the weaker anatomy and morphology of the lateral tibial condyle, with fewer and finer trabeculae compared to the medial tibial condyle. The medially femoral condyle is structurally stronger and larger than its lateral counterpart, as most of the body weight is usually transmitted through the medial femoral condyle to

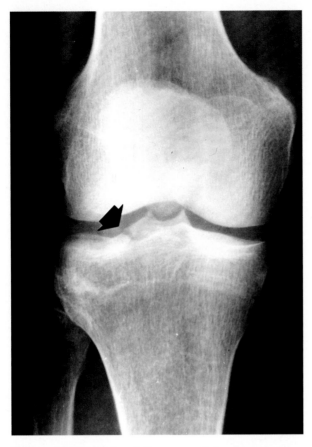

Figure 20.42. Isolated fracture of the lateral spine *(arrow)* of the intercondylar eminence.

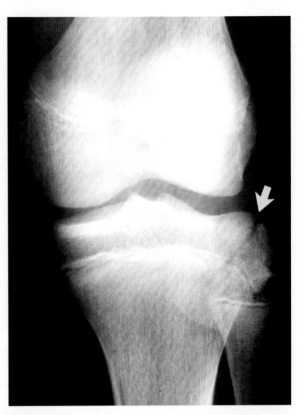

Figure 20.43. Salter-Harris III physeal injury *(arrow)* of the lateral plateau of the proximal tibial epiphysis. The vertical fracture line is confined to the epiphysis and does not cross the physis.

the medial tibial plateau. A valgus force resulting in abduction of the knee coupled with compression of the lateral tibial plateau is the usual mechanism of injury. Given that the femoral condyles are more structurally robust than the tibial plateau, a fracture of the lateral tibial plateau ensues. A summary of key information a surgeon needs from the radiologist in the assessment of a tibial plateau fracture is summarized in Table 20.5.

Schatzker Classification for Tibial Plateau Fractures

Following the identification of a tibial plateau fracture, the role of the radiologist is to determine the type of Schatzker classification the fracture conforms to. The Schatzker classification

TABLE 20.5	What the Surgeon Needs to Know in Relation to Tibial Plateau Fractures

- Is there an occult fracture?
- Depth of depressed fragment. (If the articular depression is equal to or more than 10 mm, surgery is indicated.)
- Type of Schatzker classification—this governs management.

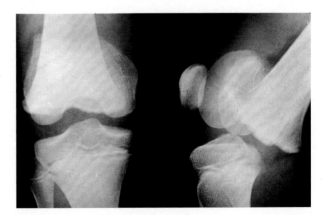

Figure 20.44. Salter-Harris type I distal femoral physeal injury. Although the distal femoral epiphysis is severely displaced, the absence of an associated fracture is consonant with the Salter-Harris type I injury.

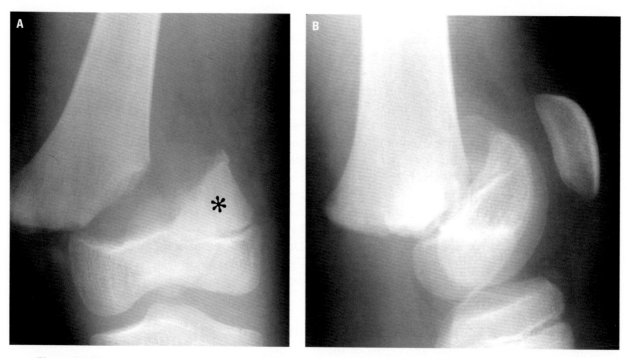

Figure 20.45. A: Type II Salter-Harris physeal injury of the distal femur, frontal projection. The large triangular metaphyseal fragment *(asterisk)*, which remains adherent through the intact physis to the epiphysis, characterizes the type II injury. **B:** Type II Salter-Harris physeal injury of the distal femur, lateral projection.

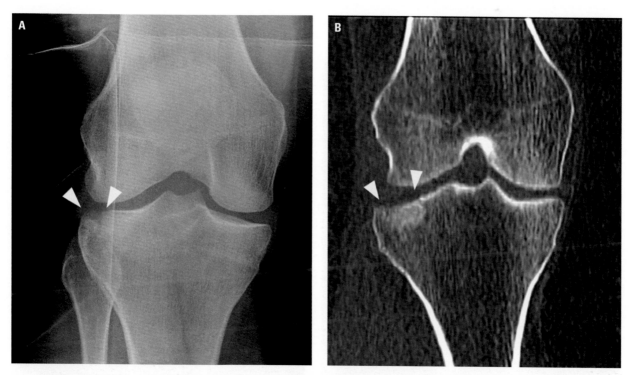

Figure 20. 46. A: Insufficiency fracture of the lateral tibial plateau *(arrowheads)*, Schatzker type II fracture, suspected in the frontal projection. **B:** Insufficiency fracture of the lateral tibial plateau *(arrowheads)*, Schatzker type II fracture, confirmed on coronal reformatted CT. There is lateral tibial plateau split and depression.

is numerical, with an ascending numeric category corresponding to increasing severity of injury, increasing energy imparted to bone on impact, and worsening of prognosis (Figs. 20.46 to 20.51). Schatzker types I to III fractures are low-energy injuries. Type I invariably occurs in young adults; type II in patients older than 30 years; and type III in osteoporotic, more elderly patients. Types IV to VI fractures are due to high-energy trauma. Schatzker IV fractures have the worst prognosis owing to their association with dislocation injury and associated neurovascular complications.

This classification system is used in assessing initial injury, surgical planning, and assessing prognosis. The Schatzker classification, its description, and associations are summarized in the Table 20.6.

The management of Schatzker I, II, and III fractures centers around evaluation and repair of the articular cartilage. Treatment of Schatzker IV fractures is with open reduction and internal fixation. Management of Schatzker IV and V is dependent on the status of the soft tissues.

Tibial Fracture Association: Popliteal Artery Injury

The popliteal artery, as it leaves the popliteal fossa, lies in a confined space bounded anteriorly by the posterior margin of the articular surface of the tibia and posteriorly by the soleus, plantaris, and medial head of the gastrocnemius muscles. In this situation, the popliteal artery is subject to laceration or occlusion by proximal tibial fractures, particularly of the "bumper" type (Fig. 20.52). Although vascular injuries associated with proximal tibial fracture are rare, the status of the peripheral circulation should be evaluated clinically. If this proves difficult, Doppler ultrasound or CT angiography may be useful in vascular assessment. Alternatively, a femoral arteriogram may be performed (Fig. 20.52).

Other Fractures

Although most fractures of the head or neck of the fibula are associated with fractures of the proximal tibia, isolated proximal fibular fractures may occur as the result of direct trauma or, indirectly,

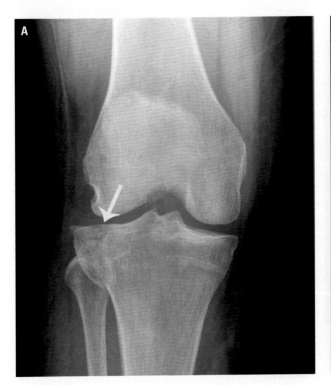
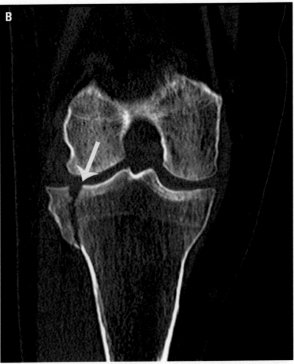

Figure 20.47. A: Schatzker I fracture with a split of the lateral tibial plateau on frontal projection *(arrow)*. **B:** Schatzker I fracture with a split of the lateral tibial plateau on coronal reformatted CT *(arrow)*.

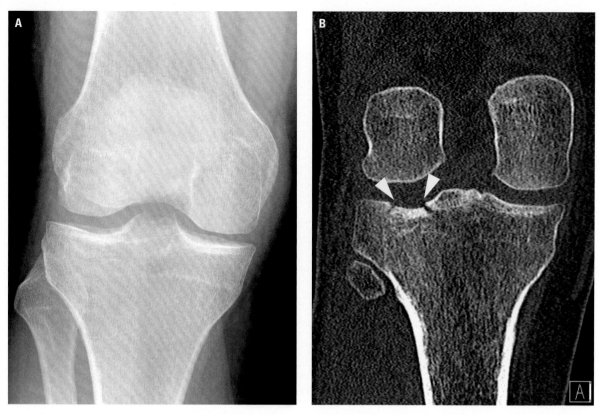

Figure 20.48. **A:** Schatzker III fracture imperceptible on the frontal projection. The patient subsequently had CT due to ongoing pain. **B:** Schatzker III fracture *(arrowheads)* not detected on plain radiographs but demonstrated on coronal reformatted CT. There is a depression of the lateral tibial plateau.

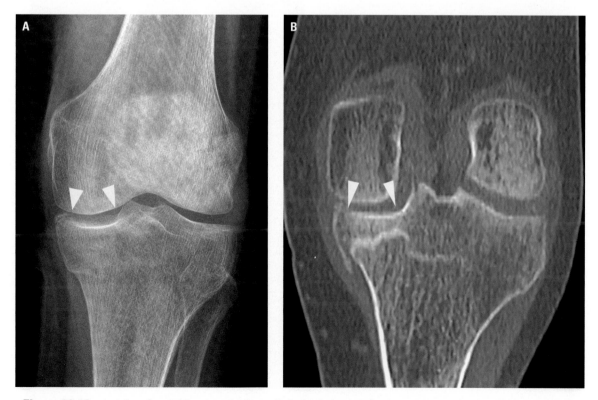

Figure 20.49. **A:** Schatzker IV fracture with medial tibial plateau depression *(arrowheads)*. **B:** Schatzker IV fracture depicted on coronal CT *(arrowheads)*.

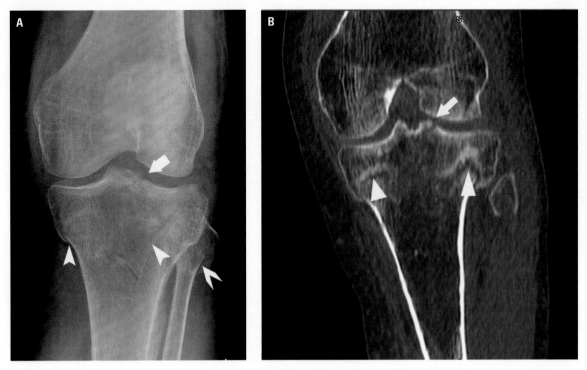

Figure 20.50. **A:** Schatzker V fracture on frontal projection. There are fractures of both medial and lateral tibial condyles *(arrowheads)*, the fibular neck *(chevron)*, and lateral tibial spine *(arrow)*. **B:** Schatzker V fracture depicted on coronal CT. Fracture of both tibial condyles *(arrowheads)* and lateral tibial spine *(arrow)* are identified.

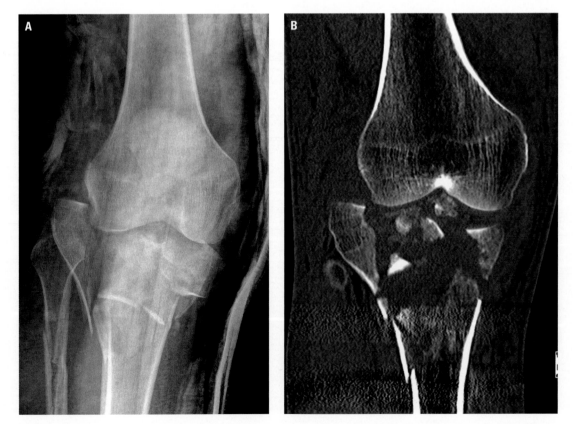

Figure 20.51. **A:** Schatzker VI fracture: Frontal projection showing the bicondylar fractures extending to the subcondylar level. Also note the longitudinal proximal fibular shaft fracture. **B:** Schatzker VI fracture depicted on coronal CT. The bicondylar fractures extend to the subcondylar region.

TABLE 20.6	Schatzker Classification of Tibial Plateau Fractures			
Schatzker Type	Description	Mechanism	Important associations and recommendations	Other Notes
I	Nondisplaced split fracture of the lateral tibial plateau	Valgus stress	MCL or ACL injury. Arthroscopy recommended to ensure lateral meniscus is not trapped by fracture.	May be very subtle on plain radiograph. 6% of all tibial plateau fractures.
II	Lateral tibial plateau split and depression	Valgus ± axial stress	MCL or medial meniscus injury.	25% of all tibial plateau fractures.
III	Pure lateral tibial plateau depression	Axial loading		36% of all tibial plateau fractures.
IV	Pure medial tibial plateau depression	Varus force + axial stress. High energy	Possible subluxation/dislocation. Lateral collateral ligament complex, posterior lateral corner, fracture-dislocation of the proximal fibula, popliteal vessel and peroneal nerve injury. **CT ± CT angiography recommended.**	10% of all tibial plateau fractures. **Worst prognosis.**
V	Bicondylar fracture	Combined valgus + varus + axial stress. High energy	Unstable knee due to disrupted collateral ± cruciate anchors.	3% of all tibial plateau fractures.
VI	Tibial metadiaphyseal fracture/transverse subcondylar fracture	Combined valgus + varus + axial stress. High energy	Increased risk of compartment syndrome.	20% of all tibial plateau fractures.

MCL, medial collateral ligament; *ACL,* anterior cruciate ligament; *CT,* computed tomography.

in association with ankle injuries (e.g., the Maisonneuve fracture).

The radiographic diagnosis of supracondylar or intercondylar fractures of the distal femur is usually obvious on the initial plain radiographs obtained in the emergency center.

Fracture of a single femoral condyle is uncommon, may be radiographically obscured, and is usually caused by direct trauma.

OVERUSE AND NONTRAUMATIC CONDITIONS

Osgood-Schlatter Disease

Osgood-Schlatter disease is a form of traction apophysitis involving the tibial tubercle. Repetitive microtrauma and traction on the tibial tubercle by the patella tendon leads to this chronic stress injury. This condition occurs most frequently in adolescent male athletes who frequently jump and kick. Clinically, the disease is manifested by pain, tenderness, and swelling over the tibial tubercle. The radiographic and CT (Fig. 20.53) signs consist of elevation of the tubercle away from the shaft, fragmentation, and irregular density of the tubercle and soft tissue swelling anterior to the tubercle. The diagnosis of Osgood-Schlatter disease is clinical. The radiographic abnormalities of the tubercle must be of major dimension and, even then, are only supportive of the clinical diagnosis.

Pellegrini-Stieda Disease

Pellegrini-Stieda disease (Fig. 20.54) is the term originally coined a century ago to denote calcification and ossification within the MCL subsequent to

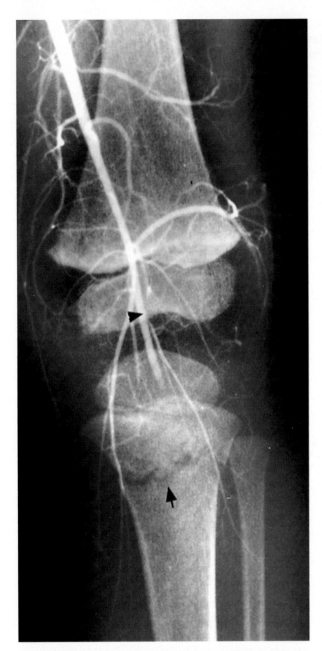

Figure 20.52. Femoral arteriogram demonstrating complete obstruction of the popliteal artery *(arrowhead)*, associated with a minimally displaced "bumper" fracture *(arrow)* in a child.

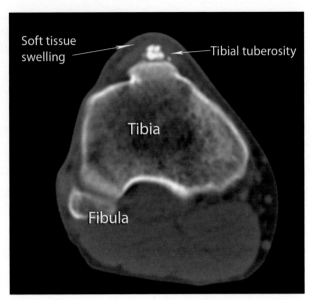

Figure 20.53. Axial CT of a 25-year-old male avid sportsman with pain over the tibial tuberosity. There is fragmentation of the tibial tuberosity and soft tissue swelling overlying it. Clinicoradiologic findings are compatible with Osgood-Schlatter disease.

injury. The MCL origin arises from the femoral epicondyle. In practice, the calcification is seen proximal to this site. A recent MRI case series has thrown light to this observation proposing the calcifications as secondary to periosteal stripping of the distal femoral metaphysis, superior to the epicondylar MCL origin, and separate from the MCL and adductor magnus origin. On radiographic follow-up, the periosteal stripping progresses to heterotopic bone formation around the medial femoral condyle, in line with the classical Pellegrini-Stieda appearance. The authors also noted an association with complete PCL disruption.

Osteochondritis Dissecans

Osteochondritis dissecans is a focal area of post-traumatic subarticular avascular necrosis that usually occurs secondary to a subchondral fracture. The lesion is usually encountered in adolescent males but can be seen in adults. The knee is the most common site of osteochondritis dissecans, and within the knee, the medial femoral condyle is the most common location. Clinically, there may or may not be a history of identifiable trauma to the knee. Symptoms are usually mild, consisting of localized pain and tenderness, some limitation of motion, gritting sensation, or even locking. It is not uncommon that a focus of osteochondritis dissecans is an incidental finding.

Radiographically, the lesion appears as a shallow, concave, subchondral defect on the articulating surface of the femoral condyle (Fig. 20.55) or tibial plateau. The margins of the concavity are smoothly sclerotic. A separate, dense, button-like piece of bone may be seen within the concavity of

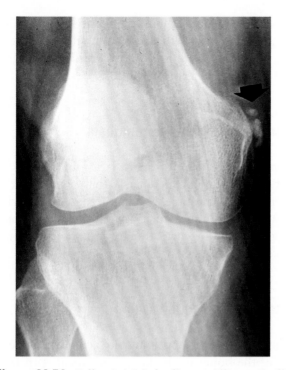

Figure 20.54. Pellegrini-Stieda disease. The vertically situated calcifications *(arrow)* are located around insertion of the medial collateral ligament on the medial femoral epicondyle. The location and orientation of the calcifications are typical of Pellegrini-Stieda disease.

the saucer-like defect or may be found free within the joint space.

Chondrocalcinosis

Chondrocalcinosis (pseudogout, calcium pyrophosphate dihydrate deposition disease) is characterized by fibrocartilage calcification, pain, and joint destruction. The pain is nonspecific and may mimic osteoarthritis or gout. The earliest radiographic sign is faint, amorphous calcification within the fibrocartilage of the knee (Fig. 20.56), hip, pubic symphysis, or elbow.

Hemophilia

Hemophilia is an X-linked recessive disorder that may either be due to factor VIII or factor IX deficiency. Either deficiency results in hemarthrosis; repeated hemarthrosis with iron deposition results in synovial irritation, synovitis, cartilage loss, and atypical osteoarthritis. Atypical osteoarthritis in this setting is evidenced by symmetrical joint space

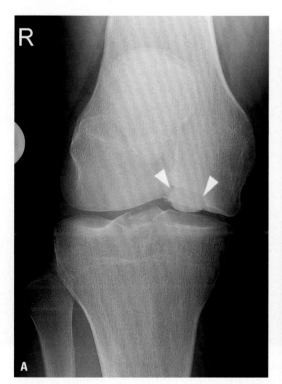
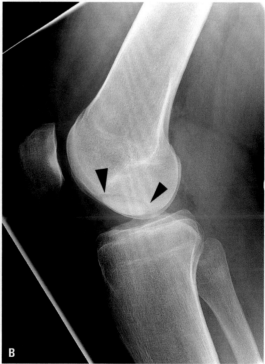

Figure 20.55. A: Osteochondritis dissecans of the medial femoral condyle *(arrowheads)* in the frontal projection. **B:** Osteochondritis dissecans of the medial femoral condyle *(arrowheads)* in the lateral projection.

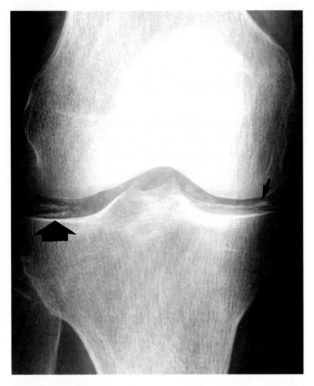

Figure 20.56. Typical faint amorphous calcifications of chondrocalcinosis *(arrows)* conform to the configuration of the medial and lateral menisci.

loss and subchondral bony irregularity. Additionally, epiphyseal overgrowth also occurs, with squaring of the patella and femoral condyles and widening of the intercondylar notch (Fig. 20.57).

Synovial Osteochondromatosis

Synovial osteochondromatosis ("joint mice") is a benign synovial metaplasia that results in the formation of multiple, varying sized loose particles (bodies) within the joint space. The loose bodies are characterized by cortical margins and central trabeculation (Fig. 20.58).

Osteomyelitis of the Knee

The radiographic appearance of acute osteomyelitis of the bones of the knee is identical with that described for other joints, in that the subchondral cortex is eroded, as are the subjacent trabeculae (Fig. 20.59). The intra-articular infection is associated with distension of the joint capsule

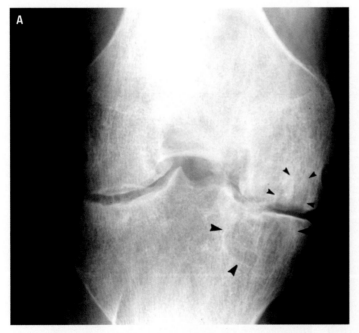

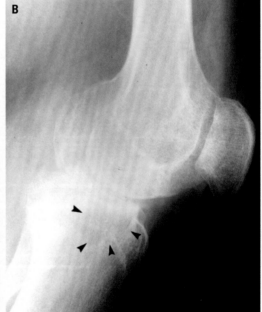

Figure 20.57. **A:** Characteristic changes of hemophilia, consisting of degenerative changes of the contiguous surfaces of the femur and tibia, including large detritus cysts *(arrowheads)* medially in the frontal projection. The intercondylar notch is also widened, which is characteristic of hemophilia. **B:** Characteristic changes of hemophilia, consisting of degenerative changes of the contiguous surfaces of the femur and tibia, including large detritus cysts *(arrowheads)* medially in the lateral projection.

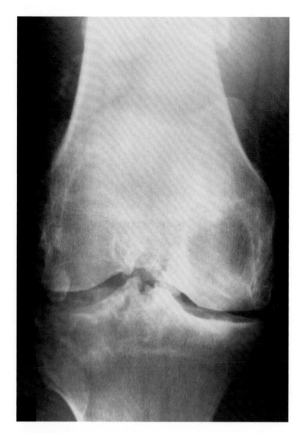

Figure 20.58. Synovial osteochondromatosis. Notice the numerous osseous bodies around the knee joint.

secondary to the pyarthrosis. Extracapsular soft tissue swelling may also be present.

Heterotrophic Ossification

Heterotrophic ossification (HO) is pathologic bone formation in a site where bone is not normally found. It is generally believed to result from mesenchymal metaplasia of unknown stimuli. Common etiologies include central nervous system trauma, other neurologic disorders particularly those associated with paralysis, burns, and direct soft tissue trauma. HO is commonly located about large joints. Radiographically, HO appears as irregularly shaped masses of heterogeneous bone in the soft tissues on large joints (Fig. 20.60). When HO is intimately involved with the periosteum, it may simulate a primary bone neoplasm. However, the clinical history—particularly one of central nervous system trauma with paralysis, burn, or an easily remembered blunt or surgical trauma to a portion of the appendicular skeleton—the multiplicity of the sites of HO, and the radiographic characteristics of the soft tissue ossification should permit a definitive radiologic diagnosis.

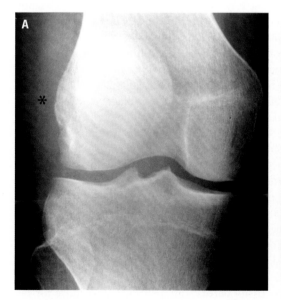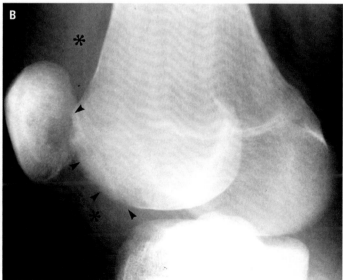

Figure 20.59. **A:** Pyarthrosis and osteomyelitis of the right knee following instrumentation. There is marked soft tissue swelling about the lateral aspect of the knee *(asterisk)* in the frontal projection. **B:** In the oblique projection, not only is an intra-articular collection evident by the increased density in the suprapatellar recess and anterior compartment *(asterisks)* but also the subchondral cortex and subchondral trabeculae are eroded and effaced *(arrowheads)*, indicating osteomyelitis.

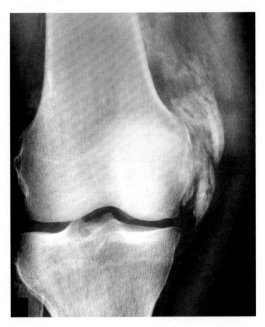

Figure 20.60. Characteristic radiographic appearance of heterotrophic ossification of the knee.

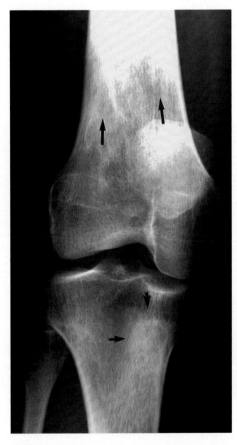

Figure 20.61. The irregular, inhomogeneous, mottled densities *(arrows)* within the medullary cavity of both the distal femur and proximal tibia are characteristic of bone infarcts of sickle-cell disease.

Sickle-Cell Disease

The infarcts of sickle-cell disease produce ill-defined areas of mottled increase in density at the sites of infarction within the medullary cavity (Fig. 20.61).

SUGGESTED READINGS

1. Verma A, Su A, Golin AM, et al. A screening method for knee trauma. *Acad Radiol.* 2001;8(5):392–397.
2. Eisenberg RL, Hedgcock MW, Williams EA, et al. Optimum radiographic examination for consideration of compensation awards: III. Knee, hand and foot. *AJR Am J Roentgenol.* 1980;135(5):1075–1078.
3. Tigges SC, Carpenter WA. Lateral radiograph of the knee: knowledge of normal anatomy aids in detection of subtle injuries. *Emerg Radiol.* 1996;3(2):56–62.
4. Huang GS, Yu JS, Munshi M, et al. Avulsion fracture of the head of the fibula (the "arcuate" sign): MR imaging findings predictive of injuries to the posterolateral ligaments and posterior cruciate ligament. *AJR Am J Roentgenol.* 2003;180(2):381–387.
5. LaPrade RF, Gilbert TJ, Bollom TS, et al. The magnetic resonance imaging appearance of individual structures of the posterolateral knee. A prospective study of normal knees and knees with surgically verified grade III injuries. *Am J Sports Med.* 2000;28(2):191–199.
6. Danzig LA, Newell JD, Guerra J Jr, et al. Osseous landmarks of the normal knee. *Clin Orthop Relat Res.* 1981;(156):201–206.
7. Gottsegen CJ, Eyer BA, White EA, et al. Avulsion fractures of the knee: imaging findings and clinical significance. *Radiographics.* 2008;28(6):1755–1770.
8. Nelson SW. Some important diagnostic and technical fundamentals in the radiology of trauma, with particular emphasis on skeletal trauma. *Radiol Clin North Am.* 1966;4(2):241–259.
9. Rieger M, Mallouhi A, Tauscher T, et al. Traumatic arterial injuries of the extremities: initial evaluation with MDCT angiography. *AJR Am J Roentgenol.* 2006;186(3):656–664.
10 Diederichs G, Issever AS, Scheffler S. MR imaging of patellar instability: injury patterns and assessment of risk factors. *Radiographics.* 2010;30(4):961–981.
11. De Nicola US, Coletti P, Monteleone G, et al. Tibial tuberosity derotation: a surgical procedure for realignment of the patellofemoral mechanism. *J Orthopaed Traumatol.* 2002;2:69–74.
12. Campos JC, Chung CB, Lektrakul N, et al. Pathogenesis of the Segond fracture: anatomic and MR imaging evidence of an iliotibial tract or anterior oblique band avulsion. *Radiology.* 2001;219(2):381–386.

13. Harish S, O'Donnell P, Connell D, et al. Imaging of the posterolateral corner of the knee. *Clin Radiol.* 2006;61(6):457–466.

14. Terry GC, LaPrade RF. The posterolateral aspect of the knee. Anatomy and surgical approach. *Am J Sports Med.* 1996;24(6):732–739.

15. Terry GC, LaPrade RF. The biceps femoris muscle complex at the knee. Its anatomy and injury patterns associated with acute anterolateral-anteromedial rotatory instability. *Am J Sports Med.* 1996; 24(1):2–8.

16. Lee J, Papakonstantinou O, Brookenthal KR, et al. Arcuate sign of posterolateral knee injuries: anatomic, radiographic, and MR imaging data related to patterns of injury. *Skeletal Radiol.* 2003;32(11): 619–627.

17. Prince JS, Laor T, Bean JA. MRI of anterior cruciate ligament injuries and associated findings in the pediatric knee: changes with skeletal maturation. *AJR Am J Roentgenol.* 2005;185(3):756–762.

18. Markhardt BK, Gross JM, Monu JU. Schatzker classification of tibial plateau fractures: use of CT and MR imaging improves assessment. *Radiographics.* 2009;29(2):585–597.

19. Stevens MA, El-Khoury GY, Kathol MH, et al. Imaging features of avulsion injuries. *Radiographics.* 1999;19(3):655–672.

20. McAnally JL, Southam SL, Mlady GW. New thoughts on the origin of Pellegrini-Stieda: the association of PCL injury and medial femoral epicondylar periosteal stripping. *Skeletal Radiol.* 2009;38(2):193–198.

Anthony Wilson ■ John H. Harris Jr.

GENERAL CONSIDERATIONS

The ankle includes the distal end of the tibia, the fibula, and the talus. The medial and lateral malleoli, together with the horizontal plate of the distal articulating surface of the tibia, constitute the ankle mortise that receives the dome-shaped superior articulating surface of the talus. Although the talus is intimately involved in the ankle joint, it is one of the tarsal bones, and primary injuries of the talus are discussed in Chapter 22, Foot and Heel. Only those talar injuries associated with primary injuries of the ankle are discussed in this chapter.

The radiographic evaluation of acute lesions of the ankle requires accurate clinical assessment of the site of the injury. Conditions affecting the heel and foot, which may produce symptoms referable to "the ankle," may not be recorded on ankle views and, thus, may be overlooked. The foot, heel, and ankle are distinct anatomic regions. Logically, then, each region requires particular radiographic projections that are usually inappropriate for the proper radiographic examination of the adjacent anatomic region.

Acknowledgement of the basic ligamentous anatomy of the ankle is fundamental to an understanding of the pathophysiology of ankle injuries and the clinical significance of the radiographic appearance of the skeletal injuries.

Ligamentous Anatomy

Laterally (Fig. 21.1), the anterior and posterior talofibular ligaments, together with the calcaneo-fibular ligament, constitute the lateral collateral ligament. The anterior and posterior talofibular ligaments extend horizontally from the anterior and posterior cortical surfaces of the fibula to the talus. The calcaneofibular ligaments extend inferoposteriorly from the tip of the lateral malleolus to the lateral surface of the body of the os calcis.

The medial collateral deltoid ligament (Fig. 21.2) is stronger and denser than the lateral collateral ligament and consists of superficial and deep fibers loosely arranged into three groups. These groups extend from the lateral malleolus to the tarsal navicular, the sustentaculum tali of the os calcis, and the talus.

Distally, the tibia and fibula are united by the anterior and posterior tibiofibular ligaments; the interosseous ligament, which is the distal extension of the interosseous membrane; and the interosseous membrane itself (Fig.21.3). Even from this brief description, it must be apparent that the ligaments of the ankle are integral to the anatomy of the ankle joint. The presence of specific ligamentous injury about the ankle is deducible from the location and orientation of malleolar fractures. Identification of the disrupted and intact ligaments should be included as part of the radiologic report of ankle injuries.

RADIOGRAPHIC EXAMINATION

The routine radiographic examination of the ankle should include anteroposterior (AP), "mortise" internally rotated oblique, and lateral projections (Fig. 21.4), unless the patient's condition

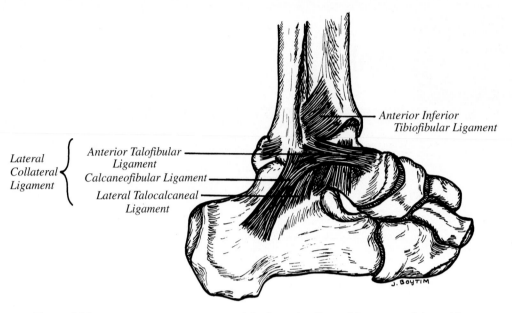

Figure 21.1. Schematic representation of the lateral collateral ligament of the ankle.

dictates a more limited AP and lateral examination. Oblique views, as included in the routine radiographic examination, can be useful in identifying minimally displaced fractures that are frequently identified or confirmed only by these projections (Figs. 21.5 and 21.6).

The oblique projections of the ankle are obtained by rotation at the hip because rotation is not a physiologic function of either the ankle or the knee. The internally rotated oblique projection (e.g., the mortise view) requires only approximately 10 degrees of internal rotation at the hip or sufficient internal rotation so that the lateral malleolus is on the

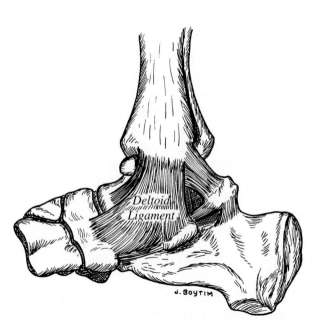

Figure 21.2. Schematic representation of the medial collateral (deltoid) ligament of the ankle.

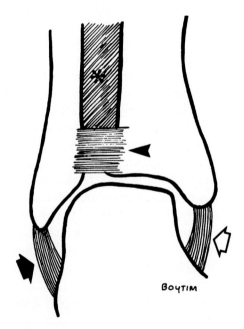

Figure 21.3. Schematic representation of the major ligaments of the ankle seen from the front. *Asterisk* indicates the interosseous ligament, the anterior tibiofibular ligament *(arrowhead)*, the medial collateral or deltoid ligament *(white arrow)*, and the lateral collateral ligament *(black arrow)*.

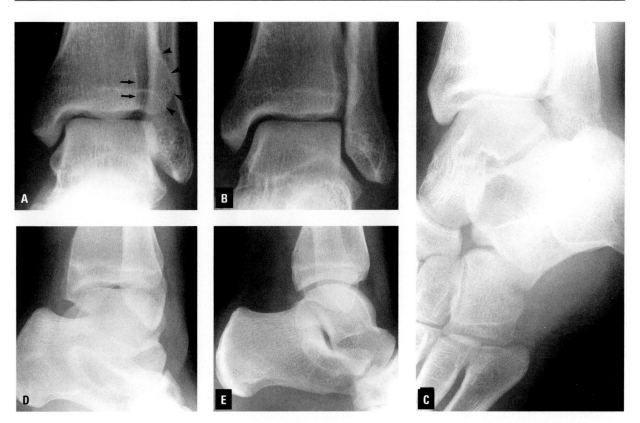

Figure 21.4. Routine radiographic examination of the ankle comprising straight AP (**A**), "mortise" (**B**), internally rotated oblique (**C**), externally rotated oblique (**D**), and lateral (**E**) projections. In the straight frontal projection (**A**), the *arrows* indicate the posterior margin, and the *arrowheads*, the anterior margin of the fibular notch of the lateral aspect of the tibia.

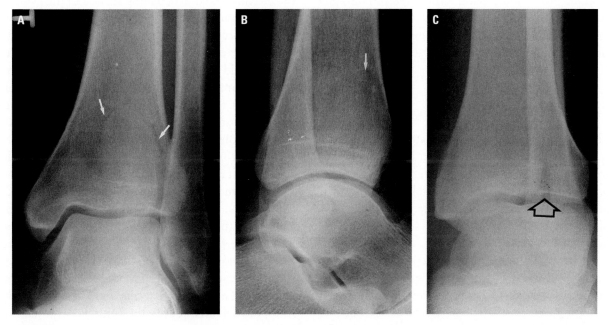

Figure 21.5. Subtle, minimally displaced fracture in the distal tibia. The fracture line is only faintly perceptible in the frontal (**A**) and lateral (**B**) projections *(white arrows)* but is clearly evident in the externally rotated oblique projection (**C**, *open arrow*).

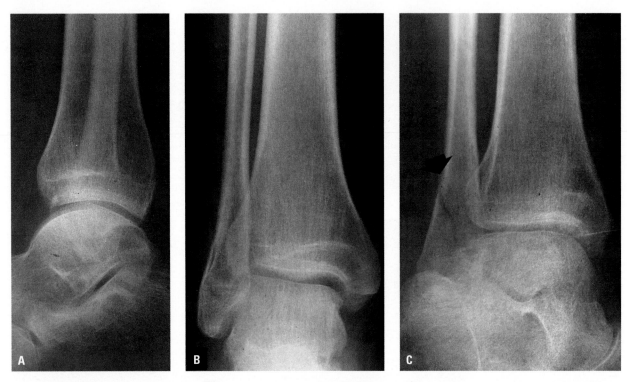

Figure 21.6. The minimally displaced fracture in the lateral malleolus (**C**, *arrow*) (eversion injury) is difficult to identify in the lateral (**A**) and frontal (**B**) projections and, consequently, could be overlooked. The fracture line is clearly perceptible in the internally rotated oblique projection (**C**).

same horizontal plane as the medial malleolus and both are parallel to the x-ray tabletop. The mortise view is the true AP projection of the ankle joint. Oblique projections,[1] plain radiograph tomography (Fig. 21.7), computed tomography (CT), or magnetic resonance imaging (MRI) may be required to identify minimally displaced ankle fractures.

RADIOGRAPHIC ANATOMY

The osseous and ligamentous anatomy of the ankle is described and illustrated earlier. It is important to remember that the ankle mortise is composed not only of the malleoli and horizontal plate of the distal articulating surface of the tibia plafond, but also of the very important ligamentous structures that are not visible on plain radiographs.

In the straight AP view of the ankle, the lateral malleolus, lying slightly posterior in the fibular notch of the lateral aspect of the distal end of the tibia, is superimposed on the lateral aspect of the body of the talus. In this projection, therefore, the talofibular joint space cannot be adequately evaluated. The need to visualize the talofibular space and to be able to

compare it with the talotibial medial space, to obtain an unobstructed view of the lateral margin of the talar trochlea dome, and to determine the relationship of the proximal talar articulating surface to the plafond have all prompted the routine use of the mortise view. In this projection, the lateral surface of the talar body and the cortex of the posterior margin of the fibular notch should normally be on approximately the same vertical plane (Fig. 21.4B). In the lateral projection (Fig. 21.4C), the concavity of the distal tibial articulating surface and the convexity of the talar trochlea are normally congruous.

The optimum lateral radiograph of the ankle results when the part is positioned so that the malleoli are directly superimposed on each other (Fig. 21.4C). This view should include the entire os calcis and the bones of the midfoot, including the base of the fifth metatarsal. Although neither the calcaneus nor the fifth metatarsal is a component of the ankle, each must be consciously studied for the presence of a fracture that may have been clinically interpreted as an injury to the ankle. For this reason, it is particularly important that the base of the fifth metatarsal be included in all radiographic examinations of the ankle. Fracture of the base of the fifth

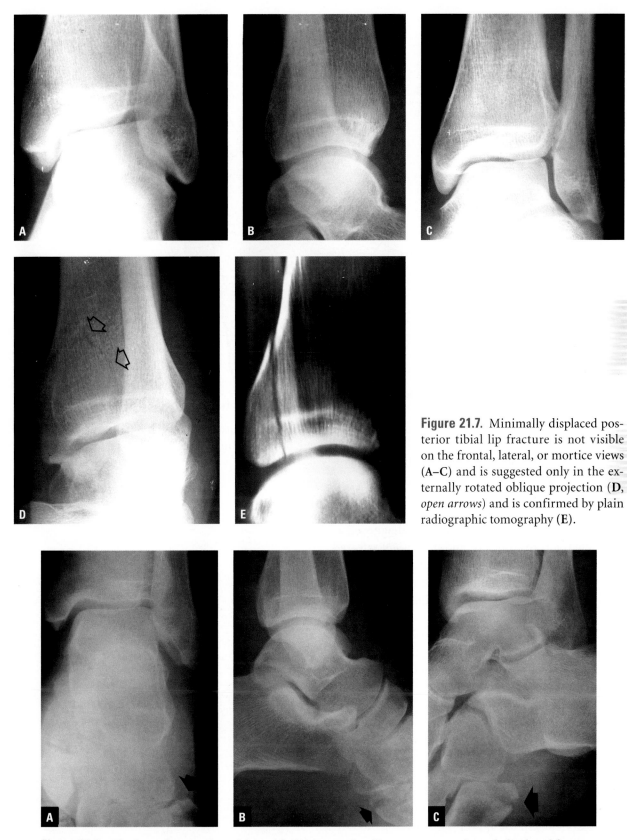

Figure 21.7. Minimally displaced posterior tibial lip fracture is not visible on the frontal, lateral, or mortice views (**A–C**) and is suggested only in the externally rotated oblique projection (**D**, *open arrows*) and is confirmed by plain radiographic tomography (**E**).

Figure 21.8. The frontal projection of the ankle (**A**) is negative. However, a comminuted, displaced fracture of the base of the fifth metatarsal *(arrow)* is visible at the edge of the radiograph. The fracture of the base of the fifth metatarsal *(arrow)* can be seen in the lateral projection of the ankle (**B**) but is seen to best advantage in the internally rotated oblique projection (**C**).

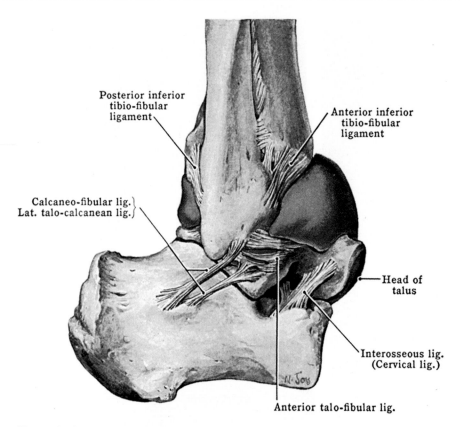

Figure 21.9. Note the anterior bulge of the distended capsule of the ankle joint. (From Anderson JE. *Grant's Atlas of Anatomy.* 6th ed. Baltimore, MD: Williams & Wilkins; 1972, used with permission.)

metatarsal (Fig. 21.8) is commonly misdiagnosed as an ankle fracture clinically, and the patient referred for radiographic examination of the ankle. In these circumstances, if the midfoot is not included on the ankle examination, the fifth metatarsal fracture could be missed.

The articular capsule of the ankle surrounds the joint. It is attached to the margin of the distal tibial articulating surface, the malleoli, and extends distally to attach onto the neck of the talus. Laterally, the capsule attaches on the fibula near the lateral malleolar fossa (Fig. 21.9).[2] Thus, posttraumatic distention of the ankle joint capsule, which may be visible on a properly exposed lateral ankle radiograph (Fig. 21.10), should be considered indicative of an intra-articular fracture of the distal tibia, the malleoli, or the talar body until specifically excluded by any of the appropriate imaging modalities, including MRI.

The radiographic appearance of the normal child's ankle is seen in Figure 21.11. The distal tibial epiphysis appears during the 2nd year of life and fuses in the

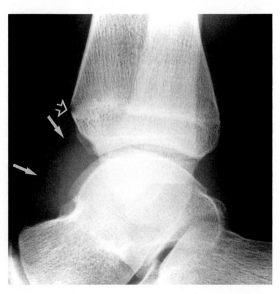

Figure 21.10. Distended ankle joint capsule *(solid arrows)* in an adolescent with a minimally displaced physeal injury *(open arrow)*.

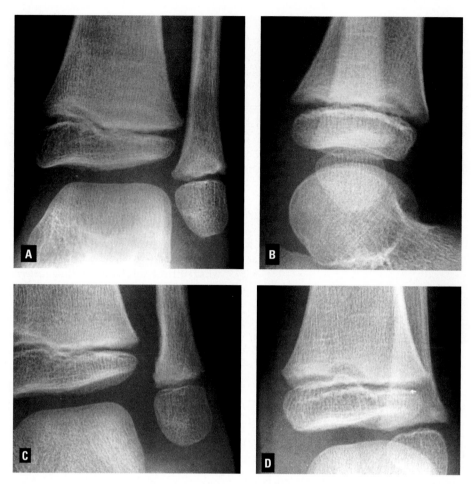

Figure 21.11. Radiographic appearance of the normal ankle of a 5-year-old boy in AP (**A**), lateral (**B**), and internally (**C**) and externally (**D**) rotated projections. The normal vagaries of the surfaces of the physes may simulate physeal injury or fracture. In that event, frontal and lateral radiographs of the opposite side should be obtained for comparison purposes.

18th year. The distal fibular epiphysis appears at age 2 and fuses at age 20. Infrequently, the tip of the medial malleolus arises from a separate ossification center. The radiographic characteristics of this apophysis, its relationship to the epiphysis, and its frequent bilaterality help distinguish this normal variant from an avulsion fracture fragment (Fig. 21.12).

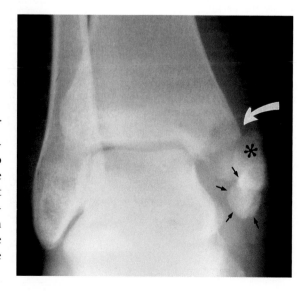

Figure 21.12. This patient sustained a comminuted fracture *(curved arrow)* of the medial malleolus secondary to direct blunt trauma. The smoothly corticated round ossicle *(small arrows)* distal to the large distal malleolar fragment *(asterisk)* represents an ununited secondary ossification center of the medial malleolar styloid process. The difference in its radiographic characteristics compared with those of the more proximal fracture fragments distinguishes it from the fracture fragments.

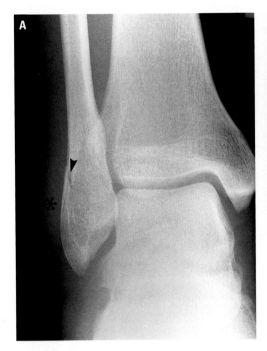

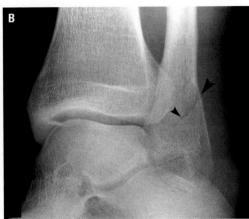

Figure 21.13. Eversion injury of the right ankle in which diffuse soft tissue swelling *(asterisk)* along the lateral aspect of the ankle (**A**) is the most obvious radiologic sign of the minimally displaced oblique fracture of the lateral malleolus *(arrowheads)*, seen best in the oblique radiograph (**B**).

RADIOGRAPHIC MANIFESTATIONS OF TRAUMA

Extracapsular soft tissue swelling about the ankle joint is discernible in a properly exposed radiograph. Although this is a nonspecific finding and is frequently present without associated skeletal trauma, it may signal a subtle fracture (Fig. 21.13). The radiographic distinction between extra-articular soft tissue swelling and joint capsular distention and its significant posttrauma is shown in Figure 21.14.

Physeal Injuries

Epiphyseal–physeal injuries, which commonly involve the ankle, are designated according to the Salter-Harris classification (Table 21.1).[3,4] The distal tibial

Figure 21.14. **A:** In the lateral projection, the *closed arrows* indicate the anterior bulge of the distended joint capsule, and the *asterisks* indicate the extracapsular soft tissue swelling. **B:** In the frontal projection, there is minor separation of the lateral portion of the distal tibial physis, and the *open arrow* indicates the subtle Salter-Harris III distal tibial epiphyseal–physeal injury.

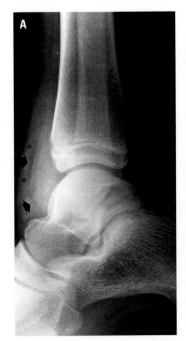

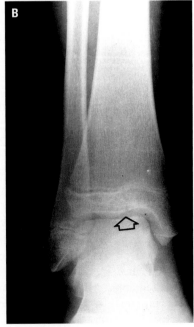

TABLE 21.1	Salter-Harris Classification of Physeal Injuries

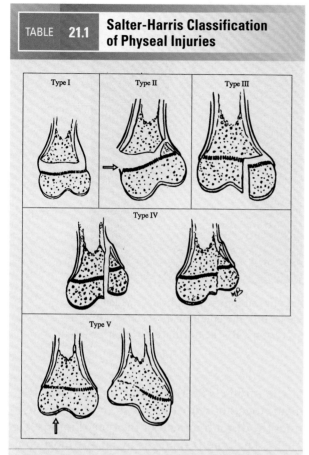

From Rang M. The growth plate and its diseases. In: Rockwood CA Jr, Wilkins KE, King RE, eds. Fractures in Children. 3rd ed. Philadelphia, PA: Lippincott–Raven Publishers; 1991:128, with permission.

epiphysis is the single most common site of physeal injury.[5] Types III and IV occur more commonly at the ankle than at any other site.

Type I epiphyseal injury, which occurs most commonly in young children, was originally described by Salter as being an epiphyseal separation without a metaphyseal or epiphyseal fracture. Typically, the momentarily separated epiphysis returns to an anatomic or type position with respect to the adjacent metaphysis by the intact periosteum. For this reason, the type I physeal injury is difficult to recognize radiographically. The most striking radiographic sign of type I injury is soft tissue swelling adjacent to the physis and minor uniform or eccentric widening of the physis itself (Figs. 21.15 and 21.16). In displaced type I physeal injuries, the periosteum is attenuated or disrupted, permitting epiphyseal displacement. The periosteum is usually disrupted on the convex side while remaining intact on the concave side of the epiphyseal displacement. Occasionally, a tiny fragment of bone is pulled off the margin of the metaphyseal or epiphyseal surface of the physis. The presence of such a fragment, usually situated in the lateral aspect of the physis between the metaphyseal and epiphyseal surfaces, together with widening of the physis and adjacent soft tissue swelling, establishes a type I physeal injury (Fig. 21.17). This tiny avulsion fracture fragment, although not included in the original Salter-Harris classification, is very commonly visible and is very helpful in the

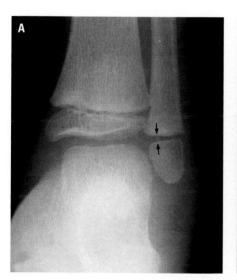

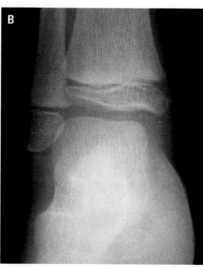

Figure 21.15. A: Salter-Harris type I physeal injury of the distal left fibula. As defined, the distal fibular metaphysis and epiphysis are intact. The injury is recognized by the soft tissue swelling lateral to the lateral malleolus and the lack of parallelism of the metaphyseal and epiphyseal margins of the physis (e.g., medial widening of the distal fibular physis) (arrows). B: Normal right ankle for comparison. Note that the metaphyseal and epiphyseal margins of the physis of the normal ankle are congruous.

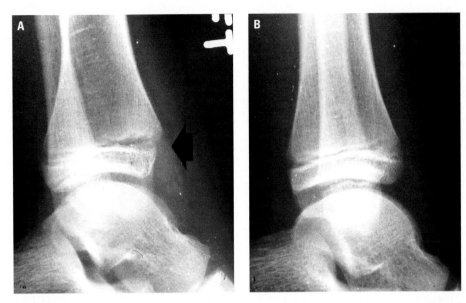

Figure 21.16. A: Salter-Harris type I distal tibial physeal injury. The physis is widened anteriorly and narrowed posteriorly, and consequently the epiphysis is eccentrically situated with respect to the adjacent metaphysis *(arrow).* **B:** The normal side has been reversed for ease of comparison.

radiologic identification of the type I physeal injury. The tiny separate fragment has none of the characteristics of the metaphyseal component of the type II physeal injury. Consequently, it seems reasonable to include this type of avulsion fracture as a variant of the type I injury.

Type II physeal injury consists of an oblique fracture extending through the metaphysis into the physis with separation through the remainder of the physis. The triangular metaphyseal fragment, together with the intact epiphysis, constitutes the distal fragment of the type II injury (Fig. 21.18). The type II injury is by far the most common of the physeal injuries and usually occurs in older children. The prognosis for normal growth is excellent. Type II injuries of the ankle are usually obvious radiographically but may be subtle and not discernible on all ankle views (Fig. 21.19).

Figure 21.17. A: Salter-Harris type I distal fibular physeal injury on the left. The physis is widened laterally, and a tiny fracture fragment *(open arrow)* has been pulled from the lateral margin of the physis. Diffuse soft tissue swelling *(asterisks)* is present about the lateral malleolus. **B:** Normal right ankle for comparison.

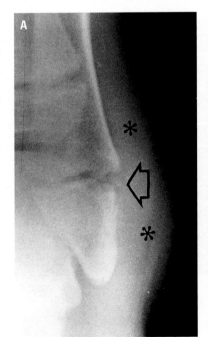
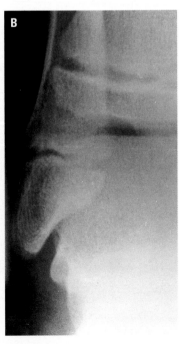

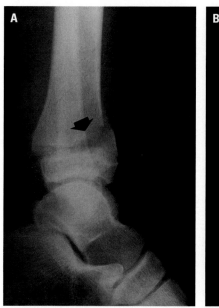
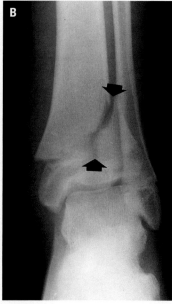

Figure 21.18. Salter-Harris type II distal tibial physeal injury. *Arrows* indicate the metaphyseal fracture in both lateral (**A**) and AP (**B**) projections. Note that the resultant triangular metaphyseal fragment is normally related to the epiphysis. The epiphysis, together with the triangular metaphyseal fragment, has been separated medially and posteriorly and is displaced anteriorly and laterally relative to the remainder of the metaphysis.

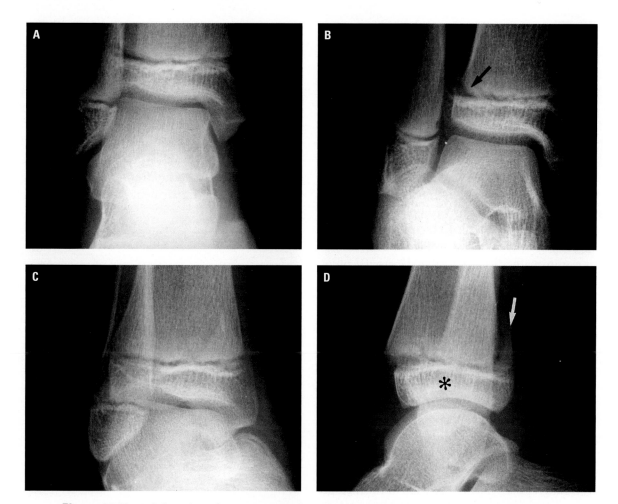

Figure 21.19. Subtle Salter-Harris type II physeal injury of the distal tibia not visible in the frontal (**A**) projection is evidenced only by the minor disruption of the lateral aspect of the tibial metaphysis *(arrow)* in the mortise view (**B**). This diagnosis is established only in the lateral radiograph (**C**), where posterior displacement of the epiphysis *(asterisk)* and attached posterior metaphyseal fragment *(arrow)* is clearly evident (**D**).

Figure 21.20. Salter-Harris type II distal tibial injury associated with a distal third fibular fracture in an eversion injury of the ankle. The metaphyseal component *(arrowhead)* is evident in both frontal **(A)** and lateral **(B)** projections.

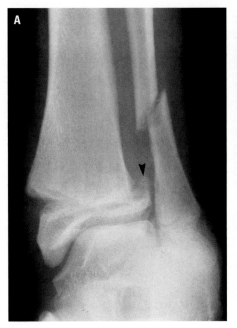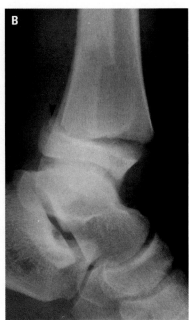

Physeal injuries are limited to a single bone but may also be associated with a fracture (Fig. 21.20) or physeal injury of an adjacent bone.

Type III injury is uncommon, is usually seen in the distal tibial epiphysis, and is entirely intracapsular. The prognosis of normal growth is good, provided the blood supply to the separated portion of the epiphysis has not been disrupted. Radiographically, the injury consists of a vertical fracture line that extends perpendicularly through the epiphysis from its articulating surface to the physis and then along the physis to its margin. Figure 21.21 illustrates a minimally displaced Salter-Harris III physeal injury in a very young child.

The biplane fracture of Tillaux[6] (Fig. 21.22) is a variant of the type III injury of the distal tibial epiphysis. The vertical epiphyseal fracture, situated in the lateral aspect of the epiphysis, occurs in older children in whom fusion of the medial portion of the distal tibial physis is more advanced than the lateral (Fig. 21.23). The mechanism of injury has been described as eversion or external rotation. The epiphyseal injury is an avulsion fracture produced by the intact anterior and posterior tibiofibular ligaments. The age of the patient usually 12 to 14 years, radiographic evidence of fusion of the medial portion of the distal tibial physis, and lateral displacement of the epiphyseal fragment distinguishes the biplane fracture of Tillaux (Fig. 21.24) from the typical type III injury of the distal tibial epiphysis.

The type IV and the rare type V physeal injuries differ in two significant aspects from the other Salter-Harris injuries, in that each is caused by a compressive rather than a shearing or rotational force and each has a high propensity for growth arrest secondary to premature or uneven physeal fusion. In both type IV and type V injuries, premature physeal closure may result from physical crushing of the physeal cells, impairment of their blood supply,

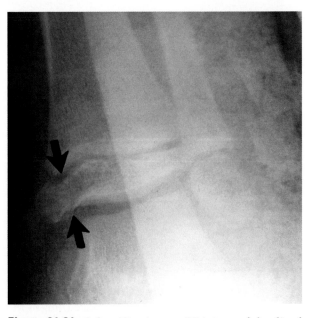

Figure 21.21. Salter-Harris type III injury of the distal tibial epiphysis *(arrows)* of an infant.

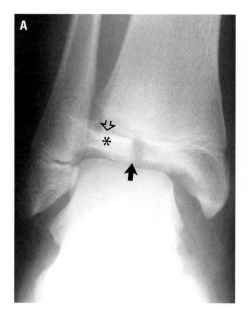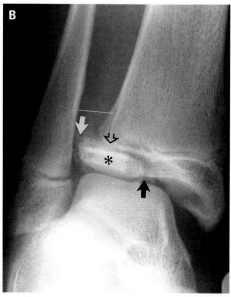

Figure 21.22. Classic biplanar fracture of Tillaux. In both the AP (**A**) and mortise (**B**) views, the vertical fracture of the epiphysis *(black arrow)* involves the junction of its lateral and middle thirds. The lateral aspect of the physis is disrupted *(open arrow)*, and the separate epiphyseal fragment *(asterisk)* is avulsed laterally by the intact tibiofibular ligaments. The normal relationship between the laterally displaced fibula and epiphyseal fragment (**B**, *white arrow*) indicates that the tibiofibular ligaments are intact, while more proximally, the interosseous membrane can be reasonably assumed to be disrupted because of the distance between the fibular metaphysis and the superior portion of the fibular groove (**B**, *white line*).

or damage to the metaphysis and epiphysis with the resultant formation.[7] Additionally, peculiar to the type IV injury is growth arrest secondary to fusion of the epiphyseal component of the separate fragment to the metaphysis of the major fragment. This is described in more detail later.

Type IV injury consists of a vertical fracture extending through the entire thickness of the medial third of the distal tibial epiphysis, across the physis, and continuing vertically through the metaphysis to exit through the medial metaphyseal cortex (Fig. 21.25). The entire separate fragment, therefore, includes the

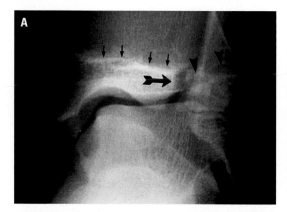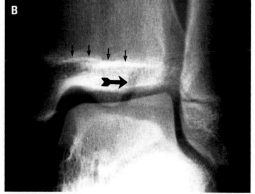

Figure 21.23. Biplane fracture of Tillaux in AP (**A**) and mortise (**B**) projections. The medial two-thirds of the distal tibial physis is fused *(small arrows)*. A vertical fracture *(large arrow)* is present in the lateral third of the epiphysis, and the physeal separation clearly extends to its lateral margin *(arrowheads)*.

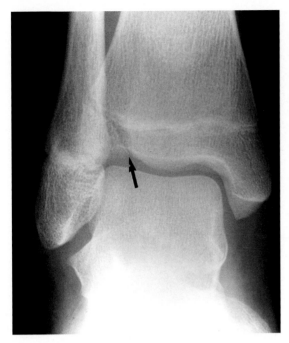

Figure 21.24. Minimally displaced biplanar fracture of Tillaux *(arrow)*.

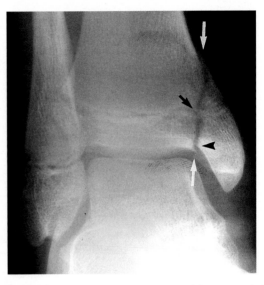

Figure 21.25. Salter-Harris IV physeal injury *(white arrows)*. Even the minimal superior displacement of the separate fragment *(arrowhead)* will permit the malleolar epiphyseal component to fuse with the distal tibial metaphysis *(black arrow)*, resulting in arrested bone growth. In this patient, it is impossible to exclude a concomitant Salter-Harris V injury of the distal tibial physis or a Salter-Harris I of the distal fibular physis.

medial malleolus with variable amounts of the medial portion of the plafond, the physis, and the metaphysis as a single unit. The mechanism of injury is primarily axial-loading vertical compression and inversion of the foot, causing the talus to impact against the medial malleolus. Continued inversion and/or vertical compression causes proximal displacement of the separate fragment (Fig. 21.26). The vertical compression component invariably results in a Salter-Harris type V injury of the physis itself. If the separate fragment remains proximally displaced and assuming there is no other distal tibial physeal injury, growth arrest will occur as the result of the epiphyseal component fusing with the metaphysis of the major fragment (Fig. 21.26B,C). "Perfect" open reduction and internal fixation[7,8] offers the best chance of healing without growth arrest. However, as mentioned earlier and as seen in the patient represented in Figure 21.26, a crushing injury Salter-Harris type V concurrently involving the distal tibial physis will contribute in large measure to the premature closure of the distal tibial physis.

The "triplanar" fracture[5,9,10] is a variant of the Salter-Harris type IV injury[7] in that it includes a fracture of the epiphysis, separation of a portion of the physis, and a fracture through the distal tibial metaphysis, as does the type IV injury. The triplanar fracture differs

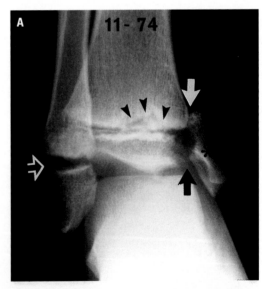

Figure 21.26. Concurrent type IV *(closed arrows)* and type V *(arrowheads)* distal tibial physeal and type I *(open arrow)* distal fibular physeal injuries, acutely **(A)** and over the ensuing 28 months **(B,C)**. **A:** On the initial AP radiograph, the type IV fragment *(asterisk)* is proximally displaced. Buckling, irregularity, and sclerosis, particularly of the metaphyseal surface of the distal tibial physis *(arrowheads)*, indicate the type V injury. *(continued)*

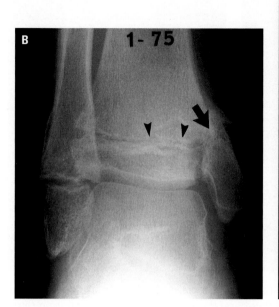
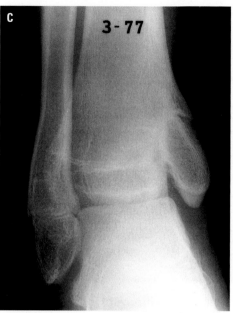

Figure 21.26. *(continued)* **B:** Within 2 months of the acute injury, the proximal portion of the medial malleolar epiphysis had fused with the metaphysis *(arrow)* of the major fragment, and signs of premature closure *(arrowheads)* of the remainder of the distal tibial physis are evident. **C:** At 28 months postinjury, the effects of distal tibial growth arrest and continued normal fibular growth are obvious.

from the type IV in that the triplanar injury occurs in three planes, whereas the type IV occurs in only one. The sites of disruption of the triplanar fracture occur in the sagittal plane epiphysis, the axial plane physis, and the coronal plane metaphysis. Triplanar fractures may occur in a two-part variety, in which all the components of the separate fragment exist as an intact unit (Fig. 21.27), or in a three-part configuration (Fig. 21.28),[5] in which the epiphyseal component is a separate fragment (e.g., the third part) (Fig. 21.29).

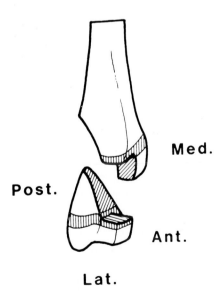

Figure 21.27. Schematic representation of a two-part triplanar fracture of the distal tibia. (From MacNealy GA, Rogers LF, Hernandez R, et al. Injuries of the distal tibial epiphysis. Systematic radiographic evaluation. *Am J Roentgenol.* 1982;138:683–689, with permission.)

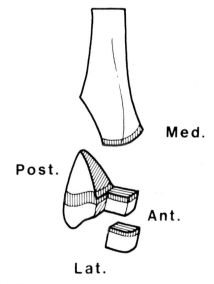

Figure 21.28. Schematic representation of a three-part triplanar fracture of the distal tibia. (From MacNealy GA, Rogers LF, Hernandez R, et al. Injuries of the distal tibial piphysis. Systematic radiographic evaluation. *Am J Roentgenol.* 1982;138:683–689, with permission.)

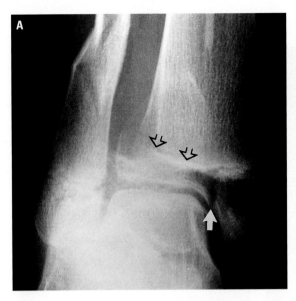
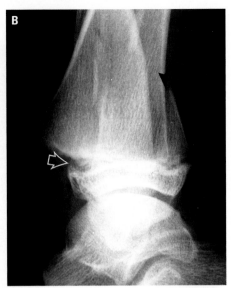

Figure 21.29. Three-part "triplanar" fracture of the distal tibia. **A:** In the frontal projection, the sagittal plane fracture *(closed arrow)* of the epiphysis and the axial plane physeal separation *(open arrows)* are visible. **B:** The lateral projection demonstrates the axial physeal separation *(arrow)* and the coronal plane metaphyseal fracture *(arrowhead)*. Note that the separated metaphyseal fragment retains its normal relationship to the distal tibial epiphysis through the intact physis.

Type V injury is a crushing axial-loading injury to the physis, most commonly the result of a fall from a height, and most commonly involves the distal tibial physis and the major physes of the knee. All reports of Salter-Harris injuries describe the type V injury as rare, probably because it is usually not identifiable in the initial posttrauma radiograph. The epiphyseal–metaphyseal relationship is normal, and there is no visible fracture. Rarely, signs of physeal crush may be evident radiographically (Fig. 21.26), but in the majority of instances, the diagnosis is only made on subsequent radiographs that demonstrate signs of growth arrest, the etiologies of which have been previously described.

Fractures

Many classifications of ankle fractures have been proposed. Of these, the Lauge-Hansen classification,[11] the Weber classification,[12] and that popularized by Edeiken and Cotler[13] are most commonly used today. In the United States, the Lauge-Hansen classification is most commonly used by orthopedic surgeons, whereas the Weber classification is most popular in Europe. The Lauge-Hansen classification has the disadvantage of being alphanumeric with terms describing ankle movements that are not part of the lexicon of most radiologists or emergency

physicians. Lucid explanations of the Lauge-Hansen system may be found in *Orthopedic Radiology* by Weissman and Sledge,[14] and in an article in *Emergency Radiology* by Wilson.[15]

The ankle joint is injured more frequently than most joints and is responsible for a significant percentage of visits to the emergency department. Although the majority of injuries are minor and purely ligamentous, many injuries include complete ligament ruptures and/or fractures, resulting in ankle instability. These patterns of injury follow predictable courses and can be readily identified by careful evaluation of the radiographs.

Before considering the injury patterns, it is best to review the normal ankle joint anatomy. This is a hinge joint comprising six major components: three ligament groups and three bones. The normal relationship between these structures provides for stability and a normal range of motion. The superior and medial articulations of the ankle joint are provided by the tibia through a horizontal surface, the plafond, and a vertical surface, the medial malleolus. The medial malleolus has two distal processes: the anterior and posterior colliculi that can be readily identified on frontal and lateral radiographs (Fig. 21.30). The more vertical anterior colliculus extends farther distal than the more horizontal posterior colliculus. Above the plafond is a groove in the lateral aspect of the distal

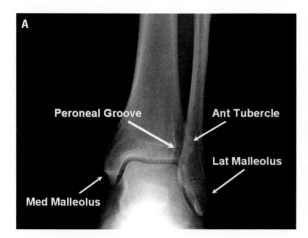

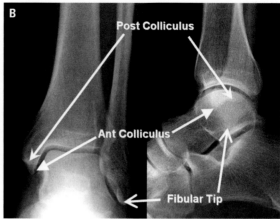

Figure 21.30. A: Mortise view of the ankle showing four important landmarks. **B:** Mortise and lateral views with additional landmarks cross-referenced between the two views.

tibia, known as the peroneal groove. The lips of the groove are known as the anterior and posterior tubercles. The larger anterior tubercle can be seen overlapping the fibula on frontal radiographs (Fig. 21.30). The distal fibula fits into the peroneal groove and extends distal to the plafond as the lateral malleolus. The medial surface of the lateral malleolus provides the lateral articular surface of the ankle mortise. The fibula is held firmly to the tibia by the ligaments of the tibiofibular syndesmosis, in and around the peroneal groove. The dome or trochlea of the talus lies between the articular surfaces of the two malleoli. The talus and ankle mortise lie in a slightly oblique sagittal plane. This means the mortise will be best profiled by a shallow (10 to 15 degrees) internal oblique view. This view not only profiles the articular cartilage between talus and medial malleolus but also profiles the floor of the peroneal groove and the medial cortex of the adjacent fibula. The apparent space between the talus and the medial malleolus has been dubbed the medial clear space, and the apparent space between the fibula and peroneal groove is known as the lateral clear space (Fig. 21.30). These apparent spaces should not measure more than 4 or 5.5 mm, respectively. Any widening of these spaces will be due to lateral shift of the talus and implies ankle instability.

The three bones of the ankle joint are held together by the lateral collateral ligaments, the medial collateral ligaments (MCLs), and the distal tibiofibular syndesmosis (Fig. 21.31). Each of these contains more than one component. The lateral collateral ligament complex comprises the anterior and posterior talofibular ligaments and the calcaneofibular ligament. The MCL complex is also known as the deltoid ligament.

It comprises deep and superficial portions. The deep fibers are much stronger and run from the medial malleolus to the talus. The weaker superficial fibers fan out and insert onto the navicular, the talus, and the sustentaculum tali of the calcaneus. The tibiofibular syndesmosis comprises anterior and posterior tibiofibular ligaments, an inferiorly located transverse ligament, and an interosseous ligament. Located just above the syndesmosis is the interosseous membrane that holds the tibia and fibula together, extending proximally, almost to the fibular neck. In order to more easily understand the mechanisms of injury, a simplified version of the anatomy is helpful. The anterior and posterior tibiofibular ligaments can

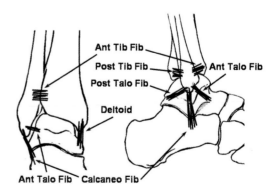

Figure 21.31. The three bones of the ankle joint are held together by ligaments arranged circumferentially around the joint. The medial collateral or deltoid ligament provides medial support. The anterior tibiofibular ligament provides anterior support. The posterior tibiofibular ligament provides posterior support. The lateral support is provided by three separate ligaments: anterior talofibular, calcaneofibular, and posterior talofibular.

TABLE	21.2	Danis-Weber Classification
Type A		Fibular fracture below syndesmosis
	A1	Isolated
	A2	With medial malleolar fracture
	A3	With posteromedial tibial fracture
Type B		Fibular fracture at or crossing the syndesmosis
	B1	Isolated
	B2	With medial injury (malleolus or ligament)
	B3	With medial injury and posterolateral tibial fracture
Type C		Fibular fracture completely above the syndesmosis
	C1	Diaphyseal fibular fracture
	C2	Complex diaphyseal fracture
	C3	Proximal fibular fracture

injury is the presence or absence of stability. This usually determines if surgery is necessary or not.

Two different classification systems are in popular use for ankle fractures. These are the Danis-Weber classification (Table 21.2) and the Lauge-Hansen classification (Table 21.3). The former was developed by orthopedic surgeons, is very helpful in surgical

TABLE	21.3	Lauge-Hansen Classification
	Supination - Adduction	
1		Transverse lateral malleolar fracture OR
2		Lateral malleolar tip avulsion OR Lateral collateral ligament rupture
	Supination - External Rotation	
1		Anterior tibiofibular ligament rupture
2		Spiral lateral malleolar fracture
3		Posterior tibiofibular ligament rupture OR Posterior malleolar fracture
4		Deltoid ligament rupture OR Medial malleolar fracture
	Pronation - Abduction	
1		Medial malleolar fracture OR Deltoid ligament rupture
2		Tibiofibular syndesmosis rupture OR Avulsion fractures at tibiofibular syndesmosis
3		Oblique, "bending" fibular fracture immediately above syndesmosis
	Pronation - External Rotation	
1		Medial malleolar fracture OR Deltoid ligament rupture
2		Anterior tibiofibular ligament rupture
3		Short oblique diaphyseal fibular fracture
4		Posterior tibiofibular ligament rupture OR Posterior malleolar fracture

be considered as anterior and posterior support struts between the bones (ignoring the other two ligaments of the syndesmosis). The medial and lateral ligament complexes can then be considered as units, providing medial and lateral support struts, respectively. Using this simple model, the fibrosseous ring of the ankle mortise has anterior, medial, posterior, and lateral support struts holding the three bones together. These support struts provide stability in all directions, in a horizontal plane.

The ankle is a hinge joint and allows normal motion in a single plane only. Any attempts to move the ankle in other planes are strongly resisted by the three bones and three groups of ligaments described in the preceding paragraph. The only normal ankle movements are plantar flexion and dorsiflexion. If excessive force is applied in an attempt to either twist (externally or internally rotate) or tilt (adduct or abduct) the talus within the mortise, ligamentous and/or bony injuries will occur. If application of the force persists after one bony or ligamentous component fails, stress will be transferred elsewhere and additional structures may fail. These failures occur in predictable sequences and the characteristic patterns can be identified on the radiographs. For this reason, a basic understanding of the various injury mechanisms and their sequence of events is very valuable for accurate ankle radiographic interpretation. The single most important feature of an ankle planning, and classifies injuries by the location of a fibular fracture (Fig. 21.32). The latter evaluates the mechanism of injury, catalogs the sequence of events, and is very helpful in accurate interpretation of the radiographs.

The Lauge-Hansen classification was developed by a Danish radiologist, after many years of careful study of the mechanisms, and presented by the original author in multiple publications over several years. Four mechanisms were initially described (Table 21.3) (Fig. 21.33). A fifth mechanism (pronation–dorsiflexion) was added later to cover vertical loading injuries. These injuries, commonly referred to as pilon fractures, are very different to the other four ankle mortise injuries and will be discussed separately.

The mechanisms and sequence of events of the four Lauge-Hansen injuries are straightforward. If these are understood, ligament injuries can be predicted from the characteristics of the fractures and the presence or absence of talar shift. The key to this understanding is the fibular fracture (Figs. 21.34 to 21.44). There are four different types of fibular fracture and each is unique to a specific mechanism (Table 21.4). Without a fibular fracture, the mechanism is not always clear. The injuries occur in a predictable sequence, dependent on the position of the foot at the time of injury (pronation or supination) and the direction of the applied force

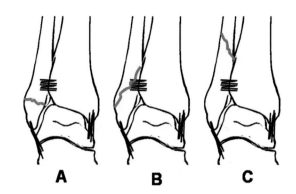

Figure 21.32. Danis-Weber classification. This system classifies an ankle injury by its location relative to the tibiofibular syndesmosis. **A,** completely below; **B,** at or crossing; and **C,** completely above the syndesmosis.

(abduction, adduction, or external rotation). The stages of each mechanism occur in order but the injury does not always progress to the final stage. When lesser force is applied, the injury may stop at stage 1 or 2. Most of these incomplete injuries will result in a stable mortise. To understand the mechanisms, it is best to think about the force applied to the lateral malleolus (push or pull, with or without a twist). When there is a straight downward pull on the malleolus (supination–adduction), the result is a transverse malleolar fracture or a lateral

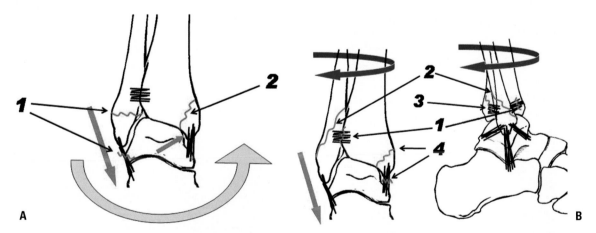

Figure 21.33. Lauge-Hansen classification. **A:** Supination–adduction mechanism. The *large curved arrow* shows the direction of motion. The *large straight arrow* denotes tensions in the adjacent ligaments. *Stage 1* is either a transverse fracture of the lateral malleolus or a lateral collateral ligament rupture. *Stage 2* is a near-vertical fracture of the tibia at the junction of the plafond and the medial malleolus. **B:** Supination–external rotation mechanism. The *large curved arrows* show the direction of rotation. The *large straight arrow* denotes tensions in the adjacent ligaments. *Stage 1* is a rupture of the anterior tibiofibular ligament. *Stage 2* is a spiral lateral malleolar fracture. *Stage 3* is a posterior malleolar fracture or posterior tibiofibular ligament rupture. *Stage 4* is a medial malleolar fracture or deltoid ligament rupture. *(continued)*

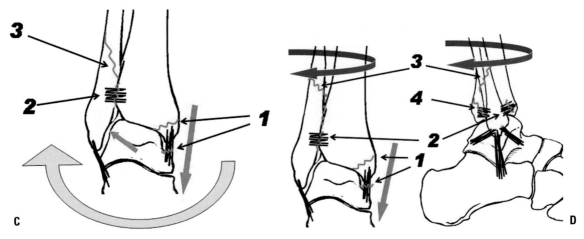

Figure 21.33. *(continued)* **C:** Pronation–abduction mechanism. The *large curved arrow* shows the direction of motion. The *large straight arrow* denotes tensions in the adjacent ligaments. *Stage 1* is a fracture of the medial malleolus or a rupture of the medial collateral ligaments. *Stage 2* is rupture of the tibiofibular syndesmosis. *Stage 3* is a fibular fracture immediately above the syndesmosis, with a bone spike that points to the proximal peroneal groove (the "bending fracture"). **D:** Pronation–external rotation mechanism. The *large curved arrows* show the direction of rotation. The *large straight arrow* denotes tensions in the adjacent ligaments. *Stage 1* is a medial collateral ligament rupture or medial malleolar fracture. *Stage 2* is an anterior tibiofibular ligament rupture. *Stage 3* is a tear through the interosseous membrane and a short oblique fibular shaft fracture, most commonly 1 to 2 inches above the peroneal groove. *Stage 4* is a posterior malleolar fracture or posterior tibiofibular ligament rupture.

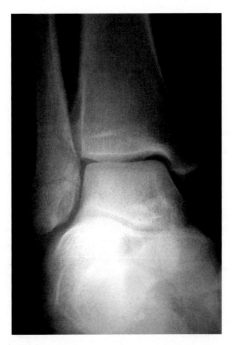

Figure 21.34. Stage 1: Supination–adduction injury. The characteristic transverse, lateral malleolar fracture is nondisplaced and there is no tibial fracture. This injury is stable.

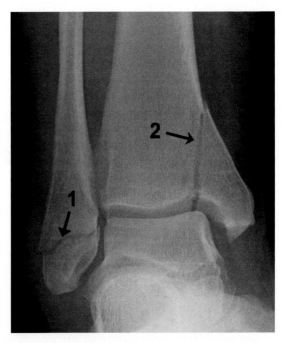

Figure 21.35. Stage 2: Supination–adduction injury. Although the transverse lateral malleolar *(stage 1)* and vertical tibial *(stage 2)* fractures are minimally displaced, this injury is unstable.

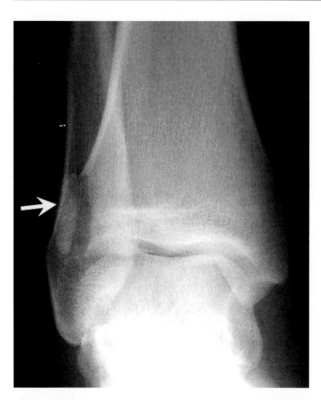

Figure 21.36. Stage 1: Supination–external rotation injury. There is a slightly displaced fracture of the anterior tibial tubercle *(arrow)* but no other injury. This injury is stable.

ligament complex tear (Figs. 21.33 to 21.35). When that pull is combined with a twist (supination–external rotation), a spiral lateral malleolar fracture is the usual result (Figs. 21.33, 21.36 to 21.40). When the force pushes straight upward of the lateral malleolus (pronation-abduction), the result is a fracture immediately above the syndesmosis. This has been referred to in the literature as the "bending" fracture. The bending fracture can be identified by a characteristic bone spike that points to the superior aspect of the syndesmosis (as marked on the frontal radiographs by the peroneal groove) (Figs. 21.33 and 21.41). When a push on the lateral malleolus is combined with a twist (pronation-external rotation), there will usually be a tear through the interosseous membrane, extending proximally. This tear usually terminates with a short oblique fracture of the fibular shaft. This shaft fracture is most commonly 1 to 2 inches above the peroneal groove (Figs. 21.33, 21.41, 21.42, and 21.44). Infrequently, the interosseous membrane tear extends all the way to the fibular neck, resulting in a fracture at that level. This complex is known as a *Maisonneuve fracture.* This fibular fracture will not be visible on the standard ankle radiographs, necessitating radiographs of the full length of the tibia and fibula (Fig. 21.43). Whenever there is evidence of talar shift and a fibular fracture

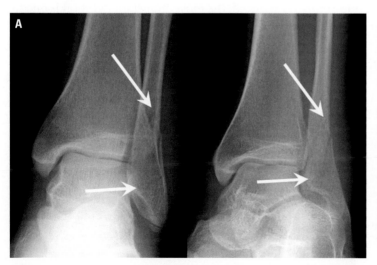
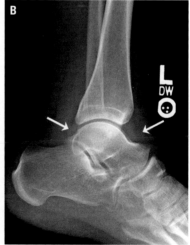

Figure 21.37. Stage 2: Supination–external rotation injury. **A:** The upper and lower extents of the characteristic spiral lateral malleolar fracture are marked with *arrows* on the mortise and AP views. There is a small unrelated ossicle at the tip of the lateral malleolus. **B:** The lateral view shows a joint effusion *(arrows)* but no posterior malleolar injury. This is a stable injury as there is no posterior or medial injury.

Figure 21.38. Stage 4: Supination–external rotation injury. *Arrows* mark the characteristic spiral lateral malleolar fracture plus fractures of the medial and posterior malleoli. This injury is unstable, as confirmed by the lateral talar shift.

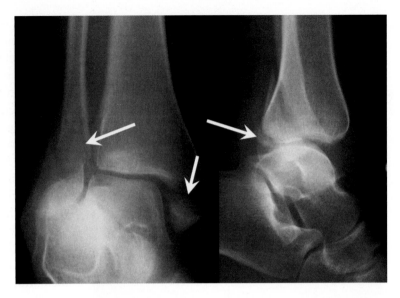

cannot be seen, the Maisonneuve complex should be suspected and the full-length images obtained.

The need to accurately identify ligament injuries cannot be overstated. An ankle that has either bony or ligamentous disruption on one side only is usually stable. An ankle with injuries on both the medial and lateral sides will usually be unstable. Although stable injuries respond well to conservative management, most unstable injuries will require surgical repair. Adequate quality radiographs obtained out of plaster are essential for reliable evaluation. The minimum series should include AP, lateral, and 15-degree oblique (mortise) views (Fig. 21.30). The observer should try

to answer the following questions: Is there a talar shift? What is the nature of the fibular fracture (if present)? Are there other fractures that do not fit into the four Lauge-Hansen patterns? Forty percent of ankles with a major fracture or ligament injury on one side have been reported to have an injury on the opposite side. If there is clinical or radiologic suspicion of injury on both sides of the ankle but no talar shift is evident, a second mortise view should be performed with eversion stress to confirm or exclude instability.

After an unstable ankle mortise injury has been reduced, the most important question is once again: Is there a talar shift? This should be assessed on both

Figure 21.39. Stage 4: Supination–external rotation injury. In this case, there is a small avulsion fracture at the tip of the medial malleolus *(arrowhead)* and a very large posterior malleolar fracture *(arrow)*, as well as the characteristic spiral lateral malleolar fracture. Because of the large posterior tibial fracture fragment, this injury will be unstable anteroposteriorly as well as mediolaterally. The large posterior fragment will need additional fixation at surgery.

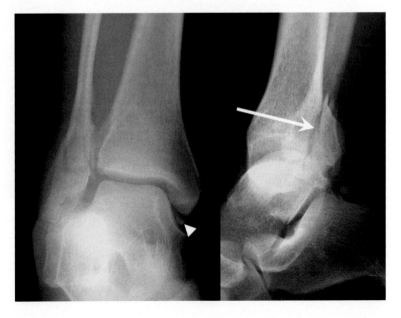

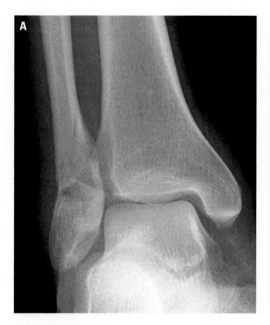
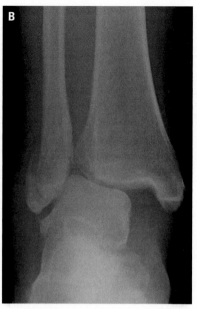

Figure 21.40. Stage 4: Supination–external rotation injury. **A:** The static mortise view reveals a spiral lateral malleolar fracture without talar shift. **B:** A second mortise view with abduction stress was performed because of medial swelling and tenderness. It shows talar shift, confirming a medial collateral ligament rupture and resultant instability.

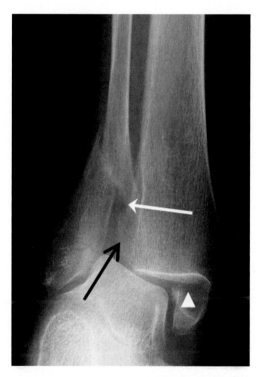

Figure 21.41. Stage 3: Pronation–abduction injury. The characteristic "bending fracture" of the fibula (stage 3) has a spike of bone *(white arrow)* pointing to the proximal portion of the peroneal groove. The syndesmosis is ruptured (stage 2) and widened *(black arrow)* and there is a displaced medial malleolar fracture (stage 1, *arrowhead*). This injury is unstable, with marked lateral talar shift.

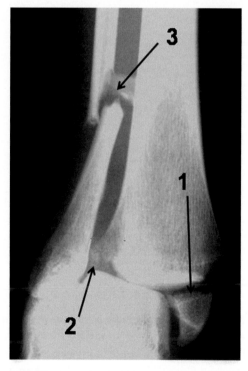

Figure 21.42. Stage 4: Pronation–external rotation injury. There is a medial malleolar fracture (stage 1), an avulsion fracture of the anterior tibial tubercle (stage 2), and a slightly comminuted oblique fracture of the fibular shaft a few inches above the peroneal groove (stage 3). The posterior injury (stage 4) was ligamentous and not visible on the lateral radiograph. This is another unstable injury, with marked lateral talar shift.

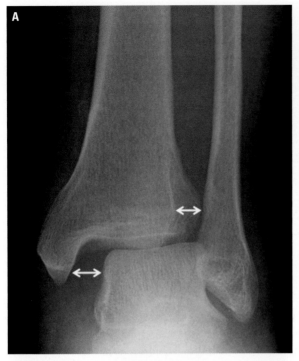

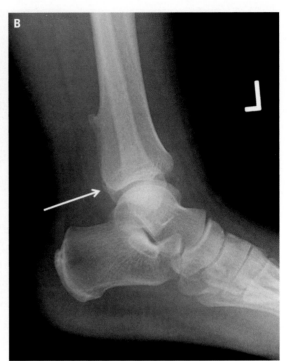

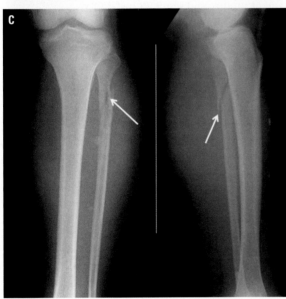

Figure 21.43. Stage 4: Pronation–external rotation injury. **A:** The mortise view shows marked lateral talar shift with widening of the medial and lateral clear spaces *(arrows)* but no fractures. **B:** The lateral view shows a small avulsion fracture of the posterior malleolus. **C:** AP and lateral views of the leg reveal a high tibial fracture *(arrows)*. This is the Maisonneuve complex with rupture of the medial collateral ligament, tibiofibular syndesmosis, and almost the entire length of the interosseous membrane.

the mortise and lateral views. Residual shift implies inadequate reduction and persistent instability.

The description of ankle injuries advocated by Edeiken and Cotler[13] is a concept rather than a classification. The concept, based on the notion that the ankle can be considered as an osseous–ligamentous circle (Fig. 21.45), is easily understood, is practical, uses common terms, and leads to precisely the same understanding of the ligamentous pathophysiology of ankle injury as the more complex classifications.

Finally, being entirely descriptive, the Edeiken–Cotler concept is easily understood by those involved in the initial management of a patient with an acute ankle fracture.

For radiographic diagnostic purposes, a pragmatic yet valid and clinically useful concept is that the majority of ankle injuries occur as the result of the foot (talus) being forcibly displaced laterally (eversion), medially (inversion), or posteriorly with respect to the ankle mortise. In both eversion

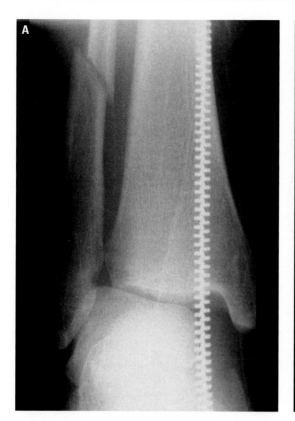 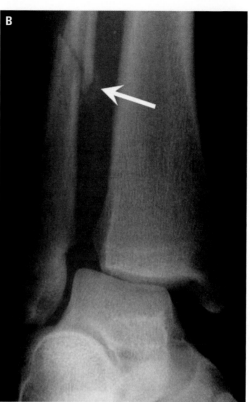

Figure 21.44. Mismanaged stage 4: Pronation–external rotation injury. **A:** The initial mortise radiograph revealed the characteristic fibular shaft fracture and lateral talar shift. Unfortunately, the treating physician did not realize how unstable this injury was and treated it conservatively, with casting alone. **B:** A follow-up radiograph obtained at 3 weeks showed increased lateral talar shift. Callus formation *(arrow)* at the fibular fracture showed healing was already well established, making the surgery more complicated and the prognosis less favorable.

and inversion injuries, one malleolus will receive an impaction force from the talus and the other malleolus will receive an avulsion force transmitted through the appropriate collateral ligament. Impaction fracture lines are characteristically obliquely oriented, whereas those caused by avulsion are typically horizontally oriented. For example, in an eversion injury, impaction of the talus on the lateral malleolus will result in an oblique fracture. The intact medial collateral deltoid ligament will cause an avulsion horizontal fracture of the medial malleolus or a cortical avulsion fracture of the medial aspect of the talus. In the example being described, if there is no medial malleolar or talar

TABLE 21.4	Fibular Fracture Types with Lauge-Hansen Mechanisms	
Mechanism	**Force on Fibula**	**Fibular Fracture**
Supination - Adduction	Straight pull	Transvere Lateral malleolar
Pronation - Abduction	Straight push	"Bending" fracture
Supination - External Rotation	Pull with twist	Spiral lateral malleolar
Pronation - External Rotation	Push with twist	Diaphyseal fracture

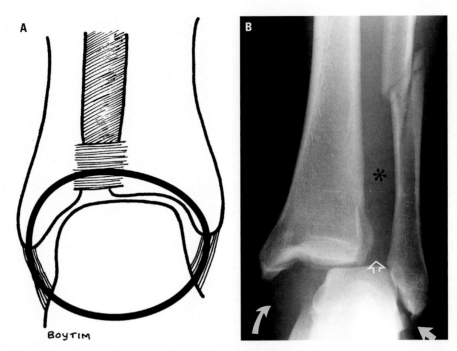

Figure 21.45. The concept of the bones and ligaments of the ankle constituting a circle from medial malleolus to medial collateral ligament, to talus, to lateral collateral ligament, to lateral malleolus, to distal tibiofibular ligaments, to the supraplafond portion of the talus, back to the medial malleolus is shown schematically (**A**) and radiographically (**B**). In the eversion injury (**B**), because of lateral displacement of the talus, the lateral collateral ligament *(straight arrow)* is compressed and remains intact; the distal tibiofibular ligaments *(open arrow)* are disrupted, as is the interosseous membrane *(asterisk)* to the level of the fibular fracture; and, in the absence of a medial malleolar or talar fracture, the medial collateral (deltoid) ligament *(curved arrow)* is torn.

fracture, it can reasonably be assumed that the MCL is disrupted. The lateral collateral ligament being compressed is, obviously, intact. Widening of the inferior tibiofibular joint indicates disruption of the anterior and posterior inferior tibiofibular ligaments and disruption of the interosseous membrane to the level of the oblique fibular fracture. The reverse occurs in the much-less-frequent inversion ankle injuries.

Forceful posterior displacement of the foot drives the talus posteriorly between the malleoli. The talar trochlea, being wider anteriorly than posteriorly, may disrupt the collateral and inferior tibiofibular ligaments, may fracture one or both malleoli, and may cause an obliquely vertical fracture of the posterior tibial lip.

The simplest eversion injury is a "sprain" of the ankle in which only a few fibers of the deltoid ligament are disrupted. Radiographically, the only abnormality is soft tissue swelling about, and distal to, the medial malleolus. The bones of the ankle are intact, and the anatomy of the ankle mortise is normally maintained (Fig. 21.46). In eversion, the intact deltoid ligament may be associated with cortical avulsion fractures of either the medial malleolus or the medial cortex of the talar body. Such fractures should not be considered insignificant "chip" fractures but indicate that some, if not all, of the MCL fibers are no longer attached to the tibia or talus (Fig. 21.47). In this instance, stress views are not required because the presence of the avulsion fracture fragment indicates the deltoid ligament is not attached to the medial malleolus. If the avulsion of the deltoid ligament is not associated with cortical fractures of the medial styloid process or talus, stress views are indicated to establish either avulsion of the ligament or ligamentous disruption. In either instance, soft tissue swelling is present at, and distal to, the level of the medial malleolus.

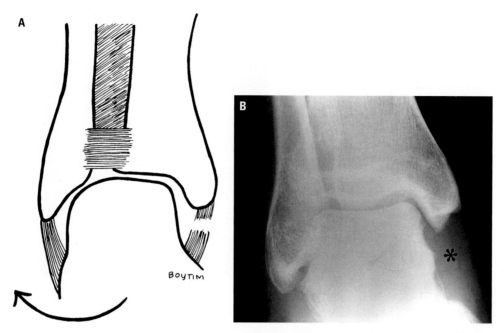

Figure 21.46. **A,B:** Eversion "sprain" of the ankle. The diffuse soft tissue swelling, principally distal to the medial malleolus *(asterisk)*, and the absence of a medial malleolar or talar fracture indicate that the deltoid ligament has been at least partially disrupted.

The eversion force expended on the medial malleolus through the intact MCL may also result in an avulsion horizontal fracture of the medial malleolus distal to the plafond (Fig. 21.48), in which event the ankle mortise is stable intact. The presence of such a fracture at or above the level of the plafond (Fig. 21.49) results in medial instability of the mortise.

Eversion injuries associated with more forceful lateral displacement and rotation of the talus within the mortise may have both an avulsion and

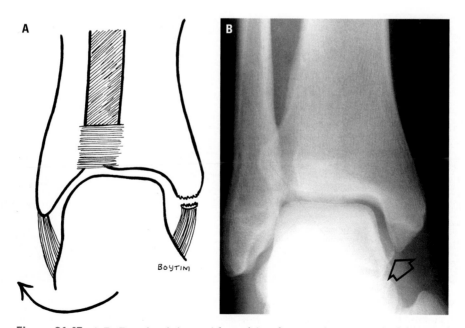

Figure 21.47. **A,B:** Eversion injury with avulsion fracture *(open arrow)* of the tip of the medial malleolus. The presence of this tiny fragment indicates that the deltoid ligament is intact but has been partially separated from the medial styloid process.

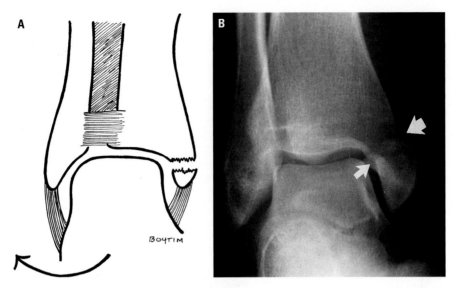

Figure 21.48. A,B: Eversion injury with an avulsion fracture of the medial malleolus *(arrows)*. The avulsion fracture line is characteristically horizontal. Its presence indicates that the deltoid ligament is intact.

an impaction component. This concept is illustrated in Figure 21.50, where the talus has clearly impacted on the lateral malleolus, producing an oblique fracture of its base. The avulsion fracture of the medial malleolus with lateral displacement of its distal fragment indicates an intact MCL. The normal relationship between the distal end of the proximal fibular fragment and the tibia indicates that the distal tibiofibular ligaments and the interosseous membrane remain intact.

The effect of both impaction and avulsion forces of eversion may result in any one of several different forms of injury, as illustrated in Figures 21.51 through 21.56. Figure 21.54 is a rare form of eversion injury in

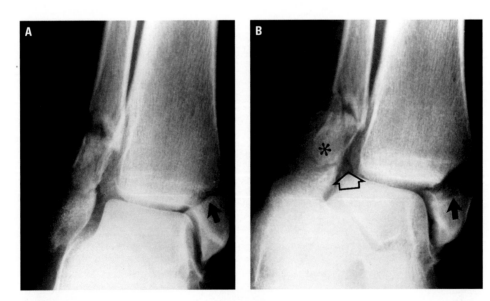

Figure 21.49. The location of the medial malleolar fracture (**A,** *arrow*) above the level of the plafond indicates instability of the mortise medially. The significance of the location of the medial malleolar fracture is seen to better advantage on the mortise projection (**B,** *black arrow*). Lateral displacement of the comminuted distal fibular fracture *(asterisk)* indicates disruption of the distal tibiofibular ligaments *(open arrow)*.

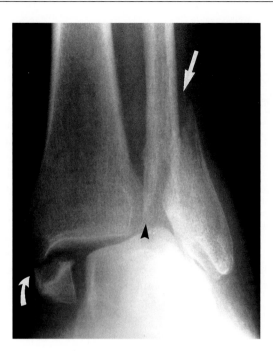

Figure 21.50. Eversion injury with an avulsion fracture of the medial malleolus *(white curved arrow)* and an oblique (impaction) fracture *(white straight arrow)* of the base of the lateral malleolus. The presence of the pointed distal end of the proximal fragment *(arrowhead)* within the fibular groove indicates that the distal tibiofibular ligaments are intact.

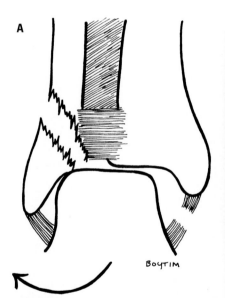

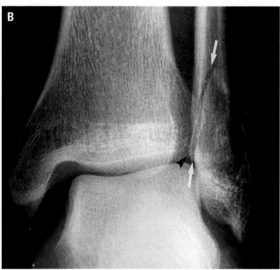

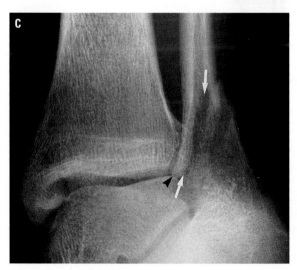

Figure 21.51. A,B,C: Eversion injury with both avulsion and impaction components **(A)**. The oblique fracture of the distal fibula (**B** and **C**, *arrows*), seen best in the internally rotated oblique radiograph **(C)**, represents the impaction force of the talus against the lateral malleolus. The normal relationship of the distal end of the proximal fibular fragment *(arrowhead)* indicates that the distal tibiofibular ligaments and the more proximal interosseous membrane are intact. The absence of a medial malleolar or talar fracture indicates that the deltoid ligament is at least partially disrupted.

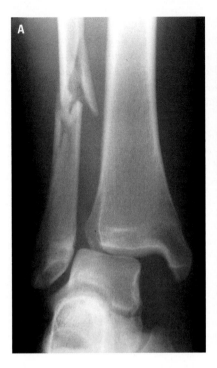

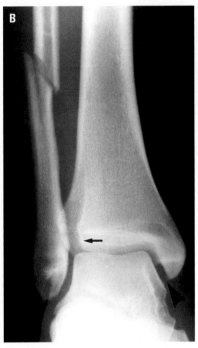

Figure 21.52. Eversion injury of the ankle with disruption of the medial collateral ("deltoid") ligament in two different patients (**A,B**). The anterior and posterior distal tibiofibular ligaments and the interosseous membrane are disrupted to the level of the fracture of the distal third of the fibula in each patient. In **A**, the displacement and rotation of the talus are obvious. However, in **B**, lateral displacement of the talus is remarkably subtle and is indicated only by lateral displacement of the talus with respect to the posterior margin of the fibular notch *(arrow)* and minimal widening of the medial talomalleolar space *(arrowhead)*.

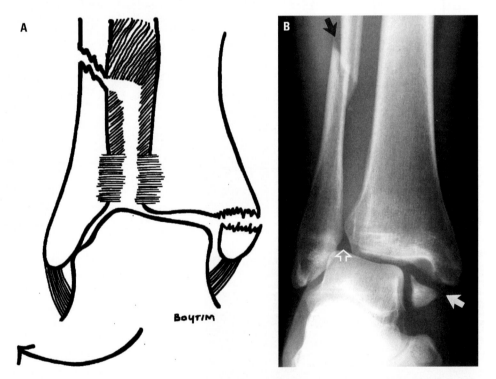

Figure 21.53. **A,B:** Eversion injury with avulsion fracture of the base of the medial malleolus and impaction fracture at the junction of the middle and distal thirds of the fibula. The presence of the medial malleolar avulsion fracture *(white arrow)* indicates that the medial collateral ligament is intact. Lateral displacement of the distal fibular fragment with widening of the distal tibiofibular joint *(open arrow)* indicates that the anterior and posterior distal tibiofibular ligaments are disrupted, as is the interosseous membrane, to the level of the fibular fracture *(black arrow)*.

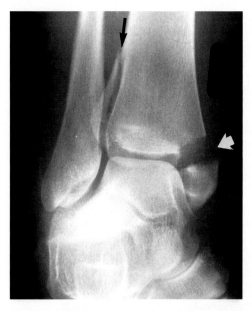

Figure 21.54. Eversion injury with avulsion fracture of the base of the medial malleolus *(white arrow)*. The impaction (lateral) component of this injury is a vertically oriented avulsion fracture of the anterior margin of the fibular notch *(black arrow)*, mediated through the intact anterior distal tibiofibular ligament.

that the talar impaction against the fibula is manifested by an avulsion fracture of the base of the anterior margin of the fibular notch mediated through the intact anterior distal tibiofibular ligament.

The Maisonneuve fracture (Fig. 21.56) is an eversion fracture in which the impaction component is an oblique fracture in the neck of the fibula. The important observation regarding the Maisonneuve fracture is lateral displacement of the fibula without a fracture in its distal third on ankle radiographs. In that circumstance, a Maisonneuve fracture must be suspected, and the entire leg including the knee must be examined radiographically to demonstrate the proximal fibular fracture.

Inversion injuries of the ankle are simply the reciprocal of those caused by eversion, that is, the oblique impacted fracture line involves the medial malleolus, and the horizontal avulsion fracture line involves the lateral malleolus. Ligamentous injuries caused by inversion are also the reciprocal of those caused by eversion, with the exception that the distal tibiofibular ligaments are not disrupted. Examples of inversion ankle injuries are illustrated on Figures 21.57 through 21.61.

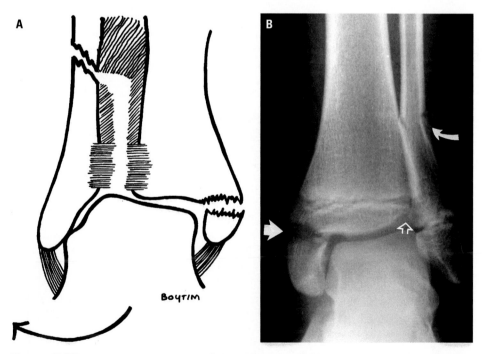

Figure 21.55. A,B: Eversion injury of the ankle of a child with an avulsion fracture of the medial malleolus at the level of the plafond *(straight arrow)* (the mortise is unstable). Widening of the distal tibiofibular joint *(open arrow)* indicates that the distal tibiofibular ligaments are torn, and a fracture in the distal third of the fibula *(curved arrow)* indicates that the distal portion of the interosseous membrane is torn. The avulsion fracture of the medial malleolus also indicates that the deltoid ligament is intact. The distal tibial and fibular physes are intact.

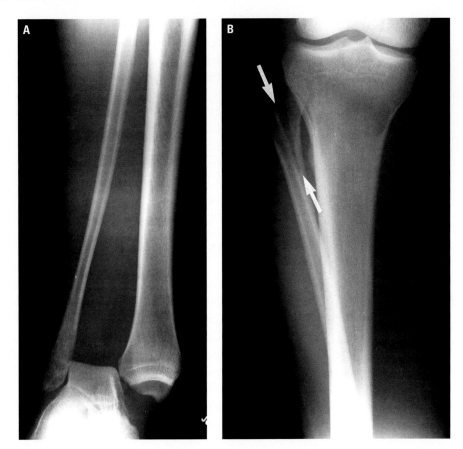

Figure 21.56. Maisonneuve fracture. The eversion mechanism of injury is obvious in the radiograph (**A**) of the leg and ankle. An injury to the ankle with lateral fibular displacement but with no fracture in the distal fibula requires radiographic examination of the proximal fibula (**B**) to document the oblique fracture *(arrows)* that must be present.

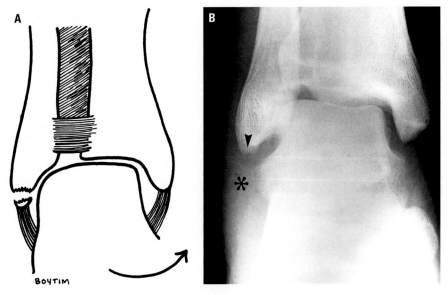

Figure 21.57. A,B: Inversion injury characterized by avulsion of the medial malleolar styloid cortex *(arrowhead)* and soft tissue swelling *(asterisk)* inferior to the malleolus. The soft tissue and skeletal anatomy on the lateral aspect of the ankle is radiographically normal.

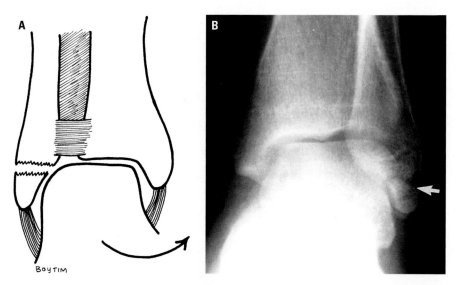

Figure 21.58. **A,B:** Inversion injury with avulsion fracture of the lateral malleolus *(arrow)* mediated through the intact lateral collateral ligament. The medial collateral ligament, the distal tibiofibular ligaments, and the interosseous membrane are all intact, as is the medial malleolus.

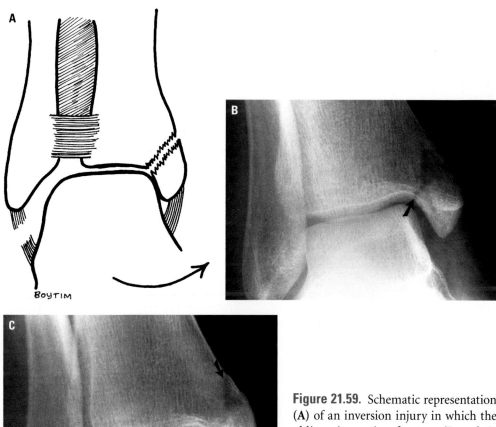

Figure 21.59. Schematic representation **(A)** of an inversion injury in which the oblique impaction fracture **(B** and **C,** *arrows)* of the medial malleolus is above the plafond in the straight frontal **(B)** and mortise **(C)** projections indicates the ankle is unstable medially.

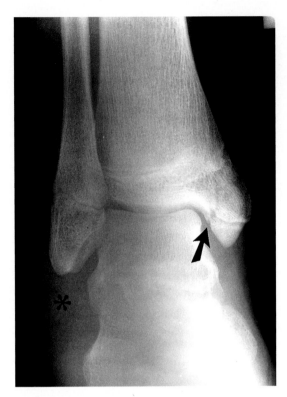

Figure 21.60. Inversion injury with oblique (impaction) fracture of the medial malleolar epiphysis *(arrow)*. Absence of an avulsion fracture of either the lateral malleolus or the lateral talar cortex indicates disruption of the lateral collateral ligament. Maximum lateral soft tissue swelling *(asterisk)* distal to the lateral malleolus is consistent with a lateral collateral ligament tear.

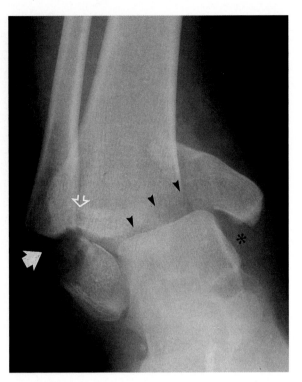

Figure 21.61. Bimalleolar fracture dislocation caused by an inversion injury. The impaction force of the dislocated talus striking the medial malleolus has resulted in the oblique fracture *(arrowheads)* of its base and the direction of displacement of the distal fragment. The distance between the medial malleolus and the medial surface of the talus *(asterisk)* indicates that the deltoid ligament is disrupted. The avulsion force transmitted through the intact lateral collateral ligament has caused the transverse fracture of the lateral malleolus *(arrow)* at the level of the plafond. The normal relationship between the distal end of the proximal fibular fracture and the tibia *(open arrow)* indicates that the distal tibiofibular ligaments and the interosseous membrane are intact.

Bimalleolar fractures or fracture dislocations may be the result of either an inversion (Fig. 21.61) or an eversion (Fig. 21.62) injury. The position of the fragments and the characteristics of the fracture lines indicate the mechanism of injury.

Although the posterior tibial lip is not a malleolus, fracture of the posterior tibial lip occurs most commonly in association with fractures of the medial and lateral malleolus or the fibula. This constellation of fractures is referred to as trimalleolar. The trimalleolar fracture may be caused by talar eversion and posterior displacement (Fig. 21.63), by talar inversion and posterior displacement (Fig. 21.64), or by essentially direct posterior displacement of the foot with the wider anterior portion of the talar trochlea causing an impaction fracture of each malleolus (Fig. 21.65).

The pilon fracture is a comminuted, intra-articular fracture of the distal tibia. Although not a fracture of the ankle joint per se because the pilon fracture involves the distal articulating surface of the tibia, it seems appropriate to consider this fracture here. Pilon fractures constitute approximately 7% of tibial fractures.[16,17] The most common mechanism of injury is axial compression of the talus against the distal tibial articulating surface, such as in a fall from a height, although infrequently a torsion injury that creates

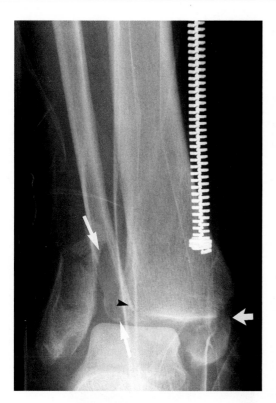

Figure 21.62. Bimalleolar fracture dislocation caused by an eversion injury. The impaction force has produced the oblique fracture in the distal fibula *(long arrows)* proximal to the level of the plafond. The normal relationship between the distal end of the proximal fibular fragment and the tibia *(arrowhead)* indicates that the tibiofibular ligaments and the interosseous membrane are intact. The avulsion force transmitted through the intact medial collateral ligament has caused the transverse fracture of the base of the medial malleolus *(short arrow)*.

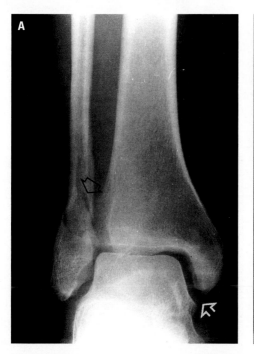

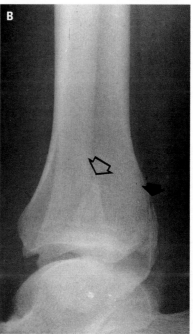

Figure 21.63. Subtle eversion trimalleolar fracture dislocation of the ankle. **A:** In the frontal projection, the talus and the distal fibular fragment are laterally displaced and the inferior tibiofibular joint is disrupted, indicating that the inferior tibiofibular ligaments are disrupted. The oblique fibular fracture *(open arrow)* above the level of the plafond indicates impaction and lateral instability of the ankle mortise. The absence of a medial malleolar or medial talar body fracture indicates disruption of the medial collateral ligament *(open arrow)*. **B:** In the lateral projection, the talus is posteriorly subluxated, and a vertical fracture involves the posterior tibial lip *(closed arrow)*. The *open arrow* indicates the distal fibular fracture.

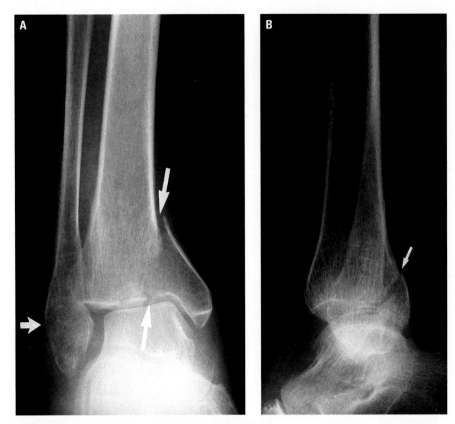

Figure 21.64. Inversion trimalleolar fracture subluxation. **A:** In the frontal projection, the orientation of the medial *(long arrows)* and lateral *(short arrow)* fracture lines, the direction of displacement of the distal fragments, and the position of the talus all indicate an inversion mechanism of injury. **B:** The lateral radiograph shows the oblique fracture of the posterior tip of the talus *(arrow)*. The talus is posteriorly subluxated with respect to the tibia.

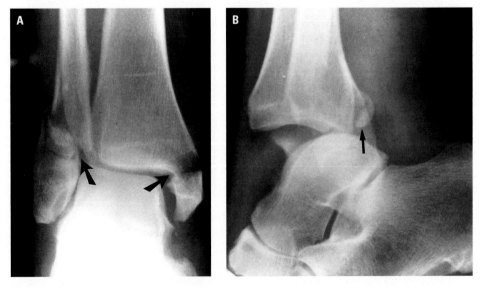

Figure 21.65. The oblique fracture of each malleolus (**A**, *arrows*) represents impaction of the talus on each malleolus associated with essentially pure posterior displacement of the foot. In lateral projection (**B**), the talus, which is almost completely posteriorly dislocated, has caused a small impaction fracture of the posterior tibial lip *(arrow)*.

a spiral fracture of the distal tibia may extend into the plafond. The magnitude of the causative force and the position of the foot at the time of impact determine the type of fracture. Pilon fractures have been classified by Ruedi and Allgower[18] into the following types: I, nondisplaced cleavage fracture into the distal tibial articulating surface with-out major displacement of the articular cartilage; II, moderate comminution of the distal tibia and incongruity of the articular surface; and III, gross distal tibial comminution and articular surface incongruity (Fig. 21.66).[19] Figure 21.67 is an example of type III pilon fracture, the most severely comminuted injury.

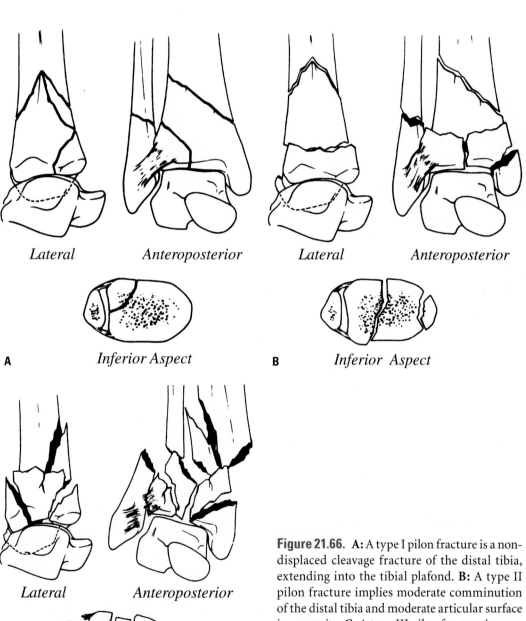

Figure 21.66. A: A type I pilon fracture is a nondisplaced cleavage fracture of the distal tibia, extending into the tibial plafond. **B:** A type II pilon fracture implies moderate comminution of the distal tibia and moderate articular surface incongruity. **C:** A type III pilon fracture is associated with gross distal tibial comminution and articular surface incongruity. (From Bourne RB, Rorabeck CH, MacNab J. Intra-articular fractures of the distal tibia: the pylon fracture. *J Trauma.* 1983;23:591–596, with permission.)

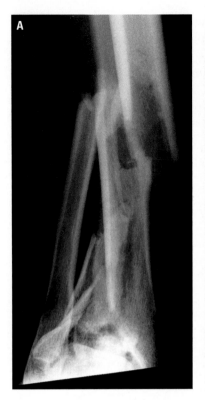
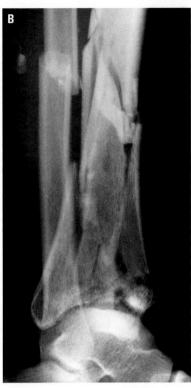

Figure 21.67. Type III (most severely comminuted) pilon fracture of the distal tibia in AP (**A**) and lateral (**B**) projections.

Old, ununited fracture fragments about the ankle, as occur at many other sites, are typically avulsion fractures, vary in size but are usually small, and are characterized by smooth, corticated margins. Commonly, their site of origin cannot be specifically identified (Fig. 21.68).

NONTRAUMATIC CONDITIONS

The os trigonum (Fig. 21.69) is a normal variant of the talus, created when the posterior process of the talus arises from a separate growth center that fails to unite. This frequently encountered anomaly may

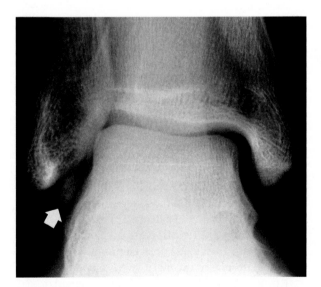

Figure 21.68. The smoothly corticated loose body (*arrow*) between the lateral malleolar styloid process and the talus is an ununited avulsion fragment, probably from the lateral malleolus.

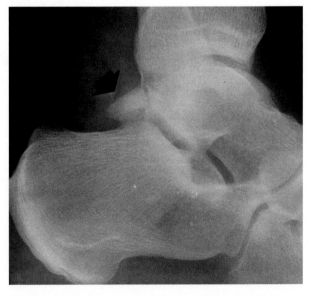

Figure 21.69. The os trigonum (*arrow*) represents the secondary ossification for the posterior talar tubercle that failed to fuse with the body of the talus.

resemble an old, ununited fracture fragment. Its location, radiographic characteristics, and the fact that it is usually bilateral should help in establishing the correct identity of this variant.

Transverse linear densities seen in the metaphyses of growing long bones are referred to by Caffey[20] as "transverse stress lines of Park," after the investigator who was primarily responsible for the present concept relative to this radiographic finding. The transverse lines may be found in healthy or sick children and never cause local signs or symptoms. The lines, which are usually bilateral, which may be found at the ends of any long bone, and which may extend partially or completely across the metaphysis, are thought to develop during periods of accelerated growth following periods of growth arrest, such as may occur during fever or starvation stress. The transverse lines may be found in both premature and full-term infants, indicating an in utero genesis (Fig. 21.70).

Acute osteomyelitis is common in infants and children, in whom the spread of infection is usually hematogenous. Acute osteomyelitis may also occur as the result of direct inoculation, as occurs in patients with penetrating injuries or in diabetics or others with soft tissue ulceration (Fig. 21.71). In infants younger than 1 year and in adults, the physis does not serve as a barrier to the spread of infection into a joint or to an adjacent bone. In children from approximately 1 year of age until physeal

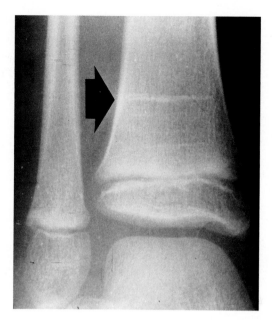

Figure 21.70. Transverse stress line *(arrow)*.

fusion, however, the physis effectively limits acute osteomyelitis to either the metaphysis or diaphysis (Fig. 21.72).

Clinically, in infants and young children, acute osteomyelitis may be manifested only by refusal to use the affected part (e.g., refusal to bear weight or walk) or by a limp. In this age group, which is prone to minor trauma as from a fall, the precedent history is of doubtful value, and the physical examination

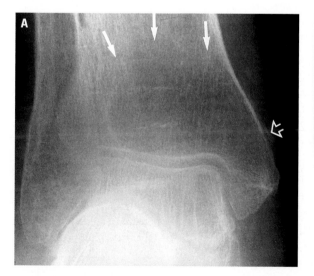
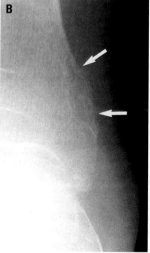

Figure 21.71. A: Acute osteomyelitis characterized in AP projection by a large area of rarefaction with loss of all but a few primary trabeculae *(solid arrows)* and very faint periosteal new bone reaction *(open arrow)*. **B:** The oblique radiograph shows frank cortical *(arrows)* and subcortical trabecular destruction.

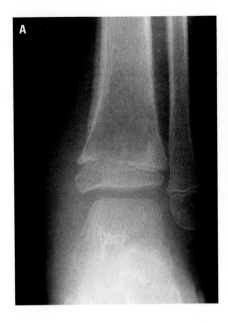
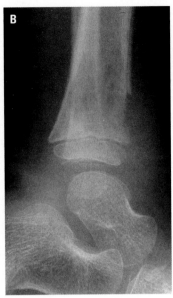

Figure 21.72. Acute osteomyelitis in the distal tibia of a 3-year-old child. The osseous lesion, characterized by an ill-defined lucent area of trabecular erosion (**A**), anterior cortical erosion (**B**), and florid periosteal reaction extending beyond the nidus of infection (**A**), is limited to the metaphysis by the physis (**A**). Diffuse soft tissue swelling of the distal portion of the leg and ankle is present both medially and anteriorly.

is usually ambiguous, including skeletal injury, osteomyelitis, pyarthrosis, or simply cellulitis. Even though the osseous signs of acute osteomyelitis usually do not become radiographically visible until 10 to 14 days after the onset of infection,[21] the initial imaging evaluation should be plain radiography. The rationale is to exclude fracture or physeal injury and, possibly, to identify localizing soft tissue swelling with loss of fascial plane delineation, which are the earliest but are nonspecific radiographic signs of acute osteomyelitis.

Scintigraphy may detect acute osteomyelitis as early as 24 hours after the onset of symptoms. In fact, a negative, or normal, radioactive bone scan obtained 24 hours after the onset of symptoms effectively excludes the diagnosis of acute osteomyelitis.

The earliest skeletal changes of acute osteomyelitis include vague demineralization resulting from hyperemia and trabecular destruction. Initially, the cortex is intact but becomes eroded (Figs. 21.71 and 21.72) as the infection extends horizontally through Howship's lacunae.

More advanced acute osteomyelitis is characterized by more extensive effacement of trabeculation over a larger area, resulting in a lytic lesion without sclerotic or definable margins but with cortical erosion. Periostitis, which may be florid in children and may extend well beyond the nidus of infection (Fig. 21.72), usually becomes radiographically visible in about 3 weeks following the onset of infection. The periostitis may have an irregular or, more commonly, smoothly laminated appearance.

Symptomatic benign and malignant neoplasms of the ankle that might precipitate an emergency center visit have the same radiographic characteristics as described in other chapters related to the appendicular skeleton and need not be repeated here.

REFERENCES

1. Mandell J. Isolated fractures of the posterior tibial lip at the ankle as demonstrated by an additional projection, the "poor" lateral view. *Radiology.* 1971;101:319–322.
2. Clemente CD. *Gray's Anatomy.* 30th ed. Philadelphia, PA: Lea & Febiger; 1985.
3. Salter RB. *Textbook of Disorders and Injuries of the Musculoskeletal System.* Baltimore, MD: Williams & Wilkins; 1970.
4. Rang M. The growth plate and its diseases. In: Rockwood CA Jr, Wilkins KE, King RE, eds. *Fractures in Children.* 3rd ed. Philadelphia, PA: Lippincott–Raven Publishers; 1991:128.
5. MacNealy GA, Rogers LF, Hernandez R, et al. Injuries of the distal tibial epiphysis. Systematic radiographic evaluation. *Am J Roentgenol.* 1982;138:683–689.
6. Hoffel JC, Lascombes P, Poncelet T, et al. Biplane fracture of Tillaux. *Eur J Radiol.* 1989;9:250–253.
7. Cass JR, Peterson HA. Salter-Harris type IV injuries of the distal tibial epiphyseal growth plate, with emphasis on those involving the medial malleolus. *J Bone Joint Surg Am.* 1983;65:1059–1070.
8. Salter RB. Injuries of the ankle in children. *Orthop Clin North Am.* 1974;5:147–152.
9. Feldman F, Singsong RD, Rosenberg ZS, et al. Distal tibial tri-planar fracture. *Radiology.* 1987;164:429–435.

10. Clemente DA, Worlock PH. Triplanar fracture of the distal tibia. A variant in cases with an open growth plate. *J Bone Joint Surg Br.* 1987;69:412–415.

11. Lauge-Hansen N. Fractures of the ankle. II. Combined experimental-surgical and experimental-roentgenologic investigations. *Arch Surg.* 1950;60:951–985.

12. Weber BG. *Die Verletzugen des oberen Sprunggelenkes.* Bern, Switzerland: Verlag Hans Huber; 1972.

13. Edeiken J, Cotler JM. Ankle trauma. *Semin Roentgenol.* 1978;13:145.

14. Weissman BN, Sledge CB. *Orthopedic Radiology.* Philadelphia, PA: WB Saunders; 1986.

15. Wilson AJ. Ankle fractures: understanding the mechanism of injury is the key to analyzing the radiographs. *Emerg Radiol.* 1998;5(1):49–60.

16. Bourne RB. Pilon fracture of the distal tibia. *Clin Orthop.* 1989;240:42–45.

17. Bartlett CS III, D'Amato MJ, Weiner LS. Fractures of the tibial pilon. In: Browner BD, Jupiter JB, Levine AM, et al, eds. *Skeletal Trauma.* 2nd ed. Philadelphia, PA: WB Saunders; 1998:2295–2301.

18. Ruedi TP, Allgower M. Fractures of the lower end of the tibia into the ankle joint. *Injury.* 1969;1:92–99.

19. Bourne RB, Rorabeck CH, MacNab J. Intra-articular fractures of the distal tibia: the pylon fracture. *J Trauma.* 1983;23:591–596.

20. Caffey J. *Pediatric X-ray Diagnosis.* 5th ed. Chicago, IL: Year Book; 1973.

21. Brown ML, Kamida CB, Berquist TH, et al. An imaging approach to musculoskeletal infection. In: Berquist TH, ed. *Imaging of Orthopedic Trauma and Surgery.* Philadelphia, PA: WB Saunders; 1989.

SUGGESTED READINGS

1. Rogers LF. *Radiology of Skeletal Trauma.* 3rd ed. New York, NY: Churchill Livingstone; 2002:1222–1317.

2. Manaster BJ, May DA, Distler DG. *Musculoskeletal Imaging.* 3rd ed. Maryland Heights, MO: Mosby; 2002:249–259.

3. Jeffrey RB, Manasrer BJ, Gurney JW, et al. *Diagnostic Imaging Emergency.* Salt Lake City, UT: Amirysis; 2007:I:4-15i–I:4-16i.

4. Greenspan A. *Orthopedic Imaging: A Practical Approach.* 4th ed. Philadelphia, PA: Lippincott Williams & Wilkins; 2004:293–347, 297–305.

5. Johnson TR, Steinbach LS. *Essentials of Musculoskeletal Imaging.* Rosemont, IL: American Academy of Orthopedic Surgeons; 2004:577–582.

6. Salter RB. *Textbook of Disorder and Injuries of the Musculoskeletal System.* 3rd ed. Philadelphia, PA: Lippincott Williams & Wilkins; 1999:538–540, 609–616.

7. Marsh JL, Salzman CL. *Rockwood and Green's Fractures in Adults.* 6th ed. Philadelphia, PA: Lippincott Williams & Wilkins; 2006:2147–2249.

8. Bittle MM, Gunn ML, Gross JA, et al. *Trauma Radiology Companion.* 2nd ed. Philadelphia, PA: Lippincott Williams & Wilkins; 2012.

9. Taylor JAM, Resnick D. *Skeletal Imaging: Atlas of the Spine and Extremities.* Philadelphia, PA: WB Saunders; 2000:692–701.

10. Pope TL, Bloem HL, Beltran J, et al. *Imaging of the Musculoskeletal System.* Philadelphia, PA: Elsevier; 2008:713–748.

CHAPTER 22

Foot and Heel

Dominic Barron ▪ K. Partington ▪ John H. Harris Jr. ▪ Thomas L. Pope Jr.

GENERAL CONSIDERATIONS

Anatomically, the foot includes all of the tarsal bones, the metatarsals, and the phalanges. The forefoot includes the metatarsals and the phalanges; the midfoot includes the three cuneiform bones, the cuboid, and the navicular bones; and the hindfoot includes the talus and calcaneus.

Injuries of the heel or midfoot commonly produce clinical signs suggesting an abnormality of the ankle, as discussed further in Chapter 21. Careful clinical evaluation is required to guide appropriate imaging of the injured area.

It is no longer routine standard of care to obtain the opposite side views in an injury involving the peripheral skeleton of a child or adolescent. Rather, the current standard is that radiographic studies of the opposite side should be obtained when specifically required to help distinguish between a developmental variant and a traumatic lesion, in the opinion of the radiologist.

Imaging Techniques

Routine radiographic study of the foot includes anteroposterior, internally rotated oblique, and lateral views (Fig. 22.1). The lateral is sometimes omitted but this does then make evaluation of subtle midfoot injuries difficult. Routine radiographs of the heel are the lateral and axial projections.[1]

Where additional information regarding the bony anatomy of these areas are required, computed tomography (CT) is indicated due to its volumetric acquisition, multiplanar reformations, and 3-D reconstructions.[2]

Magnetic resonance imaging (MRI) is becoming increasingly valuable in the assessment of the foot. The main indications are purely soft tissue injuries, stress reactions or fractures, infection, and the acute diabetic foot.

Ultrasound has a relatively limited role in this area due to predominance of bony problems. It is, however, excellent at assessment of Morton- neuroma- and plantar fascia- based pathologies.

RADIOGRAPHIC ANATOMY AND VARIANTS

In the foot, two sesamoid bones are normally present on the volar aspect of the head of the first metatarsal (Fig. 22.2). Either of these may be bifid developmentally. This variant may be distinguished from an acute fracture by the sclerotic, parallel margins of the separate ossification centers. When present, this variant is usually bilateral. Sesamoid bones are occasionally seen at the level of the interphalangeal joint of the great toe and the metatarsophalangeal joint of the second and little toes.

The tubercle of the tarsal navicular may constitute a separate bone (os tibiale externum) in approximately 4% of the population.[3] Other variants that can be diagnostically perplexing include the os intermetatarseum, os peroneum (a sesamoid bone sometimes found in the peroneus longus tendon) and the talar "beak" (Fig. 22.3).

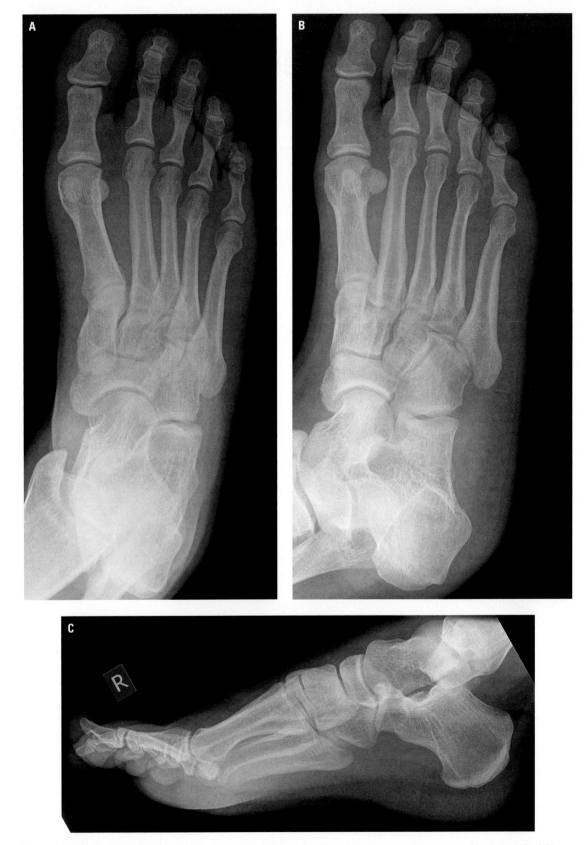

Figure 22.1. Routine radiographic examination of the foot. **A:** Frontal. **B:** Internally rotated oblique. **C:** Lateral.

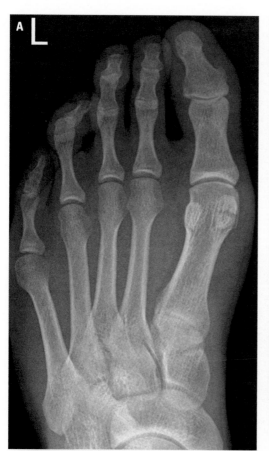

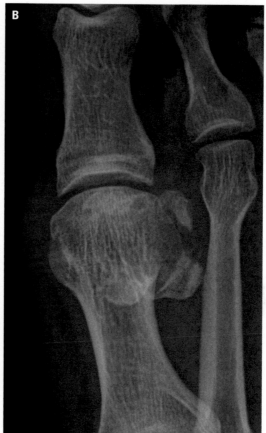

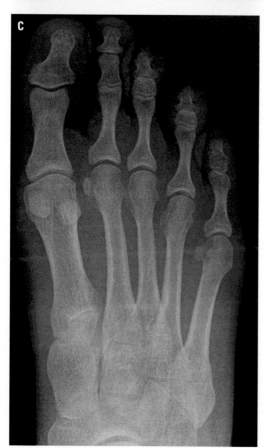

Figure 22.2. Sesamoids. **A:** AP view of tibial sesamoid. **B:** Acute fracture of both great toe sesamoids. **C:** Sesamoids to both the second and fifth toes.

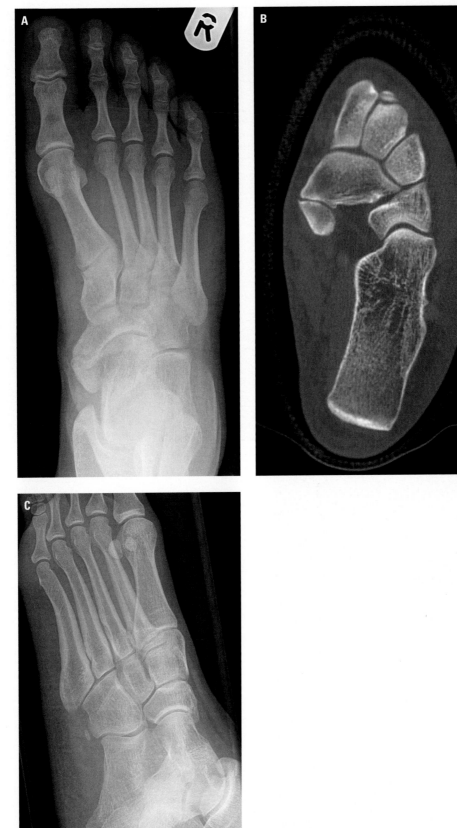

Figure 22.3. Os tibiale externum. **A:** AP radiograph of os tibiale externum. **B:** Axial CT view demonstrating the classical sclerotic smooth edges of accessory bone. **C:** Os peroneum.

Normal osseous structures that can cause diagnostic difficulty in the foot include nutrient artery canals, the calcaneal apophysis, the cone epiphyses, and the normal orientation of the epiphyses.

A nutrient artery canal should not be mistaken for an incomplete fracture or a stress fracture. The artery groove is oriented obliquely and distally in the midshaft of a metatarsal or, rarely, a proximal or middle phalanx. Its margins will be parallel, smooth, and faintly sclerotic. The nutrient canal is usually seen in only one projection, whereas the irregular, jagged margins of a fracture line should be evident in more than one projection (Fig. 22.4).

The calcaneal apophysis is typically fragmented and irregularly more dense than the calcaneus (Fig. 22.5). For a comprehensive review of normal variants that may simulate disease, the reader is referred to Keats and Anderson.[4]

Figure 22.1 is an anteroposterior view of the normal adult foot. The lateral cuneiform and cuboid are superimposed, and the anatomy of the bases of the lateral four metatarsals is obscure due to superimposition caused by the normal transverse arch of the midfoot. On this view, the lateral aspects of the

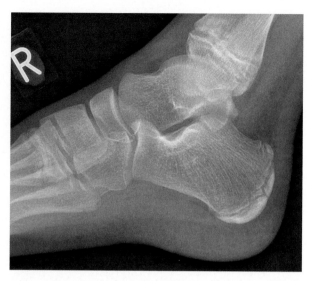

Figure 22.5. Calcaneal apophysis. Lateral view showing the typical sclerotic appearance to the calcaneal apophysis.

first metatarsal and the medial cuneiform should align, as should the medial aspects of the second metatarsal and the intermediate cuneiform.

The internally oblique view is made with the foot internally rotated and the central beam perpendicular to the tabletop centered over the third metatarsal; thus, the lateral cuneiform, cuboid, and lateral three metatarsals are projected into profile. On the internal oblique view, the medial aspects of the third metatarsal and third cuneiform should align. The lateral radiograph of the foot is essential in the radiographic evaluation of the heel and midfoot. The subtalar, talonavicular, and calcaneocuboid joints are seen well in this projection.

The externally rotated oblique projection is designed to project the medial cortical surface of the navicular, the first cuneiform, and the base of the first metatarsal in profile. This is usually omitted from the standard series and is reserved for cases where there is specific concern for injuries to this area.

The axial projection of the os calcis demonstrates the convex lateral and concave medial surfaces of the calcaneus and, in an adequately exposed radiograph, provides a clear view of the sustentaculum talus. The lateral radiograph of the heel demonstrates the subtalar joint, the sustentaculum tali, the anterior tubercle of the os calcis, and the calcaneocuboid joint (Fig. 22.6).[5]

Figure 22.7 is of a normal child's foot, where the epiphyses of the lateral four metatarsals are distally

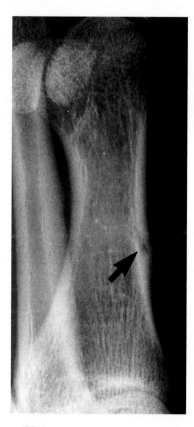

Figure 22.4. Nutrient artery canal (arrow).

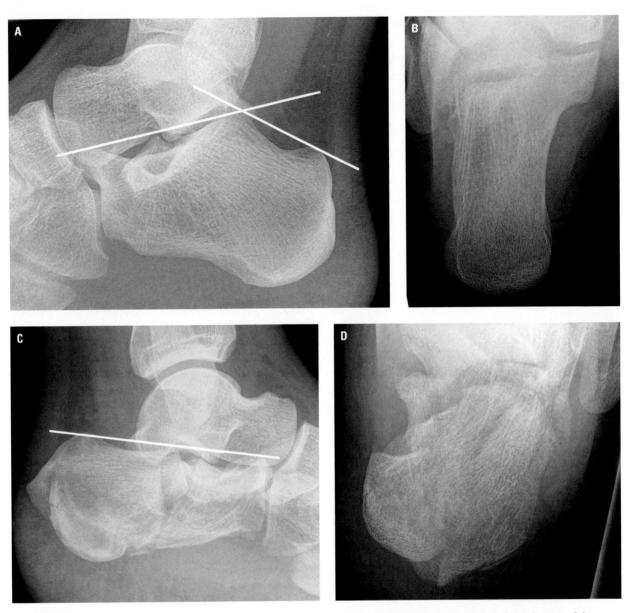

Figure 22.6. A: Normal lateral view of the calcaneus with normal Bohler angle. **B:** Normal axial view of the calcaneus. **C:** Complete loss of Bohler angle secondary to multisegmental intra-articular calcaneal fracture. **D:** Axial view of the same fracture.

located. Those of the first metatarsal and all of the phalanges are proximally situated. Cone epiphysis is another classical pitfall (Fig. 22.8).

In addition to looking for cortical disruptions and misalignment, Bohler angle should routinely be measured when assessing for calcaneal injuries. This angle is formed by the intersection of lines drawn tangentially to the anterior and posterior elements of the superior surface of the calcaneus. The normal range is between 20 and 40 degrees, with the normal average between 30 and 35 degrees (Fig. 22.6).[6]

RADIOGRAPHIC MANIFESTATIONS OF TRAUMA

Talar Injuries

The talar subluxations and dislocations usually involve the ankle mortise in association with ankle fracture dislocations and are fully described in Chapter 21.

Dislocation of the talus with respect to the ankle mortise without an associated fracture[7] and "peritalar"[8]

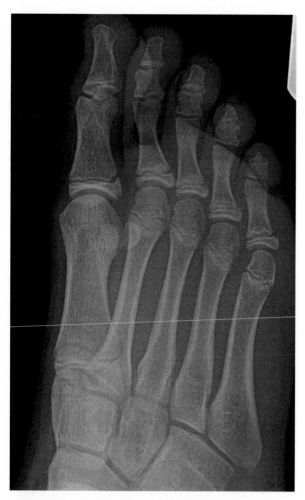

Figure 22.7. DP oblique view of child's foot showing the multiple physeal lines.

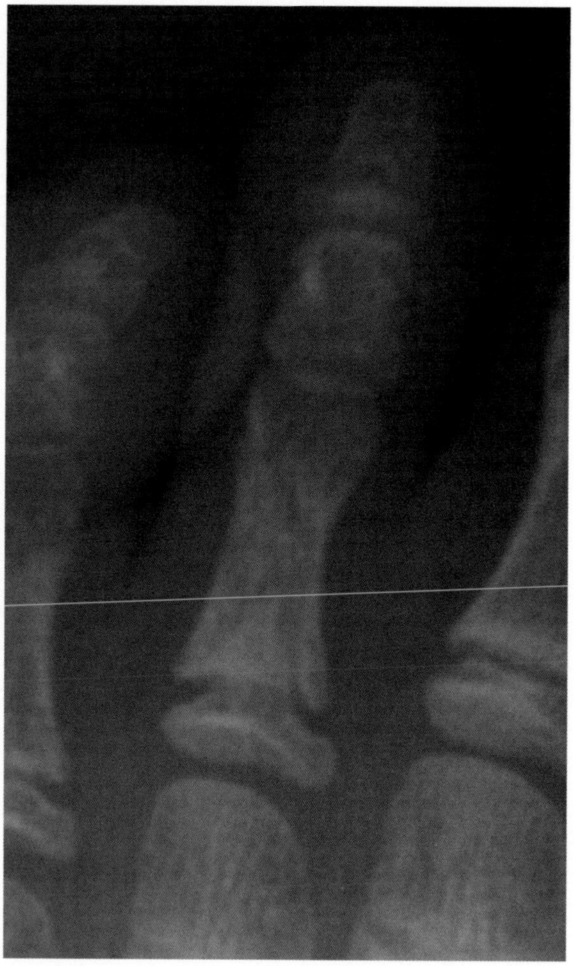

Figure 22.8. Phalangeal view demonstrating classical coned epiphysis.

and "subtalar"[9-11] dislocation—both terms for concomitant dislocation at the subtalar and talonavicular joints with a normal tibiotalar relationship—are rare. However, these can easily be overlooked, and careful evaluation of the ankle series should always include an assessment of the subtalar joint.

Talar dome (transcondylar, osteocartilaginous, or osteochondral dome) fractures are caused by impaction of the lateral or medial aspect of the talar trochlea on the ankle mortise during eversion or inversion ankle injuries (Fig. 22.9). The middle third (in the sagittal plane) of the lateral border and the posterior third of the medial border of the talar dome are the common locations. The fracture can be very subtle and is frequently not detected or not appreciated on the initial ankle radiograph.[12,13] Both CT and MRI will define the osteochondral fracture when the plain radiograph is equivocal. An MRI, however, is the imaging modality of choice for

accurate classification of an unstable osteochondral fragment. It can demonstrate cartilaginous damage, interposed fluid between the osteochondral fragment and the underlying bone, as well as size and displacement of the fragment.[14] Unstable or necrotic fragments are treated surgically.

Fractures of the talar body involving the trochlea (dome) may be obvious in one projection and subtle in the other (Fig. 22.10). Fractures of the lateral and posterior talar processes are usually avulsion fractures associated with ankle injuries (Fig. 22.11).

Talar neck fractures usually occur with only minimal displacement, and CT is frequently useful in demonstrating or confirming subtle fractures and their fragment alignment. These are described according to the Hawkin's classification (Fig. 22.12).[15] This system is based on the number of associated dislocations at the ankle, subtalar, and talonavicular joints. This has significant prognostic value because

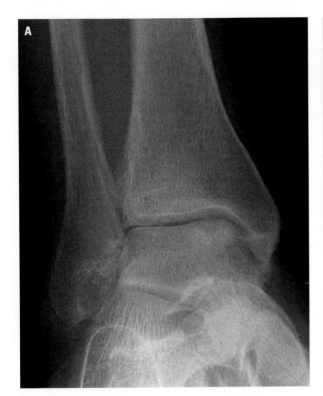

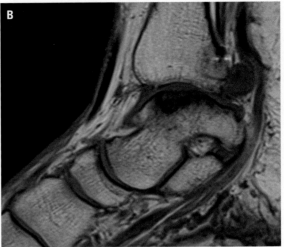

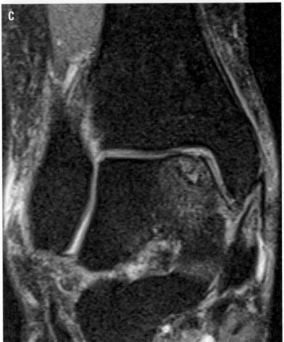

Figure 22.9. A: AP ankle view showing medial talar dome osteochondral fracture. **B:** Sagittal T1W view showing the full extent of the injury. **C:** Coronal short-tau inversion recovery (STIR) image showing the associated edema.

talar neck fractures are associated with avascular necrosis due to their distal to proximal blood supply; the greater the number of associated dislocations, the higher the risk of avascular necrosis.

Calcaneal Injuries

The calcaneus is the most commonly fractured tarsal bone and accounts for about 1% to 2% of all fractures.[16] Fractures are usually the result from axial loading, with the downward force of the body transmitted through the talus, which acts as a wedge;

crushing; and splitting the angle of the os calcis. Due to the mechanism of injury, calcaneal fractures are frequently bilateral and, in approximately 10% of cases, are associated with compression fractures of the thoracolumbar spine.[17]

Calcaneal fractures have characteristic appearances based on the mechanism of injury and are divided into two major categories: intra-articular and extraarticular. Approximately 75% are intraarticular, producing typical features including loss of height due to impaction and rotation of the tuberosity fragment, increase in width due to lateral displacement of the tuberosity fragment, and disruption of

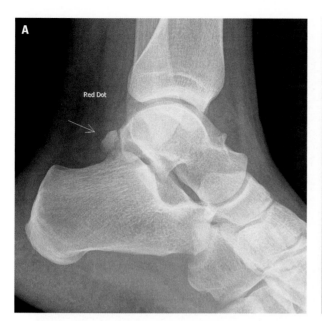 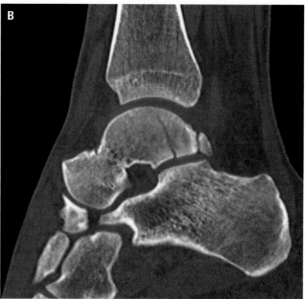

Figure 22.10. A: Lateral ankle radiograph that has unhelpfully had the normal os trigonum labeled as pathologic. Careful review of the radiograph shows the fracture through the talar body. **B:** Sagittal CT reformat unequivocally shows the fracture line.

the posterior facet of the subtalar joint.[18] They are thus readily apparent in both lateral and axial projections.

Depression of the posterior facet produces flattening of Bohler angle; however, because the normal range is from 20 to 40 degrees, it is not totally reliable as an indicator of depressed calcaneal fractures (Fig. 22.6). Calcaneal fractures that may be subtle in the lateral projection are usually readily substantiated in the axial projection because of either impaction or comminution.

Accurate description of calcaneal fractures including position and displacement of fracture fragments has significant implications for their management. CT is now routinely indicated in their

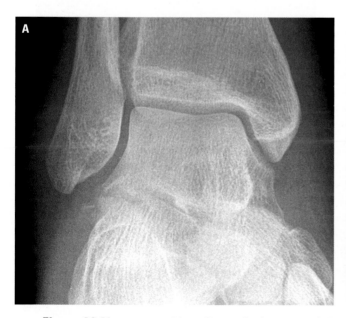 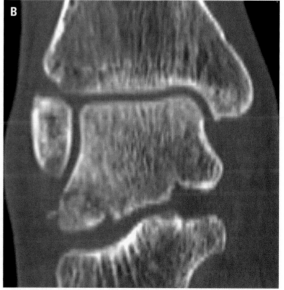

Figure 22.11. A: AP ankle radiograph showing subtle cortical irregularity to the lateral talar process. **B:** Coronal reformat showing the true extent of the lateral process fracture.

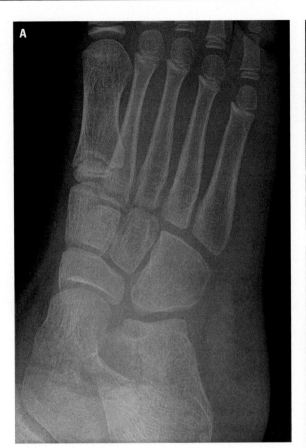

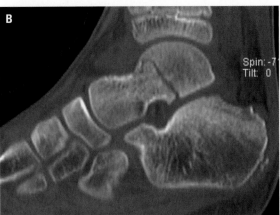

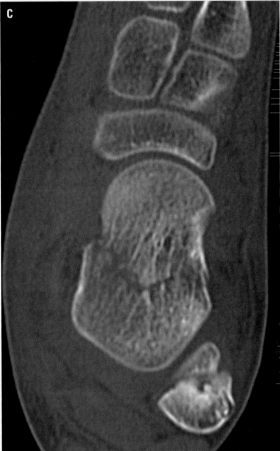

Figure 22.12. **A:** At the proximal aspect of the AP oblique radiograph, an undisplaced talar neck fracture is clearly visible consistent with a Hawkins Type 1 injury. **B and C:** CT reformats demonstrate the fracture line and confirm that there is no associated dislocation.

preoperative assessment. The key to surgical planning are the multiplanar reformations, the most important of which are the direct coronal views that are preformed tangentially to the posterior facet of the subtalar joint. These images then facilitate classification of the fractures with the Sanders or Hannover systems (Fig. 22.13).[19–21]

Extraarticular fractures are all those that do not involve the posterior facet and include fractures of the tuberosity (usually avulsion), the sustentaculum

talus, anterior process (21%), beak and avulsion fractures of the insertion of the Achilles tendon (4%), and oblique fractures that do not extend into the subtalar joint (Fig. 22.14).

Beak fractures of the calcaneal tuberosity are avulsion fractures due to the direct pull of the Achilles tendon, typically occurring in elderly osteoporotic patients (Fig. 22.15).[22]

Anterior process fractures are uncommon and often missed as they are usually very subtle with

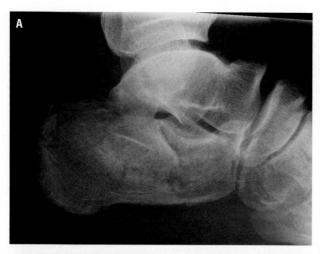

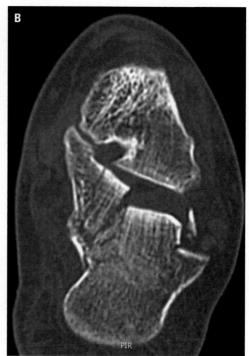

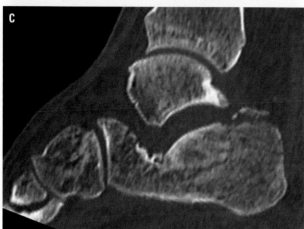

Figure 22.13. A: Lateral radiograph showing multisegmental fracture of the calcaneus with significant involvement of the subtalar joint consistent with a Sanders Type 3AC injury. **B:** Direct coronal reformat confirming significant involvement of the posterior facet. **C:** Sagittal reformat clearly shows the extent of depression of the calcaneal articular surface.

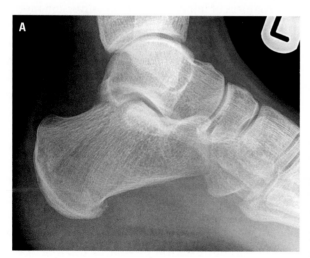

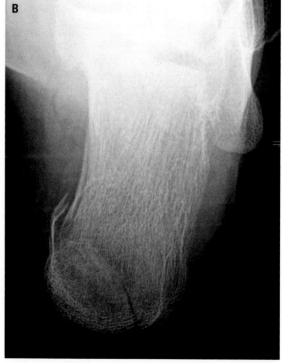

Figure 22.14. Lateral (**A**) and axial (**B**) calcaneal view demonstrate an extraarticular calcaneal fracture.

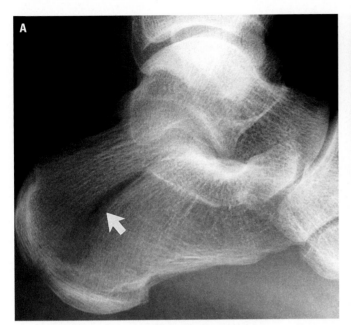
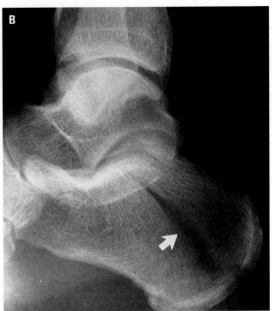

Figure 22.15. Bilateral beak (tongue) calcaneal fractures *(arrows)*.

minimal displacement. They are obscured by other superimposed bones of the midfoot or hindfoot in the lateral projection. The anterior process fracture is usually best demonstrated in the externally rotated oblique projection with CT or MRI being particularly helpful for evaluation (Fig. 22.16).[23,24]

The calcaneus is the second most common site for fatigue-type stress fractures in athletes and insufficiency fractures in the osteoporotic patient. Radiographs may be normal in the early stages, with MRI demonstrating a low T1 signal fracture line, usually in vertical orientation and surrounding marrow edema or increased uptake on radioactive bone scan within 24 to 48 hours (Fig. 22.17).[25]

Tarsal and Metatarsal Injuries

Isolated fractures of the individual tarsal bones occur rarely and should always prompt a detailed assessment of the tarsal and metatarsal bones as they are commonly associated with more complex fracture patterns. These are usually radiographically obscure and may be recognized only by subtle buckling or disruption of the cortex or a vague zone of increased density caused by impaction of the fragments. CT is being increasingly used for assessment and characterization. Fractures of

the intermediate and lateral cuneiform bones or the lateral aspect of the navicular may be hidden by the density of the superimposed tarsals in the anteroposterior radiograph (Fig. 22.18).

Fractures of the base of the fifth metatarsal are secondary to avulsion by the peroneus brevis tendon or the lateral plantar aponeurosis.[26] The common mechanism of injury is a twisting, inversion motion of the foot that is usually associated with relatively minor trauma. Commonly, the patient complains of a "twisted ankle," and it is not uncommon that the examination requested is the ankle rather than the foot. For this reason, it is advisable that at least one view of the ankle series should include the base of the fifth metatarsal.

The most common fracture of the proximal fifth metatarsal is the tuberosity avulsion fracture with most of these occurring at the tip of tuberosity where the lateral band of the aponeurosis attaches. A true Jones[27] fracture is a transverse fracture of the diaphyseal or metaphyseal portion of the fifth metatarsal without extension distal to the fourth and fifth intermetatarsal articulation and is considered to be intra-articular (Fig. 22.19).

In the skeletally immature patient, the apophysis normally present at the base of the fifth metatarsal may resemble a fracture fragment. The fracture line representing an avulsive force is transversely situated through the metatarsal bone, whereas the

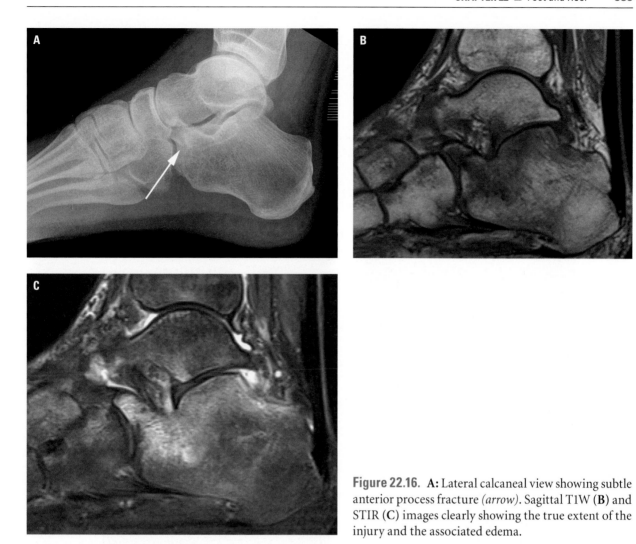

Figure 22.16. A: Lateral calcaneal view showing subtle anterior process fracture *(arrow)*. Sagittal T1W (**B**) and STIR (**C**) images clearly showing the true extent of the injury and the associated edema.

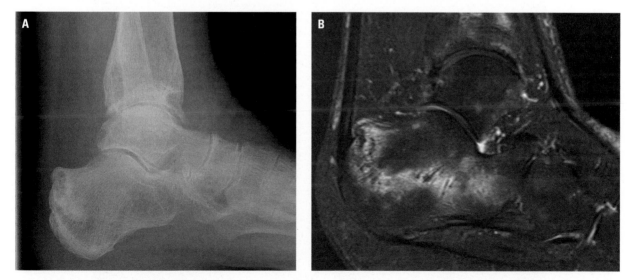

Figure 22.17. A: Lateral ankle radiograph reveals subtle sclerotic change within the calcaneus. **B:** STIR sagittal image confirms edema and developing fracture lines consistent with a calcaneal stress fracture.

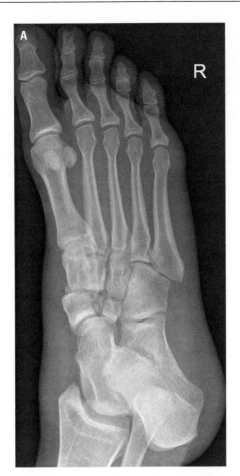

Figure 22.18. **A:** Oblique view showing a multisegmental navicular fracture. **B:** Bone scintigram in a different patient with unexplained midfoot pain showing avid uptake in the navicular secondary to a stress fracture.

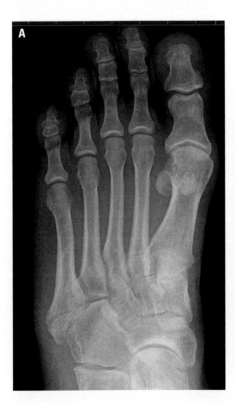

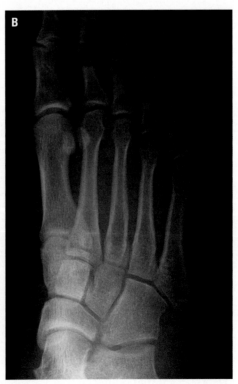

Figure 22.19. **A,B:** Peroneus brevis avulsion fractures of the base of the fifth metatarsal.

apophyseal line is typically, obliquely, and longitudinally oriented.

Stress fractures commonly involve the second or third metatarsal (March fracture). Typically, there is no history of acute injury, rather a history of prolonged chronic activity such as walking, jogging, or running. Radiographically, the metatarsal may be normal on the initial examination, whereas after 2 weeks, periosteal new bone formation, cortical disruption, and callus formation may be evident. In the acute period, a radioisotope bone scan may show increased uptake after 24 to 48 hours, or MRI may demonstrate marrow edema (Fig. 22.20).

Metatarsal neck fractures are usually obvious radiographically but may only be apparent on one projection. Freiberg infarction of the metatarsal head is characterized by fissuring, osteonecrosis, and eventual collapse of the subchondral bone with the second and third metatarsal heads most commonly affected (Fig. 22.21). Radiographs may be normal in the initial stage.

Hallux sesamoids can be involved with fractures, avascular necrosis (AVN), and sesamoiditis secondary to inflammatory arthropathies or osteomyelitis (Fig. 22.22). The medial sesamoid being more commonly involved with trauma and the lateral

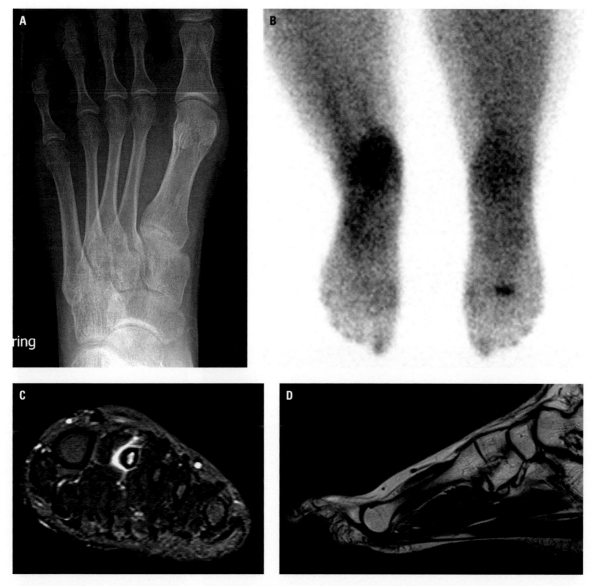

Figure 22.20. A. There is subtle cortical thickening to the second metatarsal shaft consistent with a stress fracture. **B.** Bone scintigram confirms this to be consistent with a fracture. MRI STIR (**C**) and T1W (**D**) confirm the associated edema and cortical thickening.

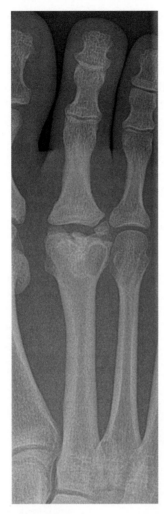

Figure 22.21. AP view of the second metatarsal with collapse and sclerosis of the metatarsal head consistent with Freiberg disease.

sesamoid AVN. A MRI is most sensitive in the acute stages, with replacement of the normal marrow fat signal with edema.

Lisfranc Injuries

Tarsometatarsal dislocations, fractures, or fracture dislocations with their nidus at the medial cuneiform–second metatarsal base relationship are referred to as Lisfranc injuries. The eponym is derived from Lisfranc's description of a midfoot amputation at the tarsometatarsal level, and this anatomic region still bears his name.[28]

The thick interosseous ligament that extends from the medial cuneiform to the base of the second metatarsal is also referred to as the *Lisfranc ligament* (Fig. 22.23). The medial cuneiform–second metatarsal relationship in the Lisfranc injury is determined by the status of the Lisfranc ligament (Fig. 22.24).

These injuries account for less than 1% of all fractures, but as many as 20% of Lisfranc joint injuries are missed on initial anteroposterior and oblique radiographs particularly in the patient who, while attempting ambulation, has spontaneously reduced the dislocation. They are mostly related to high-energy trauma, with the mechanism of injury consisting of plantar flexion with forced pronation or supination.

Lisfranc injuries have been classified as direct or indirect based on the nature of the injury,[29] uniform (convergent) or divergent,[30] and homolateral or divergent[31] based on the direction of the metatarsal

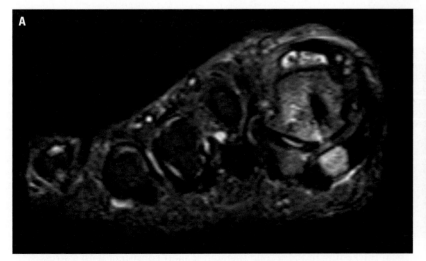
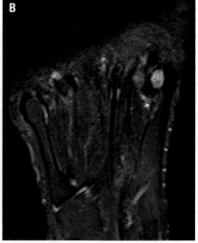

Figure 22.22. **A and B:** Axial and coronal STIR images of the sesamoids showing marked edema to the tibial sesamoid consistent with sesamoiditis.

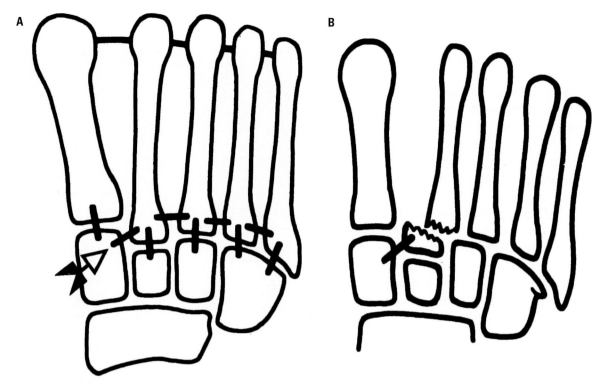

Figure 22.23. **A:** Schematic representation of the tarsometatarsal and intermetatarsal ligaments of the Lisfranc joint. *Stemmed arrow* indicates the Lisfranc ligament, which is the only obliquely oriented principal ligament at this level. **B:** Schematic representation of the pathology of a homolateral Lisfranc fracture dislocation with an intact Lisfranc ligament. (From Gross RH. Fractures and dislocations of the foot. In: Rockwood CA Jr, Wilkins KE, King RE, eds. *Fractures in Children.* 2nd ed. Philadelphia, PA: JB Lippincott Co; 1984:1078, used with permission.)

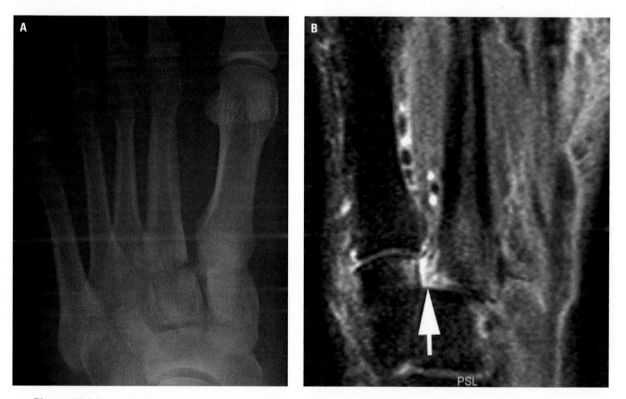

Figure 22.24. **A:** AP view showing widening of the gap between the bases of the first and second metatarsals, which is highly suspicious for injury to the Lisfranc ligament. **B:** STIR image showing gross edema to the ligament consistent with injury.

dislocation. The latter classification is the most widely accepted.

Homolateral refers to lateral dislocation of the lateral four metatarsals while the first retains its normal relationship to the medial cuneiform bone (Fig. 22.25). *Divergent* refers to the lateral displacement of the lateral four metatarsals and medial dislocation of the first metatarsal (Figs. 22.26 and 22.27).

The Lisfranc ligament plays a role analogous to the ligaments in ankle injuries in that the Lisfranc ligament either may be torn, in which event there is no associated fracture of either the medial cuneiform or the base of the second metatarsal, or may remain intact, in which event an avulsion fracture may arise from either the lateral aspect of the medial cuneiform or the medial surface of the base of the second metatarsal. The avulsion may be single or comminuted. On the lateral radiograph, the midfoot bones sublux or dislocate in a plantar direction.

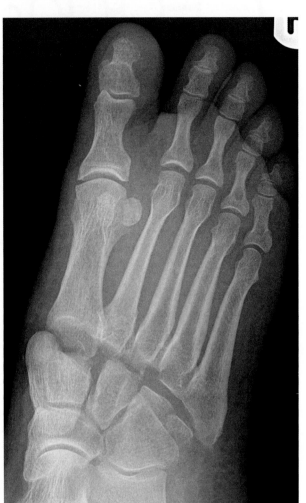

Figure 22.26. Oblique view showing dislocation across all the TMTJs with associated cuboid fracture in a diabetic patient.

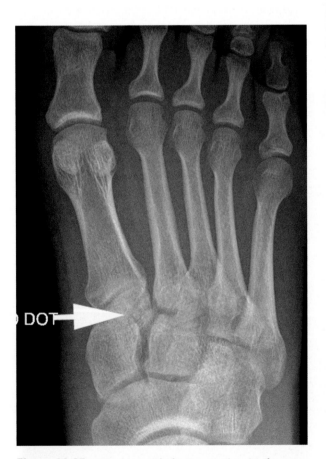

Figure 22.25. AP view with fragmentation in the two-third base interspace with disruption across the second and third tarso-metatarsal joints (TMTJs) consistent with homolateral Lisfranc type injury.

The cuboid may sustain a compression fracture secondary to impaction by the base of the dislocated fifth metatarsal. The cuboid fracture is not a component, but rather a complication, of the Lisfranc injury, as are concomitant fractures of the base of any of the dislocated lateral four metatarsals.

Variations of the homolateral Lisfranc fracture dislocation center on the third metatarsal, in which the intertarsal ligament between the second and third metatarsals is disrupted allowing the lateral three metatarsals to dislocate laterally, or, with an intact second–third intertarsal ligament, an avulsion fracture may arise from the base of the second or third metatarsal.

The other commonly missed variation of this injury is a Lisfranc fracture dislocation in the diabetic patient (Fig. 22.28). This can occur spontaneously with no significant traumatic event albeit with spectacular radiologic findings. These are often missed as they are painless due to the underlying diabetic neuropathy. The clinician should be alerted to a major injury by the associated soft tissue swelling.

Tomographic imaging methods such as CT and MRI provide excellent anatomic depiction of the tarsometatarsal joint. CT is accurate in the assessment of tarsal and metatarsal fractures and particularly of joint malalignment. It can delineate the fracture extent in particular, the degree of dorsal displacement, and the additional fractures required for surgical planning. An MRI may demonstrate the soft tissue injury more effectively than CT; however, surgical management is based largely on fracture anatomy and displacement, and CT is the imaging modality of choice.[32,33]

Chopart Injuries

The Chopart joint is the articulation between the midfoot and the hindfoot (midtarsal joint) named after the surgeon who performed amputations at the calcaneocuboid and talonavicular joint. Chopart fracture dislocations are rare according to the literature; however, with more liberal use of cross-sectional imaging, it is becoming clear that they are more common than was thought to be the case.

This injury is a midtarsal dislocation usually between the calcaneocuboid and talonavicular joints (Fig. 22.29); frequently associated with fractures of the calcaneus, cuboid, and navicular with most com-

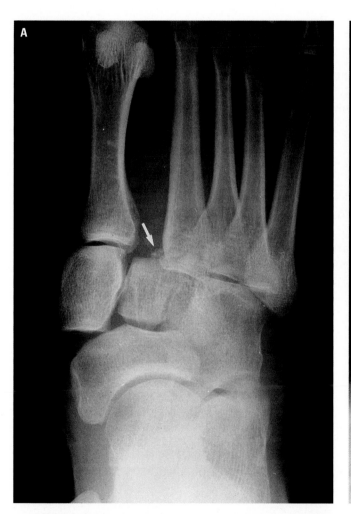
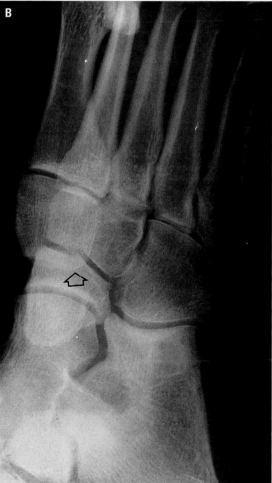

Figure 22.27. Divergent Lisfranc fracture dislocation. **A:** In the anteroposterior projection, the first cuneiform and metatarsal are medially displaced as a unit as a result of dislocation between the first and second cuneiform bones and at the naviculocuneiform joint. The lateral four metatarsals are laterally dislocated. A tiny avulsion fragment *(arrow)* arises from the medial aspect of the base of the second metatarsal. **B:** In the oblique projection, the dorsal dislocation of the first cuneiform and metatarsal *(open arrow)* is evident.

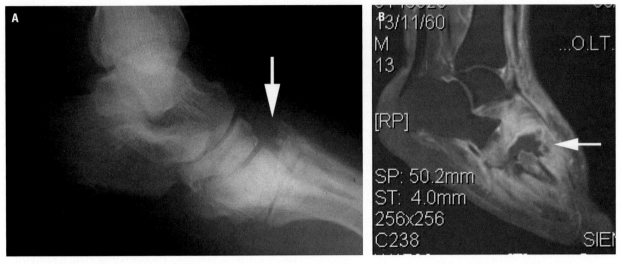

Figure 22.28. **A:** Lateral view demonstrating painless fracture/dislocation across the Lisfranc joint in a diabetic patient. **B:** T1FSGd sagittal image showing nonenhancing material within the fracture site, which was shown to be necrotic tissue at surgery.

monly medial displacement of the distal fragments (80%).[34] Although visible on plain radiographs, CT with 3-D reformats accurately demonstrates fracture fragments for surgical planning (Fig. 22.30).

Phalangeal Injuries

Dislocation at the interphalangeal joints is usually either dorsal or volar in direction, in contradistinction to metatarsal–tarsal dislocations, which are usually lateral. In the frontal projection, a loss of joint space and the increased density of the super-imposed phalanges indicate the presence of dislocation (Fig. 22.31). The direction of displacement may only be established by oblique or lateral projections of the involved digit, although these should be clinically obvious.

Fractures of the distal phalanx of the great toe are among the most common injuries of the foot and may involve the base of the phalanx or the sub-ungual tuft.

Simple phalangeal fractures are very common and require little intervention apart from immobilization but can be very easy to overlook on the standard radiographic series (Fig. 22.32).

Figure 22.29. Lateral foot radiograph demonstrating dislocation across the Chopart joint.

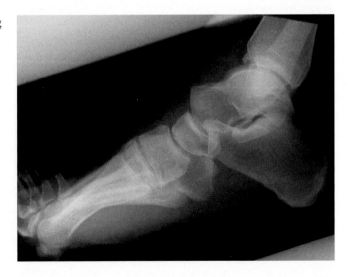

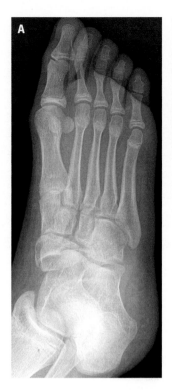

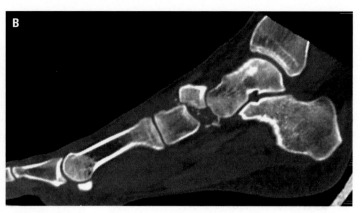

Figure 22.30. A: DP oblique view showing extrusion of the navicular. **B:** Confirms dorsal extrusion of the navicular fragment with residual fragmentation in the joint space.

Traumatic Soft Tissue Conditions

Turf toe refers to a capsuloligamentous injury of the metatarsophalangeal joint of the great toe, with the mechanism typically one of hyperextension. The abnormal forces applied at the metatarsophalangeal joint result in varying degrees of sprain or disruption of the supporting soft tissue structures that are readily evident on MRI (Fig. 22.33).[35]

Tears of the plantar fascia occur most commonly in the midportion of the fascia, more distal than the typical location of plantar fasciitis. They may be

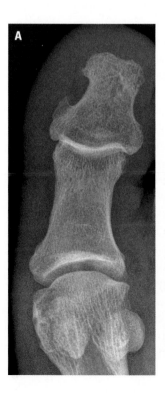

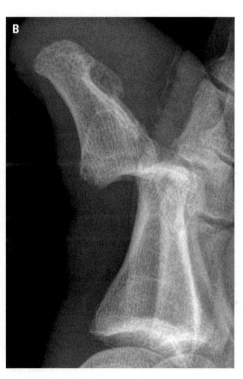

Figure 22.31. A: DP view of the great toe showing complete loss of joint space at the interphalangeal joint (IPJ). **B:** Dorsal dislocation of the distal phalanx on the lateral.

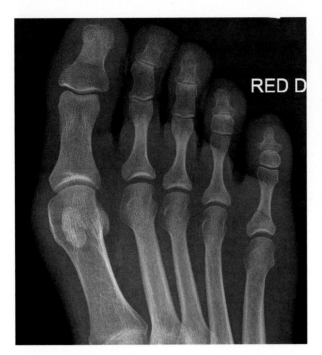

Figure 22.32. Simple undisplaced proximal phalangeal fracture of the fifth toe.

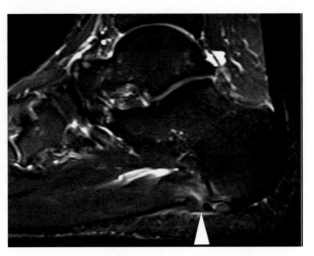

Figure 22.34. Sagittal STIR image shows disruption to the plantar fascia at its calcaneal origin consistent with a partial tear.

partial or complete, with trauma the usual etiology (Fig. 22.34). Discontinuity and waviness of the fascial cords may be seen on ultrasound with adjacent soft tissue edema on MRI.[36]

Nontraumatic Conditions

Distinguishing osteomyelitis from adjacent soft tissue infection is of paramount clinical importance because osteomyelitis can be more refrac-

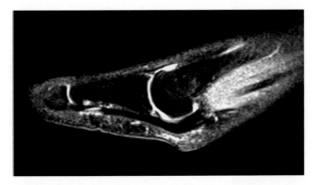

Figure 22.33. Sagittal STIR image of the great toe showing significant soft tissue injury consistent with "turf toe."

tory to treatment. Radiographs in the initial phase of acute osteomyelitis may demonstrate soft tissue swelling and irregular demineralization, progressing to periosteal thickening or elevation, cortical thickening, sclerosis, and irregularity. However, these changes may not be evident until 5 to 7 days in children and 10 to 14 days in adults; with a negative radiographic study unable to exclude the diagnosis of acute osteomyelitis, MRI is the modality of choice. With its high sensitivity and excellent soft tissue bone marrow contrast resolution, a MRI is able to define both the bony extent, seen as reduced bone marrow signal on T1, increased on T2 and fat-suppressed sequences, and associated soft tissue complications such as collections and sinus tracts (Fig. 22.35).[37,38]

The Charcot (neuropathic) joint poses a special problem in imaging, particularly when associated with soft tissue infection. Radiographs are commonly performed in the diabetic patient with concerns for osteomyelitis, with the acute Charcot joint radiographic findings simulating those of infection.[39] A MRI may demonstrate nonspecific bone marrow edema on fat suppression sequences and, in conjunction with an appropriate clinical history, can be of use in differentiating soft tissue infection, osteomyelitis, and an acute Charcot joint.[40] Radiographs of the chronic Charcot (neuropathic) joint are characterized by complete destructive disorganization with bone destruction and fragmentation, deformity, and dislocation (Fig. 22.36).

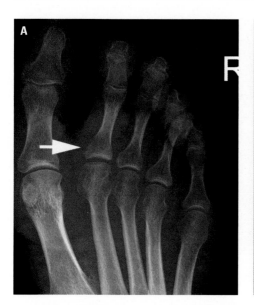 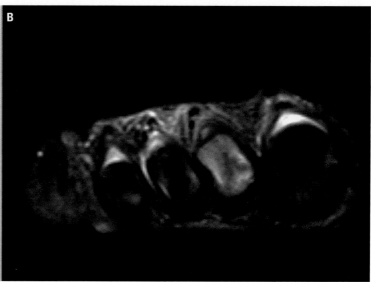

Figure 22.35. Osteomyelitis. **A:** Forefoot radiograph showing early loss of cortex to the base of the second proximal phalanx, suspicious for developing osteomyelitis. **B:** T1FSGd short axis MRI confirms enhancement of this phalanx consistent with osteomyelitis.

Indolent soft tissue conditions may be demonstrated on ultrasound. Plantar fasciitis involving inflammation and degeneration of the plantar fascia origin is readily depicted and diagnostic on ultrasound as thickening of the plantar fascia, with incidental plantar fibromas demonstrated as focal hypoechoic lesions intimately related to the plantar fascia (Figs. 22.37 and 22.38).[41] Sonography may demonstrate Morton neuroma, a nonneoplastic fusiform enlargement of the medial or lateral plantar nerves, commonly described as a hypoechoic intermetatarsal mass (Fig. 22.39).[42]

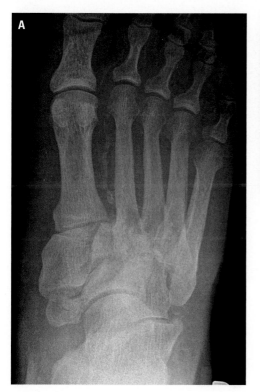 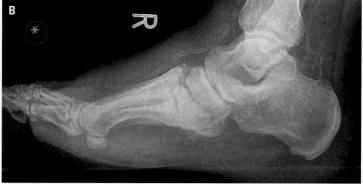

Figure 22.36. A and B : Charcot foot DP and lateral foot views showing disorganization, sclerosis, and degenerate change across the TMTJs with marked vascular calcification consistent with chronic Charcot foot.

Figure 22.37. Sagittal ultrasound image showing marked thickening of the proximal plantar fascia consistent with plantar fasciitis.

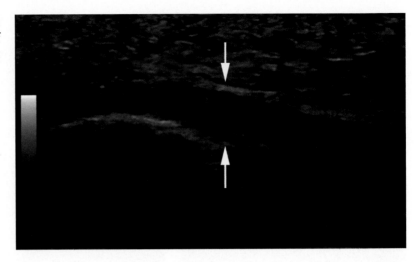

Figure 22.38. Sagittal ultrasound image showing a hypoechoic lesion *(arrowheads)* intimately associated with the plantar fascia *(arrows)* consistent with a plantar fibroma.

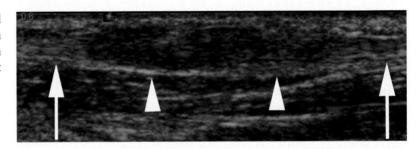

Figure 22.39. Sagittal ultrasound images demonstrating a hypoechoic lesion between the second and third metatarsal heads consistent with a Morton neuroma.

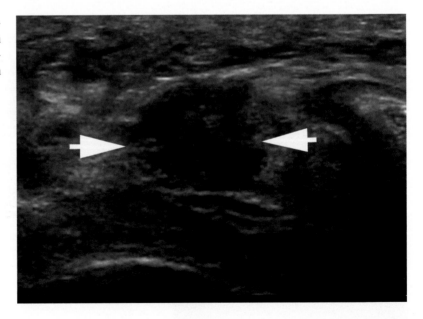

REFERENCES

1. Royal College of Radiologists. *Making the Best Use of Clinical Radiology Services. Referral Guidelines.* 6th ed. London, United Kingdom: Royal College of Radiologists; 2007:168–169.

2. Geijer M, El-Khoury GY. MDCT in the evaluation of skeletal trauma: principles, protocols, and clinical applications. *Emerg Radiol.* 2006;13:7–18.

3. Anderson JE. *Grant's Atlas of Anatomy.* 7th ed. Baltimore, MD: Williams & Wilkins; 1978.

4. Keats TE, Anderson MW. *Atlas of Normal Roentgen Variants that May Simulate Disease.* 8th ed. St. Louis, MO: Mosby-Year Book; 2007:838–978.

5. Swallow RA, Naylor E, Roebuck EJ, et al. *Clark's Positioning in Radiography.* 11th Rev ed. Oxford, United Kingdom: Butterworth-Heinemann Ltd; 1986:91–100.

6. Rogers L. *Radiology of Skeletal Trauma.* 3rd ed. Philadelphia, PA: Churchill Livingstone; 2001.

7. Segal D, Wasilewski S. Total dislocation of the talus. *J Bone Joint Surg Am.* 1980;62:1370–1372.

8. Merianos P, Papagiannakos K, Hatzis A, et al. Peritalar dislocation: a follow-up report of 21 cases. *Injury.* 1998;19:439–442.

9. Christensen SB, Lorentzen JE, Krogsoe O, et al. Subtalar dislocation. *Acta Orthop Scand.* 1977;48:707–711.

10. Monson ST, Ryan JR. Subtalar dislocations. *J Bone Joint Surg Am.* 1981;63:1156–1158.

11. DeLee JC, Curtis R. Subtalar dislocation of the foot. *J Bone Joint Surg Am.* 1982;64:433–437.

12. Schachter A, Chen A, Reddy P, et al. Osteochondral lesions of the talus. *J Am Acad Orthop Surg.* 2005;13(3):152–158.

13. Anderson IF, Crichton KJ, Grattan-Smith T, et al. Osteochondral fractures of the dome of the talus. *J Bone Joint Surg Am.* 1989;71:1143–1152.

14. Eustace S, Brophy D, Denison W. Magnetic resonance imaging of acute orthopaedic trauma to the lower extremity. *Emerg Radiol.* 1997;4(1):30–37.

15. Hawkins LG. Fractures of the neck of the talus. *J Bone Joint Surg Am.* 1970;52:991–1002.

16. Conwell HE, Reynolds FC. *Key and Conwell's Management of Fractures, Dislocations and Sprains.* 7th ed. St. Louis, MO: Mosby; 1961.

17. Moseley HF. Traumatic disorders of the ankle and foot. *Ciba Foundation Symposium.* 1965;17:26.

18. Carr JB, Hamilton JJ, Bear LS. Experimental intraarticular calcaneal fractures: anatomic basis for a new classification. *Foot Ankle.* 1989;10:81–87.

19. Sanders R, Fortin P, DiPasquale T, et al. Operative treatment in 120 displaced intraarticular calcaneal fractures: results using a prognostic computed

20. Sanders R, Gregory P. Operative treatment of intraarticular fractures of the calcaneus. *Orthop Clin North Am.* 1995;26:203–214.

21. Sanders R. Intraarticular fractures of the calcaneus: present state of the art. *J Orthop Trauma.* 1992;6:252–265.

22. Kathol MH, el-Khoury GY, Moore TE, et al. Calcaneal insufficiency avulsion fractures in patients with diabetes mellitus. *Radiology.* 1991;180:725–729.

23. Trnka HJ, Zettl R, Ritschl P. Fracture of the anterior superior process of the calcaneus: an often misdiagnosed fracture. *Arch Orthop Trauma Surg.* 1998;117:300–302.

24. Daftary A, Haims A, Baumgaertner M. Fractures of the calcaneus. A review with emphasis on CT. *Radiographics.* 2005;25:1215–1226.

25. Weber J, Vidt L, Gehl R, et al. Calcaneal stress fractures. *Clin Podiatr Med Surg.* 2005;22(1):45–54.

26. Quill GE. Fractures of the proximal fifth metatarsal. Controversies in foot and ankle trauma. *Orthop Clin North Am.* 1995;26(2):353–61.

27. Jones R. Fracture of the base of the 5th metatarsal bone by indirect violence. *Ann Surg.* 1902;35:697–700.

28. Schultz RJ. *The Language of Fractures.* 2nd ed. Baltimore, MA: Williams & Wilkins; 1990.

29. O'Regan DJ. Lisfranc dislocations. *J Med Soc N J.* 1969;66(10):575–577.

30. Lenczner EM, Waddell JP, Graham JD. Tarsalmetatarsal (Lisfranc) dislocation. *J Trauma.* 1974;12:1012–1020.

31. Rogers LF, Campbell RE. Fractures and dislocations of the foot. *Semin Roentgenol.* 1978;2:157–166.

32. Ali M, Chen TS, Crues J. MRI of the foot. *Appl Radiol.* 2006;35(12)10–20.

33. Preidler K, Peicha G, Lajtai G, et al. Conventional radiography, CT and MR imaging in patients with hyperflexion injuries of the foot: diagnostic accuracy in the detection of bony and ligamentous changes. *AJR.* 1999;173:1673–1677.

34. Main BJ, Jowett RL. Injuries of the midtarsal joint. *J Bone Joint Surg Am.* 1975;57(1):89–97.

35. Mullen JE, O'Malley MJ. Sprains-residual instability of subtalar, Lisfranc joints, and turf toe. *Clin Sports Med.* 2004;23:97–121.

36. Asham CJ, Klecker RJ, Yu JS. Forefoot pain involving the metatarsal region. Differential diagnosis with MR imaging. *Radiographics.* 2001;21:1425–1440.

37. Unger E, Moldofsky P, Gatenby R, et al. Diagnosis of osteomyelitis by MR imaging. *Am J Roentgenol.* 1988;150(3): 605–610.

tomography scan classification. *Clin Orthop Relat Res.* 1993;290:87–95.

38. Sammak B, Abd El Bagi M, Al Shahed M, et al. Osteomyelitis: a review of currently used imaging techniques. *Eur Radiol.* 1998;9(5):894–900.

39. Jones EA, Manaster BJ, May DA, et al. Neuropathic osteoarthropathy: diagnostic dilemmas and differential diagnosis. *Radiographics.* 2000;20: 279–293.

40. Devendra D, Farmer K, Bruce G, et al. Diagnosing osteomyelitis in patients with diabetic neuropathic osteoarthropathy. *Diabetes Care.* 2001;24(12):2154–2155.

41. McNally E. *Practical Musculoskeletal Ultrasound.* Philadelphia, PA: Churchill Livingstone; 2004:175–188.

42. Redd RA. Morton's neuroma: sonographic evaluation. *Radiology.* 1989;171:415–417.

CHAPTER 23

Diaphysis

Johnny U. V. Monu ■ Thomas L. Pope Jr.

GENERAL CONSIDERATIONS

Diaphyseal lesions are unique because of their location, their frequent indirect but significant bearing on related joints, and their intimate association with peripheral arteries and nerves. Lesions involving the diaphyseal region of all the long bones are considered in this chapter.

RADIOGRAPHIC EXAMINATION

The routine radiographic examination of the long bones must include both frontal and lateral projections. A single projection of a long bone is an inadequate radiographic study (Fig. 23.1) except in the severely injured patient, and then only neurologic or hemodynamic instability or possible acute traumatic aortic injury should take precedence. Prior to definitive evaluation, however, radiographs of the long bones in orthogonal planes must be obtained to provide the necessary data on which management decisions can be made.

It is equally fundamental to include the entire long bone(s) in the examination whenever possible. When not possible, for whatever reason, the joint closest to the site of injury must be included in the examination. The purpose of the "closest joint" tenet is to be able to accurately localize the injury and to identify concomitant injuries that frequently occur close to or involve the joint (Fig. 23.2).

Shortening of one of the bones of the forearm or leg as a result of angulation or overlap of fragments can be accommodated only by either a fracture or dislocation of the other bone. Therefore, when one of the bones of the forearm or leg is shortened as a result of fracture, it is imperative to examine the entire part radiographically to diagnose the fracture or dislocation that must involve the other bone (Figs. 23.3 and 23.4).

The distal fragment of midfemoral or midtibiofibular fractures may be externally rotated as much as 90 degrees. This feature may not be appreciated unless the entire part is included in the radiographic study (Fig. 23.5).

Thus, radiographic reports of diaphyseal fractures should address the fracture pattern, the bone quality, and the presence of bone loss especially if there is comminution, the amount of limb shortening, and the presence of air in the soft tissues.

The most commonly accepted convention for describing the relationship of the fragments of long or short tubular bones is to relate the position of the distal fragment to that of the proximal fragment. *Alignment* is the relationship of the longitudinal axis of the distal fragment to that of the proximal fragment. If the long axis of each fragment is parallel, alignment is said to be normal. *Displacement* refers to translation of the distal fragment in any direction with respect to the proximal fragment without angulation. "Angulation" indicates that the long axis of the distal fragment is canted (angled) with respect to the long axis of the proximal fragment. A distal fragment may be displaced, angled, or displaced and angled (Fig. 23.6) with respect to the proximal fragment. Proximal retraction of the distal fragment

Figure 23.1. **A:** The frontal radiograph of the leg could very easily be interpreted as "negative." **B:** The lateral projection clearly demonstrates the minimally displaced oblique fracture in the middle third of the tibia *(arrow)*.

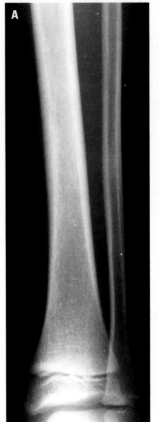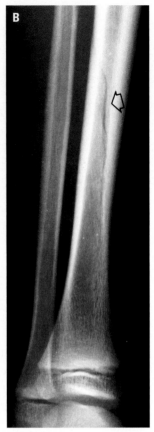

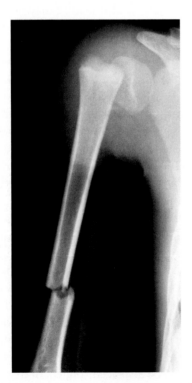

Figure 23.2. Transverse fracture in the midshaft of the humerus with an associated proximal humeral physeal injury.

with respect to the proximal is referred to as *over-riding* (Fig. 23.6).

A segmental fracture is one in which two fractures occur at disparate locations within the same long bone, resulting in a separate and discrete fragment that is not attached to either the proximal or the distal fragment. The separate fragment is the "segment" of a segmental fracture (Fig. 23.7).

Peripheral Doppler ultrasound and computed tomography angiography (CTA) play an important role in the evaluation of traumatic lesions of the extremities. Although it is the responsibility of the attending physician to specifically evaluate the circulation of an injured extremity, it is equally the responsibility of the radiologist to identify and indicate to the attending physician those injuries that, because of the normal anatomic relationship between the arteries and the bones, have the potential for associated vascular involvement. However, the "proximity of wound" alone is not an indication for emergent CTA in the presence of an otherwise clinically normal extremity. Obviously, clinical signs or symptoms of arterial compromise distal to either a penetrating injury or a displaced long bone fracture

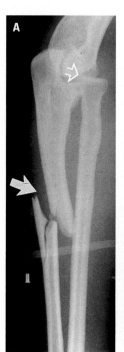
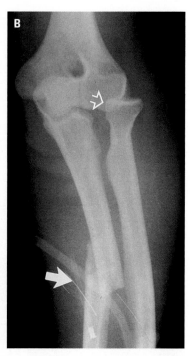

Figure 23.3. Bado type III Monteggia fracture. Shortening of the ulna due to overriding (**A**) and angulation (**A,B**) of its proximal fracture *(solid arrow)* has contributed to the anterolateral dislocation of the radial head *(open arrow)*.

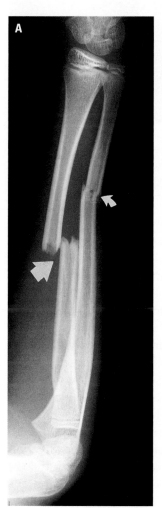
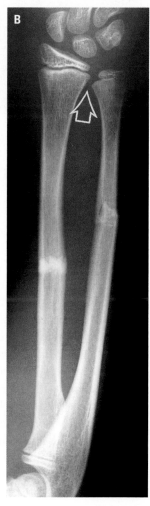

Figure 23.4. A: Complete fracture of the midshaft of the radius with shortening resulting from overriding of its fragments *(straight arrow)*. The complete ulnar fracture *(curved arrow)* is impacted. **B:** The radial shortening has resulted in distal radioulnar diastasis *(open arrow)*.

Figure 23.5. Approximately 90-degree external rotation of the distal femoral fragment. **A:** On the frontal radiograph, the hip is in the anteroposterior position, whereas the distal femoral fragment is in nearly true lateral position. **B:** On the horizontal beam lateral radiograph obtained with the patient supine, the proximal fragment is in lateral position, whereas the distal fragment is seen in frontal view.

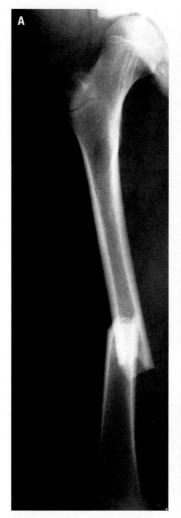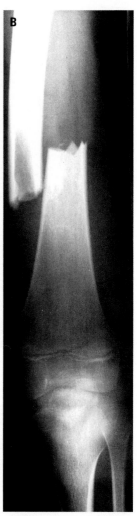

require at least consideration of CTA or peripheral angiography. The priority of the CTA or angiogram and where it is performed (e.g., the emergency center, the angiography suite, the operating room) must be determined jointly by the attending physician and the radiologist based on the patient's overall condition and the availability of angiographic facilities.

RADIOGRAPHIC ANATOMY

The contour of the part and the configuration of the soft tissues are important aspects of the radiographic evaluation of the extremities. Normally, adipose or loose areolar tissue is present adjacent to or surrounding the soft tissue structures of the extremities. In properly exposed radiographs, the muscles and fascial planes may be visible as linear or curvilinear radiolucent shadows.

RADIOGRAPHIC MANIFESTATIONS OF TRAUMA

Humerus

Fractures of the shaft of the humerus occur less frequently than fractures of the proximal end of the bone and are usually the result of direct trauma. Frequently, the humerus may be fractured by indirect force, such as a fall on the hand or elbow. Fractures of the proximal portion of the humerus caused by muscular action alone occur rarely.

Humeral shaft fractures are usually either oblique (Fig. 23.8) or transverse (Fig. 23.2). Displacement of the fragments is common, with the direction and magnitude of displacement due to (1) the direction and magnitude of force causing the injury and (2) the action of the muscles that insert on the humerus and their relation to the fracture site. Generally, if

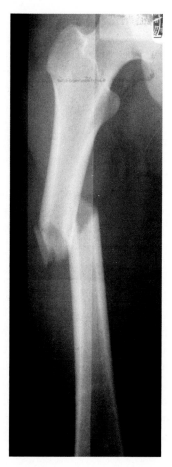

Figure 23.6. Displaced, angled fracture at the junction of the proximal and middle thirds of the femoral shaft. The distal femoral fragment is both medially displaced and angled with respect to the proximal fragment.

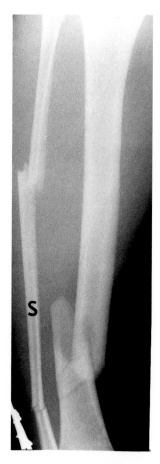

Figure 23.7. Segmental fracture. The separate fragment (S) between the proximal and distal fibular fractures constitutes the segmental fragment.

the fracture line is located distal to the insertion of the deltoid muscle, the proximal fragment tends to be retracted outward, whereas the muscles of the arm draw the distal fragment upward. When the fracture is above the insertion of the deltoid, the distal fragment will be drawn laterally, and the proximal fragment medially by the unopposed action of the pectoralis, the latissimus dorsi, and the teres major muscles.

The radial nerve lies in the musculospiral groove of the humerus. Consequently, radial nerve paralysis is the principal complication of humeral shaft fractures. Occasionally, other entrapment neuropathies may result following fractures. These fractures are typically found in the proximal to middle third of the humeral shaft (Fig. 23.9). Open fractures occur in less than 10% of humeral shaft fracture. Such injuries are often due to high-velocity trauma, and

frequently, the fracture may be comminuted and radial nerve palsy and other systemic injuries may be present.

Radius and Ulna

The pronator quadratus sign, described in conjunction with injuries of the wrist, is extremely valuable in the detection of minimally displaced fractures of the distal diaphysis of the ulna (Fig. 23.10) or of the radius.

Isolated ulnar fractures or "nightstick" fractures (Fig. 23.11) are usually the result of direct trauma. The alignment of the fragments reflects the direction of the causative force.

Monteggia fractures consist of a displaced fracture of the proximal ulna and dislocation of the radial head. Their classifications and types are described in Chapter 9.

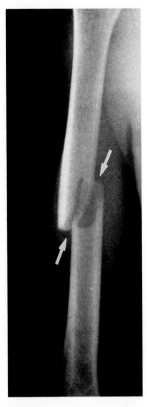

Figure 23.8. Oblique fracture *(arrows)* of the mid-humeral shaft.

Isolated fractures of the radius occur less frequently than those of the ulna and may be the result of either direct or indirect trauma, such as a fall on the outstretched hand. The displacement of the fragments reflects the pull of the muscles of the forearm and the relationship of the fracture site to the insertion of the pronator teres muscle. The Galeazzi fracture-dislocation deserves special mention because, although not a common injury, it is associated with a high incidence of complication. The Galeazzi fracture-dislocation consists of a displaced or angled fracture of the distal radius, resulting in radial shortening that must be accommodated by dislocation at the distal radio-ulnar joint (Fig. 23.12). Frequently, a fracture also occurs at the base of the ulnar styloid process. (See Chapter 10 for additional discussion and illustrations of the Galeazzi injury.)

Shortening, angulation, and rotary deformity of the fragments of forearm fractures are the result of the effects of the fracturing force and muscle pull, notably that of the biceps, brachialis, pronator teres, and pronator quadratus muscles. Displacement of the fragments is always associated with (1) soft tissue damage, including muscle tear; (2) damage to

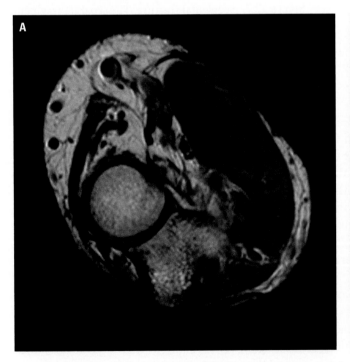

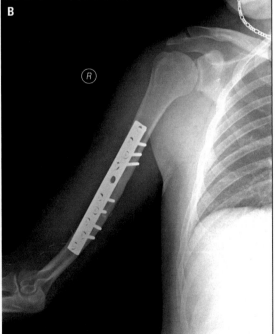

Figure 23.9. Radial nerve dysfunction syndrome. **A:** Axial proton density image at the elbow shows atrophy and fatty replacement of the supinator, brachioradialis, and the common extensors of the wrist likely due to injury to the deep branch of the radial nerve. **B:** Plain radiograph shows a compression plate and screws used to fix a midshaft fracture of the radius a few years earlier. Injury to the nerve may be due to the fracture or during manipulation of the fracture.

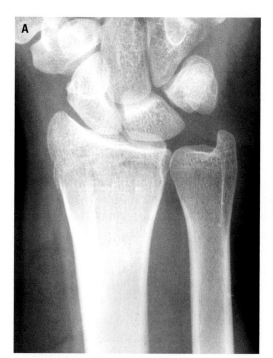
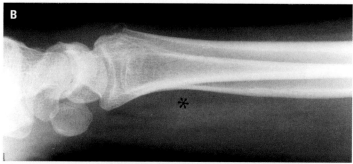
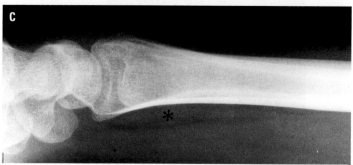

Figure 23.10. Abnormal pronator quadratus muscle shadow. **A:** The anteroposterior radiograph of the right wrist shows a subtle, minimally displaced fracture at the base of the radial styloid process. **B:** On the lateral radiograph obtained at the same time as **A**, the abnormally wide pronator quadratus muscle shadow *(asterisk)* is indicative of a subperiosteal hematoma, which supports the finding of the radial styloid process fracture in **A**. **C:** The pronator quadratus muscle shadow *(asterisk)* is normal on the follow-up lateral radiograph obtained 4 weeks after trauma.

the interosseous membrane, which may heal with excessive fibrosis or calcification resulting in limitation of pronation and supination; or (3) neurovascular disruption or compression, resulting in Volkmann ischemic contracture.

Bowing Fracture

The "bowing" fracture may occur in one (Fig. 23.13) or both bones of the forearm. The plastic deformation of one bone usually accompanies an angled fracture of the other, but bowing deformities may infrequently involve both forearm bones. Animal experiments involving the ulna of dogs have established that the mechanism of injury must be purely longitudinal; that the causative force required to produce the plastic deformity is approximately 100% to 150% of the patient's total body weight; that an equivalent force is required to reduce the bowing fracture, thereby requiring manipulation under anesthesia; and that the persistence of the plastic deformity as a result of either failure of diagnosis or inadequate reduction results in limited pronation and supination. Obviously, therefore, the bowing fracture of the forearm has significant

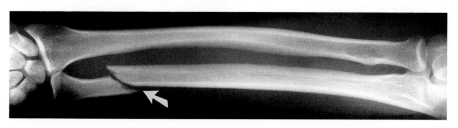

Figure 23.11. "Nightstick" fracture of the distal ulna *(arrow)*.

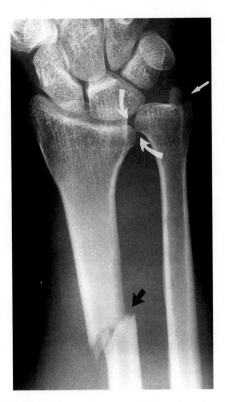

Figure 23.12. Galeazzi fracture-dislocation. Shortening of the radial fracture *(black arrow)* has resulted in diastasis of the distal radioulnar synostosis *(curved arrows)*. There is also a fracture of the ulnar styloid process *(straight arrow)*.

clinical implications, and its radiographic recognition is critical to appropriate management and optimum outcome. Histopathologically, the injury consists of microfractures extending through the entire thickness of the cortex of the concavity of the bowed bone. At this point, release of the causative force does not result in spontaneous reduction of the bowing ("plastic") deformity. If the magnitude of the force increases, the bowing deformity becomes greater until the bone actually fractures. Radiographically, the bowing deformity is a long, broad, gentle curve (Fig. 23.13) involving the shaft, which imperceptibly blends into the normal proximal and distal end of the involved bone. It is characteristic of the bowing fracture that no periosteal reaction occurs on short-term follow-up radiographs while the deformity persists. Periosteal new bone reaction develops along the concavity of the curve in young children, little new bone reaction develops in older children, and no periosteal new bone reaction occurs in orthopedically reduced bowing fractures.

Femur

Fractures affecting the femoral shaft may be subtrochanteric (up to 5 cm below the lesser trochanter or in the diaphysis). Subtrochanteric fractures tend to affect healthy young adults involved in high-velocity trauma. The fractures may also be seen in elderly osteoporotic persons. Femoral fractures are usually displaced by the force of the injury and the effect of the thigh muscles on the fragments. Both anteroposterior and lateral radiographs are mandatory to establish the degree and direction of the displacement and the degree of rotation of the distal fragment (Fig. 23.5).

Fractures of the proximal third of the femoral shaft may cause injury to the deep femoral artery or its branches. The superficial femoral artery, as it leaves the adductor canal and passes through the popliteal space, is immediately adjacent to the femur and may be injured by comminuted or displaced

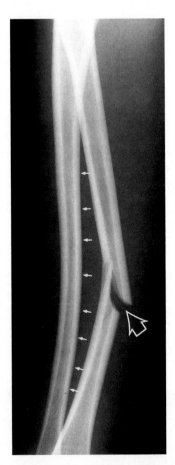

Figure 23.13. Angled fracture of the radius *(open arrow)* with a bowing fracture of the ulna *(straight arrows)*.

fractures of the middle or distal third of the femoral shaft. CTA should be considered in all patients with displaced distal femoral shaft fractures, particularly in those patients with clinical evidence of diminished or absent peripheral circulation (Fig. 23.14).

Tibia and Fibula

Fractures of the tibial shaft are the most common long bone fracture and are usually the result of direct trauma. These fractures are commonly associated with fractures of the fibula and are frequently open.

The popliteal artery and its branches may be injured by the force that causes a proximal tibial fracture or by the fracture fragments themselves. In addition, the lumina of these vessels may be compromised by the hematoma confined within the closed space of the calf (Fig. 23.15). Because clinical appraisal of the status of the anterior and posterior tibial and peroneal arteries may be difficult, CTA should be seriously considered in the evaluation of comminuted, displaced, proximal tibial shaft fractures.

Distal tibial fractures may be associated with proximal fibular fractures (Fig. 23.16). The tibial injury, being the major and most symptomatic, may mask the proximal fibular fracture. The combined injury just described, although it involves the distal tibia and proximal fibula, is not a Maisonneuve fracture. The latter, as originally described by Maisonneuve in 1812, is described and illustrated in Chapter 21.

The bowing fracture, as described earlier in this chapter, may also occur in the fibula in association with an angled fracture of the tibia (Fig. 23.17). The radiographic features of the fibular bowing fracture are identical with those described with respect to the bones of the forearm.

Isolated fractures of the fibula occur infrequently, are usually located in the distal third of the shaft, are usually nondisplaced, and are the result of a direct trauma to the lateral aspect of the leg (Fig. 23.18). The clinical signs of these fractures are commonly minimal, and the acute fracture may not be appreciated clinically.

Fracture of the fibula at the fibular neck may injure the superficial peroneal nerve, or occasionally, the nerve may become symptomatic following entrapment by healing callus.

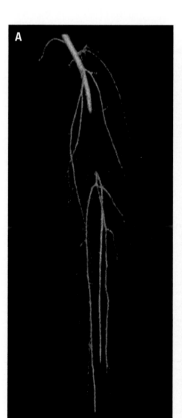 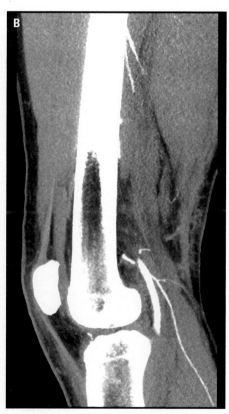

Figure 23.14. CTA of the lower leg in a patient who had a dislocation of the knee. Absent dorsalis pedis pulse (**A**) indicates interruption of the popliteal artery and reconstitution of the distal branches by collaterals flow. Reconstructed sagittal CT image (**B**) shows interruption of the popliteal artery at the level of the knee joint.

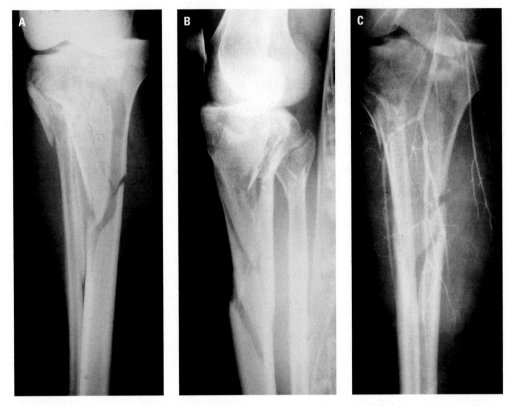

Figure 23.15. Severely comminuted, displaced fracture in the proximal third of the tibia and a nondisplaced fracture of the fibular neck seen in frontal (**A**) and lateral (**B**) projections. The femoral arteriogram (**C**) demonstrates impaired runoff of the contrast medium in the calf caused by the tamponade effect of the hematoma that developed in the confined space of the calf.

Figure 23.16. Spiral fracture of the distal third of the tibia (**A**), associated with an oblique fracture of the proximal third of the fibula (**B**, *arrow*). Because the ankle mortise is intact, the injury does not meet the criteria for a Maisonneuve fracture.

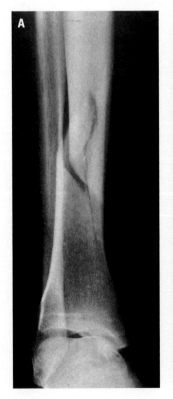

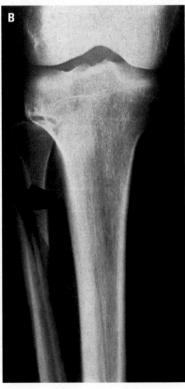

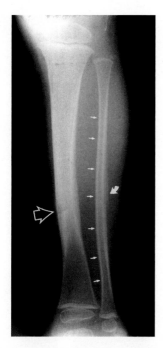

Figure 23.17. Healing fracture in the distal tibia *(open arrow)* that is associated with a bowing fracture of the fibula *(straight arrows)*. Periosteal new bone reaction *(curved arrow)* in the concavity of the fibular deformation confirms the presence of the healing fibular bowing fracture.

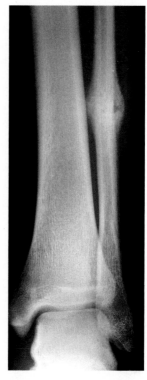

Figure 23.18. Nondisplaced, isolated, healing fracture at the junction of the middle and distal thirds of the fibular shaft. The fracture was not appreciated clinically until the callus became palpable.

Stress Fracture

"Stress" fractures are relatively common in lower extremities especially the tibia and fibula (Fig. 23.19) and usually occur in individuals who, for whatever reason, subject their lower extremities to unusual and/or repetitive stress (e.g., military recruits, long-distance runners, ballet dancers). As previously noted, the stress fracture may not be visible on the initial radiograph of the leg. If the history and clinical findings suggest a stress fracture, either a radioactive bone scan, which will be positive within 24 hours of the fracture, or MRI may be obtained immediately, or the radiographic examination may be repeated in 2 to 3 weeks, by which time the fracture should be recognizable by the presence of periosteal bone reaction and endosteal increase in density.

A recently recognized fracture in the femur is the bisphosphonate-related fracture seen most often in female patients who have been on continuous bisphosphonate treatment for more than 5 years. The fractures are provoked by little or no trauma and have a characteristic appearance and are first seen as lucency on the lateral aspect or convexity of the femur (Fig. 23.20). The fractures are often bilateral and rarely may be present at two locations in the same bone.

NONTRAUMATIC CONDITIONS

The edema associated with cellulitis results in increase in size and distortion of the contour of the involved part and in increase in soft tissue density and loss of soft tissue planes. All of these findings may be discernible on a properly exposed radiograph.

The radiographic signs of osteomyelitis are protean and depend largely on the stage of the inflammatory process. The radiographic appearance of acute osteomyelitis is illustrated elsewhere throughout this book. Sclerosis and cortical thickening of chronic osteomyelitis are seen in Figure 23.21.

Many types of dysplasias, metabolic conditions, and other systemic diseases that affect the long bones may initiate an emergency center visit. Even a listing of such conditions is beyond the scope of this text, and the reader is referred to such

Figure 23.19. Stress fracture of the proximal tibia. **A and B:** In the initial radiographs, the minimal periosteal new bone reaction, laterally and posteriorly *(arrowheads)*, and the broad, ill-defined band of increased density in the proximal third of the tibia indicate the fracture site. **C and D:** Subsequent radiographs reveal solid periosteal reaction at the fracture site and, in the lateral projection (**D**), sclerotic margins of the fracture line *(arrowheads)*.

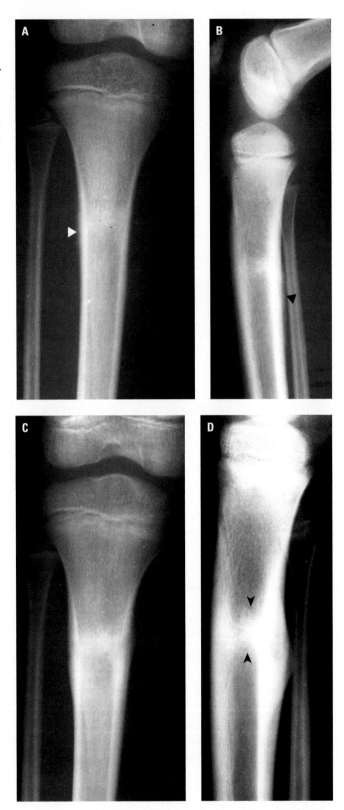

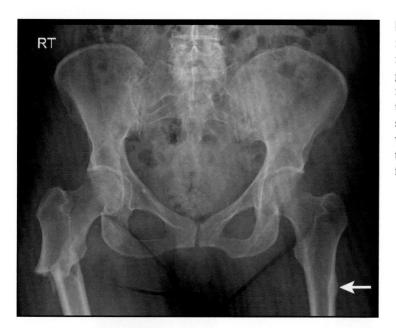

Figure 23.20. Bisphosphonate treatment-related fracture is often seen as a spontaneous fracture in the proximal femur. Plain radiograph of the pelvis shows a subtrochanteric fracture that occurred without antecedent trauma. Attention directed to the left femur shows focal cortical elevation (volcano sign) with some endosteal sclerosis and is consistent with an evolving bisphosphonate-related fracture.

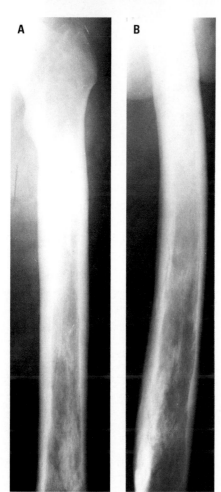

Figure 23.21. Mottled areas of increased density within the medullary cavity (**A**) and irregular endosteal and periosteal thickening (**B**) coupled with other areas of endosteal cortical resorption, with the appropriate clinical history and findings, are typical of chronic osteomyelitis of the femur.

outstanding textbooks as Edeiken's *Roentgen Diagnosis of Diseases of Bone* and Resnick's *Diagnosis of Bone and Joint Disorders*. An example is the diffuse, mottled medullary density of bone infarcts seen in sickle-cell disease (Fig. 23.22). Some chronic myeloproliferative disorders such as polycythemia vera, chronic myelogenous leukemia, idiopathic thrombocythemia, and myelofibrosis frequently involve the long bones with a characteristic, homogeneous, ground-glass increase in bone density secondary to increase in marrow fibrosis. The trabecular pattern is lost, and the marrow-cortical interface is obscured. The bone ends are typically more dense than the shaft (Fig. 23.23).

The most common benign tumor of long bones is the fibrous cortical defect (Fig. 23.24) that occurs in approximately 40% of children. This lesion usually appears after 2 years and is rarely seen beyond the age of 14 years. The cortical defect is eccentrically located in the cortex of long bones, most commonly about the knee. Radiographically, the benign cortical defect is a round or oval lytic lesion with thin sclerotic margins that expands the cortex of the diaphysis near the metaphysis. As the lesion increases in size, it may appear to be loculated as a result of endosteal irregularities. The radiographic appearance is so typical as not to require biopsy. Malignant degeneration does not occur. Fractures may occur through this area of weakened bone and the associated pain brings the lesion to attention.

A similar lesion that may be confused with "multiple fibrous cortical defects" is osteofibrous dysplasia. The lesion appears as a string of lucent defects

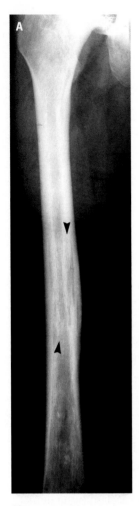

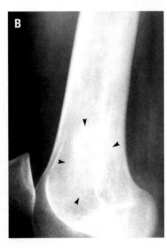

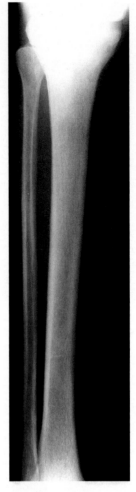

Figure 23.22. The irregular areas of increased density *(arrowheads)* within the medullary portion of the proximal (**A**) and distal (**B**) femur are consistent with infarcts of sickle-cell disease .

Figure 23.23. The diffuse increase in density throughout the tibia, which almost completely obliterates the medullary-cortical interface, coupled with the greater increase in density at each end of the tibia, is consistent with myelofibrosis.

Figure 23.24. Fibrous cortical defect (benign cortical defect, nonossifying fibroma, *arrows*) in the distal tibia in frontal (**A**) and lateral (**B**) projections.

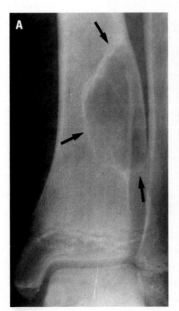

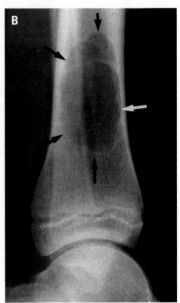

in the anterior tibia and is associated with bowing deformity of the tibial shaft.

Primary and metastatic tumors of long bones may be the cause of pain, tenderness, the presence of a mass, or a pathologic fracture.

SUGGESTED READINGS

1. Tullos HS, King JW. Lesions of the pitching arm in adolescents. *JAMA*. 1972;220(2):264–271.
2. Bingham EL. Fractures of the humerus from muscular violence. *U S Armed Forces Med J*. 1959;10(1):22–25.
3. O'Donoghue DH. *Treatment of Injuries to Athletes*. Philadelphia, PA: WB Saunders; 1962.
4. Schultz RJ. *The Language of Fractures*. 2nd ed. Baltimore, MD: Williams & Wilkins; 1990.
5. Wood B, Berquist TH. The hand and wrist. In: Berquist TH, ed. *Imaging of Orthopedic Trauma*. 2nd ed. New York, NY: Raven Press; 1992:810.
6. Borden S IV. Roentgen recognition of acute plastic bowing of the forearm in children. *Am J Roentgenol*. 1975;125(3):524–530.
7. Crowe JE, Swischuk LE. Acute bowing of the forearm in children: a frequently missed injury. *Am J Roentgenol*. 1977;128(6):981–984.
8. Chamay A. Mechanical and morphological aspects of experimental overload and fatigue in bone. *J Biomech*. 1970;3(3):263–270.
9. Chamay A, Tschantz P. Mechanical instances in bone remodeling. Experimental research on Wolf's law. *J Biomech*. 1972;5(2):173–180.
10. Salter RB. *Textbook of Disorders and Injuries of the Musculoskeletal System*. Baltimore, MD: Williams & Wilkins; 1970.
11. Salter RB, ed. *Care for the Injured Child*. Baltimore, MD: Williams & Wilkins; 1975.
12. Grusd R. Pseudofractures and stress fractures. *Semin Roentgenol*. 1978;13(2):81–82.
13. Swischuk LE. *Emergency Radiology of the Acutely Ill or Injured Child*. 3rd ed. Baltimore, MD: Williams & Wilkins; 1994.
14. Edeiken J, Dalinka MK, Karasick D. *Edeiken's Roentgen Diagnosis of Diseases of Bone*. 4th ed. Baltimore, MD: Williams & Wilkins; 1990.
15. Resnick D. *Diagnosis of Bone and Joint Disorders*. 4th ed. Philadelphia, PA: WB Saunders; 2004.
16. Clavert P, Lutz JC, Adam P, et al. Frohse's arcade is not the exclusive compression site of the radial nerve in its tunnel. *Orthop Traumatol Surg Res*. 2009;95(2):114–118.
17. Thomsen NO, Dahlin LB. Injury to the radial nerve caused by fracture of the humeral shaft: timing and neurobiological aspects related to treatment and diagnosis. *Scand J Plast Reconstr Surg Hand Surg*. 2007;41(4):153–157.
18. Rosenberg ZS, La Rocca Vieira R, Chan SS, et al. Bisphosphonate-related complete atypical subtrochanteric femoral fractures: diagnostic utility of radiography. *Am J Roentgenol*. 2011;197(4):954–960.
19. Lenart BA, Lorich DG, Lane JM. Atypical fractures of the femoral diaphysis in postmenopausal women taking alendronate. *N Engl J Med*. 2008;358:1304–1306.
20. Porrino JA, Kohl CA, Taljanovic M, et al. Diagnosis of proximal femoral insufficiency fractures in patients receiving bisphosphonate therapy. *Am J Roentgenol*. 2010;194(4):1061–1064.